Magnetic Resonance of Myelin, Myelination, and Myelin Disorders

Springer

Berlin
Heidelberg
New York
Barcelona
Budapest
Hong Kong
London
Milan
Paris
Tokyo

M.S. van der Knaap · J. Valk

Magnetic Resonance of Myelin, Myelination, and Myelin Disorders

Second Edition

With 248 Figures in 1274 Parts

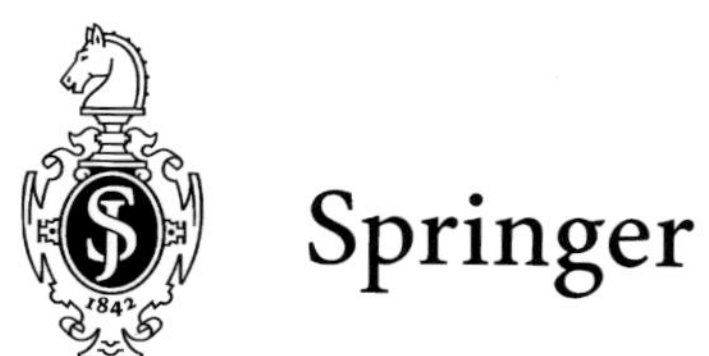

Springer

Marjo S. van der Knaap, MD, PhD
Department of Child Neurology

Jacob Valk, MD, PhD
Department of Diagnostic Radiology

Free University Hospital
De Boelelaan 1117
1007 MB Amsterdam, The Netherlands

ISBN 3-540-59277-6 2nd ed. Springer-Verlag Berlin Heidelberg New York

ISBN 3-540-50525-3 1st ed. Springer-Verlag Berlin Heidelberg New York

Cataloging-in-Publication Data applied for

Die Deutsche Bibliothek – CIP-Einheitsaufnahme
Knaap, Marjo S. van der: Magnetic resonance of myelin, myelination, and myelin disorders /
M. S. van der Knaap; J. Valk. – 2. ed. – Berlin ; Heidelberg ; New York ; Barcelona ; Budapest ;
Hong Kong ; London ; Mailand ; Paris ; Tokyo ; Springer, 1995
1. Aufl. u.d.T.: Valk, Jacob: Magnetic resonance of myelin, myelination, and myelin disorders
ISBN 3-540-59277-6 NE: Valk, Jacob:

Typesetting, printing, and binding: Universitätsdruckerei H. Stürtz AG, Würzburg
SPIN: 10481559   21/3135 - 5 4 3 2 1 0 – Printed on acid-free paper

Preface to the Second Edition

The first edition of this book was well received by readers and reviewers and we are very grateful for the positive reactions. We were convinced then, and even more now, that MRI and MRS have much to offer in diagnosis, therapy monitoring and research of hereditary and acquired myelin disorders.

In the last few years, a great deal of new information has come available, concerning the genetic basis of inborn errors of metabolism and neurodegenerative disorders, the role of subcellular structures, the enzyme biochemistry, the pathophysiological mechanisms of posthypoxic-ischemic cerebral damage, and the inflammatory processes in infectious and inflammatory disorders. MR images of many rare disorders have become available, either in our own experience or published by other groups. MR spectroscopy could confirm its role in certain clinical applications. Because of these developments, it was necessary for us to rewrite the book almost completely. In some fields developments are so fast that we may not have caught all the latest developments. The pattern of the new approaches has, however, been established, making the assimilation of newly available information easy.

We are extremely grateful for the help of colleagues to make this book as complete as possible. The positive reactions of those from whom we requested MR pictures or other forms of support were of enormous encouragement to us during our efforts to complete this project.

We hope this work will be as warmly welcomed by our colleagues as the first edition.

Amsterdam, January 1995

M.S. van der Knaap
J. Valk

Preface to the First Edition

Magnetic resonance imaging (MRI) is now considered to be the imaging modality of choice for the majority of disorders affecting the central nervous system. This is particularly true for gray and white matter disorders, thanks to the superb soft tissue contrast in MRI which allows gray matter, unmyelinated, and myelinated white matter to be distinguished and their respective disorders identified. The present book is devoted to the disorders of myelin and myelination. A growing amount of detailed in vivo information about myelin, myelination, and myelin disorders has been derived both from MRI and from MR spectroscopy (MRS). This prompted us to review the clinical, laboratory, biochemical, and pathological data on this subject in order to integrate all available information and to provide improved insights into normal and disordered myelin and myelination. We will show how the synthesis of all available information contributes to the interpretation of MR images.

Following a brief historical review of the increasing knowledge on myelin and myelin disorders, we propose a new classification of myelin disorders based on the subcellular localization of the enzymatic defects as far as the inborn errors of metabolism are concerned. This classification serves as a guide throughout the book. All items of the classification will be discussed and, whenever relevant and possible, illustrated by MR images.

We are aware of the fact that in a number of myelin disorders MRI is not a part of the usual diagnostic work up because a definite diagnosis is reached by other means, such as biochemical investigations of blood and urine, enzyme assessment or detection of specific antibodies. However, in many disorders MRI may facilitate a rapid diagnosis and early instigation of treatment, thus preventing structural cerebral damage. In other cases the role of MRI is to visualize the extent of brain damage and give an indication of the prognosis. In disorders which present in a nonspecific way, for instance with behavioral problems or learning difficulties, MRI can be one of the first-line investigations. It is important to be acquainted with the various MRI patterns of the myelin disorders, as an early diagnosis may be of major importance in young families with a view to the provision of adequate genetic counseling.

MRS has been of limited clinical importance until now, and its application in patients only has a short history. We do, however, expect it to be a promising technique in the field of myelin and myelin disorders in clinical as well as in basic, experimental research and have, therefore, devoted a separate chapter to this subject.

This volume was written by a neuroradiologist and a neurologist/child neurologist. It is the product of close cooperation, animated discussions, strong arguments, restructuring, rewriting, and editing, in which they had an equal share. If the reader finds value in this monograph, it is because of this dual effort.

Amsterdam and Utrecht, March 1989   J. Valk
                                                     M.S. van der Knaap

Contents

List of Abbreviations

ACTH	adrenocorticotropic hormone
AD	Alexander's disease
ADEM	acute disseminated encephalomyelitis
ADP	adenosine diphosphate
AHEM	acute hemorrhagic encephalomyelitis
AIDS	acquired immunodeficiency syndrome
ALD	adrenoleukodystrophy
AMN	adrenomyeloneuropathy
ANCL	adult neuronal ceroid lipofuscinosis
ASLD	argininosuccinate lyase deficiency
ASSD	argininosuccinate synthetase deficiency
ATP	adenosine triphosphate
BAEP	brain stem auditory evoked potential
CADASIL	cerebral autosomal dominant arteriopathy with subcortical infarcts and leukoencephalopathy
Cbl	cobalamin
CD	Canavan's disease
Cho	choline
CMD	congenital muscular dystrophy
CMV	cytomegalovirus
CNS	central nervous system
CoD	Cockayne's disease
CPEO	chronic progressive ophthalmoplegia
CPM	central pontine myelinolysis
CPSD	carbamyl phosphate synthetase deficiency
Cr	creatine
CS	concentric sclerosis
CSF	cerebrospinal fluid
CT	computed tomography/gram
CTX	cerebrotendinous xanthomatosis
DNA	deoxyribonucleic acid
DPHL	delayed posthypoxic leukoencephalopathy
DS	diffuse sclerosis
EAA	excitatory amino acid
ECG	electrocardiography/gram
EEG	electroencephalography/gram
EPM	extrapontine myelinolysis
ERG	electroretinography/gram
FAD	flavine adenine dinucleotide
FD	Fabry's disease
GABA	γ-amino butyric acid
GaDTPA	gadolinium-diethylene-triamine penta-acetic acid
GLD	globoid cell leukodystrophy
HIV	human immunodeficiency virus
HLA	human leukocyte antigen
HSP	heat shock protein

HTLV	human T-cell lymphotropic virus
Ig	immunoglobulin
INCL	infantile neuronal ceroid lipofuscinosis
IQ	intelligence quotient
IR	inversion recovery
IRD	infantile Refsum's disease
JNCL	juvenile neuronal ceroid lipofuscinosis
kb	kilobase
KSS	Kearns-Sayre syndrome
Lac	lactate
LHON	Leber's hereditary optic neuropathy
LINCL	late-infantile neuronal ceroid lipofuscinosis
LS	Lowe syndrome
MHC	major histocompatibility complex
MBP	myelin basic protein
MBS	Marchiafava-Bignami syndrome
MD	myotonic dystrophy
MELAS	mitochondrial myopathy, encephalopathy, lactic acidosis and stroke-like episodes
MERRF	myoclonus epilepsy with ragged red fibers
mI	myo-inositol
MLD	metachromatic leukodystrophy
MNGIE	mitochondrial neurogastrointestinal encephalomyopathy
MPS	mucopolysaccharidoses
MR	magnetic resonance
MRI	magnetic resonance imaging
mRNA	messenger RNA
MRS	magnetic resonance spectrosopy
MS	multiple sclerosis
MSD	multiple sulfatase deficiency
MSUD	maple syrup urine disease
mtDNA	mitochondrial DNA
NAA	N-acetylaspartate
NAD	nicotinamide adenine dinucleotide
NALD	neonatal adrenoleukodystrophy
NCL	neuronal ceroid lipofuscinosis
nDNA	nuclear DNA
NKH	nonketotic hyperglycinemia
NMDA	N-methyl-D-aspartate
NMO	neuromyelitis optica
OTCD	ornithine transcarbamylase deficiency
PC	pyruvate carboxylase
PCr	phosphocreatine
PDE	phosphodiesters
PET	positron emission tomography
Pi	inorganic phosphate
PKU	phenylketonuria
PLP	proteolipid protein
PME	phosphomonoesters
PML	progressive multifocal leukoencephalitis
PMD	Pelizaeus-Merzbacher disease
PNS	peripheral nervous system
PRP	progressive rubella panencephalitis
Pseudo-NALD	pseudo-neonatal adrenoleukodystrophy
Pseudo-ZS	pseudo-Zellweger syndrome
PVL	periventricular leukomalacia

RCP	rhizomelic form of chondrodysplasia punctata
RD	Refsum's disease
RNA	ribonucleic acid
rRNA	ribosomal RNA
SAE	subcortical arteriosclerotic encephalopathy
SCL	subcortical leukomalacia
SD	Sandhoff's disease
SE	spin echo
SLS	Sjögren-Larsson syndrome
SPECT	single photon emission computer tomography
SSEP	somatosensory evoked potential
SSPE	subacute sclerosing panencephalitis
T	Tesla
TE	echo time
TI	inversion time
TPD	trifunctional protein deficiency
TR	repetition time
tRNA	transfer RNA
TSD	Tay-Sachs disease
US	ultrasound
VEP	visual evoked potential
VLCFA	very long-chain fatty acids
WD	Wilson's disease
XALD	X-linked adrenoleukodystrophy
ZLS	Zellweger-like syndrome
ZS	Zellweger cerebrohepatorenal syndrome

1 Myelin and White Matter

1.1 Introduction

Myelin makes up most of the substance of white matter in the central nervous system (CNS). It is also present in large quantities in the peripheral nervous system (PNS). In both the CNS and the PNS, myelin is essential for normal functioning of the nerve fibers.

The white matter of the CNS is composed of a vast number of axons which are ensheathed with myelin. The myelin is responsible for its white color. Besides myelinated axons, white matter contains many cells of the neuroglia type, but no cell bodies of neurons. The axons it contains originate from neuronal cell bodies in the gray matter.

Two types of neuroglia are found in the white matter: astrocytes and oligodendrocytes. Among the many putative functions of glial cells, it is proposed that they contribute to the structural and nutritive support of neurons, regulate the extracellular environment of ions and transmitters, guide migrating neurons during development, and play an important role in repair and regeneration. The best known function of glial cells is the ensheathment of axons with myelin by oligodendrocytes.

Gray matter contains the nerve cell bodies with their extensive dendritic arborization. The myelin content of gray matter structures is low, but some myelin is present in the subcortical gray matter nuclei and in the cortex around intracortical fibers. The myelin content of the thalamus and globus pallidus is relatively high.

1.2 Morphology of Myelin

Myelin is a spiral membranous structure that is tightly wrapped around axons. It has a very high lipid content and is soluble in fat solvents. Hence, when ordinary paraffin sections of the brain are prepared for light microscopic examination, most of the myelin dissolves away. After staining, the sites where myelin was present appear as round spaces that are empty except for a little round dot in the center which represents a cross section of the axon. By means of fixatives that make myelin insoluble, it is possible to demonstrate it in paraffin section. Osmic acid fixes myelin so that it does not dissolve in paraffin sections. Osmic acid itself stains myelin black. When examined under very low power, the white matter appears black (Fig. 1.1). If the white matter is examined under high power, the blackened myelin will be seen to be arranged in little rings around each nerve fiber. There are several myelin stains that can be used once the tissue has been fixed by some other means. Commonly used staining methods include hematoxylin, Loyez, Luxol fast blue, and Oil-Red-O.

The information derived from light microscopic investigations is limited and insufficient when more detailed information about myelin structure is required. Analysis of the structure of myelin began in the 1930s stimulated by polarization-microscope studies and X-ray diffraction work, which led to the suggestion that the myelin sheath could be constructed from layers or lamellae. The lamellar structure was confirmed by electron microscopic studies. In electron micrographs, myelin is seen as a series of alternating dark and less dark lines separated by unstained zones. These lines are wrapped spirally around the axon (Fig. 1.2). The evidence available from studies by polarized light, X-ray diffraction and electron microscope led to the current view of myelin as a system of condensed plasma membranes with alternating protein-lipid-protein-lipid-protein lamellae as the repeating subunit.

Plasma membranes are composed predominantly of lipids and proteins, and also contain carbohydrate components. The lipid elements of the membranes are phospholipids, glycolipids, and cholesterol. A common property of these lipids is that they are amphipathic. This means that the lipid molecules contain both hydrophobic and hydrophilic regions corresponding to the nonpolar tails and the polar head groups, respectively. Hydrophobic substances are insoluble in water, but soluble in oil. Conversely, hydrophilic substances are insoluble in oil, but soluble in water. In an aqueous environment, the amphipathic character of the lipids favors aggregation into micelles or a molecular bilayer. In a micelle (Fig. 1.3), the hydrophobic regions of the amphipathic molecules are shielded from the water while the hydrophilic polar groups are in direct contact with the water. The stability of this structure lies in the fact that significant free energy is required to transfer a nonpolar molecule from a nonpolar medium to water. Likewise, much energy is required to transfer a

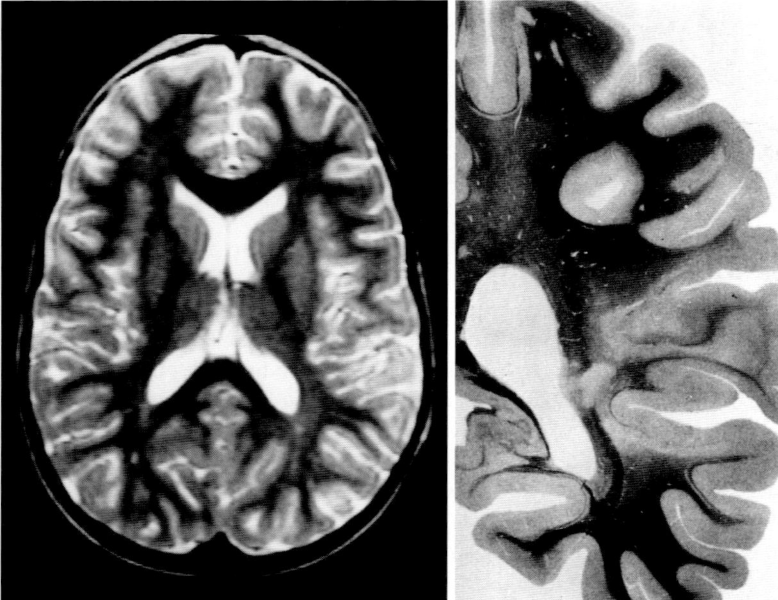

Fig. 1.1. T$_2$-weighted MR image (*left*) compared to a postmortem section (*right*) prepared with a myelin stain illustrating the capability of MRI to reflect histology

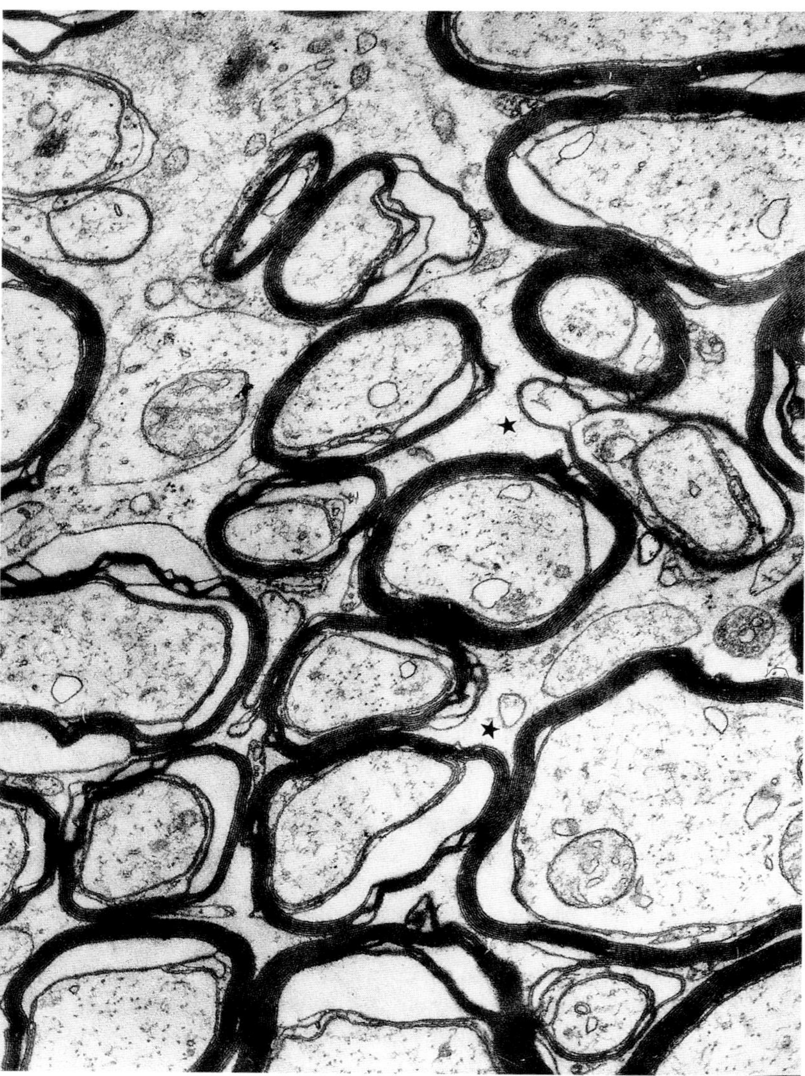

Fig. 1.2. Electron micrograph of myelin sheaths, in a case of extracellular edema. Courtesy of Cervós-Navarro (1993), with permission

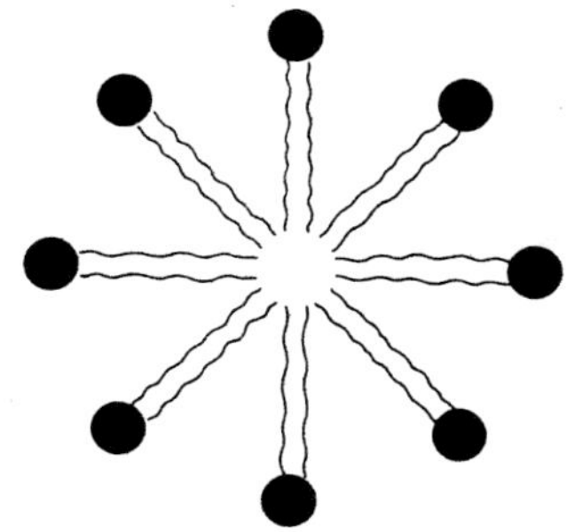

Fig. 1.3. A micelle

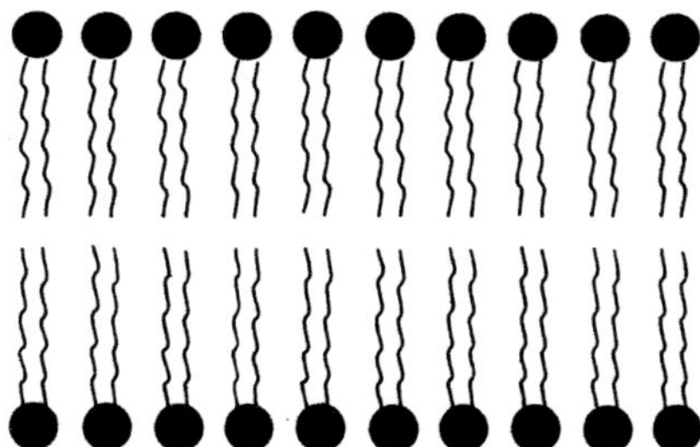

Fig. 1.4. A lipid bilayer

polar moiety from water to a nonpolar medium. Thus the micelle provides a minimal energy configuration and is accordingly thermodynamically stable. The molecular bilayer, the basic structure of plasma cell membranes, also satisfies the thermodynamic requirements of amphipathic molecules in an aqueous environment. A bilayer exists as a sheet in which the hydrophobic regions of the lipids are protected from the water, while the hydrophilic regions are immersed in water (Fig. 1.4). As the structure of the bilayer is inherent to the amphipathic character of the lipid molecules, it is evident that the formation of lipid bilayers is essentially a self-assembly process.

In comparison to other molecular bilayers, the myelin bilayer is unique in having a very high lipid content and in containing chiefly saturated fatty acids with an extraordinarily long chain length. This fatty acid composition leads to a closely packed, highly stable membrane structure. The presence of unsaturated fatty acids in a bimolecular leaflet leads to a more loosely packed, less stable structure as unsaturated fatty acid chains have a kinked, hook-like configuration. Lipids containing such unsaturated fatty acids cannot approach neighboring molecules as closely as saturated lipids can, since the latter are rod-like structures. The total interaction and the resulting binding forces between the tails of an unsaturated lipid and a neighboring molecule will be much less than that between the tails of two saturated lipids. Lipids containing long-chain fatty acids are more tightly held in a membrane structure than those containing shorter-chain fatty

acids, since the longer the hydrocarbon chain, the stronger the binding interactions between the lipid molecules. It has also been suggested that very long-chain fatty acids can form complexes by interdigitation of the hydrocarbon tail on one side with the hydrocarbon tail of a lipid on the opposite side of the bimolecular leaflet. This complex would contribute to the stability of the myelin membrane. If this lipid composition is changed, as is the case in a number of demyelinating disorders, it is clear that the stability of the myelin membrane will be diminished.

The bimolecular lipid structure allows for interaction of amphipathic proteins with the membrane. These proteins form an integral part of the membrane, with hydrophilic regions protruding from the inner and outer faces of the membrane and connected by a hydrophobic region traversing the hydrophobic core of the bilayer. In addition, there are peripheral proteins which do not interact directly with the lipids in the bilayer, but are weakly bound to the hydrophilic regions of specific integral proteins. Thus, the cell membrane is a bimolecular lipid leaflet coated with proteins on both sides (Fig. 1.5). There is inside-outside asymmetry of the lipids. Also, integral and peripheral proteins are asymmetrically distributed across the membrane bilayer.

On electron microscopic examination, a plasma membrane is shown as a three-layered structure and consists of two dark lines separated by a lighter interval. It is also revealed that the plasma membrane is not symmetrical in form as the dark line adjacent to the cytoplasm is more dense than the leaflet on the outside.

From both X-ray diffraction and electron microscope data it can be seen that the smallest radial subunit that can be called myelin is a five-layered structure of protein-lipid-protein-lipid-protein. The repeat distance is 160 to 180 Å. The dark lines seen in electron microscopic studies represent the protein layers, and the unstained zones the lipids. The uneven staining of the protein layers results from the way the myelin sheath is generated from the plasma membrane. The less dark lines (so-called intraperiod lines) represent the closely apposed outer protein coats of the original cell membrane. The dark lines (so-called major dense lines) are the fused inner protein coats of the cell membrane. High magnification electron micrographs show that the intraperiod line is double in nature (Fig. 1.6).

The myelin sheath is not continuous along the entire length of axons, but axons are covered by segments of myelin which are separated by small regions of uncovered axon, the nodes of Ranvier. The myelin lamellae terminate as they approach the node. The region where the lamellae terminate is known as the paranode. Electron micrographs of longitudinal sections of paranodal regions show that the major dense lines open up and

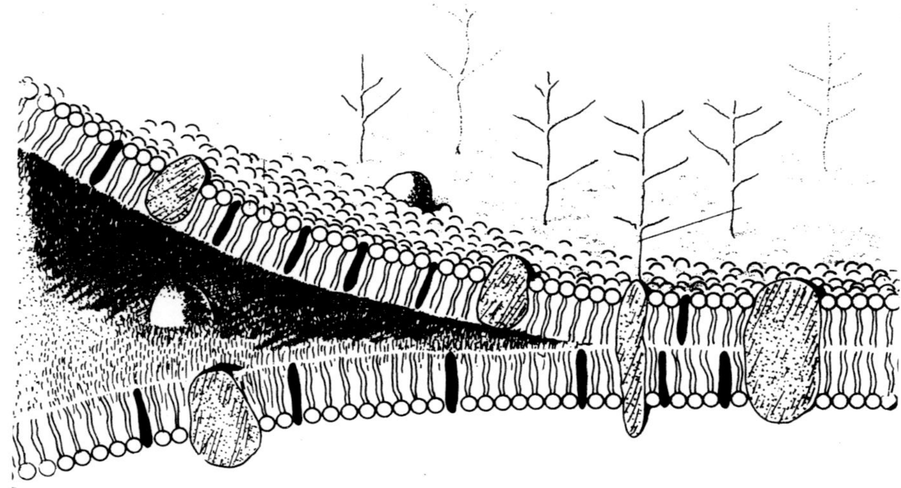

Fig. 1.5. Membrane split open to demonstrate the layers. The lipid bilayer is interrupted by proteins embedded in this layer. Glycoprotein chains rise from the surface of the membrane

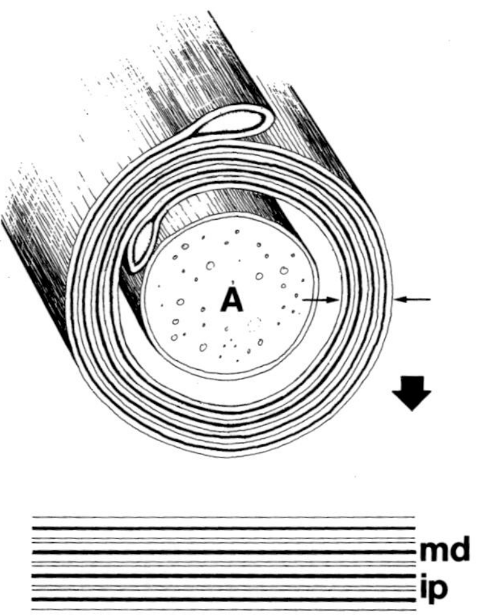

Fig. 1.6. Schematic representation of an electron microscopic picture of a myelin sheath. (*md*, major dense line; *ip*, intraperiod line; *A*, axon)

loop back upon themselves, enclosing cytoplasm within the loop (Fig. 1.7). In that part of the paranode most distant from the node, the innermost lamellae of the myelin terminate first, and succeeding turns of the spiral of lamellae then overlap and project beyond the ones lying beneath. Thus, the outermost lamella overlaps all the others and terminates nearest the node so that the myelin sheath gradually becomes thinner as the node is approached.

Schmidt-Lantermann clefts, as described in the PNS, are rare in the CNS. These are funnel-shaped clefts within myelin sheaths. They contain cytoplasm and extend from the soma of the myelin forming cell to the inner end of the myelin sheath. In a transverse section of a myelin sheath they appear as islands of cytoplasm between openings of the major dense lines.

There is considerable variation in the number of myelin lamellae in the sheaths surrounding different axons. Generally, the larger the diameter of the axon, the thicker its myelin sheath. In addition to this direct

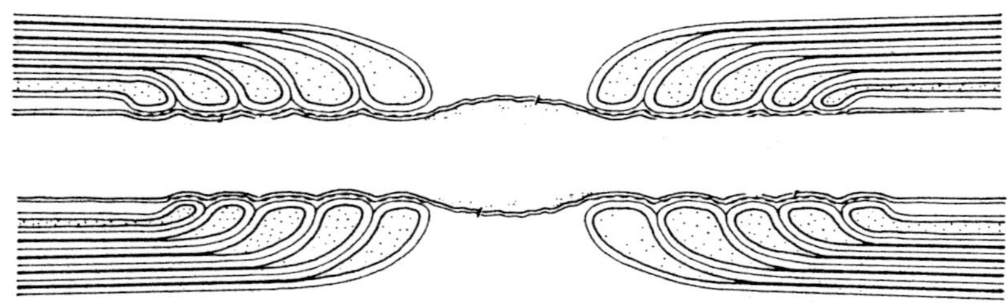

Fig. 1.7. Node of Ranvier, where the nerve fiber between two myelinated segments is bare. The outer myelin layers envelope the inner layer and cover these at the nodal junctions

relationship between axonal size and myelin thickness, it is known that the lengths of internodal segments also vary with the size of the axon. The larger the nerve fiber, the greater the internodal length.

1.3   Oligodendrocytes

Oligodendrocytes are the key cells in myelination of the CNS. They are cells of moderate size with a small number of short, branched processes. They are the predominant type of neuroglia in white matter, and are frequently found interposed between myelinated axons. Actual connections between oligodendrocytes and myelin sheaths are observed. In the gray matter they aggregate closely around neuronal cell bodies; here they are called satellite oligodendrocytes. PNS myelin is formed by Schwann cells.

The myelin membranes originate from and are part of the oligodendroglial cell membrane. The oligodendrocytes form flat cell processes which are wrapped around the nerve axon in a spiral fashion (Fig. 1.8). With the exception of the outer and lateral loops of the flat cell processes, the cellular cytoplasm disappears from these processes and the remaining cell membranes condense into a compact structure in which each membrane is closely apposed to the adjacent one. If myelin were unrolled from the axon, it would be a flat, spade-shaped sheet surrounded by a tube containing cytoplasm.

Although the myelin sheath is an extension of the oligodendroglial cell membrane, the chemical composition of myelin is quite different from it. The oligodendroglial cell membrane is transformed into myelin in processes of modification and differentiation.

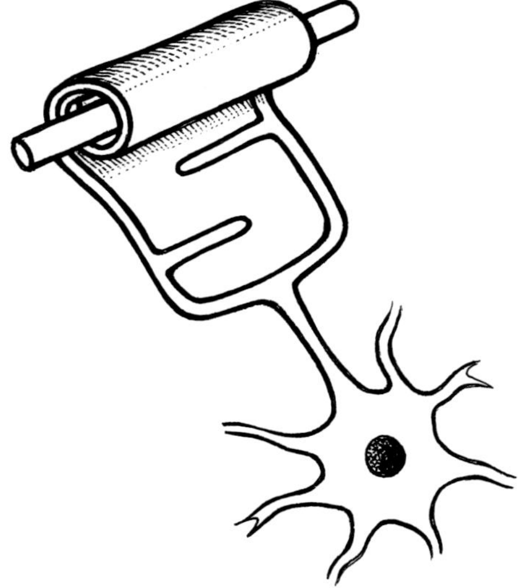

Fig. 1.8. Diagram showing the enrolling of the axon in the myelin sheath

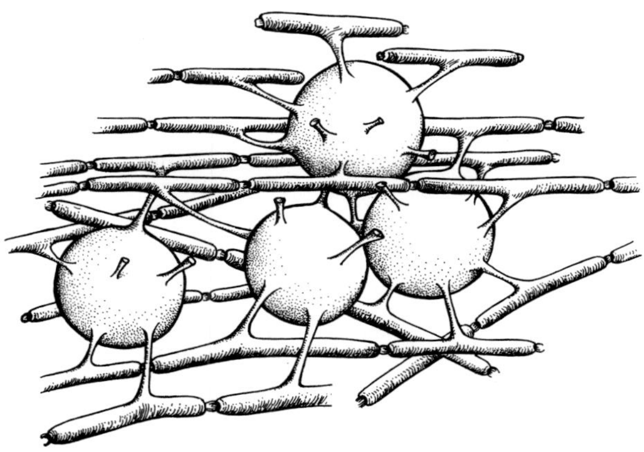

Fig. 1.9. Impression of the three-dimensional structure of oligodendrocytes with their plasma membrane extensions as myelin sheaths covering the axons which cross their region

A single oligodendrocyte provides the myelin for many internodal segments of different axons simultaneously. One oligodendrocyte may be responsible for the production and maintenance of up to 50 nerve fibers (Fig. 1.9). This has implications in disease conditions and reparative processes, as the destruction of only a few oligodendrocytes may have an extensive demyelinating effect.

Together with the Schwann cells of the PNS, oligodendrocytes are unique in their ability to proliferate vast amounts of a characteristic unit membrane. The ratio between cell body surface membrane and myelin membrane in the case of oligodendrocytes is estimated at 1:620. The deposition and maintenance of such large expanses of membrane require optimal coordination of the synthesis of its various lipid and protein components and their interaction, to ensure production of a stable membrane on the one hand and a well-regulated and controlled breakdown and replacement of worn components needed to support the myelin membrane on the other.

1.4   Biochemical Composition of Mature Myelin and White Matter

The most conspicuous feature of myelin composition compared with other membranes is the high ratio of lipid to protein. It is one of the most lipid-rich membranes, containing 70%–80% lipid by dry weight. In comparison with other membranes, the protein concentration of 20%–30% is low. For example, liver cell membranes contain 60% protein. Myelin is a relatively dehydrated structure, containing only 40% water.

CNS white matter is half myelin and half nonmyelin on a dry weight basis. Due to the high myelin content,

Table 1.1. Composition of human CNS gray matter, white matter, myelin portion and nonmyelin portion of whole white matter (from Norton and Cammer 1984)

	Gray matter	White matter	Myelin	Non-myelin [d]
Water [a]	82	72	44	82
Total protein [b]	55.3	39.0	30.0	62.2
Total lipid [b]	32.7	54.9	70.0	41.2
Cholesterol	22.0	27.5	27.7	14.6
Glycolipids	7.3	26.4	27.5	28.2
Cerebroside	5.4	19.8	22.7	19.9
Sulfatide	1.7	5.4	3.8	7.7
Phospholipids	69.5	45.9	43.1	51.9
Ethanolamine PG	22.7	14.9	15.6	6.8
Choline PG	26.7	12.8	11.2	16.5
Serine PG	8.7	7.9	4.8	20.4
Inositol PG	2.7	0.9	0.6	1.0
Sphingomyelin	6.9	7.7	7.9	5.6
Plasmalogens [c]	8.8	11.2	12.3	9.2

PG, phosphoglycerides
[a] Percentage total brain weight
[b] Figures for total protein and total lipid are percentages dry weight; all others are percentages total lipid weight.
[c] Plasmalogens are primarily ethanolamine phosphoglycerides.
[d] Figures for bovine brain, which are supposed to be in close agreement with those for human brain. (These figures are from Norton and Autilio 1966).

white matter has a relatively low water content and a high lipid content. White matter has a water content of 72%, gray matter of 82%. The nonmyelin portion of white matter contains about 80% water.

Myelin is mainly responsible for the gross chemical differences between white and gray matter. Myelin is rich in all lipid classes, although nonpolar lipids and glycolipids (galactolipids) are particularly well represented. The lipids of CNS myelin are composed of 25%–28% cholesterol, 27%–30% galactolipid, and 40%–45% phospholipid when expressed in percent total lipid weight. When lipid data are expressed as molar ratios, CNS myelin preparations contain cholesterol, phospholipid and galactolipid in a ratio varying between 4:3:2 and 4:4:2.

The biochemical composition of mature gray and white matter is shown in Table 1.1. With respect to white matter, separate figures are given for the myelin and nonmyelin portions, CNS white matter being half myelin and half nonmyelin on a dry weight basis. In Table 1.1 the lipid figures are expressed as percentages of total lipid weight. Since the water content and the dry weight lipid content of gray matter and white matter, myelin and nonmyelin, show great differences, the figures expressed in this way give no direct information about lipid concentration in either dry or wet tissue. However, from the data presented, these concentrations can be calculated.

When the lipid compositions of gray and white matter are compared, the most conspicuous difference is that white matter is relatively richer in galactolipids and relatively poor in phospholipids. Galactolipids constitute 25–30% of the lipids in white matter, whereas they are only 5%–10% of those in gray matter. Phospholipids account for two-thirds of the total lipids in gray matter, but less than half those in white matter. There are, strictly speaking, no myelin-specific lipids, which are not found elsewhere in the brain. However, the most distinguishing feature of myelin lipids is the high cerebroside content and cerebroside may be considered the most typical myelin lipid. During development, the concentration of cerebroside in brain is directly proportional to the amount of myelin present.

Ethanolamine phosphoglyceride in plasmalogen form (plasmenylethanolamine) is the major myelin phospholipid. Approximately 80% of the ethanolamine phosphoglycerides of myelin and white matter are present in the plasmalogen form, and only a small proportion is formed by phosphatidylethanolamine. Conversely, the plasmalogens, which comprise nearly one-third of the total phospholipids, are mainly of the ethanolamine type with lesser amounts of plasmenylserine. Phosphatidylcholine is the major choline phosphoglyceride; only traces of choline phosphoglyceride have the plasmalogen form.

Gangliosides are minor myelin lipids and constitute only 0.3%–0.7% of total myelin lipid. They are mainly localized in neuronal membranes, and gray matter is 10 times richer in gangliosides than white matter. Gangliosides are complex sialic acids containing glycosphingolipids. GM_1, a monosialoganglioside, is the major myelin ganglioside, and accounts for about 70 mole% of the total myelin ganglioside content. The ganglioside GM_4 (sialogalactosylceramide) is probably specific in the CNS for myelin and oligodendroglia. It is a derivate of cerebroside.

Myelin lipids contain somewhat different fatty acid constituents than other membranes. Characteristic of myelin are a-hydroxy fatty acids in cerebrosides and sulfatides and high amounts of long-chain fatty acids in the different lipid classes. There are monounsaturated fatty acids, but only low amounts of polyunsaturated fatty acids.

Table 1.2 shows the chemical architecture of the main lipid constituents of myelin. Sphingolipids of myelin are formed from sphingosine. N-acylsphingosine is termed ceramide. A phosphorylcholine group attached to ceramide forms sphingomyelin; glucose or galactose in glycosidic linkage forms cerebroside (most often: galactosylceramide). When the glucose or galactose is esterified with sulfate, sulfatide is formed. Phos-

Table 1.2. Structure of the important myelin lipids

Cerebroside	spingosine—galactose | fatty acid
Sulfatide	spingosine—galactose—sulfate | fatty acid
Phosphatidyl-ethanolamine	glycerol ⟨ fatty acid / fatty acid / phosphate—ethanolamine
Phosphatidyl-choline: =lecithin	glycerol ⟨ fatty acid / fatty acid / phosphate—choline
Phosphatidyl-serine:	glycerol ⟨ fatty acid / fatty acid / phosphate—serine
Phosphatidyl-inositol:	glycerol ⟨ fatty acid / fatty acid / phosphate—inositol
Ethanolamine plasmalogens:	glycerol ⟨ [a] fatty acid / fatty acid / phosphate—ethanolamine
Sphingomyelin:	sphingosine—fatty acid | phosphate—choline
GM_3 ganglioside:	N-acylsphingosine | glucose | galactose—N-acetylneuraminic acid
GM_2 ganglioside:	N-acylsphingosine | glucose | galactose—N-acetylneuraminic acid | N-acetylgalactosamine
GM_1 ganglioside:	N-acylsphingosine | glucose | galactose—N-acetylneuraminic acid | N-acetylgalactosamine | galactose

[a] Unsaturated ether structure

phoglycerides contain two fatty acids in ester linkage at the α and β position of glycerol and at the α^1 position a phosphate group to which the moiety definitive of the class is linked. For example, a choline group defines phosphatidylcholine. The plasmalogens are similarly formed, except that at the α position of the glycerol there is a 1:2 unsaturated ether structure. Gangliosides are synthesized from N-acylsphingosine by stepwise addition of sugars and N-acetylneuraminic acid.

The protein composition of myelin is simpler than that of other membranes. Proteolipid protein and myelin basic protein comprise 80%–85% of the total protein. Most myelin proteins are unique to myelin.

Proteolipid protein (PLP) and its isoform DM20 constitute about 50% of the total protein in CNS myelin. Their concentration is about 5 times higher in white matter than in gray matter. The proteins are encoded by the same gene and are formed by alternative splicing of the primary gene transcript. The proteins differ by a hydrophilic peptide 35 amino acids in length, whose presence generates PLP. DM20 is predominant in early development, whereas PLP is the major protein in mature myelin. The proteins are very hydrophobic.

There are multiple isoforms of myelin basic protein (MBP), arising from different patterns of splicing of the primary gene transcript. The heterogeneity is increased further by various posttranslational modifications. Myelin basic proteins account for 30%–35% of the total myelin protein. The proteins contain no extensive regions of hydrophobic residues and are hydrophilic. Myelin basic protein is the antigen which, when injected into an animal, elicits a cellular immune response, producing the CNS autoimmune disease called experimental allergic encephalomyelitis.

There are several CNS myelin glycoproteins: myelin-associated glycoprotein (MAG), myelin/oligodendrocyte glycoprotein (MOG) and oligodendrocyte-myelin glycoprotein (OMgp). These are high molecular weight proteins. They are quantitatively minor myelin components: myelin-associated glycoprotein accounts for about 1% of total protein, myelin/oligodendrocyte-myelin glycoprotein for 0.05%.

Highly purified myelin contains a number of enzymes. Two of these enzymes, 2′,3′-cyclic nucleotide 3′-phosphodiesterase (CNPase) and a cholesterol ester hydrolase, are found at much higher specific activities in myelin than in brain homogenates. It appears that these enzymes are fairly myelin specific, but probably also present in oligodendroglial membranes. Many other enzymes are found that are not specific to myelin but also present in other subcellular fractions. The exact function of the enzymes is not known. In particular, their contribution to the metabolism of myelin constituents is not known. 2′,3′-cyclic nucleotide 3′-phosphodiesterase catalyzes the hydrolysis of several 2′,3′-cyclic nucleotide monophosphates, all of which are converted to the corresponding 2'-isomer. The substrates of the enzyme are not present in nervous tissue and the protein may in fact have a structural function in the myelin membrane. 2',3'-cyclic nucleotide 3'-phosphodiesterase is one of the formerly called Wolfgram proteins, a heterogeneous group of high molecular weight myelin proteins named after the investigator who first suggested that myelin contained proteins other than proteolipid protein and myelin basic protein.

1.5　Molecular Architecture of Myelin

The currently accepted view of the myelin structure is that of a double lipid bilayer, each coated on both sides with protein. The resulting repeating subunit consists of radial protein-lipid-protein-lipid-protein lamellae. Some proteins are fully or partially embedded in the bilayer and others are attached to the surface by weaker linkages.

Both proteins and lipids have an asymmetrical distribution. Galactolipids, cholesterol, phosphatidylcholine and sphingomyelin are preferentially located in the former extracellular half of the bilayer (intraperiod line). Ethanolamine plasmalogen and myelin basic protein are preferentially located in the former cytoplasmic half of the bilayer.

Membranes are fluid structures. Lipid molecules diffuse rapidly in the plane of the membrane, as do proteins, unless anchored by specific interactions. The spontaneous rotation of lipids from one side of the membrane to the other is a very slow process. The transition of a molecule from one membrane surface to the other is called transverse diffusion, or flip-flop. Considering the asymmetry of lipids in the bilayer, the transverse mobility must be limited. The diffusion within the plane of the membrane is referred to as lateral diffusion.

Proteolipid protein consists of alternating hydrophilic and hydrophobic sequences with four stretches of hydrophobic residues that are of sufficient length to span the lipid bilayer. It is an integral membrane protein that passes through the bilayer four times. The hydrophobic transmembrane segments are linked by hydrophilic portions on both sides of the membrane. So the protein has domains in both the intraperiod and major dense lines. Probably both isoforms, PLP and DM20, are involved in stabilizing the intraperiod line. Their role is described as "adhesive struts" by some, and interpreted as "spacers", maintaining a set distance between apposed lamellae by others. It has also been proposed that the proteolipids may be organized as a multimeric complex in the lipid bilayer, forming an "adhesive pore", that is half a gap junction. When two such structures are present on ap-

posing lamellae, they may create a conduit for physiological communication between the axonal membrane and the extracellular space outside the myelin sheath. DM20 is the major product in early development, whereas PLP is the major product in mature myelin. It is believed that DM20 plays an as yet unidentified regulatory role in early oligodendrocyte progenitor development and differentiation, and that PLP plays a part later on in oligodendrocyte function, in the proper formation of the intraperiod line of myelin during its final elaboration and compaction.

Myelin basic protein is an extrinsic protein, located on the cytoplasmic face of the myelin membranes at the major dense lines. It probably stabilizes the major dense lines by keeping the cytoplasmic faces of the myelin lamellae in close apposition.

Gangliosides are located almost entirely on the external surface of membranes. They may play an important role in cell surface recognition and signal transduction processes, such as those that occur during myelination.

Myelin glycoproteins are transmembrane proteins with the polypeptide extending through the lipid bilayer and the glycosylated portion of the molecule exposed on the outer surface of the bilayer. They are all implicated in recognition and cell-cell interactions.

Myelin-associated glycoprotein is one of these proteins. Its external region contains immunoglobulin-like domains. So, myelin-associated glycoprotein is a member of the immunoglobulin superfamily. It is concentrated in the inner periaxonal membrane of the myelin sheath and probably absent from the compact multilamellar myelin sheath. The exposed, periaxonal position is compatible with its postulated involvement in oligodendrocyte-axon interaction, including maintenance of the structural integrity of the glia-axon adhesion in mature myelin. The observation, that the protein can be detected at the very earliest stages of myelination has led to the hypothesis that the protein may also play a role in mediating the oligodendrocyte-axon recognition events that precede myelination and specify the initial path of myelin deposition.

Myelin/oligodendrocyte glycoprotein is another of the myelin glycoproteins. It also belongs to the immunoglobulin superfamily. The protein is located at the outermost layer of the myelin sheath and the oligodendrocyte plasma membrane. The function of this glycoprotein is unknown. It may play a role in the adhesion between neighboring myelinated fibers and may function as a glue in the maintenance of axon bundles in the CNS.

The enzyme 2',3'-cyclic nucleotide 3'-phosphodiesterase is found in myelin and oligodendrocytes. Within the myelin sheath it is localized at the major dense lines. Several possible functions have been suggested. Its early appearance in myelin suggests a possible role in the early stages of glial differentiation. Its low concentration in myelin argues against it having a structural role here. Its presence in non-neural tissues suggests a more general function in cells or membranes.

1.6 Myelinogenesis

The time-course of appearance of newly synthesized lipids and proteins in myelin indicates that myelin is not laid down as a unit, but that different components are produced and processed on different sites in the cell and show different rates of entry into the myelin sheath. For example, myelin basic protein enters the myelin sheath with almost no lag after synthesis, whereas proteolipid protein enters myelin after a lag of 30–40 min following synthesis. Once protein synthesis is stopped with cycloheximide, the entry of myelin basic protein is halted immediately, but proteolipid protein continues to be incorporated into myelin for 30 min. These data indicate that myelin basic protein and proteolipid protein are assembled by different mechanisms with proteolipid protein taking a longer and more circuitous route through the cytoplasm. It is also interesting that lipids continue to be incorporated into myelin 4 h after protein synthesis has stopped.

Myelin basic protein is synthesized on free polyribosomes near the plasma membrane or the adjacent myelin sheath. The myelin membrane is surrounded by and infiltrated with cytoplasmic channels, called the outer loops and longitudinal incisures, respectively. There is good evidence that myelin basic protein mRNA is translocated from its site of synthesis within the cell bodies of oligodendrocytes to the myelin membrane via these cytoplasmic channels. Myelin basic protein synthesized here is rapidly sequestered into the myelin sheath and appears in the cytoplasmic leaflet of compact myelin (major dense lines). There is evidence that the enzyme 2′,3′-cyclic nucleotide 3′-phosphodiesterase is also synthesized on free polyribosomes. The synthesis of the protein within the cytoplasm is consistent with its localization at the major dense lines in compact myelin.

Proteolipid protein is synthesized on polyribosomes bound to the endoplasmic reticulum. The nascent protein is inserted into the endoplasmic reticulum and passes through the Golgi apparatus to the plasma membrane and myelin sheath via vesicular transport. Inclusion in the plasma membrane occurs by fusion of the vesicles with the plasma membrane. The inside of the vesicle after fusion becomes the outside of the plasma membrane. As a consequence, substances transported to the plasma membrane via vesicles end up in the extracellular leaflet of the myelin sheath. Myelin associated glycoprotein resembles proteolipid protein as far as site of synthesis and transport to the plasma membrane are concerned.

The same two mechanisms of synthesis and transport can be distinguished for myelin lipids, i.e., the routes of proteolipid protein and myelin basic protein, respectively. The endoplasmic reticulum is the site of synthesis of phosphotidylcholine and cholesterol. The Golgi apparatus is the site of synthesis of cerebroside, sulfatide, sphingomyelin and gangliosides. The lipids are transported from the Golgi apparatus to the plasma membrane by a vesicle-mediated process. Expression on the cell surface occurs by fusion of the vesicles with the plasma membrane. The lipids are predominantly located in the extracellular leaflet of the myelin lamellae. In contrast, the myelin phospholipids that predominantly reside on the inner leaflet, including phosphatidylserine and ethanolamine plasmalogens, are synthesized in the superficial cytoplasmic channels of the myelin sheath and enter compact myelin rapidly, possibly with phospholipid transfer proteins as carriers. Several other phospholipids are also synthesized in the superficial cytoplasmic channels.

After reaching the outermost myelin layers, substances penetrate to the deepest layers over a period of a few days. This movement of substances from outer to inner layers occurs at rates consistent with lateral diffusion along the spirally wound bilayer.

1.7 Regulation of Myelinogenesis

Elaboration of the myelin sheath involves a precisely ordered sequence of events beginning with the initial ensheathment of the axon, proceeding to formation of multiple loose wrappings and eventually compaction to form the mature multilamellar myelin sheath. These processes imply a temporally regulated program of gene expression in the oligodendrocyte to ensure that the appropriate biochemical components are synthesized in the proper proportions at each stage of myelinogenesis. It has been shown that just prior to the onset of rapid myelin membrane synthesis the genes of myelin proteins are sharply upregulated. There is evidence of a coordinated mechanism for synchronous activation of the myelin protein genes. This period of sharp upregulation of myelin genes is the most vulnerable part of the myelination process and is called the critical period.

Apparently, there are both tissue-specific and stage-specific mechanisms controlling myelin genes. Myelin genes only come to expression in oligodendrocytes and Schwann cells. The expression of the genes is developmentally regulated and probably intimately associated with the stage of differentiation of these cells. Control mechanisms are active at the transcriptional level. Regulatory regions, including promotor elements, have been identified for myelin protein genes. Key sites for tissue-specific expression of myelin proteins are clustered near the promotor areas and within these clusters are several motifs that may be involved in coordinating the regulation of myelin-specific genes. The alternative splicing patterns produced from the primary myelin protein transcripts are also developmentally regulated. The splicing patterns for the different proteins have been shown to change with development.

In both the CNS and PNS, glial cells are influenced to myelinate by both neuronal targets that they ensheath and by a range of hormones and growth factors. There is a continuous oligodendrocyte-neuron interaction. Differentiation of oligodendroglia has been shown to depend closely on presence and integrity of axons. Gene expression for myelin constituents is modulated by the presence of axons. Within oligodendrocytes, genes are translated into proteins that are thought to play roles in the induction of myelination (e.g., glial-specific surface receptors for differentiation signals), in the initial deposition of the myelin sheath (e.g., axon-glial adhesion molecules), and in its wrapping and compaction around the nerve axon (e.g., structural proteins of compact myelin). It has long been known, that a minimal axonal diameter is important for the initiation of myelination. Final myelin sheath thickness is also related to axonal size. This match is reached by local control mechanisms. Therefore, a single oligodendrocyte can be associated with several axons of different sizes, the myelin sheaths being thicker for larger axons. Larger axons also have longer internodes.

Growth hormone has a dramatic effect on myelinogenesis. A deficiency of growth hormone during the critical period leads to hypomyelination. Most of the effects of growth hormone are mediated by insulin-like growth factor I (IGF-I). Administration of this substance in early development leads to an increase in all brain constituents, but in particular and disproportionally in amount of myelin produced per oligodendrocyte. Also thyroid hormone has an effect on myelinogenesis. Hypothyroidism during early development leads to hypomyelination. Steroids have a complex influence. None of the myelin protein genes is transcriptionally regulated by steroids, but steroids probably act at the posttranslational level, stimulating the translation of myelin basic protein and proteolipid protein mRNAs and inhibiting the translation of $2',3'$-cyclic nucleotide $3'$-phosphodiesterase mRNA.

Apart from insulin-like growth factor I, many other putative oligodendrocyte growth factors have been described in recent years, that modulate oligodendrocyte proliferation and differentiation. These include glial maturation factor, oligodendroglia growth factor, fibroblast growth factor, and platelet-derived growth factor. The importance of iron in myelination has been examined. Iron and the iron mobilization protein

transferrin are localized in oligodendrocytes, and may participate in the formation and/or maintenance of myelin by complexing with enzymes involved in the synthesis of myelin components.

Myelination is vulnerable to undernourishment. If there is undernourishment during the critical period just prior to the onset of rapid myelin synthesis, myelination is more severely reduced than total brain weight, whereas the number of oligodendrocytes is unaltered. The hypomyelination is permanent. Severe undernutrition during the critical period leads to decreased levels of insulin-like growth factors and a failure in upregulation of myelin genes.

Successful myelination is also dependent upon function. It is known that myelination is diminshed by preventing the conduction of impulses in a nerve. Impulse conduction is a stimulus to myelination. Hypermyelination has incidentally been noticed in cerebral anomalies, supposedly via the stimulus of epilepsy.

After formation the myelin sheath and the axon remain mutually dependent. The myelin sheath needs an intact axon as is demonstrated by the studies on Wallerian degeneration. On the other hand, for maintenance of normal structure and function, the axon requires an intact myelin sheath.

Since myelin, once deposited, is a relatively stable substance metabolically, it is relatively invulnerable to adverse external factors. Generalized vulnerability of myelin to noxious agents and adverse influences is likely to be confined to the period just before and during active myelination.

1.8 Myelination of the Nervous System

Myelination of each of the multiple connecting fiber systems of the CNS takes place at different times in early development. Some fiber systems start to myelinate halfway through or late in gestation and rapidly attain their maximal degree of myelination, whereas other systems attain their maximal degree of myelination only slowly. One cannot, therefore, correctly refer to myelination as a singular process. There is a marked, temporal diversity in topographic patterns of myelination throughout the last half of gestation and during the first two postnatal years. Thus, at any time in early development of the human brain there are multiple separate or intermixed regions of unmyelinated, partly myelinated, or completely myelinated tracts.

Myelination of the nervous system follows a fixed pattern consisting of ordered sequences of myelinating systems, apparently governed by some rules:
1. The first rule, probably governing all other rules, is that tracts in the nervous system become myelinated at the time they become functional.

2. Myelination starts in the PNS before it starts in the CNS.
3. Myelination in central sensory areas tends to precede myelination in central motor areas.
4. Myelination in the brain occurs in areas of primary function earlier than in association areas.
5. Most tracts become myelinated in the direction of the impulse conduction.
6. Roughly speaking, myelination progresses from caudal (spinal cord) to rostral parts (brain) and spreads from central (diencephalon, pre-and postcentral gyri) to peripheral parts of the brain. However, there are many exceptions to this rule.

It is important to note that the times that will be mentioned for the myelination of the different tracts and structures of the brain are only generalizations and approximations. In the first place, there is a considerable degree of normal variation. In the second place, the onset of myelination is difficult to define. It can be defined as the first myelin tube found on light microscopic examination, as the appearance of the first myelin lamella on ultrastructural examination or as the first evidence of presence of myelin constituents in immunological investigations.

In the fourth month of gestation, myelin is first seen in the anterior motor roots and soon appears in the posterior roots.

In the fifth month of gestation, myelination starts in the dorsal columns of the spinal cord and the anterior and lateral spinothalamic tracts for conduction of somesthetic stimuli.

In the sixth month of gestation, myelination proceeds rapidly cephalad in the medial lemniscus and spinothalamic tracts in the brain stem tegmentum. Myelin begins to appear in the statoacoustic tectum and tegmentum and the lateral lemniscus for the conduction of acoustic stimuli. Myelin is seen in the inner, vestibulocerebellar part of the inferior cerebellar peduncle.

In the seventh month of gestation, myelination is still largely confined to structures outside the diencephalon and cerebral hemispheres. Progress of myelination is seen in the optic nerve, optic chiasm and tracts, inferior cerebellar peduncle, the parasagittal part of the cerebellum, the descending trigeminal tract, superior cerebellar peduncle, capsule of the red nucleus, capsule of the inferior olivary nucleus, vestibulospinal, reticulospinal and tectospinal descending tracts to the spinal cord and posterior limb of the internal capsule.

In the eighth month of gestation, myelination starts in the corpus striatum (in particular globus pallidus), anterior limb of the internal capsule, subcortical white matter of the post- and precentral gyri, rostral part of the optic radiation as well as corticospinal tracts in midbrain and pons, transpontine fibers, middle cerebellar peduncles and cerebellar hemispheres.

In the ninth month of gestation, myelination continues in the thalamus (in particular ventrolateral nucleus), putamen, central part of the corona radiata, distal part of the optic radiation, acoustic radiation, anterior commissure, midportion of the corpus callosum and fornix.

However, in a child born at term, most of the structures and tracts mentioned are not fully myelinated and, in fact, in some myelination has just started. Apart from some myelin in the central tracts of the corona radiata connected with the pre- and postcentral gyri, and the primary optic and acoustic radiations, the cerebral hemisphers are still largely unmyelinated. During the first postnatal year, myelin spreads throughout the entire brain. By the postnatal age of 12 weeks myelination is well advanced in the corona radiata, the optic radiation and the corpus callosum, but the frontal and temporal white matter are still largely unmyelinated. By the age of about 8 months, the adult state is foreshadowed in that none of the fiber systems is still completely devoid of myelin sheaths. Myelin sheaths are still sparse in the temporal and frontal areas. It is not until the end of the second postnatal year that an advanced state of myelination is seen in all subcortical areas. Histologically, myelination reaches completion in early adulthood.

1.9 Compositional Changes in the Developing Brain

The DNA content of brain is considered to be a reliable indicator of cell number. The period of cellular proliferation can, therefore, be followed by measuring the amount of DNA per brain volume. In human brain two major periods of cell proliferation have been detected by measuring DNA levels. The first period begins at 15 to 20 weeks of gestation and corresponds to neuroblast proliferation. The second period begins at 25 weeks of gestation and continues into the second year of postnatal life. This latter period corresponds to multiplication of glial cells and includes a second wave of neuronogenesis, producing mainly cerebellar neurons. The ratio of protein to DNA indicates cell size. This ratio increases after neuronal division ends, reflecting in part the arborization of neuronal processes. The maximum ratio of protein to DNA is reached at 2 years of age. The outgrowth of neuronal axons and dendrites results in a rapid increase in total ganglioside content in the brain. Increasing lipid content indicates membrane formation with, in particular, an increase in quantity of axonal, dendritic, and myelin membranes. The increasing lipid content is associated with a concomitant decrease in water content. The most rapid

Table 1.3. Lipid composition of human brain during development (from Svennerholm 1963)

	Lipid composition of (frontal) cerebral cortex			Lipid composition of (frontal) cerebral white matter		
Age	2 months	1 year	5 years	2 months	1 year	5 years
Total lipids [a]	28.4	31.3	29.5	29.5	49.6	58.2
Cholesterol [b]	21.5	19.8	19.3	26.4	25.0	24.4
Phospho- lipids [b]	76.8	77.6	75.6	66.1	53.4	49.8
Glycolipids [b]	1.8	2.6	4.1	7.5	21.6	25.8

[a] Expressed as percentage dry weight.
[b] Expressed as percentage total lipid weight.

increase in lipid content of the brain begins after the period of greatest increase of DNA and protein and is closely related to the onset of myelination.

At birth, cerebral hemispheral white matter contains very little myelin and the white matter composition of neonates is very different from the composition of mature myelinated white matter. There is an important overall decrease in water content of the brain after birth and the change in water content is larger for white matter than for gray matter. The water content of neonatal gray matter is about 89% and of neonatal unmyelinated white matter about 87%, whereas the water content of adult gray matter is estimated to be 82% and of adult myelinated white matter 72%. The lipid composition of cerebral white matter at different ages is shown in Table 1.3. A major change is an increase in total lipid content, with a relative increase in glycolipids. One of these, cerebroside, is usually considered to be a marker for myelin as it is deposited at the same rate in the brain as myelin. However, cerebroside is not restricted to myelin and as much as 30% of it may be present in membranes other than myelin. There is a relative decrease (but absolute increase) in phospholipids in the white matter, which were relatively high in concentration in unmyelinated white matter and are relatively low in concentration in myelin. The relative contribution of cholesterol to total lipids remains constant, but the absolute cholesterol content of white matter increases with deposition of myelin. The changes in gray matter composition are much less important. Myelin deposition in gray matter is minor.

The changes in white matter composition are not only caused by glial cell proliferation, growth of axons and dendrites, and myelin deposition, but also by some changes in myelin composition. The composition of myelin first deposited is somewhat different from that of the adult. The most important changes are an increase in cholesterol and glycolipids as a proportion of total lipid and a decrease in phospholipids. In immature brain significant amounts of glucose are present in the glycolipids, whereas in mature brain glycolipids are mainly present as galactolipids. In contrast to the modest decrease in total phospholipids, more marked variations in the relative contribution of individual phospholipids are found. Sphingomyelin and ethanolamine phosphoglycerides increase, whereas choline phosphoglycerides undergo a decrease. The molar ratio of galactolipids and choline phosphoglycerides appears to be a sensitive marker of myelin maturation.

In human unmyelinated white matter much of the present cholesterol is esterified. The same is true for cholesterol in newly formed myelin. During myelin maturation there is a decrease in the amount of cholesterol esters, and in adult white matter cholesterol is present almost entirely in the free form. The ratio of cholesterol to phospholipids in myelin increases after birth and reaches the adult value at about 5 years of age. The ratio of galactolipids to phospholipids reaches the adult value at about the same time.

During development the ganglioside composition of myelin becomes simplified. The polysialogangliosides decrease and the monosialoganglioside GM_1 content approaches about 90% of the total gangliosides with increasing age. The total ganglioside content remains constant.

Maturation of myelin is accompanied by an increase in hydroxy fatty acids and saturated and monounsaturated fatty acids.

Maturation of myelin is also accompanied by changes in the proteins. As the brain matures there is a change in occurrence of the major isoforms of the major myelin proteins. For example, initially, early in myelination, DM20 is the principal proteolipid protein isoform, whereas in adult brain, DM20 is present at much lower levels than the isoform PLP. With increasing development the contribution of proteolipid protein and myelin basic protein to myelin proteins shows a relative increase, whereas the high molecular weight proteins decrease.

On the whole, the differences in chemical composition of immature myelin and adult myelin are not striking, which suggests that only subtle remodeling of myelin occurs in humans once myelination commences. The major difference between white matter early in life and in adult life seems to be the quantity of myelin rather than its quality.

1.10 Myelin Turnover

The principal features of myelin metabolism are its high rate of synthesis during the active stages of myelination when each oligodendroglial cell makes more than three times its own weight of myelin per day, and its relative metabolic stability after the completion of myelination. Individual components turn over at quite different rates. There are conflicting data about the precise half-lives of the various myelin lipids and proteins. This is understandable since there are several variables in the experimental design that have considerable influence on the observed, real or apparent, half-lives. However, some general conclusions can be formulated. The concept of relative long-term metabolic stability of most myelin components has been confirmed. Some components do turn over much faster than others and all components show both a slow and a fast turning-over component. The data indicate that newly formed myelin is catabolized faster than old myelin. Hence, myelin that has been deposited early in life appears to have a higher metabolic stability than newly synthesized myelin.

1.11   Aging of Myelin

With increasing age, human brain weight decreases and water content increases. Levels of DNA and numbers of neurons in the cerebral cortex decrease significantly with aging. Little change is found in some regions, including the brain stem.

Multiple morphological changes take place with increasing age. The most prominent neuronal changes are the appearance of senile plaques (areas of degenerating neuronal processes, reactive non-neuronal cells, and amyloid), increasing deposits of lipofuscin, and areas of neurofibrillary tangles. Loss of synapses and dendrites occurs with aging. Neurotransmitter systems are also affected by aging. Acetylcholinesterase, choline acyltransferase, tyrosine hydroxylase, DOPA decarboxylase, and glutamic acid decarboxylase, enzymes involved in cholinergic, dopaminergic and GABA-ergic transmission respectively, show appreciable decreases.

The total myelin content of white matter is reduced in old age. Low myelin concentrations of white matter most probably reflect the continuous loss of neurons with degeneration of axons and of the myelin sheaths. The lipid composition of myelin is quite constant during aging, with the possible exception of galactolipids which tend to decrease. Some differences are seen in the fatty acid composition of myelin phosphoglycerides and cerebrosides during aging. Myelin proteins do not undergo distinct quantitative changes in their relative proportions during old age.

1.12   Function of Myelin

Nerve fibers transmit information to other nerve fibers and to receptors of effector organs. The information is transmitted via an electric impulse called the action potential which is conducted in an all-or-none way, i.e., the impulse is propagated or not. More detailed information is provided by temporal and spatial summation of many action potentials within one nerve. Myelin plays an important role in the impulse propagation. It is an insulator, but more important is its function to facilitate conduction in axons.

In a resting nerve fiber, polarization of the membrane exists: the inside is charged negatively compared to the outside. In an excited area the situation is reversed: the inside is charged positively compared to the outside. This is called membrane depolarization. A potential difference exists between excited and adjacent resting fiber sections due to the inversion of polarization in the excited area. In an effort to compensate this potential difference, local circuits of currents flow into the active region of the axonal membrane through the axon and out through the adjacent, polarized sections of the membrane. These local circuits depolarize the adjacent section of membrane. As soon as this depolarization reaches the threshold of excitation, an action potential arises. These local circuits depolarize the adjacent section of membrane in continuous sequential fashion. Of course, the local circuits do not only flow in the direction of the impulse conduction. However, they cause no renewed excitation in the membrane that has just been excited because a temporary state of inexcitability called the refractory period exists, which ensures that the fiber conducts the action potential in one direction and does not remain permanently excited. In unmyelinated fibers impulses are propagated in this way, and the entire membrane surface needs to be successively excited when an action potential travels along it.

In myelinated fibers, the excitable axonal membrane is only exposed to the extracellular space at the nodes of Ranvier. The remainder of the axolemma is covered by the myelin sheath which has a much higher resistance and much lower capacitance than the axonal membrane. When the membrane at the node is excited, the local circuit generated cannot flow through the high-resistance sheath, and therefore flows out through the next node of Ranvier and depolarizes the membrane there (Fig. 1.10). In this so-called saltatory conduction, the impulse jumps from node to node, whereby the conduction velocity is considerably increased. It saves energy because only parts of the membrane need to depolarize and repolarize for impulse conduction. To obtain conduction velocities in unmyelinated fibers equivalent to those in the fastest conducting myelinating fibers, one would require impossibly large unmyelin-

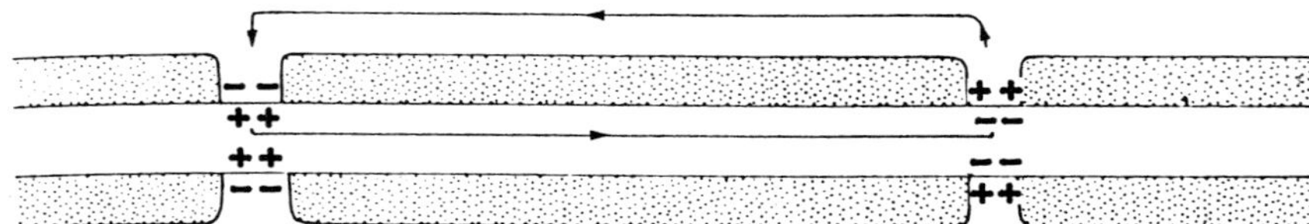

Fig. 1.10. Because of the myelin sheath, the conduction in a myelinated nerve fiber is saltatory, jumping from node to node

ated fibers and energy expenditures several orders of magnitude greater.

There are several factors which influence conduction velocity. Conduction velocity increases with increasing fiber diameter as a consequence of the smaller internal resistance, leading to an increased flow of current and thus shortening the time necessary for the excitation of the adjacent membrane section or the next node of Ranvier. Increase in myelin thickness, which accompanies increase in fiber diameter, also increases conduction velocity, mainly due to a change in myelin sheath capacitance. The internodal distance influences conduction velocity. With shorter internodal distances, the fibers behave more and more like unmyelinated fibers and with longer internodal distances the current density at the next node of Ranvier gets smaller. Consequently, there is an optimal ratio of internode distance to axon diameter. With increasing temperature conduction velocity increases, reaching a maximum at about $42\,^{\circ}$C and decreasing thereafter.

1.13 Myelin Disorders: Definitions

"Demyelination" literally means: loss of myelin and the literal interpretation of "demyelinating disorders" is: disorders characterized by loss of myelin. The term demyelination is commonly used to indicate the process of losing myelin, caused by primary affection of oligodendroglia or myelin membranes. Myelin loss that is secondary to axonal loss and simultaneous loss of axons and myelin sheaths are not usually included under the heading of demyelination.

There is, however, considerable confusion about the meaning of the terms demyelination and demyelinating disorders. Sometimes the word demyelination is used for all conditions in which loss of myelin occurs, irrespective of whether the myelin membrane was primarily affected or was broken down secondary to or at the same time as axonal loss. This is probably partly due to the fact that it is not always clear whether the loss of myelin is primary or secondary in nature. The mutual dependency of axons and myelin sheaths is an important factor in this respect. Demyelination will eventually lead to axonal loss and axonal degeneration will in the end lead to loss of myelin. Hence, using histological examination, it may be very difficult to

differentiate between primary and secondary myelin loss. Another confusing factor is that some disorders, e.g., the infantile types of the gangliosidoses and neuronal ceroid lipofuscinosis, show evidence of simultaneous occurrence of primary neuronal degeneration and primary demyelination. The random use of related terms, such as dysmyelination, myelinoclastic disorders, white matter disorders, leukoencephalopathies and leukodystrophies add to the confusion.

Poser (1957) introduced the concept of "dysmyelination". He proposed dividing the disorders characterized by primary myelin loss into "myelinoclastic disorders" and "dysmyelinating disorders" (Poser 1961, 1978). He considered the myelinoclastic disorders to be the true demyelinating disorders, in which the myelin sheath is destroyed having been normally constituted. Examples are multiple sclerosis and acute disseminated encephalomyelitis. The dysmyelinating disorders comprise those disorders in which "myelin is not formed properly, or in which myelin formation is delayed or arrested, or in which the maintenance of already formed myelin is disturbed". Examples are metachromatic leukodystrophy and adrenoleukodystrophy. The idea behind the concept of dysmyelinating and myelinoclastic disorders is to distinguish between inborn errors of metabolism leading to disturbed myelination and myelin loss, and acquired disorders characterized by primary myelin loss. However, the definition of dysmyelinating disorders, as formulated by Poser, does not exclude acquired disorders. There are many conditions characterized by a disturbance of myelination and most of these are caused by external factors.

The term "white matter disorders" and "leukoencephalopathies" are even less well defined. "White matter disorders" is a literal translation of "leukoencephalopathies". Sometimes these terms are used as if they are interchangeable with demyelinating disorders, but in other cases they are used in the context of a wider range of disorders, characterized by either primary myelin loss or aselective damage to myelin, axons and supportive tissue of the white matter. For instance, when the terms white matter disorder and leukoencephalopathy are used in elderly people, ischemic white matter lesions are also implied, which do not involve or do not only involve a selective loss of myelin.

There are several definitions of the term "leukodystrophy". Seitelberger (1984) defines leukodystrophies as degenerative demyelinating processes caused by metabolic disorders. Morell and Wiesmann (1984) state that leukodystrophies are disorders affecting primarily oligodendroglial cells or myelin. The disorders have to be of endogenous origin with a pattern compatible with genetic transfer of a metabolic defect. The clinical criterion is a steadily progressive deterioration of function. Menkes (1990) defines leukodystrophies as a group of genetically transmitted diseases in which abnormal metabolism of myelin constituents leads to progressive demyelination. Common concepts in these definitions are demyelination and inborn errors of metabolism. Heritability is implied. As such, the leukodystrophies are identical with inherited demyelinating disorders.

In this book the following definitions are used: "Demyelination" is reserved for the process of myelin loss caused by primary and selective affection of either oligodendroglia or of the myelin membrane itself. "Demyelinating disorders" are conditions characterized by demyelination. Examples: metachromatic leukodystrophy, multiple sclerosis.
"Hypomyelination" is reserved for conditions in which too little myelin is laid down. The most extreme variant of hypomyelination is amyelination. Examples: Pelizaeus-Merzbacher disease, malnutrition.
"Dysmyelination" is, as the literal translation of the name implies, reserved for conditions in which the process of myelination is disturbed, leading to abnormal, patchy, irregular myelination, sometimes but not necessarily combined with signs of myelin breakdown. Examples: some amino acidopathies, damaged structure of unmyelinated white matter after perinatal hypoxia or encephalitis.
"Retarded myelination" is reserved for disorders in which the deposition of myelin is delayed. Examples: inborn errors of metabolism with early onset, malnutrition, hydrocephalus.
"Myelin disorders" comprise all the above-mentioned conditions.
"White matter disorders" and "leukoencephalopathies" can be defined as all conditions in which predominantly or exclusively white matter is affected. Either myelin or a combination of myelin and other white matter components is involved. Hence, white matter disorders comprise all myelin disorders, but also for instance white matter infections and infarctions, which may affect various white matter components aselectively.
"Gray matter disorders" comprise all disorders in which neurons and axons are predominantly or exclusively affected. Examples: infantile neuroaxonal dystrophy, Friedreich's ataxia.

1.14 Levels of Myelin Affection

Both inherited and acquired myelin disorders can arise at the level of the myelin membranes or the oligodendroglial cells. As a consequence, the processes of myelin build-up, myelin maintenance and turnover may be disturbed.

The processes of myelin build-up and deposition are highly complex and require the activity of many genes, the presence of many substances, the activity of many enzymes, optimal coordination of processes within the oligodendrocytes and optimal cooperation with the environment. Complex and dynamic processes are particularly vulnerable and the process of active myelination is easily disturbed. Some inborn errors of metabolism lead to a shortage of myelin components and as a consequence to a disturbance of the process of myelination. An example is found in Pelizaeus-Merzbacher disease. Acquired disorders, such as hormonal disbalances and severe malnutrition may also lead to a disturbance of myelin build-up.

A disturbance of myelin maintenance and turnover may lead to demyelination. In some inborn errors of metabolism, the basic enzymatic defect involves the breakdown of one of the myelin components. This component is trapped in the myelin sheath and its concentration increases gradually. Finally, the myelin composition is altered to such a degree that the stability is lost leading to demyelination. Examples are metachromatic leukodystrophy and globoid cell leukodystrophy. Of the acquired demyelinating disorders, toxic disorders may in particular lead to a disturbance of myelin maintenance and turnover. Myelin is rich in lipids and has a long half-life. Consequently, lipophilic substances easily accumulate in myelin, disturbing the stability of the myelin membrane and leading to demyelination.

The myelin membrane may be intact and normal in appearance, biochemical composition and function, until it is attacked from the outside. This appears to be the case in several acquired demyelinating disorders, including inflammatory processes (e.g., multiple sclerosis, acute disseminated encephalomyelitis), metabolic disturbances (central pontine myelinolysis, Marchiafava-Bignami syndrome) and hypoxia (delayed posthypoxic demyelination).

Demyelinating disorders may also arise at the level of the oligodendrocytes. Damage to oligodendrocytes may lead to a disturbance of myelin build-up, maintenance, and turnover. In some inborn errors of metabolism, storage of unwanted material occurs, in the end leading to dysfunction and death of oligodendrocytes. In metachromatic leukodystrophy, storage of sulfatides may lead to oligodendroglial damage and in this way contribute to demyelination. In globoid cell leukodystrophy the toxic substance psychosine supposedly leads to oligodendroglial cell death and myelin loss. In acquired demyelinating disorders, selective oligodendroglial cell death may also occur. Such is the case, for instance, in progressive multifocal leukoencephalitis, in which viral infection of oligodendrocytes is present.

Of course, more than one mechanism of myelin affection is involved in many disorders. In disturbances of myelin build-up, the myelin that is laid down may have an abnormal composition and configuration. Delayed myelination, dysmyelination and early demyelination may occur at the same time. In other disorders, oligodendroglial cell death and myelin breakdown independent of oligodendroglial cell death occur simultaneously.

1.15 Biochemical Changes Related to Demyelination

Demyelinating disorders can be subdivided into two large categories: inherited disorders, due to an inborn error of metabolism, and acquired disorders, secondary to adverse factors in the internal or external environment.

Biochemical analysis of myelin and white matter appears to demonstrate an abnormal composition of the same type in many demyelinating disorders of diverse etiology. The concept of the nonspecific process of myelin breakdown suggests that when maintenance of normal myelin is no longer possible, it follows a stereotyped route to complete destruction, largely irrespective of the initiating causes. The etiological factors can be Wallerian degeneration, infections such as subacute sclerosing panencephalitis or intoxications such as triethyltin, but also inherited metabolic diseases like X-linked adrenoleukodystrophy, Refsum's disease, Canavan's disease, and many other demyelinating diseases. In inherited diseases affecting myelin metabolism, biochemical analysis often reveals certain abnormalities superimposed on the nonspecific compositional abnormalities. These abnormalities are specific for one particular disorder or type of disorders. For instance, an elevation of the very long-chain fatty acids of the cholesterol esters is specific for X-linked adrenoleukodystrophy, or rather a subgroup of peroxisomal disorders. An elevation of sulfatide is found in the white matter of patients with metachromatic leukodystrophy. The specific biochemical abnormalities of myelin in the various disorders are discussed in separate chapters. Here we will limit our discussion to the nonspecific myelin abnormalities. It should, however, be kept in mind that the degree of abnormality varies considerably among different diseases and among different cas-

es of the same disease depending on the stage of disease.

In degenerating myelin, the proportion of total protein to total lipid is not usually dramatically altered, but proportions of individual lipids are abnormal. The amount of galactolipids is decreased and cerebroside is usually much more severely affected than sulfatide. Moderate decreases of ethanolamine phosphoglycerides (mostly plasmalogen) are common. The amount of unesterified cholesterol is increased, often strikingly so, constituting almost half or even more than half the total lipid content, in contrast to approximately 27% in normal myelin. No esterified cholesterol is found in the degenerating myelin sheath. Such abnormal myelin is an intermediate form between normal myelin and completely catabolized myelin. The abnormalities are a result of partial degradation.

The compositional changes in white matter as a whole primarily depend on the extent of myelin loss and only secondarily on changes in myelin composition. Typical white matter changes are increased water content and reduced lipid to protein ratios, with specific decreases in major myelin constituents like cholesterol, cerebroside, sulfatide, and ethanolamine phosphoglycerides. In addition, there is an increase in cholesterol esters in whole white matter in a number of diseases, but not in all. The fatty acid composition of these esters is different from that of the small amount of esters normally present in white matter, but closely resembles the acids linked to the 2 position in phosphatidylcholine. It is assumed that these esters come from myelin cholesterol and phosphoglyceride fatty acids. The presence of cholesterol esters is taken as evidence of an active phagocytosis of myelin and, as such, as an indicator of active demyelination, but the absence of cholesterol esters does not mean that there is no active demyelination. The presence of cholesterol esters is reflected in sudanophilia on histological examination. It is probable that the mechanism of breakdown is slightly different in sudanophilic myelin destruction and nonsudanophilic breakdown.

1.16 Demyelination: Loss of Function

In normal myelinated nerve fibers conduction is saltatory and internodal conduction time is fairly regular. The conduction in demyelinated axons differs dramatically from that in normal fibers. The impulse conduction may be either saltatory or continuous. If the impulse conduction remains saltatory, the internodal conduction time varies widely from internode to internode. The internodal conduction time is prolonged by an increased leakage of current between the nodes and by a depression of excitability of the nodal membrane. There is, therefore, a decreased current generation capacity and an increased threshold for excitation. In demyelinated fibers, a very slow continuous conduction (about 5% of the conduction velocity of normal fibers) may be seen over short stretches. A so-called safety factor for impulse conduction can be calculated. If the required minimum is not reached, impulse propagation is blocked. Furthermore, the refractory period of demyelinated fibers is increased, which leads to failure to transmit high-frequency trains of impulses.

It is clear that demyelination, depending on its extent and severity, can lead to serious loss of function. However, damage to neurons, although not as prominent as destruction of myelin, may also play a role in the functional deficit. Especially in inborn errors of metabolism, substances may also accumulate in the membranes of axons and in this way axonal dysfunction may arise, contributing to the functional loss.

1.17 Remyelination

For many years it was believed that loss of myelin represented an inexorable lesion in the CNS. However, it has been demonstrated that remyelination in the CNS is possible. Remyelinated fibers can be recognized because the internodes are too short and the myelin sheath is too thin for the size of the axon. Even with time, there is no restitution of the normal axon:myelin ratio. The new myelin sheath in itself is normal with normal lamellar periodicity.

Remyelination also occurs when the demyelinated lesion is depleted of oligodendrocytes. The necessary supply of oligodendrocytes is provided by proliferation of remaining, mature oligodendrocytes and possibly also by proliferation of progenitor cells followed by differentiation into myelinating oligodendrocytes. It is often found that axons tend to be remyelinated in clusters, suggesting that a single oligodendrocyte myelinates many axons in the vicinity.

Remyelination among the demyelinating disorders is variable. The most successful examples of remyelination are found in those conditions where demyelination has occurred rapidly, irrespective of the condition being acute and monophasic or relapsing and remitting. Remyelination is much more limited in demyelinating disorders with a protracted, chronic course. Presence of additional axonal damage has an adverse effect on potential remyelination. Some local factor, when present, may stimulate remyelination. There is evidence that epidermal growth factor, interleukin-2,

immunoglobulins, platelet-derived growth factor and insulin growth factors may stimulate survival and proliferation of oligodendrocytes and remyelination. In contrast, presence of T-CD4+ immune cells interferes with remyelination.

1.18 Retarded Myelination

Myelination is a complex as well as a protracted process. This means that the process is vulnerable to adverse factors for a long period of time, namely from the second half of gestation up to the first one or two years of life. Many stress factors, that act upon the incompletely myelinated brain, interfering with the process of myelination, do not have such an adverse effect on the mature brain. For instance, in the mature brain in which myelination is complete, it is unlikely that stress factors such as malnutrition or hormonal imbalances will appreciably reduce the amount of myelin.

Well known factors potentially leading to retardation of myelination include malnutrition, hormonal imbalances (growth hormone deficiency, hypothyroidism, hypocortisolism, hypercortisolism), prenatal exposure to toxins (alcohol, anticonvulsants), chromosomal abnormalities, pre- and postnatal asphyxia, cerebral infections, hydrocephalus and inborn errors of metabolism with early onset.

It is important to realize that myelination is dependent on normal function and interaction of both oligodendrocytes and neurons and that retardation of myelination may be related to either dysfunction of oligodendroglia and myelin or to neuronal dysfunction. Cerebral infections and perinatal asphyxia may lead to disturbance of myelination through white matter damage or through neuronal damage. Also, inborn errors of metabolism may disturb the process of myelination either directly at the level of the oligodendrocyte or myelin sheath, or indirectly at the level of the neuron. In the former case, the disease is categorized as a myelin disorder, and the disturbance of myelination is expected. However, it is important to realize that a disturbance of myelination may also be seen in neuronal disorders with early onset. For instance, in Menkes disease, Alpers disease or infantile sialic acid storage disease, all three neuronal disorders, myelination is severely retarded.

It has been demonstrated that myelination is an expression of the functional maturity of the brain. Retarded myelination is an expression of immaturity or dysfunction.

2 Classification of Myelin Disorders

The history of classifications of myelin disorders shows how each classification reflects the state of scientific development of its time. Based on recent scientific insights, a revised classification is proposed at the end of this chapter.

Interest in CNS myelin dates back to the nineteenth century. In 1854, Virchow was the first to suggest the name myelin when he described the sheaths around axons in the CNS. It is not certain when Schwann (1810–1882) described the cells, which have since been named after him, that supply the myelin sheaths around the peripheral nerve fibers (1839?). In 1878, Ranvier described the nodes which have since been given his name in "*Leçons sur l'histologie du système nerveux*". He believed that the nodes prevented the essentially liquid myelin from flowing to the bottom of the nerve fiber (axon). But despite this conviction, he showed considerable insight into the functional role of the myelin sheath, both as an insulator and as a facilitatory agent in CNS functions. It was not until 1960–1961, that the role of the oligodendrocyte in the formation of myelin in the CNS became clear, due to the work of Bunge.

During the nineteenth century and the first part of the twentieth century, important progress was made with the clinical and histological description of several demyelinating disorders. Multiple sclerosis was recognized as a clinical disease entity and the characteristic histological abnormalities in the form of multiple demyelinated, sclerotic plaques within otherwise normal white matter were described. Prominent names in this development are Carswell (1838), Cruveilhier (1835–1842) and Charcot (1868).

In 1897, Heubner described a rare neurological disease in children, using the name diffuse sclerosis as opposed to multiple sclerosis. The disease was histologically characterized by diffuse demyelination of the cerebral white matter and eventually a striking hardening of the white matter. Since that time, the term "diffuse sclerosis" has been commonly used to describe cerebral diseases with diffuse demyelination and sclerotic hardening of the cerebral white matter. Pelizaeus in 1899 and Merzbacher in 1910 reported on a chronic progressive familial type of diffuse sclerosis.

In 1912, Schilder described a nonfamilial case of more acute diffuse cerebral demyelination in a child and he suggested the name encephalitis periaxialis diffusa rather than diffuse sclerosis. In this case, more prominent signs of inflammation and a less symmetrical distribution were observed than in the familial cases described until that time. Schilder considered this disease as a nosological and histological entity related to multiple sclerosis, and thought there were acute and chronic variants of diffuse sclerosis just as there were acute and chronic types of multiple sclerosis.

Since Schilder, a number of familial neurological disorders have been recognized which were histologically characterized by diffuse demyelination and which were again presented under the heading of diffuse sclerosis. In 1916, Krabbe described a familial infantile form of diffuse sclerosis. In 1925, Scholz and in 1928, Bielschowsky and Henneberg reported on another familial variant with a later onset and a less rapid progression. Scholz noted that in this case the myelin breakdown products did not show the usual (orthochromatic) staining properties, but stained metachromatically.

In 1921, Neubürger drew attention to the fact that the term diffuse sclerosis was being applied to several very different disease entities and he proposed distinguishing inflammatory and degenerative forms. In 1928, Bielschowsky and Henneberg suggested the name "hereditary progressive leukodystrophies" for the degenerative forms of diffuse sclerosis and made the following subdivision, based upon the time of onset of the disease and its clinical course:
1. Infantile type of Krabbe
2. Subacute juvenile type of Scholz
3. Chronic type of Pelizaeus-Merzbacher

Hallervorden (1940) recognized that there are endogenous and exogenous factors causing diffuse demyelination and that a distinction can be made between disorders in which demyelination is invariably present and forms a specific part of the disease and disorders in which demyelination occurs occasionally and is nonspecific. He proposed a more extended classification based on these subdivisions:
I. Endogenous central demyelination
   A. Specific demyelinating diseases
      a. Diffuse sclerosis of Krabbe and Scholz
      b. Pelizaeus-Merzbacher disease

B. Nonspecific occasional demyelination, e.g., Tay Sachs disease
II. Exogenous central demyelination
  A. Specific demyelinating diseases
    a. Inflammatory types:
      disseminated sclerosis (=multiple sclerosis)
      diffuse sclerosis (Schilder)
      concentric sclerosis (Balò)
      neuromyelitis optica (Devic)
      encephalomyelitis disseminata
      infectious encephalitis
    b. Toxic-metabolic types:
      funicular myelosis (=vitamin B_{12} deficiency)
      Marchiafava-Bignami's disease
  B. Nonspecific occasional demyelination
    a. Disturbances of blood flow, e.g., subcortical atherosclerosis (=Binswanger's disease)
    b. Edema
    c. Toxic processes (carbon monoxide)
    d. Tumors

Until that time, the distinction of different diseases had been based on neuropathological and clinical aspects of different demyelinating disorders. From about this time onwards, histochemical methods and chemical analyses were becoming increasingly important. The classification of Blackwood, proposed in 1957, is a reflection of this development. It is based not only on morphological but also on histochemical differences between various subgroups of diffuse sclerosis:

I. Disseminated sclerosis (=multiple sclerosis)
II. Diffuse demyelinating cerebral sclerosis
  1. With replacement of myelin by sudanophilic lipid
    a. With large bilateral cerebral plaques
    b. With concentric demyelination (Balò type)
  2a. With replacement of myelin by metachromatic PAS-positive lipid (Norman type or Scholz' type)
    b. With associated degeneration of interfascicular oligodendroglia (Greenfield type)

Meanwhile, the insight into normal biochemistry and into mechanisms of biochemical derangement grew. The concept of hereditary inborn errors of metabolism caused by an enzyme defect leading to dysfunction and breakdown of myelin started to emerge. Fölling (1934) reported 10 patients in the same family with mental retardation and phenylpyruvic acid in their urine. Jervis discovered in 1947 that the underlying metabolic defect in phenylketonuria is a deficiency of phenylalanine hydroxylase. In 1955, Diezel found that the lipids stored in the globoid cells in Krabbe's disease have very similar properties to those of cerebroside. In 1970, Suzuki and Suzuki were the first to propose a deficiency of galactocerebrosidase as the underlying biochemical cause of this disease. Advances in histochemistry also made it possible to discover the basis of metachromatic leukodystrophy. Metachromasia had already been found by Alzheimer in 1910, by Scholz in 1925 and later by Von Hirsch and Peiffer (1955, 1957). Edgar (1955) was the first to point out that this condition is characterized by a remarkable elevation of white matter hexosamine. In 1964, Austin et al. demonstrated a decrease in arylsulfatase A activity in metachromatic leukodystrophy.

The enzyme defect of an increasing number of hereditary diseases could be detected, whereas in other cases the precise enzyme defect was not yet discovered, but typical biochemical abnormalities could be demonstrated which characterized the disease. The increased insight into hereditary metabolic disorders and the ongoing ability to distinguish different hereditary and acquired demyelinating disorders on the basis of a combination of clinical, histological and biochemical data, were reflected in the classification proposed by Raine (1984). Raine distinguished five main categories:

I. Acquired inflammatory and infectious diseases of myelin
  1. Multiple sclerosis
  2. Multiple sclerosis variants (Schilder, Balò, Devic)
  3. Acute disseminated encephalomyelitis
  4. Acute hemorrhagic leukoencephalopathy
  5. Progressive multifocal leukoencephalopathy
II. Hereditary metabolic disorders of myelin
  1. Metachromatic leukodystrophy
  2. Globoid cell leukodystrophy (Krabbe)
  3. Adrenoleukodystrophy
  4. Refsum's disease
  5. Pelizaeus-Merzbacher disease
  6. Dysmyelinogenetic leukodystrophy (Alexander)
  7. Spongy degeneration (Canavan)
  8. Phenylketonuria
III. Acquired toxic-metabolic diseases of myelin
  1. Hexachlorophene neuropathy
  2. Hypoxic encephalopathy
IV. Nutritional diseases of myelin
  1. Vitamin B_{12} deficiency
  2. Central pontine myelinolysis
  3. Marchiafava-Bignami disease
V. Traumatic diseases of myelin
  1. Edema
  2. Compression
  3. Barbotage
  4. Pressure release

In this classification, four of the five categories involve acquired demyelinating disorders and only one category involves hereditary demyelinating disorders. The logical continuation of this development is a refinement of the classification of hereditary demyelinating disorders. For instance, in some diseases the inborn error affects the metabolism of amino acids, in other diseases the lipid metabolism. A further subdivision can be made among the disorders of lipid metabolism according to the type of lipids involved. In 1987, Poser proposed a classification of hereditary myelin disorders based on the biochemical group of compounds of which the metabolism is disturbed. He distinguished six categories:

1. Disorders of glycosphingolipid metabolism
   a. Ganglioside: GM_1 and GM_2 gangliosidoses hematoside sphingolipodystrophy
   b. Sulfatide: metachromatic leukodystrophy
   c. Galactocerebroside: globoid cell leukodystrophy
2. Disorders of phosphosphingolipid metabolism
   a. Sphingomyelin: Niemann-Pick disease
3. Disorders of fatty acid metabolism
   a. Adrenoleukodystrophy
4. Disorders of amino acid metabolism
   a. Phenylalanine: phenylketonuria
   b. Branched-chain amino acids: maple syrup urine disease
   c. Many other amino acidopathies
5. Multiple abnormalities
   a. Mucosulfatidosis
6. Unknown abnormalities
   a. Idiopathic spongy sclerosis (Canavan)
   b. Fibrinoid leukodystrophy (Alexander)
   c. Pelizaeus-Merzbacher disease
   d. Idiopathic sudanophilic leukodystrophy

An important development during the last few decades concerns the knowledge of subcellular structures, their role in normal metabolism and the consequences of their dysfunction. Major subcellular structures are nucleus, lysosomes, mitochondria, peroxisomes, cytoplasm matrix, smooth and rough endoplasmic reticulum, Golgi apparatus, ribosomes and microtubules. Demyelinating disorders have been described as resulting from nuclear, lysosomal, mitochondrial, peroxisomal and cytoplasmic enzyme dysfunctions. Classification of hereditary demyelinating disorders according to the subcellular localization of the underlying metabolic defect stresses the clinical, biochemical and neuropathological similarities within one category and the differences between the different categories. For the same reason, it is preferable to classify the acquired demyelinating disorders according to their underlying causes into noninfectious-inflammatory, infectious-inflammatory, toxic-metabolic, hypoxic-ischemic and traumatic. A number of disorders remains, of which the primary defect is largely or completely unknown.

I. Hereditary myelin disorders
   1. Lysosomal storage disorders
      a. Metachromatic leukodystrophy
      b. Multiple sulfatase deficiency
      c. Globoid cell leukodystrophy (Krabbe's disease)
      d. GM_1 gangliosidosis
      e. GM_2 gangliosidosis
      f. Fabry's disease
      g. Fucosicosis
      h. Mucopolysaccharidoses
   2. Peroxisomal disorders
      a. Zellweger cerebrohepatorenal syndrome
      b. Neonatal adrenoleukodystrophy
      c. Infantile Refsum's disease
      d. Rhizomelic chondrodysplasia punctata
      e. Zellweger-like syndrome
      f. Pseudo-Zellweger syndrome
      g. Pseudo-neonatal adrenoleukodystrophy
      h. Trifunctional protein deficiency
      i. X-linked adrenoleukodystrophy and adrenomyeloneuropathy
   3. Mitochondrial dysfunction with leukoencephalopathy
      a. Respiratory chain defects
      b. Pyruvate carboxylase deficiency
      c. Cerebrotendinous xanthomatosis
      d. Refsum's disease
   4. Nuclear DNA repair defects
      a. Cockayne's disease
   5. Defects in genes encoding myelin proteins
      a. Pelizaeus-Merzbacher disease
      b. 18q⁻ syndrome
   6. Disorders of amino acid and organic acid metabolism
      a. Phenylketonuria
      b. Glutaric aciduria type 1
      c. Propionic acidemia
      d. Hyperprolinemia
      e. Nonketotic hyperglycinemia
      f. Maple syrup urine disease
      g. Canavan's disease
      h. L-2-hydroxyglutaric aciduria
      i. Hyperhomocysteinemias
      j. Urea cycle defects
   7. Miscellaneous
      a. Galactosemia
      b. Sjögren-Larsson syndrome
      c. Lowe syndrome
      d. Wilson disease
      e. Neuronal ceroid lipofuscinosis
      f. Alexander's disease
      g. Myotonic dystrophy
      h. Congenital muscular dystrophy
      i. Infantile-onset spongiform leukoencephalopathy with a discrepantly mild clinical course
      j. Childhood ataxia with diffuse cerebral hypomyelination
      k. Leukoencephalopathy, cerebral calcifications and chronic cerebro-spinal fluid lymphocytosis (Aicardi-Goutières syndrome)

II. Acquired myelin disorders
   1. Noninfectious-inflammatory disorders
      a. Multiple sclerosis

    b. Neuromyelitis optica
    c. Concentric sclerosis
    d. Schilder's diffuse sclerosis
    e. Acute disseminated encephalomyelitis and acute hemorrhagic encephalomyelitis
2. Infectious-inflammatory disorders
    a. Subacute HIV encephalitis
    b. Subacute CMV encephalitis
    c. Progressive multifocal leukoencephalitis
    d. Subacute sclerosing panencephalitis
    e. Progressive rubella panencephalitis
    f. Other infections
3. Toxic-metabolic disorders
    a. Central pontine and extrapontine myelinolysis
    b. Vitamin B_{12} deficiency
    c. Folate deficiency
    d. Marchiafava-Bignami syndrome
    e. Malnutrition
    f. Toxic leukoencephalopathies (endogenous and exogenous toxins)
4. Hypoxic-ischemic disorders
    a. Posthypoxic-ischemic leukoencephalopathy of neonates
    b. Delayed posthypoxic-ischemic encephalopathy of maturity
    c. Subcortical arteriosclerotic encephalopathy (Binswanger's disease)
    d. Vasculitis
5. Traumatic disorders
    a. Radiation
    b. Edema

In many instances it is clear whether we are dealing with a primarily demyelinating disorder, such as metachromatic leukodystrophy, or with a primary gray matter disorder, such as Friedreich's ataxia. However, in a number of diseases there is evidence of a primary neuronal disorder as well as a variably present primary myelin degeneration. This is, for instance, the case in infantile GM_2 gangliosidosis, infantile GM_1 gangliosidosis, infantile neuronal ceroid lipofuscinosis and in some mitochondrial disorders. We agree with Hallervorden and Poser that these disorders must have a place in a classification of myelin disorders, just as they are also part of a classification of neuronal disorders. Disorders in which there is only evidence of myelin loss secondary to neuronal degeneration are not included in this classification.

The category of so-called "cytoplasmic enzyme deficiencies" is not listed in the classification. The rationale is that such a disease category would represent a very heterogeneous group of disorders as the cytoplasm contains enzymes of many different biochemical pathways. That is why it is preferable in this case to make a subdivision according to the specific metabolic pathway involved. However, the group of amino acidopathies and organic acidopathies is heterogeneous as some of the enzymes concerned are in fact mitochondrial or peroxisomal. Considering the relative homogeneity in clinical presentation, diagnostic tests and treatment strategies, we prefer to place them within one category, which is also in conformity with general practice.

Over the years this classification has been modified repeatedly. The basic defect of a steadily increasing number of hereditary myelin disorders has been elucidated and the number of "unknown" disorders is decreasing. Also the present classification of myelin disorders cannot be considered as final. However, the structure of the proposed classification allows easy integration of additional information.

3 Selective Vulnerability

Spielmeyer (1925), Meyer (1936), Vogt and Vogt (1937) and Scholz (1953) have introduced the concept that, apart from the distribution of infarctions in vascular territories and border zones, specific brain regions may be more vulnerable to ischemic injury than others. Spielmeyer tried to find an explanation for this difference by suggesting that variations in the local vascular supply facilitated vascular insuffiency in areas like the hippocampus. The Vogts (Vogt and Vogt 1937) indicated the physico-chemical properties of specific neurons as the reason for higher vulnerability to hypoxic-ischemic lesions and they coined the term "topistic areas". Scholz (1953, 1963) recapitulated these viewpoints by stating that under specific pathophysiological conditions focal ischemic brain injury could be attributed to the vascular pecularities of the anatomy, while under other conditions the pattern of brain damage could only be explained by the unique properties of the cells themselves.

There are evidently elements of the CNS which have, independently from the vascular supply, different degrees of sensitivity to oxygen deprivation. Of the cellular elements of the CNS, neurons are most vulnerable (Fig. 3.1), followed by oligodendroglia, astroglia and, finally, endothelial cells. Within the group of neurons, some neuronal types are more vulnerable to hypoxic-ischemic damage than others. Structures more liable to suffer from hypoxia-ischemia are the hippocampus, the Purkinje cells in the cerebellum, specific cells in the striatum and neocortical layers. Within these structures there is a further order of sensitivity, as indicated in Table 3.1.

Although the interest of experimental work concerning selective neuronal vulnerability was initially focused on hypoxic-ischemic conditions, selective involvement of parts of the CNS can also be observed in other conditions, such as inborn errors of metabolism, neurodegenerative disorders, inflammatory disorders, infections and in toxic encephalopathies. In some of these examples the damage may be mediated by vascular changes. A group does, however, remain where the distribution of the lesions can only be explained by unique properties of the cell.

In the context of this book, attention is paid to the concept of selective vulnerability for two reasons. In the first place the recognition of patterns of selective vulnerability contributes to the understanding of pathogenetic mechanisms of cerebral damage in the different disorders. In the second place, the recognition of patterns of selective vulnerability is of practical value and contributes to the diagnostic value of MRI. The concept of MRI pattern recognition is based on the concept of selective vulnerability.

There are several pathophysiological mechanisms to explain the selective vulnerability of certain brain areas as compared to others:

1. Level of activity is an important factor in selective vulnerability. Energy depletion by hypoxia-ischemia, toxic influences, and metabolic derangements will have the greatest effect on structures with the highest activity. Gray matter in adults has a higher level of activity than white matter and will as a rule be damaged first and most severely. In infants, active myelination zones have a high activity and are, therefore, liable to damage. Damage in primary myelination zones can be seen in asphyxiated neonates born at term (Fig. 3.2).

2. Specific chemical affinity contributes to selective vulnerability. It has been known for a long time that certain areas in the brain are especially liable to damage by certain toxic agents. Hexachlorophene intoxication exclusively involves myelin sheaths. Hexachlorophene encephalopathy, induced in preterm neonates by washing them for antiseptic reasons with hexachlorophene solutions, causes a myelinopathy with splitting of the myelin lamellae and subsequent vacuolization. Vacuolating myelinopathy in the neonate always has a special distribution, irrespective of its cause, related to the distribution of myelinated versus unmyelinated areas (Fig. 3.3). Intoxication with triethyltin, cuprizone,

Table 3.1. Hierarchy of selective vulnerability to hypoxic-ischemic conditions for different CNS structures

Degree of vulnerability	
Hippocampus	$CA_1 > CA_4 > CA_3 >$ granule cells
Cerebellum	Purkinje cells > stellate or basket cells > granule cells > Golgi cells
Striatum	Small-medium sized neurons > large neurons
Neocortex	Layers 3, 5, 6 > layers 2, 4

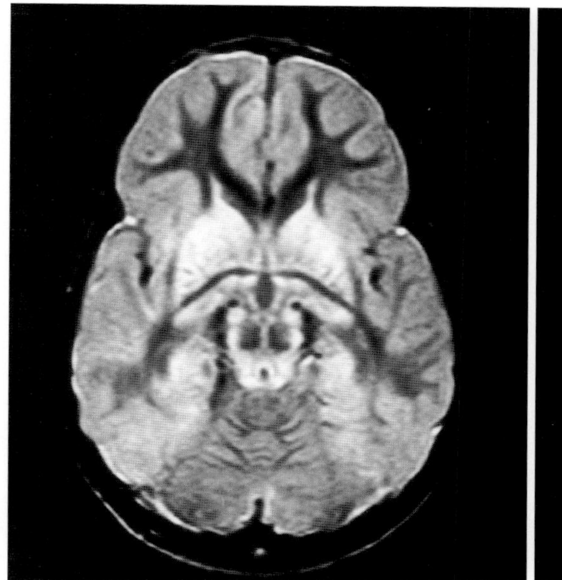 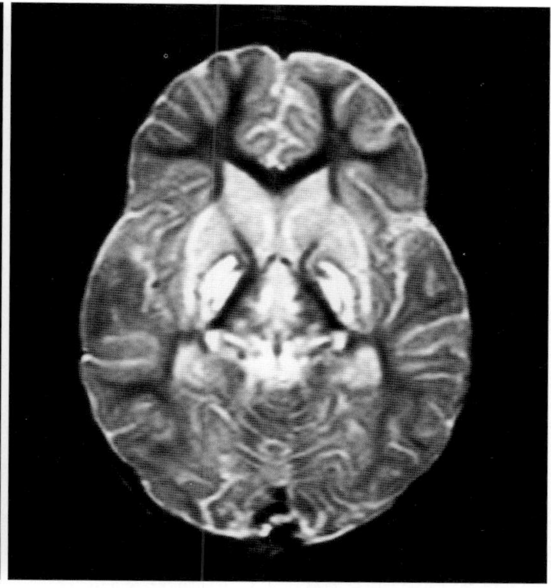

Fig. 3.1. Proton density on T_2-weighted images of a 6-year-old boy who nearly drowned. A few days after resuscitation, MR images show selective involvement of mainly subcortical gray matter structures, including the caudate nucleus, putamen, globus pallidus, thalamus, periaqueductal gray matter and hippocampus. The anterior commissure stands out in the affected gray matter

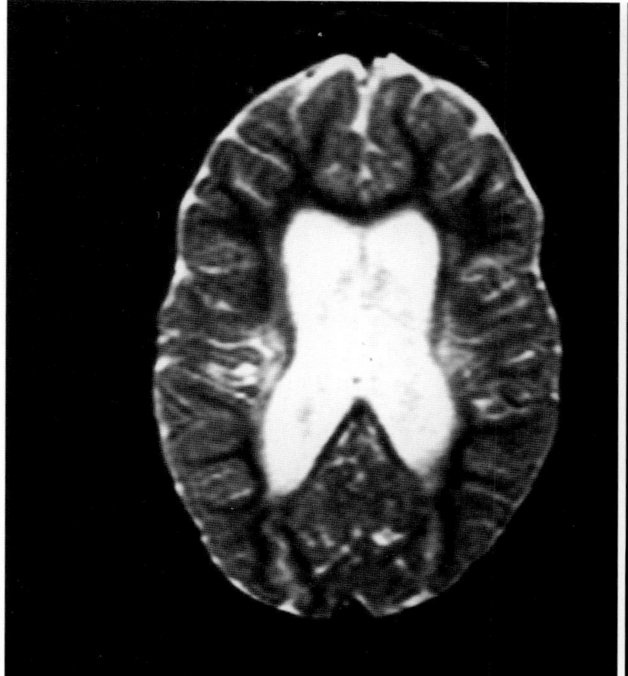 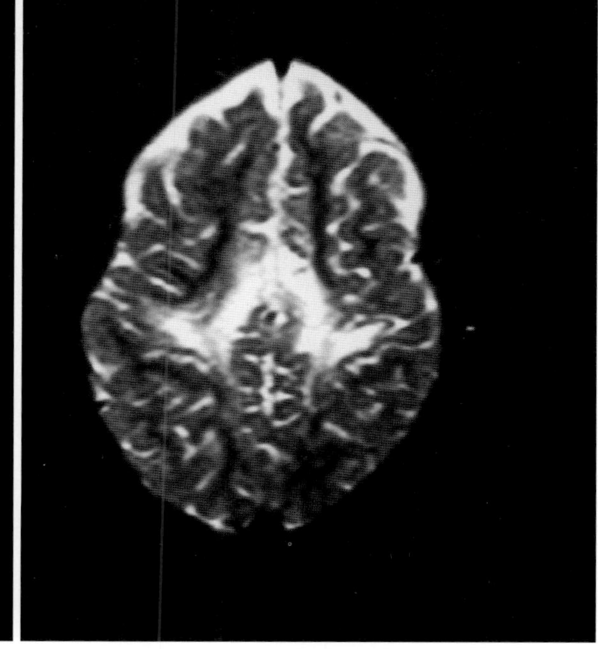

Fig. 3.2. Typical triangular pattern of involvement of white matter in a primary myelination zone, including the tracts to and from the pre- and postcentral gyri. This central cortical-subcortical pattern is seen after severe asphyxia in neonates born at term

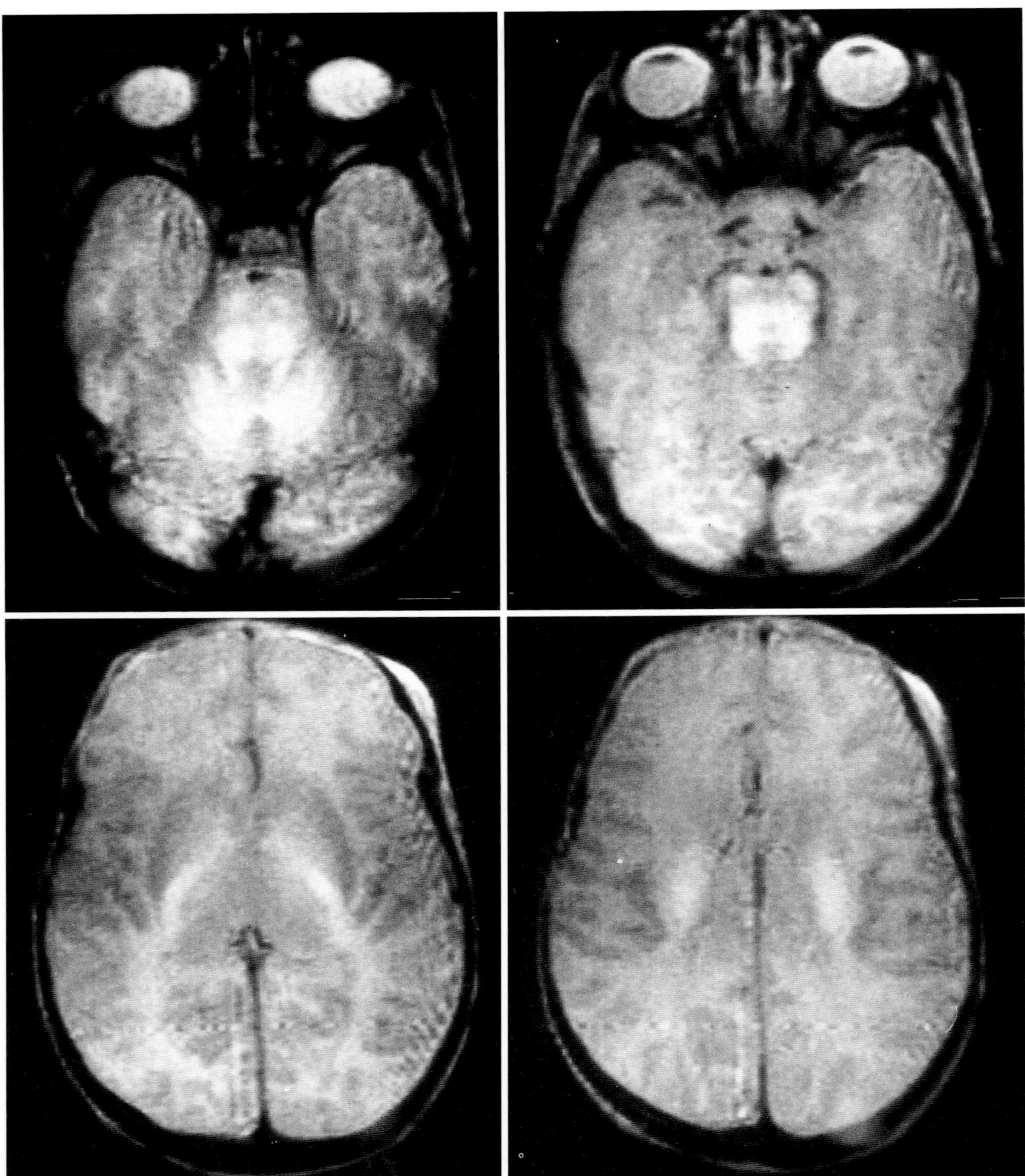

Fig. 3.3. In maple-syrup urine disease with neonatal onset, the pattern of involvement of white matter is dictated by the presence of myelin. Vacuolating myelinopathy develops in the areas that are myelinated: dorsal part of the brain stem, cerebellar white matter and dorsal limb of the internal capsule. Courtesy of Brismar et al. 1990, with permission

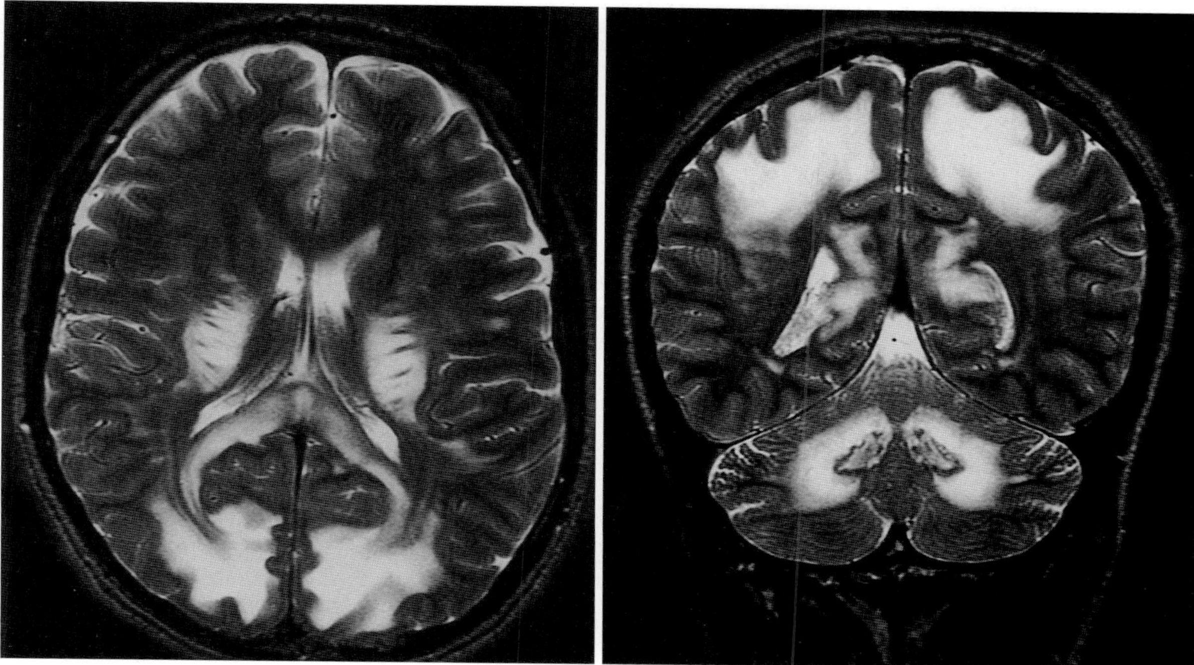

Fig. 3.4. Toxic involvement of white matter by poisoned cocaine or heroin. Histologically, a vacuolating myelinopathy has been demonstrated. (Courtesy of Dr. Tamraz, Paris, with permission)

toxic heroin or poisoned cocaine also lead to myelin splitting and vacuolation (Fig. 3.4). Furthermore, lipophilic substances accumulate preferentially in myelin. Organic solvents, as used by painters, lead to irregular, patchy demyelination and can cause the so-called house-painters dementia. Effects of demyelination have also been described in toluene sniffers.

3. Accumulation and/or deficiency of substances have different effects in different areas of the brain. In inborn errors of metabolism, the selection of primary targets and the pattern of spread of the lesions may be influenced by these factors. Differences in selective vulnerability may be explained by difference in residual activity of enzymes in the various cells, difference in importance of the enzyme function missing from different cells, differences in the effects of the accumulation of abnormal substances, differences in sensitivity to lack of substances that are not formed, and presence of other factors within the cell with synergistic or antagonistic effects. It is often very difficult, if not impossible, to define the factors responsible for well known patterns of selective involvement in inborn errors of metabolism (Fig. 3.5). Shortage of dietary nutrients may also lead to selective damage. Malnutrition of infants in the first episode of life leads to delayed myelination. Cobalamin deficiency in subacute combined degeneration leads to involvement of specific areas in the brain and spinal cord.

4. Patterns of selective vulnerability may be related to distribution of neurotransmitter systems. In some inborn errors of metabolism, some neurodegenerative disorders and some toxic-metabolic encephalopathies, selective vulnerability may result from interference with a neurotransmitter system. For instance, inborn errors of GABA metabolism have been described which lead to dysfunction of structures in which GABA-ergic neurotransmission is important. In Segawa syndrome, hereditary progressive dystonia with marked diurnal variation, disturbances of dopaminergic neurotransmission cause nigrostriatal dysfunction. In hyperammonemia, disturbance of the neurotransmission by glutamate occurs.

5. Density of synapses for excitatory amino acids determines the sensitivity to adverse effects of these substances. Excitoxicity due to overstimulation by excess excitatory amino acids (glutamate and aspartate) has recently been recognized as a final common pathway for inflicting injury upon the CNS. Many conditions can lead to the pathological accumulation of excitatory amino acids. The preferential distribution of lesions by this mechanism will basically be in areas with the highest density of related receptors. In fact this mechanism is a special form of neurotransmitter-related cerebral damage.

6. Antigen-antibody reactions may be at the root of selective CNS lesions. This is the case in a number of the paraneoplastic and parainfectious lesions of the

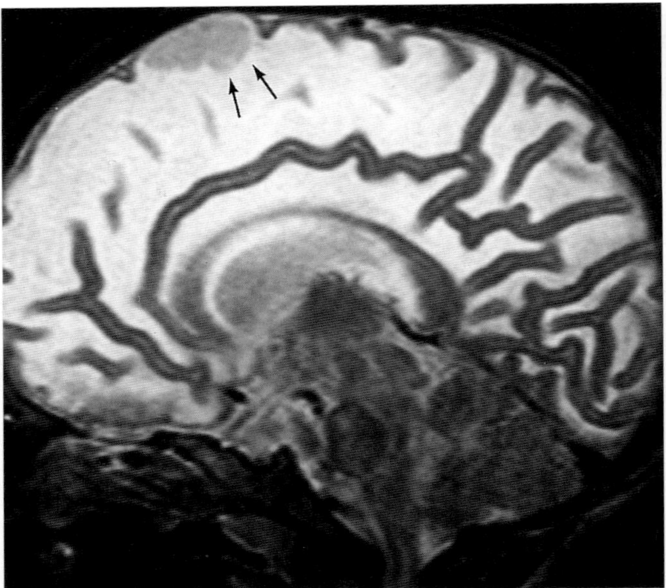
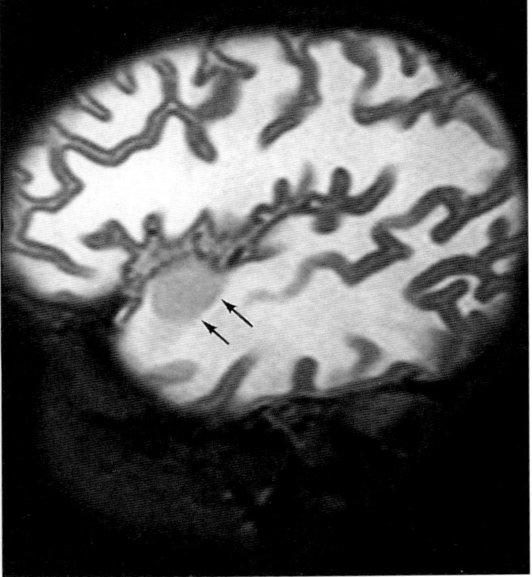

Fig. 3.5. In this disorder with autosomal recessive inheritance there is severe white matter involvement in both hemispheres. Cysts develop at highly characteristic places (*arrows*) for no known reason. See also Chap. 48 on infantile onset spongiform leukoencephalopathy with a discrepantly mild clinical course

brain. Antibodies against tumor antigens may, for example, cross-react with similar antibodies on Purkinje cells. Paraneoplastic CNS disorders such as olivopontocerebellar atrophy, limbic encephalitis, and brain stem encephalitis may be caused by this mechanism. In parainfectious disorders, for example related to Mycoplasma infections, the same mechanism may play a role and lead to myelin damage in so-called acute disseminated encephalomyelitis.

7. Bacterial, viral or fungal infection may involve specific structures in the brain. For example, progressive multifocal leukencephalitis is an infection of the oligodendrocyte, and thus predominantly involves white matter (Fig. 3.6).

8. Hyper- or hypo-osmolar conditions may cause white matter lesions in specific brain areas. In sodium intoxication in infants, unmyelinated areas appear to be most severely involved probably because of the lower "resistance" to the uptake of water. In central pontine myelinolysis, for unknown reasons, the central part of the pons is mostly involved (Fig. 3.7).

Understanding mechanisms of selective vulnerability contributes to the understanding of patterns of cerebral involvement as shown by MRI. In disorders of quite different origin, similar pathogenetic mechanisms may be important, explaining similarities in image abnormalities. On the other hand, in disorders with rather obvious similarities with regard to pathogenesis of cerebral damage, striking differences in image abnormalities are sometimes observed, indicating the insufficiency of present understanding of pathogenetic mechanisms. A few examples are given.

Independent of its cause, energy depletion will lead to failure of mitochondrial oxidative phosphorylation, ATP depletion, accumulation of glutamate and other excitatory amino acids, opening of ion channels, accumulation of Ca^{2+} in the cell, activation of polyunsaturated fatty acid cascades and finally cell death. It would be logical if all forms of cerebral energy failure, either caused by hypoxia-ischemia and hypoglycemia or by intoxications and inborn errors of metabolism mediated via mitochondrial dysfunction, would result in selective involvement of the same structures. This, however, is only partially true. Carbon monoxide intoxication leading to hypoxia preferentially affects the globus pallidus (Fig. 3.8), whereas hypoxia in cases of near-drowning or strangulation preferentially involves the putamen and caudate nucleus, cortical layers 3, 5 and 6 and Purkinje cells. In carbon monoxide intoxication, there is possibly a special, direct toxic action on the globus pallidus, whereas in other forms of hypoxia the effects follow the expected pattern. In inherited mitochondrial encephalopathies with cellular energy failure, the putamen and caudate nucleus are preferentially affected; however, exceptional cases with selective involvement of globus pallidus or other central nuclei, in the presence of preserved putamen and caudate nucleus, have been described (Fig. 3.9). The biochemical explanation for these exceptions is unclear. Outside the field of inborn errors of metabolism, toxic substances

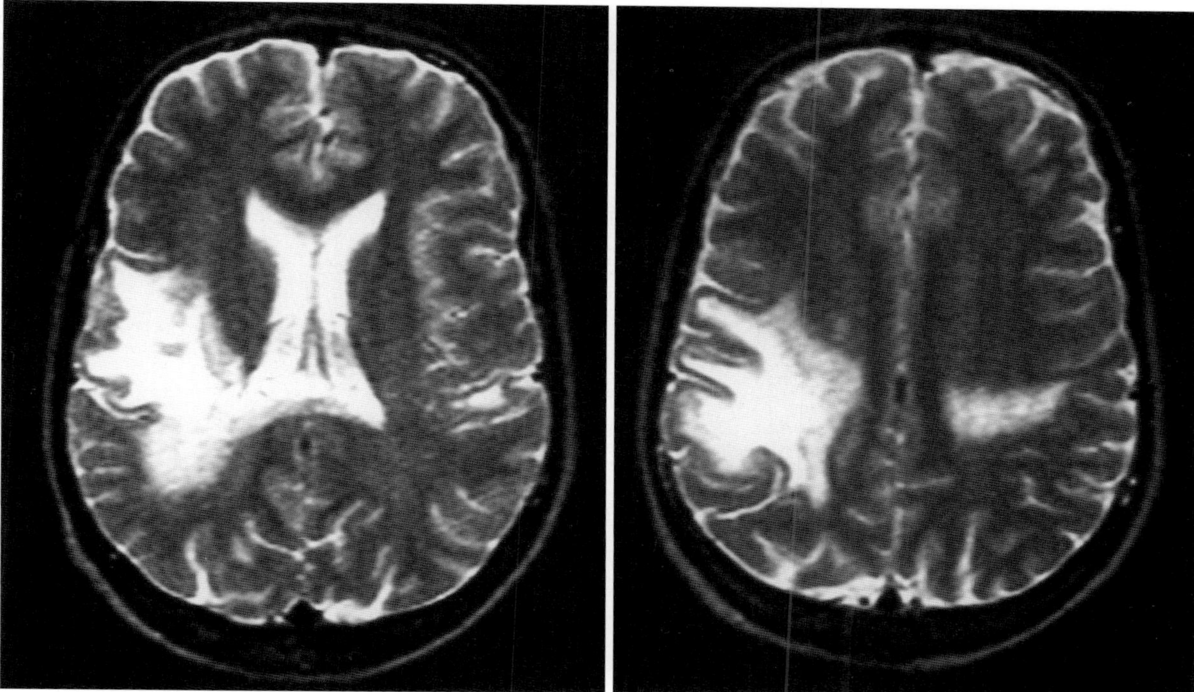

Fig. 3.6. Progressive multifocal leukoencephalitis is the result of a papova infection that attacks oligdodendrocytes. There is a rather sharp cut-off transition of the involved area towards the cortex

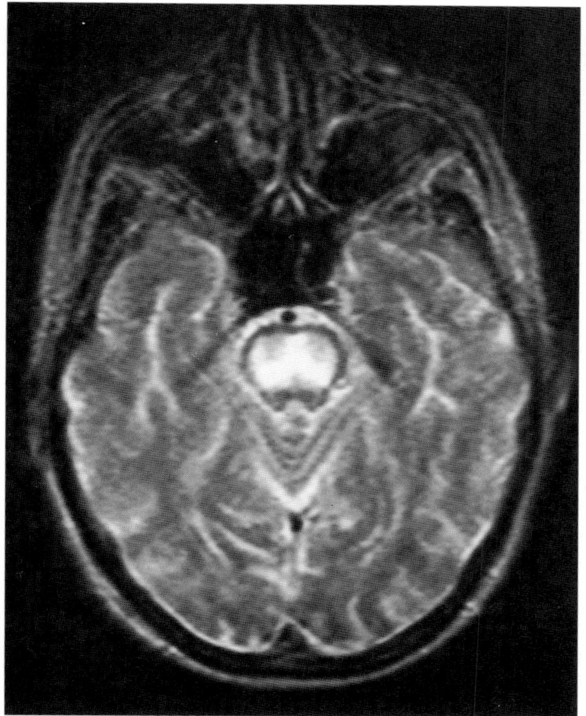

Fig. 3.7. Typical lesion in central pontine myelinolysis with central involvement of the pons, and sparing of the outer rim

and nutritional deficiencies (e.g., thiamine deficiency) may also interfere with the mitochondrial function. It is suggested that there is a close resemblance between regions involved in Leigh's disease and Wernicke's encephalopathy. This statement, however, needs critical review. In Leigh's disease there is preferential involvement of the putamen and caudate nucleus. Wernicke's encephalopathy, however, preferentially involves the phylogenetically older parts of the basal ganglia, the thalamus and the globus pallidus. But here too there are exceptions. From a diagnostic point of view, it is helpful to realize that in contrast to Leigh's disease, Wernicke's encephalopathy always involves the mammilary bodies.

Analogously, insufficiently explained differences in preferential involvement of basal ganglia have been found in other inborn errors. In glutaric aciduria type I there is typical involvement of the putamen and caudate nucleus, not, however, of the cortical layers and Purkinje cells. The neostriatal dysfunction and degeneration in glutaric aciduria type I may be due to accumulation of glutaric acid, which is toxic to striatal cells in culture. Evidence for influence of glutaric acid on glutamate receptors has also been found. In methylmalonic acidemia, as in carbon monoxide intoxication, there is preferential involvement of the globus pallidus. Putamen and caudate nucleus are usually not involved.

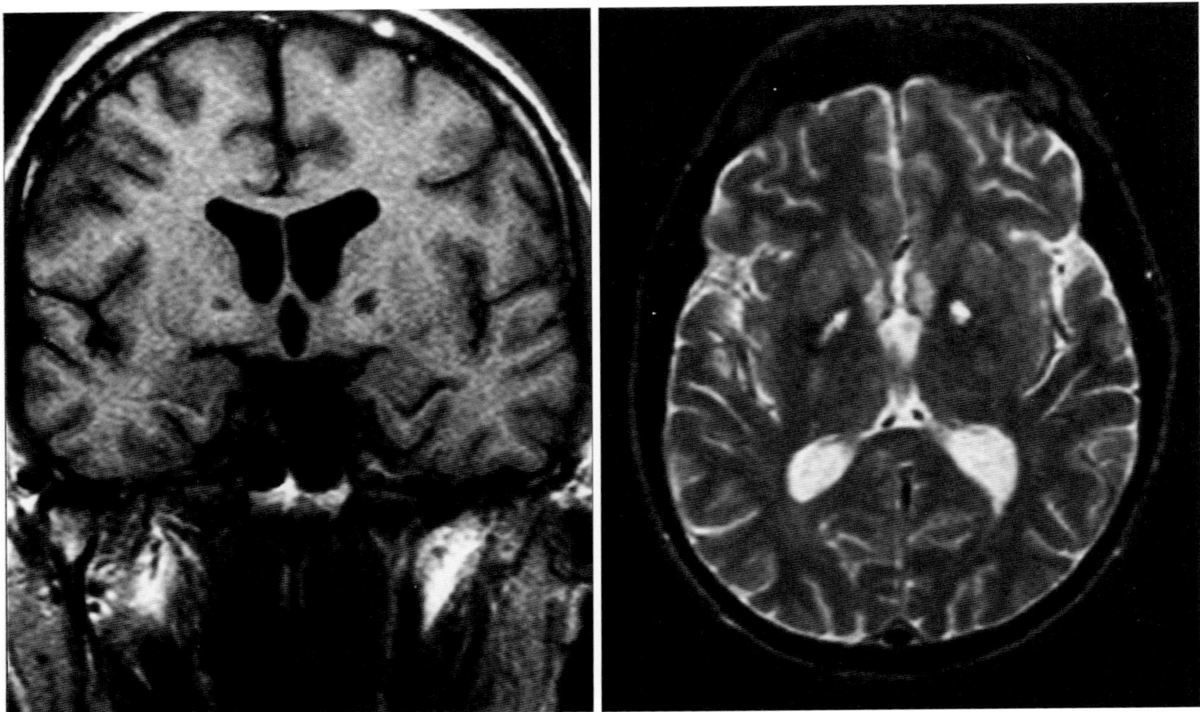

Fig. 3.8. Case of carbon monoxide intoxication with involvement of the globus pallidus on both sides

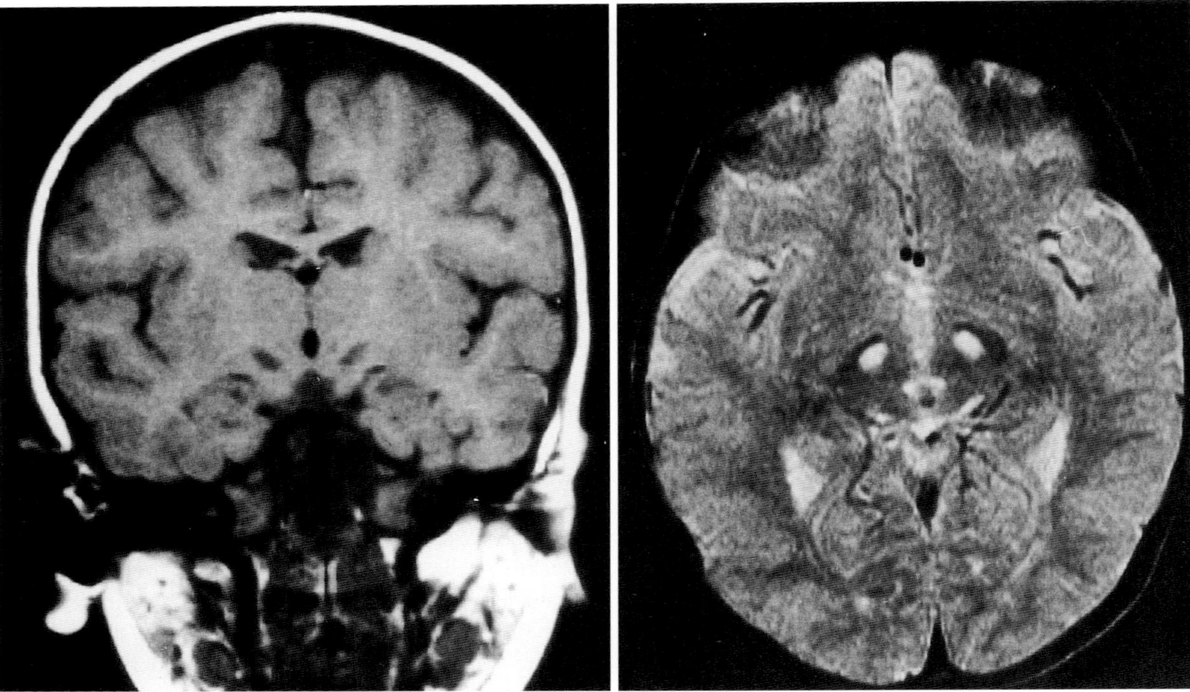

Fig. 3.9. Leigh's disease with an exceptional pattern of selective involvement of brain structures: caudate nucleus and putamen are intact, whereas the nucleus subthalamicus is selectively involved. Courtesy of M. Savoiardo, Milan, Italy, with permission

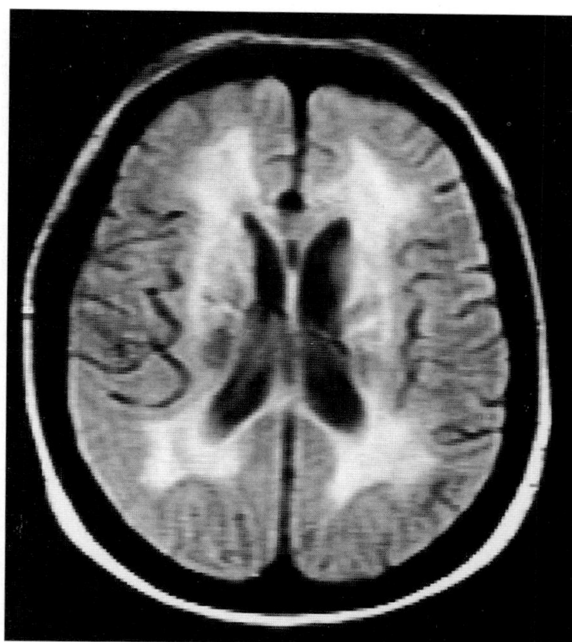

Fig. 3.10. Metachromatic leukodystrophy starts in the periventricular region, initially sparing the U fibers

This may have something to do with the specific toxic substrate accumulated in this disorder.

Impaired function of the urea cycle enzymes leads to hyperammonemia and raised concentrations of glutamine in the brain. Hyperammonemia also exists in encephalopathies due to hepatic failure. MR spectroscopy has revealed high concentrations of glutamine in the brain in these cases. Hyperammonemia also exists in Reye syndrome and in the majority of patients with methylmalonic acidemia. On the basis of similarities in the pathogenesis of encephalopathy in these disorders, similar clinical picture and similar MR images may be expected. However, the expressions, clinically and on MRI, of these disorders are unexpectedly different. In urea cycle disorders, large cerebral lesions, involving cortex and white matter are seen, with asymmetrical distribution and asymmetrical neurological signs and symptoms. In encephalopathy due to hepatic failure, the neurological symptomatology is indicative of a more generalized and symmetrical involvement of the brain. MRI shows a symmetrical T_1-shortening of the basal ganglia, including globus pallidus, putamen, caudate nucleus and other central gray matter structures. In Reye's syndrome there is generalized cerebral edema. In methylmalonic acidemia there is selective involvement of the globus pallidus with T_2-elongation.

Further analysis of these similarities and differences in patterns of selective vulnerability requires biochemical and histopathological research. Animal models and the study of effects on cell cultures may improve understanding of the mechanisms implicated in the selective involvement of CNS structures.

Selective vulnerability is not a static concept; it also refers to dynamic changes. It has become more clear with MRI than it ever was with neuropathology, that among the white matter disorders there are great differences in primary involvement of brain structures and spread in the course of time. In the lysosomal storage disorders involving the white matter, mainly the sphingolipidoses, the pattern in time is remarkably constant: the central white matter is involved first, including periventricular white matter and corpus callosum, and demyelination proceeds centrifugally from there (Fig. 3.10). The arcuate fibers are the last to be involved. An explanation for this feature could be that in these disorders abnormal substances accumulate in membranes, leading to a progressively altered myelin composition and progressively unstable myelin membrane, liable to breakdown. As the arcuate fibers are the last to myelinate they contain the youngest myelin which is altered least. Remarkably, some amino acidopathies and organic acidopathies primarily involve the arcuate fibers and the demyelination progresses in a centripetal way (Fig. 3.11). Obviously the biochemical abnormalities and interactions are completely different in these disorders as compared to lysosomal disorders: interference with energy metabolism, lack of normal myelin components, or presence of toxic metabolites are important in amino acidopathies and organic acidopathies. However, it is still difficult to explain why the arcuate fibers are first affected. MRI shows an involvement of the periventricular white matter in the occipital lobe and the splenium of the corpus callosum in the early phases of X-linked adrenoleukodystrophy. The disease spreads in a frontal direction. The reason for this occipital preference is unclear. It is noteworthy that there are cases of X-linked adrenoleukodystrophy with a completely reversed pattern, starting in the frontal lobes and the genu of the corpus callosum and progressing towards the dorsal parts of the brain. The cerebral involvement in X-linked adrenoleukodystrophy tends to be symmetrical, similar to the lysosomal disorders, but there are exceptions in which one side is far more severely involved than the other. It would be worthwhile knowing, whether the primarily involved areas have a higher vulnerability for the disease (and if so, because of what?), or whether the primarily spared areas are more resistant to the process (and if so, on which grounds?).

Symmetry of cerebral involvement can be expected to be a general rule in inborn errors of metabolism and neurodegenerative disorders, as toxic influences and deficiencies of essential substances are identical for the left and right side of the brain. In a number of disor-

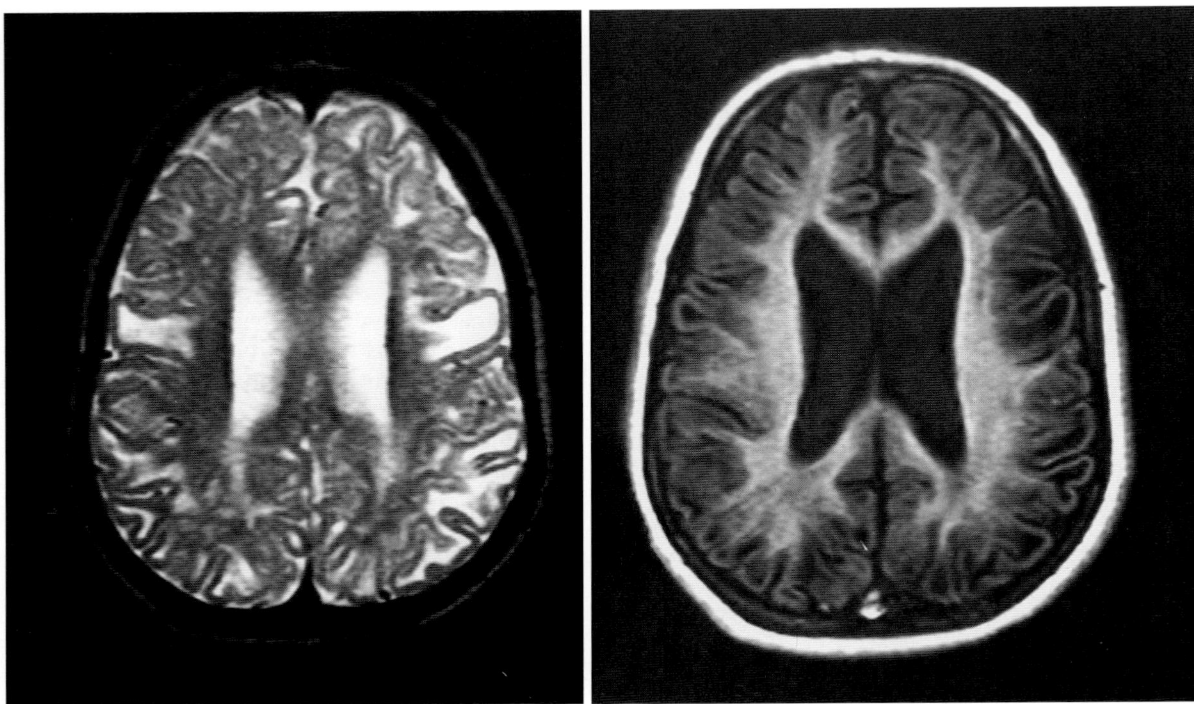

Fig. 3.11. L-2-hydroxyglutaric aciduria begins in the subcortical area, sparing the periventricular area

ders, however, asymmetrical involvement is the rule. An example is found in the urea cycle disorders. In all urea cycle disorders, metabolic derangement is characterized by the accumulation of urea precursors, notably ammonium, and by increase of glutamine in the brain. During episodes of metabolic derangement focal brain lesions may occur with myelin vacuolation and swelling of astrocytes. Neuropathological examination shows loss of neurons, cystic degeneration of the white matter and, eventually, gliosis and atrophy in the affected areas. Parallel to the asymmetry of neurological symptoms in these patients, there is a striking asymmetry in the involved CNS parts on MRI. The large lesions can involve an entire hemisphere or a large part of it. Such an MRI pattern may be misinterpreted as an infarction, because the distribution of the lesion may suggest the involvement of one or more vascular territories. The MRI characteristics of the lesion, however, are different from those of infarctions, even when both show low signal intensities on T_1-weighted images and high signal intensities on T_2-weighted images. These differences can be described by the way in which gray and white matter are simultaneously involved, the way in which the whole affected area is swollen and demar-

cated from the rest of the brain, the slightly inhomogeneous change in signal intensity, and the often "unusual" vascular territory that is occupied by the lesion. The lesions in urea cycle disorders are not mediated by vascular changes, but are probably the result of a direct toxic effect in the involved area, possibly related to the presence of elevated levels of glutamine. The asymmetrical and focal nature of the lesions is, however, unexplained. Another well known example of asymmetry is found in MELAS, a mitochondrial disorder. The lesion usually has a cortical predominance and is restricted to one part of the brain, again simulating an infarction. However, the lesion is not located in a vascular territory or a border zone area. Here too, there is no explanation for the asymmetry.

In all the chapters concerning specific disorders, one section is devoted to the description of MRI patterns in the respective disorders; another section is devoted to the description of pathogenetic mechanisms. As far as possible, these two will be connected. A separate chapter is devoted to the principles of MRI pattern recognition.

4 Myelination and Retarded Myelination

4.1 Myelination in Magnetic Resonance Imaging

Flechsig (1920) was the originator of the view that the degree of myelination of the CNS might be correlated with functional capacity. In his theory he stated that myelination started in projection pathways before association pathways, in peripheral nerves before central pathways, and in sensory areas before motor ones. Although he did modify his theory slightly because of his critics, he maintained that fibers always myelinated in the same order: first the afferent (sensory), then the efferent (motor), then the association fibers.

The histological study of fetal development has confirmed that myelination proceeds systematically and, in nerve pathways with several neurons, in the order of conduction of the impulse. The first signs of myelination appear in the column of Burdach at the gestational age of 16 weeks, growing stronger from the 24th week. The column of Goll starts to myelinate at 23 weeks gestation. Cerebellar tracts start to myelinate at about 20 weeks gestation and the amount of myelin at birth is considerable. Pyramidal tracts start to myelinate at 36 weeks at the level of the pons, but at birth the amount of myelin is still scanty. In other tracts, for example, the rubrospinal tracts, the pattern of the pyramidal tract is followed. In a full-term neonate of 40 weeks gestation, myelin stains reveal myelin in the medulla oblongata, in the central parts of the cerebellar white matter, in the cerebellar peduncles and the vermis, in the lemniscus medialis and fasciculus medialis longitudinalis in the pons and mesencephalon, in the posterior limb of the internal capsule, spreading into the globus pallidus and thalamus, and in the thalamo-cortical connections in the centrum semiovale upwards to the parasagittal parts of the postcentral gyrus, and backwards into the optic radiation. The lithographs of Paul Flechsig (1920) demonstrate this myelination pattern beautifully (Fig. 4.1).

All the mentioned structures can also be identified on MRI. On MRI, as in histology, myelination proceeds from caudal to cranial, from the afferent to the efferent areas, and in the brain centrifugally. Unfortunately, not all the areas referred to in the diagrams of progress of myelination in histological studies, as published by Keene and Hewer (1931) and Yakovlev and Lecours

(1967), can be identified on MRI, because MRI cannot match the detailed histological description (Fig. 4.2). For example, MRI cannot describe in detail the progress of myelination regarding the specific and nonspecific thalamocortical fibers, even with the knowledge that the projections of the specific "relay" nuclei – the corpora geniculata lateralia and medialia, the posteroventral and lateroventral thalamic nuclei – myelinate earlier than the projections of the nonspecific anteromedial and dorsal thalamus complex.

Although the pathway of myelination seen in MRI is similar to that found in histology, the MRI pattern lags some weeks behind when compared with the histological timetable, especially in areas with slower development of myelination. This is due to the minimal concentration of myelin required to change the signal intensity on MRI. There is, in this respect, a difference between T_1- and T_2-weighted images. On T_1-weighted images, the quantity of myelin deposited required to change the signal is smaller than on T_2-weighted images.

MRI studies of fetuses and infants have shown the presence of myelin at 23 weeks gestation in the brain stem, spreading from there to the centrum semiovale which is reached shortly before term. At 40 weeks gestational age, myelin can be seen in the central cerebellar white matter, the inferior, middle and superior cerebellar peduncles, and in a number of tracts in the pons and mesencephalon: the median longitudinal fasciculus, the medial lemniscus, the transverse pontine fibers, and in some fibers of the pyramidal tracts. The fibers in the superior and inferior vermis are well myelinated. In the region of the basal nuclei, myelination can be seen in the posterior limb of the internal capsule, in the internal fibers of the globus pallidus and thalamus, spreading to the primary sensory cortex. There is myelin in the optic tract and initial myelination in the optic radiation.

During the first month after birth, myelination progresses rapidly. It becomes more prominent in the areas mentioned. On T_1-weighted MR images myelin becomes visible in the rest of the striatum and caudate nucleus. Myelination is also seen in the optic tract, the lateral geniculate bodies and the optic radiation. From the central nuclei myelination advances in the direction of the post-rolandic sensory cortex. The corti-

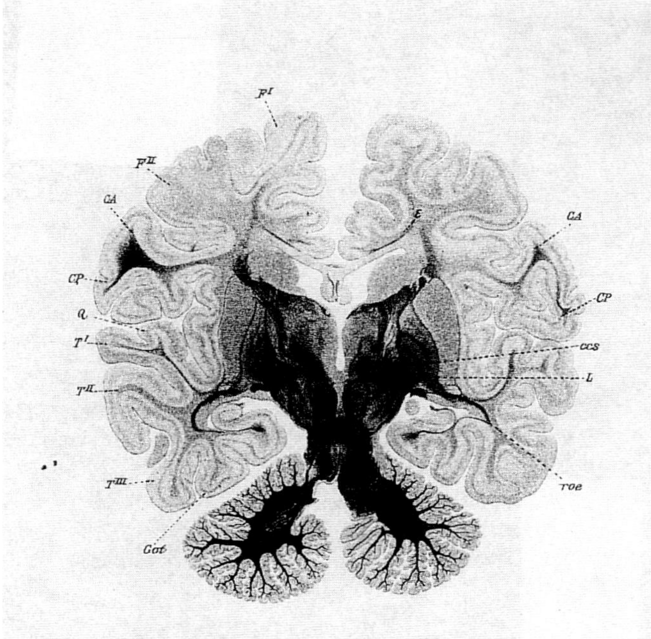

Fig. 4.1. The lithograph in the *left upper row* is reproduced from the work of Paul Flechsig (1920), who used refined histological techniques to depict the ongoing myelination in the brain. Progress of myelination of a term born neonate is presented here. Note that myelin (*dark in the image*) is already circling around the temporal horn to reach the hippocampus and parahippocampal gyrus. Also note the myelination of the auditory pathway in the superior temporal gyrus. The two T_1-weighted coronal MR images show the same features in vivo. Myelination in this case is somewhat further advanced than on the lithograph, now already spreading towards the parietal U fibers

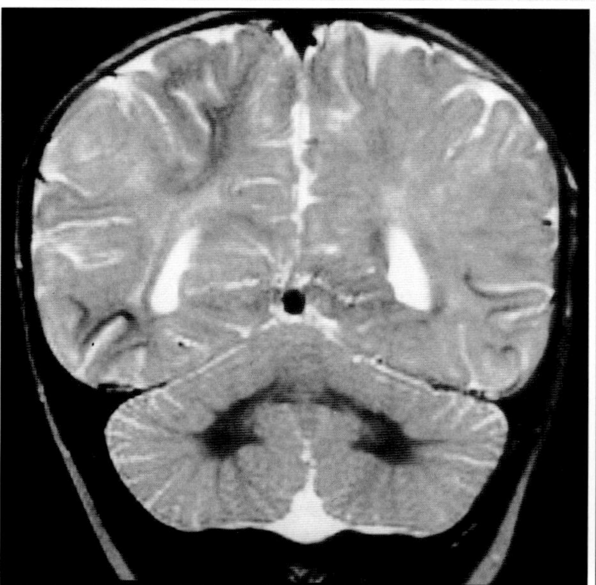

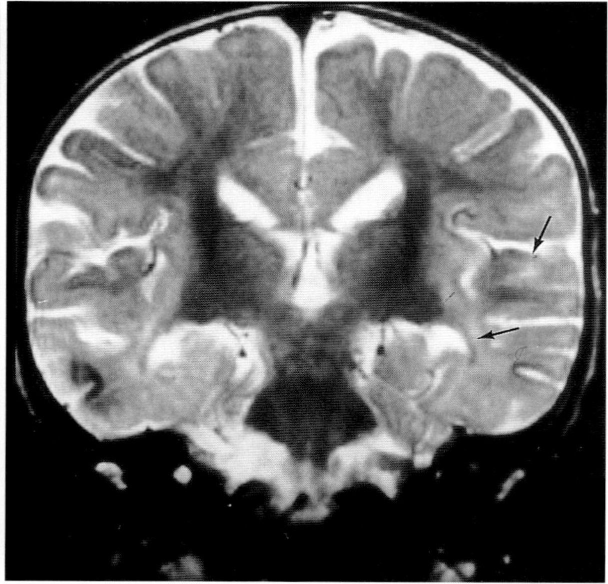

cospinal tracts from the pre-rolandic motor cortex become myelinated. From the third to fourth month onwards, myelination proceeds in the frontal direction and from the fourth to fifth month onwards, also in the temporal direction. On T_2-weighted images myelination does not reach the arcuate fibers in the frontal and temporal areas before the 12th–14th and 14th–18th month, respectively.

The corpus callosum reflects the myelination of the parts it connects. On T_1-weighted images the splenium myelinates at 3 months, the genu at about 6 months of age; on T_2-weighted images this occurs 4–6 weeks later.

Myelinated white matter gradually replaces the unmyelinated white matter. In T_2-weighted series unmyelinated white matter has a higher signal intensity than gray matter. With ongoing myelination, the white matter becomes darker and eventually can no longer be separated from the gray matter. This transition or "cross-over" period is reached in the parietal and occipital areas between 6 and 9 months after birth. After that period the myelinated white matter has a lower signal intensity than the gray matter on T_2-weighted images in this region. The frontal and temporal lobes show this cross-over at 12–14 and 14–18 months, respectively.

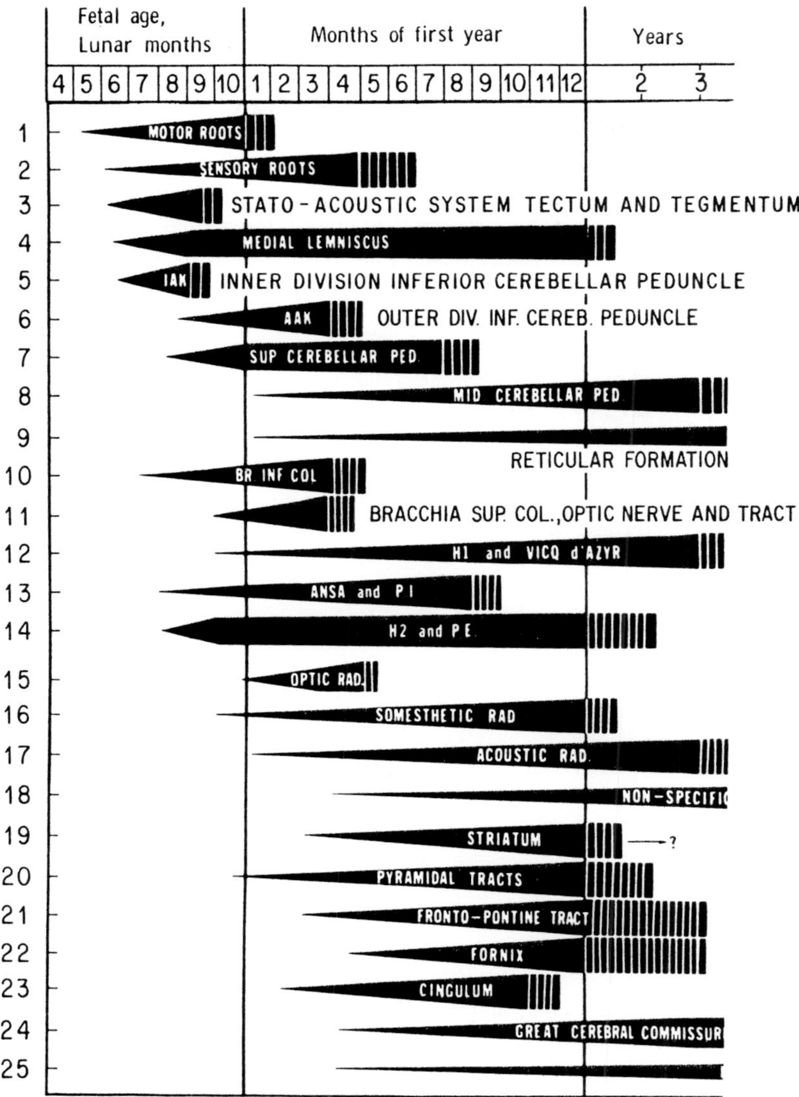

Fig. 4.2. The classical diagram of progession of myelination as conceived by Yakovlev and Lecours. Most of the structures mentioned can also be made visible on MRI. Myelination on MR images lies 1 or 2 weeks behind this schedule with conventional MR techniques. From: Yakovlev and Lecours (1967), with permission

One must, however, be careful with timetables. The visualization of myelination is strongly dependent on the pulse sequences and field strength used. Most published data are derived from SE series with relatively short TR and TE. Some series have been presented with SE 600–800/32 (McArdle et al. 1987a), others with SE 2000/84 (Dietrich et al. 1988). The features of these imaging techniques are not comparable. Differences in field strength of the magnet also play an important role. With higher field strength, T_1 becomes longer. It is important to consider the choice of pulse sequence in the assessment of progress of myelination before discussing timetables.

4.2 Pulse Sequences and Myelination

At an early stage of MRI development, the Hammersmith group advocated using IR sequences in the study of myelination. Publications from the USA emphasized the use of T_1- and T_2-weighted SE series. However, T_1-weighted SE or IR and T_2-weighted SE sequences are evidently complementary. In the first 6 months of life, IR shows the myelinated areas to better advantage, while T_2-weighted SE images, with the proper pulse sequence, differentiate more adequately the partially myelinated from nonmyelinated and completely myelinated white matter. In MRI, pulse sequences should, as a rule, be chosen so that the contrast/noise ratio is as high as possible. This is achieved if one chooses a pulse sequence that highlights the differences between tissues. It is, therefore, useful to consider the T_1 and T_2 values of gray matter, unmyelinated and myelinated white matter in order to make an adequate choice. According to Holland et al. (1986), T_1 of white matter at birth is 1615 ± 120 ms (mean $\pm$ standard deviation), at 6 months 1150 ± 60 ms and at 1 year 580 ± 50 ms; T_2 of white matter at birth is 91 ± 6 ms, at 6 months 64 ± 6 ms, and at 1 year 57 ± 5 ms. For gray matter these measurements are for T_1, at birth 1590 ± 60 ms, at 6 months 1300 ± 70 ms, at 1 year 890 ± 75 ms; for T_2, at birth 88 ± 8 ms, at 6 months 67 ± 7 ms, at 1 year 69 ± 3 ms (Table 4.1) The values are obtained at a field strength of 0.35 T. The changes observed with increasing age can be explained by the change in water content and by the progress of myelination. Protons in the myelin membrane are less mobile, water content is lower, and T_1 and T_2 are, therefore, shorter in myelinated areas. From these figures one can deduce that in T_2-weighted SE series a natural cross-over or transition in signal intensities occurs between gray and white matter.

Table 4.1. T_2 of white and gray matter at different ages

T_2 (ms)	Birth	$\frac{1}{2}$ year	1 year	3 year
Gray matter	88	67	68	62
White matter	91	64	57	53

In our SE 3000/120 series this transition or "isointense" pattern between gray and white matter is reached in the parietal and occipital lobes in normal children by the age of 6–9 months. With a different pulse sequence, SE 2000/84, Dietrich et al. (1988) found this time span to be 7–12 months. This difference might be explained by the difference in pulse sequences. Because of the heavier T_2-weighting in our series (longer TR and TE), the T_2-decay trajectories traverse each other at a somewhat steeper angle and the transition period is, therefore, more clearly marked and of shorter duration. A long TR, long TE sequence is advantageous to profit fully from the T_2-differences between gray matter, unmyelinated white matter and myelinated white matter. In an SE 3000/60,120 series, the 3000/120 images are the most important; the 3000/60 series is relatively featureless. The 3000/120 series shows unmyelinated white matter with high signal intensity, gray matter and partially myelinated white matter with intermediate signal intensity, and myelinated areas with low signal intensity. The advantage of the SE 3000/120 series is the good definition of the gray-white matter border so that migrational disorders can be assessed in the same series. The extensions of the unmyelinated white matter can be traced into the subcortical arcuate fibers.

IR series are of great importance for following the spurt of myelination during the first 6 months after birth. IR beautifully demonstrates the progress of myelination, but is less reliable for assessing the quantity of myelin deposited. The difference in T_1 between gray and unmyelinated white matter at birth gives the unmyelinated white matter a darker appearance than the cortex. With ongoing myelination the white matter will become brighter than the cortex. Between these structures again a cross-over, or contrast-inversion takes place. In T_1-weighted images, however, this is a less striking event than in T_2-weighted images. In premature neonates the unmyelinated white mattter appears much darker than the rim of cortical gray matter. Even at 40 weeks gestational age this difference is still present. Then, however, very rapidly the unmyelinated white matter starts to change its signal and becomes almost isointense with gray matter. At the same time the high intensity signal of the white matter structures in which myelin is advancing demands most of the attention in the assessment of myelination age. When comparing T_1- and T_2-weighted images it is clear that the T_1-weighted images are more sensitive for the presence of myelin. Partially myelinated structures, which are isointense or even still mildly hyperintense compared to gray matter on T_2-weighted images, are already white on T_1-weighted IR images. The reason for the higher sensitivity for myelin of T_1- compared to T_2-weighted images can be found in a number of factors at the molecular level. The special structure of the myelin membrane with a lipid:protein ratio of 70:30 (dry weight) and a cholesterol content of 30% is important. The construction of lipid layers, separated by a 40-molecule thick layer of water in which the hydrophilic phosphate polar groups of lipids and the cholesterol hydroxyls project, creates a unique lipid-water interfacial interaction, seven-fold greater than a typical protein-lipid interface. A second factor lies in the field dependent cross-relaxation between protons of myelin water and protons of myelin lipid. The apparent effect of these conditions is a shortening of T_1 induced by myelin, larger than one would expect from deposition alone of membranous structures. The long T_1 of unmyelinated white matter, in sharp contrast to the much shorter T_1 of also partially myelinated white matter, can be very well imaged with IR sequences 2400/600 (birth-3 months), 2000/500 (3–6 months), and 1400–1600/400 (older children-adults).

There are special methods for estimating progress of myelination. Anisotropic diffusion-weighted imaging has been shown to be capable of depicting myelination at an earlier stage and probably also with more accuracy than the more conventional MRI methods. Not all equipment, however, allows the application of these techniques and it will, therefore, be limited to research purposes.

4.3 Myelination: Timetables

In daily practice it is useful to have a timetable of normal progress of myelination at hand. Even with a considerable variation, it is evidently possible to provide a time scale for normal development and to assess reliably significant delay in myelination.

There are several approaches to making a timetable and each one has its own advantages and disadvantages:

1. On T_1-weighted images, preferably IR images, the progress of myelination can be followed through to its near completion. T_1-weighted sequences, in particular IR sequences, are very sensitive to relatively small quantities of myelin deposited. Partially myelinated structures already appear white on IR images. Myelination, therefore, already appears complete in the second half of the first year. T_2-weighted images, however, show that in this period myelination is still far from complete as the signal intensity of partially myelinated white matter is still higher than gray matter on T_2-weighted images. Nevertheless, the IR sequence is very useful in the first 6 months as it demonstrates progress of myelination.

At term birth, IR images show evidence of myelination in the medulla spinalis, cerebellar white matter, dorsal part of the pons, mesencephalon, posterior limb of the internal capsula, and in the postcentral parasagittal areas, as a continuation of the long ascending spino-cortical tracts. The optic radiation becomes myelinated soon after birth. The splenium of the corpus callosum is myelinated in the 3rd month, the truncus in the 4th and 5th month, the genu in the 5th and 6th month. In the 4th month myelination starts to spread to the anterior limb of the internal capsule. From the parietal parasagittal area, myelination starts to spread in anterior and posterior directions. After this stage further distinction on IR images becomes difficult.

2. Additional lightly T_2-weighted (or proton-density), and heavily T_2-weighted images can be used to refine the assessment of myelination. One can distinguish myelination of the central parts of the brain from the lobar white matter. In doing so a timetable based on signal intensities can be composed with 5 steps of progression (see Tables 4.2 and 4.3).

Some markers are useful in daily practice. On long TR, long TE SE images the splenium of the corpus callosum has a low signal by 6 months of age, the genu at 8 months of age. The cross-over in the occipital lobe, when gray and white matter uniformly and indistinguishably have an intermediate signal intensity (are

Table 4.2. Signal intensity of central white matter relative to gray matter on long TR SE images

Stage	Age	Short TE MWM	Long TE MWM
I	1st month	↑	=/↓
II	2nd month	=/↓	↓/↓↓
III	3rd–6th month	↓	↓↓
IV	7th–9th month	↓	↓↓
V	>9th month	↓	↓↓

↑↑, hyperintense; ↑ slightly hyperintense; =, isointense; ↓, slightly hypointense; ↓↓, hypointense; MWM, myelinated white matter

Table 4.3. Signal intensity of peripheral white matter relative to gray matter on long TR SE images

Stage	Age	Short TE		Long TE	
		UWM	MWM	UWM	MWM
I	1st month	↓	↑	↑	=
II	2nd month	=	=	↑↑	=
III	3rd–6th month	↑	=	↑↑	=
IV	7th–9th month		=		=
V	>9th month	↓			↓↓

↑↑, hyperintense; ↑, slightly hyperintense; =, isointense; ↓, slightly hypointense; ↓↓, hypointense; UWM, unmyelinated white matter; MWM, myelinated white matter

isointense), occurs at about 7–9 months. At about 9 months the "adult" contrast between gray and white matter starts to emerge in the occipital lobes. The anterior limb of the internal capsule is myelinated on the heavily T_2-weighted sequence at 8–11 months. At 12 months the frontal white matter starts to myelinate; it should be nearly complete at 14 months of age. The temporal lobe is the last to myelinate; this occurs between 14 and 18 months of age.

Combining methods 1 and 2 has distinct advantages and refine the assessment, in particular in the first year of life. A practical approach was suggested by Barkovich in a simplified decision tree (Fig. 4.3).

3. Use of marker sites can be helpful. For research purposes the methods under 1 and 2 do not always provide the necessary detail and quantitation. An approach defining specific targets for myelination, and scoring in a large population the time of onset and completion of myelination of such targets, leads to statistical normal values with definition of normal variation.

Another method is to use the signal intensity of one site with completed myelination as an internal standard and compare the signal intensities of other sites with this reference. The signal intensity of the posterior

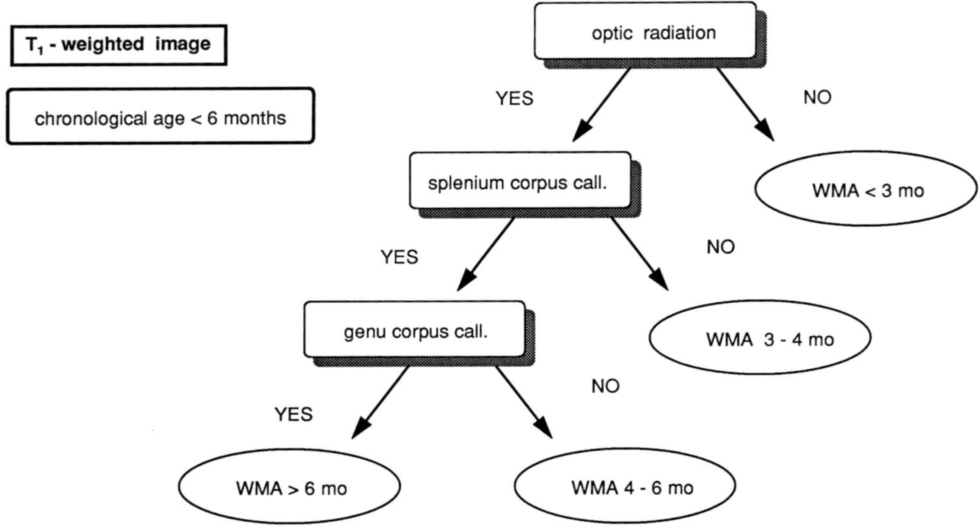

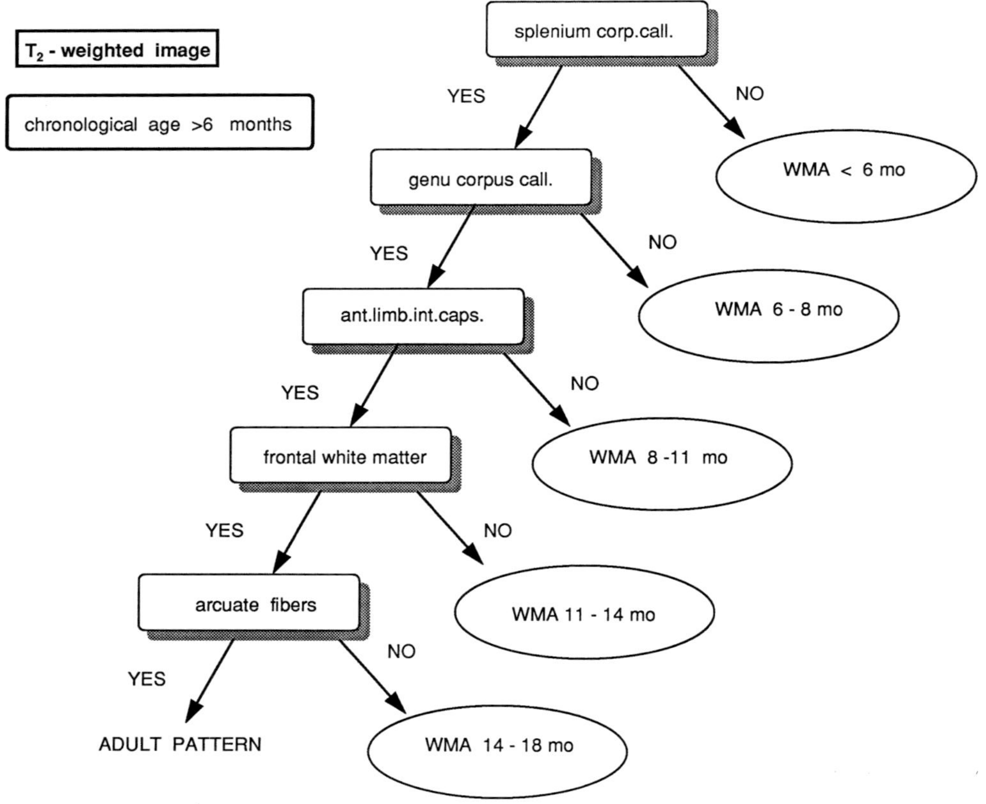

Fig. 4.3. Flow chart for the estimation of myelination age (*WMA*, white matter age). Adapted from Barkovich and Jackson (1989), with permission

limb of the internal capsule is usually chosen as reference (myelination complete at 42 weeks gestational age). A ratio of myelination per site is thus obtained, relatively independent of type of equipment and field strength. It becomes clear that there is a marked diversity in onset of changes associated with myelination of the target areas. The method allows identification of significant delays in myelination.

One can further refine the method and focus on a smaller area and a more limited time scale, for example the posterior fossa in the first two months of life, or specific tracts in the brain stem. Of course clinical relevance should be established first. As an example: one might wish to look at the development of visual functions in prematurely born children and compare this with the degree of myelination in the visual pathways. One then has to develop a scoring system for the components of this pathway: the optic nerve, chiasm, optic tract, lateral geniculate bodies, optic radiation, preferably in a ratio to an already well myelinated site, such

as the posterior limb of the internal capsule after 42 weeks gestational age. Instead of scoring myelination on a numeric scale by visual methods, one might measure the "absolute" signal intensities and obtain a myelination ratio. The drawback to this method is the possible demyelination or retarded myelination of the internal capsule, which would compromise the internal standard.

Some groups have used this more refined method of marker sites combined with the estimation of time of contrast cross-over between structures and looked at the detailed progress of myelination in the cerebellum and brain stem in the first months of life. MRI provides in such analysis astonishing detail. Stricker et al. (1990) took as target areas the cerebellar hemispheres, dentate nucleus, middle cerebellar peduncle, corpus medullare cerebelli, pontine tegmentum, basis pontis, medial lemniscus and corticospinal tracts. They defined 5 stages of progress of cerebellar myelination, depending on the relative signal intensities of these regions. Land-

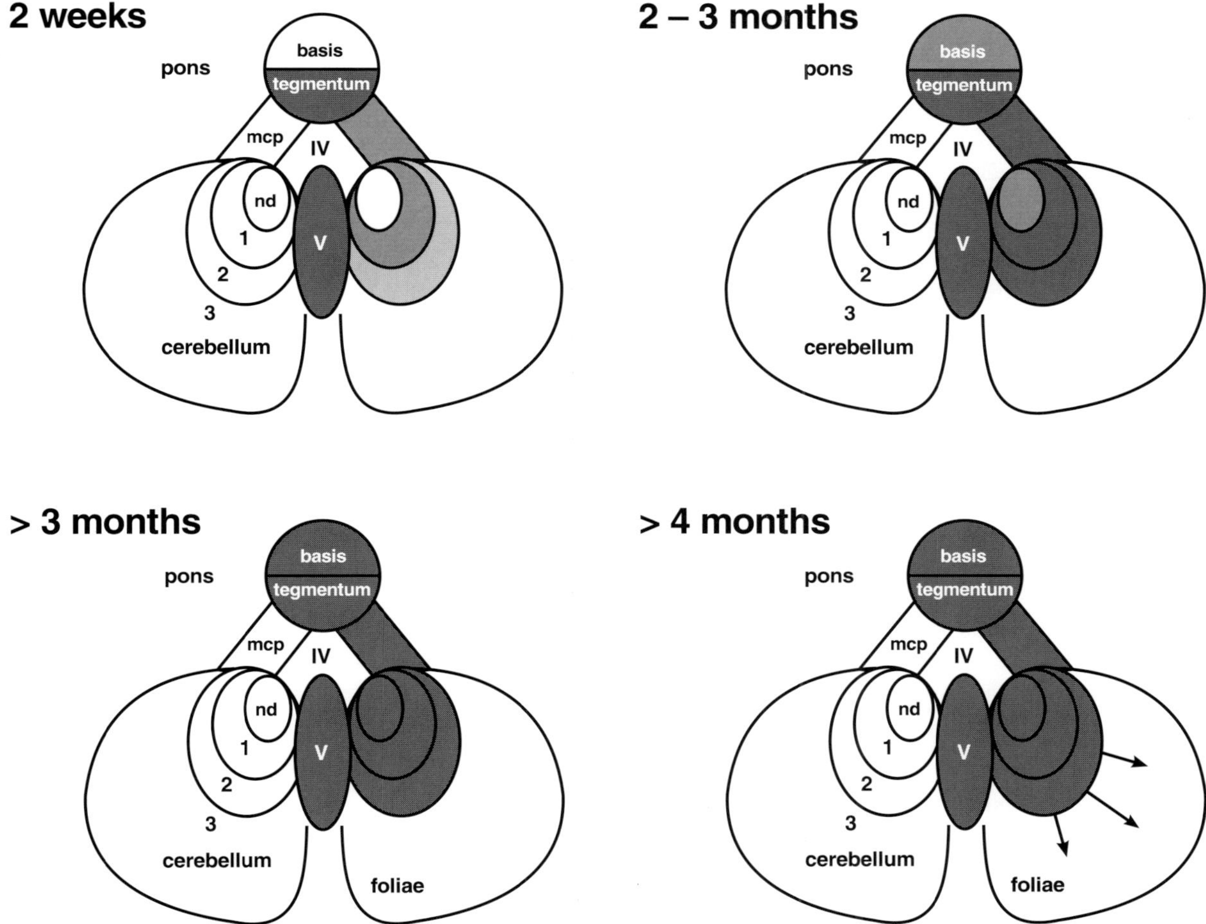

Fig. 4.4. Myelination of posterior fossa (*nd*, nucleus dentatus; *mcp*, middle cerebellar peduncle; *1*, peridentate white matter; *2*, corpus medullare; *3*, peripheral white matter; *v*, vermis cerebelli).

marks of these studies used for time-estimates were again the gradually darker appearance of myelinated areas on T_2-weighted images, the further extension of myelination towards the subcortical structures, and inversion of contrast between structures. An example of the first marker is the gradual darkening of the rim around the dentate nucleus in the first weeks of life; of the second marker the extension of myelin into the cerebellar foliae; and of the third marker, the crossover in signal intensities between the corticospinal tracts and the substantia nigra. When automatic scaling is used, which is usually the case on MR systems, it proves difficult to identify the 5 stages as described by these authors. Usually, however, 3 stages of maturation can be distinguished in the posterior fossa. The structures involved in the recognition of these 3 stages on T_2-weighted transverse images are: the basis pontis, the tegmentum pontis, the middle cerebellar peduncle, the dentate nucleus, the peridentate white matter, the corpus medullare cerebelli, and the white matter extending into the cerebellar foliae (Fig. 4.4). In stage 1 (<1 month) the basis pontis is not myelinated, there is some myelin in the tegmentum of the pons and in the middle cerebellar peduncles, the nucleus dentatus has a high signal intensity and is surrounded by a rim of lower signal intensity, followed by high signal of the cerebellar white matter. In stage 2 (>1 month, <3–4 months) myelination starts to appear in the basis pontis; the tegmentum is, however, still darker; the dentate nucleus starts to appear darker. In stage 3 (>3–4 months), tegmentum and basis pontis are now more or less equally dark; the dentate nucleus and the cerebellar white matter appear completely dark and isointense with the middle cerebellar peduncle. After the completion of these stages, myelination starts to extend towards the cerebellar foliae, gradually shaping the "arbor vitae" of the cerebellum.

One could make the assessment more detailed and add more structures: pyramidal tracts, medial lemniscus, and medial longitudinal fasciculus, structures that can be distinguished in good quality images of the brain stem and cerebellum. A similar diagram could be produced for the mesencephalic structures, where the contrast of the red nucleus, the substantia nigra, the corticospinal tracts, medial lemniscus and inferior colliculus changes with time.

4.4 Delayed Myelination, Irregular Myelination, Hypomyelination and Arrest of Myelination

Once MRI criteria for normal progress of myelination have been established (Table 4.4), it is possible to diagnose delays in this process. If indeed myelination expresses functional maturity, one might expect a correlation between delay in myelination and delayed development of psychomotor functions. Roughly speaking this appears to be the case. We could prove that in a group children with hydrocephalus, of whom MRI and neuropsychological data were obtained before and twice after shunting, there was a strong correlation between (a) the progress of myelination compared to the normal myelination standard, and (b) the progress of mental development compared to the normal developmental standard. Other evidence was collected by Dietrich et al. (1988). The follow-up of the progress of myelination in suspected cases, to see whether, and if so, when the child catches up with normal myelination, is of great importance and should be a research issue. One might assume that a longer delay in the restoration of the normal pattern would coincide with a poorer prognosis. In our follow-up studies, we have found cases of children who were catching up with normal myelination in a couple of months, and children who had not reached the normal condition 1 year after the first examination, although myelination was still progressing along the usual pattern at a slow pace. Long-term follow-up of these cases might be rewarding in establishing a relationship between these patterns and possible later disturbances in psychomotor development, behavioral disorders, and learning disabilities. These studies could demonstrate the value of early intervention.

Myelination can be delayed by many causes: hypoxia-ischemia, congenital infections, congenital malformations, chromosomal abnormalities (Down syndrome), congenital heart failure, postnatal infections, hydrocephalus, hypothyroidism, hypercortisolism, hypocortisolism, fetal intoxications, malnutrition, inborn errors of metabolism, and so on. The delay is usually bilateral and symmetrical, but unilateral delay is seen in cases with hemimegalencephaly, unilateral porencephalic cysts, cerebral hemiatrophy, or unilateral periventricular leukomalacia.

The critical period in myelin development was initially thought to coincide with the proliferation of myelin-forming cells, not with the period of membrane accumulation. The mechanism of "stunting" of oligodendroglial proliferation as a cause of hypomyelination has recently been under discussion, because in animal research no major deficits of oligodendrocytes could ever be established, other than in severely starved animals. Therefore the induction of myelin membrane formation, rather than cell proliferation seems to be the actual critical event. Damage in critical periods is often limited to areas of beginning myelination at that time. This knowledge is helpful in establishing the time of insult in infants and children.

Irregular myelination with local or generalized hypermyelination, or myelination not following the nor-

Table 4.4. Myelination on MRI: chronological table

Regions of CNS	Fetal age in months					Postnatal age in weeks					Postnatal age in months			
	24	28	32	36	40	4	8	12	16	20	6	9	12	>12 months
Cerebellar peduncles		+	+	+ +	+ + +	+ + +	+ + +	+ + +	+ + +	+ + +	+ + +	+ + +	+ + +	Further refinement of myelination in the subcortical arcuate fibers continues for several years
Tegmentum pontis				+	+	+ +	+ +	+ + +	+ + +	+ + +	+ + +	+ + +	+ + +	
Basis pontis							+	+	+ +	+ + +	+ + +	+ + +	+ + +	
Medial lemniscus						+	+ +	+ +	+ + +	+ + +	+ + +	+ + +	+ + +	
Pyramidal tracts								+	+	+	+ +	+ +	+ + +	+ + +
Optic nerve					+	+ +	+ +	+ + +	+ + +	+ + +	+ + +	+ + +	+ + +	+ + +
Optic radiation						+	+	+ +	+ + +	+ + +	+ + +	+ + +	+ + +	+ + +
Stato-acoustic system	+	+	+	+ +	+ +	+ +	+ +	+ + +	+ + +	+ + +	+ + +	+ + +	+ + +	+ + +
Intern. caps. post. limb			+	+ +	+ + +	+ + +	+ + +	+ + +	+ + +	+ + +	+ + +	+ + +	+ + +	+ + +
Intern. caps. ant. limb								+	+	+ +	+ + +	+ + +	+ + +	+ + +
Corpus call. splenium							+	+	+ +	+ +	+ +	+ + +	+ + +	+ + +
Corpus call. genu											+	+	+ +	+ + +
Parieto-occip. WM						+	+ +	+ +	+ + +	+ + +	+ + +	+ + +	+ + +	+ + +
Frontal WM													+	+ +
Temporal WM														+

WM, white matter

mal routes of progress is rare, but may be seen occasionally. General hypermyelination, or advanced myelination was observed in patients with Sturge-Weber. It has been suggested that epileptic seizures may stimulate myelination. However, advanced myelination or hypermyelination is certainly not seen in most patients with infantile forms of epilepsy. Local hypermyelination in the basal ganglia is histologically described in the so-called status marmoratus, a late sequence of perinatal hypoxia. In this case the myelination does not involve the proper targets and does not occur around axons but around astrocytic extensions. Because of the low signal intensity of the basal ganglia on T_2-weighted images and the dark appearance of myelin on this sequence, MRI has so far not succeeded in identifying this condition.

Hypomyelination or arrest of myelination occurs in Pelizaeus-Merzbacher disease, a disorder of proteolipid protein synthesis, one of the major myelin proteins. In this disorder no or very little myelin is produced. To establish a certain diagnosis of retarded or arrested myelination, at least two observations with sufficient time gap are necessary.

4.5   Iconography of Myelination

In this chapter, illustrations are presented of the progress of myelination in normal neonates and infants and a few examples of disorders of this process (Figs. 4.1, 4.5–4.20). Many other disturbances of myelination, de-, and dysmyelination are found in the other chapters of this book. In Table 4.4 the myelination of some important structures on MRI is indicated. The decision tree, as suggested by Barkovich, is a practical and rough guide, but serves its purpose as a means of quick orientation (Fig. 4.3). In some cases it is useful to look in more detail at structures in relationship to their surroundings, to see how contrast changes over time. The structures in the posterior fossa are a good example (Fig. 4.4).

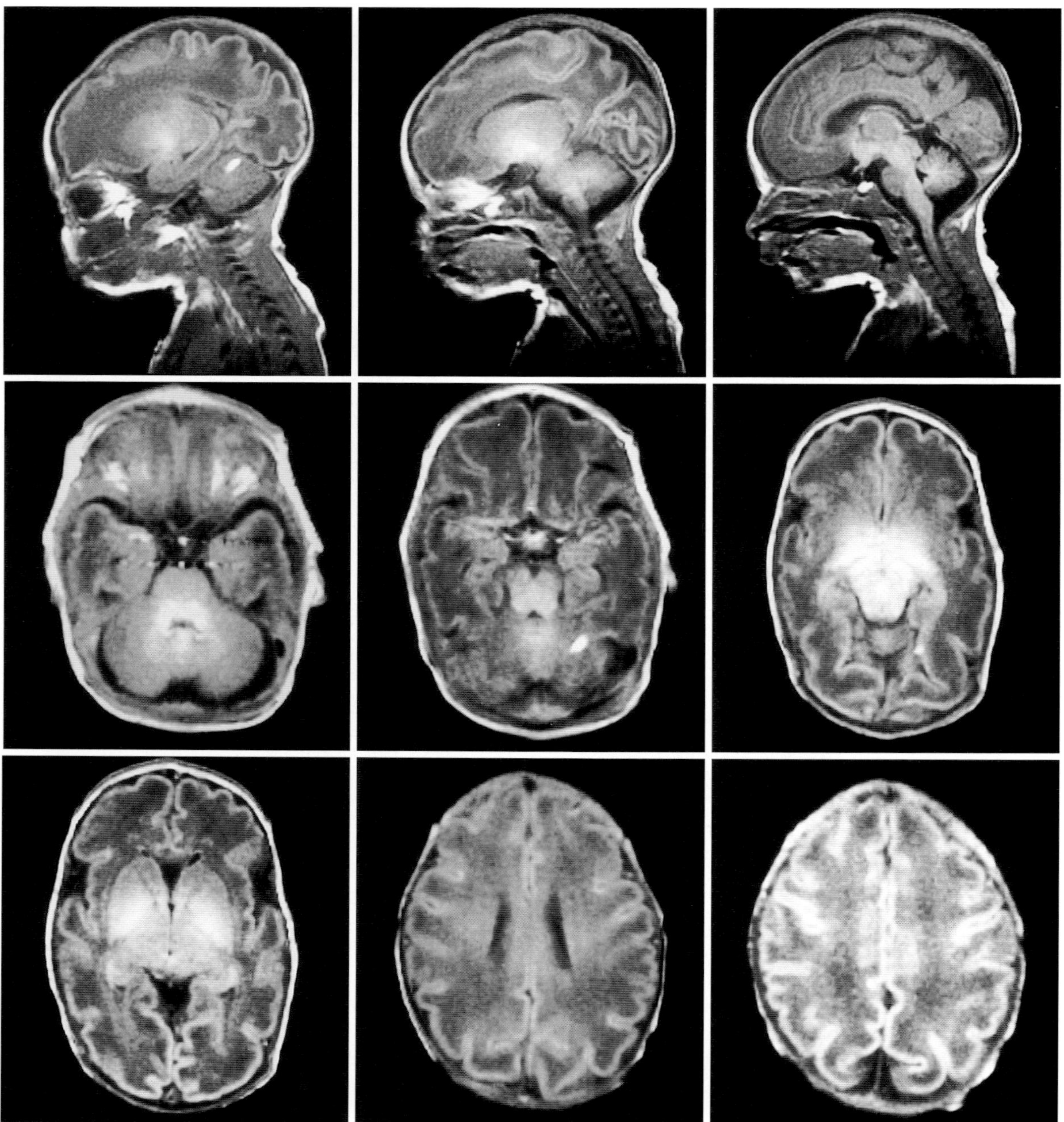

Fig. 4.5. Myelination at 32 weeks gestational age. The sagittal T_1-weighted series (*upper row*) shows nicely the features of the premature brain: the lack of gyration in the frontal areas, with some gyration in the parietal and occipital lobes. The midsagittal image (*right, upper row*) shows myelin present in the medulla oblongata, the dorsal part of the pons, the mesencephalon, and the corpus medullare of the cerebellum. The transverse T_1-weighted series (*middle and bottom row*) shows the same features and gives a good impression of the high water content of the unmyelinated white matter

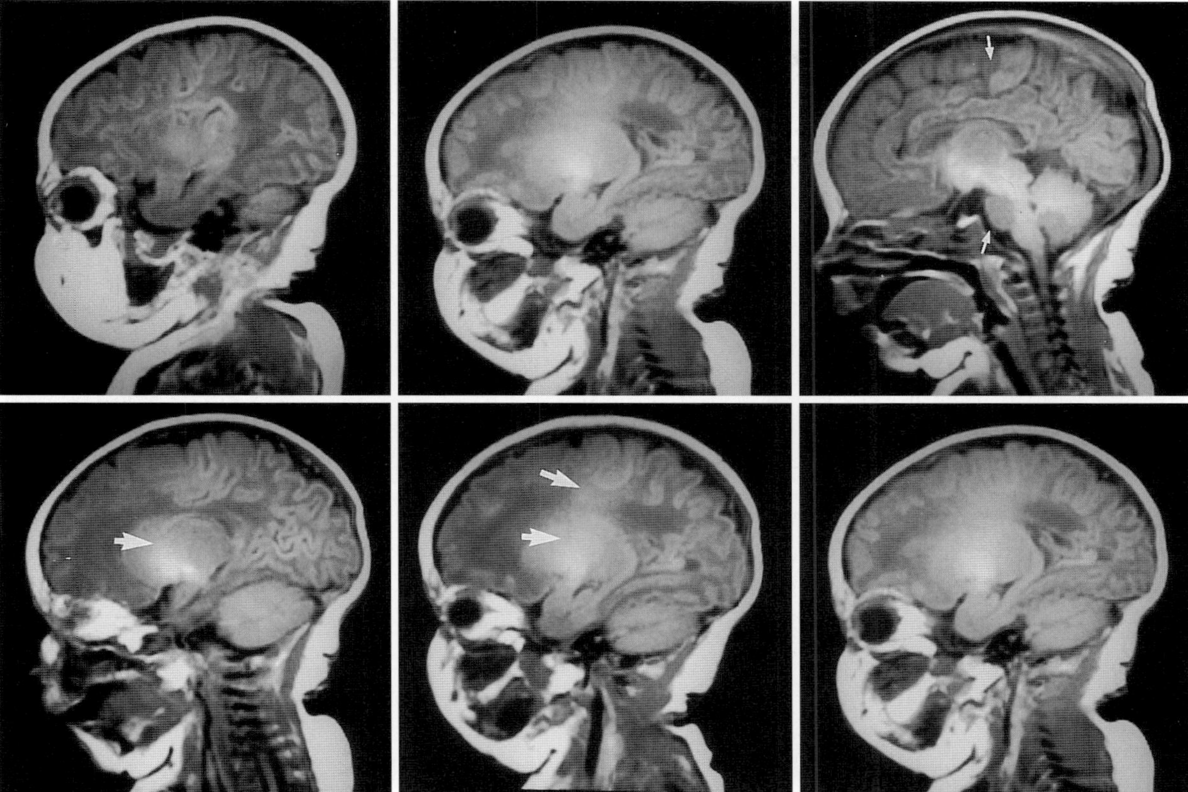

Fig. 4.6. Myelination at 38 weeks gestational age. A sagittal T_1-weighted SE series is shown *from right to left*. In the brain stem the basis pontis is still not myelinated (*arrow*). The cor-pus callosum is still thin and also unmyelinated. From the basal ganglia, myelinated white matter tracts can be followed towards the post-rolandic gyrus (*arrows, lower row*).

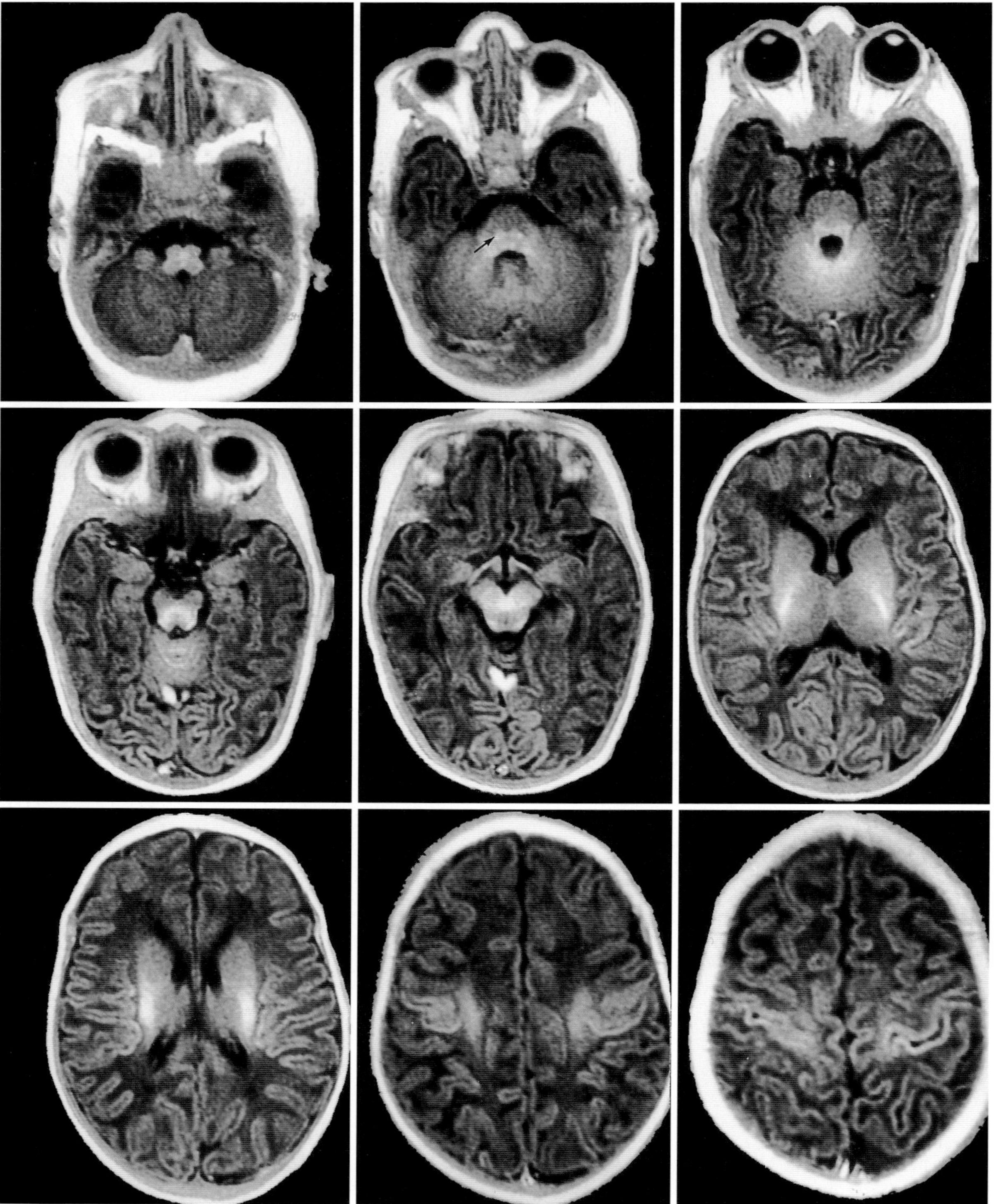

Fig. 4.7. Myelination at 2 weeks after birth at full term, as seen on a T_1-weighted transverse IR series. Myelination is seen in the medulla oblongata, the middle cerebellar peduncle, the tegmentum pontis (especially the medial lemniscus, *arrow*), the colliculus inferior, the central tegmental part of the mesencephalon, the optic tracts, the posterior limb of the internal capsule, white matter tracts in the basal ganglia and in the ascending tracts towards the postrolandic gyrus. Note that in the higher images cortical gray matter is also myelinated

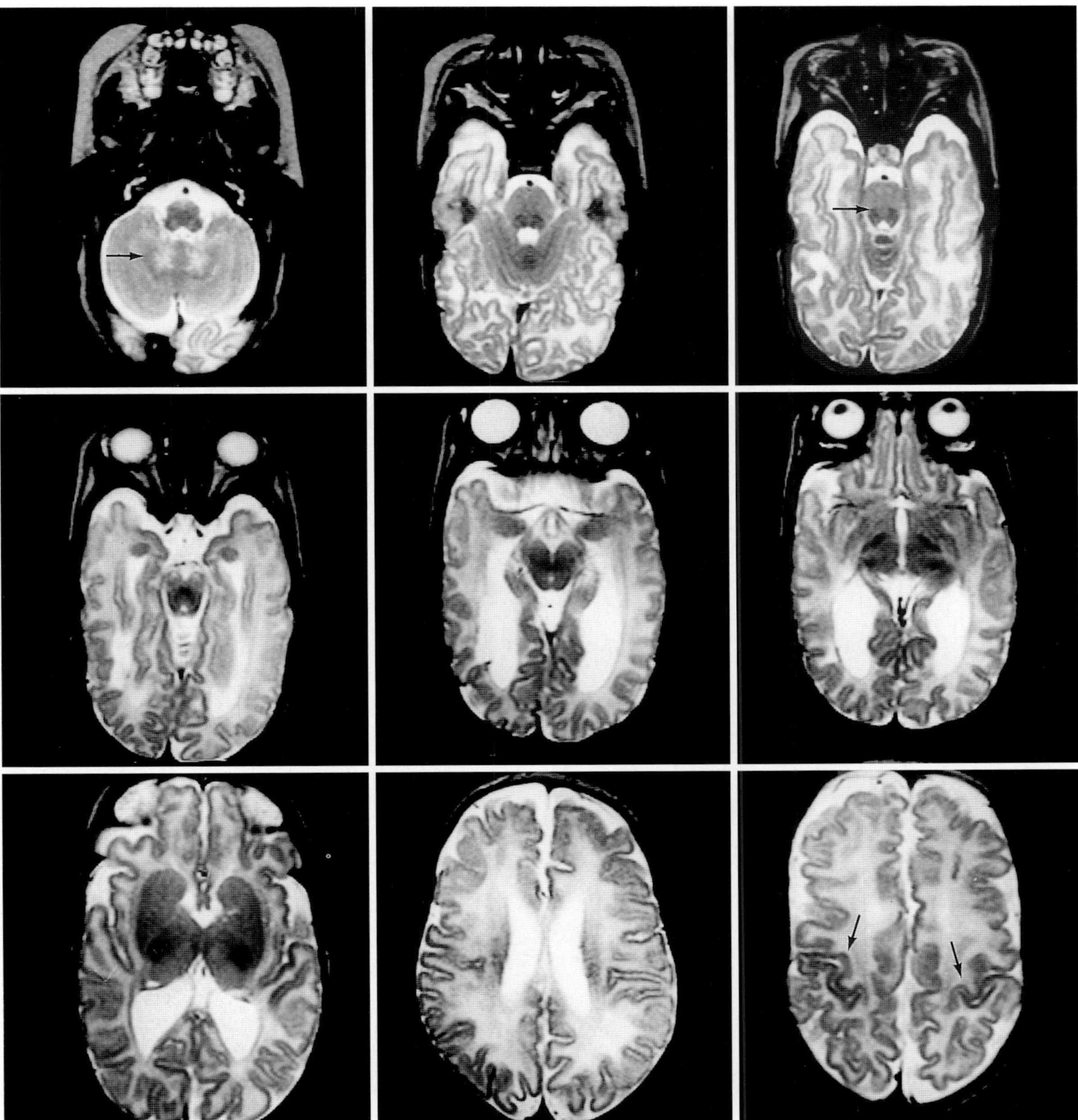

Fig. 4.8. T_2-weighted transverse series of myelination at 2 weeks after birth at full term for comparison. Cerebellar myelination is still in stage 1: the dentate nucleus is bright, surrounded by a dark band (*upper left arrow*) again followed by bright cerebellar white matter. Contrast inversion of these structures during the progress of myelination will give clues as to the age of myelination. On T_2-weighted images the tegmentum pontis and mesencephalon are darker than the ventral parts (*upper right arrow*). Myelin can be seen in the superior vermis, mesencephalon, posterior limb of the internal capsule, basal ganglia and in ascending tracts into the postrolandic gyrus (*bottom right arrows*)

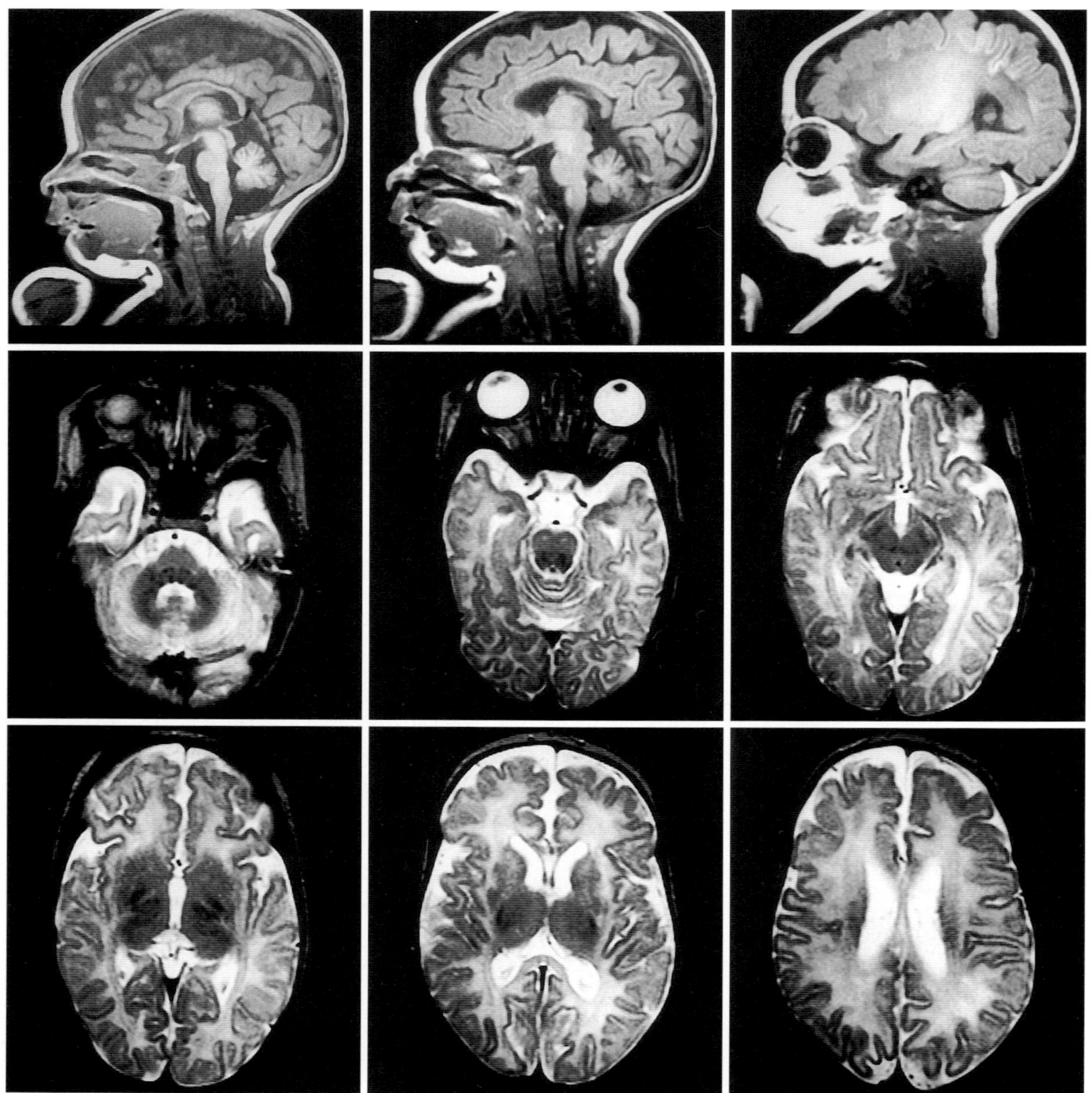

Fig. 4.9. In the posterior fossa T$_2$-weighted images show the cerebellar myelination has progressed to stage 2. The bright ring around the dentate nucleus has disappeared, but the peripheral white matter of the cerebellum is still bright. There is still a difference between the basis pontis and tegmentum pontis, although much less than before. In the mesencephalon, the pyramidal tracts and medial lemniscus can be identified. The structures will inverse contrast with the substantia nigra and nucleus ruber

Fig. 4.10. IR images at 3 months. The myelinated structures can easily be identified. Note the beginning of myelination in the pyramidal tracts in the mesencephalon (*large white arrow*) and the strongly myelinated medial lemniscus (*small black arrow*). Also the colliculus inferior and the auditory tracts are clearly myelinated (*large black arrow*). The optic tract is myelinated as is the optic radiation. The posterior limb of the internal capsule is fully myelinated at the postnatal age of 2 weeks. Myelin has now spread to the precentral gyrus and will advance dorsally and ventrally to myelinate the occipital, the frontal and finally the temporal lobes

Fig. 4.11. At the age of 5 months the genu of the corpus callosum starts to myelinate. On IR images myelination will soon appear to be complete. T$_2$-weighted images will then be more useful in providing information about maturation of the brain

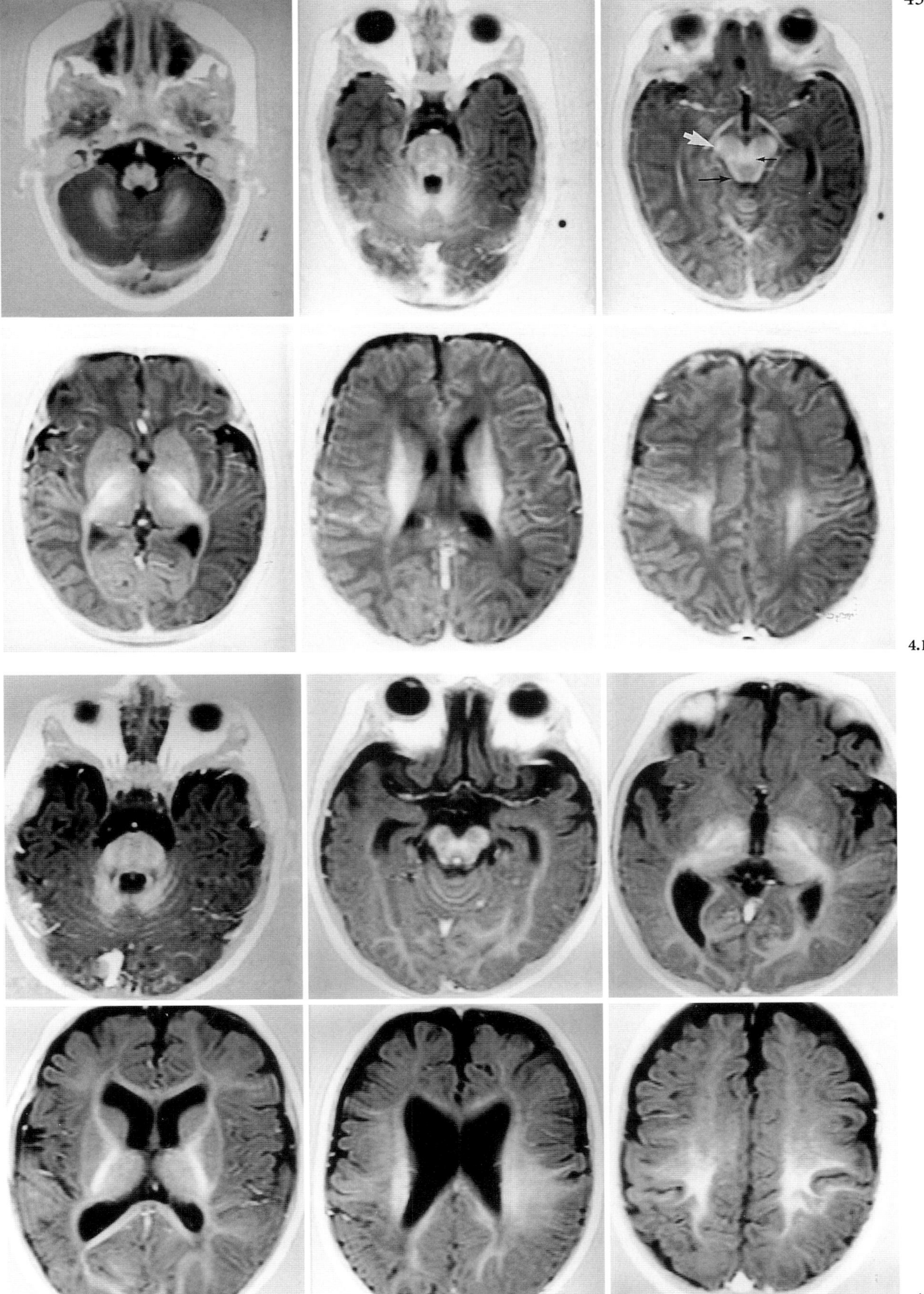

4.10

4.11

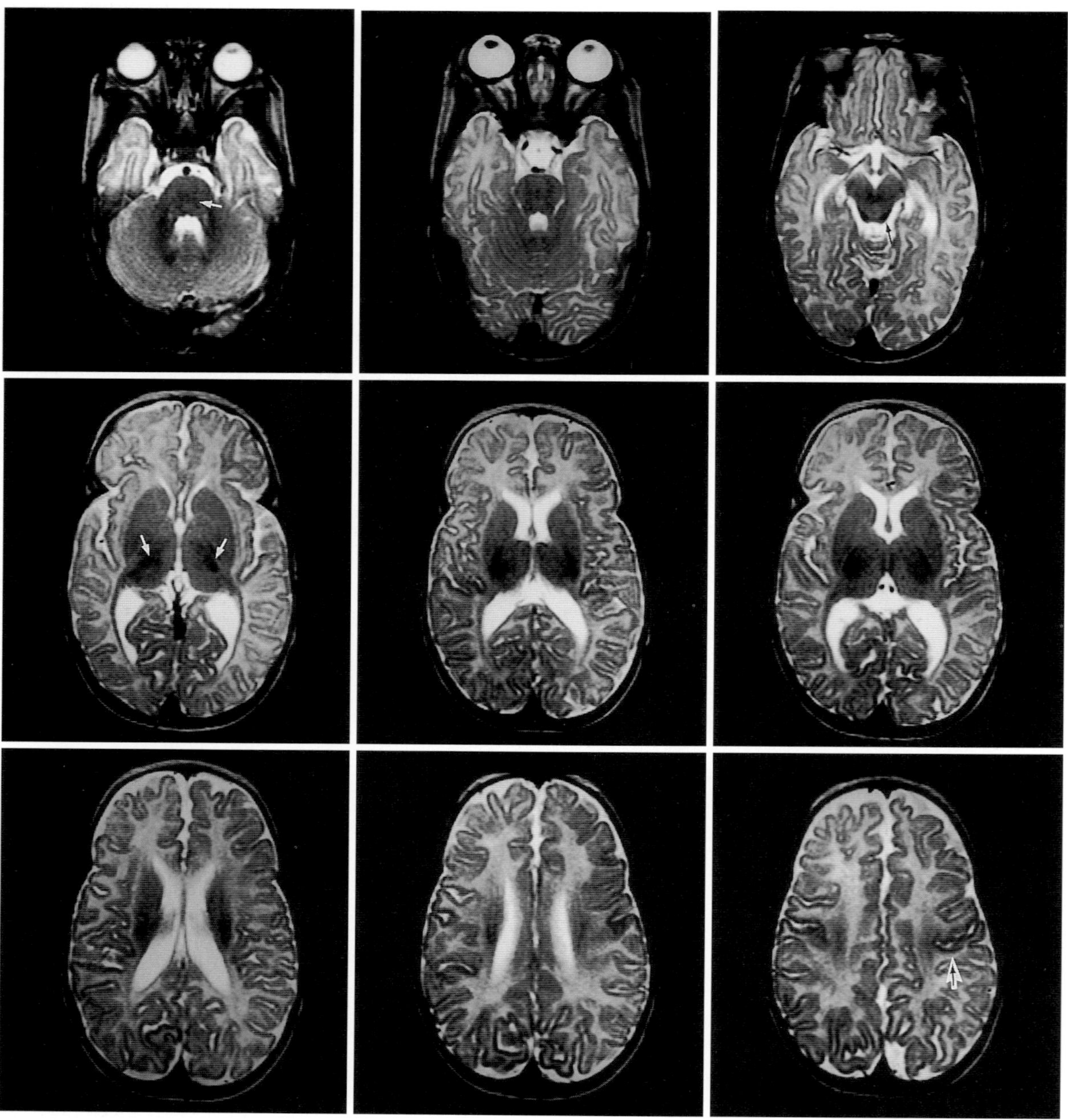

Fig. 4.12. T$_2$-weighted series at 4 months of age. In the pons, basis and tegmentum have a low signal; the medial lemniscus has an even lower signal (*white arrow*), as do the middle cerebellar peduncles. The corpus medullare of the cerebellum is myelinated, but myelination is not yet extending towards the foliae. At the level of the mesencephalon, the colliculus inferior (*black arrow*), the pyramidal tracts, the corpus mammillare and the optic tract have a low signal. The posterior limb of the internal capsule is also dark (*arrows*). Myelin is also seen in the peri-rolandic area (*arrow, bottom right*). A difference is visible between the unmyelinated white matter in the frontal and temporal region and the occipital and parietal region where myelination has started

Fig. 4.14. Myelination at 7–8 months of age. On the T$_2$-weighted images the central parts are now myelinated, including the genu of the corpus callosum. The cross-over between gray and white matter in the occipital and parietal areas has started; there is little contrast between gray and white matter. In the frontal and temporal regions this is still not the case

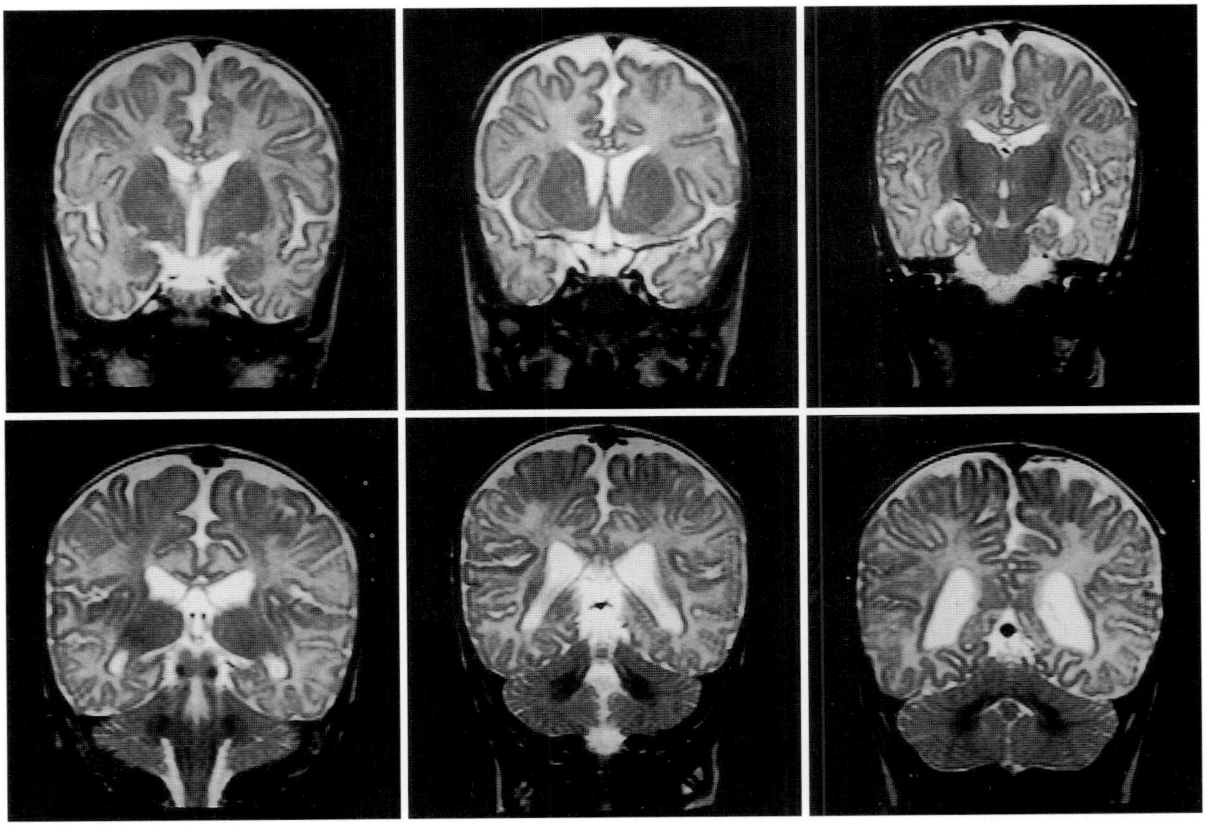

Fig. 4.13. T_2-weighted coronal images at the age of 4 months, showing the difference between still unmyelinated white matter in the frontal and temporal lobe and the more advanced myelination posteriorly

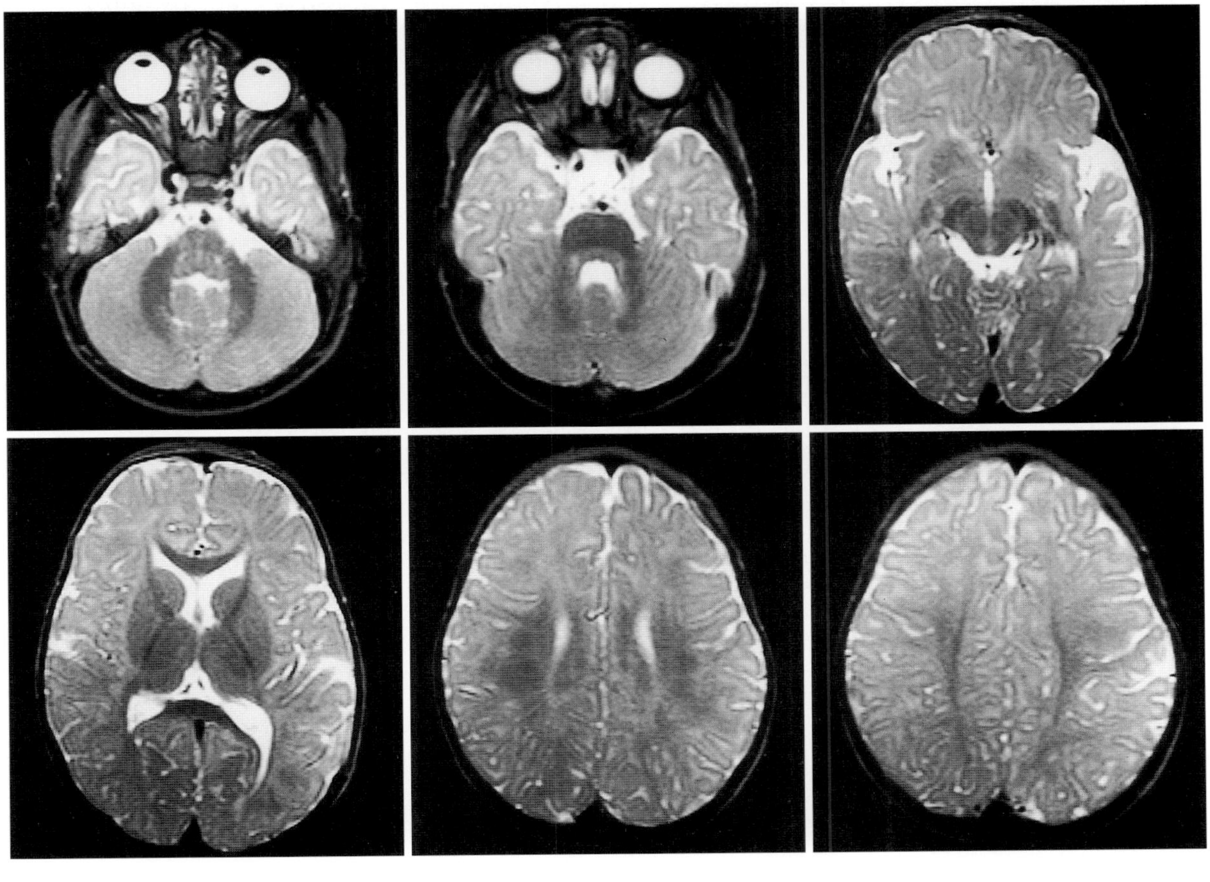

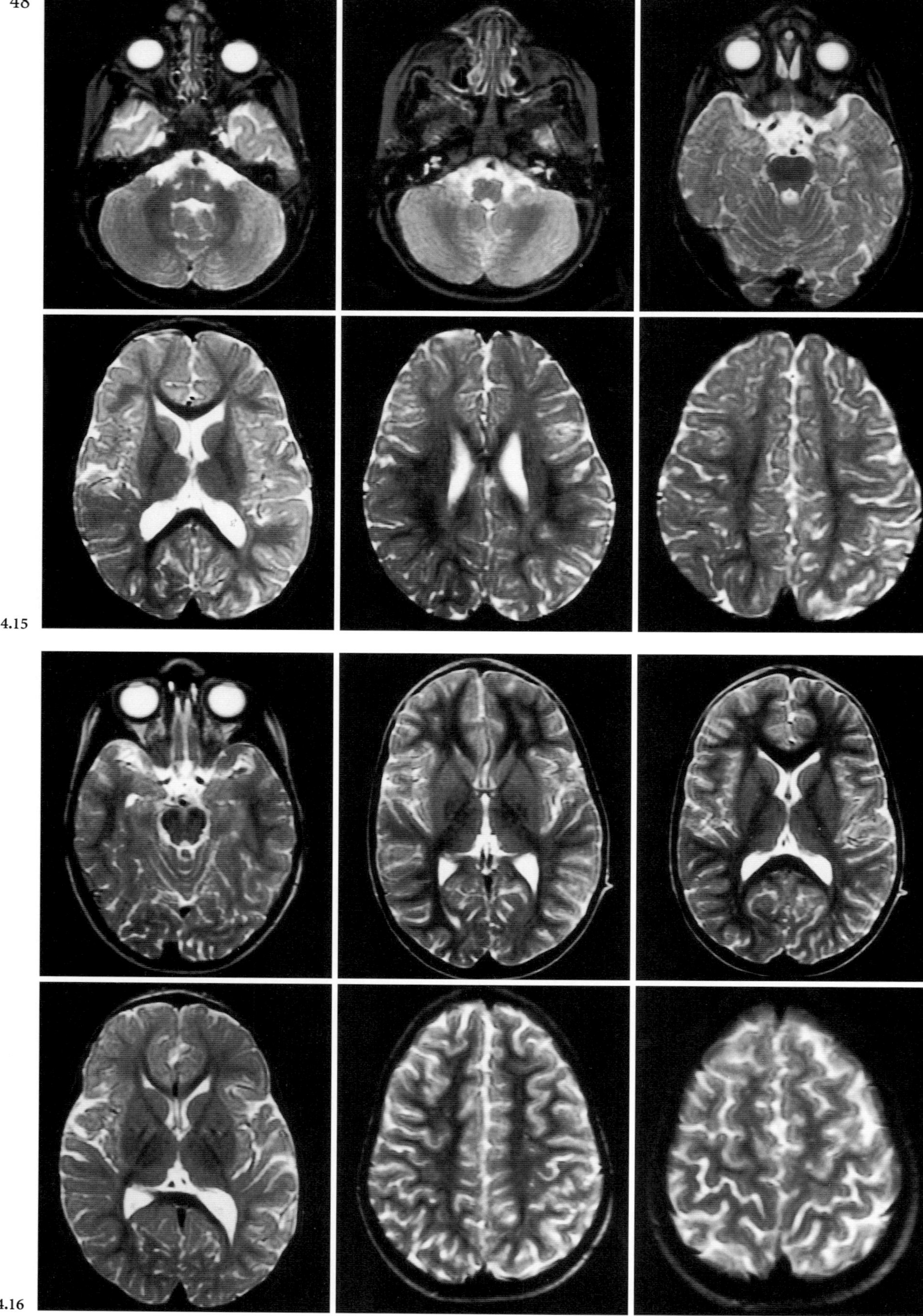

4.15

4.16

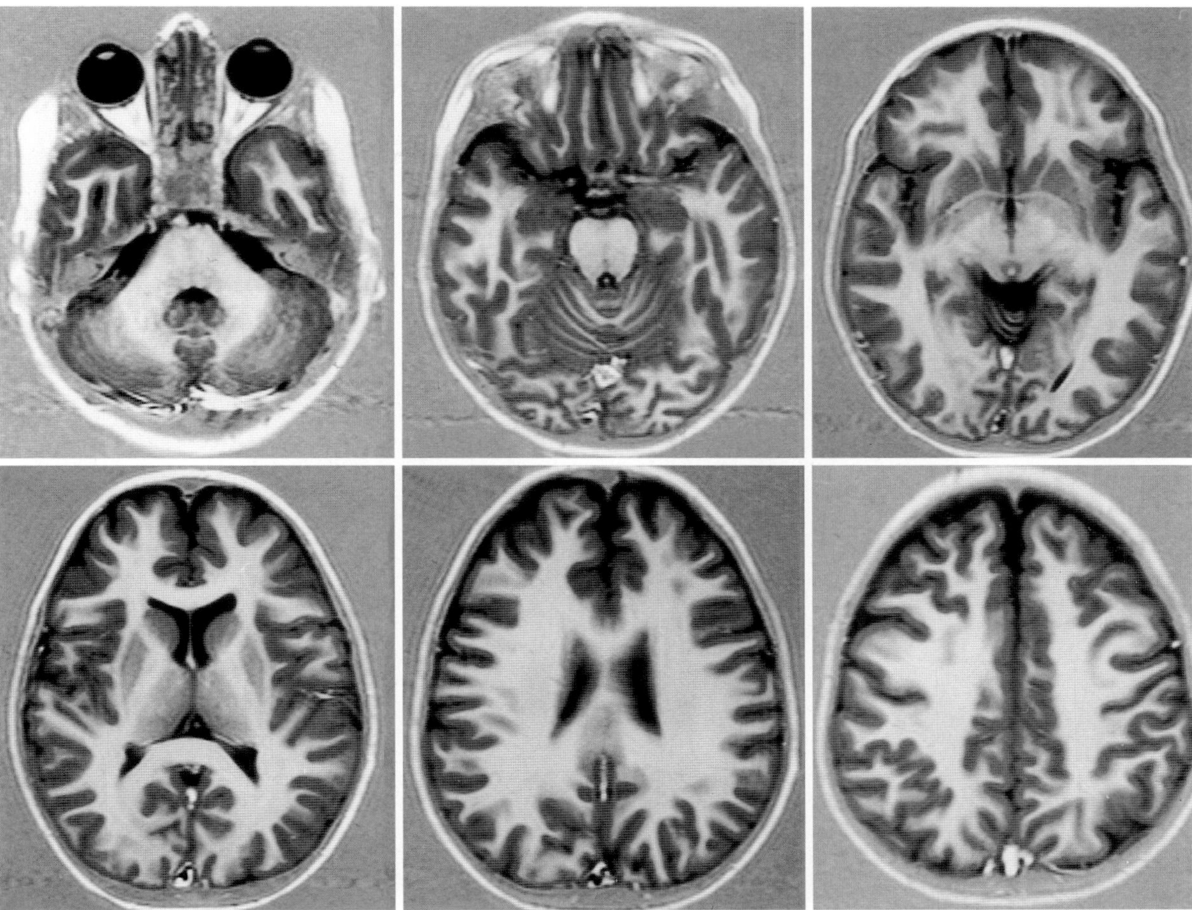

Fig. 4.17. Adult pattern of myelination on T_1-weighted (IR) images. These images were taken from a 5-year-old boy

Fig. 4.15. Myelination at 12–13 months. The adult contrast is now emerging in all lobes, except the temporal lobe, the latest to myelinate. The T_2-weighted series shows that the spread of myelin into the arcuate fibers is still not complete

Fig. 4.16. Adult pattern of myelination on T_2-weighted images in a 5-year-old child. The temporal lobes now also show the adult gray–white matter contrast

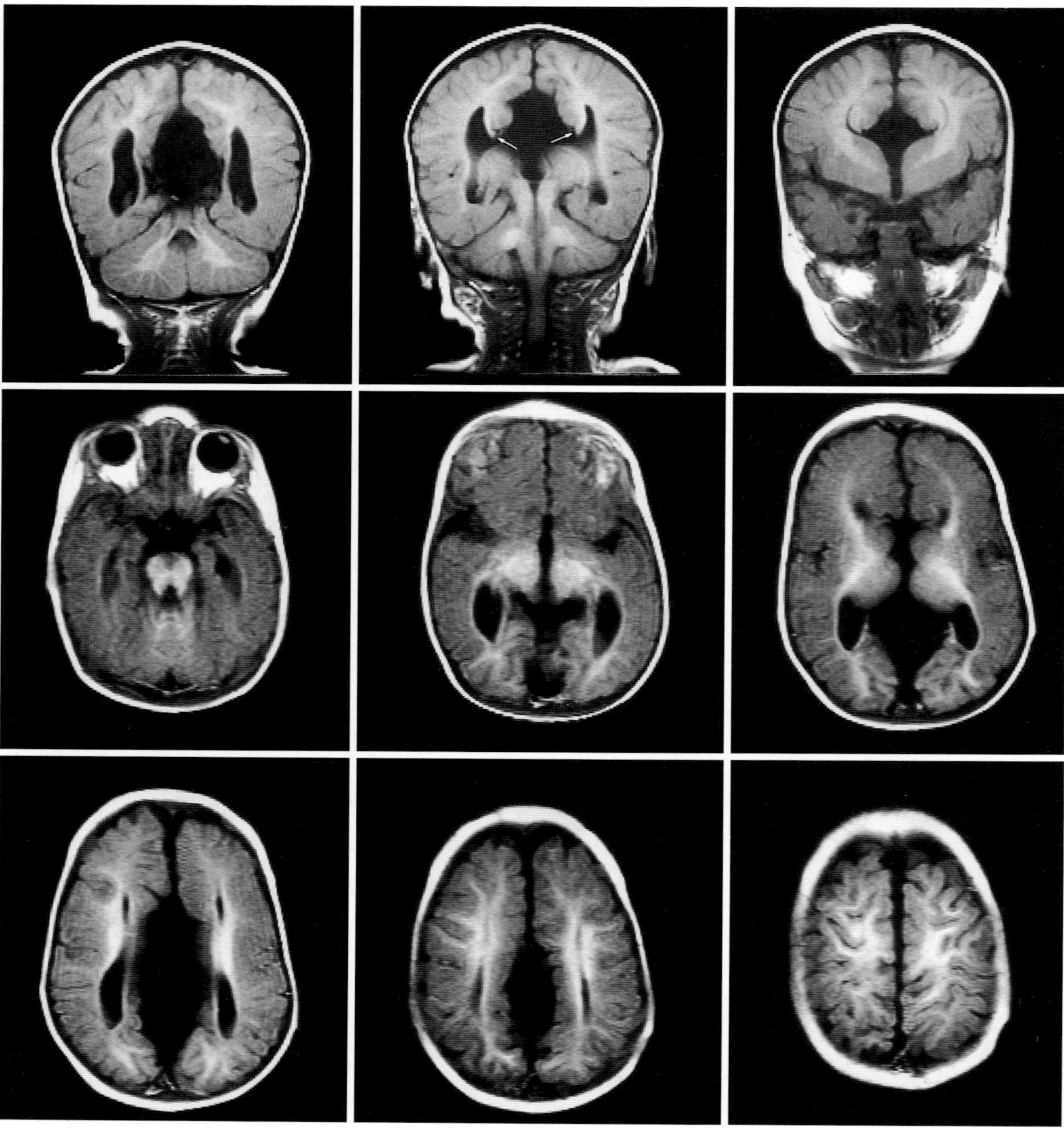

Fig. 4.18. Myelination in a baby boy at the age of 5 months with an agenesis of the corpus callosum and large midline cyst. The T$_1$-weighted coronal and transverse images show that the congenital anomaly has not influenced the progress of myelination. The images give a beautiful demonstration of the already myelinated bundle of Probst (*arrows*)

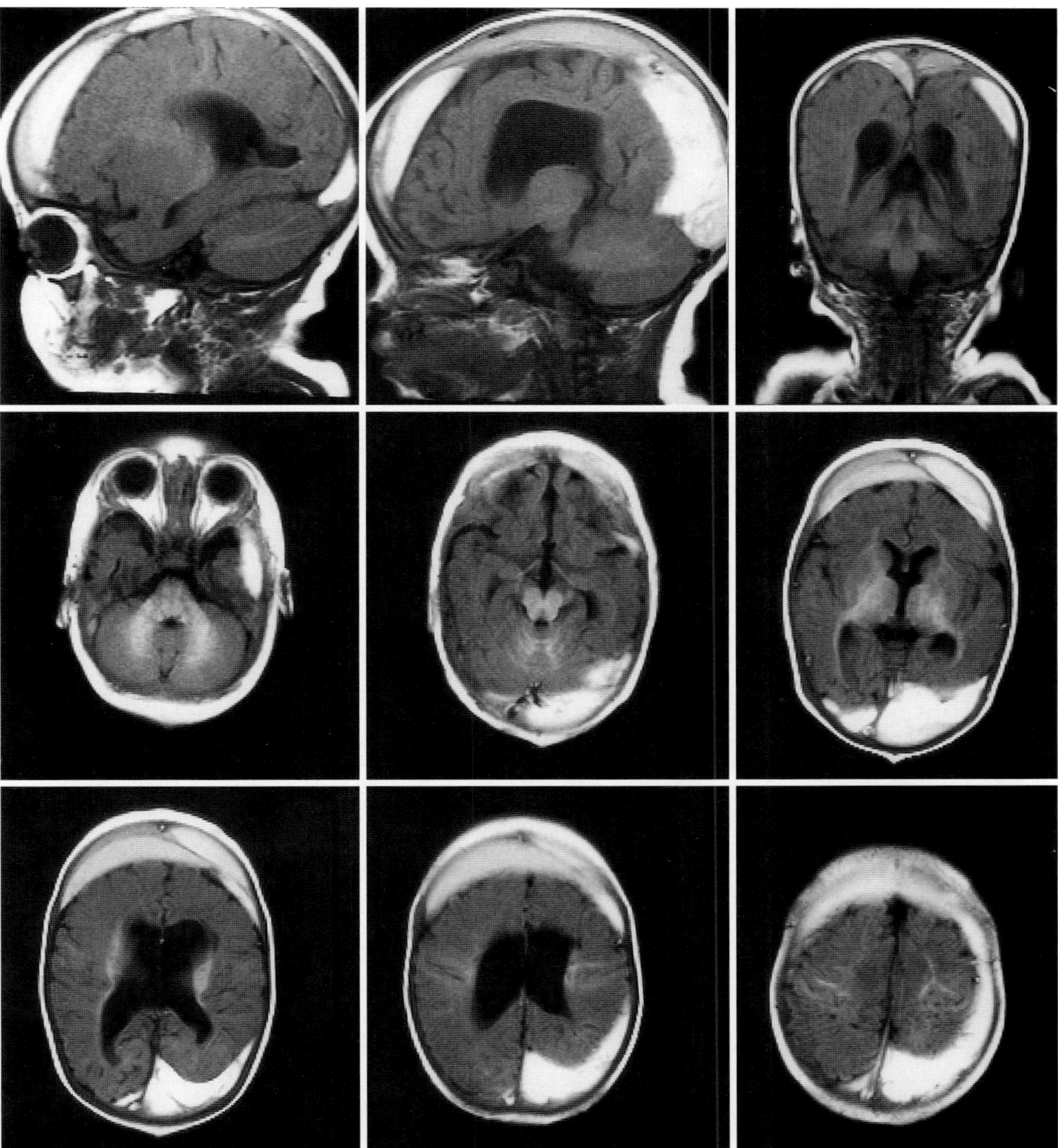

Fig. 4.19. The T_1-weighted multiplanar MR images of a 10-month-old boy show the retardation of myelination as a consequence of large subdural hematomas of various ages, the result of battering. The myelination age is about 4 months, in accordance with the severe developmental delay of the child

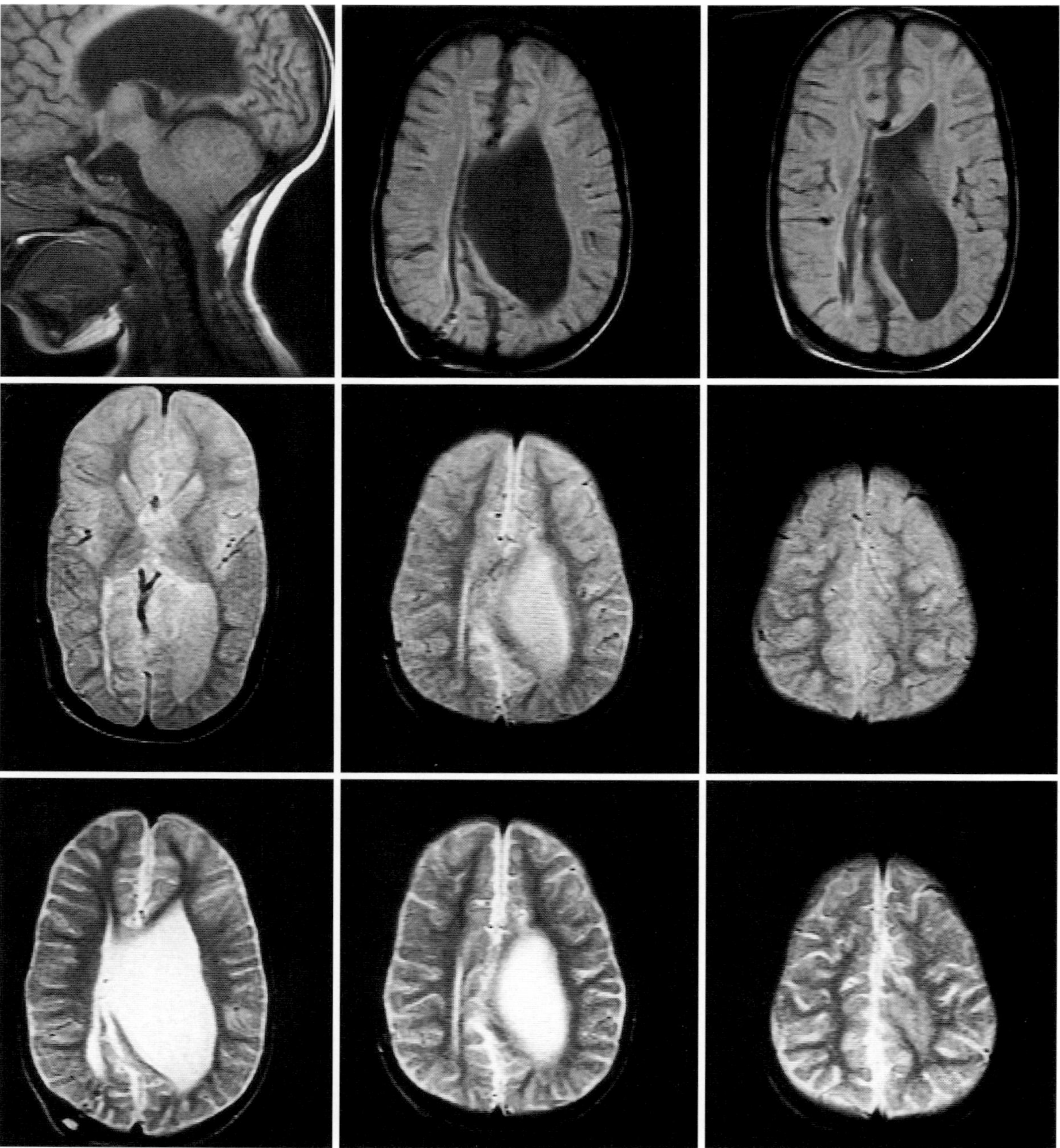

Fig. 4.20. A 5-year-old girl with spina bifida, Chiari malformation and hydrocephalus. A ventriculoperitoneal drain was installed, with insufficient drainage of the left ventricle. The MR images show that despite this long existing condition, the myelination of the left hemisphere has a normal adult pattern

5 Lysosomes and Lysosomal Disorders

Lysosomes are organelles with a single membrane. They are present in almost all types of body cells. Their number varies greatly from one cell to another, depending on its type and function. They display a considerable structural heterogeneity and appear in all shapes, sizes and densities. They have been given their name because they are small bodies (soma=body) containing various enzymes that are hydrolytic (lysis= dissolution). These hydrolytic enzymes, hydrolases, catalyze reactions in which macromolecules and macromolecular structures are broken down into smaller components. One of the hydrolytic enzymes contained in lysosomes, is acid phosphatase. This enzyme is most easily tested for using histochemical techniques, and its demonstration in a membranous organelle is usually taken as proof that the organelle is a lysosome. Other lysosmal enzymes are proteases, nucleases, glycosidases, lipases, phospholipases, sulfatases and phosphatases. Between 40 and 50 different enzymes have been identified. These give the lysosome the ability to digest almost all types of macromolecules present in biological material, such as proteins, polysaccharides, lipids and nucleic acids. The low molecular components, that are released, are transported to the cytoplasm to be reutilized. The lysosomal membrane is necessary in order to separate the hydrolytic enzymes from the rest of the cytoplasm and to prevent lysis of components of the cytoplasmic matrix. The acidic interior of lysosomes provides a favorable environment for the digestive activities of the enzymes.

Lysosomes belong to the elements of the so-called „vacuolar system", a membranous network of the cell which includes the plasma membrane, the endoplasmic reticulum, the Golgi complex, secretory vacuoles, endosomes (vacuoles formed by endocytosis of extracellular substances), lysosomes and other vesicular bodies. These elements are involved in the biosynthesis, processing, transport, storage, release and degradation of soluble and membrane-bound macromolecules.

Lysosomal enzymes, along with secretory proteins and plasma membrane proteins, are synthesized on membrane-bound polyribosomes in the rough endoplasmic reticulum. An important question is how proteins, which are destined for specific intracellular compartments, are targeted from their common site of synthesis, the ribosomes, towards their destination.

The information or signal that specifies the destination of each nascent protein, is thought to reside in its sequence or spatial structure. The cellular transport machinery that recognizes these signals distributes the proteins to the diverse cellular compartments. The first decisive information is thought to reside in so-called signal peptides. Depending on the type of signal peptide, proteins are directed to either the nucleus, mitochondria, or the endoplasmic reticulum, the latter as an entry of nascent proteins into the vacuolar system. In the lumen of the endoplasmic reticulum, the lysosomal enzyme proteins as well as most of the secretory and plasma membrane proteins, undergo glycosylation. The glycosylation step involves the transfer of a large oligosaccharide with high mannose content to selected asparagine residues of the nascent protein. Subsequently, the signal peptide is cleaved and the processing of the asparagine-linked oligosaccharide begins. The proteins then move by vesicular transport to the first (or cis) compartment of the Golgi complex. Within the Golgi complex the oligosaccharide chains are trimmed and remodeled further and it is within the Golgi complex that proteins are sorted according to their appropriate final destinations. In the cis compartment of the Golgi complex, lysosomal enzymes acquire a mannose-6-phosphate moiety. They then proceed through the remainder of the Golgi complex (from the cis to medial to trans Golgi) and it is not until they reach the trans Golgi complex, also called GERL or Golgi endoplasmic reticulum lysosome region, that they are segregated into distinct transport vesicles, away from other secretory and cell surface proteins. Receptors specific for mannose-6-phosphate-containing oligosaccharides present in the Golgi complex are important in the segregation of lysosomal enzymes from proteins with other destinations. After binding lysosomal enzymes, the mannose-6-phosphate receptor-protein complexes are collected in protein-coated pits, which bud off to form coated vesicles. These transport vesicles deliver the complexes to an acidic endosomal compartment, the so-called intermediate compartment, where lysosomal hydrolases are released. This compartment represents a prelysosome structure. The acidic content of the compartment facilitates dissociation of the lysosomal enzymes from their receptors. The mannose-6-phosphate receptors are retrieved from this compartment and returned to the trans Golgi complex. Lysosomal enzymes delivered to the intermediate compartment later appear in mature lysosomes. This step may involve maturation of an intermediate compartment into a lysosome. Mannose-6-phosphate receptors also appear briefly at the cell surface. It is likely that transport of receptors is possible from the intermediate compartment to the cell surface and back. A small amount of lysosomal enzymes, usually 5%–20%, is not transported directly to lysosomes, but is secreted at the cell surface. A portion of these enzymes binds to the mannose-6-phosphate receptors passing on the cell surface and is still internalized and delivered to lysosomes. However, the clearance of secreted enzymes is not only dependent on the recognition of mannose-6-phosphate residues, but appears to be dependent on the presence of several receptors. This secretion-recapture mechanism probably functions as a salvage pathway.

Although the mannose-6-phosphate recognition pathway is clearly important in lysosomal enzyme targeting, there is evidence that there are still other mechanisms for localizing acid hydrolases to lysosomes, independent of this recognition marker. Although it seems likely that this alternative targeting is receptor-mediated, attempts to demonstrate this receptor have been unsuccessful.

In addition to oligosaccharide processing, lysosomal enzymes undergo proteolytic processing. All enzymes are synthesized as pre-pro-enzymes. The pre-piece is the signal sequence, which is cleaved immediately after transport into the endoplasmic reticulum. The pro-piece is cleaved later. This process is initiated in the prelysosomal compartments and is completed after the enzymes arrive in the lysosomes. The biological significance of this processing is poorly understood.

The biogenesis of lysosomes and their contents involves the selective transport of soluble and membrane components. The mannose-6-phosphate receptor system, which is largely responsible for the targeting of soluble lysosomal enzymes, has been described above. Lysosomal integral membrane glycoproteins travel the same route. They are synthesized on ribosomes of the rough endoplasmic reticulum. They travel via the Golgi apparatus and endosomes to lysosomes. However, the transport of lysosomal membrane glycoproteins to lysosomes is independent of the mannose-6-phosphate receptor system. Acid phosphatase is also transported as a transmembrane protein to lysosomes in a mannose-6-phosphate receptor independent manner. After delivery to lysosomes, acid phosphatase undergoes processing of the membrane anchoring domain, resulting in conversion to a soluble form. Finally acid phosphatase is located equally in both the lysosomal matrix and membranes.

Until now the formation of new lysosomes has been a puzzling phenomenon. The lysosomal membrane differs from the endosomal and cell membrane and contains glycoproteins which are not found on the cell surface or in the endosomes. There is strong evidence that the lysosomal membrane does not originate from the cell membrane. There is some evidence that the coated vesicles budding off from the trans Golgi network form the precursors of lysosomes.

Apart from enzymes, lysosomes contain activator proteins and a protective protein. Protective protein has a protective function towards two lysosomal enzymes, b-galactosidase and N-acetyl-a-neuraminidase (sialidase), whose stability and activity depend on their interaction with the protective protein. Protective protein has been shown to be identical to the protease carboxypeptidase or cathepsin A. The cathepsin A activity and protective function are distinct and can be separated. It is not clear why one protein carries two very different functions. Activator proteins are required for the hydrolysis of sphingolipids by specific lysosomal hydrolases (see Table 5.1). They are called sphingolipid activator proteins (SAP's). SAP-1 and SAP-3 act as detergents by solubilizing their lipid substrates. They form reversible complexes with the substrates and present the substrate to the enzyme. SAP-2 and saposin A appear to act by interacting with the enzyme. They bind to the enzyme and not to the substrate and act as cohydrolases. SAP-1 and SAP-2 are formed from the same precursor protein, termed prosaposin. Two other putative activators, saposin A and saposin D, are also formed from the same precursor protein after proteolytic processing.

The acidic environment within lysosomes facilitates the digestive function. Oligomeric proteins dissociate into monomers, proteins dissociate away from protecting membrane, and stabilizing complexes (for instance receptor-substrate complexes) become split. The acidity of lysosomes is maintained by an ATP-dependent proton pump located in the lysosomal membrane. It is, however, not clear how the lysosomal pH is kept at around 5, and there are probably other controling factors besides the H^+-ATPase molecules.

Lysosomes have an important digestive function and play an essential role with regard to maintaining the health of normal cells and the body's defense against foreign invaders. The material that is to be digested enters the lysosome through autophagy, crinophagy or endocytosis. Autophagy is the process by which the cell sequesters parts of its own cytoplasm, often containing organelles. In the first step, called autophagic sequestration, a cytoplasmic membrane excises and envelops a region of cytoplasm into a closed vacuole, called an autophagosome. Through fusion, the material sequestered is transferred to lysosomes, where the final

Table 5.1. Nomenclature and function of sphingolipid activator proteins

Name	Alternative name	Substrates	Enzymes
GM$_2$-activator	SAP-3	GM$_2$ ganglioside GA$_2$ glycolipid	Hexosaminidase A
Saposin A		Glucocerebroside Galactocerebroside	β-glucocerebrosidase β-galactocerebrosidase
Saposin B	SAP-1	Sulfatides Globotriaosylceramide Sphingomyelin GM$_1$ ganglioside	Arylsulfatase A α-Galactosidase Sphingomyelinase β-galactosidase
Saposin C	SAP-2	Glucocerebroside Galactocerebroside	β-glucocerebrosidase β-galactocerebrosidase
Saposin D	component C	Sphingomyelin	Sphingomyelinase

hydrolysis step takes place. In normal cells this process is important because of its participation in cell-renewal and turnover of worn-out cell constituents. In secretory cells, there is a special kind of autophagy, called crinophagy. It occurs by direct fusion between secretory granules and lysosomes and results in the destruction of excess secretory material. Heterophagy is the uptake and digestion of extracellular materials. The exogenous material is taken up by the cell through invagination and subsequent pinching off of a part of the plasma membrane. The formed vesicle, called an endosome, fuses with a lysosome. Through heterophagy the lysosomes of polymorphonuclear granulocytes and macrophages perform their task of digestion of micro-organisms invading the body. A variety of circulating proteins and lipoproteins are taken up and digested in the lysosomes of Kupffer cells and hepatocytes. Lysosomes are also largely responsible for the profound changes that are initiated in autolysis. In the process of cell death, lysosomes liberate their enzymes and bring about the digestion of the cell and near environment. Furthermore, lysosomes may contribute to the inflammatory reaction. Apart from destruction of phagocytosed material, lysosomes may be released from leukocytes and increase the inflammation.

Lysosomes are highly dynamic structures with a high rate of substrate degradation. Due to their digestive function, lysosomes end up with an endless variety of intralysosomal structures. The number and enzymatic content of lysosomes is well regulated and depends on the activity and function of the cell. A clear example is the activated macrophage. In response to inflammatory stimuli, macrophages exhibit a severalfold increase in number of lysosomes. Apparently the assembly of lysosomes and lysosomal enzyme synthesis are regulated in a coordinated manner.

In lysosomal storage disorders the activity of one or more of the lysosomal degrading enzymes is deficient. Since undegraded substrates cannot leave the lysosomes or only very slowly, these organelles are converted into storage granules which steadily increase in size and number. Eventually they reach such a large volume that they interfere with the cell's normal function, giving rise to a storage disease.

Over the past few decades the knowledge and understanding of the biochemistry of the hereditary lysosomal storage diseases has progressed through a number of phases. In the first phase, the enzymatic defects responsible for each of the various diseases was documented. Substrates and assay conditions were identified that effectively demonstrated the profound deficiency of a particular lysosomal enzyme activity in tissues of affected persons and, in most cases, intermediate levels of activity in heterozygote carriers. The second phase resulted in the extensive characterization of the physicochemical and kinetic properties of the lysosomal hydrolases whose deficiencies were responsible for the storage diseases. There was a growing awareness that the extent of biochemical knowledge was insufficient to explain the clinical heterogeneity that characterizes most of the lysosomal storage diseases. Given the enzyme assays then available, the level of residual enzyme activity often did not correlate with the severity and age of onset of the disease, or the organ involvement (for instance, CNS versus visceral organs). In the third phase the pathophysiological significance of low molecular weight activator proteins was recognized and subclasses of particular lysosomal storage diseases due to deficiency of activator proteins were distinguished. Besides, efforts were made to identify enzyme assay conditions that more closely approximate the in vivo environment in which the lysosomal enzymes normally function in order to reach a closer estimation of the real residual enzyme activity. In the fourth phase, there was a growing insight into the genetic basis of inborn errors of metabolism. Genes coding for enzymes were identified and sequenced. It appeared that many different mutations and deletions occur involving the same gene, resulting in many different enzyme changes with different levels of remaining activity towards substrates in vivo. The extremes are formed on the one hand by no detectable enzyme with zero remaining enzyme activity, and on the other by an evidently altered enzyme but with a remaining enzyme activity in vivo that is sufficient to prevent the occurrence of storage and disease. The growing insight into the genetic and biochemical basis of lysosomal disorders has yielded improved understanding regarding clinical heterogeneity.

Lysosomal disorders can arise at different levels. In the first place there may be a gene deletion or grossly abnormal gene leading to the absence of any immunologically detectable enzyme. In the second place a more subtle gene mutation may occur leading to an altered enzyme with no or diminished catalytic activity. Thirdly, a catalytically active enzyme may be synthesized, but there is a defect in the process of transportation of the enzyme to and into the lysosome. A fourth possibility is that the enzyme is catalytically active, but unstable leading to accelerated breakdown. This may be caused by a defect in posttranslational modification or by absence of protective protein. Fifthly, activator proteins may be absent or changed. In the sixth place, the transport of substances across the lysosomal enzyme may be defective, thus preventing their departure from the lysosome.

The lysosomal storage disorders can be more or less artificially divided into five categories, depending on the class of substances stored: the sphingolipidoses, the glycoproteinoses, the mucolipidoses and the mucopolysaccharidoses. The fifth category comprises miscellaneous disorders.

In the sphingolipidoses, one of the hydrolases responsible for the degradation of one of the sphingolipids is deficient, resulting in the accumulation of this lipid in lysosomes. Apart from enzyme deficiencies, activator protein deficiencies may also form the basic defect. In multiple sulfatase deficiency, the basic defect is not known, but probably the process of posttranslational modification of all sulfatases is defective, resulting in enhanced breakdown of these enzymes.

The degradation of the oligosaccharide portions of glycoproteins involves the sequential action of several lysosomal enzymes. A deficiency of one of the enzymes in the pathway results in a glycoproteinosis.

The mucolipidoses consist of a group of lysosomal storage disorders that have clinical symptoms and biochemical characteristics of both the mucopolysaccharidoses and the sphingolipidoses. In mucolipidoses, glycolipids as well as mucopolysaccharides are accumulated in lysosomes. Mucolipidosis I has been reclassified as sialidosis. Mucolipidoses II and III are caused by a defect in the targeting of lysosomal enzymes to lysosomes. Instead, the enzymes are secreted into the extracellular space. The basic defect is a deficiency of an enzyme that is necessary in the synthesis of the mannose-6-phosphate recognition marker on lysosomal enzymes. The basic defect of mucolipidosis IV is not known.

Acid mucopolysaccharides, also called glycosaminoglycans, consist of long chains of repeating disaccharide units. The different mucopolysaccharides are characterized by the composition of their repeating disaccharide units. Mucopolysaccharides are degraded in lysosomes.

Cystinosis is an amino acid storage disease. It is characterized by intralysosomal storage of cystine, and is caused by defective carrier-mediated transport of cystine across the lysosomal membrane. In Salla disease intralysosomal storage of sialic acid occurs, also caused by a defect in the transportation of this substance across the lysosomal membrane. Pompe disease is a lysosomal glycogen storage disorder. Wolmann disease and cholesterol ester storage disease are two phenotypic forms of lysosomal acid lipase deficiency, of which cholesterol ester storage disease is the more benign variant. These disorders are characterized by intralysosomal accumulation of cholesterol esters and triglycerides.

A survey of the lysosomal storage disorders is presented here:

1. Sphingolipidoses
   a. Metachromatic leukodystrophy
   b. Multiple sulfatase deficiency
   c. Globoid cell leukodystrophy (Krabbe disease)
   d. GM_1 gangliosidosis
   e. GM_2 gangliosidosis
   f. Gaucher disease
   g. Fabry disease
   h. Schindler disease
   i. Farber disease
   j. Niemann-Pick disease
2. Glycoproteinoses
   a. Sialidosis
   b. Galactosialidosis
   c. Fucosidosis
   d. Mannosidosis
   e. Aspartylglycosaminuria
3. Mucolipidoses
   a. I cell disease (II)
   b. Pseudo-Hurler polydystrophy (III)
   c. Mucolipidosis IV
4. Mucopolysaccharidoses
   a. Hurler disease and Scheie disease (I)

b. Hunter disease (II)
c. Sanfilippo disease (III)
d. Morquio disease (IV)
e. Maroteaux-Lamy disease (VI)
f. Sly disease (VII)
5. Other lysosomal storage disorders
a. Cystinosis
b. Salla disease
c. Pompe disease
d. Wolmann disease and cholesterol ester storage disease

The following chapters only discuss those lysosomal storage disorders accompanied by a white matter disorder.

6 Metachromatic Leukodystrophy

6.1 Clinical Features and Laboratory Investigations

Metachromatic leukodystrophy (MLD) is an autosomal recessive progressive demyelinating disorder. Its incidence is estimated to be between 1:40 000 and 1:130 000. The disease can be divided into three different subtypes: the late infantile, the juvenile and the adult variant. This subdivision is based on the age of onset, the duration, and the clinical picture of the disease. Within one family only one variant of MLD occurs.

The late infantile variant is the most common variant of MLD. The age of onset varies between 6 months and 3 years. Of the different subtypes this variant is the one that shows the greatest uniformity with regard to clinical picture and course of disease. Most children learn to sit and walk with support normally, but show a delay in walking unaided. The first symptom is usually an unsteady gait due to muscle hypotonia. There are signs of a progressive polyneuropathy, ending in a generalized flaccid paresis of the arms and legs and a loss of tendon reflexes. The neuropathy may be painful. Cerebellar ataxia is also often an early sign. Nystagmus is usually present. Speech development is disturbed and dysarthria becomes manifest. Mental development stagnates and regression occurs. Gradually, involvement of the pyramidal system causes the flaccid paresis to be superseded by a spastic tetraplegia with pathological reflexes such as extensor plantar reflexes, but deep tendon reflexes are absent. Bulbar and pseudobulbar symptoms develop, including feeding difficulties. The power of speech is affected and the child eventually becomes mute. Optic atrophy with impaired vision is present. Epileptic seizures occur in about 25% of the children. Eventually the child loses all contact with his surroundings as he is blind, completely tetraplegic in a decerebrate state without purposeful movements. This final stage may last for several years. Death usually occurs about 5 years after onset of clinical symptoms.

The age at onset of the juvenile variant ranges from 4 to 16 years. The disease occurs in apparently healthy, intellectually normal children. Early signs are a gradual deterioration in school performance, language regression and clumsiness. There are usually also emotional and behavioral disturbances. These symptoms may be present several months and up to a year before the onset of other neurological signs. A spastic paresis and cerebellar ataxia gradually develop. On rare occasions the clinical picture is dominated by extrapyramidal features. Clinical symptoms of a peripheral neuropathy are often lacking and deep tendon reflexes are usually brisk. Optic atrophy develops. Seizures occur in about 50% of the patients. Eventually a complete tetraplegia with decerebration posture, brain stem dysfunction and total dementia evolves. Death usually occurs 5–10 years after onset.

Some authors prefer to divide the juvenile variant into two subgroups. An early juvenile variant has its onset between 4 and 6 years. The clinical symptomatology resembles that of the late infantile variant showing gait disturbance and other motor dysfunction as early manifestations. The late juvenile variant has its onset between 6 and 16 years. In the clinical symptomatology, behavioral abnormalities, poor school performance and language regression predominate as early abnormalities.

The adult form reveals itself usually between 16 and 30 years. Onset of the disease at 60 years or later has also been described. The patient experiences a gradual decline in intellectual abilities. At onset the clinical picture is often dominated by emotional lability, behavioral abnormalities or psychiatric symptoms like delusions and hallucinations. It is not uncommon for the patient to be treated initially for schizophrenia or a psychotic depression. After several months or years a progressive spastic paresis of the arms and legs develops with increased tendon reflexes and extensor plantar reflexes. Cerebellar ataxia and extrapyramidal features like choreiform movements and dystonia may be present. Signs of peripheral neuropathy are often absent, although a flaccid tetraparesis may occur in the terminal stage. Optic atrophy and signs of bulbar dysfunction may appear. Epileptic seizures are rare. A state of severe dementia gradually develops. The patient loses contact with the surroundings, lies in a decorticate or decerebrate posture, and eventually a persistent vegetative state is reached. The duration of the disease varies from a few years to 15 years and longer. Although a rapid deterioration is seen in some patients, in most progression is slow over a period of years.

CSF protein is elevated in the late infantile form and in most juvenile cases. In the adult form, CSF protein is increased less often. The EEG is normal at the beginning of the disease. At later stages it shows nonspecific abnormalities in the form of slowing of the background pattern, often together with paroxysmal or epileptiform activity. In the infantile and juvenile variants, the conduction velocity of peripheral nerves is markedly reduced. Particularly in adults, however, the nerve conduction velocity may be normal. In all patients urinary sulfatide excretion is increased. The activity of arylsulfatase A in urine and in peripheral leukocytes is low, but may be normal in exceptional cases of activator deficiency (see below). In all cases of MLD a decreased catabolism of exogenous sulfatide by cultured fibroblasts can be demonstrated. In this test sulfatide is radiolabeled and added to cultured fibroblasts. The uptake of label by cells with subsequent metabolism is measured at frequent intervals. This procedure is not performed routinely, but only in special situations.

During life the definite diagnosis of MLD is based on the determination of the activity of arylsulfatase A in peripheral leukocytes and fibroblasts. The diagnostic reliability of this test is hampered by the relatively frequent occurrence of so-called pseudodeficiency. In this condition low arylsulfatase A activity is found without associated clinical signs of MLD (see also under Sect. 6.4). In cases in which symptoms strongly suggest MLD, and enzyme activity in peripheral leukocytes is normal, deficiency of arylsulfatase A activator protein can be surmised. Additional tests then include the measurement of urinary sulfatide, the assessment of fibroblast sulfatide catabolism, and a sural nerve biopsy to demonstrate the deposition of metachromatic material. The determination of the enzyme activity in cultured chorionic villi, cultured amniotic fluid cells and cultured fetal fibroblasts enables prenatal diagnosis. Assessment of sulfatide catabolism can be performed in amniotic fluid cells or fetal fibroblasts. The detection of heterozygotes by determining enzyme activity in leukocytes and DNA techniques facilitates genetic counseling.

6.2   Pathology

Gross inspection of the brain reveals quite a firm consistency in most cases. The brain may be enlarged and heavier than normal, but in later stages a reduced size is usually found. The cut surface shows a discoloration of the white matter.

Initially the involvement of the white matter in MLD is patchy, but after some time all the white matter is affected, often in symmetrical fashion, so that the demyelinated lesions of the two hemispheres have a butterfly configuration. Sometimes, in cases of long duration, the white matter is reduced to a narrow strip 1–2 cm in diameter, and the shrinkage of the white matter can lead to enlargement of the ventricles. Demyelination occurs predominantly in the cerebral hemispheres, especially in the centrum semiovale. Demyelination tends to be most intense in the periventricular area, diminishes towards the surface and the arcuate fibers are relatively spared.

Microscopic examination shows demyelination with paucity or complete loss of myelin from lesion areas. Axis cylinders are relatively spared, but their density is reduced in severely affected areas. There is proliferation of astrocytes with fibrous gliosis. At the edge of affected areas and scattered throughout lesions there are macrophages that contain the specific degradation products. Usually oligodendroglia are absent from lesions and are reduced in number even in areas where the myelin is still intact. No inflammatory cells are present in the lesions.

MLD is characterized by the deposition of metachromatically staining material in the white matter. The term metachromasia designates the phenomenon that certain cationic dyes can change their color from blue to pink or brown when bound to certain anionic groups present in several organic compounds. In MLD, sulfatides are the organic compounds responsible for the metachromasia. The metachromatic material is mainly stored in the cytoplasm of the proliferated glia cells and macrophages, although some is also found in the oligodendroglia cells, in the neurons of cranial nerve nuclei, basal ganglia, and spinal cord and seemingly extracellularly as free granules in the white matter. The greatest density of metachromatic deposits is seen at sites where demyelination is complete.

The cerebral cortex is relatively intact. Loss of neurons is slight or absent. The cortical neurons contain no metachromatic material. The cerebellar cortex is normal or may show a diffuse loss of granular cells. A decrease in the number of Purkinje cells may occur. In certain areas, metachromatic granular material is stored in the neuronal perikarya, although rarely in large amounts. Neuronal metachromatic deposits are preferentially found in the globus pallidus, thalamus, subthalamic nucleus, hypothalamus, geniculate nucleus, amygdala and dentate nucleus. The cerebral and cerebellar cortex, claustrum, caudate nucleus and certain brain stem nuclei tend to be spared.

Electron microscopy demonstrates the inclusions bounded by a membrane of lysosomal origin. The morphological organization of the material varies in appearance, probably due to a difference in the lipid composition or in the physicochemical state of the lipids. In addition to the inclusions which stain metachromatically on light microscopic examination, lamellar inclusions are present in glial cells formed from fragments of degenerated myelin. The "extracellular" deposits of metachromatic material described in light microscopic studies appear to be cytoplasmic processes containing inclusions in electron microscopy.

In MLD the peripheral nerves are affected by segmental demyelination. Signs of remyelination may be found. Metachromatic material is present in Schwann cells and macrophages.

Not only are there neuropathological changes in MLD, but also visceral lesions. Outside the CNS, metachromatic material is found in the liver, spleen and lymph nodes, gall bladder, pancreas, kidneys, adrenal glands, ovaries, ganglion cells of the retina, and leukocytes of peripheral blood and bone marrow. Storage in these organs is limited to certain cell types. Visceral accumulations are not accompanied by further morphological changes or obvious clinical dysfunction. Although MLD becomes manifest only with neurological abnormalities, it is clear that it is a generalized metabolic disorder.

6.3　Chemical Pathology

Biochemical analysis of the white matter shows a greatly increased amount of sulfatide with a concomitant decrease in cerebroside as the major chemical abnormality. Whereas in normal white matter the ratio of cerebroside to sulfatide is about 4:1, in MLD it can be reversed. There is not only evidence that the membrane-bound deposits seen in this disease contain sulfatide, but also that myelin, which still appears normal ultrastructurally, has an abnormally high sulfatide content. Other biochemical changes in the white matter are a consequence of loss of myelin with a decrease in cholesterol, phospholipid, and glycolipids other than sulfatides. There is no increase in cholesterol ester. There are relatively few chemical changes in gray matter.

6.4　Pathogenetic Considerations

MLD is a sphingolipidosis caused by deficient activity of the lysosomal enzyme arylsulfatase A (=cerebroside-3-sulfate sulfatase= cerebroside-3-sulfate-3-sulfohydrolase= sulfatide sulfatase). This enzyme catalyzes the hydrolysis of sulfatide, the sulfate ester of cerebroside. Desulfation is the first step in the metabolic degradation of sulfatides. Following this sulfate cleavage, cerebroside is then degraded by cerebroside galactosidase.

The three clinical forms of the disease (late-infantile, juvenile, and adult) are due to different levels of residual enzyme activity. The locus determining the expression of arylsulfatase A activity has been mapped to chromosome 22. The gene has been cloned and sequenced. Different levels of residual enzyme activity can be explained by the existence of mutant alleles without any function (type 0 alleles) and alleles associated with some residual activity (type R alleles). Patients who are homozygous for type 0 alleles (genotype 0/0) have total lack of arylsulfatase A activity and suffer from the most severe late-infantile form. Homozygotes for type R alleles (genotype R/R) have a residual arylsulfatase A activity. In these individuals the onset of disease is usually beyond the age of 10 years (late-juvenile and adult forms). The type 0/type R compound heterozygotes have intermediate (juvenile) phenotypes. Different type 0 and type R alleles have been demonstrated.

Moreover, individuals have been found with low (approximately 10–20%) arylsulfatase A activity, but no clinical abnormalities. This is called arylsulfatase A pseudodeficiency. Genes for pseudodeficiency and MLD are allelic. Individuals who are compound heterozygotes of the pseudodeficiency (PD) allele and an MLD allele (0/PD or R/PD) have 6%–10% residual arylsulfatase A activity, but do not develop MLD. Thus, only slightly higher arylsulfase A activities than those encountered in R/R genotypes (2%–5%) are sufficient to sustain a normal phenotype.

Pseudodeficiency for arylsulfatase A is a diagnostic problem. The allele frequency for pseudodeficiency is much higher (7%–15%) than the MLD allele frequency (0.5%). Because homozygous pseudodeficiency is frequent (0.5%–2% of the population), it is not uncommon for patients with pseudodeficiency and neurological symptoms of unknown origin to be misdiagnosed as having MLD. A serious problem also exists for prenatal diagnosis of MLD in families in which the parents carry an MLD allele and a pseudodeficiency allele. MLD and pseudodeficiency cannot be distinguished on the basis of enzyme activity determinations using artificial substrates. Assays measuring the in vivo degradation of radioactively labeled sulfatide in cultured fibroblasts and measurement of sulfatide excretion in urine allow the distinction of MLD and pseudodeficiency. Both are abnormal in MLD, normal in pseudodeficiency. Demonstration of metachromatic material in a sural nerve biopsy is also diagnostic for MLD. Alternatively, the pseudodeficiency allele can be determined directly by DNA techniques, on the basis of knowledge of the underlying sequence alterations. A problem of this technique is, however, that given the high frequency of the pseudodeficiency allele, MLD mutations may also occur within the pseudodeficiency allele, rendering it nonfunctional. The frequency of MLD mutations in the normal and pseudodeficiency allele seem to be similar, so that 0.5% of the pseudodeficiency alleles will carry an MLD mutation. This assumption has been confirmed. This finding calls for caution in the diagnosis of pseudodeficiency by DNA tests detecting the mutations of the pseudodeficiency allele.

It can be anticipated that mutations in the normal arylsulfatase A allele that lower the enzyme activity but are without clinical consequences can cause MLD if they occur in the pseudodeficiency allele. Likewise, mutations which cause the milder, later onset forms of MLD when they occur in the normal arylsulfatase A allele, may lead to the severe early onset form when they occur in the pseudodeficiency allele.

A minority of MLD patients is not deficient in arylsulfatase A, but in an activator protein that is essential for the enzymatic action of arylsulfatase A. The gene for the precursor of this protein has been mapped to chromosome 10 and has been cloned and sequenced. This gene has been shown to code for a large precursor polypeptide, which is processed to yield four different activator proteins. Sphingolipid activator protein B, also called saposin B or SAP-1, activates the hydrolysis of sulfatide by arylsulfatase A. In addition it activates the hydrolysis of GM_1-ganglioside and globotriaosyl ceramide by b-galactosidase and a-galactosidase respectively. The protein interacts with the substrate and solubilizes it for enzymatic hydrolysis. The deficiency of SAP-1 causes a disease clinically resembling juvenile or late infantile MLD, but with histochemical and ultrastructural evidence of storage of gangliosides and other glycosphingolipids. Diagnosis is established in these cases by revealing metachromatic material in sural nerve biopsy, by finding an increased urinary sulfatide excretion and by demonstrating deficient turnover of sulfatide in the loading test in cultured fibroblasts, all in the presence of normal arylsulfatase A activity. It can be shown in cultured fibroblasts that the defect in sulfatide catabolism can be corrected by adding activator protein. Deficient turnover of the other glycosphingolipids can also be shown in loading tests in fibroblasts.

Sulfatides are membrane lipids. They are important constituents of cell membranes, including myelin sheaths. Within the cell they are present in the membranes of organelles. Sulfatide is predominantly present in membranes of myelin producing cells and in myelin. The amount of this substance normally present in membranes of other organs is much lower. As a result of the block in catabolism, sulfatides accumulate in tissues that normally synthesize them. In the first place, they accumulate in membranes of myelin-producing cells and myelin sheaths. The membrane buildup is basically normal in MLD. It is the membrane turnover that is abnormal. Sulfatide cannot be degraded and is trapped in the membrane. Simultaneously the cerebroside content decreases as the conversion of sulfatide to cerebroside is impeded.

A number of pathogenetic mechanisms have been mentioned to explain the demyelination in MLD. One of them is that the myelin composition in MLD becomes increasingly abnormal and therefore increasingly unstable. As soon as the disturbance of the normal physicochemical stability has reached a critical point, demyelination starts. Another explanation is that lysosomal storage of sulfatides in oligodendroglia and Schwann cells leads to cellular dysfunction and death, resulting in loss of all myelin sheaths maintained by these cells. Indeed, changes in the subcellular organelles, especially an increase in the numbers of lysosomes of these cells, have been observed before any morphological abnormalities in the myelin sheaths associated with them were detected. A third proposed mechanism is that sulfogalactosylsphingosine, a compound closely related to the cytotoxic compound galactosylsphingosine or psychosine in globoid cell leukodystrophy, might accumulate and cause the death of oligodendrocytes and Schwann cells. However, there is no evidence for the enzymatic conversion of sulfatide into sulfogalactosylsphingosine, and the concentration of this substance is not elevated in MLD.

The sulfatide accumulation in other organs (kidney, liver, pancreas, adrenal, gall bladder and intestinal tract) does not lead to impairment of functions. Only the gall bladder shows progressive functional impairment due to sulfatide accumulation, but gall bladder disease does not contribute to the fatal outcome of MLD. The tolerance of these tissues for sulfatides may be related to the fact that these organs have an excretory function and can discharge the accumulating lipid from the cell into the urine, bile, or other fluid. Another important factor is that the sulfatide content of the cellular membranes in these organs is normally much lower than that of the myelin membrane, which has a remarkably high content of galactosphingolipids (cerebroside and sulfatide).

6.5 Therapy

Various forms of therapy have been attempted in an effort to alter the natural course of disease, but with little success until now. Diets low in vitamin A or low in sulfur (both substances are necessary for the synthesis of sulfatide) have failed to bring any favorable effects. After intravenous and intrathecal infusion of arylsulfatase A, the enzyme does not enter the brain and no clinical benefit has been seen. Several patients have received bone marrow transplants in an attempt to correct their low arylsulfatase A levels and repair or retard their CNS deterioration. The results are promising, but they have to be weighed against the possibility of major complications and death after bone marrow transplantation. Especially in presymptomatic cases and in later-onset cases with no or relatively minor neurological impairment bone marrow transplantation may be ben-

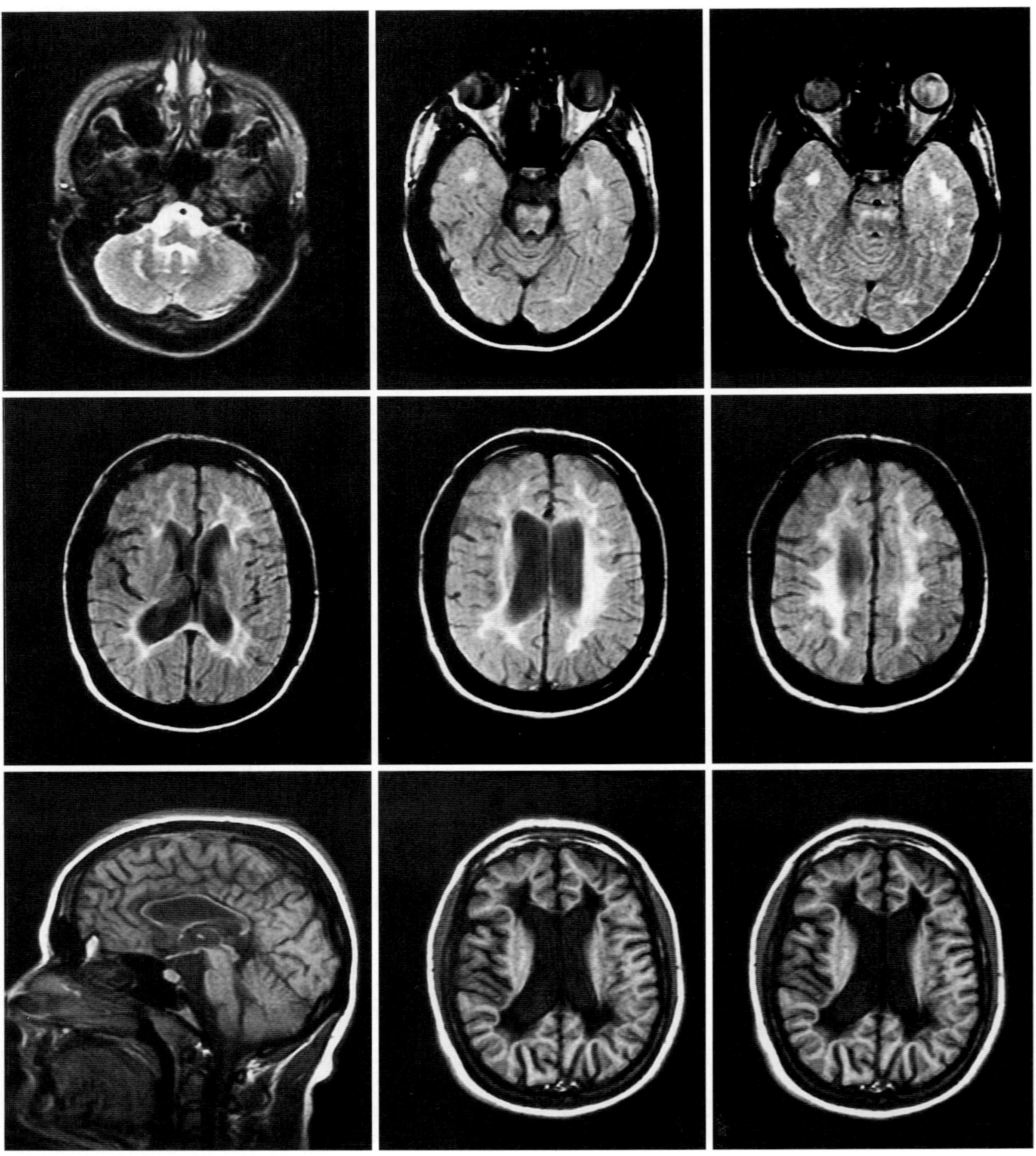

Fig. 6.1. A case of juvenile MLD in a 17-year-old girl. The *two upper rows* present transverse proton density and T_2-weighted images which show the periventricular demyelination. The cerebellar white matter is also involved, as are the cere-brospinal tracts in the brain stem. The sagittal and transverse T_1-weighted images show the involvement of the corpus callosum and the sparing of the U fibers

eficial. Stabilizaton and reversal of some of the MRI abnormalities have been described as well as clinical improvement or halt of progression. Longer term follow-up is needed to assess whether this form of therapy will halt the progression of MLD definitively and lead to lasting improvement of neurological function. Restoration of arylsulfatase A activity via retroviral-vector-mediated gene transfer has been described in human MLD fibroblasts but still has to be tested in the clinical situation.

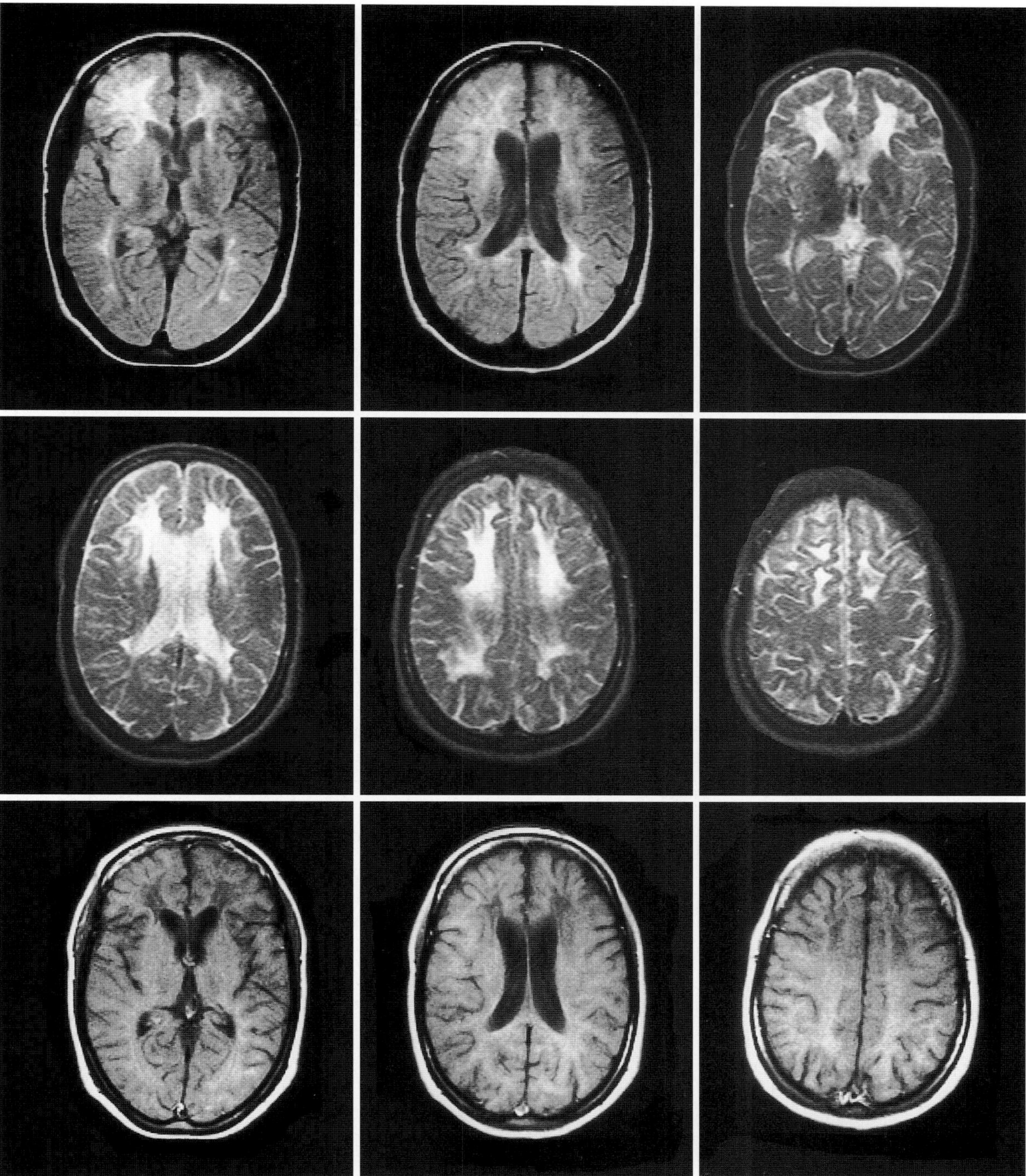

Fig. 6.2. In this MR series of a 20-year-old female with adult MLD, extensive periventricular white matter abnormalities are seen with emphasis on the frontal region. The lesions are almost symmetrical and spare the U fibers, except in the anterior frontal areas, where the U fibers are partially involved

6.6 Magnetic Resonance Imaging

The CT scan findings in MLD are well known and consist of symmetrical, diffuse decreased density of cerebral white matter with little evidence of cerebral atrophy until later stages. Hypodensity of the cerebellar white matter has been observed less frequently. No contrast enhancement has been found.

MRI discloses periventricular white matter abnormalities, essentially with a symmetrical distribution (Figs. 6.1, 6.2). In juvenile and adult cases a preferential frontal involvement has been observed (Fig. 6.2). The arcuate fibers are relatively spared, but may become involved in the later stages. The corpus callosum is invariably affected, connecting the lesions from both sides. The posterior limb of the internal capsule may be involved. In some of the patients (probably in more advanced stages) brain stem lesions are observed bilaterally in the pyramidal tracts (Fig. 6.1). Some patients show involvement of the cerebellar white matter. The white matter lesions are highly confluent but may be inhomogeneous. No contrast enhancement is seen. Atrophy occurs in advanced stages.

Gray matter lesions are never conspicuous. Subtle abnormalities in signal intensity and atrophy of the basal nuclei have been observed.

The condition has to be differentiated from globoid cell leukodystrophy, Schilder's disease and X-linked adrenoleukodystrophy. Contrast enhancement is always present in the acute stage of Schilder's disease. It is also present in patients with X-linked leukodystrophy and in some patients with globoid cell leukodystrophy. The type and extent of abnormalities in the basal ganglia, which may occur in globoid cell leukodystrophy, has never been observed in MLD. In X-linked adrenoleukodystrophy an occipital preponderance is usual, whereas MLD tends to have a frontal preponderance, especially in later-onset cases. The two zones typically present in X-linked adrenoleukodystrophy lesions, are not present in MLD. In Schilder's disease the demyelinating process is usually not perfectly symmetrical and often the cortex is not completely preserved.

7.1 Clinical Features and Laboratory Investigations

Multiple sulfatase deficiency (MSD) is a very rare disorder with an autosomal recessive mode of inheritance. The disease combines the features of metachromatic leukodystrophy and mucopolysaccharidosis. It is also called mucosulfatidosis, Austin's variant or variant O. Three different types of MSD have been described: a neonatal form, an early-childhood form and a very rare juvenile form.

The early-childhood form is the usual or classical form of MSD. The clinical features are those of infantile metachromatic leukodystrophy with mild features of mucopolysaccharidosis. Early development may be normal or delayed. Affected children usually acquire the ability to stand and to say a few words, but their development is less well advanced in the presymptomatic period than that of children with infantile metachromatic leukodystrophy. During the second year of life the children develop signs of a progressive encephalopathy with loss of acquired abilities, progressive dementia, spasticity, microcephaly, blindness, hearing loss and difficulties in swallowing. Tendon reflexes are variable. In the final stages there is often areflexia caused by the peripheral neuropathy. Mucopolysaccharidosis-like features may occur early or later in the course of the disease. These include ichthyosis, mild coarsening of the facial features, hepatosplenomegaly, stiff joints, growth retardation and skeletal anomalies. Hydrocephalus may occur. There is no corneal clouding. Optic atrophy, cherry-red macula and retinal degeneration may occur. Death usually occurs when the patient is aged between 10 and 18 years.

The neonatal form presents at birth with severe mucopolysaccharidosis-like features, such as facial dysmorphism, short neck, cloudy cornea, ichthyosis, cardiac valvular involvement, hepatosplenomegaly and severe dysostosis multiplex. The children are macrocephalic due to hydrocephalus. They have signs of a severe encephalopathy with early death, before the end of the first year.

A Saudi variant of the neonatal type of MSD has been described with mild to moderate mental retardation, cranial synostosis and consequent deformities, and cervical cord compression or transection due to vertebral abnormalities. Severe facial dysmorphia, corneal clouding, hepatosplenomegaly, dwarfism, severe dysostosis multiplex and hirsutism are present, but no ichthyosis, no retinal degeneration, no deafness and no progressive dementia. Some patients are macrocephalic, rarely hydrocephalic. Some suffer from cardiac valvular involvement.

A rare juvenile type of MSD has been reported with onset at the age of about 5 years. The disease is characterized by short stature, ichthyosis, hepatomegaly, moderate dysostosis multiplex and slowly progressive neurological abnormalities consisting of dementia, ataxia, quadriplegia, retinal degeneration and blindness. Corneal clouding is not present.

Additional investigations show changes on bone X-ray, such as a J-shaped sella turcica, structural changes in vertebral bodies, scoliosis, gibbus, flaired ribs, broad phalanges, abnormal metacarpals and, in the Saudi variant, synostosis of cranial sutures. Large basophilic to azurophilic granules are seen in lymphocytes of bone marrow and peripheral blood. There is an increased urinary content of sulfatide and mucopolysaccharides, including dermatan sulfate and heparan sulfate. CSF protein is increased. Nerve conduction velocity is slowed. Diagnosis is established by demonstrating a deficiency of arylsulfatases A, B and C and a number of sulfatases necessary in the degradation of mucopolysaccharides.

7.2 Pathology

Pathological findings have only been described in the classical form of MSD. The basic findings are those of late-infantile metachromatic leukodystrophy in combination with widespread neuronal lipid storage in cortex and subcortical gray matter structures. The storage is lysosomal. The neuronal deposits are finely granular, PAS-positive, with a slight reddish-purple metachromasia. On electron microscopy, neuronal inclusions range in configuration from membranous cytoplasmic bodies, typical for neuronal gangliosidoses, to the zebra bodies, often seen in mucopolysaccharidoses. There is loss of neurons in cerebral and cerebellar cortex and cortical atrophy. The white matter shows demyelination with deposition of metachromatic material, oligodendroglial loss, relative axonal preservation and marked gliosis. The U fibers are relatively spared. There is storage of mucopolysaccharides in perivascular mesenchymal tissue up to the formation of macroscopically visible pseudocystic cavities. Meninges are thickened and cloudy. Obliteration of the subarachnoid spaces may lead to hydrocephalus. Abnormalities in peripheral nerves are typical of metachromatic leukodystrophy.

7.3　Chemical Pathology

Chemical analysis of the brain has shown an increase in sulfatide, sulfated steroids (e.g., cholesterol sulfate), gangliosides and mucopolysaccharides. The lipids stored in the white matter are predominantly sulfatides, those stored in the gray matter predominantly gangliosides and mucopolysaccharides.

7.4　Pathogenetic Considerations

In MSD a deficiency of multiple enzymes is found: arylsulfatase A (metachromatic leukodystrophy), arylsulfatase B (N-acetylgalactosamine-4-sulfatase; Maroteaux-Lamy syndrome), arylsulfatase C (steroid sulfatase; X-linked ichthyosis), N-acetylgalactosamine-6-sulfate sulfatase (Morquio syndrome type A), heparan sulfate sulfatase (Sanfilippo A), iduronate-2-sulfate sulfatase (Hunter syndrome), N-acetylglucosamine-6-sulfate sulfatase (Sanfilippo D) and some other sulfatases. The residual activities of the sulfatases vary considerably in fibroblast lines from different patients. The lysosomal storage of sulfatides, mucopolysaccharides and sulfated steroids is a direct consequence of the enzyme deficiencies mentioned. The accumulation of gangliosides may be caused by the inhibition of other lysosomal hydrolases due to the present lysosomal storage. It is probable that the different phenotypic expressions of MSD are due to differences in relative residual activity of the various enzymes.

The gene for MSD and those for metachromatic leukodystrophy or any other single sulfatase deficiency are nonallelic. The genes coding for the various deficient sulfatases are intact. The basic defect of MSD has not been identified and the question of how a single genetic defect can result in the deficiency of so many sulfatases has not been answered. Evidence has been found that the rate of synthesis of various sulfatases is normal in MSD, but that they are degraded at an enhanced rate. The studies with MSD cells are consistent with a defect in cellular regulatory processes for the expression of sulfatases. It has been suggested that in normal cells a gene product exists that affects the activ-

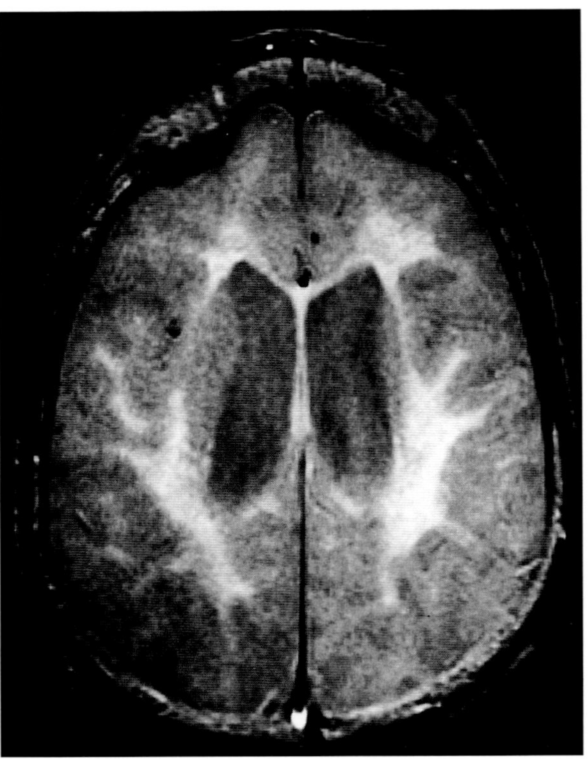

Fig. 7.1. This proton density image of a 4-year-old child with classical MSD show the symmetrical periventricular white matter abnormalities, also involving the corpus callosum. Courtesy of Harbord et al. (1991), with permission

ity or stability of sulfatases. It has been proposed that the primary defect in MSD is a mutation of such a gene product which activates or modifies the sulfatases post-translationally. This factor would be common to all sulfatases and confer catalytic and/or stability properties to the sulfatases.

7.5　Therapy

No effective form of treatment is known.

7.6　Magnetic Resonance Imaging

Imaging findings in MSD are scarce and limited to the classical and Saudi variants. In the classical variant, images are indistinguishable from those of infantile metachromatic leukodystrophy with severe white matter abnormalities consistent with a demyelinating disorder (Fig. 7.1).

In the Saudi variant a variable white matter involvement has been described. Myelination is always de-

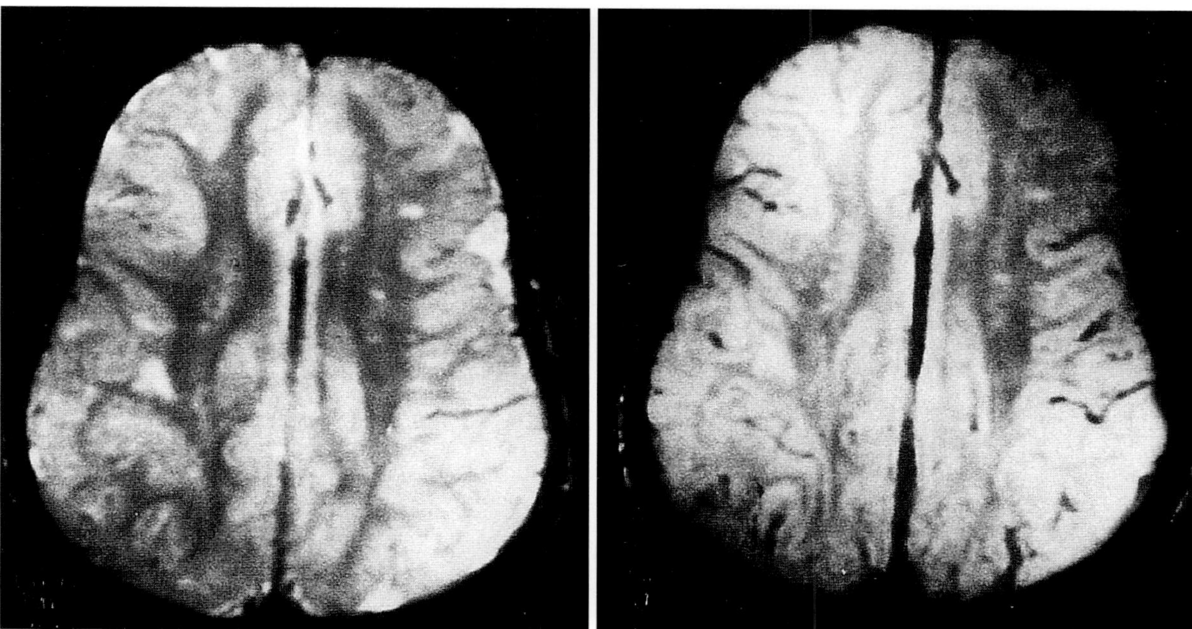

Fig. 7.2. 4.5-year-old child with the Saudi variant of MSD. Note the multiple small high signal intensity spots in the centrum semiovale bilaterally. Courtesy of Aqeel et al. (1992), with permission

layed. In addition, in most children, scattered, small high signal intensity spots are seen in the subcortical white matter which are more suggestive of mucopolysaccharidosis than metachromatic leukodystrophy (Fig. 7.2). In some of the children, white matter abnormalities are more extensive and more confluent. Severe, highly confluent white matter disease has also been found. Some prominence of ventricular system and sulci may be present. On the cranial-cervical junction signs of cervical cord compression may be found caused by atlantoaxial abnormalities.

8 Globoid Cell Leukodystrophy: Krabbe's Disease

8.1 Clinical Features and Laboratory Investigations

Globoid cell leukodystrophy (GLD), also known as Krabbe's disease, is a disorder of myelin metabolism with autosomal recessive inheritance. A number of clinical types can be distinguished, which differ in age of onset and in the more or less rapid course of symptomatology. The early-infantile type or classical type is most well known. The other types are: congenital, late-infantile, juvenile and adolescent-adult. Early and late onset forms of GLD may occur within the same family.

Clinical features and course of disease are fairly uniform in early-infantile GLD. Hagberg distinguished three clinical stages. During the first few months of life the infants are healthy and their psychomotor development is normal. The onset of clinical symptoms occurs between 1 and 6 months of age. Stage I is characterized by hyperirritability and periods of unmotivated crying, particularly when handled and nursed. The infants seem to be extremely sensitive to light and noise and often have excessive startle responses. Periods of fever often occur without signs of infection. The muscular tone increases. At the onset of the disease the deep tendon reflexes are normal. There is a stagnation of mental and motor development, soon followed by regression. In sporadic cases convulsions, hemiplegia or predominant signs of peripheral neuropathy are the presenting abnormalities.

Within 2–4 months of onset most patients reach stage II. This stage comprises the subsequent period of rapid and severe motor and mental deterioration. There is a permanent opisthotonus, a hypertonic flexion in the arms and extension in the legs. The deep tendon reflexes can no longer be evoked. There are extensor plantar signs. Achieved abilities are lost. At the same time the general condition deteriorates with more frequent hyperpyretic periods, often accompanied by intense sweating. The patient suffers from hypersalivation and hypersecretion from the lungs, often complicated by infections. Myoclonic irregular jerks of the arms and legs, startle myoclonus, hypertonic fits, and other atypical seizures occur as well as typical, generalized tonic-clonic seizures and infantile spasms. The signs of visual failure and optic atrophy begin to appear.

Stage III is the vegetative, burned-out stage. The children seem to have no mental activity and lie in a decerebrate posture. They are blind and make no voluntary movements. Touching may elicit primitive generalized reflex movements. The children lack sucking abilities and have to be fed by nasogastric tube. The muscular tone often changes again. The opisthotonic posture disappears and is followed by a tendency to hypotonicity. The children become cachectic and if they do not die of an intercurrent respiratory infection or aspiration, they gradually succumb. Death occurs between 5 months and 3 years of age.

In sporadic cases GLD is already manifest at birth during the neonatal period in the form of unspecific feeding difficulties, irritability, twitchiness or respiratory problems. Both floppy and hypertonic neonatal variants have been described.

The later onset forms of GLD are clinically more heterogeneous and progress more slowly. A subdivision in late-infantile onset (6 months to 3 years), juvenile onset (4–10 years) and adolescent-adult onset has been proposed, but the subdivision is arbitrary. Adolescent-adult onset is very rare and in most children the onset of disease occurs before the age of 5 years. There is no significant difference in symptomatology according to the age at onset. The initial signs of the late onset forms of GLD are quite variable: spastic paraparesis, hemiplegia, cerebellar ataxia, peripheral neuropathy, isolated visual failure, either as a result of optic atrophy or as a result of bilateral involvement of the optic radiations, dystonia, epileptic seizures, psychosis or mental deterioration. Among these signs increasing difficulties in walking caused by spasticity or ataxia and isolated visual failure constitute the most frequent first manifestations. Irritability is not infrequently noted early in the disease. The pace and duration of the disease are quite variable. Some of the patients, in particular patients younger than 3 years, have a very rapid course of disease, in which the child becomes bed ridden, tetraparetic and demented in less than 3 months. Most children, especially with later onset, have a more chronic course of disease. Death occurs after a highly variable period ranging from 18 months to more than 14 years. Bronchopulmonary infections are the most frequent cause of death.

In early onset GLD, an abnormally high protein level is always found in CSF and a normal cell count. Only occasionally are there more than 10 cells/ml, the majority of these being mononuclear leukocytes. The increase in CSF protein level is less constant in later onset forms of GLD, and occurs in about 50% of the patients.

EEG findings have been described most extensively for early onset GLD. At the beginning of the disease, the EEG is normal, sometimes even after some months of manifest clinical symptoms. Pathological findings tend to appear at the end of stage I. The pattern then becomes increasingly pathological, characterized by marked slow activity of high voltage. In the terminal stage the background activity is often disturbed by numerous fast, sharp-wave activities, episodic dysrhythmias or epileptiform episodes. Sometimes a picture of hypsarhythmia is found.

Nerve conduction velocity is markedly reduced in all patients with early onset GLD. In later onset forms the reduction in nerve conduction velocity is more variably present; conduction velocity may also be normal.

The diagnosis of GLD is established by showing a deficiency of galactocerebroside β-galactosidase in white blood cells or cultured fibroblasts. It is not possible to distinguish early onset GLD and late onset variants by comparing their residual enzyme activities. Rare cases of pseudodeficiency have been reported, meaning that in healthy people low (less than 10%) galactocerebroside β-galactosidase activity can be found. Unfortunately the ^{14}C-sulfatide loading test which will produce ^{14}C-galactosylceramide after removal of the sulfatide moiety by arylsulfatase A does not result in significant accumulation of ^{14}C-galactosylceramide in cells from patients with adult GLD. Therefore, the diagnosis of adult GLD is based on low enzyme activity coupled with clinical findings and other studies, such as MRI and measurement of nerve conduction velocity. The diagnosis of GLD will be helped by applying additional methods, in particular DNA analysis. GLD can be diagnosed prenatally by assaying the enzyme activity in chorionic villi samples or amniotic fluid cells.

8.2 Pathology

Gross examination of the brain reveals a moderate to marked reduction in size. On section the cortex appears to be relatively spared, but there is a marked reduction in the amount of white matter, which shows a brownish discoloration. Microscopic examination confirms that there is no or minimal involvement of cortical gray matter. The cerebral, cerebellar and brain stem white matter shows diffuse demyelination. The process occurs throughout the brain, although there are regional variations in intensity. There is a distinct tendency for arcuate fibers to be preserved. The extent to which tracts in the brain stem and cord are affected varies. Long tracts, in particular the spinocerebellar tracts, the dorsal columns and corticospinal tracts are usually severely damaged. In the areas of demyelination axonal degeneration is observed, but axons are relatively preserved in comparison to the degree of myelin loss. There is an early and marked loss of oligodendrocytes. There is a diffuse fibrillary gliosis throughout the white matter with proliferation of astrocytes. In the central nuclei of the brain moderate neuronal loss may be observed and sometimes intense gliosis.

The pathognomonic feature of GLD is the accumulation of globoid cells. These cells are multinucleated giant cells with ballooned cytoplasm containing finely fibrillar to granular material. Their cytoplasm stains eosinophilic in HE, moderately positive in PAS and negative or faintly positive in Sudan black preparations. There are also smaller rounded cells with single nuclei and accumulation of identical material in their cytoplasm. These are called epitheloid cells by some, included as globoid cells by others. Globoid cells are present as single cells or, more often, as groups of cells in the affected white matter. They show a tendency to accumulate around blood vessels. Considerable variations occur in the distribution and number of globoid cells present in the individual case, depending on the duration of the disease and the intensity of the histopathological process. Their number decreases in older burned-out cases. In exceptional cases no globoid cells can be found. At an ultrastructural level the globoid cells appear to contain specific straight and twisted tubular-like inclusions. The tubular inclusions are usually dispersed throughout the cytoplasm, rarely membrane bound. The profile of the straight tubules on cross section is angular or crystalloid, of the twisted tubules rectangular or oval. Sometimes myelin figures and lipid droplets are found in the cytoplasm of globoid cells. Globoid cells are considered to stem from phagocytic mesenchymal cells.

In GLD the peripheral nerves also undergo pathological changes. Light-microscopic examination reveals segmental demyelination and variable axonal degeneration. Usually no typical globoid cells are found. Electron microscopy shows that Schwann cells and endoneurial macrophages contain cytoplasmic inclusions similar to the inclusions of the globoid cells of the CNS.

8.3 Chemical Pathology

Chemical analysis of the brain shows that the gray matter is only moderately abnormal, while severe changes are present in the white matter. The white matter has an increased water content and its lipid content is greatly diminished. Although both cerebroside and sulfatide are greatly decreased, as might be expected from the myelin loss, there is a significant change in the cerebroside: sulfatide ratio from the normal value of 4:1 to as much as 10:1. Proportional to the total loss of myelin there is a decrease in the white matter content of total lipids, cholesterol, glycolipids and ethanolamine phosphoglycerides. There is a relative increase (though an absolute decrease) of other phospholipids such as choline phosphoglycerides, serine phosphoglycerides, and sphingomyelin. No elevation of cholesterol esters is found. Galactosylsphingosine, also called psychosine, accumulates in considerable amounts in the white matter of GLD patients. Concentrations of up to 100 times the normal value have been found. Galactosylsphingosine is not normally detectable in gray matter, but is elevated in GLD patients, though not nearly to the same extent as in white matter.

Analysis of isolated myelin in GLD reveals a relatively normal lipid composition. The cerebroside content of myelin is not elevated. A relatively high concentration of cerebroside is found in globoid cell-enriched fractions from the diseased white matter. It is concluded that there is storage of cerebroside in globoid cells, while there is no storage in the white matter as a whole or in the myelin membrane.

8.4 Pathogenetic Considerations

The primary defect in GLD is a deficiency of galactosylceramidase, also called galactocerebroside β-galactosidase. This is a lysosomal enzyme, that catalyzes the first step of cerebroside (galactosyl ceramide) degradation and splits cerebroside into galactose and ceramide. Also sulfatide is normally degraded through cerebroside into ceramide and galactose. The gene encoding for galactocerebroside β-galactosidase is localized on chromosome 14. Complementation studies by somatic cell hybridization suggest that the early and late forms of GLD arise from allelic mutations in the same gene.

Mammalian tissues contain two genetically distinct lysosomal β-galactosidases with different, though overlapping substrate specificities: galacto-cerebroside β-galactosidase and GM$_1$-ganglioside β-galactosidase. It has been demonstrated that under certain assay conditions GM$_1$-ganglioside β-galactosidase can also hydrolyse cerebroside. Psychosine (galactosyl sphingosine) is hydrolyzed by galactocerebroside β-galactosidase, but not by GM$_1$-ganglioside β-galactosidase. This difference in substrate specificity explains why psychosine accumulates to high levels in GLD brain, whereas cerebroside is moderately increased in relative concentration, but decreased in absolute concentration.

Cerebroside is almost exclusively a constituent of oligodendrocytes, Schwann cells and myelin sheaths. Metabolism of cerebroside is closely related to the metabolism of myelin. In immature brains, prior to myelination, cerebroside is practically absent and, therefore, lack of galactocerebroside β-galactosidase is of little consequence. As soon as myelination begins, the normal turnover of myelin starts. This coincides with a rapid rise of galactocerebroside β-galactosidase activity in normal brain. In GLD brains cerebroside from catabolized myelin cannot be disposed of sufficiently because of the lack of the enzyme. GM$_1$-ganglioside β-galactosidase may be responsible for part of the cerebroside breakdown and prevent real accumulation of cerebroside. Excess of cerebroside in phagocytic cells leads to the transformation of these cells into globoid cells. In experimental studies the relationship between cerebroside and globoid cells has been confirmed. Intracerebral injection of cerebroside into rat brain elicited a globoid cell reaction, whereas the injection of many other substances did not lead to this response.

Psychosine is a deacylated form of cerebroside. However, a potential route for psychosine formation, deacylation of cerebroside, could not be demonstrated. There is evidence that psychosine is synthesized from UPD-galactose and sphingosine by UDP-galactose sphingosine galactosyltransferase. Psychosine is a highly cytotoxic substance. It exerts its effect by inhibiting mitochondrial function. It cannot be disposed of in GLD. It is probable that psychosine generated within oligodendrocytes during the period of active myelination accumulates until it reaches a toxic level. Oligodendrocytes are selectively destroyed because psychosine formation occurs primarily in these cells. This explains the early and marked loss of oligodendrocytes, resulting in loss of the myelin sheaths maintained by these cells. In GLD brains the concentration of psychosine correlates well with the severity of pathological changes. When the stage of massive death of oligodendroglial cells is reached, rapid myelin breakdown occurs, contributing more cerebroside which may enhance the globoid cell reaction. The death of oligodendroglia prevents further myelination.

The sequence of events is well illustrated in the Twitcher mutant mouse, which has the same defect as in the human disease. Initial myelin development is normal, highlighting the point that myelin build-up is essentially normal in GLD. Subsequently, there is a declining rate of myelination, followed by demyelination and the appearance of globoid cells. It is myelin turnover, which brings the enzymatic defect to expression.

The difference in tissue reaction between CNS and PNS is difficult to explain. Phagocytic cells in the PNS contain abnormal inclusions similar to those in the brain, and it is not clear why they are not transformed to the typical multinucleated globoid cells. The almost obligatory involvement of the CNS and the, in particular in later onset forms of GLD, variable involvement of the PNS suggests that oligodendrocytes are more vulnerable to psychosine than Schwann cells.

In the brain there is a regional variation in vulnerability to pathological changes. In particular, the U fibers are typically spared. As in GLD the process of myelin build-up is normal and the defect involves myelin turnover and breakdown, the areas of the brain that myelinate last can be expected to be involved in later stages of the disease than the early myelinating areas. The U fibers are the last in the order of myelination, which may explain their relative preservation. In addition, in animal research the in vivo turnover rate of cerebroside appears to be higher in those areas of the white matter which are consistently more severely affected in GLD; this may furnish another part of the explanation for regional variation in white matter involvement.

GLD is a primary myelin disorder and there are no morphological or functional abnormalities outside the nervous system. This is explained by the fact that cerebroside is almost exclusively present in nervous tissue. The amounts in organs outside the nervous system are quantitatively negligible.

Although GLD and metachromatic leukodystrophy (MLD) are both caused by a genetic defect in the catabolism of myelin constituents and initial myelin build-up is normal in both disorders, there are interesting dissimilarities between GLD and MLD. MLD is characterized by extreme storage of sulfatide, whereas GLD hardly deserves the name storage disorder. In MLD the composition of the myelin membrane is altered with excessive sulfatide within the myelin sheath. In GLD, myelin is compositionally normal, and the relative rise in cerebroside compared to other lipids in the analysis of whole white matter appears to be related to an excess of cerebroside in globoid cells. An acceptable hypothesis explains these differences by a difference in rate of oligodendroglial cell death. In GLD these cells disappear rapidly, early on in the local disease process. This early cell death is probably caused by psychosine toxicity. With oligodendroglial cell death myelin membranes are lost simultaneously, before the defect in turnover can trap cerebroside or other abnormal constituents within the myelin sheath. In MLD oligodendroglial cells disappear later, slower and not as completely. Sulfatide is trapped in the myelin membrane and its content increases until the composition of the myelin sheath is so abnormal that the normal stability of the membrane is lost and demyelination ensues.

8.5 Therapy

To date, GLD has been inevitably fatal. There is no specific treatment other than supportive care. The problem of, in particular, early onset forms of GLD is that neuropathological changes have been shown to start in fetal life. In later onset forms bone transplantation has been performed in a very limited number of patients. It is too early to evaluate the results of this treatment. Carrier detection, genetic counseling, prenatal diagnosis and early abortion of affected fetuses is currently the strategy of choice.

8.6 Magnetic Resonance Imaging

In cases of early onset GLD, CT findings have been described more often than MRI findings. The abnormalities reported are related to the stage of the disease. In stage I, there are no changes, or symmetrical increased density in the thalami, corona radiata, and, less often, posterior limb of the internal capsule, caudate nucleus, globus pallidus and putamen. Sometimes more extensive hyperdensity areas are noted, also in the brain stem, cerebellar cortex, optic radiation, subcortical white matter and cortical gray matter (Fig. 8.1). Autopsy has confirmed the presence of calcium deposits in hyperdense areas. In stages II and III, symmetrical low-density areas in the periventricular white matter and corpus medullare of the cerebellum become obvious. The low density of the white matter is relatively less marked than in other leukodystrophies. The low density represents demyelination and increased water content. The severe fibrous astrogliosis which occurs in GLD may be responsible for the less intense hypodensity. In stage III diffuse brain atrophy, both central and peripheral, is observed. Sulci become widened, there is flattening of the head of the caudate nuclei and widening of the ventricles, including the 3rd due to atrophy of the thalamus. In a number of cases an enhancing rim at the border between the deep white matter and the arcuate fibers has been described, but absence of contrast enhancement has also been found.

MRI has confirmed the presence of periventricular white matter abnormalities with relative sparing of the arcuate fibers in early onset GLD (Fig. 8.2). The posterior limb of the internal capsule, corpus callosum, cerebellar white matter and brain stem tracts are also involved. A linear pattern of white matter abnormalities along the fibers of the corona radiata has been described (Fig. 8.3), but this pattern is not obligatory. The areas of high density on CT may not be so clearly abnormal on MRI. These areas often have a relatively low signal intensity on T_2-weighted images and may have a normal, decreased or increased signal intensity

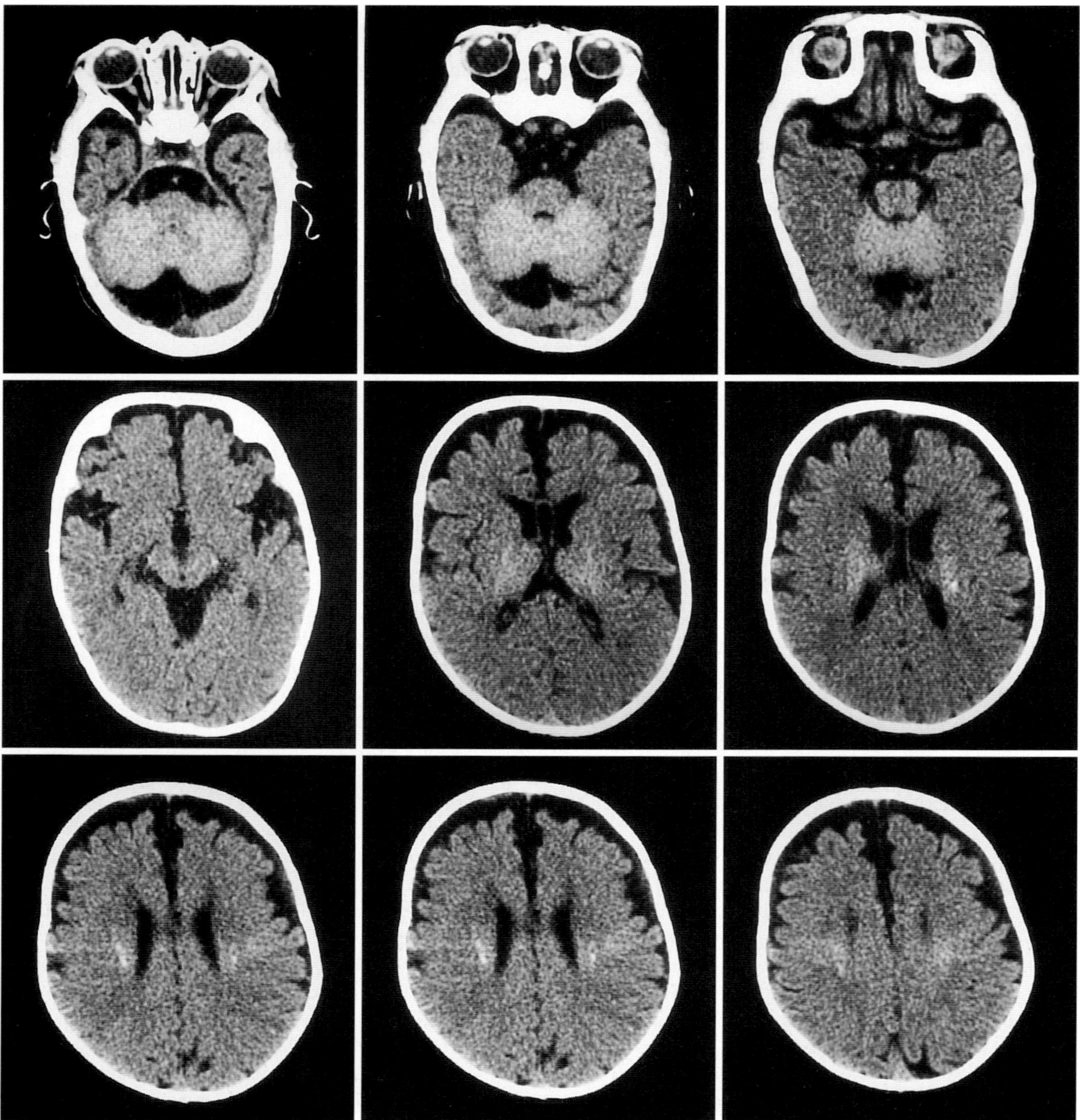

Fig. 8.1. CT findings in a boy, 4 months of age with early-infantile GLD. The series demonstrates the hyperdensities in the primary myelination zones: brain stem, cerebellum, internal capsule, basal ganglia and corona radiata. At this stage the CT appearance is almost diagnostic and more characteristic than the MRI findings

on T_1-weighted images. It has been suggested that both the presence of calcium and the accumulation of fatty material in globoid cells may contribute to the changes in T_1 and T_2. With progression of the disease, the subcortical white matter also becomes involved and global atrophy ensues. In many patients MRI and CT provide complementary information, CT showing the characteristic hyperdensities and MRI showing the extent of the demyelination.

In cases of late onset GLD, MRI reports are more frequent than CT descriptions. Hyperdensities in the thalamus and basal ganglia have been found with CT. Both CT and MRI show a predominant involvement of the occipital periventricular white matter with extensions in the parietal and temporal direction and associated involvement of the splenium of the corpus callosum. The arcuate fibers are relatively spared (Fig. 8.4). The posterior limb of the internal capsule may be in-

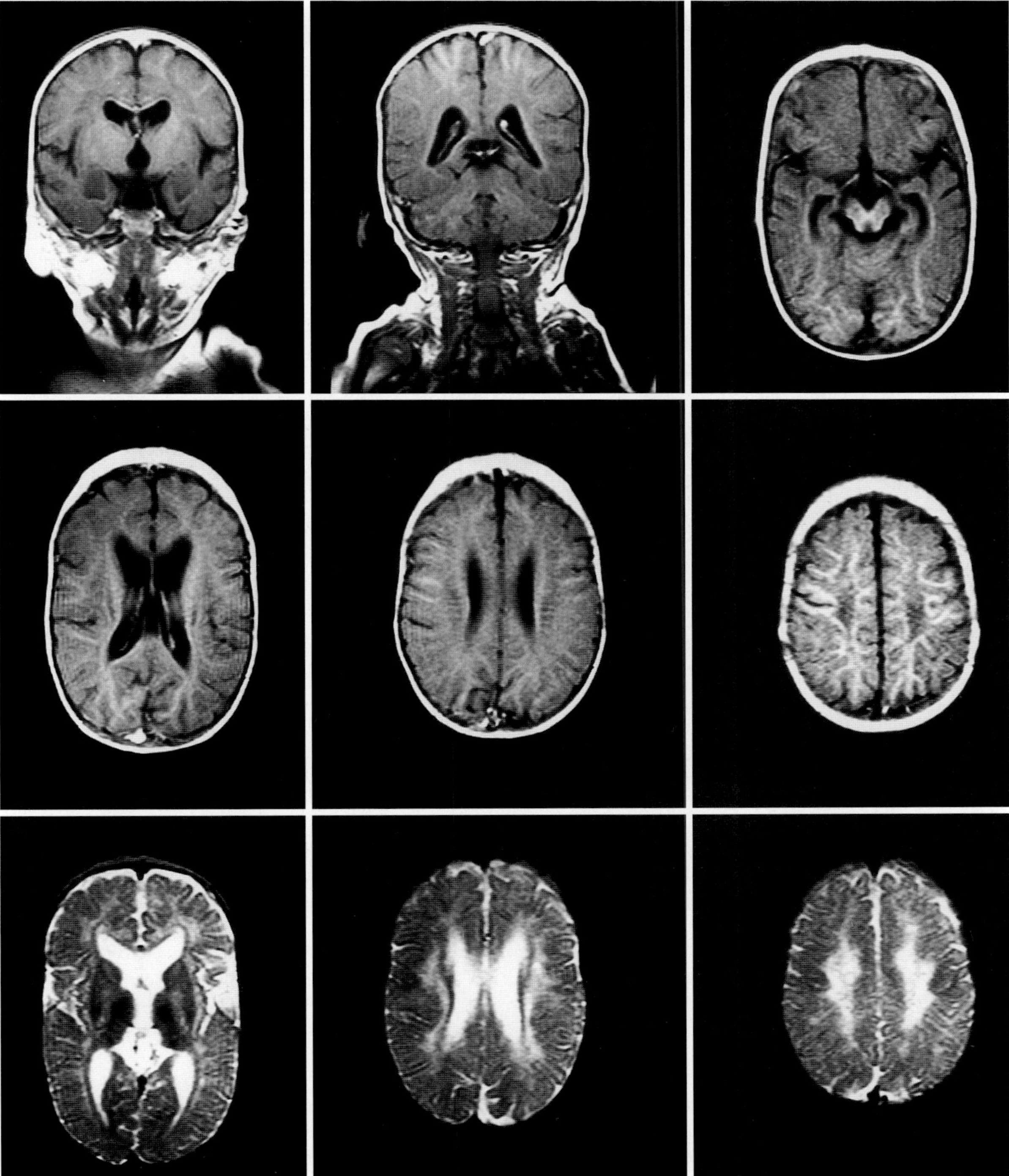

Fig. 8.2. Early-infantile GLD in a 7-month-old boy. The *two upper rows* show coronal and transverse T_1-weighted images. The myelin that had already been formed starts to disappear in the periventricular area, where there is some tissue loss. The more peripherally located myelin is still spared. An indication of the stripe-like pattern is seen in the periventricular area. The T_2-weighted transverse images (*lower row*) indicate the extent of white matter involvement and the relatively late inclusion of the arcuate fibers

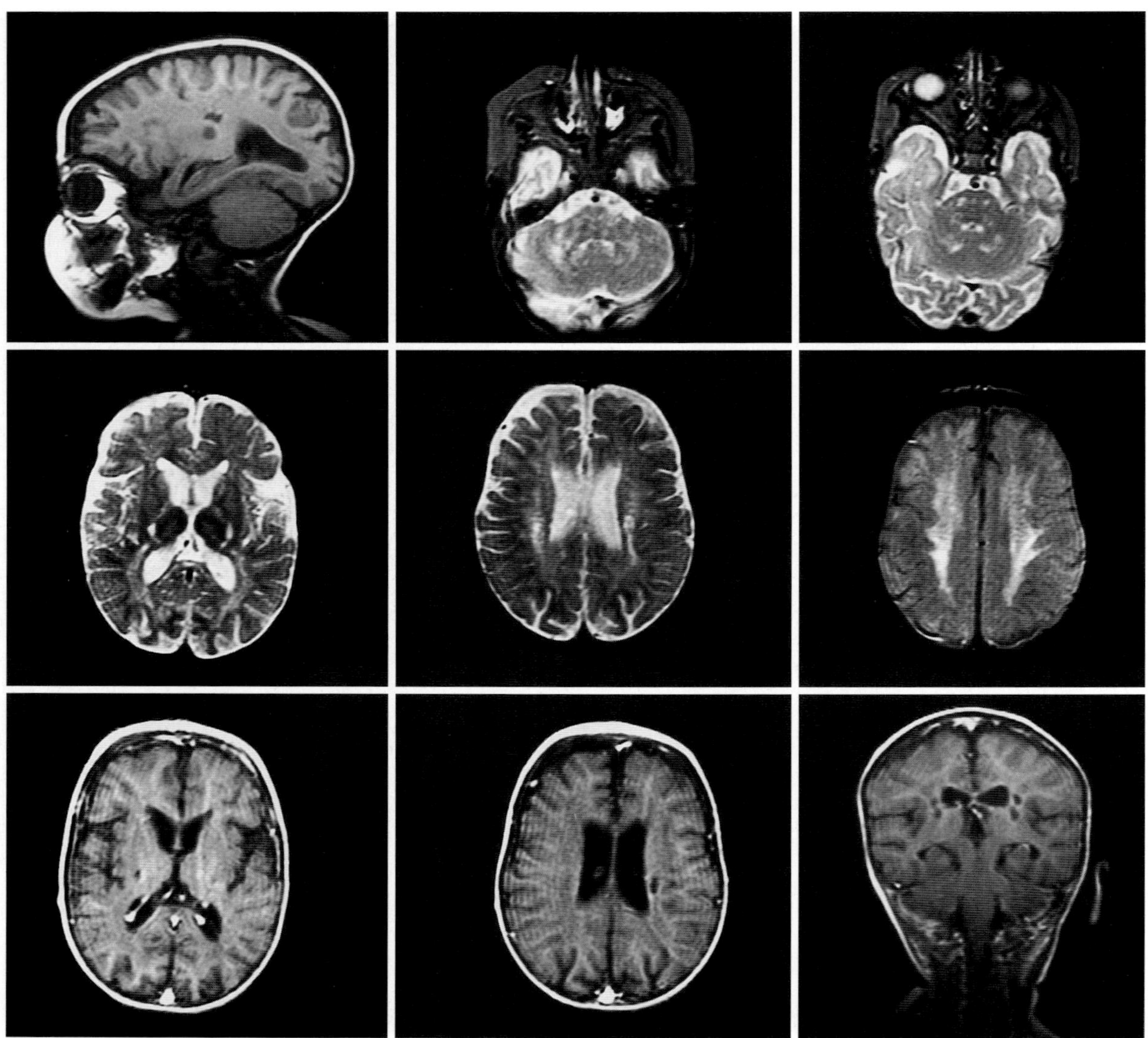

Fig. 8.3. Early-infantile GLD in a boy 9 months of age. There is generalized atrophy and cavities have developed in the periventricular region. Tracts in the brain stem, including the dentato-rubral tracts, are also involved. Following contrast injection (*lower row*) there seems to be a faint contrast uptake around the cavities and the lateral border of the lesions. Also in this case the internal capsule is affected. The periventricular lesions have a stripe-like radiating appearance

volved. Again the white matter abnormalities may have a high density on CT due to deposition of some calcium. On MRI the white matter abnormalities have the usual high signal intensity on T_2-weighted images, low signal intensity on T_1-weighted images. The pattern strongly resembles that of X-linked adrenoleukodystrophy. However, the characteristic two zones present in the white matter abnormalities in X-linked adrenoleukodystrophy with a rim of contrast enhancement in between, have never been described in GLD. In late onset GLD, contrast enhancement of the splenium of the corpus callosum has been described, as well as absence of any contrast enhancement. More extensive white matter lesions affecting the whole centrum semiovale probably represent a more advanced stage of disease. In the later stages atrophy becomes obvious.

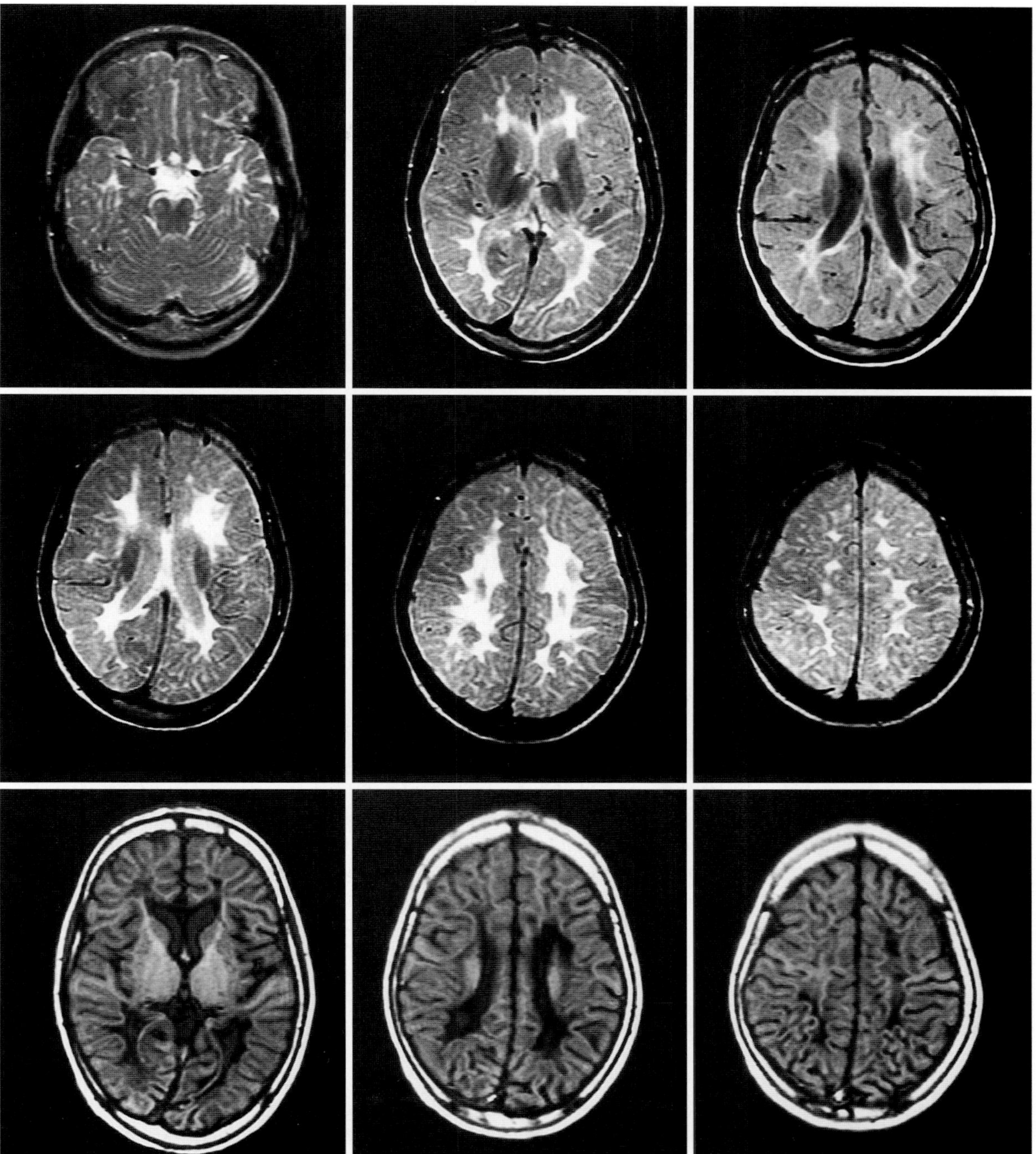

Fig. 8.4. MRI series of a juvenile form of GLD in an 8-year-old girl. The *upper two rows* show a series of T$_2$-weighted and proton density images, to demonstrate the periventricular white matter involvement, spreading to the arcuate fibers, which are already partially affected. The T$_1$-weighted transverse series in the *lower row* shows the partial sparing of the U fibers and the loss of white matter volume

9 GM₁ Gangliosidosis

9.1 Clinical Features and Laboratory Investigations

GM_1 gangliosidosis is an autosomal recessive disorder of GM_1 metabolism, resulting in variable neural and visceral accumulations. Three forms can be distinguished: infantile, generalized or type 1 GM_1 gangliosidosis, juvenile or type 2 GM_1 gangliosidosis, and adult, chronic or type 3 GM_1 gangliosidosis.

Infantile GM_1 gangliosidosis presents at or soon after birth, signs being poor sucking and feeding. The child is hypotonic and hypoactive and soon develops facial and peripheral edema. At times neonatal ascites and hydrocele are seen, sometimes generalized edema. There are characteristic coarse facial features similar to those found in mucopolysaccharidoses. Facial abnormalities include frontal bossing, wide and depressed nasal bridge, long philtrum and large low set ears. The gums and tongue may appear hypertrophied. The cornea is, however, clear. Hepatomegaly is present and the spleen may also be enlarged. The dysmorphic features and hepatosplenomegaly gave the disease its name: pseudo-Hurler disease. The skin is usually thick and rough. Exceptional cases of angiokeratoma corporis diffusum have been described. Failure to thrive and severe psychomotor retardation are present from birth onwards. Bilateral, cherry-red spots at the maculae are found in about half of the patients. Early blindness occurs which is of cortical or retinal origin. The child remains hypoactive and is weak. An exaggerated startle response to noise is frequently present. Movements are poorly coordinated. Reflexes are hyperactive. Macrocephaly may develop, but less markedly than in Tay-Sachs disease. As the child gets older, broadness of the hands and shortness of the fingers become apparent. Joints are stiff. The wrist and ankle joints are often enlarged, but not tender. Flexion contractures occur frequently at elbows and knees. Kyphoscoliosis is frequently found. After a year neurological deterioration is rapid, with occurrence of epileptic fits, progressive spasticity and eventually decerebrate rigidity, deafness, blindness, and loss of social contact. In rare cases cardiomyopathy with cardiac failure and generalized myopathy occur. Flexion contractures of arms and legs may become extremely severe. Respiratory problems are common with frequent infections. Bronchopneu-

monia is a frequent cause of death, which usually occurs around the age of 12–24 months.

In type 2 GM_1 gangliosidosis the clinical course is slower and the onset insidious. The children initially appear normal. The first clinical signs begin between 6 months (late-infantile form) and 2 years (juvenile form) of age. They usually consist of developmental arrest and gait disturbances. The subsequent course is characterized by progressive dementia, lethargy, epilepsy, increased startle response to noise, spastic tetraplegia, cerebellar ataxia, loss of speech and extrapyramidal features like choreo-athetosis. Blindness is of late occurrence. Retinal degeneration and a cherry-red spot are not seen. The patients lack organomegaly and coarsening of facial features suggestive of mucopolysaccharidosis. Skeletal deformaties are relatively mild. The average life span varies between 3 and 10 years. Death is usually caused by recurrent bronchopneumonia.

Type 3 GM_1 gangliosidosis is the adult or chronic variant. The clinical signs usually emerge in the second decade, but onset in the first decade has also been described. Gait disturbance and speech disturbance are early signs of the disease. Extrapyramidal features are usually most prominent and may take the form of slowly progressive dystonia, choreoathetotic movements, facial grimacing, blepharospasmus, dysarthria, rigidity, parkinsonism with immobile face, bradykinesia, and typical gait abnormalities. Infrequently ataxia, pyramidal signs, mild intellectual impairment and seizures occur. Bony abnormalities are minimal, if present. Cherry-red spot, visceromegaly and facial dysmorphism do not occur.

In type 1 GM_1 gangliosidosis vacuolated lymphocytes are found in the peripheral blood smear, but these are not present in types 2 and 3. Large, foamy sea-blue histiocytes are present in the bone marrow in type 1; these cells are fewer in number in types 2 and 3. Rectal biopsy shows neuronal lipidosis in Meissner's plexus. Ultrastructurally, membranous bodies similar to those seen in GM_2 gangliosidosis are seen within neurons. The membranous bodies consist of spirally wound lamellae enclosed within a membrane of lysosomal origin. Other inclusions are more pleomorphic in nature. Evidence of neuronal lipidosis on rectal biopsy can be found in all types of GM_1 gangliosidosis.

Also clear vacuoles in visceral histiocytes and parenchymal cells of visceral organs and in epithelial cells can be found in all types, but are less abundant in the later onset forms.

Biochemical investigations demonstrate an abnormal urinary oligosaccharide excretion. The concentration of the urinary oligosaccharides appears to correlate with the severity of the disease, the excretion being highest in type 1, lowest in type 3 GM_1 gangliosidosis. CSF protein is normal. In types 1 and 2 an increased concentration of GM_1 ganglioside may be found in plasma and CSF. Demonstration of a deficiency of β-galactosidase activity in leukocytes or cultured fibroblasts is the most effective means of establishing the diagnosis. A decreased hydrolysis rate of GM_1 ganglioside can be demonstrated in cultured skin fibroblasts. Prenatal diagnosis is established by enzyme analysis in cultured amniotic fluid cells.

Radiological abnormalities in type 1 may be minimal at birth but become progressively more pronounced with time. By 6 months there is usually little difficulty in identifying them. The abnormalities include kyphoscoliosis and hypoplasia and beaking of one or more vertebrae. The long bones are wide in the center and taper at both ends. There is a generalized rarefaction of the cortex of most bones. With increasing age the externally thickened cortical wall is removed by expansion of the medullary cavity. The metacarpalia are wedge-shaped, expanded distally and constricted proximally. The sella turcica is shoe-shaped, shallow and elongated. In type 2, radiological changes are mild and involve mainly the vertebral bodies. In type 3 the radiological changes are minimal or absent. Flattening of vertebral bodies may be seen. In types 1 and 2 the EEG shows progressive deterioration, but epileptic discharges are rare. The ERG remains normal.

9.2 Pathology

External examination of the brain in type 1 GM_1 gangliosidosis usually reveals no abnormalities, sometimes some cortical atrophy. The consistency of the white matter may be increased.

Light microscopy reveals neuronal storage throughout the nervous system, mainly in cerebral and cerebellar cortex, but also in basal ganglia, brain stem, spinal cord, and Meissner's plexus. The neurons have a ballooning, foamy cytoplasm and the nucleus is displaced to the periphery. Accumulation of storage material in proximal nerve cell processes results in the formation of meganeurites and megadendrites. There is degeneration and loss of neurons. Storage bodies are also present in glia.

Electron microscopy demonstrates that the neuronal inclusion bodies are identical to the membranous cytoplasmic bodies seen in GM_2 gangliosidosis. They consist of spirally wound membranous lamellae enclosed within a limiting membrane of lysosomal origin.

The white matter in type 1 GM_1 gangliosidosis is gliotic and there is a diffuse paucity of myelin. The white matter abnormalities are too severe to be accounted for by Wallerian degeneration only. They are probably the result of a combination of disturbed myelination, myelin loss in the process of Wallerian degeneration and primary demyelination.

In type 1 GM_1 gangliosidosis visceral storage is found. The liver is enlarged and storage material is present in hepatocytes and in histiocytes in liver sinusoids. The renal glomerular epithelium shows marked vacuolization of the cytoplasm. The spleen, lymph nodes, thymus and intestinal mucosa contain many foamy histiocytes. Large foamy histiocytes are present in bone marrow aspirates. Skin biopsies show foamy vacuolization of sweat gland epithelium, histiocytes, fibroblasts, and endothelium cells. The vacuoles appear empty. The stored oligosaccharides in visceral organs are extremely water soluble and are lost on fixation.

In types 2 and 3 GM_1 gangliosidosis, identical neuronal storage is seen. In type 3 the neuronal storage is predominantly present in the basal ganglia. White matter is either not affected at all, or only to a minimal extent. The visceral storage varies considerably. There may be no storage at all, or sparse histiocytes may be seen in spleen and liver. There may be foam cells in bone marrow, lymphatic tissue and vacuolization of hepatic and renal cells, similar in form to but less severe than in type 1.

9.3 Chemical Pathology

In type 1 GM gangliosidosis a severe accumulation of the normal monosialoganglioside GM_1 occurs, accompanied by a minor accumulation of its asialo derivative GA_1, and other minor glycolipids and glycopeptides. The total ganglioside content of the brain is increased with an approximately 10-fold increase of GM_1 in gray matter and a twofold increase in white matter. In gray matter GM_1 ganglioside constitutes 70%–90% of total ganglioside, which is normally about 25%. The level of total lipid in gray matter is slightly decreased, mainly due to a moderate decrease of phospholipids and glycolipids. In white matter a marked decrease of major myelin constituents is found, like cholesterol, phospholipids, cerebrosides, sulfatides and proteolipid protein. A marked increase in free fatty acids and in cholesterol esters is found in most cases. The white matter chemical abnormalities are compatible with moderately severe myelin destruction. In the myelin membrane itself the concentration of GM$_1$ ganglioside is also several times the normal concentration. Other abnormalities in the composition of isolated myelin are a very high concentration of cholesterol, a low level of glycolipids, especially cerebroside, and a low concentration of phosopholipids, especially ethanolamine phospholipids. These myelin abnormalities represent the transitional state of myelin undergoing nonspecific breakdown.

The neuronal inclusion bodies, the so-called membranous cytoplasmic bodies, have an extremely high ganglioside content. GM$_1$ accounts for approximately 95% of the total ganglioside content. Other components are proteolipid protein, phospholipds and cerebroside. One of the glycolipids, cerebroside, consists mainly of glucocerebroside, which is an unusual cerebral constituent after the infantile period.

There is a 20- to 50-fold accumulation of GM$_1$ ganglioside in liver and spleen. Furthermore, there is visceral accumulation of galactose-containing oligosaccharides, which by far exceeds the accumulation of gangliosides. Some oligosaccharide fractions contain sialic acid. The oligosaccharide accumulation rather than the ganglioside storage is the chief cause of the visceral histiocytic vacuolation.

Storage of galactose-containing partially degraded derivatives of keratan sulfate has been demonstrated in liver and brain. These compounds are glycopeptides.

In type 2 GM$_1$ gangliosidosis the concentration of GM$_1$ ganglioside and its asialo derivative are moderately elevated in the brain, considerably less than in type 1 GM$_1$ gangliosidosis. The myelin lipids like cholesterol, phospholipids, sulfatide and cerebroside are moderately decreased, but much closer to normal than in type 1 GM$_1$ gangliosidosis. Visceral accumulation of oligosaccharides is less marked.

In type 3 GM$_1$ gangliosidosis the accumulation of GM$_1$ ganglioside in the brain is more focal. Accumulation is most marked in the putamen and caudate nucleus, where GM$_1$ accounts for 50% or more of all gangliosides, whereas GM$_1$ accounts for about 30% of all gangliosides in the white matter and only a slight increase, if any, in the proportion of GM$_1$ ganglioside is noted in the cerebral cortex. Abnormal accumulation of asialo GM$_1$ is only noted in the basal ganglia. There are no abnormalities in concentration of other lipids, such as cholesterol, phospholipids and glycolipids. Visceral accumulation of oligosaccharides is minor.

9.4 Pathogenetic Considerations

GM$_1$ gangliosidosis is caused by a deficiency of the lysosomal degradative enzyme acid β-galactosidase. This enzyme is an acid hydrolase catalyzing cleavage of terminal β-linked galactose from a variety of substrates, including GM$_1$ ganglioside, asialo GM$_1$, lactosylceramide, lactose, the galactose containing oligosaccharides and mucopolysaccharides, particularly keratan sulfate.

The gene encoding for β-galactosidase is located on chromosome 3. Expression of the β-galactosidase gene is regulated by a functional protein, called protective protein or carboxy peptidase. This protein is encoded by a gene on chromosome 22. Protective protein stabilizes the enzyme molecule intracellularly and protects it against the action of intralysosomal proteases. Substrates cleaved by β-galactosidase differ in their requirement of natural activators. Sphingolipid activator protein 1 (called SAP-1 or saposin B) is required for the cleavage of GM$_1$ ganglioside by β-galactosidase. SAP-1 acts on GM$_1$ as a kind of solubilizer. SAP-1 has a common larger precursor protein with some other SAP's. This precursor protein is encoded by one locus on chromosome 10. SAP-1 not only activates β-galactosidase to cleave GM$_1$ ganglioside, but also activates the cleavage of sulfatide by arylsulfatase A and globotriaosylceramide by α-galactosidase.

GM$_1$ gangliosidosis is caused by a deficiency of β-galactosidase. A number of different mutations of the gene on chromosome 3 have been identified. Compound heterozygotes have two different abnormal alleles. The age of onset and rate of progression of the disease depend on the residual activity of the mutant enzyme.

Deficiency of the protective protein by a protective protein gene mutation causes the disease galactosialidosis. Deficiency of the protective protein gives rise to a secondary deficiency of both β-galactosidase and neuraminidase activity.

SAP-1 deficiency results in a form of metachromatic leukodystrophy, with -apart from sulfatide storage – a variable concomitant accumulation of gangliosides and other glycosphingolipids.

β-Galactosidase deficiency occurs in a number of disorders caused by different gene mutations: GM$_1$ gangliosidosis, variant form of metachromatic leukodystrophy, galactosialidosis, I cell disease and in mucopolysaccharidosis type IV B, also called Morquio disease type B. In I-cell disease, or mucolipidosis III, deficiency of β-galactosidase is caused by a defect in posttranslational processing of the enzyme molecule. With respect to GM$_1$ gangliosidosis and Morquio disease type B being the result of the same single enzyme deficiency, it has been suggested that this multiplicity of phenotypes can be explained by different alterations in the catalytic activity of the mutant enzyme which differentially alters its activity on a variety of substrates. There is evidence that patients with Morquio disease type B retain a higher catalytic activity for GM$_1$

ganglioside than for oligosaccharides and mucoplysaccharides.

The phenotypic variability in clinical symptomatology of GM_1 gangliosidosis may be explained in the same way. The early infantile form is characterized by neurological dysfunction in combination with bony abnormalities and visceral storage. In later onset forms, progressive neurological symptoms are present but visceral and bony abnormalities are minimal or absent. Differences in residual enzyme activity, different types of mutations affecting different catalytic functions of the enzyme, different rates of turnover of the enzyme and substrates in brain, viscera and bone may be responsible for these phenotypic variations. An attractive hypothesis would state that in some cases the mutant enzyme possesses about the same low residual activity for each natural substrate (infantile type), whereas the mutant enzyme possesses significantly different residual activities for different natural substrates in other cases (juvenile and adult types).

In GM_1 gangliosidosis, GM_1 ganglioside and its asialo derivative accumulate in lysosomes due to the impairment of normal degradation. GM_1 is a normal component of cellular membranes and its content is especially high in neuronal plasma membranes. Accumulation occurs predominantly in neurons, resulting in neuronal dysfunction and eventually neuronal cell death. There are several factors which may contribute to neuronal dysfunction and death. The accumulated GM_1 ganglioside and its asialo derivative are relatively insoluble in water and aggregate within lamellated membranous bodies in lysosomes. Expanding lysosomes with increasing amounts of stored products may disturb intracellular transport, in this way disturbing cellular metabolism. Leakage of toxic intralysosomal products of enzymes into the cytoplasm during the process of intralysosomal storage may cause damage. The accumulation of gangliosides may lead to exhaustion of precursor pools for the biosynthesis of cellular components. Accumulation of GM_1 ganglioside in the neuronal membrane results in alterations of membrane structure. Gangliosides contain long, saturated fatty acids which increase the packing density of the membrane and reduce its fluidity. GM_1 ganglioside, specifically, has a pronounced effect on reducing membrane fluidity as the carbohydrate moieties of GM_1 reduce the rotational freedom within the hydrophobic regions of the membrane. The increased cholesterol content also contributes to the reduction of membrane fluidity. The altered membrane fluidity may influence the synaptic transmission and the activity of membrane-bound enzymes. GM_1 gangliosidosis is also characterized by inappropriate proliferation of secondary neurites and aberrant formation of synapses. This abnormal sprouting may lead to changes in neuronal connectivity, resulting in specific functional impairment. Evidence has also been found for neurotransmitter dysfunction with disturbed neurotransmitter release and re-uptake, and specific dysfunction of GABAergic neurons.

The later-onset forms of GM_1 gangliosidosis have more focal neuronal pathology especially marked in basal ganglia and spinal cord, whereas the infantile form has more generalized neuronal pathology but especially pronounced in cerebral and cerebellar cortex. The explanation for this phenomenon is speculative. The regulation of substrate and enzyme synthesis and turn-over may not be identical in different types of cells and may not be the same at all ages, changing the distribution of cells in which saturation of the residual enzyme occurs earliest and most prominently.

Significant white matter changes are only present in type 1 GM_1 gangliosidosis. There is a severe myelin deficiency, which is mainly caused by a disturbance of myelinogenesis with hypomyelination and delayed myelination. Other factors which may contribute to the myelin deficiency, are Wallerian degeneration with myelin loss secondary to degeneration of neurons and primary myelin loss due to altered myelin composition and myelin instability.

Galactose containing oligosaccharides accumulate in the viscera, particularly in type 1 GM_1 gangliosidosis. These oligosaccharides are derived from the incomplete degradation of glycoproteins in lysosomes. The accumulation of these water-soluble compounds is responsible for the cytoplasmic vacuolation of visceral cells, the foamy histiocytosis in bone marrow and the vacuoles in circulating lymphocytes.

Storage of galactose containing partially degraded derivatives of keratan sulfate occurs in liver and brain, especially in type 1. Storage of these compounds is probably responsible for the bony deformities.

9.5 Therapy

At present there is no effective treatment for GM_1 gangliosidosis. Bone marrow transplantation may be attempted in the future, especially in the later onset forms, but with the limited amount of experience so far, it has proved unsuccessful.

9.6 Magnetic Resonance Imaging

In type 1 GM_1 gangliosidosis MRI shows severely delayed and disturbed myelination with persistent high signal intensity of the white matter on T_2-weighted images after the first year of life (Fig. 9.1).

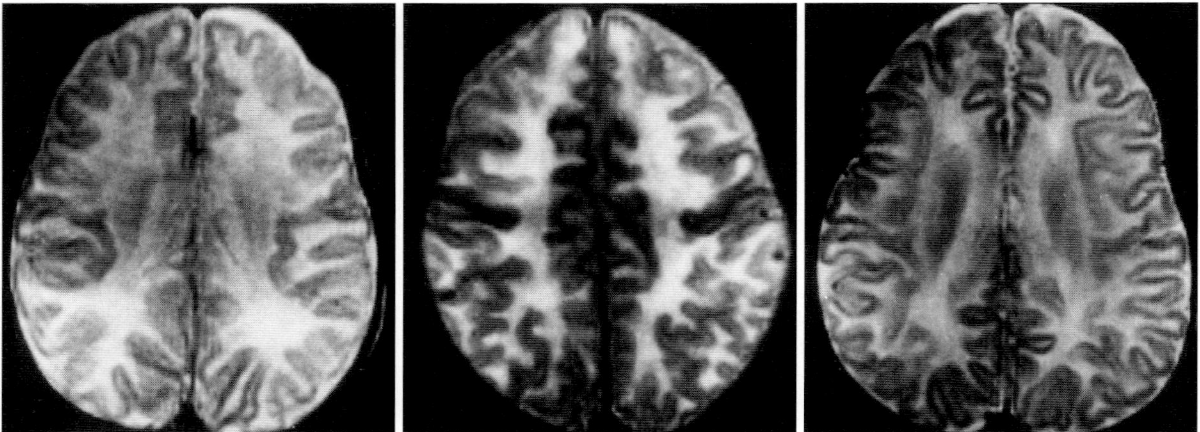

Fig. 9.1. Serial T$_2$-weighted MR images performed in a patient with type 1 GM$_1$ gangliosidosis at 2, 5 and 13 months of age, respectively. MRI demonstrates that the white matter fails to develop an increasingly low signal intensity; this is indicative of poor myelin formation. Courtesy of Kaye et al. (1992), with permission

In type 2 GM$_1$ gangliosidosis, progressive atrophy of the cerebral hemispheres has been described with enlargement of the ventricular system and subarachnoid space, and atrophy of cerebellum and brain stem. No focal abnormalities in signal intensity were found, but imaging experience in type 2 is very limited.

In type 3 GM$_1$ gangliosidosis, abnormal signal intensity is found in the caudate nucleus and putamen on both sides. The caudate nucleus is atrophic resulting in absence of the normal bulging contour. In addition, some cerebral atrophy can be found. The images are identical to those of adult GM$_2$ gangliosidosis.

10 GM$_2$ Gangliosidosis

10.1 Clinical Features and Laboratory Investigations

GM$_2$ gangliosidoses are inherited disorders of GM$_2$ ganglioside metabolism. Inheritance is autosomal recessive. There are three major, biochemically distinct types: B, O, and AB. Among the B and O types, infantile, juvenile and adult forms can be distinguished; the AB variant is known only as an infantile form. Infantile type B is the classical Tay-Sachs disease (TSD) and infantile type O is equivalent to Sandhoff's disease (SD).

TSD is common in Ashkenazi Jews of eastern European origin. In the United States the gene frequency is 1 in 30 among Ashkenazi Jews and only 1 in 380 among other groups. However, in Britain most of the affected families are non-Jewish. TSD infants seem normal at birth and their early development apparently follows a normal pattern. The disease begins in the first year of life. An exaggerated startle response is often the earliest symptom, although frequently only recognized in retrospect. It is provoked by sudden noise and consists of extension, abduction, and elevation of the arms. Listlessness and irritability usually occur early in the course of disease. Gradually, psychomotor retardation and deterioration with loss of skills becomes evident. After 6 months of age, vision noticeably deteriorates and hypotonic motor weakness becomes obvious. The infant may crawl, sit unaided, and pull himself up to a standing position, but does not usually manage to walk. By 1 year of age the deterioration of mental and motor capacities is obvious. The child no longer sits, holds or transfers objects, loses interest in the surroundings and usually lies placidly in bed. In the second year hypotonic motor weakness progresses and by the end of the second year a generalized flaccid paralysis has developed. The tendon reflexes are increased at all stages and plantar responses may be extensor. In the later stages of the disease signs of spasticity, dystonia, rigidity, chorea and athetosis may be variably present. Blindness becomes obvious after the first year of life. Ophthalmoscopic examination reveals a cherry-red spot in one or both maculae in about 90% of the patients. Optic atrophy is also seen. Feeding becomes a problem in the second year because of ineffective swallowing. Seizures are rare before the age of 1 year, but frequent thereafter. The epileptic manifestations may consist of tonic-clonic seizures, myoclonic epilepsy and also gelastic epilepsy. A characteristic sign in TSD is megalencephaly which usually becomes prominent at about 2 years of age. By the age of 2, most patients are completely paralyzed, retarded, blind, and deaf with frequent seizures. Decerebrate posturing may be present. Most patients die of bronchopneumonia and emaciation. Death usually occurs between 2 and 3 years of age, survival after the age of 4 being rare.

The clinical features of SD are similar to those of TSD, with the exception of hepatosplenomegaly which does not occur in TSD. Occasionally there are bony deformities similar to those associated with infantile GM$_1$ gangliosidosis. Infantile GM$_2$ gangliosidosis type AB is also clinically similar to TSD. These disorders have no racial predilection.

In addition to the severe infantile forms of GM$_2$ gangliosidosis, later onset forms are known. The so-called juvenile form usually has its onset between 2 and 6 years of age. The adult form, or, rather, chronic form, has its onset between the end of the first decade and the third decade of life. Even later onset has been described. However, the age of onset is difficult to determine because of the very slow progression of the disease. While the juvenile form has no ethnic predilection, the adult B form is more frequent among Ashkenazi Jews than in other ethnic groups.

The main systems affected in the juvenile and adult variants are the cerebellum, the pyramidal cells, the lower motor neurons, and less frequently basal ganglia. Atypical spinocerebellar ataxia syndromes are common as modes of presentation of late-onset GM$_2$ gangliosidosis. They are charaterized by slowly progressive ataxia, spasticity, dysarthria and muscle atrophy. Such cases have been diagnosed as atypical variants of Friedreich's ataxia, with one major difference, namely the lack of sensory involvement. In some patients additional abnormalities in the form of supranuclear or internuclear ophthalmoplegia, and sensory neuropathy have been described, but these are rare. Another relatively frequent presentation is as motor neuron disease. Clinical features include weakness, cramps, proximal muscle wasting and fasciculations. This clinical picture closely resembles the Kugelberg-Welander phenotype of spinal muscular atrophy or bulbospinal neuronopathy. Amyotrophic lateral sclerosis-like syndromes present with involvement of both lower and upper motor neurons. Apart from paresis, atrophy and fasciculations, high reflexes and extensor plantar reflexes are found. Upper limb postural tremor may occur, as in other disorders of the lower motor neuron. Various extrapyramidal features have been described in late-onset GM$_2$ gangliosidosis, either in isolation or in combination with the more common motor neuron and cerebellar syndromes. Dystonia, rigidity, choreiform movements and athetoid posturing have been noted. Another clinical characteristic of late-onset GM$_2$ gangliosidois is the high incidence of recurrent psychosis. In addition, psychic changes include anxiety, depression, insomnia, aggressiveness, severe behavioral troubles and personality disintegration. The psychic changes may precede all other manifestations or may appear later. Neurovegetative disorders are common, and consist of sweating impairment, loss of libido, impaired esophagus motility, fixed cardiac frequency and orthostatic hypotension. Intellectual deterioration is frequent. Epilepsy may occur, but is not obligatory. Blindness occurs late in the course of the disease. On ophthalmoscopic examination, optic atrophy and retinitis pigmentosa may be seen at that time, but a cherry-red spot is not a consistent finding and of late appearance. In the juvenile variant death occurs between 5 and 15 years of age, often secondary to bronchopneumonia. Patients with the adult form usually live for decades.

In the infantile variants, EEG is either normal or shows slight changes during the first year of life. In the second year, one sees paroxysmal discharges of high voltage, slow wave activity with single and multiple spikes and sharp wave complexes. In the vegetative state of the disease, there is a marked decrease in spike discharges. These findings are not specific for infantile GM$_2$ gangliosidosis. In later-onset variants, the EEG shows variable, nonspecific findings. Nerve conduction velocities are usually normal in the first stage of the disease, followed by a decrease. EMG shows fasciculations, in particular in the proximal muscles and signs of loss of motor units with collateral reinnveration. Muscle biopsy shows signs of neurogenic atrophy with type grouping and increase in connective tissue. Sural nerve biopsy demonstrates decreased fiber density. A histogram of counted nerve fibers shows a decrease in the number of large myelinated fibers and an increase in small myelinated fibers, indicative of active regeneration. Rectal biopsy reveals swollen ganglion cells with vacuolated cytoplasm. Ultrastructurally, the ganglion cells contain membranous cytoplasmic bodies, typically found in neurons in GM$_2$ gangliosidosis.

A definite diagnosis is established by assaying hexosaminidase A and B in serum, leucocytes or cultured skin fibroblasts. In the case of variant B, hexosaminidase A is deficient. In the case of variant O, both hexosaminidase A and hexosaminidase B are deficient. In the case of variant B$_1$, the activities of hexosaminidase A and B are found to be normal when tested with the conventional synthetic substrate. There is a profound deficiency of hexosaminidase A activity when tested with the natural substrate GM$_2$ ganglioside or a sulfated artificial substrate. In the case of type AB, the activities of hexosaminidase A and B are found to be normal, since in this type the defect is a deficiency of the activator of hexosaminidase. In type AB the diagnosis requires either the demonstration of accumulating GM$_2$ ganglioside in the presence of normal hexosaminidase A and B activities or the demonstration of the activator protein deficiency. GM$_2$ ganglioside accumulation can be demonstrated in brain biopsy tissue or alternative sources of nervous tissue (rectum, conjunctiva) and probably also in CSF (although the sensitivity and specificity of the latter test is not known). The deficiency of activator protein can be demonstrated directly in fibroblasts or indirectly by feeding radiolabeled GM$_2$ ganglioside to cultured fibroblasts and correcting the disturbed degradation of this substance by the addition of purified activator protein to the culture medium.

Accurate and inexpensive screening tests for detection of GM$_2$ gangliosidosis carriers are available. These tests determine total serum hexosaminidase and hexosaminidase A activity. The leucocyte hexosaminidase assay is used for confirmation. These screening tests are applied in populations with a high risk. Prenatal diagnosis of all variants of GM$_2$ gangliosidosis is possible in the first trimester of pregnancy in cultured amniotic fluid cells or chorionic villi.

10.2   Pathology

In infantile GM$_2$ gangliosidoses, the gross changes in the brain vary with the duration of the patient's life. The weight and volume of the brain increase massively during the second year of life. The brain frequently weighs over 2000 g (normal weight 1000 g). Enlargement of the brain causes the gyri to become broadened. The cerebellum, however, is usually atrophic. On sectioning, the cut surface is abnormally firm. The hemispheric white matter may be gelatinous with local cavitation. The ventricles are variably enlarged.

Light microscopy shows a ubiquitous involvement of the nerve cells throughout the brain, with a predilection for the neurons in the cerebral hemispheres over the ganglion cells of the motor cranial nerves or other brain stem nuclei. There is a diffuse disturbance of the cytoarchitecture of the gray matter with a reduction in the number of nerve cells, an unusual increase in size of the remaining neurons, and a concomitant augmentation in the number of glial elements. The neurons are large and distorted due to depositon of lipid material. They have a distended, rounded outline; their nuclei are displaced to the circumference of the cell and are often shrunken and pyknotic. Cortical neuronal cells have swellings in the proximal axon segment or in the apical dendrite, resulting in so-called meganeurites. As the disease progresses, the neurons gradually disappear. There is a decrease in the number of axons seen within the white matter of the brain which parallels the process of degeneration of the cerebral cortical nerve cells. With progression of the disease there are profound disturbances in myelination which exhibit a tendency to symmetric distribution. Demyelination may be very extensive. In some patients the demyelination predominantly affects the centrum semiovale with sparing of the subcortical U fibers, but in other patients it involves almost the entire white matter, including the U fibers. The internal capsule is usually well preserved. The preserved myelin sheaths frequently appear thinner than normal. Complete absence of myelin throughout the hemispheric white matter can occur if the patient survives for a long time. There is evidence that the white matter changes cannot be attributed to Wallerian degeneration only. There is evidence for an additional role of failure of myelination and active demyelination: the severity of myelin loss is often greater than the neuronal loss; the tendency to softening and cavitation in the most severely affected areas is consistent with active demyelination, but not with Wallerian degeneration only. As the disease progresses, the glial reaction increases, and eventually large numbers of microglia as well as numerous proliferating astrocytes can be observed. The glial cells are swollen and filled with large globules. The contents of these glial cells show similar properties to those observed in neurons. The cerebellum shows extensive degenerative changes. Narrowing or reduction in size of the cerebellar folia is associated with decreased numbers of cells in the cerebellar cortex. The Purkinje cells show extensive damage and those remaining are filled with the same material that is present in the neurons of the cerebral cortex. The neurons of the cerebellar nuclei also show the typical ballooning due to deposition of lipids. The spinal cord neurons undergo changes similar to those seen elsewhere in the CNS. The neurons of the anterior horns are more intensely affected than those of the posterior and lateral horns. The spinal cord white matter frequently shows rarefaction of the nerve fibers, particularly in the lateral columns and in the pyramidal tracts, but they are normally myelinated. Microscopic examination of the retina reveals extensive degeneration and loss of ganglion cells. The cytoplasm of the remaining cells is filled with lipid material similar to that seen in the neurons of the brain. These changes are particularly conspicuous in the area of the macula.

Electron-microscopic studies have shown that the cytoplasm of the distended neurons contains so-called membranous cytoplasmic bodies. These are membrane-bound structures which contain closely packed lamellae, frequently arranged concentrically in a regular fashion. The lipid material, which is seen under light microscopy, is located in these membranous cytoplasmic bodies. They occupy a considerable proportion of the nerve cell cytoplasm. Their accretion within the neuronal cytoplasm causes the enormous ballooning of the cell and the displacement of the nucleus to the periphery. Accumulation of these storage bodies in proximal nerve processes leads to the formation of meganeurites and megadendrites. It has been shown that these storage bodies are lysosomal in origin. They are also found in axons and glial cells. In glial cells the deposits are more pleomorphic than in neurons.

In infantile GM_2 gangliosidoses, extraneuronal storage of lipids can be found, especially in SD. Cells containing stored material are discovered in the spleen, in renal tubular cells, and in liver cells. The deposited material appears to be similar to that of the neurons.

In juvenile and adult GM_2 gangliosidoses pathological changes predominantly affect the anterior horn cells of the spinal cord, the cerebellar cortical neurons, brain stem nuclei and basal ganglia. In these areas prominent neuronal storage and degeneration is present. The cerebral cortex is less severely or minimally involved. This is the reverse of what occurs in infantile gangliosidoses. The cerebellum is atrophic. Slight but diffuse demyelination of cerebral and cerebellar white matter has been described. In other patients almost complete demyelination of the posterior columns was found.

10.3 Chemical Pathology

GM_2 ganglioside is accumulated in abnormally large amounts in GM_2 gangliosidoses. In the brain, the increase in concentration of gangliosides ranges from 100 to 300 times that found in normal brain. The storage patterns of the gangliosides exhibit some characteristic differences in the three variants of GM_2 gangliosidosis. In all cases the accumulation of the ganglioside GM_2 is most pronounced. It is accompanied by minor storage of its sialic acid-free derivative, GA_2. Variant 0 is characterized by the fact that the nervous tissue contains – in relative terms – the lowest amount of GM_2 and the highest amount of GA_2. Variant B and variant AB differ from each other in the extent to which GM_2 and GA_2 are accumulated, the accumulation being higher in the AB variant. The gangliosides are mainly stored in the neuronal cells, but the ganglioside concentration of white matter is also increased. In late-onset forms of GM_2 gangliosidosis, cerebral levels of GM$_2$ and GA$_2$ are markedly increased above normal but not to the extent seen in infantile forms. A regional variation in ganglioside accumulation in the brain can be seen, depending on the variation of neuronal storage in the different types of GM$_2$ gangliosidosis.

Some 30%–40% of the lysosomal inclusion bodies consists of GM$_2$ ganglioside. Other components are proteolipid protein, cholesterol, phospholipids, and glycolipids.

Except for a high concentration of GM$_2$ ganglioside, the change in chemical composition of the white matter is nonspecific and reflects the extent of demyelination. The main findings are a decrease of proteolipid protein, total lipids, glycolipids as well as phospholipids, and the presence of significant amounts of cholesterol in esterified form.

In the B variant and the AB variant, GM$_2$ ganglioside is not stored in large amounts outside the nervous system. In the O variant there is an extensive storage of globoside in the visceral organs, besides storage of GM$_2$ and GA$_2$ ganglioside. The level of globoside is approximately normal in the visceral organs in the B variant and the AB variant.

10.4 Pathogenetic Considerations

GM$_2$ gangliosidosis is caused by a deficient activity of the lysosomal enzyme β-hexosaminidase, also called GM$_2$ gangliosidase or β-N-acetylgalactosaminidase. This enzyme hydrolyses the terminal N-acetylgalactosamine from the ganglioside GM$_2$. Hexosaminidase is composed of two subunits. The α- and the β-chain can associate in different combinations to produce isoenzymes of different structure and catalytic activity. Isoenzyme αβ is called hexosaminidase A, isoenzyme ββ hexosaminidase B, isoenzyme αα hexosaminidase S. Hexosaminidase A cleaves the substrates ganglioside GM$_2$, the asialo derivative GA$_2$, globoside, neutral oligosaccharides and negatively charged substrates, such as terminal β-linked N-acetylglucosamine-6-sulfate contained in keratan sulfate, chondroitin sulfate or dermatan sulfate. Hexosaminidase B has an overlapping substrate-specificity and cleaves GA$_2$, globoside and neutral oligosaccharides. Hexosaminidase B does not posses any significant ganglioside GM$_2$-cleaving activity. Hexosaminidase S has only negligible catalytic activity. Apart from the α- and β-chains of hexosaminidase, a third protein is necessary for in vivo catabolism of GM$_2$ ganglioside: an activator protein. This activator protein is termed GM$_2$ activator or sphingolipid activator protein 3 (SAP-3). The GM$_2$ activator has an isoenzyme specificity for hexosaminidase A, not for hexosaminidase B or S. Interaction of the activator protein with GM$_2$ ganglioside or related compounds results in the formation of a water soluble dimer. The activator-lipid complex binds to a specific recognition site of hexosaminidase A in such a way that the glycosidic bond is positioned at the active site in the α-subunit. Thus the GM$_2$ activator functions as a transport protein rather than as an activator of the enzyme.

The different types of GM$_2$ gangliosidosis are characterized by the isoenzyme which is missing. In type B, there is a deficiency of hexosaminidase A (isoenzyme αβ), resulting from a mutation at the α-chain locus on chromosome 15. In type O, both hexosaminidase A (αβ) and hexosaminidase B (ββ) are deficient. This is the result of a mutation in the β-chain locus on chromosome 5. Type AB is caused by a deficiency of the activator protein. A fourth variant of GM$_2$ gangliosidosis has been described, the B$_1$ variant, in which a mutation affects a specific α-chain site to which the activator -substrate complex binds. The mutant enzyme has an almost normal activity towards substrates that are split at the active site located on the β-subunit. It is virtually inactive towards the substrates that are exclusively or preferentially cleaved at the active site on the α-subunit (GM$_2$ ganglioside and also synthetic substrates containing a sulfate group). The B$_1$ mutation is allelic to the B mutation. The B$_1$ variant appears to be rare in the homozygous form, but may be more commonly encountered in the B/B$_1$ compound heterozygous form. However, the recent application of the sulfated substrate in enzyme testing may reveal the B$_1$ variant to be a more common disorder than previously thought.

The time of onset and clincial severity of the disease are related to the rate of ganglioside accumulation, which is inversely related to the residual activity of hexosaminidase in the patient's tissues. The most common mutation in the α-subunit gene is the TSD allele, which in its homozygous state causes total absence of hexosaminidase A. In contrast, adult α-subunit mutations cause a severe, but not complete, deficiency of hexosamindase A. Both the infantile and adult α-subunit mutations occur with enhanced frequency among Askenazi Jews. Compound heterozygotes, carrying an infantile and an adult α-subunit mutation on homologous chromosomes, have adult-onset GM$_2$ gangliosidosis. The variable residual enzyme activity among adult-onset GM$_2$ gangliosidosis probably explains the considerable clinical variation. It has been confirmed that patients homozygous for the adult mutation have clinical symptoms that closely resemble those of compound heterozygotes, but that the onset of the disease is later, that the patients are less severely affected and that the progress of the disease is slower than in compound heterozygotes. The patients homozygous for the B$_1$ mutation generally belong to the juvenile category. The clinical severity of compound heterozygotes depends on the other allele. When the other allele is totally inactive, a late-infantile phenotype results. Compound heterozygosity in which the other allele carries an adult GM_2 gangliosidosis mutation, is probably responsible for the very rare patients with a chronic form of B_1 variant with survival into the third decade of life.

The β-subunit mutations have not yet been studied as extensively as the α-subunit defects. Different mutations have been identified and also here compound heterozygotes have been described. Likewise, the variations in residual enzyme activity will explain the different clinical phenotypes.

Gangliosides are typical components of the outer leaflet of plasma membranes and are particularly abundant in the neuronal plasma membranes. An accumulation of these lipids will therefore occur predominantly in neurons. The accumulation of lipids occurs primarily inside the lysosomes, where they fail to be broken down in the absence of adequate hexosaminidase activity. The accumulating amphipathic lipids will precipitate and form lamellar structures. Although the stored compounds are normal, nontoxic components of the cell, their excessive storage will interfere with normal cell function. In cells with extreme storage a mechanical destruction of the neurons may occur. Undegraded storage material is not completely confined to the lysosomes but can to some extent be recycled and reach other compartments such as Golgi and plasma membrane via normal membrane flow. This may lead to changes in the content and pattern of gangliosides in the neuronal plasma membrane. Gangliosides are implicated in cell-cell recognition phenomena including synaptogenesis. Presence of abnormalities in gangliosides in neuronal plasma membranes interferes with the establishment of proper connections and leads to aberrant synaptogenesis. Inappropriate proliferation of secondary neurites, a tremendous increase in synaptic spines on neurons, and formation of meganeurites and megadendrites occurs. Increased ganglioside content in plasma membranes results in markedly reduced membrane fluidity. Evaluation of neurotransmitter metabolism has shown reduced high-affinity uptake of glutamate, GABA and norepinephrine by synaptosomes. Other studies have suggested abnormal calcium homeostasis and interference with second messenger systems.

In the infantile form, mechanical storage is responsible for the megalencephaly and may be a major cause of neuronal dysfunction and death. In the late-onset forms the lipid accumulation is much less pronounced and the other mechanisms mentioned may be more important in explaining the neuronal dysfunction.

It is difficult to explain why in different variants of the disease neurons from different locations are preferentially involved. It may have something to do with the relative contribution of pathogenetic mechanisms mentioned in each particular variant. Besides, the regulation of substrate and enzyme synthesis and turnover may not be identical in different types of cells, and may not be the same over the years, altering the distribution of cells in which saturation of the residual enzyme occurs most prominently. Impairment of cellular functions can occur at different threshold values of accumulated gangliosides in different types of cells at different times.

The white matter disease in infantile forms of GM_2 gangliosidosis can probably be explained by a combination of hypomyelination, Wallerian degeneration and demyelination. The hypomyelination may be secondary to neuronal dysfunction, as a normal neuron-myelin interaction is necessary for normal myelin deposition. The demyelination might be explained by altered myelin composition, structure and stability. The myelin membrane fluidity is decreased by the increased content of GM_2 ganglioside. GM_2 gangliosides contain long, saturated fatty acid moieties, which increase the packing density of the lipid matrix, resulting in reduced fluidity.

10.5 Therapy

No effective treatment is available at present to halt the inexorable deterioration or to improve function in any of the GM_2 gangliosidoses. Attempts at enzyme replacement have been made by intravenous as well as intrathecal and intraventricular injection of hexosaminidase preparations. These attempts have been unsuccessful. More recently, it has been suggested that bone marrow transplantation might be successful in halting the disease.

At present, treatment is largely restricted to supportive care and appropriate management of intervening problems. Psychoactive drugs, which may be necessary in psychotic episodes, require extra attention as they are potentially harmful. Phenothiazines and tricyclic antidepressants may aggravate the clinical condition, since they induce lysosomal lipidosis by inhibiting the activity of lysosomal enzymes and the uptake of the enzymes by lysosomes in vitro.

10.6 Magnetic Resonance Imaging

Most neuro-imaging reports, which are scarce, relate to the infantile forms of GM_2 gangliosidosis. A characteristic abnormality in infantile GM_2 gangliosidosis is a homogeneously and symmetrically increased density within the thalami on CT scans (Fig. 10.1). Sometimes, also the caudate nucleus, putamen and globus pallidus are also hyperdense (Fig. 10.2). Thalami are hy-

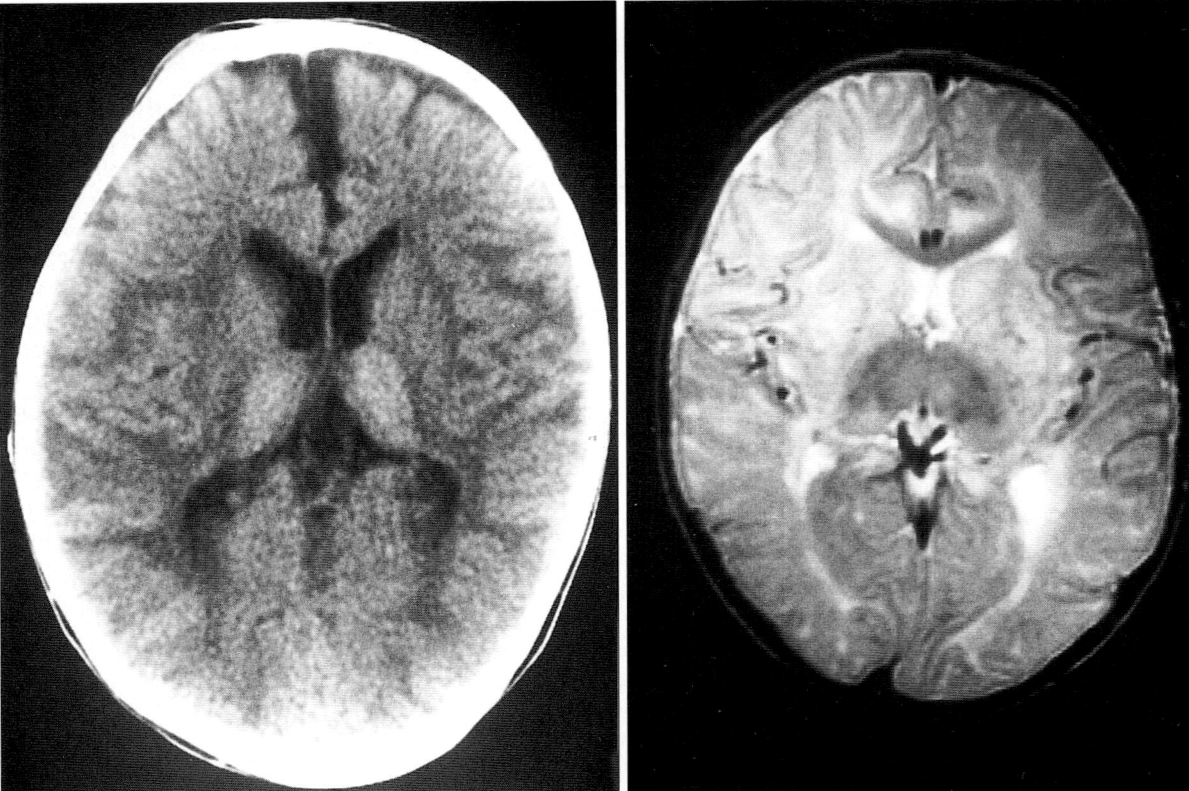

Fig. 10.1. The CT scan of this 12-month-old girl with SD shows the hyperdensity of the thalamus on both sides. The T_2-weighted MR image shows hypointensity of the thalamus. The caudate nucleus, globus pallidus and putamen have an abnormally high signal intensity. The white matter has a high signal intensity, consistent with abnormal and delayed myelination. Only the corpus callosum is well-myelinated. Courtesy of Brismar et al. (1990), with permission

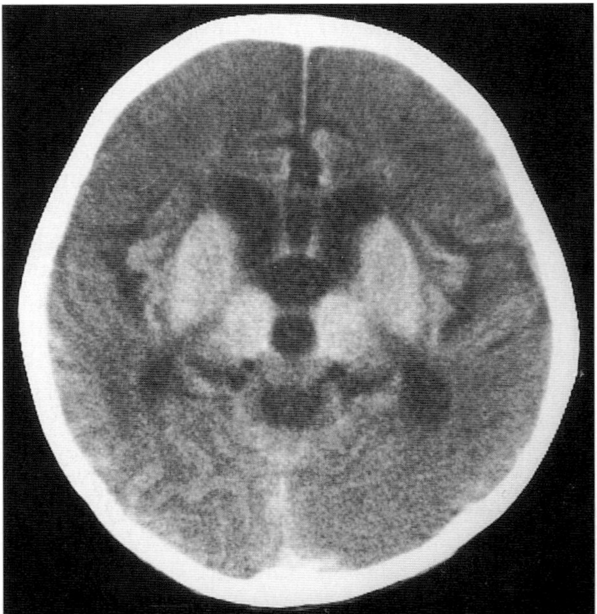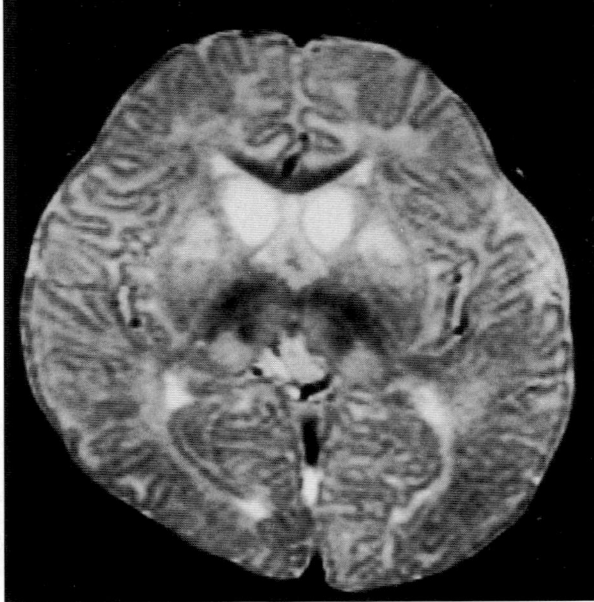

Fig. 10.2. The CT scan of a 5-year-old child with TSD shows hyperdensity of thalamus, globus pallidus, putamen and caudate nucleus together with some diffuse white matter hypodensity and cerebral atrophy. The MR image of an 11-month-old patient with TSD shows abnormal thalami, the signal intensity being partially too low and partially too high. The caudate nucleus has a very high signal intensity and is swollen. Also the putamen and globus pallidus have a high signal intensity. The signal intensity of the cerebral white matter is diffusely abnormally high, with the exception of corpus callosum and internal capsule. Courtesy of Fukumizu et al. (1992), with permission

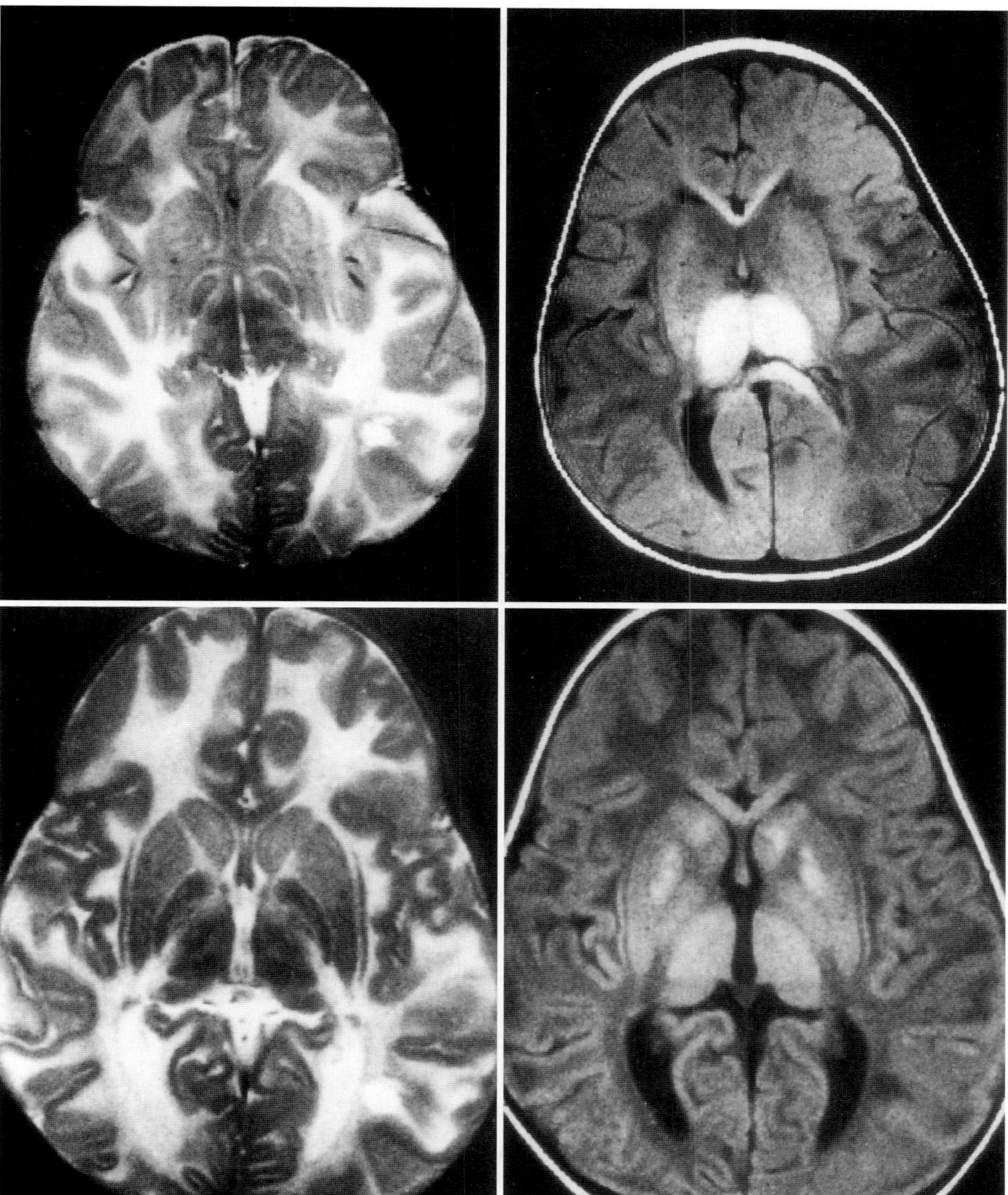

Fig. 10.3. Patient with SD at the ages of 19 months (*upper row*) and 27 months (*lower row*). The T_2-weighted MR images show a persistent high signal intensity of all supratentorial white matter structures, except for the corpus callosum. The T_1-weighted image at the age of 19 months shows a high signal intensity in the thalamus, which has been lost at the age of 27 months. At 27 months, new foci of high signal intensity are seen in the head of the caudate nucleus and the globus pallidus. Courtesy of Koelfen et al. (1994), with permission

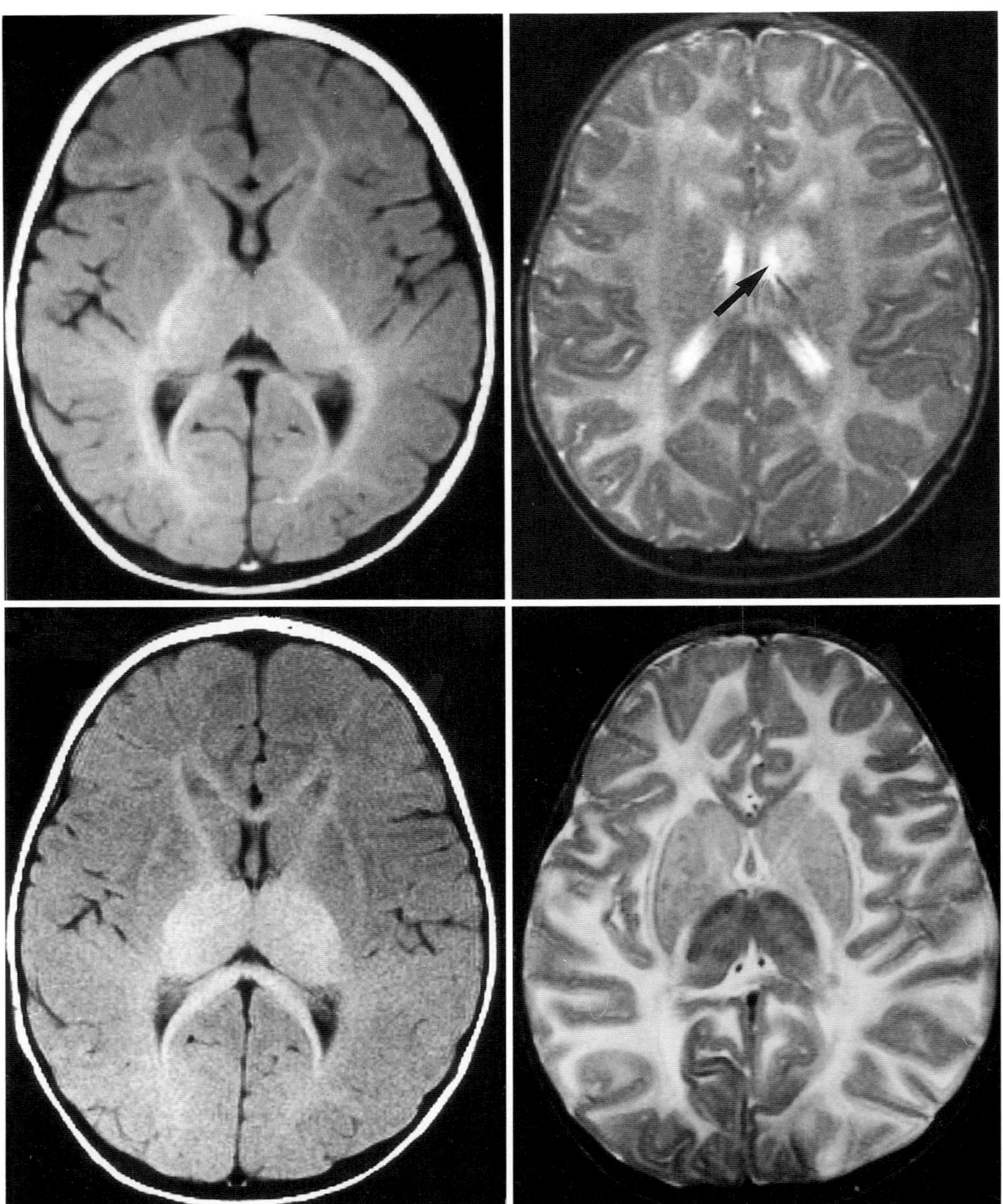

Fig. 10.4. Patient with SD at the ages of 9 months (*upper left*), 15 months (*upper right and lower left*) and 23 months (*lower right*). At the age of 9 months, the patient was clinically presymptomatic, but the T$_1$-weighted image shows a delay in myelination. At 15 months of age, myelination has not advanced any further and possibly some myelin has been lost in the frontal and occipital area. Note the increase in signal intensity of the thalamus on the T$_1$-weighted image and the lesion in the caudate nucleus on the T$_2$-weighted image (*arrow*). The T$_2$-weighted images show a progressively increased signal intensity of the cerebral white matter between the ages of 15 and 23 months. Courtesy of Koelfen et al. (1994), with permission

pointense on T_2-weighted MR images; hyperintense on T_1-weighted images (Fig. 10.4), probably due to calcium deposition. In addition, MRI may show high signal intensity abnormalities on T_2-weighted images in the caudate nucleus, globus pallidus and putamen on both sides (Figs. 10.1, 10.2). If calcium depositions are also present in these areas, the signal intensity may be low on T_2-weighted images, high on T_1-weighted images (Fig. 10.3). The cerebral white matter shows homogeneous or patchy high signal intensity, suggestive of a combination of disturbed and abnormal myelination (Figs. 10.1, 10.2) and myelin loss (Fig. 10.4). In all cases reported, the corpus callosum is well myelinated and intact. In later stages cerebral and cerebellar atrophy ensues.

The finding of high density of the thalamus on CT scans and low signal intensity of the thalamus on T_2-weighted MR images is also seen in Krabbe's disease. However, in Krabbe's disease many more brain structures may show similar high density on CT, white matter disease is more extensive, more homogeneous and does not spare the corpus callosum. The images in infantile GM_2 gangliosidosis do not resemble those of exclusively neuronal degenerative disorders, which may show delayed myelination or hypomyelination, but not a picture suggestive of demyelination. The striking combination of gray and white matter disease in imaging should suggest the possibility of GM_2 gangliosidosis.

In late-onset GM_2 gangliosidosis, CT and MRI findings of cerebellar atrophy have been described. Considering the histopathological findings, one might expect abnormalities in signal intensity on MR images of basal ganglia and brain stem nuclei.

11 Fabry's Disease

11.1 Clinical Features and Laboratory Investigations

Fabry's disease (FD) is an X-linked recessive disorder. The onset of clinical symptoms usually occurs during childhood or adolescence, but may be as late as the third or fourth decade. Early manifestations consist of episodic pain in the extremities and a teleangiectatic scaly maculopapular rash called angiokeratoma corporis diffusum. The angiokeratomas usually appear between the ages of 7 and 10 years and are dark red to black nonblanching macules and papules that range in size from punctate to 4 mm in diameter. They increase in number with time. They have a predilection for the genitals, the upper thighs and the lower trunk, and spare the face, scalp, palms and soles.

Pain is a predominant symptom of FD, both chronic acral paraesthesias with burning discomfort in the hands and feet and episodes of excruciating pain, especially of the extremities and abdomen. The pain crises, which last from minutes to several days, are often accompanied by fever and an elevated erythrocyte sedimentation rate. These episodes can easily be mistaken for rheumatic fever, appendicitis or renal colic. The attacks are triggered by exercise, temperature change, fatigue and emotional stress. The painful crises persist throughout life and are often the most debilitating aspect of the disorder.

Hypohydrosis begins at puberty and progresses to an absence of sweating by the third decade of life.

Ophthalmological abnormalities occur in more than 90% of the patients and often predate skin changes. Whorled corneal opacities, posterior linear lenticular cataracts with narrow wavy spokes, and dilatation and tortuosity of conjunctival and retinal vessels are frequent; anterior lenticular deposits, periorbital edema and retinal edema are less frequent. The corneal and lenticular opacities do not impair the visual acuity. Central retinal artery occlusion may cause acute blindness.

With increasing age, the major morbid symptoms result from the cardiovascular system. Cardiac disease is characterized by mitral regurgitation or aortic stenosis, left ventricular hypertrophy, dysrhythmias, hypertrophic obstructive cardiomyopathy and finally angina pectoris, myocardial ischemia and infarction and congestive heart failure. Cardiac disease is worsened by systemic hypertension caused by renal vascular disease.

Cerebrovascular disease results mainly from small vessel involvement with transient ischemic attacks, ischemic infarctions and aneurysm formation with cerebral hemorrhage. Clinical symptomatology includes hemiplegia, hemianaesthesia, aphasia, and seizures. Dementia, personality changes and psychosis may appear in older patients.

Less prominent clinical signs and symptoms include decreased pulmonary function, episodic diarrhea, vomiting, and growth retardation.

Over the years, the patients develop symptoms of chronic progressive renal failure with proteinuria, signs of tubular dysfunction and development of azotemia. Death usually results from chronic renal failure by the fourth or fifth decade, unless chronic dialysis or renal transplantation is performed.

Atypical variants have been described with mild single symptomatology at ages when the patients with classical disease are severely affected.

In heterozygous female patients, clinical expression is variable. Especially with increasing age, some minor symptoms of the disease may become manifest. The typical whorled corneal opacities can be found in 70%–80% of the female carriers and are often the only disease manifestations. A few angiokeratomas are found in 20%–30% of the females. Renal and cardiac disease is usually mild, if present. Cerebral infarction has been described, but is rare. A small percentage of the female carriers suffer from the characteristic FD pain.

Maximal motor and sensory nerve conduction velocities are normal. In contrast, quantitative assessment of thermal thresholds reveals small fiber neuropathy in some of the patients.

The diagnosis of FD is established by demonstration of a deficiency of α-galactosidase activity in plasma, leukocytes, urine, cultured skin fibroblasts or single hair roots. Plasma or cells can also be assayed for their content of accumulated glycosphingolipids. In female heterozygotes 25%–40% have levels of α-galactosidase within the normal range. High performance liquid chromatography of urinary sediment glycolipids is a more sensitive test for the detection of carriers.

Prenatal diagnosis can be made by fetal sex determination and enzyme assay in cultured amniotic fluid cells or chorionic villi. In some pregnancies with a female carrier fetus, enzyme activity may be very low or deficient in cultured amniotic fluid cells, when they are derived from only a few cell clones which predominantly express the mutant X-chromosome. Without knowledge of fetal sex, this result can be misinterpreted as being indicative of an affected male fetus. In chorionic villi, an intermediate enzyme activity could either indicate an unaffected female carrier or could result from some maternal tissue contamination of the sample from an affected male pregnancy. Hence, it is necessary to combine enzyme analysis with chromosome analysis.

11.2 Pathology

The pathology of the brain is mostly related to vascular changes. Pathological lipid storage occurs in vascular endothelium throughout the brain and spinal cord leading to thickening of vessel walls and obstruction of vessels resulting in infarcts. In particular small vessels are involved. Lacunar infarcts are seen in the basal nuclei and central white matter. Larger infarcts may also be seen.

Apart from vascular endothelium, lipid accumulation occurs in the leptomeninges and the choroid stroma, in astrocytes, and in neurons in layers V and VI of the cerebral cortex, hypothalamus, amygdala, subiculum, entorhinal cortex, substantia nigra, periaqueductal gray, dorsal motor nucleus of the vagus, midline raphe nuclei in the medulla oblongata, intermediolateral cell column, dorsal root ganglia, anterior horn of the spinal cord, dorsal horn of the spinal cord, Meissner's and Auerbach's plexuses, and peripheral autonomic ganglia. Neurons in other areas of the CNS, including thalamus, subthalamic nucleus, caudate nucleus, putamen, red nucleus and cerebellar cortex and nuclei do not show signs of lipid accumulation. Neurons of the more superficial layers of the cortex contain some lipid but are relatively spared. Quantitative studies of peripheral sensory neurons and spinal ganglia have shown preferential loss of small myelinated and unmyelinated fibers as well as small cell bodies of spinal ganglia.

Many organs other than the CNS are also affected. FD is characterized by widespread deposits of lipids, occurring predominantly in the lysosomes of endothelial, perithelial and smooth muscle cells of blood vessels and, to a lesser degree, histiocytes and reticular cells of connective tissue. The deposits are also present in epithelial cells of the cornea, in renal glomeruli and tubuli, and in cardiac muscle fibers.

Histochemical studies of the deposits show that they are PAS-positive, positive with Sudan black, show birefringence, and stain with Luxol fast blue. Electron microscopic examination reveals that the inclusions are composed of tightly packed lipid lamellae, which may be concentric or parallel.

11.3 Chemical Pathology

FD is characterized by the accumulation of glycosphingolipids, in particular trihexosylceramide, dihexosylceramide and, to a lesser extent, of other galactolipids. In the CNS an increased content of trihexosylceramide is found in FD patients, but no evidence has been found of an increase in dihexosylceramide. The most dramatic increases in trihexosylceramide are found in the dorsal root ganglia, choroid plexus and leptomeninges, where they can exceed 150-fold. Furthermore, trihexosylceramide is present in CSF of FD patients, in contrast to normal CSF.

11.4 Pathogenetic Considerations

The basic defect in FD is a deficient activity of α-galactosidase, leading to a progressive accumulation of glycosphingolipids with terminal α-galactosyl residues in lysosomes. The gene encoding for the enzyme has been localized on the long arm of the X-chromosome and has been sequenced. Different mutations have been identified. In the male patients with classical FD (classical hemizygotes) there is no detectable enzyme activity and either no detectable enzyme protein or normal or decreased amounts of enzyme protein. In the latter case, presumably, the enzyme is altered and kinetically defective. In mild, atypical hemizygotes, some residual enzyme activity is found.

Glycosphingolipids are important constituents of plasma cell membranes and of some intracellular membranes including lysosomal membranes. The glycosphingolipids that accumulate in FD are neutral glycosphingolipids and have a terminal α-galactosyl moiety. The highest increase is found in trihexosylceramide or globotriaosylceramide and dihexosylceramide or digalactosylceramide. FD hemizygotes and heterozygotes, who have blood group B or AB, also accumulate B and B_1 glycosphingolipids, which are normal human erythrocyte antigens. Another neutral glycosphingolipid that can accumulate in FD is the P_1 blood group antigen.

The pattern of glycosphingolipid accumulation in FD differs from that in other glycosphingolipidoses. There is a very special cellular and tissue distribution of accumulated glycosphingolipids with particular involvement of vascular endothelium, smooth muscles and neurons. Within the nervous system the pattern of involved neurons is also very special. A number of explanations have been given for this distribution of neuronal storage. Site-specific differences in trihexosylceramide metabolism have been proposed. Absorption of high levels of trihexosylceramide from blood has been suggested as the source of glycosphingolipids in cells, as concentrations of this substance are much elevated in the blood of patients with FD. Anatomical location in areas of reduced blood-brain barrier could potentially promote neuronal absorption from blood, but not all involved neuronal groups are in such areas. Absorption of trihexosylceramide from the CSF into adjacent neurons could be a possible mechanism. Many of the involved neuronal groups are located adjacent to the CSF. There is, however, selective sparing of neighboring neuronal groups, similarly exposed to CSF. Selective uptake and transfer of trihexosylceramide by neurons could play a role.

The correlation of neurological complaints and lipid storage is hampered by the presence of a combination of neuronal storage, angiopathic infarcts in nervous tissue and deposition of glycosphingolipids in end-organs such as the sweat glands in the skin. The episodic limb pain typical of FD has been ascribed to dorsal root ganglia neuropathy, peripheral small fiber neuropathy, involvement of substantia gelatinosa neurons and peripheral nerve ischemia due to involvement of the vasa nervorum. Autonomic dysfunction could arise from involvement of the autonomic nevous system at either central or peripheral level but anhydrosis could also be explained by dysfunction of sweat glands. The episodic fever may be related to lesions of the hypothalamus. The clinical correlate of the cerebral neuronal glycosphingolipid deposition is unclear. Psychosis, personality changes and dementia have been described in FD but are not prominent phenomena. Seizures are rare. Apparently the accumulation of the glycosphingolipid in neurons is a problem of lesser importance than the accumulation in endothelial cells producing an occlusive angiopathy and cerebral infarction.

The white matter involvement in FD is of hypoxic-ischemic origin and not demyelinating in nature. However, in many cases the MR images demonstrate a predominant white matter involvement and resemble those of a demyelinating disorder.

11.5 Therapy

The pain in FD can in many cases be reduced by phenytoin and carbamazepine, alone or in combination. Care with regard to cardiac, pulmonary and central nervous system manifestations is only symptomatic. Renal insufficiency requires chronic hemodialysis and/or renal transplantation. In addition to correcting the chronic renal failure, kidney transplantation provides a source of α-galactosidase. Although a transient or sustained biochemical and/or clinical improvement has been reported in several patients, in others no positive effect could be demonstrated. Significant lipid deposition and allograft dysfunction have been reported several years after transplantation. Several patients, who underwent successful engraftment, expired after 10–15 years from complications of cardiac disease.

11.6 Magnetic Resonance Imaging

MRI in FD changes with the course of time. In older patients lesions tend to be more extensive and more confluent. In cases of mild cerebral affection multiple bilateral lacunar infarcts are seen (Fig. 11.1). These may occur anywhere in the brain, in both gray and white matter structures. In some patients an additional small rim of periventricular signal abnormality is seen. In older patients extensive confluent periventricular white abnormalities are seen in combination with small lacunar infarcts elsewhere in the brain, especially the basal nuclei. This pattern closely resembles the pattern of Binswanger's disease. Dilatation of the ventricles and cortical sulci may occur in severe disease.

In female heterozygotes, MRI is often normal. However, cases with periventricular white matter abnormalities in combination with lacunar infarctions elsewhere in the brain have also been described.

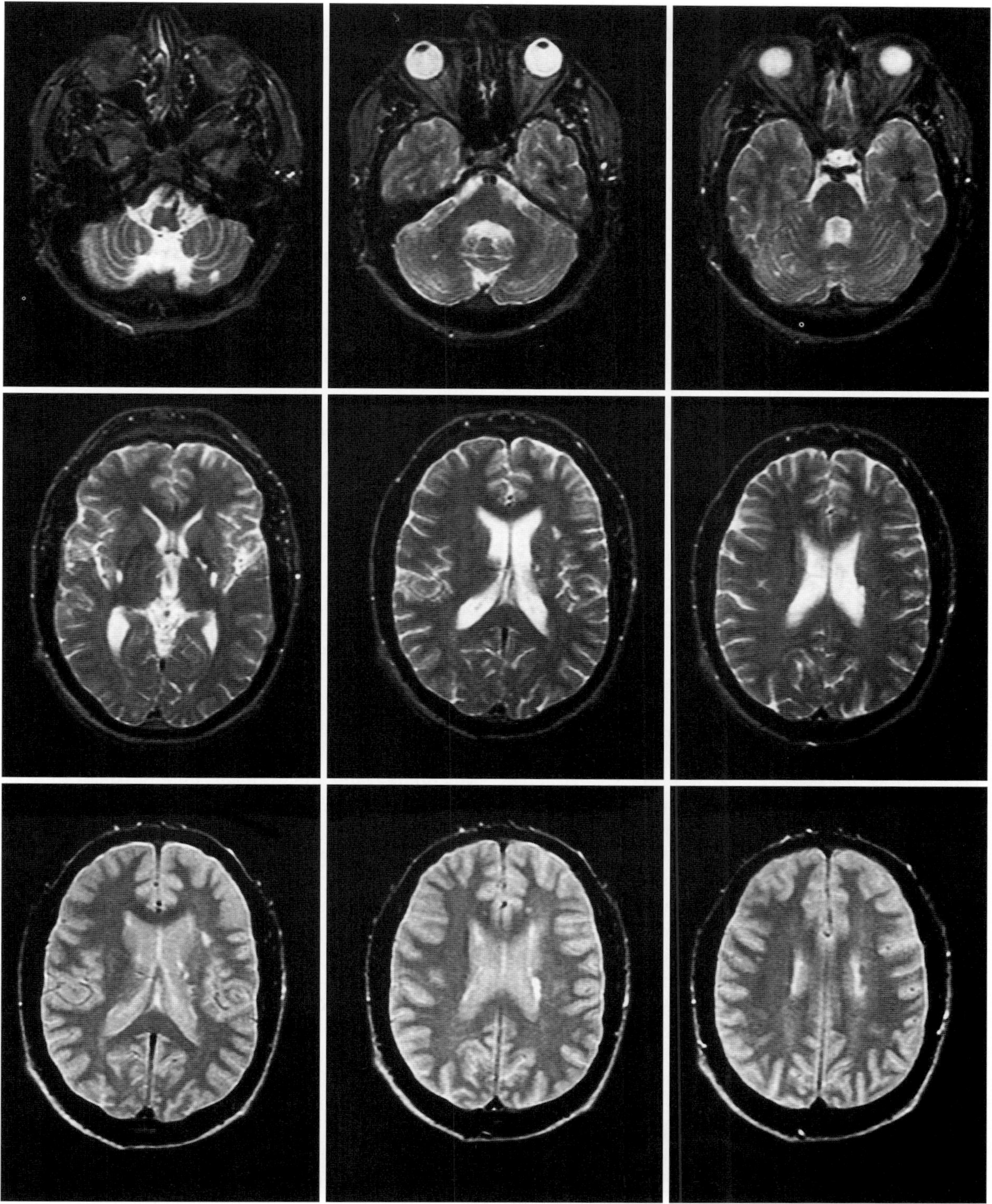

Fig. 11.1. T$_2$-weighted (*two upper rows*) and proton density (*lower row*) images of a 36-year-old male with FD. There are a few small isolated lesions, probably infarctions, in the cere-bellar hemispheres, in the putamen, the globus pallidus, and a small rim of hyperintense signal is seen around the ventri-cles

12 Fucosidosis

12.1 Clinical Features and Laboratory Investigations

Fucosidosis is a very rare, autosomal recessive neurovisceral storage disorder. Two clinical variants have been described.

Type I manifests before the end of the first year of life with frequent respiratory infections. From the age of about 1 year, mental and motor regression occurs. Initially, the children show signs of hypotonic weakness, but later hypertonia and spasticity develop. Seizures may occur. Neurological deterioration is progressive. In the end stage decorticate and decerebrate postures are seen. The children's facial appearance resembles that seen in mucopolysaccharidosis type I, with coarse features and a protruding tongue. Other similarities between these disorders are growth retardation and a mild to moderate dysostosis multiplex. Hepatosplenomegaly, cardiomegaly and anhydrosis with a marked increase in the sodium chloride content of sweat are present. Death occurs in the first decade of life.

Type II has a milder and more prolonged course. Mental retardation becomes evident between the ages of 1 and 2 years. The coarse facies, growth retardation and skeletal deformities are very similar to those seen in mucopolysaccharidosis type I. Angiokeratoma corporis diffusum is a very special characteristic of this type and is identical to that occurring in Fabry's disease. The content of sodium chloride in sweat is normal, although anhydrosis may be present. The patients suffer from similar but milder neurological signs than in type I. These patients survive much longer and often reach adulthood.

In the urine of patients with fucosidosis, an increased level of fucose-containing glycoconjugates is found, including fuco-oligosaccharides and fucoglycopeptides. There is evidence that fucosidosis types I and II can be distinguished by the pattern of urinary excretion. Cytoplasmic vacuolation in circulating lymphocytes is common in type I, less frequent in type II. Definite diagnosis is established by the demonstration of a deficiency of the lysosomal enzyme α-fucosidase in leukocytes, cultured fibroblasts or other tissue cells. Prenatal detection is possible by assessing enzyme activity in amniotic fluid cells.

12.2 Pathology

The brain may be enlarged or small, depending on the stage of the disease. The most striking feature is diffuse neuronal ballooning and neuronal loss. The cytoplasm of remaining neurons is packed with small vacuoles. These neuronal changes are seen everywhere in the gray matter. There are prominent white matter abnormalities, variably described as deficient myelination or severe demyelination reminiscent of a leukodystrophy. The white matter is gliotic.

Electron microscopy demonstrates that the vacuoles present in brain cells are membrane-bound. Many vacuoles are empty, but they may contain sparse floccular material or parallel lamellae. The vacuoles are present in neurons, astrocytes, and oligodendroglia.

Enlargement of many internal organs is found, including liver, spleen, heart, pancreas, thymus, thyroid and kidneys. Marked vacuolar storage is present in hepatocytes, Kupffer cells, and bile duct epithelium. The gall bladder may be "strawberry like" and nonfunctioning and the adrenals may be small and atrophic. Granulovacuolar storage is seen in almost all organs, including kidney, spleen, lymph nodes, lungs, heart, endocrine glands, and sweat glands. In addition, vacuoles are present in vascular endothelial cells, fibroblasts, bone marrow cells, and circulating lymphocytes.

12.3 Pathogenetic Considerations

Fucosidosis is caused by a deficiency of the lysosomal enzyme acidic α-L-fucosidase. This enzyme hydrolyzes α-fucose from glycolipids and glycoproteins. Fucose is a normal sugar constituent of many tissue mucopolysaccharides, plasma glycoproteins and tissue mucolipids. In the condition fucosidosis, tissues store fucose-rich glycolipids, sphingolipids, glycoproteins, oligosaccharides and mucopolysaccharides. The major part of the stored material consists of ceramide containing fucose and other hexoses. This material is derived from secretor antigens and blood group antigens which are fucose-rich glycolipids and glycoproteins. In the liver, there is a major accumulation of glycolipids. These are only present to a minor extent in

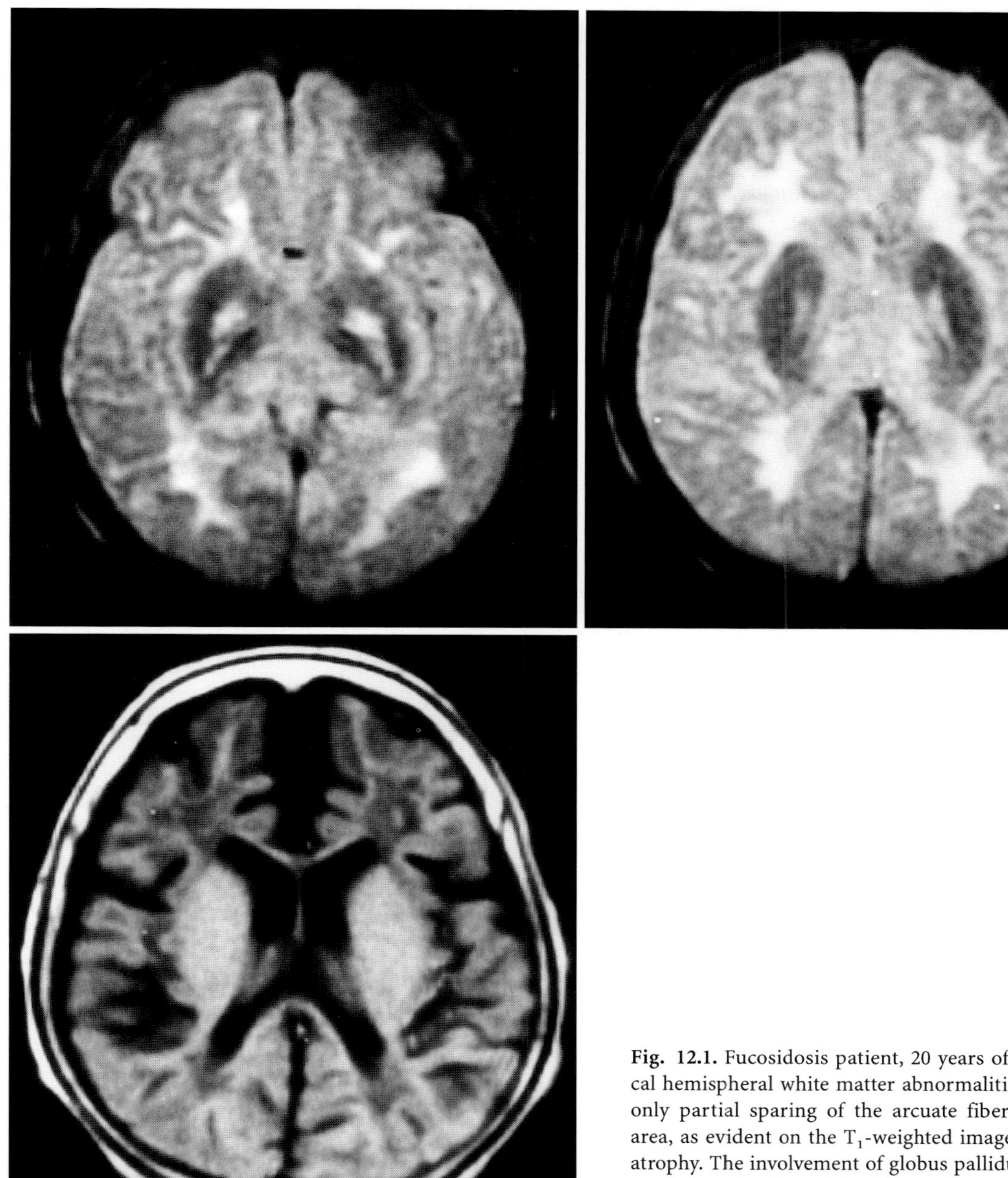

Fig. 12.1. Fucosidosis patient, 20 years of age. Symmetrical hemispheral white matter abnormalities are seen with only partial sparing of the arcuate fibers in the frontal area, as evident on the T_1-weighted image. There is some atrophy. The involvement of globus pallidus and thalamus is seen on the T_2-weighted images. Courtesy of Dr. N.R. Altman, Department of Radiology, Miami Children's Hospital, Miami, with permission

the brain, where oligosaccharides predominate as storage material.

The locus for α-fucosidase has been assigned to chromosome 1 at position 1p34.1–36.1 and is designated FUCA1. Fucosidosis mutations reside in FUCA1. A number of mutations have been identified. In addition, a region showing homology to the fucosidase gene was identified on chromosome 2 and designated FUCA1L. The FUCA1L region does not encode for fucosidase enzyme activity and is a so-called pseudogene. Because of the wide variation in clinical severity of fucosidosis, even within families, it is of interest to know whether the FUCA1L locus could encode for a protein product that might affect fucosidase enzyme activity. A third locus, FUCA2 on chromosome 6, is thought to regulate the fucosidase activity, although it does not encode for the fucosidase enzyme.

12.4 Therapy

Until now therapy has been entirely supportive. Bone marrow transplantation has been performed in fucosidase deficient animals. Following successful bone marrow engraftment, increased levels of fucosidase activity were found in leukocytes, plasma, neural and visceral tissue. The enzyme reaches viscera and peripheral nerves rapidly via phagocytes, but it takes months to achieve substantial levels of enzyme activity in the CNS. Long-term engraftment from an early age reduced the severity and slowed the progression of clinical neurological disease. Transplantation after the onset of clinical signs was not effective. To date, it is still uncertain whether early treatment will completely prevent the clinical signs of disease.

12.5 Magnetic Resonance Imaging

The MR images obtained in a fucosidosis patient show symmetrical white matter abnormalities, as was expected on the basis of neuropathological findings (Fig. 12.1). In addition, the white matter is atrophic with gliotic retraction of the cortex, and enlargement of CSF spaces. The subcortical arcuate fibers are only partially preserved. The globus pallidus and thalamus, nuclei relatively rich in myelin, have an abnormal signal intensity. The involvement of a combination of cerebral hemispheral white matter, globus pallidus and thalamus is reminiscent of Canavan disease and later onset variants of maple syrup urine disease, but in the latter two conditions the white matter is swollen, whereas it is atrophic in fucosidosis.

13 Mucopolysaccharidoses

13.1 Clinical Features and Laboratory Investigations

The mucopolysaccharidoses (MPS) are a family of heritable disorders caused by the deficiency of specific lysosomal enzymes involved in the degradation of mucopolysaccharides (glycosaminoglycans). The MPS are classified into six groups, which are further subdivided on the basis of genetic, biochemical and clinical findings (Table 13.1). These disorders share a number of characteristic clinical features, although there is considerable variability among the MPS types and within one type of MPS.

MPS type I, inherited as an autosomal recessive disease, can be divided into three subtypes: Hurler syndrome, Scheie's syndrome and Hurler-Scheie syndrome. The clinical phenotype in Hurler-Scheie disease is intermediate between the severe presentation of Hurler disease and the mild presentation of Scheie disease.

Children with Hurler syndrome appear normal at birth. They may be unusually large in infancy, but subsequent growth is retarded, finally resulting in dwarfism. During the first year of life mental retardation becomes evident, and after several years this is followed by progressive deterioration. Most children with Hurler syndrome manage to walk, but develop only limited language skills. They have a characteristic appearance. Prominent features are a relative macrocephaly, prominent forehead, coarse facial features, hypertelorism, flat nasal bridge, prominent bushy eyebrows, thick and dry hair, hirsutism, thick skin, enlarged tongue, hypertrophic gums, short and broad hands with stubby fingers, short and broad feet, exaggerated lumbar lordosis, thoracic kyphosis and a protuberant abdomen frequently with umbilical and inguinal hernias. On physical examination hepatosplenomegaly is found. Patients experience increasing joint stiffness and limitation of joint mobility, which may begin in early infancy. The preferentially affected joints are shoulders, fingers and wrists. Deformities become apparent with claw hands and flexion contractures of elbows and knees. Vision becomes impaired by progressive corneal clouding. Glaucoma, optic atrophy and pigmentary retina degeneration can contribute to the loss of vision. The majority of children have some degree of hearing loss, usually caused by a combination of conductive and neurosensory problems. Most patients have recurrent upper respiratory tract infections, copious nasal discharge and ear infections. Valvular heart disease is common. Occasionally patients have progressive communicating hydrocephalus caused by dysfunction of arachnoid villi and some patients have overt signs of increased intracranial pressure. Signs of spinal cord compression may occur but are infrequent.

Not all mentioned signs and symptoms are obligatory and there is a considerable clinical variability. However, progressive physical and neurological deterioration is the rule. Patients with Hurler syndrome rarely survive beyond the age of 16 years. Obstructive airway disease caused by deposition of mucopolysaccharides in soft tissue, respiratory infections and cardiac disease are the usual causes of death.

Scheie syndrome represents a mild variant of Hurler syndrome. Intelligence is normal. Common abnormalities are restricted mobility of joints, development of claw hands, hirsutism, variable deafness, corneal clouding and aortic valve disease. Stature is normal. Glaucoma and pigmentary retina degeneration may occur, which together with cornea opacities lead to impaired vision. Neurological problems may occur in the form of carpal tunnel syndrome and cervical cord compression by the thickened dura. Psychosis has been described in adults with Scheie syndrome. First abnormalities are usually noted in the second half of the first decade of life and the disease is slowly progressive.

Hurler-Scheie syndrome represents a variant with intermediate severity with onset of clinical signs and symptoms between 3 and 8 years. Most patients have normal or near-normal intelligence, but slowly progressive loss of mental capacities may occur. Coarsening of facial features, corneal clouding, joint stiffness and valvular cardiac disease are frequent. Cervical spinal cord compression may occur. Development of communicating hydrocephalus is rare. Psychosis may occur in adulthood. Most patients survive well into adulthood. Cardiac complications and upper airway obstruction are the most common causes of death.

MPS type II or Hunter syndrome is an X-linked disorder with two clinical phenotypes, a severe type and a mild type. The mild type is rarer than the severe type.

Table 13.1. Classification of the mucopolysaccharidoses

Number	Eponym	Enzyme Deficiency	Urinary glycosaminoglycan
MPS I H	Hurler	α-L-iduronidase	DS, HS
MPS I S	Scheie	α-L-iduronidase	DS, HS
MPS I H/S	Hurler-Scheie	α-L-iduronidase	DS, HS
MPS II	Hunter	Iduronate sulfatase	DS, HS
MPS III A	Sanfilippo A	Heparan N-sulfatase	HS
MPS III B	Sanfilippo B	α-N-acetylglucosaminidase	HS
MPS III C	Sanfilippo C	Acetyl-CoA: α-glucosaminide acyltransferase	HS
MPS III D	Sanfilippo D	N-acetylglucosamine 6-sulfatase	HS
MPS IV A	Morquio A	Galactose 6-sulfatase	KS, C-6-S
MPS IV B	Morquio B	β-galactosidase	KS
MPS V	no longer used	–	–
MPS VI	Maroteaux-Lamy	N-acetylgalactosamine 4-sulfatase	DS
MPS VII	Sly	β-glucuronidase	DS, HS, C-4-S, C-6-S
MPS VIII	no longer used	–	–

DS, dermatan sulfate; HS, heparan sulfate; KS, keratan sulfate; C-4-S, chondroitin-4-sulfate; C-6-S, chondroitin-6-sulfate

The most important distinguishing feature is the presence or absence of mental deterioration. In the severe type progressive intellectual decline occurs, whereas intellectual performance remains normal or relatively normal in the mild type. The age of onset of the severe form is usually between 1 and 4 years of age. Early abnormalities are coarse facial features, enlargement of the tongue, growth retardation, mental retardation, severe behavioral problems, joint stiffness, gibbus formation and skeletal deformities. Head growth is abnormally rapid initially, but slows down after several years. Retinal degeneration may occur, but there is no corneal clouding. Occasionally characteristic skin changes are found. They consist of pebbly, ivory-colored patches over the lower angle of the scapulae and sometimes over the pectoralis area, in the neck and on the lateral sides of upper arms and thighs. Progressive neurological impairment dominates the course of the disease. By the age of 6 years, developmental skills begin to plateau and to regress. By the age of 10 years, 90% of the patients are bed-ridden. The neurological deterioration may be worsened by progressive communicating hydrocephalus. This problem usually arises between 7 and 10 years. Upper and lower respiratory tract disease is common. Trachea stenosis may occur. Ear infections and progressive hearing impairment occur in most patients. There is a high incidence of hepatosplenomegaly and inguinal and umbilical hernias. Chronic and intractable diarrhea is a troublesome problem in many of the patients. Cardiac disease is present with valvular dysfunction, myocardial thickening, cardiac failure, pulmonary hypertension, coronary artery narrowing and myocardial infarction. In end-stage disease convulsions may occur. Respiratory problems in the form of infection or obstruction or cardiac problems superimposed on a condition of emaciation

are the usual causes of death. Death usually occurs between 8 and 15 years of age.

In the mild variant of Hunter syndrome, onset of disease is usually between 2 and 6 years. Coarse facial appearance is the commonest presenting feature. Intelligence is preserved and there are no behavioral problems. There are, however, obvious somatic problems: hepatosplenomegaly, cardiac symptoms primarily valvular in origin, upper and lower respiratory tract disease, tracheal stenosis, and inguinal and umbilical herniae. Diarrhea is less frequent than in severe Hunter syndrome. Hearing impairment is common. Subtle corneal opacities have been found. Retinal degeneration is much less marked than in severe Hunter syndrome. The picture of chronic papilledema has been observed in about 60% of the patients probably due to the deposition of glycosaminoglycans within the sclerae. The occurrence of hydrocephalus is exceptional. Head growth is, however, abnormally rapid with evident macrocephaly. Carpal tunnel syndrome is common. Death usually occurs in early adulthood, although survival into the fifth and sixth decade has been described. Death results primarily from cardiac problems, respiratory infections and upper respiratory airway obstruction.

Sanfilippo syndrome comprises four different diseases, MPS III A, B, C and D, which are caused by different enzyme deficiencies. Clinically, however, they are indistinguishable. Sanfilippo syndrome presents with great inter-and intrafamiliar heterogeneity. The clinical characteristics of the disease are relatively mild somatic features and severe, progressive mental deficiency. Early psychomotor development is usually slightly or moderately delayed. Speech development, in particular, is often slow and poor. Intellectual deterioration is usually evident by school age. Dementia occurs early and progresses rapidly in some patients, but is more gradual in others. Behavioral disturbances are often dramatic with extreme restlessness and hyperkinesis. Some patients are withdrawn and lose contact with their environment. Aggression is often present in stressful situations. Most of the children are too mentally disabled to attend nursery school, but some are able to attend primary school. Speech deteriorates, becomes slurred, the patient begins to stutter and eventually loses speech altogether. Motor functions are less frequently and less severely affected, but in some patients the gait becomes unstable with frequent falling. Facial changes are mild or absent in most of the patients. Height is usually normal and may even be above average in young patients. Some patients are macrocephalic, but most older patients have a normal head circumference and may even be microcephalic. Hepatomegaly is usual in younger patients, but is less frequent in older patients. Splenomegaly is rare. Other features that can be found are inguinal and umbilical herniae, coarse hair, hirsutism, hearing loss, kyphosis, scoliosis, and mild contractures of joints. Neurological findings are inconsistent; they may include hypotonia, hypertonia, hyporeflexia, hyperreflexia, tetraparesis and muscular atrophy. Corneas are usually not cloudy, but pigmentary degeneration of the retina may occur. Some patients develop epilepsy. Many patients develop swallowing difficulties with time, necessitating tube feeding at later stages. Infections and unexplained diarrhea are frequent problems. Cachexia and aspiration pneumonia are common causes of death. Death usually occurs in the second or third decade.

Morquio syndrome is characterized by marked skeletal involvement and preserved intellectual capacities. Two types can be distinguished, MPS IV A and MPS IV B, characterized by different enzyme deficiencies. Presenting features of Morquio syndrome are growth retardation with dwarfism, short neck and trunk, pigeon breast deformity, kyphosis, hyperlordosis, scoliosis, genua valga, valgus deformity of the elbow, and ulnar deviation and broadening of the wrist. The tone appears to be decreased due to ligamentous laxity. Decreased joint mobility may occur in the large joints. The teeth are usually widely spaced and there are numerous minute pits in the abnormally thin enamel causing the surface of the teeth to be rough and discolored. Facial features are usually coarse and the mouth wide. Corneal opacities may be present but are usually mild. Hepatomegaly, cardiac valvular abnormalities and inguinal and umbilical hernias may occur. Intelligence is usually normal or just below normal. Neurological complaints are caused by compression of the medulla or spinal cord due to atlantoaxial subluxation and diffuse thickening of the cervical dura. The signs of cervical myelopathy are usually slowly progressive, but occasionally acute tetraplegia occurs. Car-

diac valvular disease and cervical myelopathy contribute to death, which usually occurs in late childhood or early adulthood. Survival into the fourth and the fifth decade has been described. As a rule, MPS IV B has a later onset and slower course than MPS IV A, but severe forms of MPS IV B and mild forms of MPS IV A have been described. A variant of MPS IV B has been described with progressive mental handicap.

Maroteaux-Lamy syndrome or MPS VI clinically resembles Hurler disease, but intelligence is preserved. The disease usually presents in the third year of life and is characterized by growth retardation, coarse facial features similar to but milder than those seen in Hurler syndrome, corneal clouding, joint contractures, claw hand deformities, kyphosis, protrusion of the sternum, hepatosplenomegaly, umbilical and inguinal hernias and mild hirsutism. Nerve entrapment syndromes may occur, in particular carpal tunnel syndrome. Myelopathy secondary to thickening of the cervical dura occurs frequently with the insidious development of spastic tetraparesis. Exceptional cases with mental retardation have been described. Cardiac valvular dysfunction resulting in cardiac failure is the most common cause of death. In the severe forms death usually occurs in the second or third decade, but patients with milder variants of the disease have a longer life expectancy.

Sly syndrome or MPS VII is also characterized by considerable clinical variation. In the severe neonatal form, hydrops foetalis and dysostosis multiplex are prominent early features; the course is rapidly fatal. The other end of the clinical spectrum is formed by patients with very mild clinical symptomatology with normal intelligence, normal height, absent coarse facial features and minimal skeletal abnormalities. The classical form of the disease is characterized by coarse facial features, hepatosplenomegaly, diastasis recti, umbilical and inguinal herniae, thoracolumbar gibbus, short stature, metatarsus adductus, and variably present corneal clouding. Respiratory infections are frequent. Early psychomotor development is normal, but after 2 or 3 years of life retardation becomes evident. Retardation is usually moderate, but severe mental deficiency has also been reported. Epilepsy is rare.

Radiograms show skeletal changes in all MPS variants, but the dysostosis multiplex varies in severity. Typical findings are cortical sclerosis and thickening of the skull which may involve the base and the vault. The pituitary fossa is often elongated and J-shaped. Teeth are widely spaced. The head is often scaphocephalic and there is early closure of cranial sutures, in particular the sagittal and lambdoid sutures. Orbits are shallow. Basilar impression may occur. In MPS IV odontoid dysplasia is a universal finding with a tendency for atlanto-axial subluxation. Various types of vertebral dysplasia are seen. Clavicles are short and stubby. There is anterior flaring of the ribs, hypoplasia of the inferior portion of the iliac bones, flared iliac wings, oblique acetabular margins and a valgus deformity of the hips. Long bones are short and broad with metaphyseal and epiphyseal deformities. Cortical margins are wavy and scalloped. Metacarpals and phalanges are widened and shortened.

The MPS variants were originally classified according to the types of glycosaminoglycans excreted in the urine in addition to consideration of clinical features. In MPS I and II dermatan sulfate and heparan sulfate are excreted, but inheritance is autosomal recessive in MPS I and X-linked in MPS II. MPS III is associated with excretion of heparan sulfate. MPS IV is characterized by excretion of keratan sulfate, MPS VI by excretion of dermatan sulfate. MPS VII is associated with excretion of dermatan sulfate, heparan sulfate and chondroitin sulfate. A problem in the diagnosis of MPS IV is that keratosulfaturia can be fairly easily missed. Special sensitive techniques are required for the detection of urinary keratan sulfate excretion. An additional problem of diagnosis in MPS IV is that keratan sulfate excretion may be diminished both early and late in the disease process.

Peripheral blood cells may also show changes related to the specific type of MPS. Alder-Reilly granulation, a coarse reddish-violet granulation present in neutrophils in blood films stained with May-Grünwald-Giemsa or Wright stain, is found in MPS VI and MPS VII. Vacuolated lymphocytes may be present in MPS IV B. Occasionally vacuolated lymphocytes with basophilic inclusions can be seen in any of the MPS variants. Metachromatic inclusions in lymphocytes are most prominent in MPS III. On the whole, however, vacuolation of lymphocytes is not usually prominent in MPS. Bone marrow aspirates will reveal the presence of storage cells.

Definitive diagnosis of the MPS is established by enzyme assays. Prenatal diagnosis is possible for all MPS variants on cultured amniotic fluid cells or chorionic villus cells. Prenatal diagnosis poses a problem in Hunter syndrome because of the X-linked mode of inheritance. When the cells obtained are derived from only a few cell clones which predominantly express the mutant X-chromosome, a very low enzyme activity may be detected in a carrier female fetus. Hence, sex determination is essential in prenatal diagnosis of Hunter syndrome.

13.2 Pathology

Mental deficiency is an important clinical characteristic of MPS I H, MPS II, MPS III, and MPS VII. Neuropathological findings in the syndromes causing mental deficiency are similar. In particular neuronal storage is confined to the MPS variants with intellectual problems.

The skull is sometimes grossly thickened. The leptomeninges are thickened and opalescent. There is a marked increase in connective tissue elements and there are numerous mononuclear cells containing large cytoplasmic vacuoles. These cells stain positive for glycosaminoglycans. The blood vessels running over the surface of the brain are prominent and enveloped by the thickened leptomeninges which extend deep into the brain parenchyma.

The weight of the brain is usually at the upper limit of normal or even slightly increased. The external surface is normal or the gyri are slightly atrophic. At the cut surfaces increased perivascular spaces with increased volumes of connective tissue are evident. Hydrocephalus is a common finding caused by impaired circulation of CSF through the subarachnoid spaces or dysfunction of the arachnoid granulations.

Within the brain there are two main pathological abnormalities which may occur in MPS: increase in perivascular connective tissue and neuronal storage.

The neuronal changes are ubiquitous but their extent varies in different parts of the brain. Generally, the large nerve cells in the cerebral cortex and brain stem are the most severely affected. The cytoplasm of neurons is distended by an excessive amount of accumulated material, which stains positively with various Sudan dyes and PAS, corresponding to the presence of gangliosides. Variable numbers of neurons are in various stages of degeneration and shrinkage. Loss of nerve cells is usually mild. Electron microscopic examination of neurons shows several types of inclusions. The most characteristic are the zebra bodies. Zebra bodies are single membrane-bound vacuoles filled with stacked transverse lamellae, separated at intervals by larger clear spaces. In rare instances the lamellae have a concentric arrangement and look very similar to the membranous cytoplasmic bodies seen in the gangliosidoses. Granular inclusions are less common than zebra bodies. Transitional forms between zebra bodies and bodies with granular material may occur. Inclusions resembling lipofuscin granules are infrequent. All inclusion bodies have acid phosphatase activity indicative of their lysosomal origin.

In MPS the formation of meganeurites has been reported as well as the formation of ectopic secondary neurites. These are identical to those described in GM_1 and GM_2 gangliosidosis.

The cerebral white matter and basal ganglia are characterized by perivascular lacunation. Radially oriented, round to oval cystic white matter abnormalities are found at cut surfaces. On microscopic examination, the adventitia of vessels is abnormally thick and consists of a delicate fibrous network with numerous large cells containing large clear inclusions caused by storage of glycosaminoglycans. On electron microscopy they appear empty except for a variable amount of granular dispersed material. A few lamellar-lipid inclusions resembling the zebra bodies are also observed. Loss of myelin may occur in the cyst walls but is not conspicuous. On occasion, focal areas of demyelination have been described. Oligodendrocytes contain some abnormal, clear inclusions.

In visceral organs a variable degree of cellular vacuolation is seen caused by glycosaminoglycan accumulation. Hepatocytes and Kupffer cells store glycosaminoglycans, in particular in MPS I, II and III, in which hepatic fibrosis may occur. In addition to glycosaminoglycans, Kupffer cells may store gangliosides. Glycosaminoglycan storage is found in lymph nodes, spleen, kidney and the heart. Cardiac valvular dysfunction is caused by the presence of large foamy cells and an increase of connective tissue. Fibroblasts in skin, cornea and conjunctiva, endothelial cells of the vascular system, smooth muscle cells, skeletal muscle cells, macrophages, epithelial cells of distal and collecting tubules of the kidney, chondrocytes, osteoblasts and periosteal cells of bone and cartilage show glycosaminoglycan storage. There are irregularities in enchondral ossification with variations in size and shape of the diaphyses of the long bones, periosteal fibrosis and various degrees of fibrosis and lipid storage in marrow tissue.

13.3 Chemical Pathology

Chemical analysis of the brain and leptomeninges reveals a highly increased concentration of glycosaminoglycans. The level of glycosaminoglycans is much higher in the meninges than in brain tissue, where the largest amounts of glycosaminoglycans are found in vascular and perivascular tissue. In MPS I and MPS II, it is mainly dermatan sulphate that is stored, whereas in MPS III it is mainly heparan sulphate.

In MPS I, MPS II and MPS III, chemical studies demonstrate that in neuronal perikarya glycosaminoglycans and gangliosides are increased. Ganglioside storage involves the gangliosides GM_2, GM_3 and GD_3. These substances together amount to 65% of the gangliosides stored in neurons. The ganglioside storage is comparable in magnitude to the amounts stored in the gangliosidoses.

13.4 Pathogenetic Considerations

Glycosaminoglycans, formerly called mucopolysaccharides, are degradation products derived by proteolytic cleavage of proteoglycans. Many enzymes are necessary in the intralysosomal stepwise degradation of each of the glycosaminoglycans, dermatan sulfate, heparan sulfate, keratan sulfate and chondroitin sulfate. The respective enzyme deficiencies in the various forms of MPS are listed in Table 13.1. α-L-Iduronidase the enzyme that is deficient in MPS I, hydrolyzes terminal α-L-iduronate residues from dermatan sulfate and heparan sulfate. Iduronate sulfatase, the enzyme that is deficient in MPS II, removes a sulfate group from L-iduronate present in dermatan sulfate and heparan sulfate. In a concerted action, the four enzymes related to MPS III accomplish removal of the variably substituted α-linked glucosamine residues from heparan sulfate. Heparan-N-sulfatase, the enzyme that is deficient in MPS III A, removes sulfate groups linked to the amino group of glucosamine. The enzyme is important in the breakdown of heparan sulfate. The enzyme is also called sulfamate sulfohydrolase or sulfamidase. α-N-Acetylglucosaminidase, the enzyme deficient in MPS III B, removes N-acetylglucosamine residues in heparan sulfate. Acetyl-CoA: α-glucosamide acetyltransferase is deficient in MPS III C. It catalyzes the acylation of glucosamine amino groups that have become exposed by the action of heparan N-sulfatase. After the acylation of glucosamine amino groups, α-N-acetylglucosaminidase removes the N-acetylglucosamine group. N-acetyl-glucosamine 6-sulfatase is deficient in MPS III D. This enzyme desulfates 6-sulfated N-acetylglucosamine residues of heparan sulfate and keratan sulfate. Since hexosaminidase A can bypass the block in the degradation of keratan sulfate, only the block in the degradation of heparan sulfate is important. Galactose 6-sulfatase is deficient in MPS IV A. It cleaves sulfate from 6-sulfated galactose residues of keratan sulfate and 6-sulfated N-acetylgalactosamine residues of chondroitin 6-sulfate. β-Galactosidase is deficient in MPS IV B. It removes galactose residues of keratan sulfate. N-acetylgalactosamine 4-sulfatase, also called arylsulfatase B, is deficient in MPS VI. It hydrolyzes the sulfate groups in the 4-position of N-acetylgalactosamine residues in dermatan sulfate and chondroitin 4-sulfate. Urinary chondroitin 4-sulfate is not elevated in MPS VI, probably because the enzymatic block is bypassed by the action of lysosomal hyaluronidase. β-Glucuronidase, the enzyme deficient in MPS VII, removes β-glucuronate residues present in dermatan sulfate, heparan sulfate and chondroitin sulfate.

All MPS types have autosomal recessive inheritance, with the exception of MPS II which is X-linked. The loci for several genes encoding enzymes of glycosaminoglycan degradation have been determined. The relevant gene for MPS I has been localized on chromosome 22, for MPS II the distal region of the X-chromosome, for MPS IV B (as well as GM_1 gangliosidosis) chromosome 3, for MPS VI chromosome 5, and for MPS VII chromosome 7.

There is a striking clinical variability within all MPS subtypes. An example is found in MPS I, in which Hurler syndrome is the most severe variant, Scheie syndrome the mild variant and the Hurler-Scheie syndrome in between. The Scheie syndrome was previously classified as a separate disease entity, MPS V, until it became known that deficiency of the same enzyme underlies both Hurler syndrome and Scheie syndrome. It is probable that the clinical heterogeneity is caused by the presence of different mutant alleles, the Hurler patients being homozygous for a "severe" allele, Scheie patients being homozygous for a "mild" allele. Hurler-Scheie patients could be compound heterozygotes. It is, however, improbable that there are only two mutant alleles. It is reasonable to assume that there are multiple mutations and deletions with homozygosity and compound heterozygosity with variable residual enzyme activities, which are responsible for a wide clinical variation within well as between clinical subgroups. A multiplicity of alleles has already partly been detected in each of the other MPS types. Environmental factors and modifying genes may also play a role in clinical severity, being in particular responsible for intrafamilial variability. On the other hand, when different mutations are present in the same family, this may also lead to differences in clinical severity within one family. A special phenomenon is the presence of clinical disease in female MPS II carriers, caused by unbalanced inactivation of the normal X-chromosome.

The same enzyme deficiency underlies MPS IV B and GM_1 gangliosidosis. β-Galactosidase hydrolyzes terminal β-linked galactose residues found in GM_1 ganglioside, glycoproteins, oligosaccharides as well as keratan sulfate. Deficiency of enzyme activity toward all substrates causes GM_1 gangliosidosis. A mutation that predominantly impairs catalytic activity towards keratan sulfate results in MPS IV B.

In the absence of specific enzymes, non-degraded or partially degraded glycosaminoglycans accumulate in lysosomes and are partially excreted in urine. Glycosaminoglycans normally constitute the "ground substance" of connective tissue. They are attached to protein in proteoglycans, the macromolecular forms in which they exist in connective tissue. In MPS mainly bone and connective tissue are affected, causing the most characteristic clinical signs and symptoms: growth retardation, dysostosis multiplex, coarse facial features, joint stiffness, corneal opacities, valvular heart disease and upper airway narrowing. In the CNS storage of glycosaminoglycans also occurs in connective tissue elements. Thickening of the leptomeninges may lead to hydrocephalus, and to compression of the spinal cord in the cervical region resulting in cervical myelopathy. Subluxation of the odontoid process can contribute to spinal cord compression. Storage in perineural tissue may lead to entrapment neuropathy.

Within the brain, glycosaminoglycans are stored in the tissue around vessels.

In addition to glycosaminoglycans, there is evidence of accumulation of gangliosides (GM_2, GM_3 and GD_3) in the brain of MPS patients, especially in MPS I, II and III. Intralysosomal storage of gangliosides leads to the formation of zebra bodies and membranous cytoplasmic bodies, similar to those seen in GM_1 and GM_2 gangliosidoses. The question is what causes the storage of gangliosides. Apart from β-galactosidase none of the enzymes involved in MPS plays a role in ganglioside breakdown. It has been demonstrated, however, that the activity of several additional lysosomal enzymes is reduced in the MPS, probably as a result of inhibition by the accumulating glycosaminoglycans and this decreased enzyme activity may lead to ganglioside storage. The accumulation of gangliosides is probably responsible for the formation of meganeurites and ectopic secondary neurites, as these are also seen in GM_1 and GM_2 gangliosidoses. It is striking that the ganglioside storage is only found in MPS subtypes characterized by mental deficiency. These phenomena are most probably related.

13.5   Therapy

Until now the results of enzyme replacement therapy have been disappointing. Infusion of plasma or leukocytes has had no persisting beneficial effects; at most, some transient improvement of joint mobility. Fibroblast transplantation or human amnion membrane implantation were not effective. There is evidence that bone marrow transplantation may result in an improvement of somatic complaints with decrease in joint stiffness, decrease in hepatosplenomegaly, clearing of the cornea and prevention of (further) skeletal abnormalities. There is evidence that in disorders asociated with intellectual deterioration, further deterioration can be halted or retarded by bone marrow transplantation, but already existing pathology cannot be reversed. This observation forms an argument for transplantation at an early age. Gene transfer is still in an experimental stage.

Symptomatic treatment is very important in MPS. Corneal transplantation can be performed in cases of corneal clouding, however, poor vision caused by retina degeneration or optic atrophy cannot be reversed. Hearing aids may be helpful in cases of significant hearing loss. Exercise to optimize joint mobility should be started early. Airway obstruction may be alleviated by tonsillectomy and adenoidectomy, tracheostomy sometimes being required. Cardiac valve replacement is occasionally performed in cases of valvular disease. Progressive hydrocephalus may require ventriculoperitoneal shunting. Cervical fusion to prevent atlantoaxial

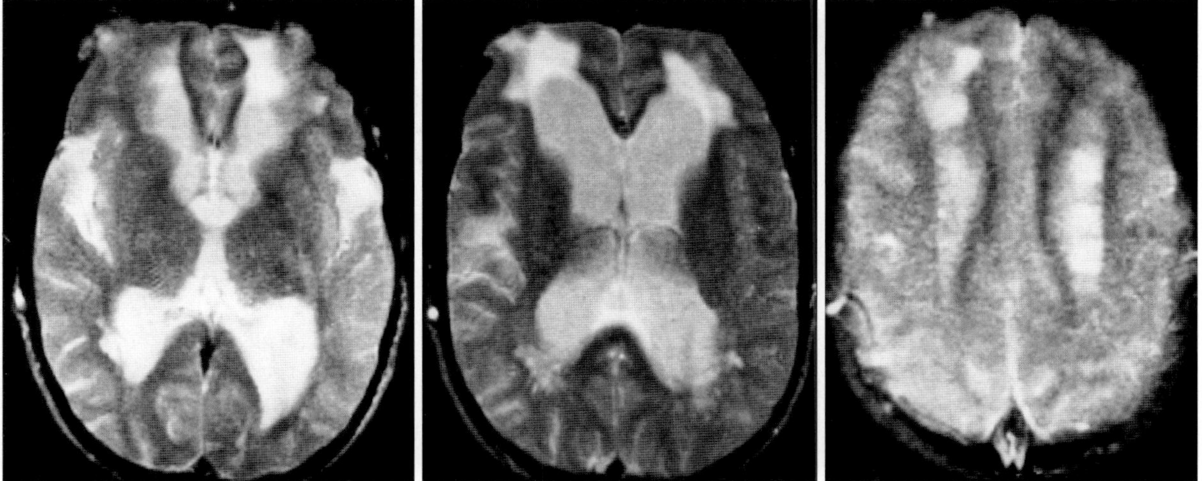

Fig. 13.1. 17-year-old male with Hurler-Scheie syndrome (MPS I). T$_2$-weighted MR images show extensive involvement of the white matter in the frontal periventricular region and in the centrum semiovale. The ventricles are greatly enlarged. Courtesy of Paolo Tortori Donati, Genua, Italy, with permission

subluxation is performed to prevent or treat cervical spinal cord compression, especially in MPS IV. Anesthesia poses a particular problem in MPS. Atlantoaxial instability requires careful positioning and avoidance of hyperextension of the neck. Another problem may be difficulty in maintaining an adequate airway during anesthesia and postoperative airway obstruction. Sudden cardiovascular collapse may be caused by a combination of valvular disease, myocardial thickening, systemic and pulmonary hypertension and narrowing of coronary arteries, all contributing to congestive heart failure.

13.6 Magnetic Resonance Imaging

The MRI abnormalities found in MPS vary greatly in severity from absent or negligible to severe, with a marked variation among sibs. However, in themselves, the abnormalities are fairly homogeneous.

Over the years many patients develop white matter abnormalities. These consist of multiple small spot-like lesions dispersed in the white matter with a predilection for the parietal and occipital white matter. The signal intensity follows the signal intensity of CSF, indicative of the cystic nature of the lesions. The cystic areas often have a radial orientation from the subependymal region toward the cortex (Fig. 13.2). Also, in the corpus callosum punched-out cystic areas are often present, best visualized on the sagittal images (Fig. 13.4). These cystic white matter lesions represent the perivascular lacunae seen on histopathological examination. In addition, T$_2$-weighted images may show spot-like hyperintense areas, of which the signal inten-

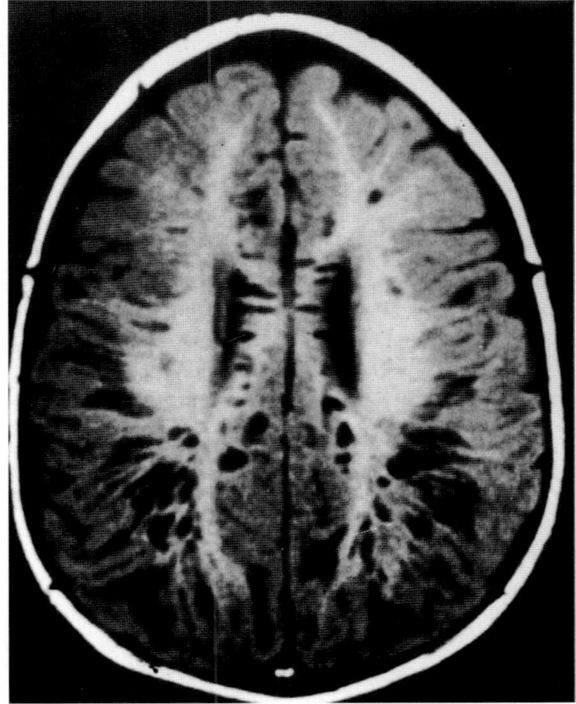

Fig. 13.2. Patient with Hurler syndrome (MPS I). The MR shows the characteristic widening of the Virchow-Robin spaces, where mucopolysaccharides accumulate in phagocytic cells. Courtesy of Harwood-Nash and Blaser (1991), with permission

sity does not parallel that of CSF on any sequences (Fig. 13.1). These areas may become more extensive and confluent, and probably reflect demyelination and gliosis, also seen on histopathological examination.

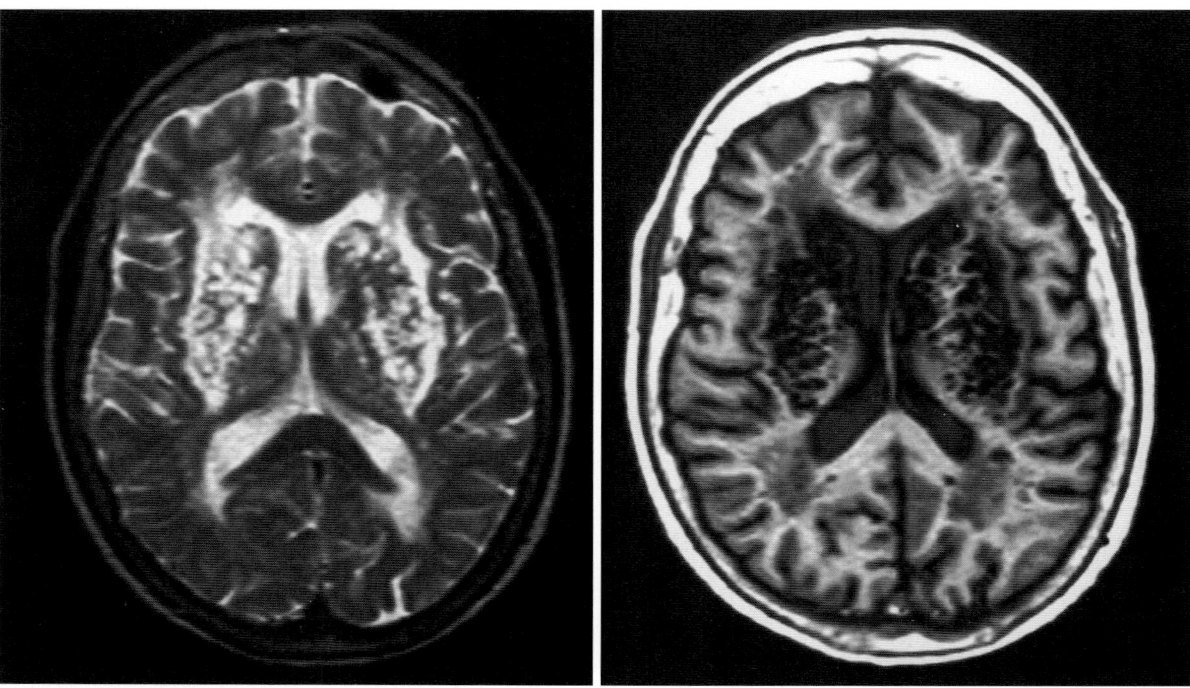

Fig. 13.3. A 44-year-old male with Hunter syndrome (MPS II). The MR images show the typical honeycomb structure of the basal ganglia

MRI and CT have demonstrated that white matter abnormalities may occur in all MPS variants. MRI may show a delay in myelination in young children.

A second frequent observation consists of ventricular enlargement (Fig. 13.1), with or without accompanying enlargement of subarachnoid spaces. The ventricular enlargement is of variable severity and is in some cases progressive. Some of the patients appear to have enlarged CSF spaces on the basis of diffuse atrophy of the brain parenchyma. In many cases the enlargement of the CSF spaces is caused by hydrocephalus, as a consequence of disturbed CSF resorption. Signs of hydrocephalus are upward bulging of the lateral ventricles, depression of the floor of the third ventricle and elevation of the corpus callosum. Progressive hydrocephalus may contribute to the periventricular white matter abnormalities. Enlargement of CSF spaces may occur in all MPS variants.

In exceptional cases abnormalities are seen in the basal ganglia. A honeycomb-like appearance of thalamus and basal ganglia has been reported in MPS I and MPS II (Fig. 13.3).

MRI of the cervico-occipital region (Fig. 13.4) often shows thickening of the dura at the cranio-cervical junction which causes subarachnoid space narrowing and spinal cord compression in some patients. In MPS IV, atlantoaxial subluxation may contribute to the spinal cord compression. This subluxation is the result of dysplasia or absence of the odontoid process and laxity of the transverse odontoid ligament. Gibbus formation, most marked in MPS IV, may cause thoracic cord compression.

The images may also show airway compression due to soft tissue thickening around the pharynx.

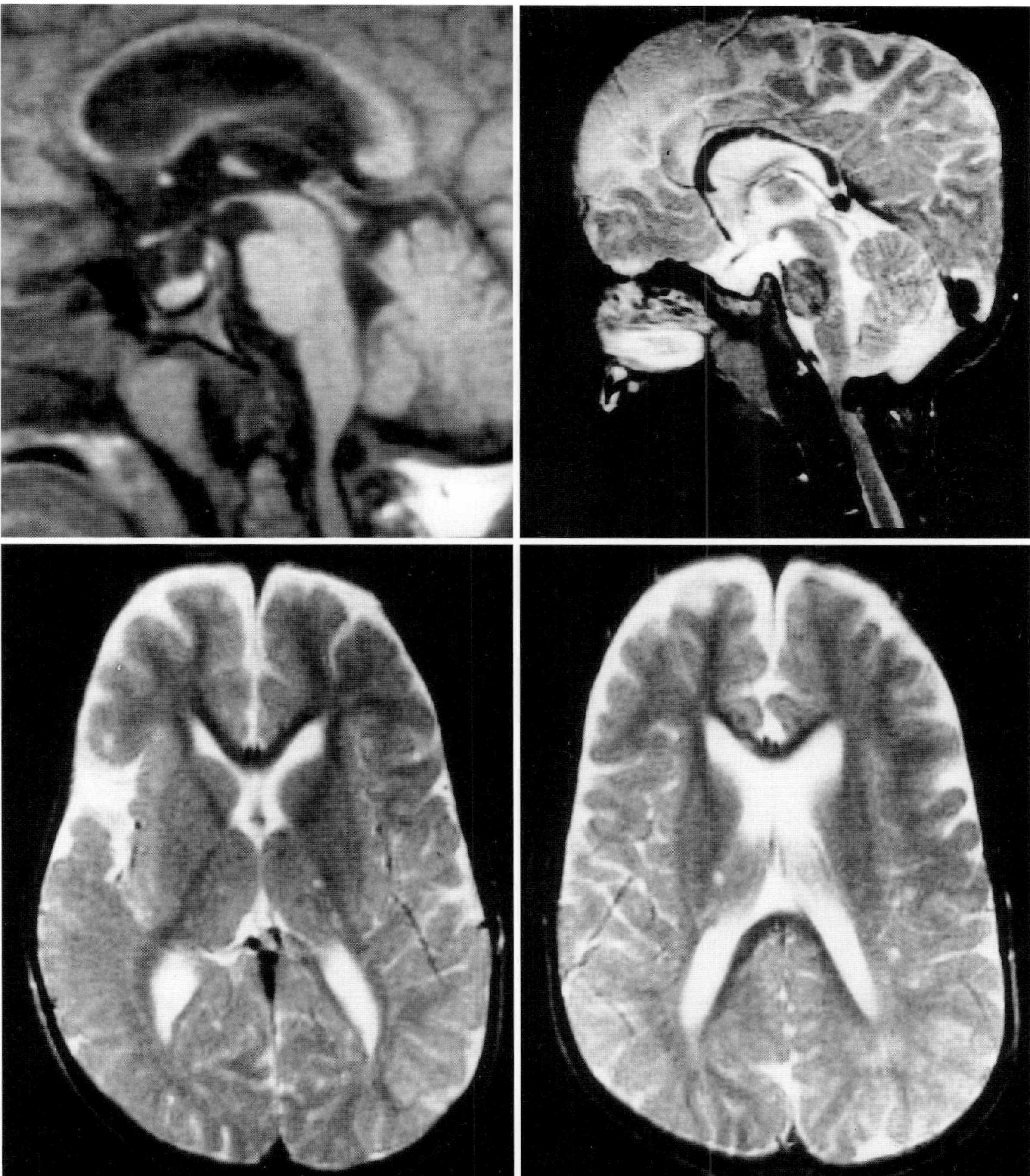

Fig. 13.4. 5 year old boy with Morquio's syndrome (MPS IV). The midsagittal image shows the intradural mucopolysaccharide deposits, leading to severe narrowing of the arachnoid space at the level of the cranio-cervical junction. The T_2-weighted transverse images at the ventricular level show some small hyperintense spots, indicative of widened perivascular spaces. The lower border of the corpus callosum is irregular due to the presence of cystic spaces. Courtesy of Paolo Tortori Donati, Genua, Italy, with permission

Peroxisomes are organelles that are present in virtually all human cell types. Their diameter varies between 0.5 and 1.5 μm. Morphologically, peroxisomes are differentiated from mitochondria by their single membrane, electron-dense fine granular and homogeneous matrix and absence of cristae. They can also be differentiated from lysosomes, which often contain vacuoles and various inclusions, and have a positive acid phospatase reaction on histochemistry, whereas peroxisomes are positive in reactions which show the presence of catalase. The size and abundance of peroxisomes and their enzyme content vary considerably. A striking feature of peroxisomes is that their enzymes can be induced and that the whole organelle can proliferate in response to many stimuli including dietary, hormonal and other physiological changes. The most profound proliferations are caused by hypolipidemic drugs. In liver and kidney, peroxisomes are normally present in high numbers, whereas in skin fibroblasts relatively few peroxisomes are present. Peroxisomes are also numerous in cells specialized in lipid metabolism. In the nervous system peroxisomes are more abundant in the early postnatal period than in adults. Oligodendrocytes contain peroxisomes during the period of active myelination and the organelles can be demonstrated in the cellular processes that form the myelin sheath. Peroxisomes are required for the synthesis of essential myelin constituents.

Both peroxisomal membrane proteins and peroxisomal matrix proteins are encoded for by nuclear genes and synthesized on free polyribosomes in the cellular cytosol. The newly synthesized proteins are imported into preexisting peroxisomes. This leads to progressive enlargement of the organelle, which then divides to form new peroxisomes. Most peroxisomal enzymes are located inside the organelle; some, including the enzyme involved in activation of fatty acids for subsequent β-oxidation and enzymes involved in the biosynthesis of ether lipids, are located in the peroxisomal membrane. A number of integral peroxisomal membrane proteins has been identified. The function of most of these proteins remains to be elucidated. Some of them are probably necessary for the assembly of functional peroxisomes. There is evidence that several proteins are involved in transmembrane transport. The

bulk of evidence suggests that peroxisomes have a nonpermeable membrane and that there are energy requiring uptake systems for both small molecules and larger proteins.

Peroxisomal proteins are generally synthesized in their final form, without cleavable amino-terminal targeting sequences as found on most secretory and mitochondrial proteins. The topogenic information directing proteins to peroxisomes is present in the mature polypeptides. The best known targeting signal which directs proteins to the peroxisome, is contained in a sequence of three amino acids present in the carboxy-terminal of the protein, serine-lysine-leucine (SKL). There is evidence that only a limited number of substitutions can be made within the SKL sequence without eliminating its activity. Many, but not all, peroxisomal proteins contain a carboxy-terminal SKL or SKL variant. It is evident that the SKL sequence is not the only peroxisomal targeting signal and several proteins are targeted to the peroxisome via another mechanism. Enzymes lacking the SKL sequence are very long-chain fatty acyl-CoA synthetase and thiolase. Thiolase is exceptional as it is produced as a larger precursor carrying an amino-terminal peptide extension. There is evidence that this presequence has peroxisomal targeting information. This presequence is cleaved on maturation. Peroxisomal integral membrane proteins also lack the SKL targeting sequence. The topogenic signals for these proteins are unknown. Also cytosolic factors are probably involved in the transport of peroxisomal proteins as binding proteins.

Originally peroxisomes were thought to play only a limited role in human cells. At least 40 enzymes have now been shown to have a peroxisomal localization, and it has been demonstrated that peroxisomes play an essential role in a large variety of anabolic and catabolic reactions. Peroxisomes have a variable enzymatic composition depending on the tissue, stage of development, and presence of substrates and chemical agents.

Peroxisomes contain enzymes for a simple respiratory pathway: oxidases and catalase. Oxidases use oxygen to oxidize a variety of substrates and thereby produce hydrogen peroxide as a reaction product, which is highly toxic. The hydrogen peroxide is efficiently converted to water and oxygen by catalase, which is present in a high concentration. The organelle was called peroxisome because of the presence of these peroxide-based reactions. These reactions protect cells against hydrogen peroxide by compartimentalization of most hydrogen peroxide metabolism within the organelle.

One of the major functions of peroxisomes is the β-oxidative chain-shortening of fatty acids. The fatty acids are activated by acyl-CoA synthetase, also called acyl-CoA ligase, at the site of the peroxisomal membrane. Fatty acids are converted to their corresponding acyl-CoA esters, which are transported into the peroxisomal matrix. Subsequently, acyl-CoA oxidase produces double-bonded, enoic fatty acids and hydrogen peroxide. The enoic acids are then hydroxylated and oxidized to keto acyl acids by trifunctional protein, an enzyme which has both 2-enoyl-CoA hydratase and 3-hydroxy acyl-CoA dehydrogenase activities necessary for these conversions. The enzyme 3-ketoacyl-CoA thiolase then splits the keto acyl-CoA, formed by trifunctional protein, into a molecule of acetyl-CoA and fatty acyl-CoA which is two carbon atoms shorter than the original acid.

The peroxisomal fatty acid β-oxidation system functions in a manner similar to that of the mitochondrial system with respect to degrading of fatty acids by two carbon units (acetyl-CoA) per cycle. However, the two β-oxidation systems differ with respect to substrate specificity, sensitivity to electron transport inhibitions, enzyme composition and requirement for carnitine. The peroxisomal oxidases are free of the constraints imposed by respiratory control which regulates mitochondrial activity. Consequently, they may function relatively independently of cellular energy status and may be active even when the intracellular ATP/ADP ratio is high. Import of fatty acids into peroxisomes is not dependent upon carnitine, whereas in mitochondria carnitine is required for the passage of fatty acids through the mitochondrial membrane. With respect to energy conservation, mitochondrial β-oxidation is much more advantageous than peroxisomal β-oxidation. Mitochondria transform energy released in respiration into ATP, whereas peroxisomal respiration is thermogenetic, as all energy produced is released as heat. The most important difference between the mitochondrial and peroxisomal β-oxidation systems is the difference in substrate specificity. The mitochondrial system is capable of handling oxidation of short-chain, medium-chain (C6-C14) and long-chain (C15-C22) fatty acids with a chain length of up to 22 C atoms. In contrast, peroxisomes have little or no activity with respect to fatty acids with a chain length shorter than 8 C atoms. Medium-chain and long-chain fatty acids can be degraded by the peroxisomal β-oxidation system, but the bulk of the catabolism of these compounds

occurs in mitochondria. Oxidation of very long-chain fatty acids with a chain length of 24 or more C atoms appear to take place mainly, if not exclusively, in the peroxisome. Although the pattern of substrate specificity of the peroxisomal and mitochondrial β-oxidation overlaps, peroxisomes preferentially oxidize fatty acids greater than C22, whereas fatty acids shorter than C22 are preferentially oxidized in mitochondria. Since peroxisomal acyl-CoA oxidase is only reactive towards fatty acyl-CoA esters containing 8 C atoms or more, very long-chain fatty acids cannot be oxidized to completion in peroxisomes, but only chain-shortened to yield shorter acyl-CoA esters and acetyl-CoA. The chain-shortened acyl-CoAs enter the mitochondrial β-oxidation pathway, where the oxidation is completed. The import of fatty acids into peroxisomes is independent of carnitine. However, peroxisomes contain medium-chain carnitine acyltransferase and acetyltransferase activity. These enzymes probably play a role in the transfer of end-products of peroxisomal β-oxidation, acetyl-CoA and medium-chain acyl-CoA esters out of the peroxisome into the mitochondria.

The peroxisomal β-oxidation system not only acts upon saturated very long-chain fatty acids, but is also capable of catalyzing chain shortening of monounsaturated and polyunsaturated long-chain fatty acids. Peroxisomal enzymes involved in oxidation of unsaturated fatty acids are 2,4-dienoyl-CoA reductase and Δ^3,Δ^2-enoyl-CoA isomerase. In addition to enoyl-CoA hydratase and 3-hydroxyacyl-CoA dehydrogenase activity mentioned above, trifunctional protein also has Δ^3,Δ^2-enoyl-CoA isomerase activity and is as such involved in the β-oxidation of both saturated and unsaturated fatty acids.

Peroxisomes have also been implicated in β-oxidation of cholestanoic acids, pristanic acid, dicarboxylic acids, certain prostaglandins, certain leukotrienes and xenobiotic compounds.

Bile acid synthesis is partly dependent upon the peroxisomal β-oxidation system. The conversion of the bile acid precursors, trihydroxycholestanoic acid and dihydroxycholestanoic acid, into cholic acid and chenodeoxycholic acid, respectively, takes place in peroxisomes via a sequence of reactions similar to the β-oxidation of fatty acids, leading to oxidative cleavage of the cholesterol side chain.

Phytanic acid is a saturated, branched-chain fatty acid of dietary origin. Because of the presence of a β-methyl group it cannot undergo direct β-oxidation. Instead, phytanic acid is first subjected to α-oxidative decarboxylation, yielding pristanic acid and CO_2. This conversion takes place in mitochondria. Subsequently, pristanic acid can be β-oxidized in peroxisomes. In fact, recent evidence has been provided that the conversion of phytanic acid to pristanic acid occurs in two steps, the first step being an α-hydroxylation and probably mitochondrial, the second step a decarboxylation and probably peroxisomal.

Long-chain and medium-chain dicarboxylic acids can be chain-shortened by the peroxisomal β-oxidation pathway.

Peroxisomal β-oxidation is of major importance for chain-shortening of certain prostaglandins. Prostaglandins E_2 and $F_{2\alpha}$ are β-oxidized in peroxisomes, which also play a role in the degradation of the carboxyl side-chain of thromboxane B_2. The metabolic inactivation of leukotrienes is mediated by ω-oxidation and subsequent β-oxidation. The latter reaction takes place in peroxisomes.

Peroxisomes play an important role in the degradation of xenobiotics with an acyl side-chain. The β-oxidation of the acyl side-chain allows these compounds to be excreted as shortened, more polar substances.

It is clear that peroxisomes catalyse the β-oxidative chain-shortening of a variety of compounds. The question arises, whether the same set of β-oxidative enzymes is responsible for the β-oxidation of all these diverse compounds. There is evidence that multiple enzymes are involved. In the first place it has been shown that activation of a substrate to its CoA-ester, destined to be β-oxidized in peroxisomes, need not necessarily occur at the peroxisomal membrane. In the case of di- and trihydroxycholestanoic acid, dicarboxylic acids and prostaglandins, activation occurs in the endoplasmic reticulum, followed by transport of the CoA-esters to the peroxisome. A number of distinct synthetases has been demonstrated to be involved in the activation of different metabolites. There is evidence for a separate fatty acyl-CoA synthetase, cholestanoyl-CoA synthetase and pristanyl-CoA synthetase. There is also evidence that very long-chain fatty acyl-CoA synthetase, also called lignoceroyl-CoA synthetase, is distinct from long-chain acyl-CoA synthetase, also called palmitoyl-CoA synthetase. Furthermore, at least three distinct oxidases are present: very long-chain fatty acyl-CoA oxidase, cholestanoyl-CoA oxidase and pristanyl-CoA oxidase. One and the same acyl-CoA oxidase is involved in the β-oxidation of very long-chain fatty acids and prostaglandins. Current information suggests that the subsequent reactions in the β-oxidation of the various compounds are catalyzed by a single trifunctional protein and a single thiolase.

Another important peroxisomal function concerns the biosynthesis of ether phospholipids, such as plasmalogens and platelet activating factor. Plasmalogens constitute 5%–20% of the phospholipids of cell membranes and are especially abundant in the ethanolamine phospholipid class. Plasmalogens are present in high concentrations in the brain, especially in myelin. Platelet activating factor induces both platelet and leukocyte aggregation and degranulation and is important in several pathological processes including inflammation and anaphylaxis. Peroxisomes are involved in the introduction of ether bonds in ether phospholipids via the catalytic activity of acyl-CoA: dihydroxyacetone phosphate actyltransferase and alkyl dihydroxyacetone phosphate synthetase. All subsequent steps are catalysed by enzymes in the endoplasmic reticulum.

Peroxisomes are involved in a number of different processes. They contain pipecolate oxidase, important in the breakdown of pipecolic acid, which is an intermediate product in the catabolism of lysine. Degradative enzymes of glutaric acid are located both in mitochondria and in peroxisomes. Peroxisomes have furthermore been implicated in the oxidation of polyamines, purines, and glyoxylate. They play a role in the transamination reactions in gluconeogenesis from amino acids via glyoxylate amino transferase and D or L amino acid oxidase. Peroxisomes are capable of de novo cholesterol synthesis, but its contribution to the overall cholesterol synthesis is unclear.

Disturbance of normal peroxisomal function is associated with far-reaching and devastating consequences. Depending on the extent of peroxisomal dysfunction, peroxisomal disorders can be classified into three groups.
1. Generalized loss of peroxisomal functions:
   a Zellweger cerebrohepatorenal syndrome
   b Neonatal adrenoleukodystrophy
   c Infantile Refsum disease
2. Loss of multiple peroxisomal functions:
   a Rhizomelic chondrodysplasia punctata
   b Zellweger-like syndrome
3. Loss of a single peroxisomal function:
   a Pseudo-neonatal adrenoleukodystrophy
   b Trifunctional protein deficiency
   c Pseudo-neonatal adrenoleukodystrophy
   d Pseudo-Zellweger syndrome
   e X-linked adrenoleukodystrophy
   f Glutaryl-CoA oxidase deficiency
   g Acatalasemia
   h Hyperoxaluria type I

In the first category peroxisomes are either absent or very reduced in number and have an abnormal structure. In fibroblasts remnant structures may be seen, which are called "peroxisomal ghosts". The disorders are characterized by a generalized loss of peroxisomal functions. They are also called disorders of peroxisome biogenesis, because the organelle fails to be formed normally. The import of peroxisomal matrix proteins is grossly defective leading to generalized peroxisomal dysfunction. The defective import may be explained by a number of possible defects. There may be a defect in the targeting sequence – receptor interaction, for instance caused by a primary defect in receptors located at the peroxisomal membrane or by a primary defect in the targeting sequence. Another possibility is that the structure of the peroxisomal membrane is altered by absence or abnormality of one of the integral membrane proteins, to such an extent that transmembrane transport is secondarily disturbed. A third possibility is that mutations affect the structure of one of the cytosolic proteins (binding or stabilizing proteins) which are indispensible for the import of proteins into the peroxisome.

In the second category, peroxisomes are intact, but more than one peroxisomal enzyme is lacking. The basic problem could be a more limited defect at the level of targeting signal or receptor required for the import of the absent enzymes.

The peroxisomal disorders of the third category are similar to classical inborn errors of metabolism, in that there is defective activity of a single enzyme.

In recent years several patients have been described with an as yet unclassified peroxisomal disorder. A few examples are mentioned. In 1989 Guerroui et al. described a patient diagnosed as having neonatal adrenoleukodystrophy, who had biochemical evidence of generalized peroxisomal failure, absence of catalase-positive organelles on electron microscopy of liver tissue, but normal presence of all three enzymes involved in β-oxidation in immunoblotting studies. In 1990 MacCollin et al. described a 5-year-old boy with mild neurological dysfunction, but biochemical evidence of generalized peroxisomal dysfunction and absence of catalase-positive organelles on electron microscopy.

The clinical picture of the child, characterized by hypotonia, ataxia and signs of a peripheral polyneuropathy, but normal intelligence, vision and hearing, and absence of dysmorphic features and epilepsy, was unusually mild for a generalized peroxisomal dysfunction. In 1993, Molzer et al. reported on a leukodystrophy in three sisters with onset of disease between 4 and 8 years and death 9–15 months later. Postmortem biochemical analysis of the affected white matter revealed a marked increase in very long-chain fatty acids, but the biochemical basis of the disease was not elucidated further. The onset and course of disease could be compatible with X-linked adrenoleukodystrophy, but the sex of the patients could not. In 1993, Tranchant et al. described four patients with a disease clinically resembling adult Refsum disease. Postmortem examination of the brain of one patient, however, showed diffuse severe spongy degeneration of the white matter never seen in adult Refsum disease. Biochemically, an elevation of both phytanic acid and pipecolic acid was found with evidence of a deficiency of phytanic acid and pipecolic acid oxidase activity, whereas adult Refsum disease is characterized by an isolated accumulation of phytanic acid. It is apparent from these unclarified cases that the classification of peroxisomal disorders has not yet been completed and will no doubt alter in the near future as insight into mechanisms of peroxisomal dysfunction increases.

The following chapters will discuss the peroxisomal disorders that affect the white matter of the CNS either by dysmyelination or by demyelination.

15 Zellweger Cerebrohepatorenal Syndrome, Neonatal Adrenoleukodystrophy, and Infantile Refsum Disease

15.1 Clinical Features and Laboratory Investigations.

Zellweger syndrome (ZS), also called cerebrohepatorenal syndrome, belongs to the same category of disorders as neonatal adrenoleukodystrophy (NALD) and infantile Refsum disease (IRD). The clinical picture of these disorders is very similar. The most important difference is a difference in severity, the clinical course being most severe in ZS and mildest in IRD. All three disorders have an autosomal recessive mode of inheritance.

After birth children with ZS show profound muscular hypotonia or even atonia. Most patients lie motionless with weak or absent Moro reflex, tendon reflexes and sucking and swallowing reflexes. Gavage feeding is necessary. Typically, the children have craniofacial dysmorphia with a high and bulging forehead, flat occiput, upslanting palpebral fissures, puffy eyelids, hypoplastic supraorbital ridges, low and broad nasal bridge with hypertelorism and epicanthus folds, giving them a mongoloid appearance. In addition, Brushfield spots, peripheral pigmentary retinopathy, optic atrophy or hypoplasia, glaucoma, corneal clouding, cataracts, low-set malformed ears, high arched palate, micrognathia, and widely patent sutures and fontanelles are present. There may be macrocephaly. Some children have a cleft soft palate. Nystagmus is often present. The children have a severe visual and hearing deficit. Hepatomegaly, prolonged neonatal or later-onset icterus, and hemorrhages due to hypoprothrombinemia are common. Limb anomalies include cubitus valgus, camptodactyly, single transverse palmar creases, and talipes equinovarus. Failure to thrive and severe psychomotor retardation are conspicuous. Convulsions are frequent. Cardiac defects are not frequent, but ventricular septum defect, patent ductus arteriosus, and patent foramen ovale may occur. Cryptorchidism is frequently observed in boys, clitoromegaly and labial hypoplasia in girls. About 90% of the patients die within the first year of life, death occurring in the majority within the first few months.

NALD is not related to the other forms of adrenoleukodystrophy and it has never been observed in the same kindred with X-linked adrenoleukodystrophy or adrenomyeloneuropathy. Most children have neurological abnormalities at birth, but some are described as being initially near normal. Hypotonia is moderate to severe, reflexes are hypoactive. Craniofacial dysmorphism is milder than in ZS. Widely patent fontanelles are uncommon. The affected children show major feeding problems, a failure to thrive, hepatomegaly, and sometimes jaundice. Furthermore, the disease is characterized by convulsions, sensorineural hearing loss, decreased vision with nystagmus, optic atrophy or dysplasia, and pigmentary retina degeneration. The posterior eye segment abnormalities are identical to those of ZS, but anterior segment abnormalities are lacking. Macrocephaly may be present. Within the first year of life severe developmental retardation becomes apparent, although most infants reach some milestones before neurological deterioration occurs. The age at which regression begins, varies from 12 months to more than 7 years. Progressive neurological dysfunction is characterized by cerebellar ataxia, spasticity, increased deep tendon reflexes, extensor plantar reflexes and sensory defects. If not present from birth onwards, convulsions usually occur in this period. Marked truncal hypotonia remains present. Visual dysfunction progresses to blindness. Adrenal insufficiency is rarely clinically manifest. The course of disease is more protracted in NALD compared to ZS, death occurring between the ages of 1.5 and more than 10 years.

IRD is the mildest variant of the 3 mentioned disorders. The disease is not manifest at birth but presents itself within the first 6 months of life with severe psychomotor retardation, minor facial dysmorphism, mild hypotonia, sensorineural deafness, visual impairment with retinal pigmentary degeneration and optic atrophy, hepatomegaly, and failure to thrive with growth retardation. Convulsions occur but epilepsy is not as severe as in ZS. There are no clinical signs of adrenal insufficiency. Some patients are able to sit and walk independently after several years, whereas others never acquire this ability. Signs of spasticity and ataxia may develop. Life expectancy is considerably longer than in ZS and NALD, up to more than 12 years.

In ZS, laboratory investigations may reveal many different, in themselves nonspecific biochemical abnormalities, such as hyperbilirubinemia, elevated liver enzymes, hypoprothrombinemia, reduced albumin level, hypocarnitinemia, hypocholesterolemia, generalized amino aciduria and elevated CSF protein. These abnormalities are not all necessarily present. Elevated serum iron, iron saturation and transferrin may be found, but these findings are inconsistent and transient. As a rule, an abnormally low cortical response to ACTH stimulation is found despite normal basal cortisol level.

More specific abnormalities are directly related to generalized deficiency of peroxisomal function. Serum and plasma levels of very long-chain fatty acids are increased with an elevation of the C26:C22 and C24:C22 fatty acid ratio. Saturated as well as monounsaturated and polyunsaturated very long-chain fatty acids are increased. Plasma pipecolic acid and phytanic acid may be normal initially but increase with age. Plasma dicarboxylic acids are raised. Abnormal bile acids such as dihydroxycholestanoic acid and trihydroxycholestanoic acid are elevated. In urine elevated levels of dicarboxylic acids, dihydroxycholestanoic acid and trihydroxycholestanoic acid are present. In platelets and red blood cells a deficiency of the peroxisomal enzyme dihydroxyacetone phosphate acyltransferase can be shown. The plasmalogen content of red blood cells is decreased in the first few months of life. The plasmalogen level of the red blood cells increases with age and may be normal in patients who are 4 months or older. The synthesis of platelet activating factor by leukocytes is deficient. In cultured fibroblasts a decreased content of plasmalogen and increased levels of very long-chain fatty acids can be demonstrated. The β-oxidation of very long-chain fatty acids, the de novo biosynthesis of plasmalogens, the activity of dihydroxyacetone phosphate acyltransferase, alkyl dihydroxyacetone phosphate synthetase and phytanic acid oxidation can be shown to be deficient in fibroblasts. Finally, in fibroblasts catalase activity is not found in organelles, but in the cellular cytoplasm.

Laboratory abnormalities are essentially the same in NALD and IRD, but less pronounced than in ZS. In ZS the accumulation of very long-chain fatty acids includes the saturated and monounsaturated C26 fatty acid and is associated with a decrease in the C22 saturated fatty acid concentration. In NALD the rise in very long-chain fatty acids is not associated with an increase in monounsaturated C26 fatty acid and the C22 fatty acid is on average higher than normal. In NALD, mild adrenal insufficiency and low cortisol response in ACTH stimulation is found although apparently normal adrenal function is not incompatible with the diagnosis. In IRD adrenal function is normal.

X-ray examinations in ZS often reveal calcific stippling of bony epiphyses. Stippled, irregular calcification of particularly the patellae, greater trochanters, triradiate cartilages, acetabulum, scapula and sternum is seen in 50 to 70% of the ZS patients. Ultrasound may detect multiple small renal cortical cysts, but they are often difficult to find. ERG is extinguished at a very early age. EEG is highly abnormal with epileptic discharges. BAEP shows reduced potentials.

In NALD and IRD no calcific stippling of bony epiphyses is present. No renal cysts are found. ERG becomes extinguished. BAEP is abnormal. Nerve conduction velocity may be decreased in NALD; it is normal in IRD.

Prenatal diagnosis can be performed with help of various biochemical investigations in chorion villus fibroblasts and cultured amniocytes. DNA techniques are being developed.

15.2 Pathology

Brain weight in ZS is normal or may exceed normal. External examination reveals abnormalities in the cerebral convolutional pattern with areas of pachygyria and polymicrogyria. Polymicrogyria is typically present in the opercular regions of the frontal, parietal and temporal lobes and within the insular region, with an increased number of gyri and decreased amplitude of the gyri. In the superior region, over the frontoparietal convexities, the polymicrogyric cortex merges with a pachygyric cortex, where convolutions are abnormally broad and reduced in number. There is a failure of full opercularization of the insulae and the Sylvian fissure is abnormally vertical in orientation. Otherwise the gyral pattern of the cerebral hemispheres is normal. Often the cerebellum is hypoplastic and the cerebellar cortex has areas of polymicrogyria. External appearance of the brain stem is normal.

On sectioning the gyral abnormalities are confirmed with moderate thickening of the cortical plate in the areas of abnormal gyration. The lateral ventricles are mildly enlarged and have a mildly colpocephalic configuration. There is a moderate symmetrical decrease in volume of the white matter. Olfactory bulbs and tracts and optic nerves are thin, as is the corpus callosum. Periventricular subependymal cysts, called germinolytic cysts, are often present over the heads of the caudate nucleus. In the brain stem hypoplasia and dysplasia of the inferior olives is apparent.

Microscopic examination reveals that the cerebral cortex has a normal cytoarchitectonic pattern in the normally convoluted areas. The cytoarchitecture of polymicrogyric and pachygyric cortex is abnormal and heterotopias in the subcortical white matter underlie the regions of cortical abnormality. The migrational abnormality has principally affected neurons destined for the outer cortical layers. Many cells normally found in the outer cortical layers (layers II and III) are distributed in heterotopic position within the deep cortical layers (layers V and VI) and in the white matter below the cortex. The impediment to migration appears to be only partially effective in that a portion of the neurons destined for the deep cortical layers are in their normal laminar positions. The difference between the pachygyric and polymicrogyric cortices is related to differences in intracortical cell patterns. The outer cortical layers are relatively more cellular in polymicrogyric cortex than in pachygyric cortex, whereas the reverse is true with regard to the deeper cortical layers. Within the cortex a marked astrocytic gliosis is present. Within the proliferated astrocytes, an excess of sudanophilic lipid material is seen. PAS-positive deposits are seen in the cortex of some of the patients related to glycogen deposition in the cytoplasm and nucleoplasm of neurons and astrocytes. Clusters of unusual histiocytes and multinucleated giant cells have been described with partly homogeneous PAS-positive and partly foamy and sudanophilic cytoplasm.

The white matter is characterized by deficiency of myelin and presence of gliosis. Myelin deficiency is caused by delayed and disturbed myelination. Active loss of myelin cannot be demonstrated. Throughout the white matter many astrocytes are present which are hypertrophic and contain sudanophilic lipid material in their cytoplasm. Lipid deposits are also seen in histiocytes and macrophages. No perivascular infiltration with inflammatory cells is present. The white matter abnormality is usually diffuse and generalized. In some cases the periventricular white matter is most severely involved with no myelin left in that area. Oligodendrocytes are reduced in number. There is a decrease of axons in the white matter corresponding to an area of pachygyria or polymicrogyria. The ventricles are partially denuded of ependyma and regionally the ependyma is a pseudostratified columnar epithelium resembling midfetal life. In many patients germinolytic cysts are present in subependymal areas.

The basal ganglia have a normal configuration, but in microscopic examination pathological changes similar in nature to those in the cortex are seen, with an increase in astrocytes and presence of lipid-laden cells. The optic nerves, chiasm and optic tracts may show diffuse deficiency of myelin and presence of gliosis. The brain stem is normal in architecture, except for hypoplasia and dysplasia of the inferior olives, which lack the usual delicately convoluted pattern. The brain stem is poorly myelinated. A diffuse increase in the number of astrocytes is found in gray and white matter and lipid-laden foam cells are present. The cerebellum is often hypoplastic and its convolutional pattern abnormal. Areas of polymicrogyria are common and microscopic examination shows that cortical lamination is markedly abnormal at these points. Many heterotopic Purkinje cells are present in the subcortical white matter. A marked increase in astrocytes is present in the cerebellar cortex and many glial cells and macrophages have vacuolated foamy cytoplasm filled

with lipid droplets. The changes in the cerebellar white matter are similar to those in the white matter of the cerebral hemispheres. The dentate nuclei may be hypoplastic and dysplastic, showing the same lack of convolutions as observed in the inferior olivary nuclei.

Electron microscopy reveals that the lipid-laden cells contain typical trilamellar inclusions along with heterogeneous material. These inclusions are intralysosomal. The trilamellar structures are composed of two parallel electron-dense lines separated by an electron-lucent zone. They are identical to those encountered in other peroxisomopathies and may contain very long-chain fatty acids. Structurally abnormal mitochondria have been reported in some cases.

Following birth hepatic cirrhosis may develop rapidly, although not invariably. The liver is enlarged in most patients. Histological findings vary from near normal to diffusely abnormal, dependent on the age of the ZS patient. In the first 2 months of life, microscopic abnormalities are absent or mild and include fibrosis, cholestasis and intrahepatic bile duct hypoplasia. In older patients fibrosis and distortion of liver architecture is more severe, ending in micronodular cirrhosis. Inconstant excess of hemosiderin in hepatocytes and in particular in Kupffer cells and macrophages may be related to age with the greatest prominence between 5 and 18 weeks of age. In exceptional cases, accumulation of glycogen is found. On ultrastructural examination, no peroxisomes are seen in hepatocytes, where they are normally found in abundance. Invariably abnormal mitochondrial morphology is seen. Intralysosomal trilamellar inclusions are present in Kupffer cells and macrophages. In the kidney multiple small cysts are present in the cortex, especially in the subcapsular region. The average diameter is 3 mm, with some reaching 8 mm. They are predominantly of tubular, occasionally of glomerular origin. Ultrastructural examination reveals no peroxisomes in renal tubular epithelium, where they are normally found in large numbers. Adrenal glands are either normal in size or small. The medulla is unremarkable. In the zona reticularis and inner-fasciculata large striated cells are seen with dense inclusions. On ultrastructural examination, these cells contain trilaminar inclusions. Hyperplasia of pancreatic islets and pancreatic fibrosis have been observed in isolated patients. In muscle tissue myopathic changes and presence of abnormal mitochondria are occasionally observed.

In NALD brains, the gyrational abnormalities are much milder than in ZS. Small areas of polymicrogyria, pachygyria and a few islands of heterotopic neurons are seen within the white matter. The cerebral cortex is otherwise normal. Few cerebellar heterotopias are seen. Inferior olives may be dysplastic.

White matter degenerative changes are, however, much more severe in NALD than in ZS. Diffuse demyelination involves cerebral hemispheres, cerebellar white matter and brain stem. Demyelination tends to be more diffuse than in X-linked adrenoleukodystrophy. The process is most severe in the occipital region, cerebellar white matter and descending tracts in internal capsule, brain stem and spinal cord. One atypical patient with frontal demyelination and sparing of occipital and cerebellar white matter has been described. The cerebral arcuate fibers are relatively spared. In the areas of demyelination, the axons are relatively intact, but if demyelination is severe, axons may also be destroyed and cavitation may occur. In the affected areas gliosis is present and there is an accumulation of lipids predominantly in histiocytes and macrophages, and little, if any, in astrocytes. Perivascular infiltration with mononuclear inflammatory cells is present, but less severe than in X-linked adrenoleukodystrophy. On ultrastructural examination trilamellar inclusions have been found in vacuoles within histiocytes and macrophages in areas of demyelination. A demyelinating polyneuropathy has been found in some of the patients.

Liver disease in NALD is less severe than in ZS. Hepatic fibrosis and micronodular cirrhosis occur, but are not obligatory. Evidence of glycogen deposits may be present. Mitochondria have been described as either normal or abnormal in morphology. In most cases, absence or a marked reduction in number and size of peroxisomes has been reported, but enlarged hepatic peroxisomes have also been found. In contrast to ZS, the liver is infiltrated with abundant histiocytes and macrophages that contain lipid storage material. On ultrastructural examination these cells are shown to contain the typical trilamellar inclusions. No renal cortical cysts are present. The adrenal cortex is atrophic and contains ballooned, lipid-laden cells. Electron microscopy reveals trilamellar inclusions in adrenocortical cells and in macrophages. Myopathic changes and mitochondrial abnormalities have been found in muscle tissue.

NALD is characterized by a generalized, systemic infiltration by lipid-laden macrophages, not seen in ZS. The storage cells harbor trilamellar inclusions and heterogeneous material. They are seen in multiple sites of the reticulo-endothelial system and are not confined to sites of active degeneration such as the CNS. They occur in liver, spleen, lungs, lymph nodes and gastrointestinal mucosa.

In IRD no malformations of the cerebral cortex are present and no neuronal heterotopias within the white matter. The white matter may be hypoplastic. White matter changes are mild. Myelin content is diminished, but there are no signs of active demyelination. In the areas of myelin deficiency and gliosis, one finds macrophages surrounding vessels and containing trilaminar lamellae.

The liver in IRD is either normal or fibrotic changes may be present. Trilamellar lipid inclusions have been described in macrophages, Kupffer cells and hepatocytes. Peroxisomes are absent or reduced in number and size. No cortical renal cysts are seen. No adrenal degeneration is present.

15.3 Pathogenetic Considerations

In ZS, histochemical examination with staining for the peroxisomal enzyme catalase, and electron microscopy fail to demonstrate peroxisomes in the liver or renal tubular epithelium, tissues in which they are normally abundant. However, studies utilizing antibodies to peroxisomal membrane proteins show that cultured skin fibroblasts contain structures consisting of peroxisomal membrane proteins. Ultrastructural examination reveals these structures to be largely empty. They sediment at a density significantly lower than normal peroxisomes, and are referred to as peroxisomal ghosts. The number of ghosts in ZS fibroblasts is usually smaller than the number of peroxisomes in control cells. However, all results concerning the membrane ghosts are obtained in cultured fibroblasts and on ultrastructural examination of liver tissue, no vesicles have been found corresponding to peroxisomal ghosts. Searches for peroxisomal ghosts with antibodies to peroxisomal membrane proteins have not revealed labelled structures in ZS liver cells. Many laboratories have reported discrepancies in findings between liver and cultured fibroblasts.

In ZS the absence of normal peroxisomes is associated with a defective function of multiple peroxisomal enzymes. The primary defect is generally thought to involve one of the steps in the biogenesis of peroxisomes, leading to a defective import system for a variety of peroxisomal proteins. Peroxisomal proteins are synthesized on free polyribosomes and transported through the cytosol into the target organelle. In ZS several of the enzyme proteins which are normally located in the peroxisomal matrix, are localized free in the cytosol and are stable and biologically active. This is the case with catalase, D-amino acid oxidase, alanine glyoxylate aminotransferase, polyamine oxidase and L-α-hydroxy acid oxidase. The total activity per cell of these enzymes is not reduced in liver or cultured fibroblasts. In contrast, other peroxisomal enzymes are synthesized normally, but are unstable in the cytosol and are rapidly degraded. Their enzyme activity is decreased to less than 10% of control value. This is the case with the peroxisomal β-oxidation enzyme proteins, alkyldihydroxyacetone phosphate synthetase and dihydroxyacetone phosphate acyltransferase, and the plasmalogen synthesizing enzymes.

Initially, the peroxisomal ghosts were described as being empty. However, it has recently been shown that these structures contain the unprocessed precursor form of thiolase, unprocessed acyl-CoA oxidase and the residual dihydroxyacetone phosphate acyltransferase activity. It is clear that the enzyme proteins contained in these structures are not only membrane-bound enzyme proteins, since acyl-CoA oxidase and thiolase are predominantly localized in the matrix of these structures. Some catalase has also been found in the interior of peroxisomal remnant structures.

The discovery of peroxisomal ghosts has focused attention on the probability that the basic defect in ZS resides in a defect in the peroxisomal membrane. A number of separate mechanisms for the abnormality in peroxisomal biogenesis have been described in ZS. One of the known ZS mutations concerns so-called peroxisome assembly factor I (PAF-1). PAF-1 is a peroxisomal integral membrane protein with a relative molecular mass of 35 000. The point mutation in the PAF-1 gene causes a premature termination of PAF-1 and the ZS phenotype. Addition of PAF-1 restores the normal assembly of peroxisomes in fibroblasts. In another subset of ZS patients a mutation has been found in a gene coding for the peroxisomal membrane protein with a relative molecular mass of 70 000 (PMP70). PMP70 is an important component of peroxisomal membranes and plays a role in peroxisomal biogenesis. PMP70 is a member of the ATP-binding cassette (ABC) transporter family. Members of this family are involved in the transmembrane transport of a variety of molecules ranging in size from ions to proteins. One possibility is that PMP70 is directly involved in importing proteins into peroxisomes. The consequences of altering this transport system would be that peroxisomal membrane proteins and certain matrix proteins which do not use the affected system would be expected to integrate into peroxisome-like structures. The organelles would be defective owing to the failure of the majority of the matrix enzymes to be imported. Alternatively, the primary function of PMP70 may involve the transport of small molecules (ions and metabolites) across the peroxisomal membrane. In that case the observed abnormalities of peroxisomal morphology and matrix protein import in ZS would all be secondary effects. Lastly, PMP70, despite its homology with ABC transporter proteins, may not have a role in transport, but rather serve a necessary structural function in the peroxisomal membrane.

Complementation analysis studies have confirmed that mutations in different genes can lead to the biochemical phenotype characteristic of ZS, indicating that several proteins are involved in the structural integrity and import machinery of peroxisomes. Also a cytoplasmic factor appears to be required for peroxisomal biogenesis. There is evidence that not only a defect or absence of a peroxisomal protein important in peroxisomal assembly or transport may lead to ZS, but that also some other cytoplasmic factor may be missing. It is not clear whether this cytoplasmic factor is some form of primordial membranous peroxisomal ghost or a smaller component, required for binding or stabilizing peroxisomal proteins en route to the peroxisome.

The defect in import of proteins across the peroxisomal membrane can also be located at the level of the targeting process. A tripeptide sequence (SKL) located at the carboxy terminal end of certain peroxisomal proteins is able to direct them to peroxisomes. Changes in the tripeptide sequence abolishes transport into the peroxisome. Several proteins, among which thiolase, lack a carboxy terminal tripeptide sequence, suggesting that the tripeptide sequence is not the only perosixome targeting signal. It is possible that a subset of ZS patients is caused by a defective targeting signal.

It has been shown that there are variations in abundance of peroxisomal membrane proteins and in numbers of peroxisomes in different ZS cell lines. These variations are probably related to the clinical severity of the disease. Different mutations in a gene and mutations in different genes may lead to quantitative differences in the ability to assemble a peroxisome or maintain a functioning peroxisome due to differences in the residual biological activity of the protein in question. In certain ZS cell lines particle-bound activity of the peroxisomal β-oxidation enzymes was observed, suggesting that peroxisomal dysfunction is only partial in these cells.

There is recent evidence that most of the structures referred to as peroxisomal ghosts are found in vacuoles, presumably autophagic vacuoles, as lysosomal compartments. There are also indications that peroxisomal membrane proteins are mainly present in lysosomes. In several ZS cell lines the presence of a few normally assembled peroxisomes has been shown. The reduction in number of peroxisomes in ZS cell lines was found to be associated with the presence of peroxisomes in vacuoles. This evidence from studies in ZS fibroblasts, suggests that peroxisomes are synthesized in ZS, but that they are rapidly degraded by autophagic proteolysis. The autophagy of peroxisomes may reflect a cellular response to altered peroxisomal membrane constituents.

ZS, NALD and IRD are the so-called disorders of peroxisomal biogenesis. In NALD absence of hepatic peroxisomes or presence of small and sparse peroxisomes has been found. Incidental patients have been described with abnormally enlarged hepatic peroxisomes. In IRD hepatic peroxisomes are either absent or reduced in number and small. The NALD and IRD peroxisomes have a variable cytochemical staining for catalase.

The classification of the disorders of peroxisome biogenesis is being advanced by complementation analysis. In complementation studies cultured skin fibroblast cell lines from different patients are fused with polyethylene glycol, and the resulting multinucleated cells are collected. Complementation is said to have occurred when the multinucleated cells show a restoration of function or structural features that were deficient in the unfused cell lines. A growing number of different complementation groups has been identified among the disorders of peroxisomal biogenesis. The presence of so many complementation groups in ZS, NALD and IRD indicates that an equal number of different genes are involved in the assembly and transport systems of peroxisomes. One problem of the complementation studies is that the absence of complementation between two cell lines does not provide absolute proof that the same gene loci are concerned in the two mutants. Absence of complementation after fusion of two cell lines might also be due to the absence of preexisting peroxisomes, since new peroxisomes arise by budding or fission of preexisting ones. Complementation can occur only if peroxisomal membranous structures (incomplete or abnormal) are present in at least one of the fused parental cells and act as a framework for peroxisomal assembly.

Now that a number of complementation groups has been identified, it is clear that the genetic classification does not reflect the clinically defined entities and that the clinical categories do not reflect the genetic heterogeneity of the diseases. Among the clinically and biochemically typical ZS patients several complementation groups have been identified. On the other hand, ZS, IRD and NALD cell lines have been shown to belong to the same groups of complementation. Apparently, different genes code for a similar phenotype and one defective gene may lead to variant phenotypes. Possibly, the phenotypic differences reflect differences in the degree of peroxisomal dysfunction, with ZS being the most severe, NALD being intermediate and IRD being the least severe.

Hyperpipecolic acidemia was formerly considered to be a separate disease entity, but this view is no longer held and the patients are assigned to the ZS or NALD category depending upon severity of disease.

In the disorders of peroxisomal biogenesis an impairment of metabolic processes is found in which peroxisomes are normally involved. In addition, disturbances of mitochondrial function are found. Morphological mitochondrial abnormalities are often noted. Evidence of a defect in electron transport chain prior to the cytochromes and a loosened coupling between oxidative phosphorylation and electron transport has been provided. Whether the mitochondrial abnormalities are of primary significance or secondary to the peroxisomal abnormality is not known, but it is generally assumed that they are secondary. Deficiency of peroxisomal function can lead to a disturbance in structure of mitochondrial membranes, causing defects in the mitochondrial electron transport chain. There is also a metabolic interdependence of mitochondria and peroxisomes. Participation in fatty acid metabolism is a property of both organelles. Peroxisomes shorten very long-chain fatty acids prior to their oxidation by mitochondria. Phytanic acid is converted to pristanic acid by mitochondria, and pristanic acid is catabolized further by peroxisomes. Defects in peroxisomal β-oxidation lead to accumulation of long-chain fatty acyl-CoAs, which have regulatory effects on a number of mitochondrial enzymes. Whether primary or secondary, the mitochondrial abnormality might contribute to the disease. The glycogen accumulations which are occasionally seen, are ascribed to a generalized mitochondrial abnormality. In some patients muscle pathology with abnormal mitochondria is observed, suggesting a mitochondrial myopathy. However, no changes in lactate, pyruvate, 3-hydroxy butyrate and acetoacetate have ever been reported in patients indicating that in vivo the proposed mitochondrial dysfunction is usually of no or only minor importance.

The disorders of peroxisomal biogenesis are histopathologically characterized by a combination of malformative and degenerative abnormalities. The dysontogenetic or malformative changes include facial dysmorphia, renal cortical cysts, gray matter migrational disturbances and abnormal myelinogenesis. The degenerative, regressive changes include the pigmentary retinal degeneration, the liver fibrosis and cirrhosis, the adrenal cortical atrophy, and storage, demyelination and neuronal degeneration in the nervous system. In ZS the dysontogenetic abnormalities predominate in the CNS. In NALD there are some malformative changes, but CNS pathology is dominated by degeneration and storage phenomena. In IRD both are mild or absent in the nervous system.

Mechanisms which interfere with migration in ZS and NALD do so to a partial degree only, as portions of neurons are in their normal position and only a portion of the neurons of a given class fail to complete their migrations. The fact that many of the neurons destined for layers II and III in the polymicrogyric cortex and of layers II, III and IV, perhaps even V, of pachygyric cortex are affected, implies that the mechanism of migration is disturbed continuously from a relatively early stage of cortical histogenesis. The migrational derangement is probably caused by circulating toxic substances which are not adequately cleared from the circulation of fetuses by the placenta. Neuronal migration is not disturbed in rhizometic chondrodysplasia calcificans punctata. This observation makes a disturbance of plasmalogen synthesis or phytanic acid oxidation improbable as causes of the migrational defect. The disturbance of neuronal migration in the patient with pseudo-Zellweger syndrome directs attention to the very long-chain fatty acid and bile acid abnormalities. Neuronal migrational abnormalities may reflect the effect of accumulated very long-chain fatty acids, since elevations consistently accompany the peroxisomal disorders with disturbed migration. The exception is X-linked adrenoleukodystrophy, in which very long-chain fatty acids are elevated and no migrational disturbance is present. However, in X-linked adrenoleukodystrophy the increase in very long-chain fatty acids is not as severe as in ZS or NALD, and is more restricted. In ZS, saturated, mono-unsaturated and polyunsaturated fatty acids are increased. In NALD and IRD, saturated and mono-unsaturated fatty acids are elevated, whereas in X-linked adrenoleukodystrophy, only saturated fatty acids are elevated. A possible role of bile acid intermediate accumulation must also be considered. It is hypothesized that an accumulating substance interferes with the cell adhesion molecule interactions and linkages which are necessary for normal migration of neurons along radial glial fibers. In ZS, ependymal abnormalities are found which are qualitatively similar but quantitatively less extensive than those found in classical lissencephaly. Shared features include persistent pseudostratified columnar arrangement resembling the normal condition of midgestation, discontinuities in ependymal lining disproportionate to the minor degree of ventricular dilatation, and persistence of high fetal concentrations of S-100 protein. The abnormal ependyma may be a primary factor in the pathogenesis of migrational disturbances. The pathogenesis of subependymal cysts and their relation to the ependymal abnormalities are uncertain.

The white matter abnormalities vary among the disorders of peroxisomal biogenesis from predominantly deficient and disturbed myelination in ZS, predominantly demyelination in NALD to some white matter gliosis in IRD. In ZS myelin is severely deficient, but no signs of active demyelination are seen; in NALD the process of myelination is initially relatively normal, but demyelination follows. The difference between the two may be related to the degree of abnormality of membrane composition. Abnormal membrane composition is related to decreased availability of plasmalogens, and accumulation of very long-chain fatty acids and phytanic acid in the various membrane lipids. The abnormality being more severe in ZS results in disturbed myelin formation, whereas in NALD myelin is laid down but subsequently broken down as a consequence of increasing instability. In IRD the biochemical abnormalities are mildest and white matter pathology only mild or minor. The inflammatory response in NALD may be related to the liberation of lipids containing very long-chain fatty acids in the process of myelin breakdown. These may be immunogenic and elicit an inflammatory response, as seen in X-linked adrenoleukodystrophy.

ZS, NALD and IRD are all characterized by the presence of trilamellar inclusions in lysosomes, the amount of which increases with age. They consist of cholesterol-bound very long-chain fatty acids. An increase in very long chain-fatty acids is a necessary, but probably not a sufficient condition for their occurrence. The storage is, as a rule, more abundant in macrophages than in parenchymal cells.

Hypotonia is a central clinical feature in all disorders of peroxisomal biogenesis. The hypotonia is of cerebral origin, but may be aggravated in some instances by muscle pathology. Pipecolic acid can produce muscular hypotonia in experimental animals. It has been conjectured that the hyperpipecolic acidemia could be responsible for the extreme hypotonia. However, in hyperlysinemia, which is also accompanied by elevated pipecolic acid levels, no hypotonia is observed.

Hepatic fibrosis and cirrhosis are probably related to abnormal bile acid oxidation. Bile acid intermediates, such as trihydroxycholestanoic acid with known hepatic toxicity may be important pathogenetically for both the development of bile duct paucity and hepatocellular injury.

No biochemical explanation is present for the cystic renal lesions.

The adrenal cortex is affected in all peroxisomal disorders with an elevation of very long-chain fatty acids. The increase in these fatty acids causes an increase in membrane viscosity in adrenocortical cells, which in turn results in a decreased number of hormone receptor sites, subsequently leading to a decreased ability to respond to ACTH. Adrenal insufficiency followed by atrophy is due to the lack of response to ACTH.

15.4   Therapy

In treating patients with a disorder of peroxisomal biogenesis, it would seem rational to try to compensate as far as possible for the biochemical abnormalities that have been brought about by the peroxisomal dysfunction. Treatment would include oral supplementation of ether lipids and bile salts and dietary restriction of very long-chain fatty acids and phytanic acid. The treatment has so far not resulted in definite clinical improvement or prolongation of life. Recently, treatment with docosahexaenoic acid was advocated on the basis of improvement of biochemical parameters and some neurological improvement in one of the two treated children. The rationale of the treatment was the observation of severe docosahexaenoic acid deficiency in tissues of children with disorders of peroxisomal biogenesis, while this substance is known to be an important constituent of brain membrane phospholipid and of photoreceptor cells.

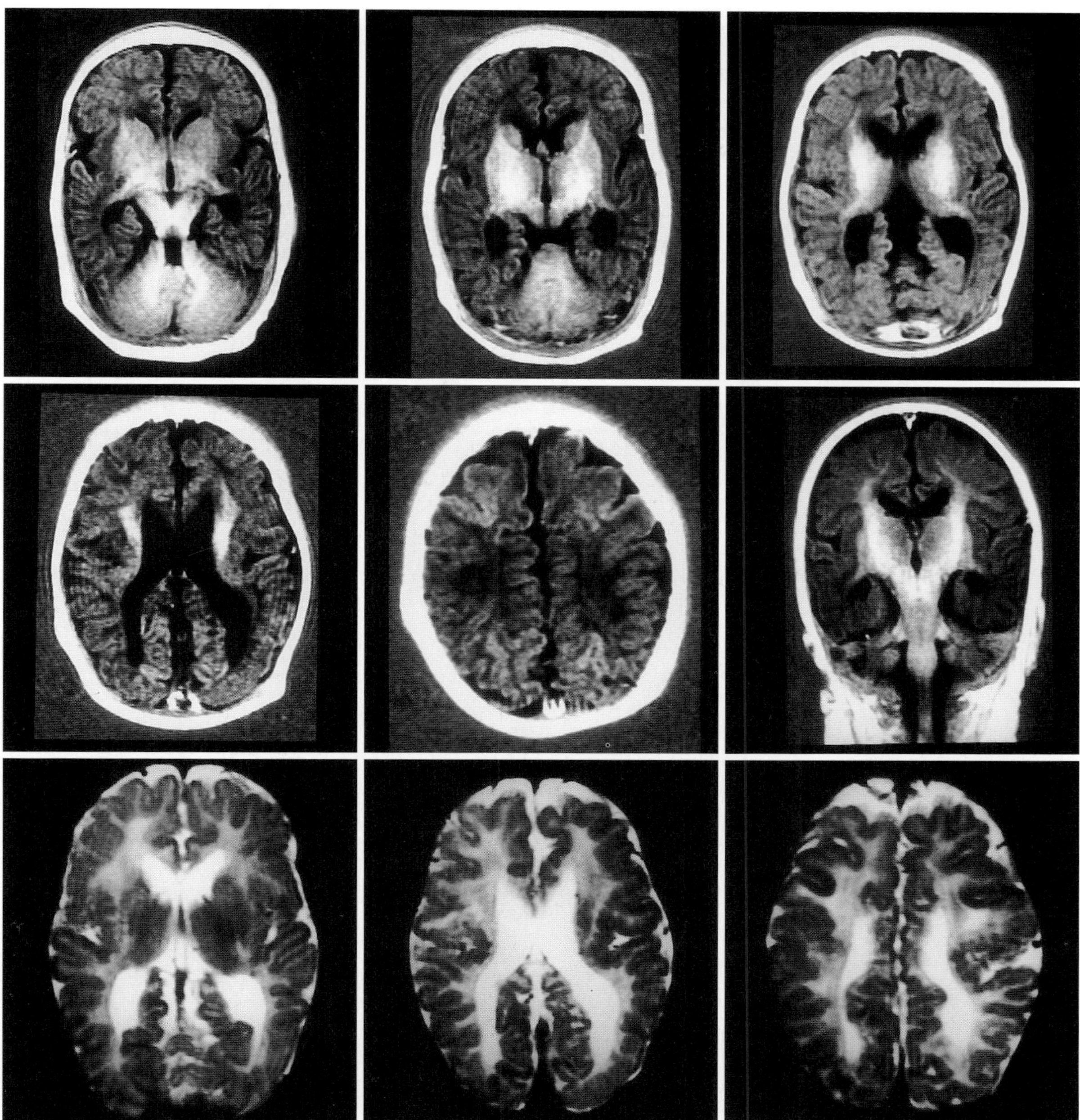

Fig. 15.1. T$_1$ (*upper two rows*) and T$_2$ (*lower row*) weighted images in a 2-month-old boy with ZS. The images show some ventricular enlargement. Myelination is adequate in the central areas, but sparse in the peripheral white matter. Cortical dysgyria is seen in the T$_2$-weighted images. In the frontal area the gyri are too coarse (pachygyria), whereas there is evidence of polymicrogyria in the perisylvian region. There are several minor neuronal heterotopias in the periventricular region

The problem of any therapeutic trial in the disorders of peroxisomal biogenesis is that the dysontogenetic abnormalities cannot be changed by treatment and that only the degenerative changes acquired postnatally can be hoped to be prevented.

Supportive care is essential. Administration of corticosteroids may be considered, especially during stress, considering possible borderline adrenal function.

15.5 Magnetic Resonance Imaging

In ZS the migrational derangement is well depicted by MRI. A very characteristic abnormality is the perisylvian polymicrogyria, which appears as a thickened cortical mantle consisting of many little dots (Figs. 15.1, 15.2). The dots are cross-sections of the microgyri. The polymicrogyric cortex merges with pachygyric cortex

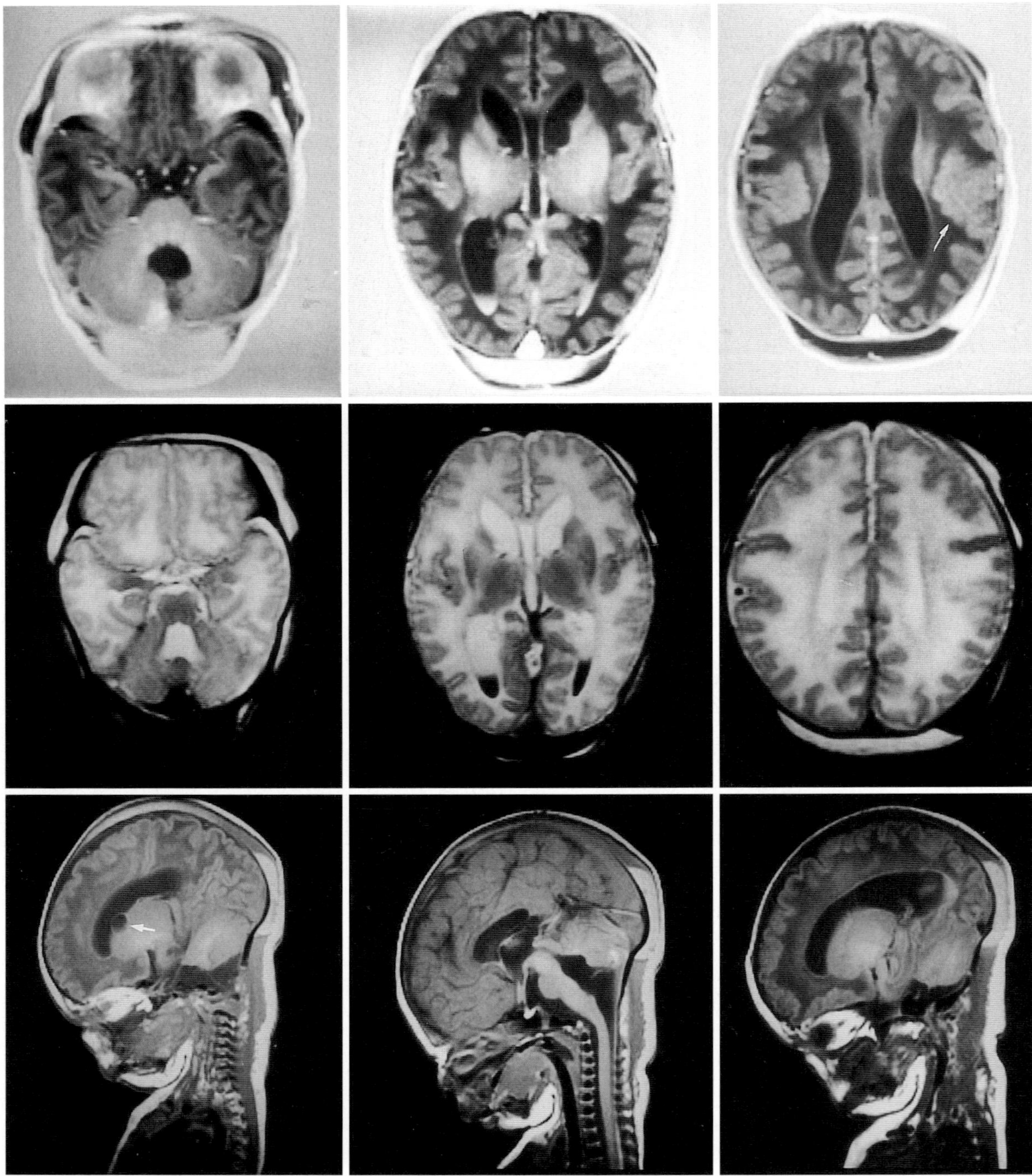

Fig. 15.2. A 1-week-old baby boy with ZS. The *upper row*, T_1-weighted transverse images, shows the mildly enlarged ventricles, the absence of a large part of the vermis and the gyral deformity with evidence of polymicrogyria in the insular region (*arrow*). The *middle row*, T_2-weighted, comparable series shows presence of some blood in the occipital horns and confirms the observations on the T_1-weighted images. The *lower row* of T_1-weighted sagittal images shows a germinolytic cyst over the caudate nucleus (*arrow*), and agenesis of the inferior vermis, with an abnormally shaped fourth ventricle

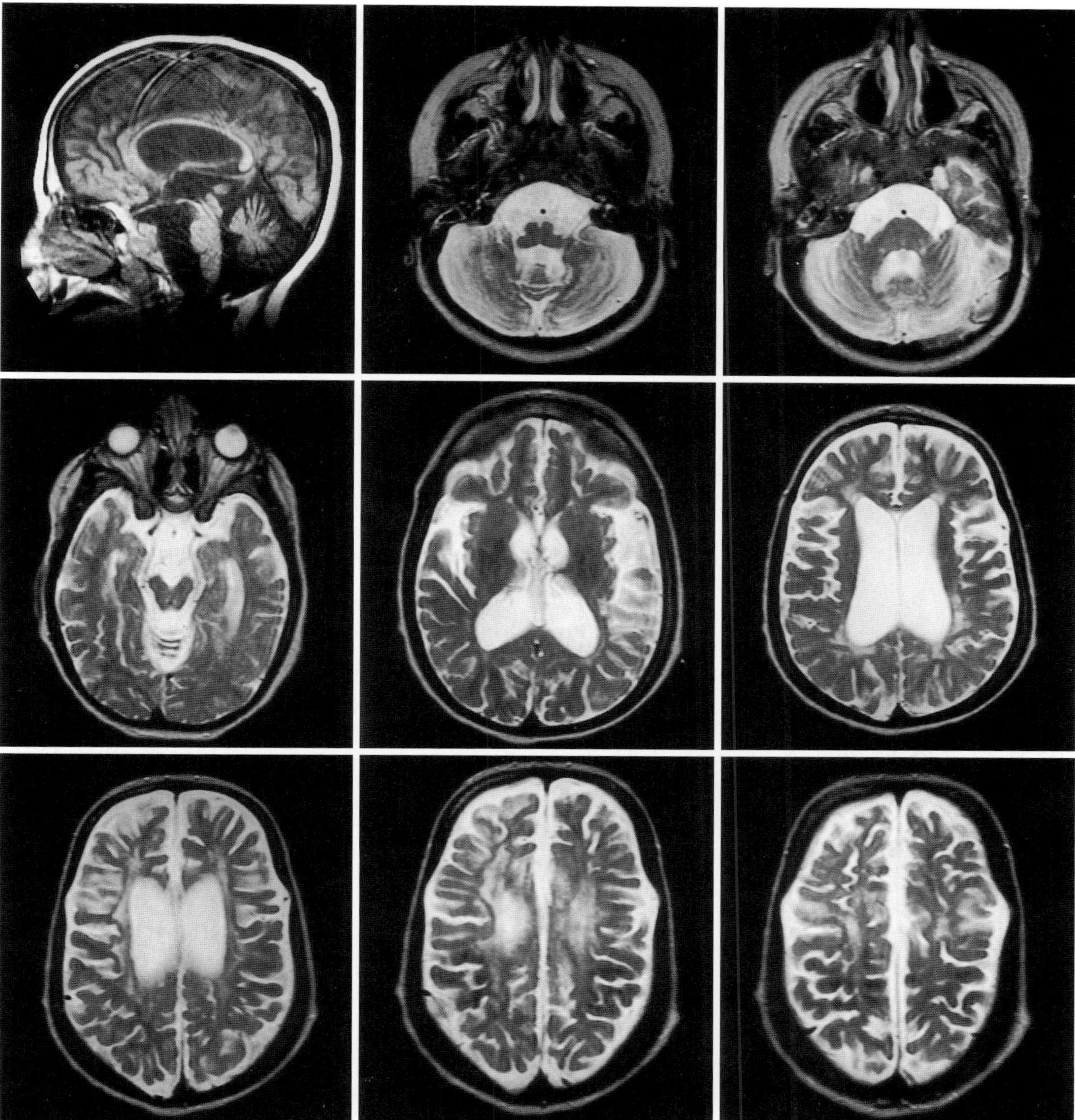

Fig. 15.3. One sagittal T_1 (*upper left*) and a series of transverse T_2-weighted images of a 14-year-old boy with IRD. The sagittal image shows the dilated ventricles with thin corpus callosum and the severe cerebellar atrophy. The T_2-weighted images show dilated ventricles, cortical and cerebellar atrophy and bilateral involvement of the hilus of the dentate nucleus. There are abnormalities in signal intensity in the periventricular white matter and the white matter of the centrum semiovale. The white matter abnormalities are symmetrical and extend into the arcuate fibers. There is cortical atrophy

in the frontoparietal region (Fig. 15.1). The pachygyric cortex is visualized as broad convolutions of mildly thickened cortex. The cortex bordering the interhemispheric fissure and the occipital cortex are relatively normal. Small dots of ectopic gray matter may also be seen under the cortex and in the subependymal region. The ventricular system is mildly enlarged and tends to have a primitive form with mildly enlarged occipital horns which have a squared-off configuration. The corpus callosum is thin. The width of the white matter is markedly reduced. Myelination is delayed and may be patchy, consistent with a disturbed myelination.

In NALD, CT has been shown to reveal progressive white matter hypodensities consistent with demyelination, particularly in the periventricular area, centrum semiovale and cerebellum. The presence of extensive contrast enhancement in centrum semiovale, internal capsules and cerebral peduncles has been reported. No MRI findings have been reported until now. MRI would visualize the extent of the migrational abnormalities and the distribution of the white matter abnormalities in more detail than CT. Diffuse, symmetrical, progressive white matter abnormalities would be visualized by MRI with most severe involvement of occipital white matter, internal capsule, cerebellum and brain stem tracts. Subcortical arcuate fibers would be shown to be preserved.

In IRD no migrational disturbances are seen on MRI. Subtle white matter abnormalities have been described histologically. Normal MRI findings have been reported in one patient. In another patient, a pattern of symmetrical abnormalities in signal intensity in the area of the dentate nuclei has been described. In two further patients, a pattern of abnormal signal intensity in the periventricular area, in particular in the occipital region, in the posterior limb of the internal capsule and in pyramidal tracts of midbrain and pons was described. There was no contrast enhancement in these two patients. In our patient, we found cerebral and cerebellar atrophy in combination with mild periventricular white matter changes (Fig. 15.3).

16 Rhizomelic Chondrodysplasia Punctata

16.1 Clinical Features and Laboratory Investigations

The rhizomelic form of chondrodysplasia punctata (RCP) is a rare autosomal recessive disorder. Clinical signs are present from birth onwards and consist of proximal shortening of the limbs (rhizomelia), microcephaly and in some of the neonates also a low weight and/or height. Contractures of large joints are often present and feet may show equinovarus or calcaneovalgus deformities. Some patients have a characteristic facies with flat nasal bridge, hypertelorism, anteverted nares and a long philtrum. Respiratory distress is occasionally present in the neonatal period. Feeding is usually poor due to poor sucking and swallowing. Erythematous and scaling skin lesions (ichthyosiform erythroderma) are observed in 25% of the patients. In 75% cataracts are found, but optic fundi are normal.

The course of the disease is characterized by persistent feeding difficulties and growth deficiency affecting weight, height and head circumference. Hypertonicity of extremities and trunk is present. Developmental delay is severe. Some patients develop epileptic seizures but these are not severe. Hearing loss and optic atrophy have been reported.

Most affected children die within the first year of life, apparently from recurrent respiratory infections. However, some do survive into childhood, the oldest reported patient being 16 years. Exceptional cases without rhizomelic shortening of the limbs and with a much better psychomotor development, but biochemically indistinguishable from classical RCP, have been reported.

In laboratory investigations, usually, but not invariably, an elevated level of phytanic acid is found in plasma. Phytanic acid oxidation in cultured skin fibroblasts is reduced to the same extent as in adult Refsum disease, infantile Refsum disease and Zellweger syndrome. The level of plasmalogens in erythrocytes is decreased. Plasmalogen synthesis in cultured fibroblasts is deficient due to deficient activity of the enzymes, dihydroxyacetone phosphate acyltransferase and alkyldihydroxyacetone phosphate synthetase. The defect in plasmalogen synthesis is more severe than in Zellweger syndrome or other variants of generalized peroxisomal dysfunction.

The plasma levels of very long-chain fatty acids, pipecolic acid, pristanic acid and bile acid intermediates are normal. Peroxisomal β-oxidation of very long-chain fatty acids in fibroblasts is normal.

In liver and in cultured fibroblasts, catalase is present in normal amounts and is particle bound. A special finding is that the peroxisomal enzyme 3-keto-acyl-CoA thiolase is present in normal quantity, but most of it in its larger precursor form.

Skeletal X-ray survey confirms shortening of the proximal limb bones with disturbed ossification, and epiphyseal and extra-epiphyseal punctate calcific stippling of the ankle, knee, hip, elbow and shoulder joints. The calcific stippling may disappear after 1 or 2 years of age. Metaphyseal flaring may be present. In the vertebral column paraspinous stippling may be seen. Kyphoscoliosis occurs in some of the patients. Vertebral coronal clefts are often multiple, but their presence is not invariant. They can be seen in lateral spinal radiographs as a radiolucent band running superinferiorly through one or more vertebral bodies. They are the results of an arrest of chondrification and ossification during gestation leading to incomplete fusion of the anterior and posterior halves of the vertebral body. They are present in up to 5% of the normal newborns, but they normally do not persist beyond infancy or early childhood. Multiple vertebral coronal clefts have been particularly associated with RCP, but they can also occur in several other conditions.

Prenatal diagnosis can be performed by measurement of plasmalogen biosynthesis and phytanic acid oxidation in cultured chorionic villus samples or amniocytes.

16.2 Pathology

Only very limited data are present on histopathological findings in postmortem examination of the brain. In all cases reported, the brain is too small. The convolutional pattern of cerebrum and cerebellum and the configuration of the brain stem are normal. Mild ventricular dilatation may be present due to cerebral atrophy.

Within the cortex the number of neurons is decreased, but their orientation and stratification are normal. Also in other areas of the brain the number of neurons is reduced. In the few reports present, no or little reference is made to the condition of the white matter, apart from the observation that myelination is poor.

In electron microscopy of liver tissue moderately to markedly enlarged peroxisomes are found. In one patient peroxisomes were absent in some hepatocytes, whereas other hepatocytes displayed an increased number of enlarged peroxisomes. The enlarged peroxisomes have a relatively low level of catalase as indicated by cytochemistry and immunocytochemistry, but the total content of catalase is unchanged. In some RCP patients peroxisomes have normal morphology, size and abundance.

Histopathological examination of the skeletal system shows that the growth plates of the proximal limbs are disrupted and that foci of calcification, ossification, cyst formation and zones of inflammation are present throughout the epiphyses.

16.3   Pathogenetic Considerations

In RCP an impairment of multiple peroxisomal functions is found. The activities of dihydroxyacetone phosphate acyltransferase and alkyldihydroxyacetone phosphate synthetase are deficient, resulting in a deficient synthesis of ether phospholipids, including plasmalogens. Phytanic acid oxidation activity is deficient leading to phytanic acid accumulation. Finally, 3-ketoacyl-CoA thiolase is mostly present in its larger precursor form.

Although the first step in breakdown of phytanic acid is probably mitochondrial, the second step is probably peroxisomal explaining the accumulation of phytanic acid in several disorders of peroxisomal dysfunction. It has recently been shown that the conversion of phytanic acid to pristanic acid is a two-step process with 2-hydroxyphytanic acid as an obligatory intermediate. The first step in the degradation of phytanic acid is an α-hydroxylation which probably occurs in mitochondria; the second step is a decarboxylation, which probably requires peroxisomes. In RCP the second step could be deficient.

In RCP, the enzyme 3-ketoacyl-CoA thiolase is largely present in its unprocessed precursor form. Processing of the enzyme normally takes place in peroxisomes. Only a small fraction of the thiolase precursor is present in the peroxisomes in RCP. Evidence for presence of some mature thiolase has also been found. Most of the thiolase precursor present is associated with particles similar to peroxisomal ghosts observed in Zellweger syndrome. The precursor enzyme present in peroxisomal ghosts is not enzymatically active. Although thiolase is one of the β-oxidation enzymes, in RCP no evidence of impairment of β-oxidation is found. Very long-chain fatty acids do not accumulate. Apparently, the residual capacity of thiolase is sufficient to prevent accumulation of substances that normally undergo peroxisomal β-oxidation.

Thiolase is special with respect to its targeting signal. All peroxisomal proteins are synthesized in their final form on free polyribosomes within the cytoplasm and subsequently transported into preexisting peroxisomes. Most enzymes are targeted towards peroxisomes by the presence of a carboxy-terminal tripeptide (SKL). In contrast to most peroxisomal proteins, thiolase is synthesized as a larger precursor protein with an amino-terminal peptide extension that is cleaved upon maturation of the enzyme. There is evidence that the targeting signal of thiolase is present in this amino-terminal pre-piece.

The basic defect in RCP is unknown. One possibility is that the mutation in RCP involves a receptor or another component of the import machinery, which is specific for a limited number of peroxisomal proteins, including dihydroxyacetone phosphate acyltransferase, alkyldihydroxyacetone phosphate synthetase, and an enzyme involved in phytanic acid oxidation. The defect in processing of thiolase inside the peroxisome may be caused by a lack of a proteolytic enzyme required for this reaction.

The relationship between abnormalities and clinical consequences requires futher elucidation. As chondrodysplasia calcificans punctata is a feature of both RCP and Zellweger syndrome, it seems plausible that the bone lesions are related to a deficiency of plasmalogens. As calcific stippling occurs only in RCP and Zellweger syndrome, and not in neonatal adrenoleukodystrophy or infantile Refsum disease, probably the plasmalogen deficiency has to be severe before skeletal abnormalities occur. A few patients have been described who had all the features of RCP, but whose biochemical abnormalities were limited to a deficiency of dihydroxyacetone phosphate acyltransferase and de novo plasmalogen biosynthesis. Apparently, an impairment of the de novo synthesis of plasmalogens and other ether phospholipids plays a key role in the pathogenesis of the clinical phenotype RCP.

Ichthyosiform skin changes are also seen in Refsum disease, and may thus be ascribed to accumulation of phytanic acid. Some authors ascribe them to a disturbance in utilization of fatty alcohols in RCP, analogous to Sjögren-Larsson syndrome. Alkyldihydroxyacetone phosphate synthetase requires fatty alcohol as a substrate to form the ether-linked alkyl bond. Indeed it has been shown that RCP patients accumulate fatty alcohol in plasma and cultured fibroblasts.

The pathological findings in the CNS consist of retardation of development, including delay in myelina-

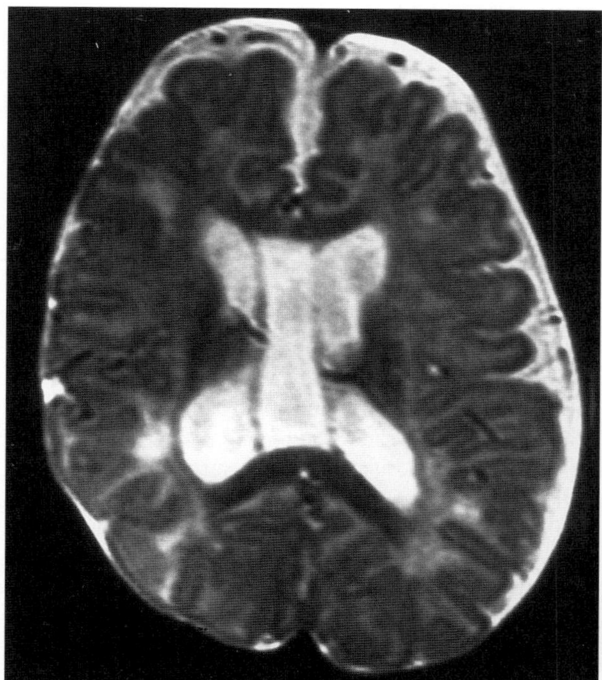
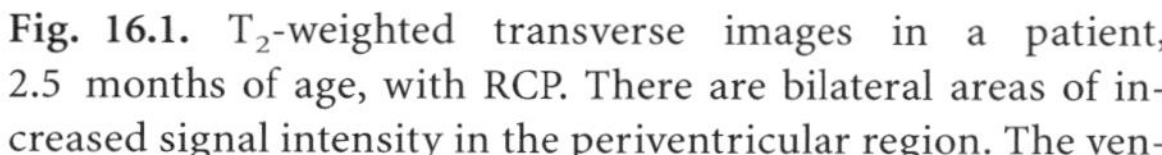
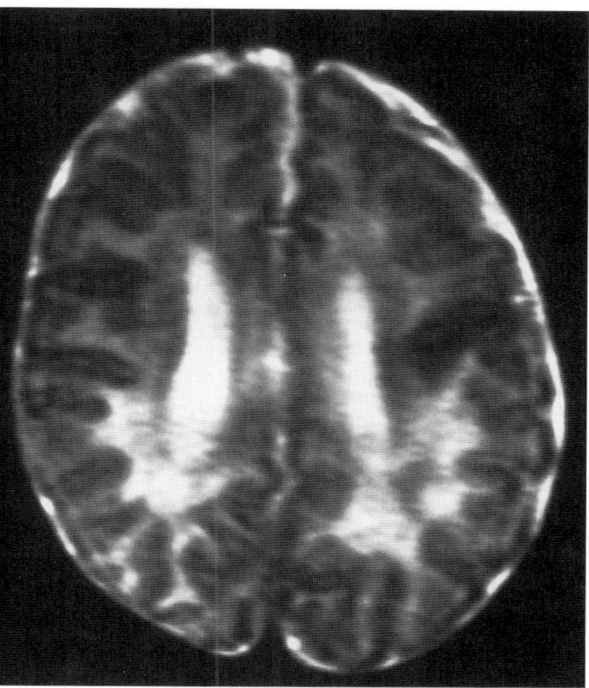

Fig. 16.1. T_2-weighted transverse images in a patient, 2.5 months of age, with RCP. There are bilateral areas of increased signal intensity in the periventricular region. The ventricles are enlarged; there is a prominent cavum septi pellucidi and cavum Vergae. Courtesy of Williams et al. (1991), with permission

tion, and neuronal degeneration. Contributing pathogenetic factors may be the severe undernutrition, deficiency of plasmalogens, which are normally present in all membranes and especially in high concentration in myelin, accumulation of phytanic acid and accumulation of fatty alcohols.

16.4 Therapy

A diet reduced in phytanic acids has been shown to result in reduction of plasma phytanic acids levels and some transient clinical improvement. Plasmapheresis can achieve the same results more rapidly and has been reported to result in improvement of mood and appetite. However, no definitive treatment is as yet possible. Prenatal diagnosis may prevent the birth of a second affected child.

16.5 Magnetic Resonance Imaging

Recently MRI findings were reported in one patient. At the age of 2.5 months a slightly enlarged ventricular system was found in combination with a mild enlargement of the subarachnoid spaces, a very large cavum septi pellucidi and a cavum Vergae. A high signal intensity was found in the parieto-occipital white matter on T_2-weighted images (Fig. 16.1). In a follow-up study at the age of 8.5 months, patchy areas of increased signal intensity were still apparent in the same white matter region, but the abnormalities were less pronounced. At that time the white matter still appeared to be largely unmyelinated. The enlargement of the subarachnoid spaces was slightly more pronounced. The described white matter changes would appear to be consistent with delayed and disturbed myelination.

Zellweger-like syndrome (ZLS) is a very rare disorder which has only been described in a few patients. The clinical and biochemical findings are typical of Zellweger syndrome. The children show profound hypotonia and severe epileptic convulsions from birth onwards. There is the characteristic facial dysmorphia with a large fontanelle, frontal bossing, shallow supraorbital ridges, a low nasal bridge and hypertelorism. Hepatomegaly is present. The neurological condition is poor. The children lie virtually motionless and have weak or absent Moro reflex, sucking and swallowing reflexes. Ocular findings include retinopathy and nystagmus. The patients described died within a few months.

Laboratory findings include signs of liver dysfunction, elevated serum iron, and increased levels of very long-chain fatty acids, dihydroxycholestanoic acid, and trihydroxycholestanoic acid. Phytanic acid level is normal. In urine increased dicarboxylic levels are found. Tissue concentration of plasmalogens is decreased.

In liver tissue deficient activity of peroxisomal β-oxidation and plasmalogen biosynthesis can be demonstrated. The activity of dihydroxyacetone phosphate acyltransferase, the enzyme that catalyzes the first step in plasmalogen synthesis, is deficient. In immunoblotting studies all 3 peroxisomal β-oxidation enzymes, acyl-CoA oxidase, trifunctional protein and 3-ketoacyl-CoA thiolase, appear to be deficient.

In electron microscopic examination of liver tissue, peroxisomes are demonstrated in normal amounts and with normal morphology. Catalase, a peroxisomal matrix protein, is present within these peroxisomes in normal amounts and with normal configuration.

The etiology of the multiple peroxisomal enzyme defects in patients with ZLS apparently differs from that in classical Zellweger syndrome. As peroxisomes are present in normal amounts and have a normal morphology in ZLS, their biogenesis and assembly must be intact. The basic defect in ZLS possibly involves one component of the protein import machinery, specific for a limited number of peroxisomal proteins. The basic problem may concern one of the targeting systems, may concern a cytoplasmic factor (a binding protein of stabilizing protein) or may concern a peroxisomal receptor.

 Pseudo-neonatal Adrenoleukodystrophy, Trifunctional Protein Deficiency, and Pseudo-Zellweger Syndrome

This chapter concerns the peroxisomal disorders with the isolated deficiency of one of the peroxisomal enzymes involved in β-oxidation. Only X-linked adrenoleukodystrophy and adrenomyeloneuropathy are discussed in a separate chapter.

A very small number of patients has been described with *pseudo-neonatal adrenoleukodystrophy* (pseudo-NALD). The first two siblings were reported by Poll-The et al. (1988). The name of the disease was chosen, because clinical features were very similar to those of neonatal adrenoleukodystrophy. The parents were first cousins, which makes an autosomal recessive mode of inheritance probable. The disease had its onset in the neonatal period with severe hypotonia and seizures. Neonatal reflexes were absent. No craniofacial dysmorphism was present. In one of the sibs no hepatomegaly was present, mild hepatomegaly in the other. In both children psychomotor development was severely retarded, but several motor milestones were reached and one of the sibs could crawl and walk with support at the age of 2 years. From about the age of 2 years onwards, neurological deterioration became evident. The hypotonia gradually changed into hypertonia with pyramidal tract signs. In one of the children epilepsy became very severe with almost continuous epileptic seizures. Sensorineural hearing deficit was noted. Whereas ophthalmological examination initially revealed normal pupillary light responses and normal fundi, increasing abnormalities were subsequently noted with nystagmus, strabismus, optic atrophy, tapeto-retinal degeneration and absent pupillary light responses. After a few years a vegetative state was reached, followed by death.

Neurophysiological investigations revealed increasing EEG abnormalities with epileptic discharges; the ERG became flattened, and VEP became almost entirely absent. Motor and sensory nerve conduction velocities were normal. Skeletal X-ray examination and echography of the kidneys were normal.

Laboratory investigations showed signs of slight liver dysfunction. Serum cortisol level was low, with an increased ACTH value. In serum and fibroblasts, very long-chain fatty acids were elevated, but no increase was found in plasma levels of phytanic acid, pipecolic acid and bile acids like dihydroxycholestanoic acid and trihydroxycholestanoic acid. The activity of dihydroxy-acetone phosphate acyltransferase was normal in fibroblasts.

Liver tissue was investigated in both patients, in one patient twice. Soon after birth (in one patient), peroxisomes were found to be abundant and increased in size. The catalase reaction was weak and variable. At the age of about 2.5 years (both patients) the number of peroxisomes was normal, but they were still enlarged in size. In one patient the peroxisomes had an unusual configuration.

Immunoblotting studies showed that trifunctional protein and thiolase were present. No immunologically cross-reactive material was found for acyl-CoA oxidase. The biochemical findings were also consistent with an isolated deficiency of fatty acyl-CoA oxidase, as an isolated accumulation of very long-chain fatty acids was found in the absence of abnormal bile acid intermediates. Bile acid intermediates have their own CoA oxidase, whereas trifunctional protein and thiolase are active for all substances β-oxidized in peroxisomes.

Recently two siblings were described by Mandel et al. (1992), who presented at birth with a poor start, severe hypotonia, absence of neonatal reflexes, presence of hepatomegaly and facial dysmorphism with wide open fontanelles, high forehead, shallow supraorbital ridges, long philtrum and thick lips. The synacthen test elicited a normal cortisol response at that time. Severe epilepsy occurred. Both infants died after a few months. Laboratory investigations revealed an elevation of very long-chain fatty acids in plasma and cultured fibroblasts but normal bile acid intermediates. In fibroblasts a normal dihydroxyacetone phosphate acyltransferase activity was found with a normal de novo plasmalogen biosynthesis. Electron microscopic examination of liver tissue revealed the presence of normal, catalase containing peroxisomes. Thus far, the clinical and biochemical findings are similar to the cases described by Poll-The et al., with the exception of the presence of facial dysmorphism and the severity of clinical course. However, immunoblotting studies revealed the normal presence of all three peroxisomal β-oxidation enzymes. A mutation affecting the catalytic site of acyl-CoA oxidase but sparing the synthesis of its protein may explain the enzyme protein to be immunologically detectable, but functionally inactive.

No postmortem examination of the brain has been performed in patients with pseudo-NALD.

In three patients CT scan of the brain was performed at birth and found to be unremarkable. No evidence of cortical malformation was seen, although minor or mild gyrational abnormalities and heterotopias can easily be missed on CT. In one child CT was repeated at the age of 4 years, when neurological deterioration was advanced. The images revealed symmetrical white matter hypodensities in the centrum semiovale and the occipital area with contrast enhancement of the border of the lesions. The CT findings are reminiscent of those reported in neonatal adrenoleukodystrophy.

A very limited number of patients has been described with isolated *trifunctional protein deficiency* (TPD). Watkins et al. (1989) described a male infant, who was very hypotonic at birth, with minimal spontaneous movements and depressed neonatal reflexes. He was macrocephalic with large fontanelles, but no signs of facial dysmorphism were found. From the beginning he suffered from severe epilepsy. There was no hepatosplenomegaly. Repeated funduscopic examinations revealed no retinal changes. He died at the age of 5 months.

Neurophysiological studies were performed. EEG was severely abnormal with epileptic discharges. VEP and BAEP were grossly abnormal. Nerve conduction velocity was normal. Skeletal X-ray survey and renal ultrasound were normal.

Laboratory examinations revealed an elevation of very long-chain fatty acids in plasma and fibroblasts. The plasma levels of phytanic acid and pipecolid acid were normal, but the level of trihydroxycholestanoic acid was elevated. Plasmalogen synthesis in fibroblasts was normal.

In liver tissue peroxisomes were found to be present and positive for catalase. In immunoblotting studies acyl-CoA oxidase and thiolase were found to be present, but trifunctional protein was not detectable. As trifunctional protein is involved in the β-oxidation process of both very long-chain fatty acids and bile acids, a deficiency of the protein results in accumulation of very long-chain fatty acids and abnormal bile acid intermediates.

Since that time a number of patients has been described with evidence of TPD. All children presented at birth with severe hypotonia and depressed neonatal reflexes. In some children a relatively large head was noted. Although some had no facial dysmorphism, the majority of the reported patients had the typical facial characteristics seen in patients with generalized peroxisomal dysfunction. Epilepsy had an early onset and was severe. Some patients had ocular abnormalities, including optic atrophy, pigmentary retinal degeneration and cataract. Auditory dysfunction was present in some, as was hepatomegaly. Psychomotor development was severely delayed. Death occurred between 4 and 12 months of age, with the exception of one child who died at the age of 3 years.

Laboratory investigations revealed signs of adrenal insufficiency in some of the patients. In all patients very long-chain fatty acids were elevated in plasma and fibroblasts. The plasma level of bile acid intermediates was also elevated. Plasma pipecolic acid, plasma phytanic acid and the de novo plasmalogen synthesis were normal. In liver tissue peroxisomes were present and positive for catalase. In immunoblotting studies all three peroxisomal β-oxidation enzymes were present. However, in complementation studies evidence of a defect at the level of trifunctional protein was found in all patients. Apparently, the enzyme is present but functionally inactive.

Postmortem examination of the brain has been reported in two TPD patients. In both cases the brain was relatively large. A combination of malformative and destructive abnormalities was found. In both cases polymicrogyria was present, in one case in particular over the lateral aspects of the frontal lobes. Scattered heterotopic neurons were found in the centrum semiovale and the subcortical white matter. Mild dysplasia of the inferior olivary nucleus was noted. In one patient, who died at 5 months, demyelination was reported in the cerebral white matter and corticospinal tracts of the spinal cord. A few foamy macrophages were seen in perivascular spaces and cystic degeneration of the periventricular white matter was found. In the second case, who died at the age of 14 months, decreased myelin stainability was found in the centrum semiovale, in particular in the frontal lobe, with relative sparing of the arcuate fibers. Active demyelination was most pronounced in the occipital lobe and cerebellar white matter. Axons were spared. Lipid-filled macrophages, occasionally striated, and astrocytosis were seen in the areas of demyelination, cerebral cortex and basal nuclei. In both cases, adrenocortical atrophy was found with presence of lipid-containing, ballooned, striated cells, which electron microscopy revealed to contain trilamellar lipid inclusions. In one case microscopically minute, glomerular cysts were seen in the kidney; in the other case no renal microcysts were found.

A number of CT scans have been reported. Most were described as normal, some as showing white matter hypodensity and slight enlargement of the occipital horns of the ventricular system. Considering histopathological findings, MRI is expected to show a characteristic pattern of polymicrogyria, especially over the lateral aspects of the frontal lobes, and white matter abnormalities. Most probably, there is a combination of dysmyelination, leading to myelin paucity, and, in particular in the older children with more advanced myelination, active demyelination. The demyelination is probably most pronounced in the occipital and cerebellar white matter, comparable to the demyelination in neonatal adrenoleukodystrophy and X-linked adrenoleukodystrophy. The combination of gyrational abnormalities and demyelination with predilection for the occipital and cerebellar white matter is also seen in neonatal adrenoleukodystrophy. In TPD no inflammatory reaction is seen in the area of active demyelination. In conformity with this observation, no contrast enhancement was found on the CT of the child who had active demyelination at autopsy, unlike the situation in neonatal adrenoleukodystrophy, where extensive contrast enhancement is seen.

The third disorder with an isolated deficiency of one of the peroxisomal enzymes involved in β-oxidation is the *pseudo-Zellweger syndrome* (pseudo-ZS), of which a few patients have been reported. The first patient was reported by Goldfisher et al. (1986). The infant was severely hypotonic at birth and lay almost immobile. Neonatal reflexes and tendon reflexes were absent. She had an expressionless face, but no facial dysmorphia was reported. Hepatosplenomegaly was present. She developed severe epilepsy soon after birth. She made no developmental progress in any field. She died at the age of 11 months.

Neurophysiological investigations included an EEG, which showed multifocal epileptic activity, nerve conduction velocity studies which were normal, and a VEP which was absent. X-ray examination revealed no calcificic stippling of the patellae.

Laboratory investigations revealed an elevation of very long-chain fatty acids in serum and an accumulation of trihydroxycholestanoic acid in duodenal aspirate. Phytanic acid levels in plasma were normal. The activity of the enzyme dihydroxyacetone phosphate acyltransferase was normal.

In liver tissue peroxisomes were abundant and many were larger than normal. They were reactive for catalase. In immunoblotting studies acyl-CoA oxidase and trifunctional protein were present in normal amounts, but 3-ketoacyl-CoA thiolase was absent. As this enzyme is involved in β-oxidation of both very long-chain fatty acids and bile acid intermediates, these substances accumulate in pseudo-ZS.

On postmortem examination of the CNS, malformative and destructive changes were noted. The most impressive abnormalities were found in the cerebellum. Within the cerebellar subcortical white matter scattered heterotopic neurons were found. The cerebellar white matter was involved in a process of demyelination, most pronounced in the area surrounding the dentate nucleus. Some perivascular infiltration with mononuclear cells was found. In the cerebral hemispheral white matter a lack of myelin was shown, with the exception of the arcuate fibers which were well myelinated. The internal capsule was normal and myelinated. The brain stem was preserved. In the

spinal cord the anterior and lateral corticospinal tracts and dorsal spinocerebellar tracts showed loss of axons and myelin. The liver showed signs of a mild fibrosis. Lamellar inclusions were present in hepatocytes and Kupffer cells. Microscopic renal cortical cysts were common. Adrenal cortex was atrophic and contained ballooning striated cells.

Neuroimaging findings have not been reported. Considering histopathological findings, evidence of a combination of dysmyelination and demyelination with most severe abnormalities in the cerebellar white matter is expected to be found on MRI.

A number of patients have been described in whom the diagnosis is either TPD or pseudo-ZS, as both very long-chain fatty acids and bile acid intermediates are accumulated. However, in immunoblotting studies both trifunctional protein and thiolase are present. In these patients complementation studies have (not yet) been performed to establish the precise enzyme defect. The clinical picture of these patients is variable.

The patient described by Van Maldergem et al. (1992) and Espeel et al. (1991) had the most severe course of disease, characterized by extreme hypotonia, myoclonia, facial characteristics resembling Zellweger syndrome and death at the age of 3 months. Postmortem examination revealed heterotopic neurons within the cerebellum. The olivary nuclei were dysplastic. No gyral abnormalities of the cerebral cortex were found. Myelination was normal.

The patient described by Barth et al. (1990) had a somewhat milder course of disease. She had a marked hypotonia from birth onwards, and suffered from severe epilepsy. No facial dysmorphia was present. She developed a progressive visual failure due to pigmentary retina degeneration and progressive deafness. Development was grossly delayed. She died at the age of 3 years. Initially MRI showed a delay in myelination. On follow-up examination at the age of 3 years (Fig. 18.1), signs of demyelination were found. There were symmetrical abnormalities in the pyramidal tracts in the brain stem, the cerebellar white matter, the posterior limb of the internal capsule, the corona radiata and the radiatio optica. There was no evidence of gyral abnormalities.

The patient reported by Santer et al. (1993) is highly unusual in his mild course. There was marked hypotonia in the postnatal period and some facial dysmorphism. At the age of 1 year sensorineural hearing impairment was noted. Psychomotor development was retarded, but walking with one hand held was possible at 2 years. He started talking at 2.25 years. He developed a hepatosplenomegaly. He never had convulsions. Examination at the age of 15 years revealed gross mental retardation, muscular hypertonia and normal findings at funduscopy. MRI showed mild widening of the ven-

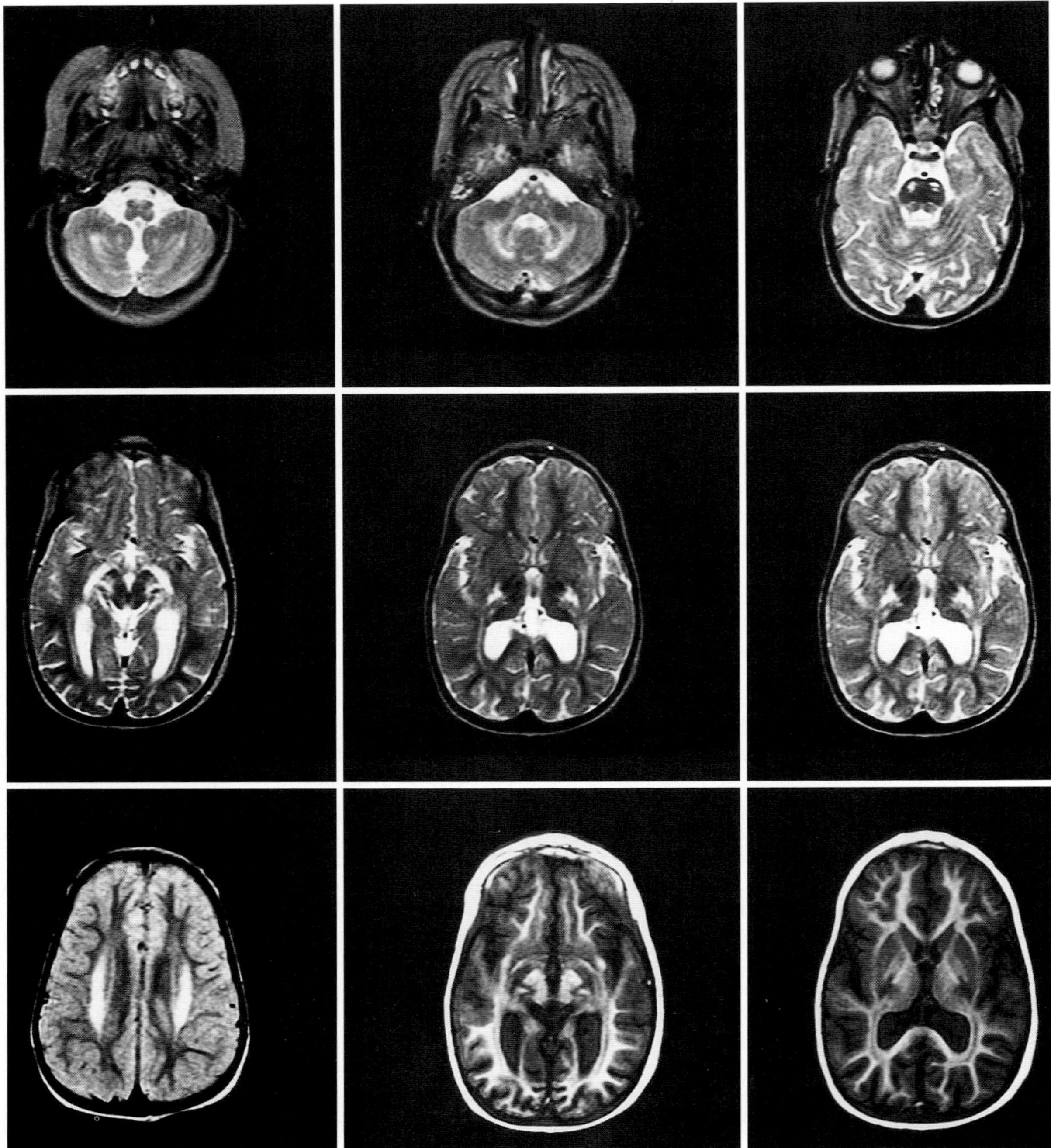

Fig. 18.1. In the T_2-weighted transverse series, the abnormalities in the cerebellar white matter, the dentatorubral tracts, the corticospinal tracts, the posterior limb of the internal capsule and paraventricular white matter are well depicted. The two T_1-weighted IR images (*two images right bottom row*) show the involvement of the corticospinal tracts and the dorsal part of the posterior limb of the internal capsule

tricular system, but no signs of demyelination or gyral abnormalities.

It is striking that diseases, caused by an isolated deficiency of one of the peroxisomal β-oxidation enzymes, can have clinical symptomatology that is indistinguishable from Zellweger syndrome or neonatal adrenoleukodystrophy. This observation indicates the pathophysiological significance of accumulation of very long-chain fatty acids and possibly also of the accumulation of abnormal bile acid intermediates, although these are lacking in pseudo-NALD. However, on the other hand, both pseudo-NALD and X-linked adrenoleukodystrophy/adrenomyeloneuropathy are characterized by an isolated accumulation of very long-chain fatty acids, whereas the first has a neonatal onset and early death and the second an onset varying from childhood to adulthood and a variably progressive course. Evidently, the relationship between biochemical abnormalities and clinical symptomatology requires further elucidation.

19 X-linked Adrenoleukodystrophy

19.1 Clinical Features and Laboratory Investigations

X-linked adrenoleukodystrophy (XALD) is a genetically determined disorder that mainly involves the adrenal cortex and white matter structures of the CNS. Inheritance is X-linked recessive. The disease has a wide phenotypic variability. The childhood cerebral form is the most frequent and accounts for about half of the cases. The second most common form is adrenomyeloneuropathy (AMN), which accounts for about a quarter to one-third of the patients. The less frequently occurring forms are the adolescent cerebral form, the adult cerebral form and the Addison-only form. In addition, there are asymptomatic cases and cases with unusual presentation. These different phenotypes may occur within one affected family.

In the childhood cerebral form of XALD, the age at onset of neurological symptoms is usually between 5 and 9 years. Features of adrenal insufficiency may occur before overt neurological symptoms or may follow. In some cases a diagnosis of Addison disease is made 1–3 years before any neurological disorder is evident, on the basis of increased pigmentation, fatigue, episodes of vomiting and catastrophic reactions to intercurrent infections. In others, neurological deterioration may have continued for some years without endocrine symptoms, and sophisticated investigations may be needed to reveal evidence of adrenocortical dysfunction. Adrenocortical dysfunction is present in at least 80% of the patients. The neurological symptoms appear rarely in the acute form of seizures or clouding of consciousness. Usually they are slowly progressive. The earliest neurological symptoms are often vague and frequently consist of behavioral changes. The changes vary from withdrawn to bizarre hyperactive and aggressive behavior and are often accompanied by poor school performance. Many boys receive psychiatric treatment until deteriorating learning capabilities and other neurological symptoms force recognition of the organic nature of the disease. Early neurological abnormalities are disturbances of gait and loss of vision. Walking problems are caused by a spastic diplegia. Decreased vision is caused by optic atrophy or bilateral occipital white matter lesions or, more often, a combination of the two. Initially, neurological findings are often asymmetrical with hemiparesis or hemianopia. Frequently noted subsequent problems are dysarthria, dysphagia, hearing loss, clumsiness and disturbed motor performance due to spasticity of the upper extremities. Cerebellar ataxia or sensory disturbances may be present, but are not usually prominent. There are no clinical signs of peripheral nerve dysfunction. Progressive dementia occurs. Epileptic seizures occur and are often multifocal in origin. The disease is always progressive, but the pace of deterioration is variable. In the final stage a spastic quadriplegia is present and a variable degree of decorticate posturing. The affected boys are blind, deaf and mute. A vegetative state or death is reached in 1–5 years.

The usual age at onset of AMN is within the third or fourth decade, but ranges from 14 to 60 years. Most patients with an adult onset form of XALD have AMN. Affected males have a slowly progressive paraparesis, cerebellar ataxia and signs of a distal polyneuropathy. There are sphincter disturbances and a variable degree of sexual dysfunction. About half of the patients has evidence of some cerebral involvement, with usually mild cognitive dysfunction of the "subcortical dementia" type. It is visual memory which is affected most. Psychological dysfunction may also ocur with emotional disturbances and depression. Approximately two-thirds of the patients have overt or biochemical signs of adrenocortical insufficiency which may precede or follow neurological dysfunction. Twenty percent of the patients has signs of hypogonadism with infertility. The disease is slowly progressive through decades.

In up to 50% of the female carriers some, usually minor, signs of neurological dysfunction can be detected. In 10%–20% of the female carriers the neurological signs are more serious and these patients have an AMN-like clinical picture, similar to that of male AMN patients. The only differences are that the neurological abnormalities are milder and of later onset in females. Average onset of clinical disease in females is within the fourth to sixth decade. Cerebral involvement and adrenocortical insufficiency are very rare among female carriers. Only 5% of the female carriers have mild intellectual impairment which is only detected by detailed psychological tests.

The adolescent (onset at 10–21 years) and adult (onset after 21 years) cerebral forms resemble the childhood cerebral form, except for the later onset. Just like the childhood from, the adolescent and adult cerebral forms have a rapidly progressive course. The disease is often misdiagnosed. It may present as a psychosis or dementing illness, or as a single focal brain lesion that can be mistaken for a tumor.

In the Addison-only form no neurological dysfunction is found. However, one cannot be sure about the future and all patients are considered at risk of developing over neurological symptoms later. Cases have been reported of Addison disease in childhood and finally development of neurological abnormalities in adulthood.

The asymptomatic group includes males in whom the typical biochemical abnormalities of XALD are found and who are completely healthy. Most of the males included in this group are small boys who were investigated because of clinically evident XALD in an older brother. The group also includes adolescents and a few older males. The oldest asymptomatic male ever mentioned was 62 years old.

There are few patients with an unusual form of XALD. Patients have been reported with predominantly cerebellar ataxia. Some AMN patients develop fulminating cerebral demyelination in their last few years, identical to the cerebral forms of XALD. One patient, aged 57 years, has been reported with rapid neuropsychiatric deterioration and signs of cerebral demyelination at the site of a severe cerebral contusion suffered several months previously. An adult female has been described with a lethal cerebral leukodystrophy.

Laboratory testing usually reveals signs of adrenocortical dysfunction. Urinary excretion of 17-hydroxycorticosteroids and 17-oxysteroids may be reduced. Primary adrenocortical insufficiency is further evidenced by impaired cortisol responsiveness to adrenocorticotropic hormone (ACTH) in the presence of elevated baseline ACTH levels. Evidence of primary testicular insufficiency is provided by low testosterone levels and elevated luteinizing hormone (LH) or follicle stimulating hormone (FSH) levels. CSF protein is elevated in the majority of the patients, sometimes combined with an elevation of gamma-globulin level or moderate increase in lymphocytes.

Diagnosis of XALD depends upon the demonstration of abnormally high levels of saturated very long-chain fatty acids (VLCFA) in plasma, serum, cells or tissue. For routine purposes plasma or serum is used. The concentration of C26:0 fatty acids is investigated as well as the ratios of C26:0/C22:0 and C24:0/C22:0 fatty acids. In over 90% of XALD patients all threer parameters are abnormally elevated. In a minority of the patients only one or two of the three parameters are abnormal. VLCFA analysis and C26:0 fatty acid β-oxidation measurements in cultured skin fibroblasts are used for definite diagnosis. Patients with XALD already

show the characteristic elevations in blood VLCFA during the first 2 weeks of life and even in cord blood.

Neurophysiological investigations are often used to establish the extent of disease in XALD. Nerve conduction studies usually show a normal conduction velocity in cerebral forms, but may also show a decreased velocity. In AMN the conduction velocity is decreased. In cerebral forms of ALD the EEG is as a rule abnormal, although nonspecifically, with diffuse slowing of the rhythm and a maximum usually in the posterior regions. Evoked potential studies may show abnormalities reflecting the central white matter involvement.

Investigation of the level of VLCFA is also a sensitive test in carrier detection. Ninety three percent of heterozygotes can be identified when the results of VLCFA assays in plasma and cultured fibroblasts are combined. Antenatal diagnosis can be established by measuring VLCFA in cultured amniocytes and chorionic villi, or by measuring the activity of peroxisomal β-oxidation. DNA techniques are becoming increasingly important. A problem in genetic counseling and prenatal diagnosis is that the demonstration of the biochemical defect does not provide information about whether the patient will develop severe childhood XALD or the milder AMN or remain neurologically asymptomatic.

19.2 Pathology

At autopsy the surface of the brain of a patient with childhood XALD is either normal or shrunken, depending on the degree of tissue loss. The central white matter is grayish and indurated, sometimes cystic and cavitated. The thickness of the cortex is normal. The atrophic external appearance is, if present, secondary to loss of white matter. In cases of extensive loss of myelin the ventricular system is enlarged.

Histologically there is widespread demyelination of the white matter. The demyelinating lesion constitutes one large area extending across the corpus callosum and involving both hemispheres. In most cases of childhood XALD the demyelinating process starts bilaterally in the occipital region and the splenium of the corpus callosum. Gradually the process spreads outwards and forwards as a confluent lesion until most of the cerebral white matter is involved. The frontal white matter is generally affected less severely and often asymmetrically. The subcortical U fibers are preserved until a far-advanced stage, and usually the U fibers in the occipital area are affected before those elsewhere.

Other areas of the brain that are usually heavily involved are the fornix, the hippocampal commissure, the posterior limb of the internal capsule, the lateral two-thirds of the cerebral peduncles including the occipitoparietotemporopontine and pyramidal tracts, and the lemniscus lateralis. In some patients the cerebellar white matter is involved, sometimes the cerebellar peduncles as well.

In a minority of the patients with childhood XALD the distribution of the demyelinating lesion differs from the pattern described above. Sometimes the demyelination starts bilaterally in the frontal area, also involving the anterior part of the corpus callosum. In these cases the anterior limb of the internal capsule and the medial third of the cerebral peduncles containing the frontopontine tracts are affected. In the minority of the patients the demyelinating lesions are highly asymmetrical.

Within the white matter lesion three zones can be distinguished on histopathological examination. The outer zone shows evidence of active destruction of myelin with axonal sparing. Scattered PAS-positive and sudanophilic macrophages are present. The middle zone shows signs of active inflammation with marked perivascular mononuclear cell infiltration. This zone contains many large ballooned macrophages laden with lipids. There are many preserved demyelinated axons and little myelin remains. The large central area is destroyed and burnt-out. There is no evidence of an active process. Axons, myelin sheaths and oligodendroglia are absent. There are few lymphocytes and only occasional macrophages surrounding blood vessels. This area is filled with a dense mesh of glial fibrils and scattered astrocytes. Sometimes cavitation or calcium depositions are seen in this area.

In the brain stem and spinal cord degeneration of the tracts appears to proceed at the same rate throughout, with no evidence of a dying back phenomenon. Here too the demyelinating process occurs in a continuous fashion. No small independent foci of demyelination are seen. Perivascular accumulations of inflammatory cells may well be noted.

The cytoarchitecture of the cerebral cortex is normal. Only in more advanced cases neuronal loss and gliosis may be seen, especially in the deeper cortical layers. The cerebral cortical damage is mainly found in the occipital region where the demyelinating lesion may not spare the U fibers and may be contiguous with the deep layers of the cortex.

Electron-microscopic examinations show that many macrophages and microglia contain distinctive cytoplasmic inclusions, consisting of linear lamellae. An individual lamella has a trilaminar structure, compared of paired electron-dense leaflets separated by an electron-lucent space. These trilamellar structures are often closely associated with lipid droplets. They are not found in oligodendroglia or astrocytes. In addition, macrophages contain myelin debris.

Microscopic examination of peripheral nerves reveals either no abnormalities or demyelination. On ultrastructural examination abnormal cytoplasmic inclusions may be seen in Schwann cells and in endoneurial macrophages. These inclusions have the characteristic linear, trilamellar appearance.

The pathological abnormalities of adolescent and adult cerebral XALD are similar to those described in childhood XALD.

Pathological studies in AMN demonstrate demyelination of corticospinal, spinocerebellar and dorsal tracts in the spinal cord and demyelination of peripheral nerves. In the brain, demyelination is predominantly seen in brain stem corticospinal and spinocerebellar tracts, medial lemniscus, posterior limb of the internal capsule, cerebellar white matter and cerebellar peduncles. Some patchy, poorly defined areas of demyelination may be seen scattered throughout the cerebral hemispheres or moderate diffuse demyelination may be observed but cerebral hemispheral involvement is milder than in the cerebral forms and of late occurrence. Only the optic radiations are more consistently and more severely affected. Inflammatory infiltrates are less prominent in AMN than in the cerebral forms of XALD. The characteristic trilamellar cytoplasmic inclusions in macrophages, microglia and Schwann cells are also present in AMN.

The adrenal glands in XALD show gross atrophy of the cortex, the medulla being normal. The zona reticularis and fasciculata are particularly affected with ballooned cortical cells in which a striated appearance of the cytoplasm may be seen. These striated cells are specific for XALD. Ultrastructurally the striations are shown to consist of linear, trilamellar accumulations within the adrenal cortical cell cytoplasm. Lymphocytic infiltrates are found in approximately 25% of the patients. Light-microscopic examination of the testis often reveals no abnormalities, although fully developed Leydig cells may be lacking. Interstitial cells, presumptive Leydig cell precursors, may contain the characteristic trilamellar profiles.

19.3 Chemical Pathology

XALD is a lipidosis, in which accumulation of saturated VLCFA occurs in all tissues, especially in CNS white matter, peripheral nerve, adrenal cortex and testis. Substantial quantities of these VLCFA are deposited as cholesterol esters, which appear as the characteristic lamellated cytoplasmic inclusions. These VLCFA vary in chain length from C23 to C32 with a peak at C25-C26. Also several other lipids contain an increased percentage of saturated VLCFA.

The changes in lipid composition of myelin and whole white matter have been investigated separately for regions with different stages of myelin breakdown.

In morphologically normal white matter, only subtle changes in lipid composition are found. Phospholipids are increased, whereas galactolipids and cholesterol are slightly decreased. Only traces of cholesterol esters are found in histologically intact white matter. The fatty acid composition of cholesterol esters, cerebroside and sulfatide in intact white matter is relatively normal, whereas phospholipids in the same area contain increased VLCFA, with the most striking increase in VLCFA in phosphatidylcholine. A moderate increase in VLCFA is seen in gangliosides.

The area of active demyelination shows major changes in lipid composition. The water content is increased, the amount of total lipids is decreased and there is a large increase in cholesterol esters, whereas unesterified cholesterol is severely decreased. Galactolipids are decreased, whereas phospholipids are stable as a proportion of total lipids. The fatty acid composition of cerebroside and sulfatide shows a slight elevation in VLCFA, whereas the VLCFA content of phospholipids, gangliosides and cholesterol esters is highly increased. The most striking rise in VLCFA among the phospholipids is seen in phosphatidylcholine and sphingomyelin.

In the area of gliosis, the amount of remaining lipids is small, and the water content is high. The amount of galactolipids is relatively very low, whereas phospholipids and cholesterol are low in absolute content but constitute a relatively normal proportion of total lipids. Cholesterol esters are present in small but measurable amounts. Also significant amounts of triglycerides and free fatty acids can be measured. In gliotic tissue the VLCFA content of cerebroside, sulfatide and phospholipids is hardly elevated, whereas the VLCFA content of gangliosides and cholesterol esters is still mildly to markedly elevated.

The adrenal and testicular content of cholesterol esters is abnormally high. The cholesterol esters contain an abnormally elevated amount of saturated VLCFA.

19.4   Pathogenetic Considerations

The basic metabolic defect in XALD is an impaired capacity to degrade VLCFA, caused by a defect in peroxisomal β-oxidation. The impairment is due to a single enzyme deficiency and the morphology of peroxisomes is normal. The first step in β-oxidation of VLCFA is conversion to fatty acyl-CoA, catalyzed by the enzyme VLCFA-CoA synthetase or ligase, present on the peroxisomal membrane. The enzyme is more specifically called lignoceroyl-or hexacosanoyl-CoA synthetase or ligase. There is evidence that the primary defect in XALD does not reside in the ligase enzyme itself, but in an ATP-binding transporter in the peroxisomal membrane. The gene has been mapped to a specific locus on the distal long arm of the X-chromosome. Probably this membrane protein is necessary to import VLCFA-CoA ligase, or a protein that is functionally associated with VLCFA-CoA ligase, into the peroxisome. The impaired degradation of VLCFA leads to enrichment of these fatty acids in various lipids at the expense of the normally degraded short-chain fatty acids. The accumulating fatty acids are saturated and have a chain length varying between C24 (lignoceroyl acid) and C32 with a peak at C26 (hexacosanoic acid). It is possible that there is a fatty acyl-CoA ligase specific for saturated VLCFA, as only saturated VLCFA accumulate in XALD.

VLCFA are derived both from the diet and from endogenous synthesis by a microsomal system that elongates long-chain fatty acids. There is evidence that in XALD not only the oxidation of VLCFA is decreased but that also the fatty acid chain elongation activity is elevated contributing to the accumulation of VLCFA. It has been shown that the addition of monounsaturated fatty acids to culture medium has a dramatic effect in lowering the content of VLCFA in XALD fibroblasts. These monounsaturated fatty acids appear to inhibit the synthesis of VLCFA without having any effect on the degradation of VLCFA. The mechanism of enhanced activity of the fatty acid elongation system in XALD is still unclear.

VLCFA-CoA ligase is also present in the endoplasmic reticulum. This enzyme is not deficient in XALD. Available evidence suggests that the two enzymes possess different functions in the cell. The peroxisomal enzyme generates VLCFA-CoA esters for β-oxidation in the peroxisome. The microsomal enzyme generates CoA esters for incorporation in cholesterol esters and triglycerides. Apparently, the VLCFA-CoA esters synthesized in the endoplasmic reticulum are not available for β-oxidation in the peroxisome.

The pathogenesis of the demyelinating process in XALD has remained elusive until now. There is evidence for a role of biochemical and immunological mechanisms. Evidence for immunological mechanisms in the pathogenesis of XALD is found in the observation of an intense inflammatory reaction in the CNS in the cerebral forms of the disease, occasionally signs of intrathecal immunoglobulin production, increased levels of IgA and IgG in XALD tissues and high levels of myelin antibodies in serum of XALD patients. The perivascular cell infiltrates in the CNS consist of T4, T8 and B-cells as well as macrophages compatible with an immune response to a CNS antigen. Occasionally, one encounters XALD patients who concurrently suffer from an autoimmune disease. An argument against a major role of immunological mechanisms is formed by the lack of improvement on immunosuppressive treatment. It is also noteworthy that in the destruction of other cell types, like adrenocortical cells, Leydig cells and Schwann cells, there is little inflammatory reaction and that in the AMN variant of the disease inflammatory infiltrates are much less prominent than in the cerebral variants. A more plausible hypothesis states that saturated fatty acids are toxic and their toxicity increases with chain length. Due to increasing levels of toxic VLCFA in myelin, instability and breakdown of myelin occurs. Most probably the cytotoxic properties of VLCFA also affect oligodendroglia, and oligodendroglial cell death contributes to the myelin loss. Breakdown of myelin leads to liberation of VLCFA containing myelin moieties. These might be antigenic and elicit an immune response. The VLCFA containing substances may also stimulate nearby astrocytes, microglia and macrophages to initiate a cytokine cascade resulting in further myelin destruction by T-cells, B-cells and complement. This two-stage hypothesis explains why the zone of active inflammation is found behind the zone of active demyelination. This location of the inflammation contrasts with the situation in multiple sclerosis, and Schilder disease, with which XALD has been compared in the past. In multiple sclerosis the inflammation is most intense at the edges of the lesion with little or no inflammatory response in the inner zones of the lesion. The location of the inflammatory cells in the second zone of the lesion in XALD provides evidence that inflammation is secondary rather than primary. It has been shown that VLCFA containing phosphatidylcholine is in particular increased in intact white matter and at the active edge of the demyelinating lesion. Phosphatidylcholine may be involved in antigen formation or in activation of the cytokine cascade. The normal level and fatty acid composition of cholesterol esters in intact white matter in XALD indicates that the accumulation of VLCFA-containing cholesterol esters in the advanced XALD lesion is a secondary phenomenon. VLCFAs released during myelin breakdown are readily incorporated into cholesterol esters and they are poor substrates for esterases. As a result they easily accumulate in the cholesterol esters. This concept is consistent with the finding that the amount of cholesterol ester increases primarily at the expense of nonesterified cholesterol.

Adrenal cortical cells, Leydig cells and Schwann cells are also involved in the disease process. They accumulate VLCFA incorporated in cholesterol esters in the form of lamellar cytoplasmic inclusions. A cytotoxic pathogenesis has been proposed for the adrenal, testicular and Schwann cell lesions. Furthermore, it has been shown that accumulation of VLCFAs in adrenal cortical cell membranes leads to increased membrane microviscosity and can interfere with ACTH responsiveness. Impaired ACTH receptor function has been found, probably contributing to the adrenocortical insufficiency. It is noteworthy that the destruction of these cells is accompanied by little or no inflammation.

All forms of XALD have the same basic defect and all forms may occur within the same family. No differences in fatty acid abnormality could be established in fibroblasts, erythrocyte membranes and blood in repeated investigations. There is one report about the presence of a correlation between the level of VLCFA in mononuclear cells and phenotype, the levels being higher in childhood forms of XALD than in adult XALD, but this finding still requires confirmation. There is evidence that there is an autosomal modifier locus, which can explain the phenotypic variability of XALD within pedigrees. This modifier gene probably has an influence on the immune response, considering the marked difference in immune reaction between childhood XALD and later-onset AMN.

Some female heterozygotes suffer from a slowly progressive neurological disorder. Cultured skin fibroblast clones of female carriers are of two types: one type has normal VLCFA levels and the other has levels similar to those of patients with XALD. This means that part of the normal X-chromosomes and part of the X-chromosome with the XALD mutation are inactivated. The majority of the clones are of the XALD type, which is unusual. The observation that selection appears to favor the mutant type may be a factor in the relatively frequent occurrence of symptoms in female carriers.

Why cerebral XALD and AMN frequently show a characteristic pattern of spread of the demyelinating lesion in the CNS, and why in some cases exceptional patterns are seen, has still not been explained. The relative sparing of the U fibers may be explained by the fact that these fibers myelinate last and contain the youngest myelin in which the effects of VLCFA accumulation will be expressed latest.

19.5 Therapy

Many therapeutic trials have been performed in XALD with disappointing results. Hormonal substitution is often necessary to correct the adrenocortical insufficiency, but it does not influence the progress of neurological changes. Testosterone administration can be of help in the AMN patients who have testicular insufficiency. Immunosuppresive therapy in order to suppress the inflammatory reaction and high-dose intravenous immune globulin were ineffective. Therapeutic strategies aiming at the lowering of VLCF have been clinically unsuccessful until now. Dietary restriction of VLCFA was insufficient to lower blood VLCFA. Monounsaturated fatty acids compete with saturated fatty acids for the microsomal fatty acid elongation system and diets enriched in monounsaturated fatty acids were more effective in lowering blood VLCFA. Diets restricted in saturated VLCFA with addition of oleic acid (a C18 monounsaturated fatty acid) and erucic acid (a C22

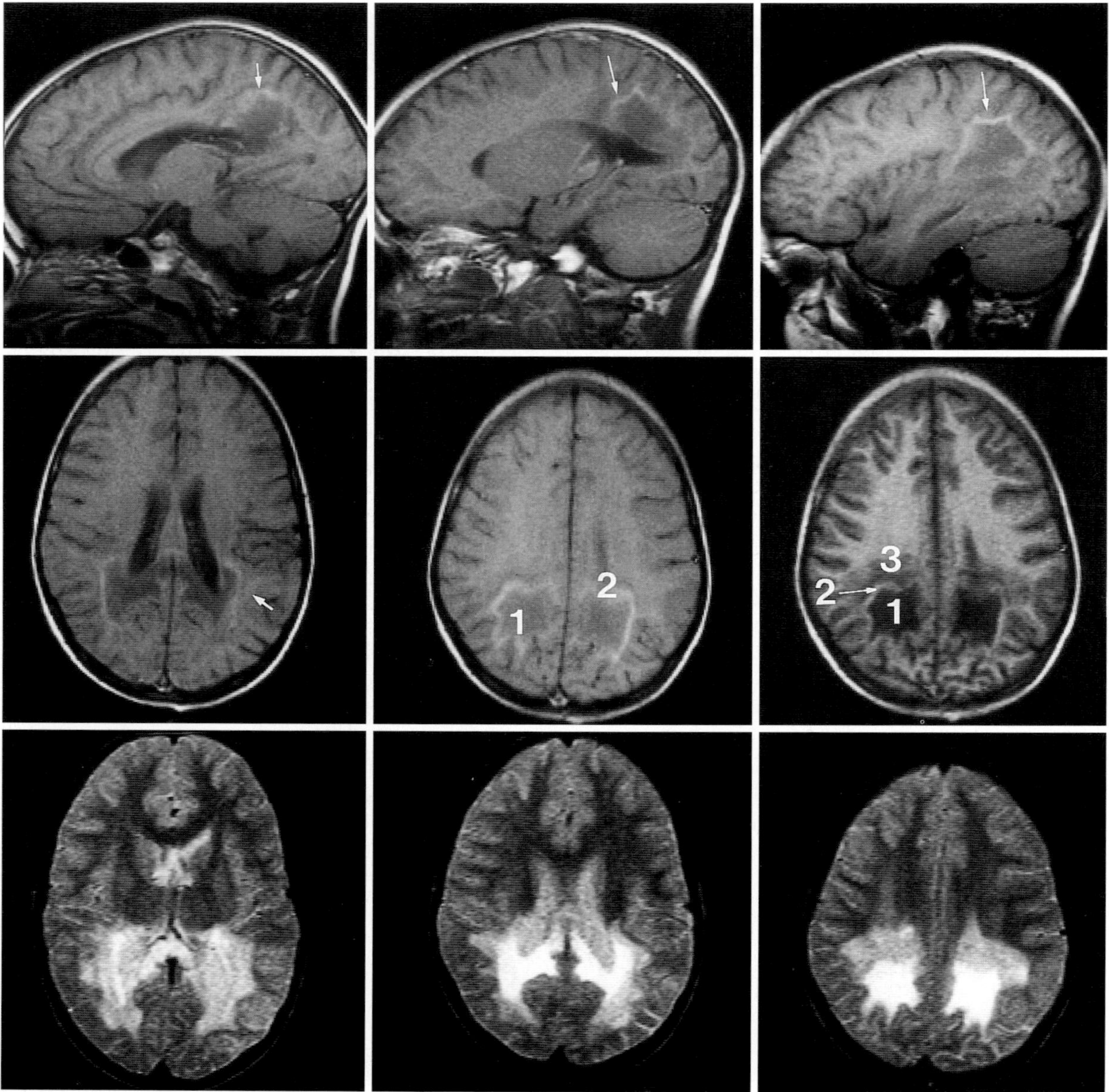

Fig. 19.1. Five-year-old boy with XALD. T_1-weighted sagittal images (*upper row*) with contrast show bilateral parieto-oc-cipital lesions, with an enhancing rim after injection of con-trast, the active border of the disease (*arrows*). The *second row* with two T_1-weighted SE images and one IR image also shows the enhancing ring around the lesion. The three zones of the disorder can be visualized this way: zone *1* being inactive and completely demyelinated, zone *2* showing marked inflamma-tion and advanced demyelination, and zone *3* representing the start of demyelination. Zone *1* and zone *3* can be distin-guished on T_2-weighted images (*lower row*)

Fig. 19.2. A 6-year-old boy with XALD. The *upper two rows* show a mixture of proton density and T_2-weighted transverse images of the disease in its classic form. The *lower rows* show the IR images, depicting better the involvement of the spleni-um of the corpus callosum, the corpora geniculata lateralia and the optic radiation. The corticospinal tracts show typical involvement (*arrows*)

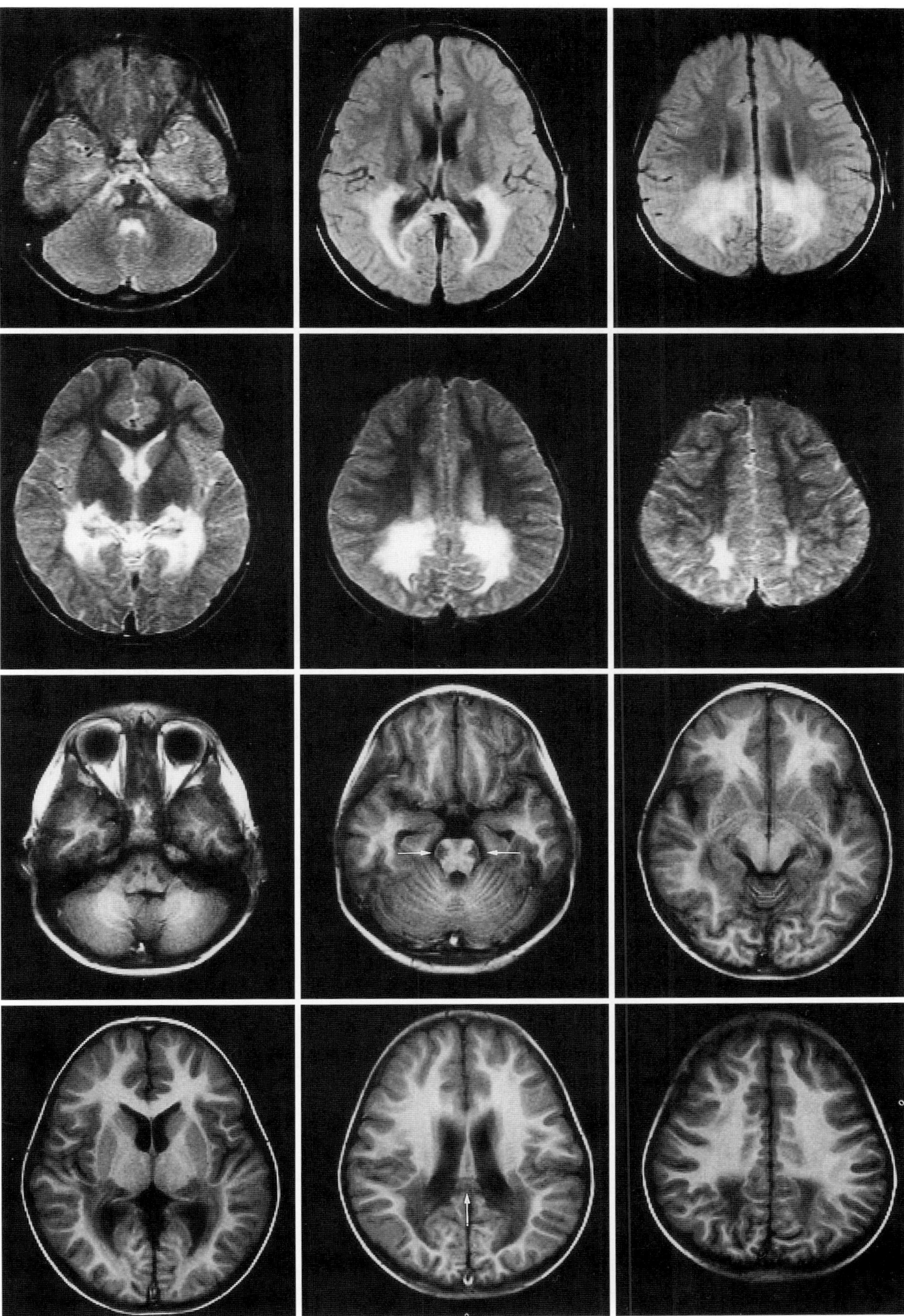

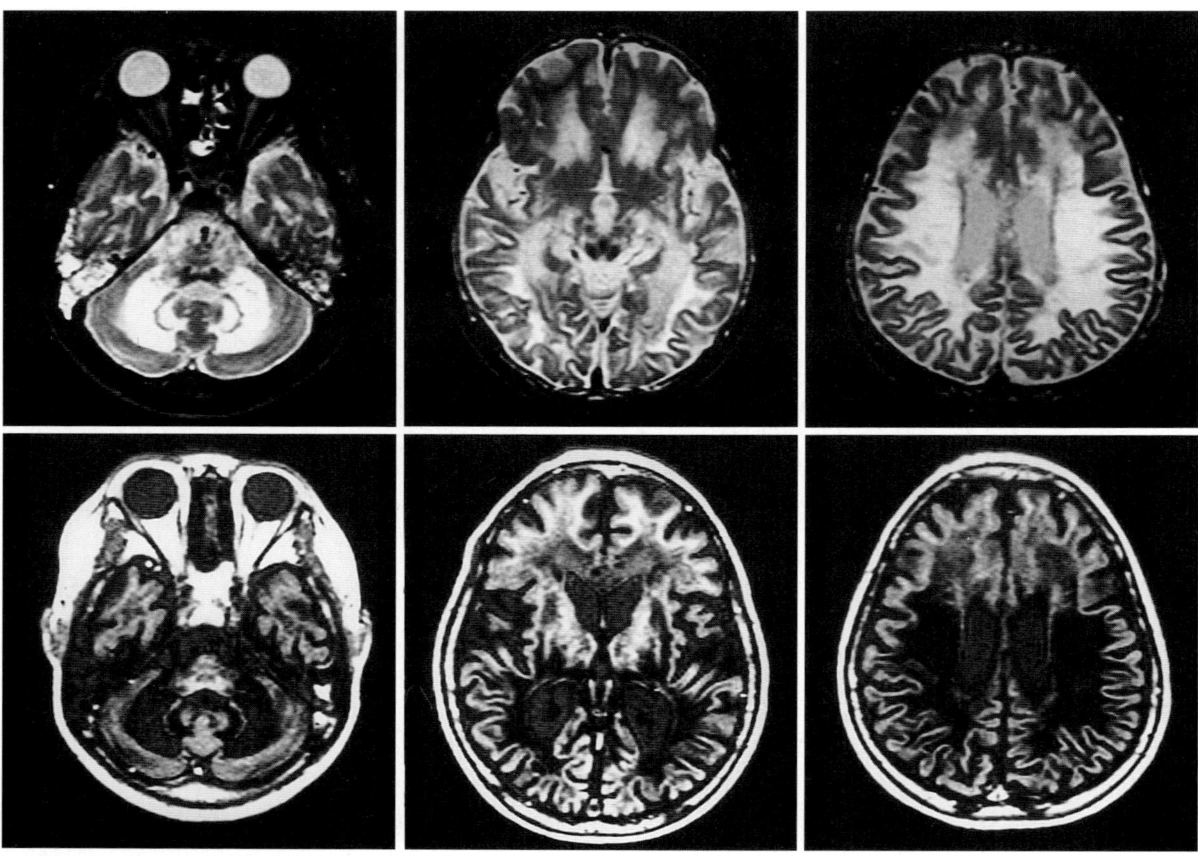

Fig. 19.3. Same patient as in Fig. 19.2, 3 years later. The disease has spread throughout the entire brain. These images are now end-stage and aspecific

monounsaturated fatty acid) led to complete normalization of blood levels of VLCFA and constituted a highly promising therapy. Reduction in platelet count occurred as a side-effect in 40% of the patients but did not lead to hemorrhages. There is definite evidence that these diets have no substantial beneficial effect on the course of disease in childhood XALD and in AMN. The results of the studies in asymptomatic and presymptomatic patients must be awaited.

A few promising cases of treatment with bone marrow transplantation have been reported. Ultimately, gene therapy in combination with bone marrow or oligodendrocyte transplantation may hold the greatest hope for the treatment of symptomatic patients.

Family counseling, carrier detection and prenatal diagnosis is important in preventing the occurrence of further cases in known families.

19.6 Magnetic Resonance Imaging

The most commonly occurring pattern of MRI abnormalities in symptomatic childhood XALD is diagnostic for the disease. This pattern is present in about 80% of the patients with childhood XALD. Extensive white matter lesions are seen in the occipital region with concomitant involvement of the splenium of the corpus callosum (Figs. 19.1, 19.2). The occipital arcuate fibers are relatively or completely spared, which is most easily seen on T_1-weighted images. In most patients two zones can be distinguished, the anterior zone where demyelination advances being less severely affected than the posterior zone. After administration of gadolinium-DTPA, a rim of enhancement can be seen surrounding the most severely affected area and separates this area from the less severely affected and normal white matter (Fig. 19.1). These three zones are in accordance with the three zones recognized histologically. The outer and advancing zone is in the process of active demyelination without inflammation. The middle zone shows signs of prominent inflammation. The innermost and most posterior region is completely demyelinated and burnt-out. In this latter area, cavitation and calcification may be present. The lesions are essentially symmetrical. Demyelination advances in the frontal direction (Fig. 19.3). Structures which are affected relatively early on are the lateral and medial

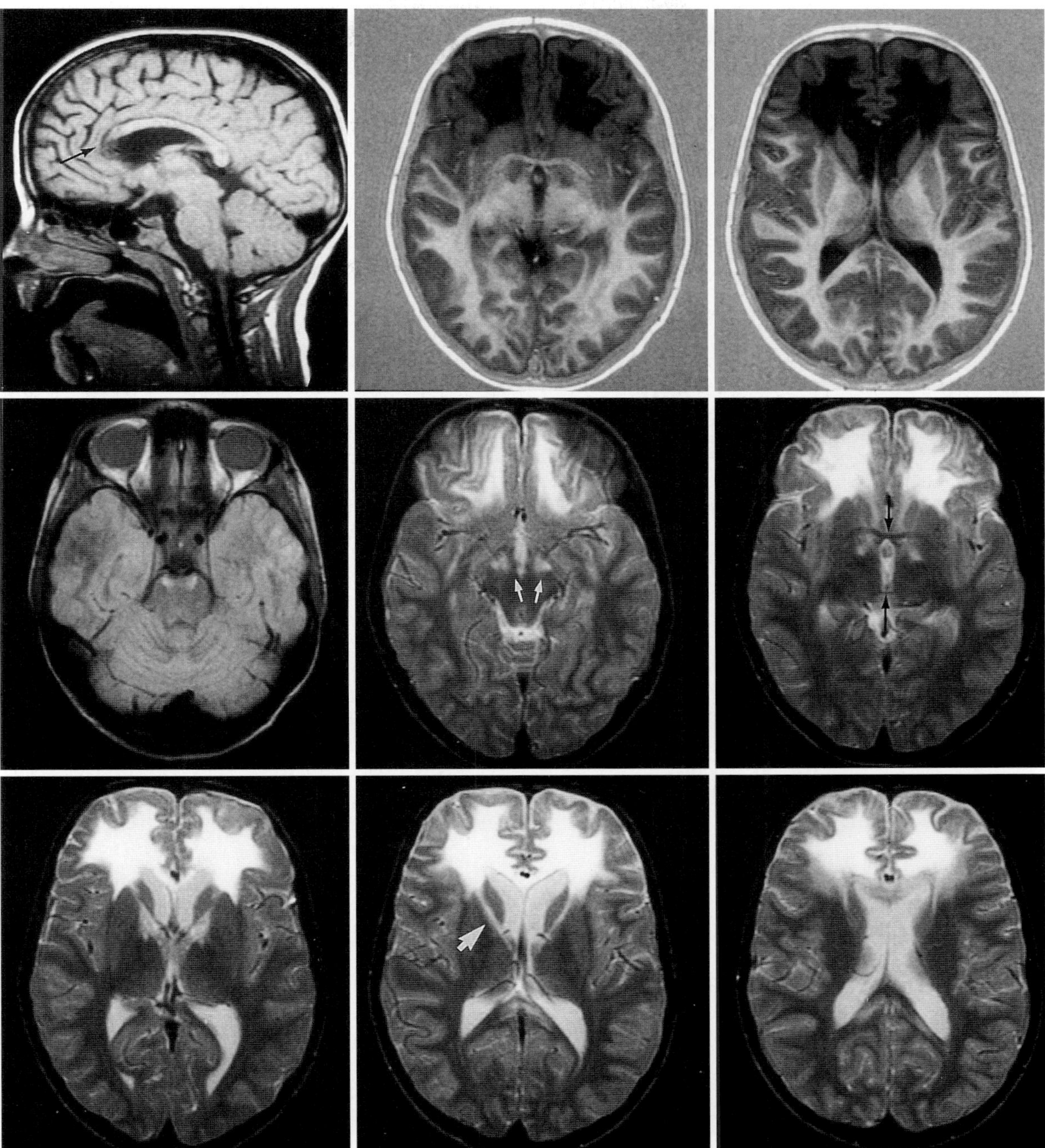

Fig. 19.4. Parasagittal and transverse T_1-weighted images (*upper row*) and a series of T_2-weighted transverse images of a 6-year-old boy with XALD are shown. The pattern of white matter involvement is the reverse of the usual pattern, affecting the frontal white matter, genu of the corpus callosum, geniculate bodies, in some cases the lateral-inferior part of the thalamus, the posterior limb of the internal capsule and the external capsule. The frontal lobe is affected last and more variably. The cerebellum is not usually involved early in the course of disease, in con-

anterior limb of the internal capsule (*large white arrow*) and frontopontine tracts (*small white arrows*) in the brain stem. The anterior and posterior commissures are spared (*black arrows*). Courtesy of P. Hoogland and W.F.M. Arts, The Hague, The Netherlands, with permission

trast to the brain stem. Typically the involved tracts are the occipitoparietotemporopontine and pyramidal tracts, the brachium of the inferior colliculus, the brachium of the superior colliculus and the lateral lemniscus. The frontopontine tracts are preserved.

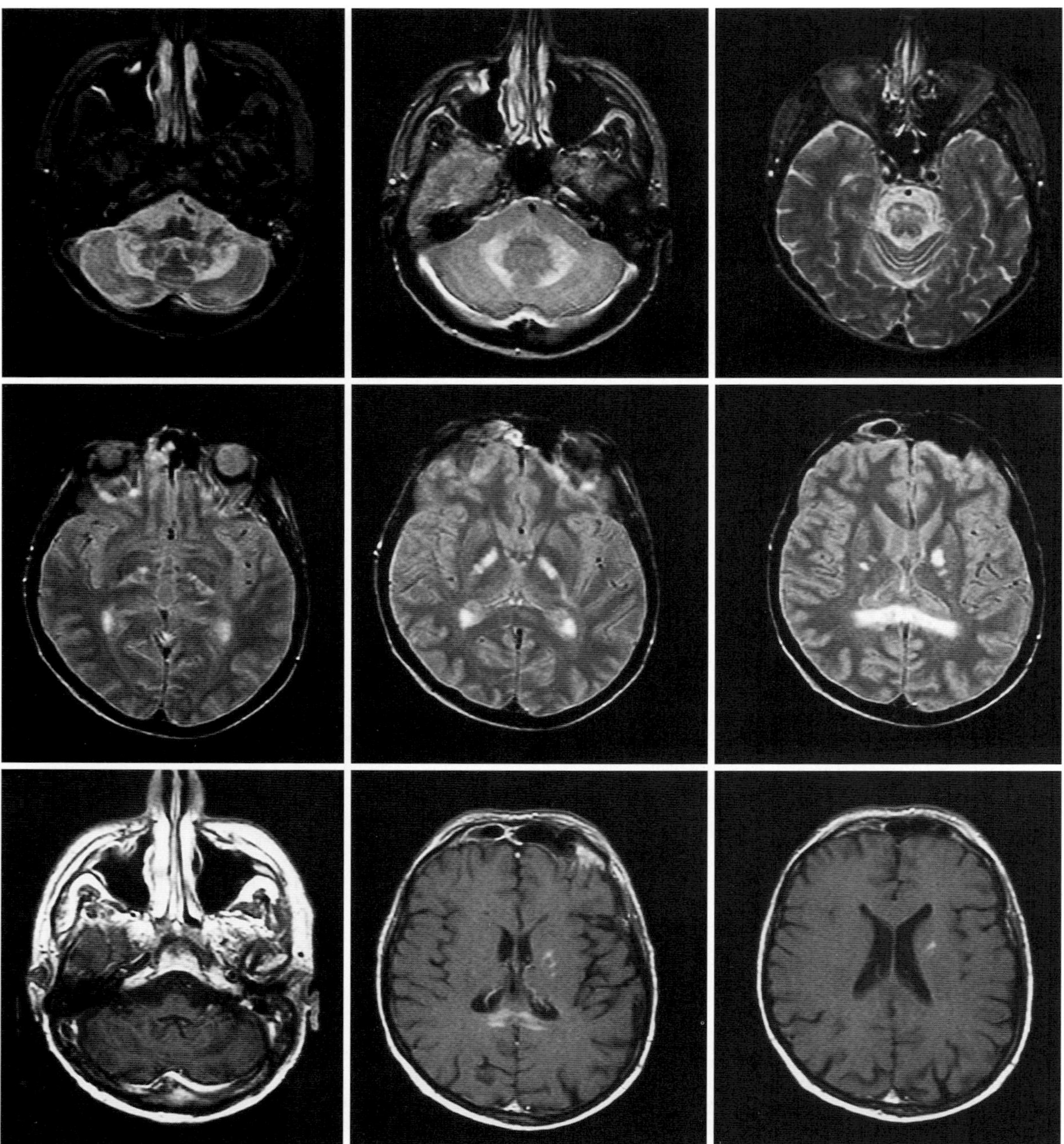

Fig. 19.5. A 45-year-old male with AMN. The T$_2$-weighted images (*upper rows*) show the involvement of the cerebellar white matter, the brain stem tracts, the splenium of the corpus callosum and the posterior limb of the internal capsule. Some enhancement occurs after injection of Gadolinium (*lower row*)

Exceptions to the rule are not rare. The pattern may be reversed, starting bilaterally in the frontal area with concomitant involvement of rostrum and genu of the corpus callosum (Fig. 19.4). In such cases the anterior limb of the internal capsule is involved instead of the posterior limb, and the frontopontine brain stem tracts instead of the occipitoparietotemporopontine tracts. This pattern is seen in about 10% of the patients with childhood XALD. In about 5% of the cases the parietal area is the site involved first.

Other exceptional cases have unilateral disease initially and bilateral but markedly asymmetrical disease in later stages. The presence of two zones in the lesion on unenhanced images and contrast enhancement of the rim in between these zones are helpful diagnostic clues. In one child presenting with initially predominant signs of cerebellar ataxia, MRI showed symmetrical involvement of cerebellar white matter and middle cerebellar peduncles only. The course of disease was rapid and otherwise indistinguishable from the common form of childhood cerebral XALD.

Much less is known about the pattern of adolescent and adult cerebral XALD. From the scanty reports in the literature, one obtains the impression that the pattern of abnormalities is more variable. One asymptomatic, adult patient suffered a severe cerebral contusion in the left temporal area after which the course was downhill. Demyelination started in the area of the contusion, and proceeded to affect both hemispheres, but asymmetry remained. Marked contrast enhancement was seen and extensive inflammation on brain biopsy. Another adult patient had changing lesions. The frontal bilateral lesions that were seen initially cleared, and the peritrigonal lesions became more pronounced. Subsequently, all abnormalities disappeared spontaneously. Cases have also been described with images identical to those of childhood XALD.

In half of the symptomatic AMN patients, abnormalities are noted on brain MRI. During the course of the disease, this percentage will probably increase. The pattern we found consists initially of abnormalities in the posterior limb of the internal capsule. Subsequently, abnormalities become visible in the cerebral peduncles including occipitoparietopontine, frontopontine and pyramidal tracts. With progression of disease ab-

normalities occur in cerebellar white matter and the splenium of the corpus callosum (Fig. 19.5). Following contrast administration, some contrast enhancement is seen in the advancing area, probably in the region just behind the most advanced zone, analogous to the findings in cerebral XALD.

In the literature, several observations on MRI in AMN are in accordance with our experience. In the "minimally" abnormal MRI's, involvement of the posterior limb of the internal capsule and cerebral peduncles in the brain stem are mentioned, whereas a minority of the patients has extensive demyelinating lesions in the frontal, occipital, temporal and parietal lobes and in the corpus callosum. Cerebellar lesions are noted in only some patients. Cerebellar atrophy and atrophy of the spinal cord are reported. One study mentions a much higher relative percentage of hemispheral white matter abnormalities, but these patients were probably in a more advanced stage of disease. Here too, the hemispheral lesions are described as being more subtle than in childhood XALD, and a predilection for the parieto-occipital area is found.

Only a minority of the symptomatic female heterozygotes shows abnormalities on MRI of the brain, although the pattern of full-blown cerebral demyelination has also been observed.

In asymptomatic or rather presymptomatic cases minor cerebral abnormalities have been found.

Mitochondria are membranous organelles that are responsible for providing most of the energy required for the cell in the form of adenosine triphosphate (ATP). They are termed mitochondria because of their thread-like appearance (mitos= thread) on light microscopy. On electron microscopy they appear as vesicles bounded by two membranes. The inner membrane is thrown into folds that project like shelves into the mitochondria. These projections are called cristae. Mitochondria consist of four compartments: the outer membrane, the intermembrane space, the inner membrane and the mitochondrial matrix. Mitochondria vary considerably in size in any one cell type, but most have a diameter of between 0.1 and 1.0 μm. In different cell types the size, shape, and number of cristae vary considerably. Most cells contain many mitochondria, the actual number differing in relation to the energy requirements of the type of cell. Mitochondria undergo continual renewal; they divide by fission.

The main role of mitochondria is to synthesize ATP, the universal source of energy for the cell. Mitochondria convert the energy derived from oxidation of substrates into the high-energy bond of ATP, which is then transported into the cytosol in exchange for adenosine diphosphate (ADP). The process of production and storage of energy by mitochondria is called oxidative phosphorylation. In addition to this process, mitochondria also perform many other functions, including the first two reactions of the urea cycle, the synthesis of ketone bodies, and propionate metabolism.

Pyruvate and fatty acids are the most important substrates for energy production, although amino acids may also contribute in certain conditions, for instance during fasting. Pyruvate represents the metabolic end point of glycolysis, which occurs in the cytoplasm and yields a small amount of ATP. Pyruvate is carried across the mitochondrial membrane into the mitochondrial matrix space by monocarboxylate translocase. Subsequently it is oxidatively decarboxylated by the pyruvate dehydrogenase complex (PDHC), which produces CO_2 and acetyl-CoA, while reducing one nicotinamide adenine dinucleotide (NAD^+) to NADH + H^+. The pyruvate dehydrogenase complex contains five components, three of which (E_1 or pyruvate dehydrogenase, E_2 or dihydrolipoyl transacetylase, and E_3 or dihydrolipoyl dehydrogenase) subserve a catalytic function, and two (pyruvate dehydrogenase phosphate phosphatase and pyruvate dehydrogenase kinase) a regulatory role. The E_3 component is shared by α-ketoglutarate dehydrogenase in the citric acid cycle, and by branched chain α-keto acid dehydrogenase (see maple syrup urine disease). Pyruvate dehydrogenase complex is located at the inner border of the inner mitochondrial membrane. Acetyl-CoA enters the Krebs cycle (also called citric acid cycle, tricarboxylic acid cycle, or TCA cycle).

Fatty acids with more than 8 or 10 carbon atoms require a specific carrier system to enter the mitochondrial matrix space (see Fig. 20.1). They are activated to acyl-CoA by acyl-CoA ligase (=acyl-CoA synthetase) on the mitochondrial outer membrane. Fatty acyl-CoA is subsequently converted to fatty acyl carnitine in the intermembrane space by carnitine palmitoyl transferase 1 (CPT 1), which is located in the outer mitochondrial membrane. Fatty acyl carnitine is then translocated across the inner mitochondrial membrane in exchange for free carnitine, a reaction catalyzed by carnitine: acylcarnitine translocase, located in the inner mitochondrial membrane. On the inner surface of the inner membrane a second carnitine palmitoyl transferase, CPT 2, converts fatty acyl carnitine to acyl-CoA and free carnitine. Shorter chain fatty acids (10 or fewer carbons) enter the mitochondria independently of the carnitine requiring transport system, and are activated by short- and medium-chain acyl-CoA ligase to the respective acyl-CoA esters in the mitochondrial matrix. Acyl-CoA is the primary substrate for mitochondrial β-oxidation. This β-oxidation spiral involves four successive reactions, mediated by acyl-CoA dehydrogenase, 2-enoyl-CoA hydratase, 3-hydroxyacyl-CoA dehydrogenase, and 3-ketoacyl-CoA thiolase. The products of each turn of the spiral are acetyl-CoA and acyl-CoA now 2 carbons shorter, under conversion of flavine adenine dinucleotide (FAD) to $FADH_2$ and NAD^+ to NADH + H^+. An acyl-CoA can recycle through β-oxidation spirals as many times as it can yield acetyl-CoA fragments. With each turn of the spiral, as the acyl-CoA becomes shorter, it encounters enzymes with different substrate specificities. An example of this is the series of chain-length-specific acyl-CoA dehydrogenases: long-chain acyl-CoA dehydrogenase mediates the reaction for acyl-CoA compounds

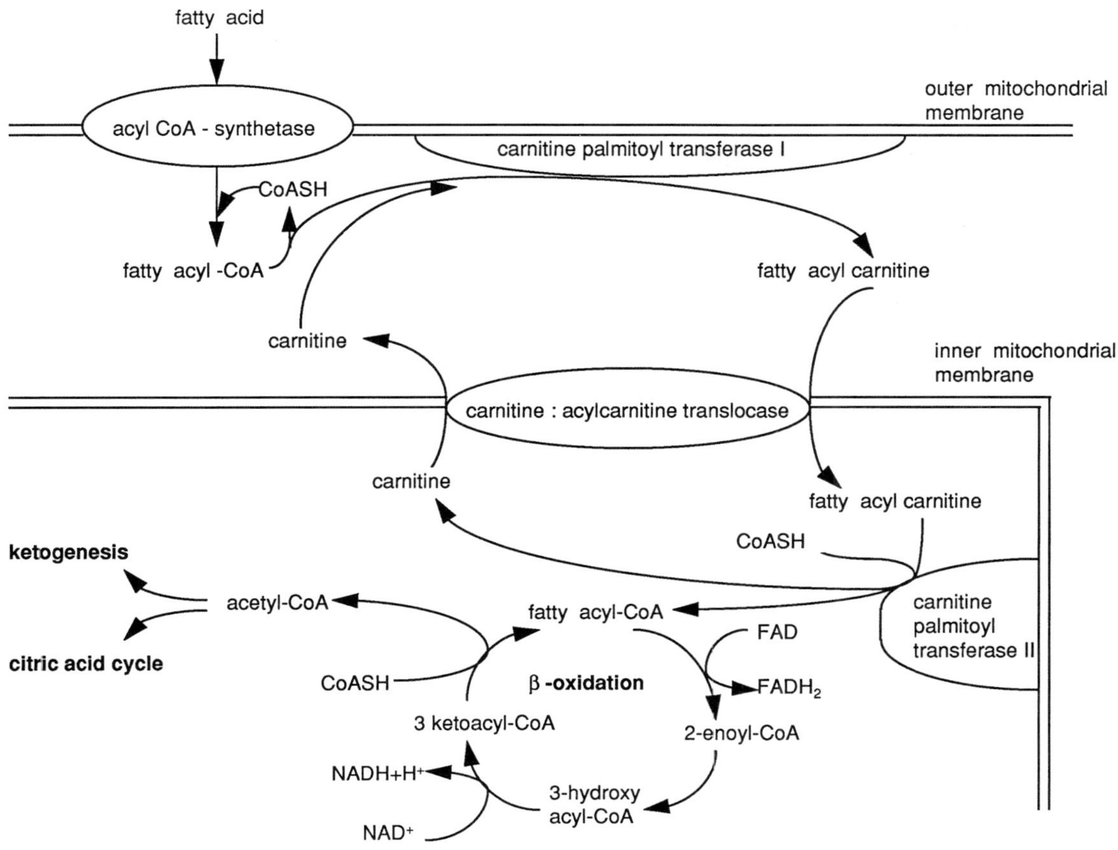

Fig. 20.1. Import and β-oxidation of fatty acids in mitochondria

from 8 carbons to 18 carbons; medium-chain acyl-CoA dehydrogenase from 4 to 12 carbons; and short-chain acyl-CoA dehydrogenase from 4 to 6 carbons. Fatty acids with double bonds require additional enzymes: Δ^3, Δ^2-enoyl-CoA isomerase and 2,4-dienoyl-CoA reductase. In the liver, the metabolic end-product of each cycle of β-oxidation, acetyl-CoA, is primarily converted to ketone bodies, while in other tissues acetyl-CoA is completely oxidized via the citric acid cycle. Electrons from the acyl-CoA dehydrogenase-mediated reactions are transferred to electron transfer flavoprotein to the electron transport chain.

Carboxylation of pyruvate yields oxaloacetate and decarboxylation of pyruvate yields acetyl-CoA. Acetyl-CoA is produced in the β-oxidation of fatty acids and can also be derived from breakdown of certain amino acids (for instance leucine and isoleucine). Oxaloacetate and acetyl-CoA condense to form citrate. Citrate is decarboxylated in the citric acid cycle (see Fig. 20.2), yielding CO_2 and reducing equivalents in the form of $NADH + H^+$ and $FADH_2$. Certain amino acids can be converted to citric acid cycle intermediates, such as glutamate, aspartate, alanine, proline and glutamine.

The reducing equivalents produced by β-oxidation of fatty acids and the citric acid cycle are reoxidized to NAD^+ and FAD by the respiratory chain. This oxidation sequence is tightly coupled to the phosphorylation of ADP to yield ATP. This process of so-called oxidative phospharylation is responsible for the main production of ATP in most cells. Oxidative phosphorylation (see Fig. 20.3) is achieved by means of five multi-subunit enzyme complexes (complexes I–V) plus the adenine nucleotide translocator, all located within the mitochondrial inner membrane. Complexes I–IV constitute the electron transport chain. Complex I (NADH ubiquinone reductase = NADH-coenzyme Q reductase) oxidizes NADH to NAD^+ and the electrons of the hydrogen are transferred to ubiquinone (CoQ) to yield ubiquinol (reduced CoQ). Complex II (succinate ubiquinone reductase) accepts reducing equivalents from succinate and also passes electrons down the chain to ubiquinone to yield ubiquinol. The electrons from ubiquinol are transferred to complex III (ubiquinol: cytochrome c reductase), subsequently to cytochrome c, then to complex IV (cytochrome c oxidase), and finally to oxygen which combines with pro-

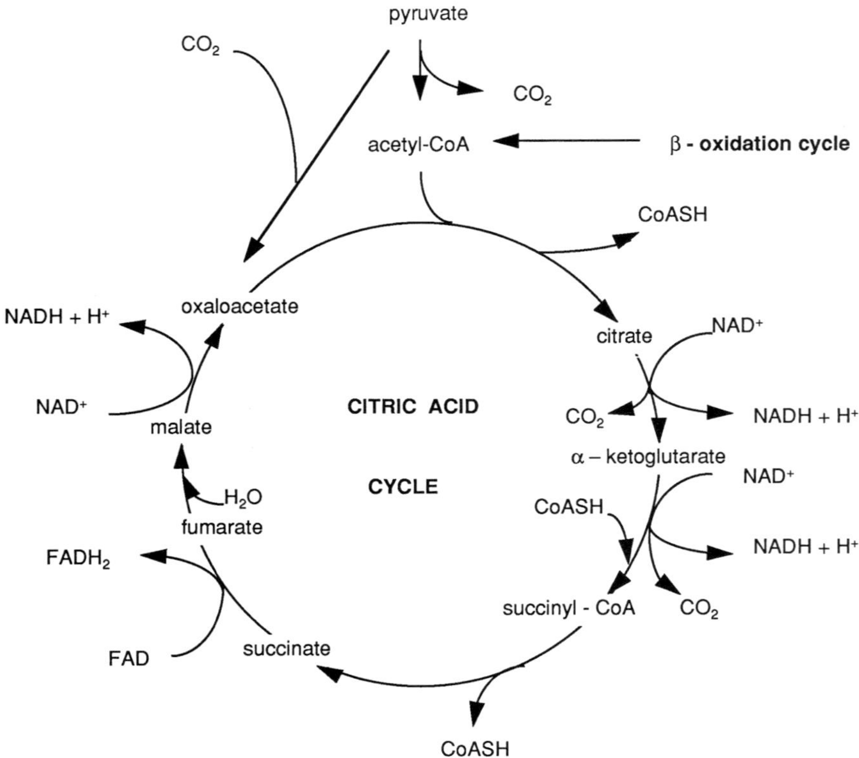

Fig. 20.2. Citric acid cycle in the mitochondrial matrix

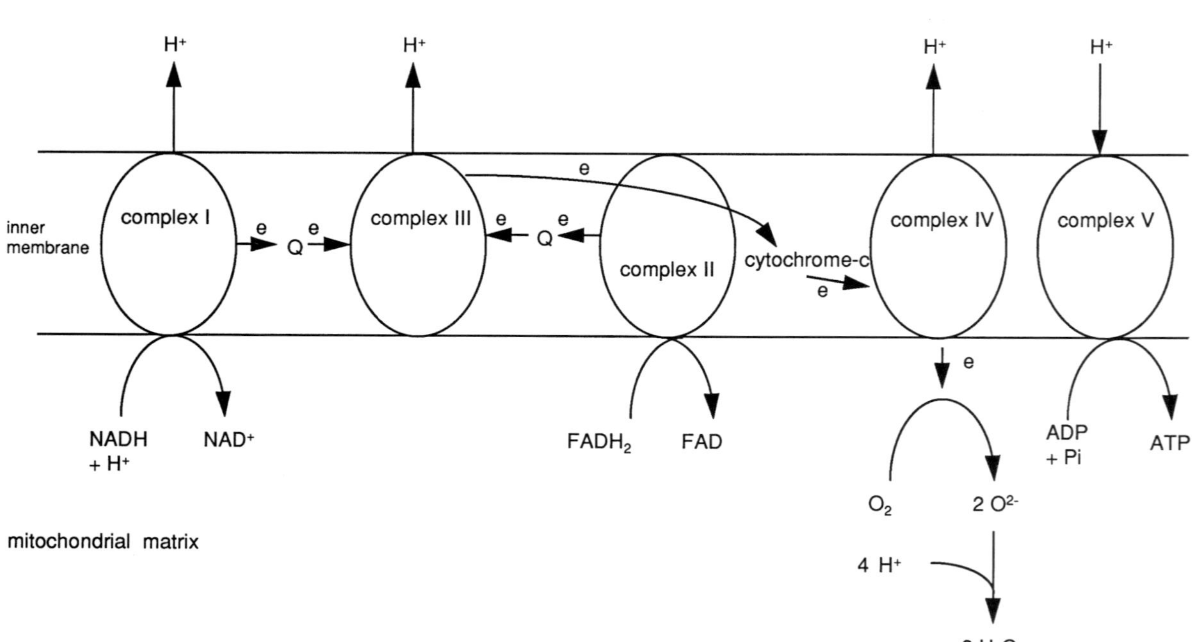

Fig. 20.3. Electron (*e*) transport chain in mitochondrial inner membrane

tons to form water. The energy released in the electron transport is used to pump hydrogen ions out of the mitochondrial inner membrane through complexes I, III and IV. The resulting electrochemical gradient is exploited by complex V (ATP synthetase= ATPase). Complex V allows some of the protons to flow back into the mitochondria and uses the energy so generated for the synthesis of ATP from ADP and inorganic phosphate. ATP formed in the matrix space is then transported out of the mitochondria by adenine nucleotide translocase in exchange for ADP. The production and storage of energy by mitochondrial oxidative phosphorylation is a very efficient process with a high ATP yield. The rate of mitochondrial substrate oxidation is finely geared to the needs of the cell. The main control mechanism is the ratio of ATP to ADP. ADP is an activator of mitochondrial respiration.

Each complex of the respiratory chain is made up of a number of protein components. Complex I contains at least 41 polypeptides and has as prosthetic groups flavin mononucleotide and several nonheme iron-sulfur clusters. Complex II consists of 4 subunits. Complex III is composed of 10 subunits including cytochrome b, cytochrome c_1, and a nonheme iron protein. Complex IV is composed of 13 different protein units, 2 cytochromes (a and a_3) and two copper atoms. Complex V is composed of 12 different polypeptides. Ubiquinone (coenzyme Q) and cytochrome c (a low molecular weight hemoprotein) act as shuttles between the complexes.

Human cells possess two different genomes: nuclear DNA (nDNA), a 3×10^9 base pair-long genome, present in two copies in each cell; and mitochondrial DNA (mtDNA), a 16,569 base pair-long genome, present in 2–10 copies per mitochondrion and, therefore, in several hundred or thousand copies per cell. Mitochondria are dependent upon the coordinated expression of these two seperate genetic systems. Most mitochondrial membrane and matrix proteins are coded by nuclear genes and synthesized in the cellular cytoplasm on free polyribosomes and have to be imported from the cytoplasm into the mitochondria through a complicated translocation machine, which is under the control of the nuclear genome. In addition, nDNA encodes several factors that control mtDNA replication, transcription and translation.

Most nuclear encoded mitochondrial proteins destined for the inner three mitochondrial compartments (intermembrane space, inner membrane and matrix) are synthesized as larger precursors containing an amino-terminal extension (presequence). The presequences are the targeting signals of the precursor proteins and direct these proteins to mitochondria. The presequences consist of 20–80 amino acid residues. There is no apparent sequence identity among the dif-

ferent mitochondrial protein presequences, but a characteristic common to all of them is a relatively high content of positively charged and nonpolar residues and an almost complete absence of negatively charged residues. This finding suggests that the specificity of the presequences resides in a structural configuration rather than a particular biochemical motif. Most of the presequences probably adopt an α-helical structure. Most mitochondrial proteins, in particular matrix proteins, contain their targeting signal in a presequence, but there are a few exceptions. A few proteins do not have presequences and apparently contain a targeting signal in their mature form.

Presequences are recognized by specific receptors on the mitochondrial surface (a special class of mitochondrial outer membrane or MOM proteins). The receptors directly interact with another protein, the general insertion protein (GIP), and thereby donate the precursor proteins to this membrane insertion site. The further transport of precursor proteins occurs through contact sites, where the mitochondrial outer and inner membranes are closely apposed. The inner membrane has a translocation channel distinct from, but in dynamic interaction with, the translocation channel of the outer membrane. Import across the inner mitochondrial membrane requires ATP and the presence of a membrane potential across this membrane.

The configuration of proteins is important in the process of import across the mitochondrial membrane. Completely folded polypeptides are unable to transverse the membrane. Premature folding in the cellular cytoplasm of the precursor proteins is prevented by stabilization of the proteins in a translocation competent, unfolded conformation with help of so-called molecular chaperones in an ATP-dependent manner. Molecular chaperones bind to interactive protein surfaces and prevent folding of the polypeptide chain. Appropriate peptide folding is attained after the chaperone has released the polypeptide substrate in a stepwise ATP-dependent manner. Molecular chaperones do not form part of the final folded or assembled protein structure but prevent nondesired folding and interactions of the substrate protein along its transport, folding and assembly pathways. The majority of the currently identified molecular chaperones belong to the class of so-called "heat shock proteins", or "stress proteins". As their name implies, these proteins were first noticed because of their specific induction during the cellular response to heat shock. However, the majority of the family members are expressed constitutively and abundantly in the absence of any stress. Subsequent studies have shown that many of these proteins are essential for cell viability under normal conditions of growth. Many heat shock protein family members, including those that do not respond significantly to heat shock, are induced under a variety of other stress conditions, whose common denominator may be the accumulation of unfolded or malfolded proteins in cells. They play a role in the stabilization or generation of unfolded or partially folded protein precursors before assembly in the cytosol or before translocation into organelles, in the stabilization of newly translocated polypeptides before folding and assembly, in the rearrangement of protein oligomers, and in the dissolution or disentanglement of malfolded or aggregated proteins. A different kind of molecular chaperones involved in mitochondrial precursor proteins consists of the so-called "presequence binding factors". These proteins, by means of their interaction with the presequences of mitochondrial precursors, are also essential in the import pathway of proteins into mitochondria.

After import across the mitochondrial membrane presequences are proteolytically removed in the mitochondrial matrix. This cleavage is necessary for further assembly of the newly imported polypeptides into functional proteins and complexes. Two different proteins are required for full protease activity, namely mitochondrial processing peptidase (MPP) and processing enhancing protein (PEP). The MPP component contains the catalytic activity, which is stimulated by PEP. MPP is completely soluble in the matrix, PEP is partly associated with the inner surface of the inner membrane.

Chaperone molecules are not only essential prior to and for translocation of precursor proteins across the mitochondrial membrane, they also play a role inside the mitochondrion. Some have a direct interaction with the import site, suggesting that binding to the translocating protein is an early event in intramitochondrial sorting of different precursors. Others are apparently important in the intramitochondrial chaperone-mediated folding pathway in which the newly imported polypeptides reach their final structures. The substrate polypeptide is released from the chaperone in a step-wise, ATP requiring manner, which leaves the product in a progressively more compact configuration. In many cases, the proteins are assembled into multisubunit complexes.

Finally, the proteins are sorted to their respective mitochondrial subcompartments. Allocation to the intermembrane space may involve a number of routes. Some proteins lack cleavable presequences and appear to use a different import machinery across the outer membrane than most mitochondrial precursor proteins. Other proteins have presequences and are translated completely into the matrix, and from there they are translocated to the intermembrane space. The third class of proteins has a bipartite presequence containing an amino-terminal matrix-targeting signal, followed by a stretch of hydrophobic amino acids that is a targeting signal for the intermembrane space. This hydrophobic stretch may function as a stop-transfer sequence for the inner membrane, by means of which the protein remains in the intermembrane space. These proteins may also pass entirely into the matrix and then be re-exported across the inner membrane. Some protein components of the inner membrane are initially targeted to the matrix or the intermembrane space before being assembled into oligomeric complexes in the inner membrane. Proteins can also be targeted directly to this membrane. Proteins are sorted to the outer membrane by many different mechanisms, sometimes but not always requiring the common translocation machinery in the outer membrane. They lack the typical targeting presequences.

The outer and inner mitochondrial membranes differ in permeability. The transport of metabolites and inorganic ions across the inner membrane is highly regulated. This relative impermeability is important in maintaining a membrane potential and pH gradient across the membrane necessary for oxidative phosphorylation. The permeability of the outer membrane is less restricted. The outer membrane contains pore-forming proteins, called porin or voltage-dependent, anion-selective channel (VDAC). Whether the pore is open or partially closed is dependent on the membrane potential. In addition to VDAC, other types of channels are present in the outer membrane. Probably the outer membrane has several permeability pathways differing in selectivity, regulation, and function.

Each mitochondrion also contains a piece of its own mitochondrial DNA encoding for different proteins of the respiratory chain and the structural RNAs (transfer and ribosomal RNAs) necessary for expression of these genes. The mitochondrial DNA is a circular genome formed by two complementary strands: one filament is rich in guanine nucleoticle residues, while the other is rich in cytosine residues. They are conventionally called heavy (H) and light (L) strands, respectively. Mitochondrial DNA encodes for 2 ribosomal RNAs (rRNA), 22 transfer RNAs (tRNA), and 13 messenger RNAs (mRNA). The 13 mRNAs specify as many polypeptides of the respiratory chain: 7 subunits of complex I, the cytochrome b subunit of complex III, 3 subunits of complex IV and 2 subunits of complex V.

There are a number of special features that characterize the mitochondrial genome:

1. The gene organization is highly compact. All of the coding sequences are continuous with each other; there are no introns. The only noncoding stretch of DNA is the displacement-loop (D-loop), a region of 1123 base pairs that contains the origin of replication of the H-strand and the promotors for L-and H-strand transcription. The D-loop is an important area of interaction of mitochondrial DNA with nuclear encoded

proteins regulating mitochondrial DNA housekeeping functions.

2. The genetic code used in mitochondria differs from the universal code, making nuclear DNA and mitochondrial DNA reciprocally untranslatable.

3. The entire mitochondrial genome of each individual, either male or female, is (almost) exclusively inherited from the mother, although it is not excluded that a small contribution of the mitochondrial genotype may be of paternal origin. This is due to the fact that during egg fertilization the sperm cell contributes almost no cytoplasm to the zygote.

4. The rate of spontaneous mutations of mitochondrial DNA genes is much higher than that of nuclear DNA genes and repair mechanisms are limited and less efficient.

5. The mitochondrial genome is present in two to ten copies per mitochondrion and, therefore, in several hundred or thousand copies per cell. In normal individuals all of these copies of mitochondrial DNA are identical (homoplasmy), but in disease there may be more than one distinct population of mitochondrial DNA (heteroplasmy), one being normal and the other being mutant.

6. Replication and expression of mitochondrial DNA are controlled by nuclear genes. The nuclear genome furthermore encodes for most of the mitochondrial proteins and cooperates with the mitochondrial genome in the assembly of the multisubunit enzyme complexes of the oxidative phosphorylation apparatus. The D-loop region is an important area of interaction between nuclear and mitochondrial DNA.

Inborn errors of mitochondrial function constitute a heterogeneous group of disorders, caused by a defect in either nuclear or mitochondrial genome. Considering the central role of mitochondria in cellular metabolism, it is no surprise that mitochondrial disorders are often multi-organ disorders with predominant involvement of brain and muscles.

Multiple classifications of mitochondrial disorders have been proposed. One of the earlier classifications stems from Morgan-Hughes (1982):

1. Defects of mitochondrial substrate transport (e.g., monocarboxylate translocase deficiency, defects of the carnitine: acylcarnitine carrier system)

2. Defects of mitochondrial substrate utilisation (e.g., pyruvate decarboxylase deficiency, β-oxidation defects)

3. Defects of the respiratory chain (e.g., deficiency of one of the cytochromes)

4. Defects of energy conservation and transduction (e.g., "loose" coupling of oxidation and phosphorylation, deficiency of ATPase).

Zeviani et al. (1989) extended this classification:

I. Defects of energy metabolism
　1. Defects of transport
　2. Defects of substrate utilization
　3. Defects of the citric acid cycle
　4. Defects of oxidation-phosphorylation coupling
　5. Defects of the respiratory chain
II. Defects of other mitochondrial pathways
　1. Defects of the urea cycle
　2. Defects of propionate metabolism and ketone bodies utilisation.

A recent classification by DeVivo (1993) is based on a genetic framework. The major subdivision is into nuclear DNA defects, mitochondrial DNA defects and intergenomic signaling defects:

I. Nuclear DNA defects
　1. Substrate transport defects
　2. Substrate utilization defects
　3. Citric acid cycle defects
　4. Oxidation-phosphorylation defects
　5. Respiratory chain defects
　6. Protein importation defects
II. Mitochondrial DNA defects
　1. Sporadic large-scale rearrangements
　2. Point mutations affecting structural genes
　3. Point mutations affecting synthetic genes
III. Intergenomic signaling defects
　1. Autosomal dominant multiple mitochondrial DNA deletions
　2. Autosomal recessive mitochondrial DNA depletion.

In the following chapters only those disorders are discussed that may lead to significant white matter changes. One chapter is devoted to disorders related to defects in mitochondrial DNA. Separate chapters deal with the disorders related to deficiency of a nuclear-encoded enzyme. One chapter is devoted to Leigh syndrome, which may be caused by both mitochondrial DNA mutations and nuclear DNA mutations.

21 Defects of Mitochondrial DNA

21.1 General Considerations

Human mitochondrial DNA is small (16.5 kb compared to 3 million kb of nuclear DNA). Each mitochondrion contains multiple genomes. Per cell there are hundreds or thousands of copies of mitochondrial DNA. In normal persons all mitochondrial DNA molecules are identical (homoplasmy). If there is a mutation in the mitochondrial DNA, this may affect all genomes (homoplasmy), or part of the genomes, resulting in the presence of two types of mitochondrial DNA, normal and mutant (heteroplasmy). In most cases of mitochondrial genomic defects, heteroplasmy is present. At cell division mitochondria (and mitochondrial DNA) distribute haphazardly between daughter cells. As a consequence, the proportion of mutant genomes may shift in daughter cells. The percentage of mutant DNA versus normal DNA may, therefore, be very different in different tissues and may shift in the course of time. Whether or not the mitochondrial DNA mutation is actually expressed, is largely determined by the relative proportion of normal versus mutant genomes in a given tissue. A minimum critical number of mutant DNAs is necessary to impair energy metabolism severely enough to cause dysfunction of that particular organ or tissue. This phenomenon is known as the threshold effect. The number of mutant genomes needed to cause cell dysfunction varies from tissue to tissue depending on the vulnerability of any given tissue to impairments of oxidative phosphorylation. The relative reliance of tissues on oxidative phosphorylation energy decreases in the following order: CNS, skeletal muscle, heart, kidney and liver. The presence of a mutation in a particular percentage of mitochondrial genomes may lead to signs of encephalopathy and/or myopathy, without any sign of dysfunction of other organs. The metabolic vulnerability may also vary in the same tissue with time and according to functional demands. As the proportion of mutant mitochondrial genomes may shift in daughter cells, this may also be the cause of a change in phenotype. Finally, there is a decline in oxidative phosphorylation capacity with age. The most likely mechanism for this phenomenon is the accumulation of damage to mitochondrial DNA in the face of insufficient ability to repair DNA alterations. This phenomenon may explain the late age of onset of clinical signs and symptoms in some patients, and the increase in severity of the disease with age.

Many mitochondrial disorders follow maternal inheritance. While at fertilization the same amount of nuclear DNA is contributed by oocyte and spermatocyte, virtually all mitochondrial DNA is derived from the mother. A mother carrying a mitochondrial DNA mutation will transmit it to all her children, males and females, but only her daughters will pass it on to their progeny. At a clinical level maternal transmission may be difficult to detect. Due to heteroplasmy, unequal mitotic segregation and threshold effect, different individuals in the matrilinear lineage may differ in symptomatology, differ in organ involvement or may even be asymptomatic.

Mitochondrial DNA is particularly sensitive to alterations. For a 16.5-kb DNA strand, it is a tremendous source of genetic alterations, which finds no counterpart in the nuclear genome. A rapid rate of spontaneous mutation and the presence of a poor repair system are probably important in this respect.

Different defects in mitochondrial DNA can be distinguished: point mutations, deletions and duplications. The DNA defects can involve genes coding for proteins of the respiratory chain or genes coding for transfer RNA (tRNA) or ribosomal RNA (rRNA).

Different point mutations in genes coding for complex I of the respiratory chain have been observed in Leber's hereditary optic neuropathy (LHON). In neurogenic muscle weakness, ataxia and retinitis pigmentosa (NARP), there is a mutation in the gene coding for ATP synthetase (complex V). Two pedigrees have now been described in which high proportions of the heteroplasmic NARP mutation are associated with Leigh syndrome (LS). In cases of mitochondrial DNA mutations affecting genes coding for proteins of the respiratory chain, biochemical analysis reveals a defect restricted to one respiratory enzyme.

A number of point mutations in tRNA genes have been identified. Each mutation is generally associated with a distinctive phenotype, although phenotypic overlap between pedigrees with tRNA defects is common. Well known clinical phenotypes include myoclonic epilepsy with ragged-red fibers (MERRF), mitochondrial encephalomyopathy, lactic acidosis and stroke-like episodes (MELAS), and variable combinations of myopathy, cardiomyopathy, progressive external ophthalmoplegia, diabetes mellitus and hearing loss. Despite the overlap in clinical symptoms between the different syndromes mentioned, the association of different tRNA mutations with clinical syndromes is still surprisingly specific, if one considers that these mutations all act on the same mitochondrial function, i.e., the ability of mitochondria to translate their own genes. Since mutant tRNA is unavailable for translation, a decrease in all mitochondrially encoded proteins is present. Among the different clinical phenotypes the abnormalities at biochemical level are vitually indistinguishable, usually characterized by multiple partial defects of the mitochondrial DNA-dependent respiratory complexes.

Large, single deletions of a substantial proportion of mitochondrial DNA have been described in chronic progressive external ophthalmoplegia (CPEO), Pearson syndrome, and Kearns-Sayre syndrome (KSS). These syndromes are clinically overlapping: muscle weakness and chronic progressive external ophthalmoplegia form part of the symptomatology in KSS; most patients with Pearson syndrome die in early childhood from a combination of pancreatic, hepatic, renal and bone marrow insufficiency with pancytopenia, but the few patients that improve and survive, develop the KSS and histological signs of a mitochondrial myopathy in later childhood. Although the size of the large, single deletions ranges from 1.8 to 8 kb, the same 4.9-kb deletion is known to occur more often and is therefore known as "the common deletion". In most cases the deletions encompass not only many of the genes encoding for proteins of the respiratory chain, but also several tRNAs. This explains the decrease in presence of all mitochondrial translation products demonstrated by immunological analyses. Biochemical analysis reveals decreased activity of complexes I, III and IV, individually or in combination. The percentage of deleted mitochondrial DNA is similar in muscles of both CPEO and KSS patients, but deletions are restricted to skeletal muscle in CPEO and widely distributed in extramuscular tissue in KSS. In Pearson syndrome mitochondrial DNA defects are present in a high amount in bone marrow precursor cells. This proportion probably falls with age if the patient survives, whereas conversely an increase in proportion of deleted mitochondrial DNA has been shown in repeated investigation of muscle tissue. Most (or all) of the cases associated with single DNA deletions are sporadic. This means that the deletion probably occurs after egg fertilization and by means of unequal mitotic segregation is spread over part of the cells. Replication of deleted genomes occurs more rapidly and as a consequence selection of respira-

tory-deficient cells may occur in the rapid turnover tissues.

Duplications of mitochondrial DNA are very rare in man. Sporadic cases of KSS heteroplasmic for mitochondrial DNA duplications have been described. In the cases described the duplicated region includes the D-loop, genes encoding for several proteins of the respiratory chain and the genes for several tRNAs and both rRNAs. As a result of the insertion of a duplication, one gene is interrupted or two genes have an in-frame junction. There is a second normal and complete copy of these genes. The DNA abnormality results in the production of an abnormal truncated protein of the respiratory chain or chimeric peptides which consist of two different truncated subunits, but the normal proteins are also present. It is possible that abnormal peptides impair mitochondrial function by competing with the normal gene products or, alternatively, that an imbalance of normal gene products from the duplicated regions could be harmful through relative deficiency of tRNAs or excess of products from the duplicated region.

The mitochondrial genome depends heavily on the nuclear genome, which encodes several factors involved in mitochondrial DNA replication, transcription and translation. Faulty communications between nuclear and mitochondrial genomes lead to either multiple mitochondrial DNA deletions or DNA depletion. These disorders are transmitted by mendelian inheritance, because the primary genetic defect resides in nuclear DNA.

Multiple deletions of mitochondrial DNA have been described in a number of clinical syndromes: autosomal dominantly inherited chronic progressive ophthalmoplegia plus variable additional symptoms, several case descriptions with variable symptomatology and evidence of autosomal dominant or autosomal recessive inheritance, and so-called mitochondrial neuro-gastrointestinal encephalomyopathy (MNGIE) with autosomal recessive inheritance. Although the molecular mechanisms leading to multiple deletions are still obscure, one possibility is that the abnormal product of the nucleus encoded gene acts by facilitating or amplifying an intrinsic propensity of mitochondrial DNA to undergo rearrangements.

Depletion of mitochondrial DNA underlies a number of rapidly fatal mitochondrial disorders in infancy. Quantitative analysis of the mitochondrial DNA reveals a severe depletion, varying from 50% up to 98% when compared to normal controls. Depletion of mitochondrial DNA correlates with presence of multiple respiratory chain defects. Clinically three syndromes are distinguished: fatal infantile hepatopathy, congenital myopathy with or without nephropathy, and later-onset infantile or childhood progressive encephalomyopathy.

Inheritance is autosomal recessive, suggesting that the genetic defect may involve a nuclear gene controling mitochondrial DNA replication.

The relationship between mitochondrial DNA changes, biochemical defects of the respiratory chain and clinical phenotype remains difficult to understand. One point mutation can be associated with different clinical phenotypes (for instance, the same mutation is present in both NARP and in some cases of Leigh syndrome; the same mutation in a tRNA gene is found in MELAS, in maternally inherited myopathy and cardiomyopathy and in maternally inherited diabetes mellitus). The phenotype related to the same abnormality in mitochondrial DNA may also vary within a single kindred. The same disease can be caused by different point mutations (see LHON). Combined features of different syndromes have been observed in one patient (KSS combined with MELAS; MERRF with MELAS, Pearson syndrome progressing into KSS). Part of the relationship between genotype and phenotype can be explained by heteroplasmy with different percentages of mutant mitochondrial DNA in different tissues and changes of percentages with course of time.

The following sections of the chapter are confined to those diseases that are associated with significant white matter involvement: MELAS, LHON, KSS and MNGIE. Leigh syndrome is described in a separate chapter.

21.2   Clinical Features and Laboratory Investigations

Mitochondrial myopathy, encephalopathy, lactic acidosis and stroke-like episodes constitute the MELAS acronym. The disease shows maternal inheritance with considerable intrafamilial variation in expression of disease. The age of onset varies between 3 months and 40 years but in most cases first signs and symptoms occur before adulthood. Early development is normal in the majority of patients. The first manifestations of disease usually belong to the group of general features of encephalomyopathies. A growth disturbance and epileptic seizures are the most frequent first symptoms. The disease is progressive with increasing symptomatology. Learning disabilities, cognitive regression, exercise intolerance and limb weakness are frequent manifestations of the disease. The myopathic features are rarely very prominent in MELAS. Stroke-like episodes are rarely early signs of the disease but have occurred before the age of 40 years in almost all patients. The stroke-like events give rise to both reversible and permanent neurological deficits. Hemiparesis and hemianopia or cortical blindness are seen most frequently. Episodic migranous headaches with nausea and vomiting are common and often precede the stroke-like episodes. In some patients focal seizures progress to epilepsia partialis continua. All patients eventually develop cognitive impairment. In those with early-onset neurological impairment, development is generally delayed from early on in life, whereas in patients with later-onset impairment, the rapidity of disease progression and the number of cerebral infarcts have a direct impact on the presence and severity of cognitive impairment. Sensorineural hearing loss is frequent. Delayed puberty, infertility and hypogonadism may be present. Less frequent findings, noted in less than half of the patients and by some considered to be "overlap symptoms", include myoclonus, cerebellar ataxia, peripheral neuropathy, pigmentary retinopathy, ophthalmoplegia, ptosis, optic atrophy and Wolff-Parkinson-White electrocardiographic syndrome. In relatives of typical MELAS patients a "partial" syndrome may be seen instead of the full-blown MELAS picture. Short stature, sensorineural hearing loss or myopathy may be the only clinical manifestation of disease.

On laboratory examination, CSF protein is often found to be elevated. Most patients have a lactic acidosis, although in some resting serum lactate is normal. CSF lactate is often also elevated. In EMG a myopathic pattern may be found. Some patients have ECG abnormalities with evidence of a cardiomyopathy, a Wolff-Parkinson-White abnormality or conduction block. In most patients ragged red fibers are seen in muscle biopsy.

Leber's heretidary optic neuropathy (LHON) is a maternally inherited disorder that causes acute or subacute loss of bilateral central vision. The onset is usually asymmetrical, but the interval between involvement of the two eyes is usually less than a few months. Men are affected much more frequently than women. The male preponderance ranges from 80% to 90% in most white pedigrees to approximately 60% in Japanese families. The onset of visual loss typically occurs between the ages of 15 and 35 years, with a maximal reported age range of 5–70 years. In most patients visual acuities deteriorate to worse than 2/20 in the course of several months, stabilizing thereafter. Visual field defects are typically central or cecocentral, but may also be bitemporal. Headache, eye discomfort, and flashes of light may occur at the time of vision loss. Transient worsening of vision with exercise or heat may occur (Uhthoff's symptom). Color vision is affected severely, often early on in the course of vision loss. In most patients visual loss is permanent, but improvement may occur. At the onset of visual loss, the optic disc is swollen and has a marked dilatation and tortuosity of vessels, initially interpreted as signs of inflammation. However, vessels do not leak fluorescein on fluorescein angiography. The typical ophthalmoscopic findings may also be present in asymptomatic family members, but some patients with LHON never exhibit these characteristics, even if examined at the time of acute vision loss. After the development of visual loss, a capillary-poor retina with attenuated arterioles and a pale optic disc remain.

In the majority of patients with LHON, visual dysfunction is the only significant manifestation of the disease. In some pedigrees additional cardiac conduction abnormalities are seen, in particular pre-excitation syndromes such as Wolff-Parkinson-White syndrome. Minor neurological abnormalities, such as hyperreflexia, Babinski signs, mild ataxia or distal sensory neuropathy have been reported. Several pedigrees have been described in which some of the patients experience more severe neurological problems. An extrapyramidal movement disorder with bilateral lesions of the basal ganglia on MRI has been reported in several patients. Association with a progressive polyneuropathy (Charcot Marie Tooth-like disease) has also been observed. Probably the most frequently observed association is with a multiple sclerosis-like disease. Episodic neurological abnormalities occur with partial or complete recovery. Apart from optic neuropathy frequently observed signs include spasticity, cerebellar ataxia, sensory disturbances, vertigo, diplopia, internuclear ophthalmoplegia, and urgency of micturition. The clinical features are indistinguishable from multiple sclerosis, as defined by the Poser criteria, however, occurring in the context of a family history of LHON.

Laboratory tests are of limited use in LHON. Fluorescein angiography is helpful in illustration and confirmation of the LHON funduscopic features. VEP studies confirm the absence of any response or presence of responses with prolonged latencies and decreased amplitudes. ERG is typically normal. In cases in whom the disease course resembles that of multiple sclerosis, an elevation of CSF immunoglobulin production is often found. ECG may reveal conduction abnormalities. Until recently, a definitive diagnosis depended on a positive family history, age of onset of the vision loss and the characteristic circumpapillary microangiopathy of the optic disc in the acute stage. Demonstration of a point mutation in mitochondrial DNA in affected individuals means that confirmation of the diagnosis can now also be obtained in atypical or sporadic cases.

Kearns-Sayre syndrome (KSS) is a rare, sporadic disorder, that affects the sexes equally. The onset of disease is prior to the age of 20 years. The sequence of manifestations is not constant, but the signs and symptoms in themselves are consistent. Early development is normal. Ptosis and chronic progressive external ophthalmoplegia are usually the initial signs. Apart from progressive external ophthalmoplegia the typical clinical triad includes a pigmentary degeneration of the retina and cardiac conduction block. The fine salt-and-pepper type of atypical retinitis pigmentosa is usually associated with good visual function and follows a benign course. Presence of choroideremia instead of pigmentary retinopathy has also been described. Most common cardiac conduction blocks are complete atrioventricular block, bundle branch blocks and fascicular blocks. Other frequently noted signs are short stature due to progressive growth failure, delayed psychomotor development, neurosensory hearing loss, cerebellar ataxia, proximal myopathy, cardiomyopathy and sensory neuropathy. Less frequent are pyramidal dysfunction and dementia. Endocrine disease is often present and includes primary gonadal failure, delayed puberty, diabetes mellitus, hypopituitarism, hyperaldosteronism, hypothyroidism, and hypoparathyroidism. Cardiac arrhythmias and congestive cardiomyopathy may be the cause of death.

Incidentally, patients have been reported, who suffered from Pearson syndrome in infancy followed later by KSS. Pearson syndrome comprises refractory sideroblastic anemia requiring transfusion, thrombocytopenia, neutropenia, pancreatic insufficiency and hepatic dysfunction. Onset is in infancy and many patients die before the age of 3 years. Some children survive the infantile period and no longer need repeated blood transfusions. These patients subsequently developed KSS syndrome.

Laboratory investigations almost invariably reveal an increased CSF protein level, usually above the level of 1 g/l. CSF lactate and pyruvate are mostly elevated. Signs of variable endocrine dysfunction are frequently found. EMG may reveal signs of a myopathy. ECG shows evidence of a disturbance of cardiac conduction. In echocardiography and chest X-ray cardiomegaly may be found.

Another multisystem mitochondrial disease has been described by a number of acronyms: *mitochondrial neurogastrointestinal encephalomyopathy* (MNGIE), myo-neuro-gastrointestinal encephalopathy (also MNGIE), polyneuropathy, ophthalmoplegia, leukoencephalopathy and intestinal pseudo-obstruction (POLIP), oculogastrointestinal muscular dystrophy (OGIMD), mitochondrial encephalomyopathy with sensorimotor polyneuropathy, ophthalmoplegia, and pseudo-obstruction (MEPOP), and chronic intestinal pseudo-obstruction (CIPO) with myopathy and ophthalmoplegia. The disease has an autosomal recessive mode of inheritance. In the majority of the patients symptoms begin before the age of 20 years. Initial symptoms are most frequently gastrointestinal, ocular or both. Gastrointestinal signs include recurrent nausea, vomiting, diarrhea, malabsorption, diverticulosis, and pseudo-obstruction. In most of the patients studies, delayed gastric emptying and dysmotility of small intestine, esophagus and/or pharynx are found. The gastrointestinal dysmotility is caused by visceral myopathy or visceral neuropathy. Ocular signs include chronic progressive external ophthalmoplegia, ptosis and pigmentary retinopathy. Other common clinical features include thin body habitus, short stature, sensorineural hearing loss, and sensorimotor peripheral neuropathy. Limb weakness is either distal, proximal or diffuse. Areflexia may be present. There is rarely evidence of CNS involvement. Mental retardation and cerebellar ataxia have been reported incidentally.

Laboratory investigations may reveal an elevated blood lactate and pyruvate. CSF protein level is often raised. Nerve conduction velocity is decreased moderately to markedly and EMG reveals signs of denervation consistent with a combination of demyelination and axonal loss. Some patients have abnormal ECGs with evidence of conduction disturbances.

21.3 Pathology

On light microscopic examination of muscle biopsies, application of the modified Gomori trichrome stain often reveals the presence of ragged red fibers. With this stain the abnormal fibers demonstrate a mottled and irregular appearance with red staining peripheral and intermyofibrillar zones. Histochemistry for oxidative enzymes, such as NADH dehydrogenase and succinate dehydrogenase, may yield abnormal staining patterns. On electron microscopy, the ragged red fibers display large aggregates of mitochondria, generally under the sarcolemma, but also between myofibrils. The mitochondria are frequently abnormal in size and structure. The mitochondrial cristae are often increased in number and irregularly oriented. The mitochondria may contain different abnormal inclusions such as crystalline or paracrystalline structures or globular bodies. Ragged red fibers are usually present in cases of single large deletions or duplications of mitochondrial DNA, in multiple deletions, in depletion of mitochondrial DNA, and in point mutations affecting tRNA genes, all conditions that interfere with intramitochondrial protein synthesis. In contrast, point mutations affecting mitochondrial DNA coding for single proteins of the respiratory chain are not generally associated with ragged red fibers.

Postmortem examination of the brain of deceased *MELAS* patients often reveals atrophy on external examination. Also the cerebellum may have an atrophic aspect. Major blood vessels are normal. Microscopic examination reveals areas of extensive cortical laminar necrosis, usually in the occipital and posterior temporal areas. The cortical lesions usually have an asymmetrical distribution and are not related to vascular supply areas. The three deepest cortical layers are affected most severely. The gyral crests and sulcal depths are equally affected. The severity of the cortical damage varies from fractional neuronal loss to microcystic

destruction. Gliosis is present. The cortical damage may have a spongiform aspect. In the area of cortical damage, there is a proliferation of capillaries. The lesions vary in age, the patient often having lesions of different ages. The adjacent white matter is involved with loss of myelin and presence of fibrous gliosis. The white matter damage may be spongiform. The deep white matter is not usually involved. Calcium deposits are frequently present in the globus pallidus, less frequently in the caudate nucleus, lateral thalamus, dentate nucleus, subthalamic nucleus, substantia nigra and red nucleus. The calcium granules are mostly deposited in and around capillary and small arterial walls. Otherwise the basal nuclei are intact and no neuronal loss is seen. Within the cerebellum pathological changes consist of some variable loss of Purkinje cells and granule cells. Brain stem and spinal cord may also contain spongiform lesions.

In *LHON* severe axonal degeneration with myelin loss of the central part of the optic nerve and pregeniculate pathway is found. The nature of the cerebral multiple sclerosis-like white matter lesions has not yet been investigated.

In *KSS* the main finding on postmortem examination that has been reported is a spongy state of the cerebral white matter due to splitting of myelin sheaths. The axons are generally preserved. The white matter changes are diffusely observed in the frontal, parietal, temporal and occipital lobes of both hemispheres. It is the hemispheral white matter that is involved, whereas corpus callosum and internal capsule tend to be preserved. Some authors mention particular involvement of the U fibers; sparing is rarely mentioned. The cerebral cortex is intact. The basal ganglia are involved, in particular the globus pallidus and caudate nucleus, but also the putamen, thalamus, hypothalamus, subthalamic nuclei, and substantia nigra may be affected. The basal ganglia lesions are characterized by loss of nerve cells, spongiosis, gliosis and capillary proliferation. Within the globus pallidus perivascular depositions of calcium and intracellular depositions of iron may be seen. The same type of depositions may be seen within the caudate nucleus. Within the cerebellar cortex, loss of Purkinje cells may be seen, as well as spongiosis and gliosis of the cerebellar white matter. In the brain stem spongiosis and gliosis have been reported in white matter structures, in the tegmentum and other gray matter nuclei. In addition, presence of cardiomyopathy with ragged red fibers and fatty infiltration of the pancreas have been reported.

In *MNGIE* cerebral gray matter structures are all intact. However, striking myelin pallor is found in cerebral hemispheres extending from the periventricular area into the arcuate fibers, and into the internal capsule. The white matter is also pale in axonal preparations, but myelin pallor is relatively more marked. The corpus callosum is well myelinated. There are no signs of active myelin breakdown, no necrosis and no significant astrogliosis. Electron microscopy provides some evidence of loosening and thinning of myelin sheaths. Similar changes are present in the cerebellar white matter. Myelin pallor is also seen in the central part of the pons. The optic nerves show myelin pallor, some vacuolation, and some axonal loss. In the cranial nerves myelin pallor and fibrosis is seen. In the spinal cord, tracts are either normal or also show some myelin pallor and vacuolation. Within the spinal roots a marked endoneurial fibrosis and myelin pallor is present, the changes being more severe in the dorsal than in the anterior roots. Within peripheral nerves a combination of scanty presence of myelin sheaths, axonal loss and excessive endoneurial fibrosis is seen. Visceral nerves show axonal loss.

21.4 Pathogenetic Considerations

Two point mutations have been discovered in most cases of *MELAS*. In 80%–90% of the patients a mutation is present in nucleotide 3243 of mitochondrial DNA, which affects a nucleotide position in the dihydrouridine loop of the tRNA specific to leucine (UUR codon). In addition, another mutation has been found in the same tRNA$^{leu(UUR)}$ gene at nucleotide 3271. Only a few MELAS patients lack one of these mutations. A mutation at nucleotide 11084 leading to an alteration in subunit 4 of complex I has been reported in a MELAS patient with a classical clinical picture. Another patient with migranous headaches and stroke-like episodes had a 5-kb deletion of mitochondrial DNA. On the other hand, the 3243 mutation has also been found in some non-MELAS patients, most of whom have chronic progressive external ophthalmoplegia with other neurological complaints, but no stroke-like episodes.

In muscle mitochondria an isolated defect of complex I or combined defects in complexes I, III and IV are found in MELAS. The link between mutation and biochemical defect is not quite clear, although it is apparent that the presence of a mutant tRNA disturbs the mitochondrial gene translation machinery and leads to a decrease in all mitochondrially encoded proteins. Potential mechanisms include incorrect post-translational processing of tRNA^{leu}, mischarging of tRNA synthetase, or aberrant recognition of tRNA by elongation factors or ribosomal proteins.

The cause of the large cerebral lesions is a matter of debate. One hypothesis is that the relationship between mitochondrial dysfunction and cerebral pathology is explained by a mitochondrial vasculopathy of small arteries, observed in the "infarcted" areas. There is a marked increase in number of mitochondria in endothelial cells, smooth muscle cells and pericytes of arterioles. The mitochondria are abnormal and enlarged. The vascular abnormalities may result in decreased blood supply. However, in SPECT and PET scan studies, evidence of patency of blood vessels is found in the acute stage with presence of a well preserved blood flow. Hence, it is more probable that the metabolic demands exceed the potential of energy provision by the disturbed oxidative phosphorylation leading to cell damage and edema.

Among MELAS patients and their maternal relatives there is a clear relationship between percentage of mutant mitochondrial DNA and severity of disease. Asymptomatic relatives have the lowest percentage, oligosymptomatic relatives an intermediate percentage and MELAS patients the highest. Among patients it has been found that the higher the percentage of mutant DNA, the earlier the appearance of symptoms of stroke-like attacks.

An increasing number of mitochondrial DNA mutations has been described in association with *LHON*. The mutations can be distinguished into high risk mutations, called class I or primary mutations, and low risk mutations, called class II or secondary mutations. Class I mutations include a mutation at position 11778 in the mitochondrial gene encoding subunit 4 of complex I, present in 40%–60% of all LHON pedigrees; a mutation at nucleotide position 3460 in the gene encoding subunit 1 of complex I, present in about 20% of all LHON pedigrees; a mutation at position 15275 in the gene encoding cytochrome b of complex III; a mutation at nucleotide 4160 in the gene encoding for subunit 1 of complex I; and a mutation at position 14484 in the gene encoding for subunit 6 of complex I. Known class II mutations affect nucleotide positions 4216 (in the gene encoding subunit 1 of complex I), 4917 (in the gene of subunit 2 of complex I), 5244 (in the gene of subunit 2 of complex I), 13708 (in the gene of subunit 5 of complex I), 15812 (in the gene of cytochrome b, complex III), 7444 (in the gene of subunit 1 of cytochrome c oxidase, complex IV) and 3394 (in the gene of subunit 1 of complex I). Generally, only one class I mutation occurs in a LHON pedigree and individuals harboring one of these mutations have a relatively high probability of vision loss. These mutations are not observed in the normal population. The pathogenic significance of class II mutations is less clear. They occur at a much higher frequency among LHON patients than among the normal population. When present in LHON patients, they occur in combination with other class I or II mutations. They may serve as additional predisposing or exacerbating genetic factors that increase the probability of expressing LHON. It is probably the synergistic effect of multiple mitochondrial DNA mutations that, by their accumulative effect on the oxidative phosphorylation, produces a pathogenic reduction in ATP generating capacity.

For all class I mutations variable penetrance is observed among apparently homoplastic LHON pedigrees. Some family members carrying the mutation remain unaffected. In spite of sharing the same mutations, males have a four times higher risk of being affected than females. Some families appear to be heteroplasmic for a class I mutation, but heteroplasmy is not sufficent to explain the observed phenotypic variation. Therefore, class I mutations appear to be necessary but not sufficient for the clinical manifestation of LHON. Additional genetic (nuclear or mitochondrial), environmental or physiological factors may play a significant role in the expression of LHON. Both internal and external environmental factors may play a role. Systemic illnesses, nutritional deficiencies and toxins that stress or inhibit the body's mitochondrial respiratory capacity could conceivably initiate or increase phenotypic expression of the disease. Adverse effects of tobacco smoke (cyanide present in tobacco smoke inhibits cytochrome c oxidase activity) and alcohol have been suggested but never been proven. The male preponderance and later onset for females suggest an X-linked predisposition to the disease. Susceptibility to LHON expression has been tentatively linked to an X-chromosomal marker (DXS7). Affected females, heterozygous for the X-chromosomal marker, may be involved because of unfortunate X-chromosome inactivation.

The relationship between the mitochondrial DNA mutations and optic neuropathy is difficult to explain. Mutations affecting complexes I, III and IV can underlie LHON. Biochemical abnormalities in mitochondrial function have been hard to demonstrate, but have been shown. It is suggested that the decline in oxidative phosphorylation capacity caused by a combination of influences (class I and class II mutations, X-linked nuclear factor, other genetic factors, environmental factors, effects of aging) results sequentially in optic atrophy, cardiac conduction abnormalities and neurological disease. With regard to those pedigrees with LHON with neurological disease, it would appear that certain mitochondrial DNA mutations may be particularly responsible.

In *KSS* large single deletions of mitochondrial DNA are present. These are sporadic and not inherited. The deletions are not present in mothers of patients or in children of affected mothers. Apparently, the deletions occur in the zygote and affect somatic rather than germ cells. Another possible explanation is that oocytes containing mitochondrial DNA deletions are not viable for gametogenesis and/or fertilization. The size and position of the mitochondrial DNA mutation is variable, but part of the deletion is fairly constant and referred to as a common deletion. As a rule a 13 base pair repeat is present at the breakpoint, suggesting that a recombination event is responsible for the deletion. Deleted genomes are usually competent for replication and transcriptionally active and they accumulate in the ragged red fibers. Most frequently the deleted segment encompasses part of the genes encoding the 13 proteins of the respiratory chain, but also several genes encoding tRNAs. This explains the decrease in all mitochondrial translation products demonstrated in immunological and biochemical analyses, leading to respiratory chain dysfunction. In all patients the deletions are heteroplasmic. An increase with time of the mutated mitochondrial DNA fraction has been reported, paralleling the progression of the disease. In patients surviving Pearson syndrome it is likely that the patient initially had a high percentage of mitochondrial DNA with a deletion in blood cells. The spontaneous recovery indicates that selection favoring normal cells may occur in vivo. In incidental KSS patients, a duplication of mitochondrial DNA is found rather than a deletion. The pathogenetic mechanism of mitochondrial dysfunction is in these cases probably related to interruption of normal genes and/or imbalance of mitochondrial gene products.

MNGIE has an autosomal recessive inheritance. In some of the patients multiple deletions of mitochondrial DNA are found. The multiple deletion breakpoints have sequence repeats identical to those of patients with single mitochondrial DNA deletions. The disease is probably caused by a mutation in a still unknown nucleus-encoded gene, which has a deleterious interaction with the mitochondrial genome. However, precise mechanisms have not yet been elucidated. Biochemical analyses have revealed variable respiratory chain dysfunction with single or combined complex deficiencies. A special problem in MNGIE is the nature of the nervous system pathology. In both CNS and PNS, myelin and axons are involved, but myelin more so than axons. The myelin paucity in CNS and PNS is impressive. It is remarkable that in PNS histopathological abnormalities are associated with evident signs of dysfunction (peripheral polyneuropathy, visceral neuropathy), whereas patients rarely have overt signs of CNS dysfunction. This and the nature of the histopathological findings form arguments for disturbed myelination (dysmyelination), rather than demyelination.

21.5   Therapy

Various therapeutic strategies are possible in respiratory chain defects. In particular administration of cofactors is often applied in an attempt to ameliorate the course of disease. Riboflavin is a precursor of both flavin monophosphate and flavin adenine dinucleotide (FAD), which are part of NADH-coenzyme Q reductase (complex I) and of complex II. Nicotinamide is a pre-

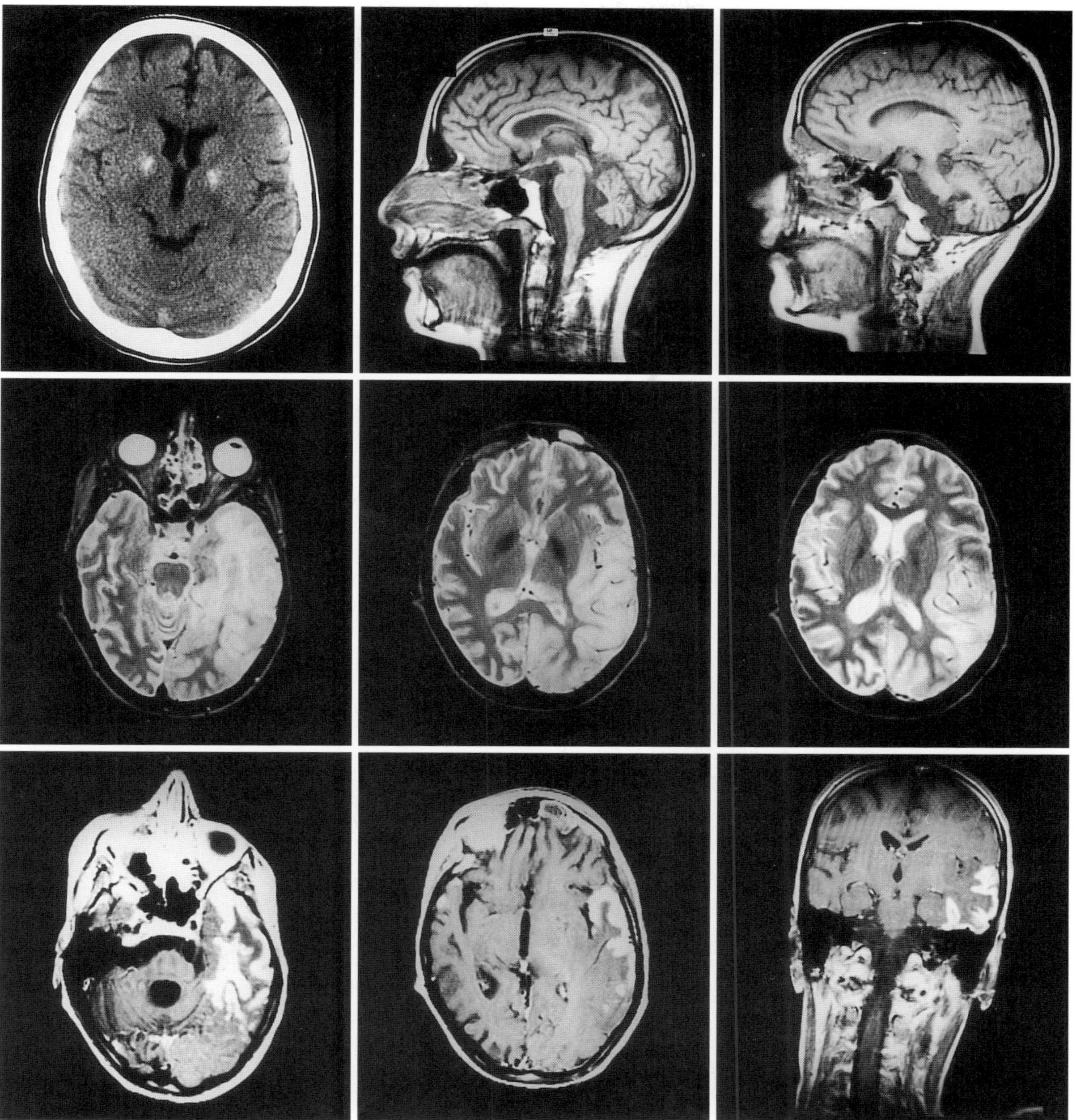

Fig. 21.1. Female patient, 21 years, with MELAS and a recent stroke-like episode. In the left upper corner, CT shows calcification in the globus pallidus. The two sagittal images in the *upper row* show atrophy of the inferior vermis and cerebellar hemispheres. The T_2-weighted images in the *second row* show the large area of abnormal signal on the left side, involving gray and white matter not respecting arterial territorial zones. The *lower row* shows cortical enhancement after Gadolinium injection

cursor of NAD. Coenzyme Q10 can be given to substitute and supplement for endogenous coenzyme Q. Vitamin C and vitamin K_3 (menadione) can be given to bridge a defect in the electron transport chain, as they accept and transport electrons. These drugs are given alone or in varying combinations. In patients with MELAS and KSS variable improvement has been reported, ranging from none to remarkable. Endocrine dysfunction in KSS can be treated symptomatically. In a case of cardiac conduction block a pacemaker should be implanted.

Antenatal diagnosis is very difficult in defects of mitochondrial DNA. As a consequence of heteroplasmy a chorionic villus sample may not be representative of the level of mutant mitochondrial DNA in the embryo.

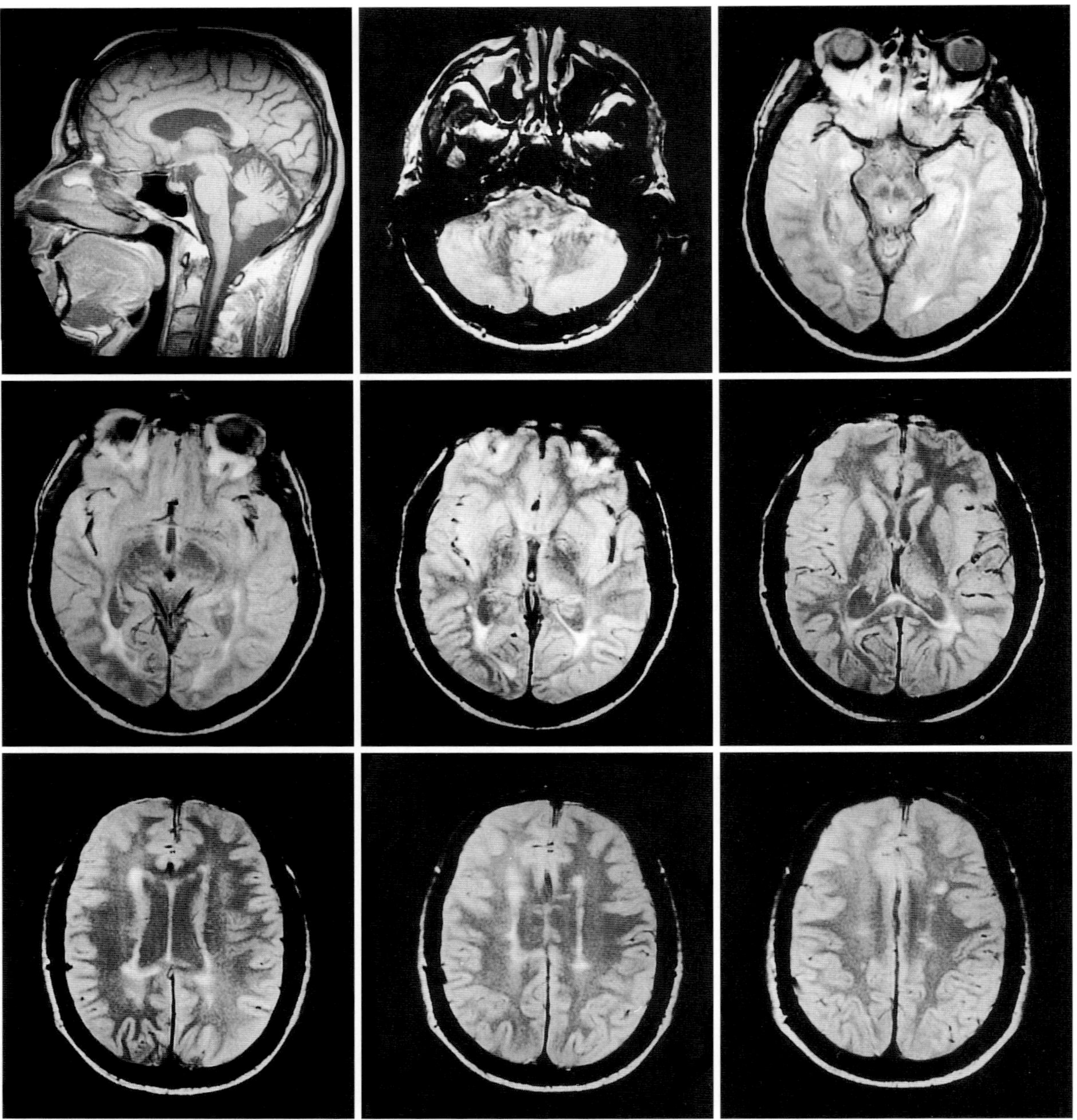

Fig. 21.2. Male patient, 43 years of age, with LHON. The sagittal image shows some vermis atrophy. The transverse proton density series shows a white rim around the ventricles with involvement of the corpus callosum and some isolated spots in the centrum semi-ovale. The ventricles are somewhat enlarged

21.6 Magnetic Resonance Imaging

In *MELAS* CT often shows the presence of calcium deposits in the globus pallidus and caudate nucleus (Fig. 21.1). During the acute phase of stroke-like episodes, one or more large hypodense areas are seen (Fig. 21.1). The areas are swollen. They have, as a rule, an asymmetric distribution. In MRI the calcium deposits in the basal nuclei are more difficult to see. The signal intensity in those areas may be low. MRI shows the precise distribution of the lesions occurring during the stroke-like episodes. From MRI it is clear that the cortex is often more severely involved than the underlying white matter. It is also the cortex that enhances after contrast injection. The lesions are large and confluent, sometimes single, often multiple and usually asymmetrical. The distribution of the lesions does not follow vascular supply or vascular border zones. The

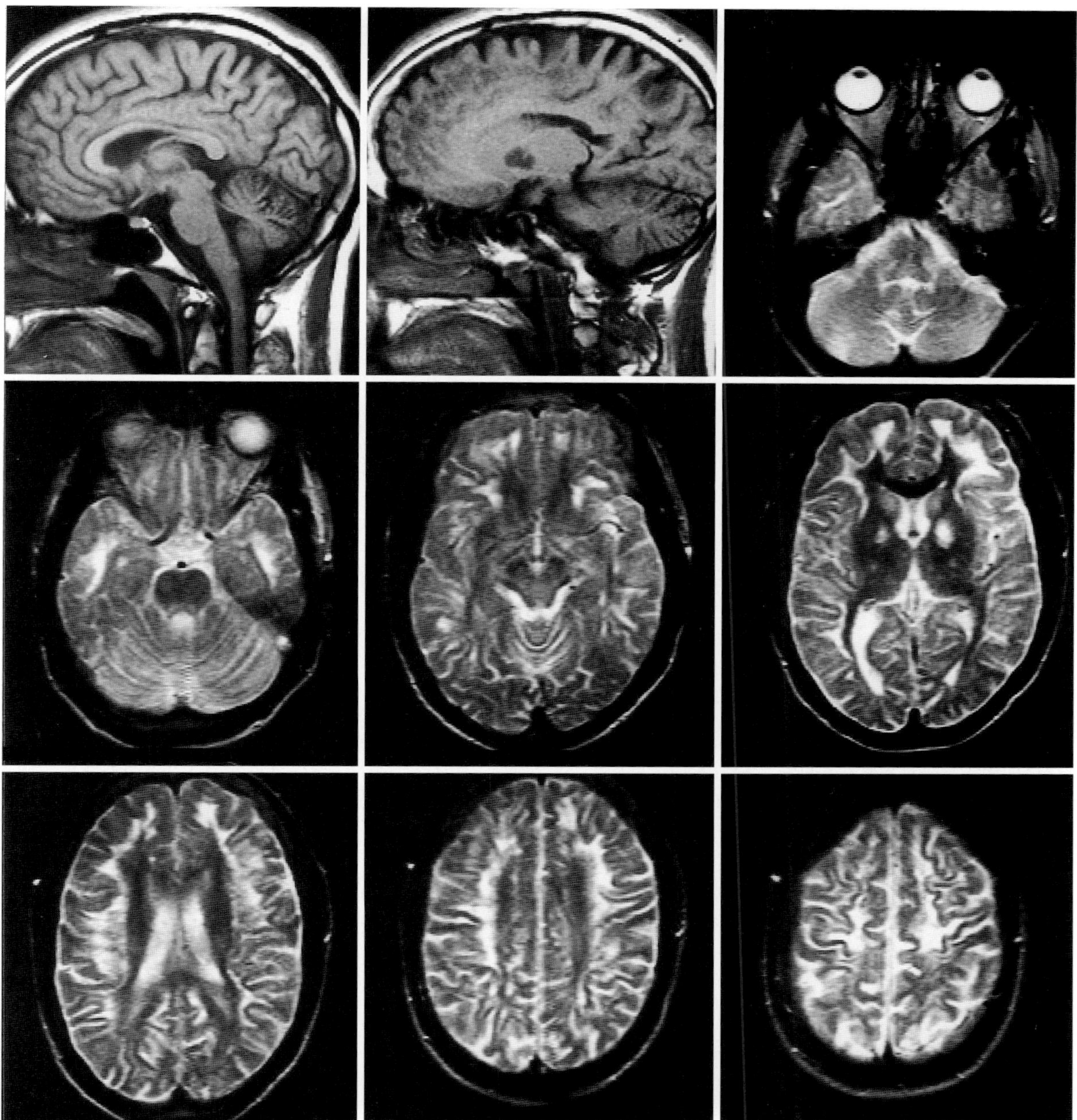

Fig. 21.3. Male patient, 29 years, displaying the features of KSS. The two sagittal T_1-weighted images show the lesions in the basal ganglia and the cerebellar atrophy. The T_2-weighted transverse series shows the symmetrical involvement of the white matter in the arcuate fibers, with extensions in the lobar white matter. Brain stem and cerebellum seem intact. The lesions in the globus pallidus and caudate nucleus are conspicuous

occipital and posterior temporal areas are preferentially involved. Diffuse cerebellar involvement has also been described. In the acute stage the lesion may be swollen. In the course of a few weeks, the lesions may either resolve or leave behind an area of atrophy and altered signal intensity, in particular in the cortex. Over the years MRI may show "migrating infarcts" that leave their traces in progressive atrophy with enlargement of the ventricular system and subarachnoid spaces. In particular diffuse cerebellar atrophy may be present.

The acute lesions can be differentiated from infarctions by their different distribution. The calcium deposits which are almost invariably present in the basal ganglia may help in differentiation. Cerebral angiography, xenon-enhanced computed tomography and SPECT demonstrate patency of vessels and, in fact,

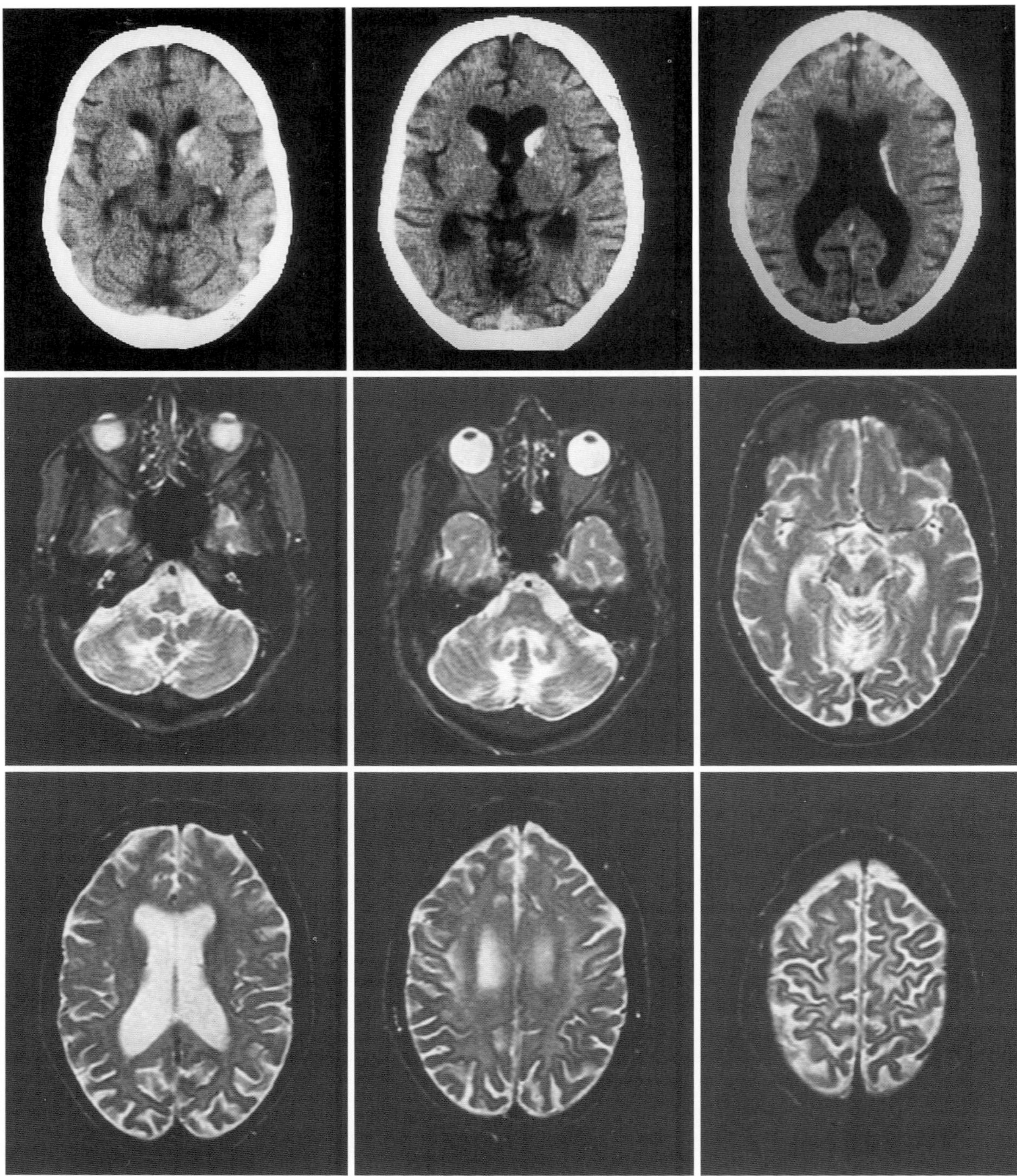

Fig. 21.4. Male patient, 30 years, with KSS. The CT scans in the upper row show calcification in the nucleus caudatus (head and tail) and globus pallidus. The T_2-weighted series shows involvement of cerebellar white matter, and frontal and parietal arcuate fibers in the cerebral hemispheres. The ventricles are mildly enlarged

vasodilation. In a case of predominantly temporal location of the acute lesion, herpes simplex encephalitis may be suspected. However, the raised serum lactate suggests mitochondrial dysfunction rather than herpes encephalitis. Single and multiple large areas of abnormal signal intensity in the cortex and white matter are also seen in urea cycle defects. In MRS, however, findings are very different with raised lactate in MELAS

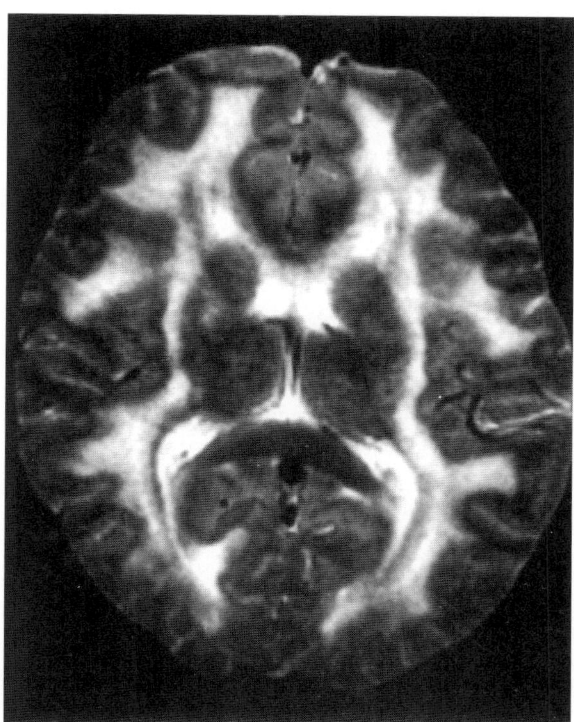

Fig. 21.5. A 17-year-old patient with MNGIE. Note the diffusely high signal intensity of the hemispheral white matter on this T_2-weighted MR image. The corpus callosum, internal capsule and optic radiation are spared. Courtesy of Simon et al. (1990), with permission

and raised glutamine in urea cycle defects. Assessment of blood lactate and ammonia levels produces the same difference.

In patients with *LHON* optic nerve abnormalities can be shown with STIR (short time inversion recovery) sequences. An increased signal intensity of the mid and posterior intra-orbital section is seen, sparing the anterior portion. In most patients brain MRI is normal. In LHON associated with dystonia, bilateral putamen lesions have been found. In patients with a multiple sclerosis-like disease, multiple small white matter lesions are seen as in multiple sclerosis (Fig. 21.2). The lesions are found in the periventricular and lobar white matter of the cerebral hemispheres, in the brain stem and in the cerebellum. The periventricular white matter is predominantly involved. On the basis of MRI only, differentiation between LHON and multiple sclerosis is not possible. In MRS we found no elevation of lactate in LHON, and so MRS also fails to provide a means of differentiation.

In *KSS* CT scan often reveals calcium deposits in the globus pallidus and caudate nucleus in addition to low density of the cerebral white matter and progressive atrophy (Fig. 21.4). In the absence of calcium deposition, low density of the globus pallidus may be apparent. MRI often shows a very characteristic pattern with symmetrical lesions of the globus pallidus and caudate nucleus and subcortical white matter abnormalities (Figs. 21.3, 21.4). Other central nuclei that may be involved include the thalamus and substantia nigra. The white matter abnormalities are symmetrical and tend to involve all subcortical white matter in a patchy or confluent way, sparing the periventricular white matter, corpus callosum and internal capsule. The cerebellar white matter may also be involved. This pattern of abnormalities is specific. When the complete picture is present, it is diagnostic.

In *MNGIE* CT reveals diffuse hypodensity of cerebral and cerebellar white matter. MRI shows diffuse high signal intensity of cerebral and cerebellar white matter on T_2-weighted images with sparing of the corpus callosum and internal capsule (Fig. 21.5). The brain stem may show patchy involvement. On its own this MRI pattern only suggests diffuse dysmyelination rather than demyelination, but it is not specific.

22 Leigh Syndrome

22.1 Clinical Features and Laboratory Investigations

Leigh syndrome, also called subacute necrotizing encephalomyelopathy, is a neurodegenerative disorder of infancy and childhood. In most cases the disease has an autosomal recessive inheritance; in some cases inheritance is maternal. Both sexes are affected, but among infants there is a 3:2 male predominance. The disease usually starts before 1 year of age and leads to death within months or years. Juvenile and adult-onset forms have also been described. The course can be acute, subacute, episodic or chronically progressive. Generally, the later the onset, the slower the progression of the disease.

Although Leigh syndrome is a multisystem disorder, the clinical picture is dominated by signs of CNS dysfunction. In patients with neonatal onset, frequent signs are respiratory problems (irregular respiration, apnea, sighing and hyperventilation), ocular abnormalities (strabismus, bizarre eye movements, external ophthalmoplegia, ptosis, optic atrophy, nystagmus, loss of vision, impaired pupillary reaction, retinal pigmentary degeneration), hypotonia, pyramidal signs (spastic paresis, hyperreflexia, extensor plantar reflexes), weakness, easy fatiguability and feeding problems (anorexia, difficulty in swallowing or sucking, vomiting, weight loss and retarded growth). Episodes of lethargy, seizures, deafness, renal tubular dysfunction, and cardiac problems (cardiomyopathy and disturbances of cardiac rhythm with periods of tachycardia and bradycardia) may also be present. The same problems are frequent in later-onset forms of the disease, in addition to presence of mental and motor retardation or deterioration, exercise intolerance, cerebellar signs (ataxia, dysarthria) and extrapyramidal signs (rigidity, hypokinesia, chorea, athetosis, myoclonus, tremor, ballism). Sometimes there are signs of a peripheral polyneuropathy. In cases of acute onset, coma and convulsions, sometimes status epilepticus, may dominate the clinical picture. Causes of death are neurogenic disturbances of respiration, status epilepticus, sudden coma, pneumonia, hyperpyrexia and cardiac problems.

Laboratory investigations reveal blood levels of lactate and pyruvate to be typically but not invariably elevated. In CSF, lactate and pyruvate are usually elevated. CSF protein is increased in about half of the patients. EEG shows normal findings or nonspecific abnormalities including diffuse or focal slowing, and epileptic phenomena. EMG is either normal, or shows signs of denervation or signs of a myopathy. Nerve conduction velocity is either normal or reduced. On biochemical analysis of intact mitochondria in muscle biopsy tissue, variable defects are encountered (see under Sect. 22.3).

22.2 Pathology

The brunt of histopathological abnormalities in Leigh syndrome is borne by the central gray matter. The most consistent site of lesions is the brain stem gray matter. The lesions are usually bilateral, although not necessarily symmetrical. They are sharply delineated and not confined to the gray matter structures but often spread into the white matter. Preferential sites of affection are periaqueductal region and brain stem tegmentum, posterior colliculi, substantia nigra, floor of the fourth ventricle, red nuclei, inferior olivary nuclei, dentate nuclei, putamen, caudate nucleus and globus pallidus. Thalamus, hypothalamus and subthalamic nuclei may also be involved but less often. In the spinal cord lesions are mainly located in the anterior horns, dorsal columns and pyramidal tracts. Lesions rarely occur in the cerebral or cerebellar cortex or mammillary bodies. Exceptional cases with predominant cerebral and cerebellar cortical damage have been described. Microscopic examination of the lesions shows a marked sponginess with loosening and rarefaction of the neuropil. There is a characteristic intense capillary proliferation. Astrocytosis and microglia proliferation are present and macrophages may occur. Nerve cells are remarkable well preservated, although there may be some nerve cell loss. The spongy lesions contain numerous vacuoles, enclosed by single or double membranes. Evidence has been provided for myelin splitting underlying the vacuolation. Cavitation and tissue collapse is the end-result in most severe lesions.

In the majority of the cases the white matter is well preserved, but sometimes there is also extensive involvement of cerebral and cerebellar white matter with sparing of corpus callosum and internal capsule. The white matter changes are characterized by sponginess, myelin degeneration, myelin loss, abundant presence of lipid-laden macrophages, marked capillary proliferation, prominent gliosis and eventually also axonal loss. In all areas there is a gradient of damage, so that myelin sheaths and dendrites degenerate prior to axons and cell bodies. Optic nerves and tracts are often affected by demyelination and gliosis. In the sural nerve signs of demyelination and remyelination have been found as well as loss of myelinated and unmyelinated axons. Ragged red fibers are found in muscle tissue of some of the patients.

22.3 Pathogenetic Considerations

Leigh syndrome is caused by a number of inborn errors of energy metabolism. In particular, deficiency of cytochrome c oxidase and deficiency of pyruvate dehydrogenase complex are strongly associated with Leigh syndrome. Less frequently, Leigh syndrome is related to deficiency of NADH coenzyme Q reductase, or pyruvate decarboxylase. In some patients the elevation of lactate and pyruvate in blood and CSF indicates a disturbance of energy metabolism, but the basic defect has not been found. It was recently shown that in a substantial number of the unsolved cases, a mutation could be found in mitochondrial DNA, nucleotide position 8993, affecting the gene encoding subunit 6 of ATP synthetase (complex V of the respiratory chain). The same mutation has repeatedly been shown in NARP (neurogenic weakness, ataxia and retinitis pigmentosa). Both in Leigh syndrome and in NARP patients the mitochondrial DNA mutation is heteroplasmic, but the percentage of mutated genome is much higher in Leigh syndrome than in NARP. A few patients with Leigh syndrome were found to harbor the point mutation in the tRNA gene encoding lysine, associated with MERRF (myoclonus epilepsy and ragged red fibers). The common mechanism in all these defects causing Leigh syndrome is obscure, but evidently related to a disturbance in the energy producing system of the brain.

In this respect the clinical and morphological similarity between Leigh syndrome and thiamine deficiency (beriberi) is striking. Thiamine is part of the pyruvate dehydrogenase, ketoglutarate dehydrogenase and branched-chain keto acid dehydrogenase complexes. Thiamine deficiency leads to a disturbance in oxidation of pyruvate and consequently to energy failure. The only histopathological differences between thiamine deficiency and Leigh syndrome are that in thiamine deficiency the corpora mammillaria are mostly involved and the substantia nigra not, whereas in Leigh syndrome the substantia nigra is often involved and rarely the corpora mammillaria. These differences, however, are not absolute.

Considering the basic defects, the inheritance of Leigh syndrome is variable. In most cases it is autoso-

mal recessive. Although cytochrome c oxidase contains subunits encoded by both nuclear DNA and mitochondrial DNA, cytochrome c oxidase deficiency in Leigh syndrome has an autosomal recessive mode of inheritance. One of the subunits of the pyruvate dehydrogenase complex is encoded by a gene on the X-chromosome (the $E_{1\alpha}$ subunit), and so transmission of deficiency of pyruvate dehydrogenase may be autosomal recessive or X-linked. The X-linked inheritance in some patients contributes to the male preponderance in infants, but cannot be held totally responsible for it.

22.4 Therapy

Therapeutic success is limited in Leigh syndrome. In deficiency of the pyruvate dehydrogenase complex, a low carbohydrate, high fat ketogenic diet may be beneficial. Decreased glycolysis results in a lowered production of lactate. The β-oxidation of fatty acids generates acetyl-CoA, which enters the citric acid cycle, thus bypassing the block at the level of pyruvate dehydrogenase. Furthermore, administration of thiamine (a cofactor of the first enzyme of the pyruvate dehydrogenase complex) and α-lipoic acid (a cofactor of the second enzyme of the pyruvate dehydrogenase complex) can be considered, and may prove beneficial. L-carnitine supplementation may have a nonspecific beneficial effect, in particular if toxic organic acid intermediates are present. Variable favorable results have been reported following the use of riboflavin (vitamin B_2), nicotinamide, coenzyme Q10, vitamin C and menadione (vitamin K_3) in respiratory chain defects (see previous chapter).

22.5 Magnetic Resonance Imaging

The most commonly reported abnormalities on CT and MRI in Leigh syndrome involve the basal nuclei. The putamen and caudate nucleus are usually affected, but globus pallidus, dentate nucleus, substantia nigra, brain stem tegmentum, red nuclei are also frequently involved, and less often the thalamus, hypothalamus, subthalamic nucleus and cortex. Although the lesions are often symmetrical, they may also be asymmetrical. In young children delay in myelination may be noted (Figs. 22.1, 22.2). Incidentally, focal or more often diffuse white matter lesions are seen on MRI (Figs. 22.1, 22.2). The white matter changes may become polycystic. Atrophy may ensue with, in particular, enlargement of the ventricular system.

In combination with clinical history and presence of high lactate, the MR images are often diagnostic.

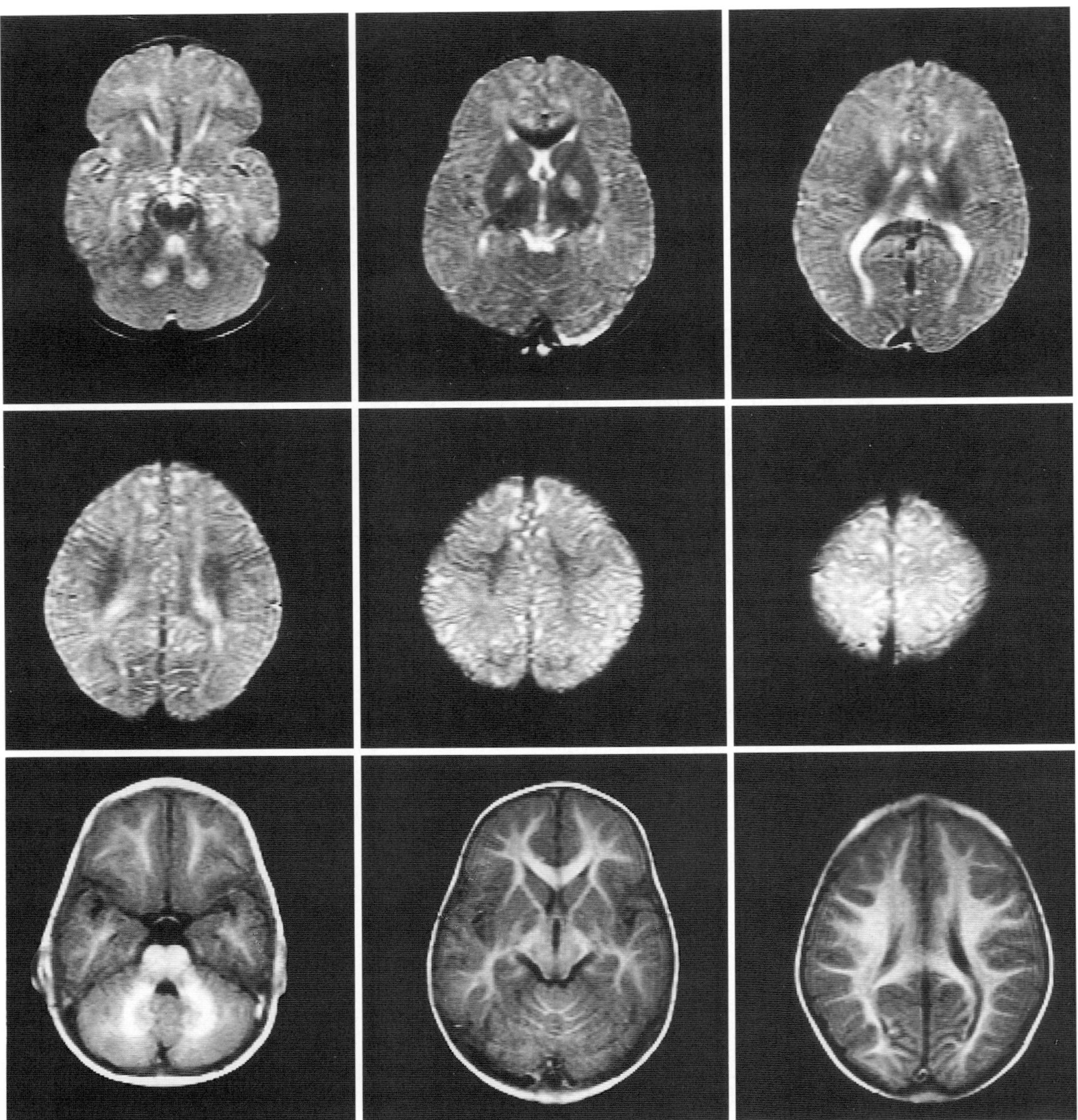

Fig. 22.1. Boy, 14 months of age, with Leigh syndrome. Note the symmetrical lesions in the globus pallidus and dentate nucleus. Myelination is somewhat irregular and severely delayed, considering the high signal intensity on the T_2-weighted images

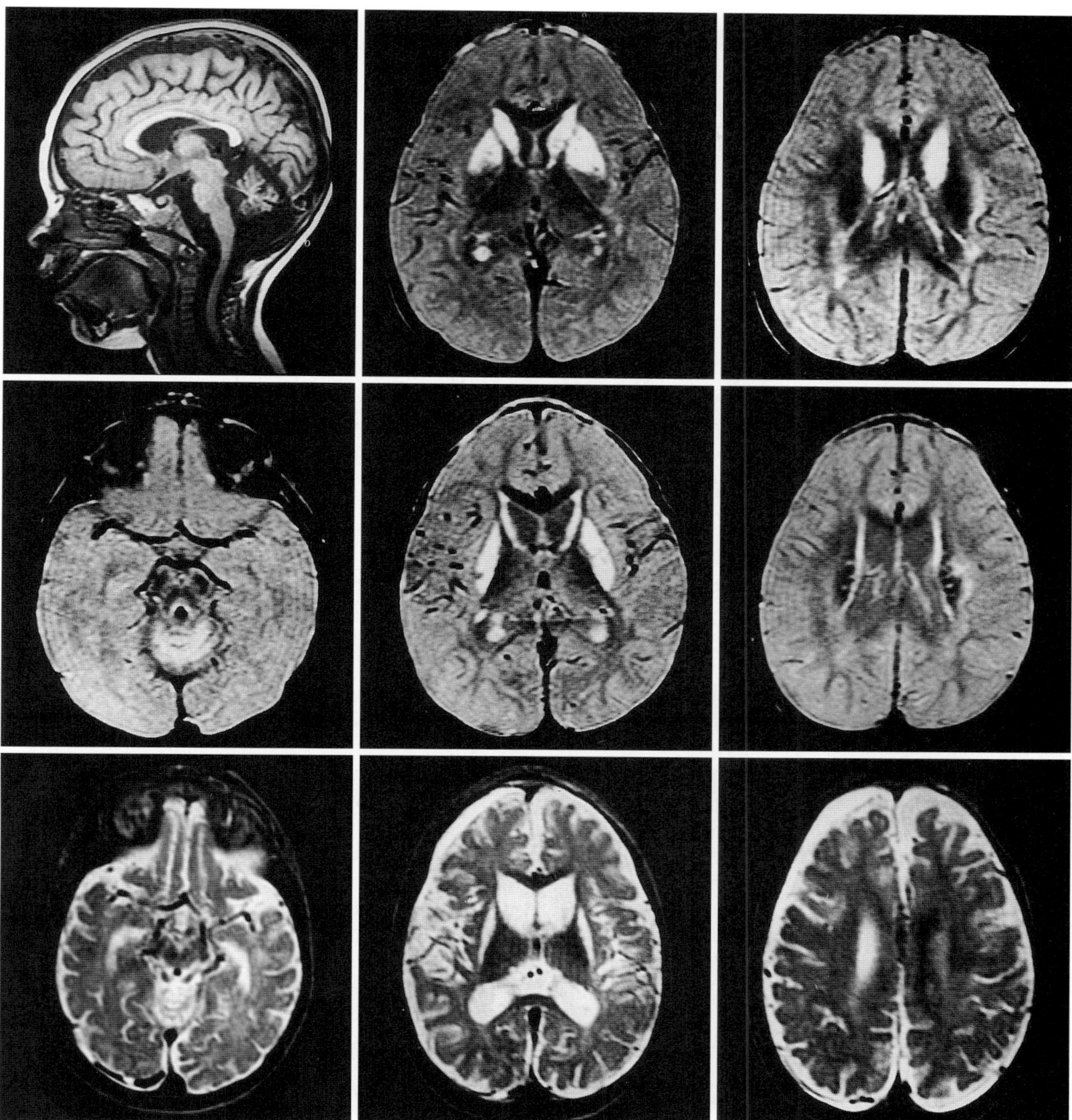

Fig. 22.2. Boy with Leigh syndrome. The child was normal up to the second half of the first year of life, after which progressive neurological deterioration set in. The *upper row* of images was made at the age of 1 year and 3 months, showing cerebellar atrophy. The caudate nucleus and globus pallidus are swollen. The *second row* of images, made at the age of 2 years, shows the high signal intensity in the cerebellar cortex, the periaqueductal gray matter and the caudate nucleus and puta-men. The latter two nuclei show signs of atrophy. The *third row* of images, made at the age of 3.5 years, just prior to death, shows the generalized atrophy. In all images the delay in myelination is evident, particularly as a lack of contrast between cortex and subcortical white matter. From the beginning there are slight white matter abnormalities in the parieto-occipital lobar white matter

23 Pyruvate Carboxylase Deficiency

23.1 Clinical Features and Laboratory Investigations

Pyruvate carboxylase (PC) deficiency is a rare disorder with autosomal recessive inheritance. Generally, two clinical and biochemical phenotypes of isolated PC deficiency can be distinguished. The so-called French phenotype presents in the neonatal period with severe lactic acidemia and is clinically characterized by failure to thrive, anorexia, vomiting, weak cry, convulsions, stupor, hyporeactivity, hypotonia, tachypnea, dyspnea, respiratory failure, and subsequently hypertonia, extrapyramidal tract signs and severely retarded development. Most children die within the first few months of life. The North American phenotype is less severe. Patients become symptomatic between 2 and 5 months of age with developmental delay, failure to thrive, apathy, hypotonia, spasticity, ataxia, nystagmus and convulsions. Episodes of vomiting, tachypnea, tachycardia, ataxia and lactic acidosis occur, precipitated by metabolic or infectious stress. Some patients die in the infantile period, while most of the survivors are grossly retarded. A few exceptional patients have been reported who despite the episodic metabolic derangement have a normal or near normal motor and mental development. Formerly, Leigh syndrome was thought to represent another clinical phenotype of PC deficiency, but this could not be confirmed.

In the French phenotype, laboratory investigations reveal lactic acidemia with a highly elevated lactate/pyruvate ratio and a lowered 3-hydroxybutyrate/acetoacetate ratio. There is a ketoacidosis, a moderate hyperammonemia, and blood levels of alanine, citrulline, proline and lysine are elevated. The level of aspartate is often decreased but normal levels have also been reported. In the North-American phenotype lactic acidemia is associated with a normal lactate/pyruvate ratio. There is no hyperammonemia. Alanine is elevated.

Diagnosis is established by demonstrating a deficiency in PC activity in fibroblasts, white blood cells or liver cells. The activity of propionyl-CoA carboxylase is normal, excluding multiple carboxylase deficiency. Prenatal diagnosis can be performed by enzyme assessment in amniocytes.

23.2 Pathology

In all reported cases, whether of French or North-American phenotype, the brunt of abnormalities is borne by the white matter of the CNS. The brain may be swollen. The hemispheral white matter is sometimes grossly cystic, the cysts being located either in the periventricular or in the lobar white matter. Cystic degeneration tends to be symmetrical, but is not always symmetrical in detail. On microscopic examination myelin paucity, sponginess and gliosis of the white matter are found, involving diffusely cerebral and cerebellar white matter and sometimes also the base of the pons. The myelin paucity is variably described as hypomyelination or demyelination. Probably, both are important. Perivascular accumulation of foamy macrophages is an argument in favor of a component of active myelin breakdown. The white matter is decreased in volume in cases of longer duration resulting in enlargement of the ventricular system. The corpus callosum is thin.

The condition of the gray matter is variable, but gray matter pathology never dominates. In some cases all gray matter structures are completely normal. Some have noted that the globus pallidus, a nucleus rich in myelin, is involved in the process of myelin abnormality and loss. Some describe a cystic degeneration of the deep gray nuclei. In one report ectopic neurons are seen in the subcortical white matter.

23.3 Pathogenetic Considerations

PC is a mitochondrial matrix enzyme, encoded by nuclear DNA. The gene is localized on the long arm of chromosome 11. PC is a homotetramer consisting of four identical polypeptides, each with a covalently bound biotin molecule. There are four major biotin dependent carboxylases: PC, propionyl-CoA carboxylase, methylcrotonyl-CoA carboxylase, and acetyl-CoA carboxylase. PC deficiency can occur as isolated PC deficiency, presumed to be due to a mutation involving the PC gene and as multiple carboxylase deficiency related to biotin deficiency. PC is expressed in many tissues, including brain, liver, kidney, white blood cells, fibroblasts and other tissues. Low activity is found in skeletal muscle. Tissue-specific isoenzymes are not known.

PC catalyzes the conversion of pyruvate into oxaloacetate. This step serves two important functions: it is the first step in gluconeogenesis and it replenishes oxaloacetate for the citric acid cycle. Availability of oxaloacetate is essential for citric acid cycle activity. Oxaloacetate is in equilibrium with aspartic acid.

In PC deficiency there is a defect in the conversion of pyruvate to oxaloacetate. Availability of this metabolite is essential for citric acid cycle activity. When oxaloacetate synthesis from pyruvate is limited, aspartate is converted to oxaloacetate and depletion of aspartate occurs. Aspartate is an important component of the shuttle mechanism transfering reducing equivalents across the mitochondrial membrane. Depletion of aspartate leads to accumulation of reducing equivalents (NADH) in the cytosol and mitochondrial NADH becomes more oxidized. This altered redox state results in an increase in the lactate to pyruvate ratio and a decrease in the β-hydroxybutyrate to acetoacetate ratio. Depletion of aspartate also interferes with urea cycle activity. Aspartate is a nitrogen donor for the urea cycle and depletion of aspartate leads to hyperammonemia, citrullinemia and hyperlysinemia. Accumulation of acetyl-CoA may also occur under these circumstances and result in overproduction of ketone bodies. Despite the fact that PC is an important enzyme in gluconeogenesis, hypoglycemia is not a consistent finding in PC deficiency.

The different phenotypes of PC deficiency are related to the severity of enzyme deficiency. Many patients with the French phenotype have no immunologically detectable enzyme at all, but some have. In all patients with the North-American phenotype, the PC enzyme protein can be shown to be present with immunological techniques, although deficient in activity. Presumably, the French phenotype is related to absent or almost absent residual enzyme activity, whereas in the North-American phenotype the residual activity is enough to ameliorate the most severe symptoms of PC deficiency.

This is the situation with the straightforward cases. However, a number of cases has been described, which do not exactly fit this picture. Despite the fact that tissue-specific isoenzymes have never been shown, one patient has been reported (Hansen et al. 1983) in whom PC activity was zero in liver tissue and 50% of normal activity in cultured fibroblasts. In another patient (Baal et al. 1981), an unusual late onset, slow and mild course, well preserved intellectual capacities and long survival were noted. PC activity was very low in liver tissue, but normal in leukocytes and fibroblasts. The normal intelligence was thought to be incompatible with a severe cerebral enzyme deficiency, but cerebral activity was not determined. A similarly mild affected patient with normal mental and motor abilities was recently described (Van Coster et al. 1991). A profound PC deficiency was found in fibroblasts. The preserved cerebral functions were thought to exclude a severe PC deficiency in the brain. In all these cases tissue heterogeneity would provide an explanation, although this has not been shown up to now.

23.4 Therapy

Treatment has proven to be quite difficult and disappointing in PC deficiency. Metabolic acidosis must be corrected by bicarbonate therapy. Aspartate supplementation has been recommended to increase oxaloacetate concentrations and overcome aspartate depletion, and some patients have actually shown some improvement. Unfortunately, aspartate does not freely cross the blood-brain barrier. Glutamine, also a precursor of oxaloacetate, has also been mentioned as having some beneficial effect. Thiamine has been advocated to stimulate the pyruvate dehydrogenase complex. Administration of biotin to stimulate PC has no effect.

23.5 Magnetic Resonance Imaging

Reports on neuroimaging findings are very scarce in PC deficiency. In one case it was reported that MRI demonstrated dysmyelination of cerebral hemispheral and brain stem structures. In another case T_2-weighted MR images showed high signal intensity of the hemispheral white matter, particularly pronounced in the periventricular region, in combination with a lesion in the basis of the pons. In a third case severe, diffuse hypodensity of the cerebral and cerebellar white matter was found on CT. The white matter was moderately swollen.

Considering histopathological findings high signal intensity of cerebral, cerebellar and pontine white matter is expected to be found on T_2-weighted MR images (Fig. 23.1). In most cases the white matter changes will be diffuse, but probably more focal lesions may also occur. In some patients the white matter degeneration is cystic. The white matter is either swollen or atrophic, depending on the stage of disease. The abnormalities are usually symmetrical, although this may not be an obligatory feature.

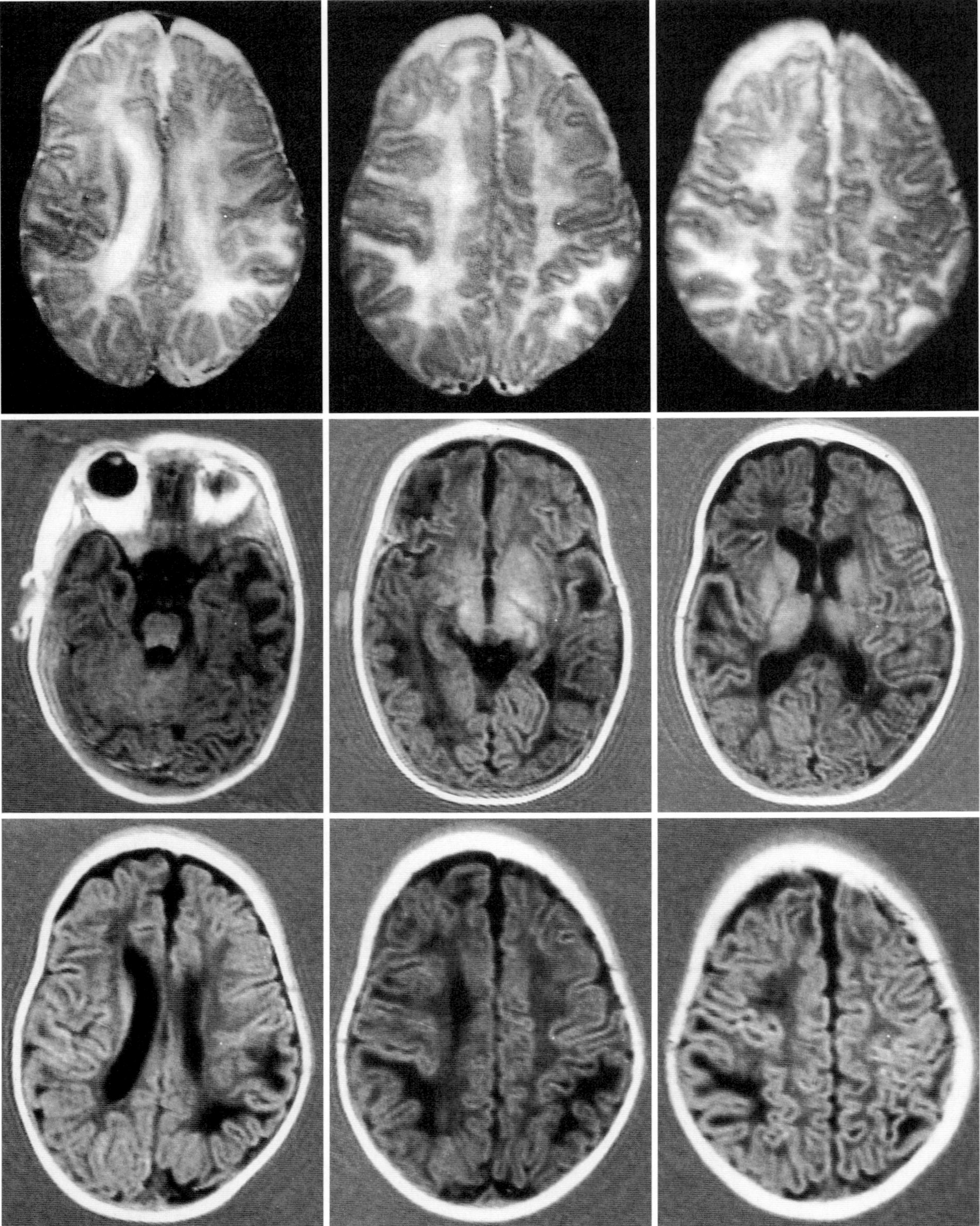

Fig. 23.1. Baby girl, 3 months of age, with PC deficiency. The upper row of T_2-weighted transverse images shows the enlarged ventricles and the irregular areas on left and right side with increased signal intensity, some local swelling of the white matter and some stretching of cortical gyri. The T_1-weighted IR series demonstrates the affected areas where signal intensity is too low. The images suggest presence of spongiform white matter changes, confirmed at brain biopsy. Myelination is delayed, considering the insufficient myelin presence in the posterior limb of the internal capsule and optic radiation

24 Cerebrotendinous Xanthomatosis

24.1 Clinical Features and Laboratory Investigations

Cerebrotendinous xanthomatosis (CTX) is a rare neurometabolic disorder with an autosomal recessive mode of inheritance. Most patients are of borderline or low intelligence from the beginning and their school performance is poor. The more specific clinical manifestations usually appear in late childhood or early adolescence, or even later. The most commonly noted early manifestations of the disease include cataracts and xanthomas of tendons, especially the Achilles tendons, but also the tendons of the quadriceps muscle, the triceps muscle and the finger extensors. During the second or third decade, neurological problems gradually become manifest with signs of cerebellar ataxia, spastic paraparesis and tetraparesis, signs of dysfunction of the posterior columns, and signs of a peripheral polyneuropathy. Tendon reflexes are generally hyperactive. Vibratory and position senses are diminished whereas the superficial sensory modalities remain relatively intact. Foot deformity, in particular pes cavus, is often noted. About 40% of the patients develop epilepsy with generalized tonic-clonic seizures. In most cases a decline of mental function occurs in the third decade but there is a large diversity in the rapidity of the decline. Changes in personality and psychiatric problems may be present. Premature atherosclerosis may lead to angina pectoris, myocardial infarction and cardiac failure. Less frequent complaints are chronic unexplained diarrhea, pharyngeal and palatal myoclonus, mask-like facies, bulbar and pseudobulbar paresis, visual loss due to optic atrophy, generalized muscular wasting, parkinsonism, bone fractures due to osteoporosis, impaired lung function due to pulmonary xanthomas, and signs of endocrine dysfunction. In untreated cases death usually occurs between the fourth and sixth decades.

The problem with the diagnosis of CTX is that there are no obligatory symptoms and that the development of symptoms varies markedly in nature and degree of progression, even within one family. In particular, in the absence of the typical tendon xanthomas, the diagnosis can be easily missed.

Laboratory investigations reveal a normal or only moderately elevated serum cholesterol but a markedly increased level of serum cholestanol. CSF protein may be increased. CSF cholestanol levels are elevated. Low serum levels of 25-hydroxy vitamin D_3 and 24,25-dihydroxy vitamin D_3 may be found. The measurement of the serum cholestanol: cholesterol ratio has been advocated as a means of establishing the diagnosis, but elevated levels can also be found in patients suffering from various liver diseases. A preferable method to establish the diagnosis is the demonstration of abnormal bile alcohols in urine. The diagnosis can be confirmed by demonstration of the lack of 27-hydroxylase activity in cultured fibroblasts.

X-ray examination may reveal the swelling of the Achilles tendons and, less frequently, of the tendons of the hamstrings, quadriceps and finger extensors. Calcification of these soft tissue masses may be seen. Motor and sensory nerve conduction is often slowed. Evoked potentials, in particular SSEPs, are as a rule delayed. EEG shows diffuse slowing of background activity with poorly organized theta and delta waves.

Carriers of CTX can be identified by observing an abnormal increase in bile alcohols in their urine after administration of cholestyramine, a drug that leads to intestinal loss of bile acids and as a consequence an increased endogenous synthesis. Normal controls fail to produce the unusual bile alcohols. Carrier detection can also be performed by analysis of 27-hydroxylase activity in cultured fibroblasts. DNA techniques for carrier detection are becoming available.

24.2 Pathology

On external examination of the brain, mild atrophy is found, especially of the cerebellum. Sometimes xanthomas are seen in the choroid plexus.

On microscopic examination the cerebral cortex and hemispheral white matter usually appear normal. Sometimes gliosis and perivascular collections of large mononuclear cells with foamy cytoplasm are found. However, more prominent demyelination has occasionally been found at the level of the corona radiata, periventricular white matter, and globus pallidus. Demyelination of the optic nerves is common, where fibrillary gliosis with perivascular lipid-laden mononuclear cells may be seen. Mononuclear cells with foamy cytoplasm are also found in the basal nuclei and thalamus.

The most conspicuous abnormalities are found in the cerebellum. Xanthomatous tissue sometimes replaces most of the white matter. On microscopic examination extensive demyelination of cerebellar white matter is seen with most severe myelin loss in the outflow tract of the dentate nucleus and the superior cerebellar peduncles. In the demyelinated areas there are many small and large cystic spaces and needle-like clefts. Large quantities of neutral fat accumulate in the cysts and in perivascular spaces within large mononuclear cells with foamy cytoplasm. The needle-shaped clefts contain crystalline deposits with staining properties of sterols. The crystalline deposits are surrounded by inflammatory cells and reactive multinucleated foreign-body giant cells. These cells represent the tissue reaction to deposition of sterols. There may be an extensive loss of Purkinje cells and a destruction of the dentate and fastigial nuclei.

In the brain stem the pyramidal tracts, transverse pontine fibers and the fiber tracts emerging from the inferior olives are demyelinated. At the higher levels of the brain stem, in particular in the red nucleus and substantia nigra, deposits of neutral lipids and crystalline sterols are present. Gray matter changes in the brain stem include loss of neurons, particularly in the inferior olives and other nuclei. In the spinal cord the pyramidal tracts and posterior columns are demyelinated.

In the peripheral nerves signs of segmental demyelination and remyelination with onion bulb formation are seen. Others, however, also find evidence of a component of primary axonal degeneration. Histological examination of muscle tissue discloses some signs of denervation and reinnervation with mild type grouping. There are also primary myopathic changes consisting of increased variability of fiber size and randomly distributed atrophic fibers. On electron microscopy, large aggregates of mitochondria are seen, mainly in the subsarcolemmal region. The mitochondria show mild morphological abnormalities such as increased size and irregular cristae.

Microscopic examination of Achilles tendon xanthoma reveals islets of mononuclear cells with foamy cytoplasm and clefts filled with crystalloid material surrounded by multinucleated giant cells. The clefts are scattered in fan-shaped clusters without any relation to blood vessels. Under polarized light birefringence of the clefts is shown, suggesting presence of sterols. The cells filled with neutral fat are mainly present around blood vessels but also throughout the tissue. Similar xanthomatous tissue can be found in the lungs and bones.

In liver tissue fatty lipofucsin-like pigment granules have been reported in hepatocytes and Kupffer cells.

Crystals are found in the cytoplasm of hepatocytes. Mitochondria are hypertrophied and peroxisomes are increased in size and number.

Premature atherosclerosis of coronary arteries can be found.

24.3 Chemical Pathology

In CTX patients the lipids stored in the brain and in xanthomas consist of free and esterified cholestanol and cholesterol. Free cholestanol is found not only in the evidently affected areas of the brain, but also in portions which appear normal on histological examination. Cholestanol is not only found in myelin but in all other membrane structures in the brain, including cell membranes and membranes of subcellular structures. The concentration of unesterified cholesterol is normal or only slightly increased. In demyelinated areas the concentrations of esterified cholestanol and cholesterol are elevated. Concentrations of cholesterol esters are nonspecifically elevated in many actively demyelinating disorders, but esterified cholestanol is not present in any of these disorders.

24.4 Pathogenetic Considerations

In CTX the basic defect is located in the mitochondrial enzyme 27-hydroxylase. This enzyme catalyzes the initial steps in the side-chain cleavage of sterols. The enzyme hydroxylates a spectrum of sterol substrates, including cholesterol and vitamin D_3. The sterol 27-hydroxylase gene has been mapped to the distal portion of the long arm of chromosome 2. The gene has been cloned, its structure has been determined and a number of different mutations have been characterized.

The most important pathway for the metabolism and excretion of cholesterol in humans is the formation of bile acids. The two major bile acids, cholic acid and chenodeoxy cholic acid, are formed in the liver and secreted in bile into the intestine. The enzymes involved in modifying the steroid nucleus of cholesterol are mainly located in the endoplasmic reticulum and the cytosol. The enzymes involved in the side-chain degradation are mainly located in mitochondria and peroxisomes. The major pathway for side-chain cleavage is the 27-hydroxylase pathway.

Deficient activity of 27-hydroxylase results in a defect in bile acid biosynthesis. The formation of normal bile acids, in particular chenodeoxycholic acid, is reduced. Large amounts of unusual C27-bile alcohols are excreted in bile, faeces and urine. As bile acids are involved in a feedback regulation of the hepatic cholesterol production, the decrease in bile acids leads to enhanced cholesterol production and an excessive production of bile alcohols.

Cholestanol is the 5α-dihydro derivative of cholesterol. It normally represents about 0.1%–0.3% of cholesterol in tissues and plasma. In CTX cholestanol is increased 10- to 100-fold so that it accounts for 2% of plasma and tissue sterols with even greater enrichment in the brain (20%–50%), tendon xanthomas (10%) and bile (10%). There is evidence that at least part of the cholestanol accumulating in CTX is formed by a pathway involving bile acid intermediates as precursor. Accumulation of bile acid intermediates has been shown to result in an increased synthesis of cholestanol.

Like cholesterol, cholestanol is transported by low-density lipoproteins (LDL) and high-density lipoproteins (HDL). Despite the enhanced production of both sterols, plasma LDL concentrations are low and HDL cholesterol levels are also diminished. The role of LDL is to transport cholesterol from the liver to peripheral tissues. LDL turnover is exceedingly rapid in CTX. The catabolism of LDL by the augmented expression of LDL receptors is sufficiently great to maintain low plasma concentrations, despite enhanced cholesterol production. The role of HDL is to transport cholesterol from peripheral tissues to the liver. HDL cholesterol levels are subnormal in many CTX patients. This may account for the accumulation of tissue sterols in atheromas and xanthomas by hindering reverse sterol transport.

Neurological dysfunction apparently results from the deposition of cholestanol and cholesterol in the nervous system and the replacement of cholesterol by cholestanol. It is likely that the incorporation of cholestanol into the myelin membranes makes myelin unstable and liable to breakdown.

24.5 Therapy

Treatment in CTX aims at breaking the vicious circle of defective endogenous bile acid synthesis leading to absence of negative feedback, which in turn leads to increased production of cholesterol, abnormal bile alcohols and cholestanol. Treatment with oral bile acids, in particular chenodeoxycholic acid, repairs the negative feedback and leads to decreased production of cholesterol, cholestanol and abnormal bile alcohols. The progression of CNS damage is retarded or halted. It has been reported that a number of patients receiving therapy with chenodeoxycholic acid showed reversal of their neurological disability, with clearing of dementia, and improved motor function. There is also evidence of improved results of paraclinical tests, such as nerve conduction velocity, evoked responses, EEG and CT.

Combined treatment with chenodeoxycholic acid and inhibitors of cholesterol synthesis leads to the most important redcution of cholesterol and cholestanol. The clinical efficacy of this treatment compared to therapy with bile acids alone still has to be proven.

Some patients experience a more important improvement than others. As the effects of therapy depend largely on the extent of irreversible structural damage of nervous tissue, early diagnosis and early treatment is important. If the disease is detected in early childhood, treatment of the patient not yet clinically affected can prevent occurrence of complaints. It is a treatment for life.

24.6 Magnetic Resonance Imaging

CT scan of the brain has been reported to show cerebellar hypodensity and in some cases also moderate hypodensity of cerebral hemispheral white matter.

The most important and earliest MRI abnormalities are noted in the cerebellum. On T_2-weighted images the cerebellar hemispheral white matter has a high signal intensity, consistent with demyelination (Fig. 24.1). The cerebellar foliae are prominent, indicative of atrophy. In some patients the cerebellar white matter lesions are surrounded by a rim with markedly low signal intensity, probably reflecting the presence of macroscopic xanthomas (Fig. 24.2). Symmetrical demyelinating lesions may be present in the pyramidal tracts in the brain stem (Fig. 24.1).

In the supratentorial region variable abnormalities may be noted, but in many patients no abnormalities are found. Slight enlargement of ventricular system and subarachnoid spaces may be seen. In a few patients, focal round or ovoid masses with low signal intensity on T_2-weighted images are noted within the ventricles, probably reflecting the presence of xanthomas within the choroid plexus (Fig. 24.2). Bilateral high signal intensity lesions may be seen in the globus pallidus. There may be variable periventricular white matter abnormalities with a symmetrical distribution. The lesions may be confluent or more patchy. The white matter changes often have a moderately abnormal signal intensity and blend with the normal white matter without a sharp demarcation between the two. U fibers and corpus callosum are spared.

The full-blown MRI pattern of CTX with presence of the typical lesions in the cerebellar hemispheres with central high signal intensity and a low signal intensity rim on T_2-weighted images has a high diagnostic value. When only high signal intensity lesions are present in the cerebellar (and also cerebral) white matter, other diagnoses should be considered, including adrenomyeloneuropathy and Refsum disease.

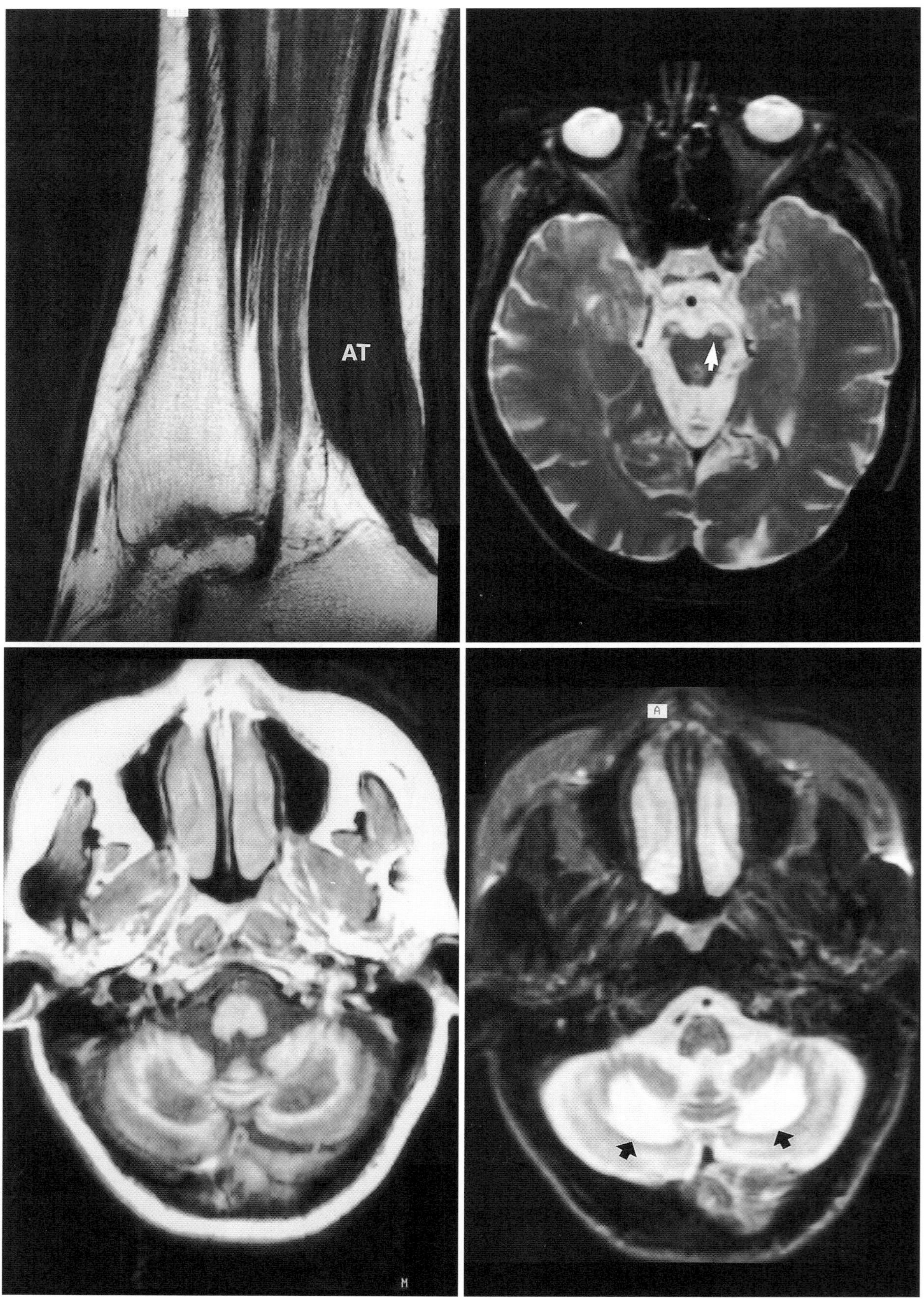
AT
A
M

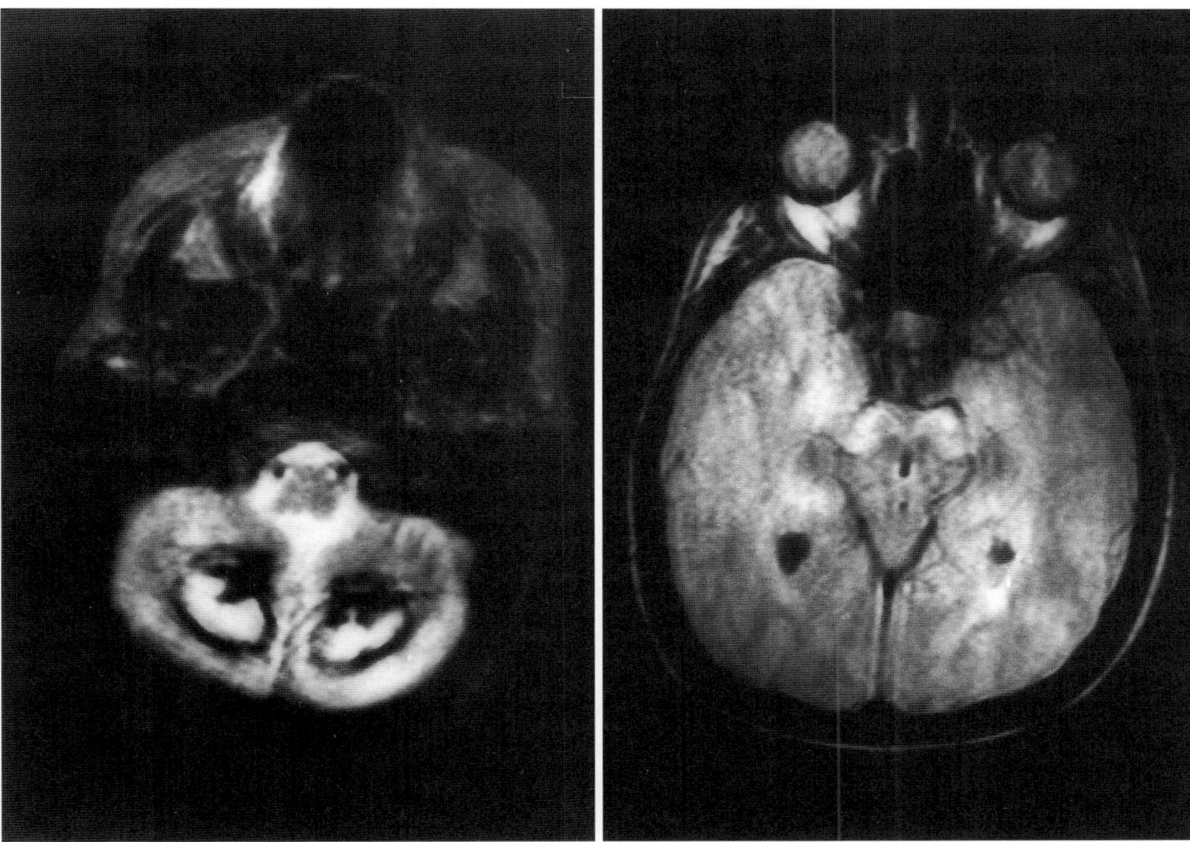

Fig. 24.2. Female, 43 years of age, with CTX. On the T_2-weighted image on the left, the cerebellar white matter has a high signal intensity surrounded by a rim of very low signal intensity. The moderately T_2-weighted image on the right shows the involvement of the corticospinal tracts in the mesencephalon. Note the round masses with low signal intensity in the choroid plexus of the lateral ventricles. Courtesy of Fiorelli et al. (1990), with permission

Fig. 24.1. Male, 51 years of age, with CTX. The *left upper image* shows the typical swelling of the Achilles tendon (*AT*). The images through the brain demonstrate involvement of the corticospinal tracts in the mesencephalon, and the T_1- and T_2-weighted images in the *lower row* show the involvement of the cerebellar white matter. Courtesy of F. Barkhof, Amsterdam, The Netherlands, with permission

25 Refsum Disease

25.1 Clinical Features and Laboratory Investigations

Refsum disease (RD), also called heredopathia atactica polyneuritiformis, is a rare disorder with an autosomal recessive mode of inheritance, characterized by accumulation of phytanic acid. The age at onset of clinical signs and symptoms varies from early childhood to the fifth decade. The onset is insidious and may be difficult to determine precisely. Symptoms are sometimes precipitated by infections. Dramatic exacerbations and remissions of symptoms may also occur spontaneously, without obvious antecedent cause.

The main clinical features are visual disturbances, peripheral polyneuropathy and cerebellar ataxia.

Initial visual disturbances include night blindness, which may be present for years before the diagnosis is established. Gradually, concentric constriction of the visual fields develops and finally only a tubular field of vision remains. Central vision may be intact or only minimally disturbed for years. In some cases optic atrophy, cataract or vitreous opacities occur contributing to visual failure and blindness. The funduscopic appearances are variable, also depending on the stage of disease. Typical pigmentary retinal degeneration is rare and usually pigmentation looks like fine, small granules or has a salt and pepper appearance. In the majority of the patients pigmentation occurs in the peripheral retina and macula pigmentation is exceptional. In rare cases, no pigmentary degeneration is seen on funduscopy. The pupils are often small and reaction to light, convergence and acccommodation is often minimal or absent.

Chronic progressive polyneuropathy is the second major manifestation of RD. The visual symptoms sometimes precede the polyneuropathy by several years. When the polyneuropathy develops gradually, it is usually symmetrical and initially distal, causing muscular weakness, atrophy, cutaneous hypesthesia, painful paresthesia and disturbed position sense. Peripheral nerves are sometimes palpably enlarged. There is a progressive lowering and loss of myotatic reflexes. The plantar responses are as a rule flexor or absent. Over a period of years the muscular weakness can become widespread and disabling, involving not only distal but also proximal musculature. Acute exac-

erbations are observed frequently in RD patients. Then the weakness is not limited to distal muscles of the extremities but also proximal muscles are paretic and cranial nerves may be involved. Periods of exacerbations may be followed by remissions in which the acutely developed weakness disappears.

Cerebellar ataxia forms the third major manifestation of RD. Ataxia is more marked than can be explained by the degree of weakness and sensory loss present. Nystagmus may be present as a sign of cerebellar dysfunction.

Other frequently observed abnormalities are cardiac problems, skin changes, skeletal abnormalities, anosmia and sensorineural deafness. Psychoses, particularly of paranoid type, occur more frequently than one would expect on the basis of pure coincidence.

Cardiomyopathy is present in most patients, as demonstrated by cardiac enlargement, tachycardia, conduction disturbances and ECG abnormalities. Sudden death is common during acute exacerbations and is probably caused by cardiac arrhythmias.

Skin changes vary from a dry, scaly skin to a condition of full-blown ichthyosis. The skin abnormalities change rapidly with the clinical state and are well correlated with plasma phytanic acid level. The skin problems tend to be more severe in children than in adults.

Bony deformities are frequently present. The skeletal manifestations include abnormalities of the metacarpal and metatarsal bones, which may be short or elongated, pes cavus, hammer toes, and epiphyseal dysplasia of the shoulders, elbows and knees.

The signs and symptoms of RD can be divided according to liability to rapid change following changes in blood phytanic acid levels. Bony abnormalities are stationary. Visual disturbances, anosmia, sensorineural deafness and testicular atrophy develop gradually, do not worsen rapidly on increasing phytanic acid levels and do not improve on lowering of phytanic acid levels. Only stabilization at the same level of impairment can be achieved by low blood phytanic acid levels. Peripheral neuropathy, cerebellar ataxia and cardiomyopathy are slowly progressive but liable to deteriorate rapidly if phytanic acid levels rise. The component of rapid deterioration responds well to lowering of phytanic acid levels, while the more chronic component responds slowly and often incompletely. Skin abnormalities are closely related to actual blood phytanic acid levels.

During the last few years it has become apparent that a considerable number of patients do not manifest all major characteristics of the disease, and that several patients manifest atypical signs. A case of RD has been described with Babinski signs, optic atrophy and absent retinitis pigmentosa. Also in other studies, a considerable number of the patients, otherwise typical RD cases, showed no signs of retinitis pigmentosa. Cases with isolated polyneuropathy have been reported. Children have been discovered with mental impairment in addition to other RD signs. In a considerable proportion of the affected children, hepatic problems have been reported, which are highly exceptional in adults. Renal dysfunction with amino aciduria and hypokalemia has occasionally been mentioned.

The clinical diagnosis of RD is difficult as no symptom is pathognomonic for the disease and the various signs and symptoms may develop in succession at different times. The demonstration of excessive amounts of phytanic acid in serum is the most valuable aid in the diagnosis of RD. Phytanic acid is not normally present in detectable amounts and the absence of phytanic acid in the serum of an untreated patient suspected of suffering from RD makes the diagnosis highly improbable.

The protein in CSF is increased to levels between 1 and 7 g/l or even higher. The cell count is normal. Neurophysiological studies show a greatly reduced motor and sensory nerve conduction velocity and signs of denervation and reinnervation in EMG. The nerve conduction velocity improves in conjunction with clinical improvement. The ERG shows absent or reduced reaction. ECG may reveal a prolonged QT segment and a widened QRS complex. When the urinary sediment of a patient with RD is stained for lipids, large amounts of fatty material can be detected.

A deficiency of phytanic acid oxidase can be shown in cultured fibroblasts. In RD patients the rate of oxidation of phytanic acid is less than 5% of normal, whereas in parents from RD patients the oxidation rate is about 50% of normal, indicating a heterozygous state. Phytanic oxidase activity can be determined in cultured amniotic cells, allowing prenatal diagnosis.

25.2 Pathology

In RD the site of major involvement is the PNS, whereas the CNS shows more subtle abnormalities. On gross examination of the brain, the leptomeninges appear thickened, but the brain appears normal. On microsocpic examination, deposition of fat is noted in the leptomeninges, ependymal cells, choroid plexus epithelium and cells of the pallidum. The cerebral hemispheres are otherwise intact with normal cytoarchitecture of the cortex.

In the brain stem variable demyelination occurs mainly affecting the pontocerebellar tracts, medial lemniscus, olivocerebellar tracts, cerebellar peduncles and corticospinal tracts. Axons are relatively spared. A variable number of fat-filled macrophages and hypertrophic astrocytes are present. Diffuse loss of neurons in the inferior olivary nuclei is commonly observed.

The cerebellar cortex is usually normal, although some neuronal loss may occur. The white matter within and surrounding the dentate nucleus is affected. Lipid-laden macrophages and hypertrophic astrocytes are present. Important loss of neurons is present within the dentate nucleus.

In the leptomeninges surrounding the spinal cord large amounts of fat are present. Sudanophilic granules of variable size are deposited in endothelial cells, histiocytes and macrophages. Within the spinal cord there is a marked demyelination of the posterior columns and demyelination of less severity in both spinocerebellar tracts. Retrograde changes and loss of motor neurons are observed in the anterior horns at all levels. In the spinal roots, especially at the level of the cauda equina, severe demyelination is observed together with complete destruction of some axons and axonal swellings. Onion-bulb formations are present.

The peripheral nerves, both the somatic and the autonomic nerves, show macroscopic thickening. The changes in the peripheral nerves are constant, but their intensity varies greatly between cases. Nerve hypertrophy is usually most conspicuous in the lumbar and brachial plexuses. The hypertrophy is often irregular, forming localized swellings. Histological study of these swellings indicates that myelinated nerve fibers are reduced in number, and Schwann cell processes have given rise to typical onion-bulb formations. Many unmyelinated axons are present within the onion bulbs. The myelin sheaths are often abnormally thin and of unequal thickness, and segmental demyelination has been found. Axonal destruction is also present. In some onion bulbs the whorls are closely packed, but in others they are more loosely disposed and separated by large extracellular spaces of variable width. In the cytoplasm of the whorl-forming Schwann cells, several types of inclusion can be seen with help of electron microscopy: large crystalline inclusions and rounded osmiophilic bodies which are probably lipid in nature.

In the kidney, fat is accumulated in large amounts in the epithelial cells of the convoluted tubules. In the liver, fat is stored in mesenchymal and parenchymal cells. There are no or only slight signs of fibrosis. In cultured fibroblasts, the presence of normal or somewhat elevated numbers of peroxisomes has been demonstrated.

25.3 Chemical Pathology

RD is a disorder of phytanic acid metabolism. Phytanic acid is a C20 multibranched fatty acid. It has been isolated in the brain and has been found to be present in much larger amounts in the white matter than in the gray matter. The presence of substantial proportions of phytanic acid can be demonstrated without any appreciable alteration in total amounts of fat. Analysis of the lipid composition of the CNS reveals that the proportions of the remaining lipids are nearly normal. Phytanic acid is mainly present in phosphoglycerides, with higher proportions of phytanic acid in the choline phosphoglycerides than in the other phosophoglycerides. Lower concentrations are present in the galactolipids. Phytanic acid accumulates mainly in myelin and is found in higher concentrations in the choline phosphoglycerides from myelin than from gray matter or whole white matter. The proportions of phytanic acid in peripheral nerve myelin are even higher.

In several organs other than the nervous system there are accumulations of neutral lipids, especially in liver and spleen. A high proportion of the fatty acids consists of phytanic acid, incorporated in cholesterol esters and triglycerides. Also the heart muscle and blood contain a large amount of phytanic acid.

25.4 Pathogenetic Considerations

Phytanic acid is a C20 multibranched fatty acid: 3,7,11,15-tetramethylhexadecanoic acid. The basic defect is a defect in α-oxidation of phytanic acid. The defect results in an excessive accumulation of phytanic acid in blood and various tissues.

The common pathway for fatty acid degradation is formed by the β-oxidation pathway in mitochondria and peroxisomes. The presence of a β-methyl group in phytanic acid prevents it from undergoing β-oxidation. Instead, phytanic acid first undergoes α-oxidation to pristanic acid, which is further degraded by β-oxidation. Pristanoyl-CoA oxidase is localized in peroxisomes.

The subcellular organelle responsible for the oxidation of phytanic acid has not yet been established with certainty. For many years it has been thought that peroxisomes are involved, because accumulation of phytanic acid was not only observed in RD, but also in disorders characterized by generalized loss of peroxisomal functions. In all these disorders an impairment of phytanic acid α-oxidation was found. However, there has been doubt about the peroxisomal location of the defect in RD. In contrast to the disorders with generalized peroxisomal dysfunction and lack of morphologically normal peroxisomes, the peroxisomes in RD are morphologically normal. Evidence that the first step of phytanic acid oxidation has a mitochondrial location has been accumulating. Based on the evidence of α-oxidation of phytanic acid in mitochondria and the identification of pristanoyl-CoA oxidase in peroxisomes, cooperation of the two subcellular organelles in the breakdown of phytanic acid has been proposed and explanations have been sought for the accumulation of phytanic acid in disorders with generalized peroxisomal dysfunction. A possible explanation is found in product inhibition of phytanic acid oxidation by pristanic acid which accumulates in these latter disorders as a result of deficient peroxisomal β-oxidation. Product inhibition could, however, not be demonstrated. Another explanation states that abnormalities in lipid metabolism, including decreased synthesis of plasmalogens in generalized peroxisomal dysfunction, lead to alterations in the mitochondrial membrane and as a consequence to disturbance of α-oxidation of phytanic acid. Probably, the solution to the problem has been found recently. It has been shown that the conversion of phytanic acid to pristanic acid is a two-step process with 2-hydroxyphytanic acid as an obligatory intermediate. The first step in the degradation of phytanic acid is an α-hydroxylation, resulting in formation of 2-hydroxyphytanic acid and this step probably occurs in mitochondria. The second step is a decarboxylation, resulting in pristanic acid. The second step probably requires peroxisomes, explaining the accumulation of phytanic acid in disorders with generalized peroxisomal dysfunction.

Phytanic acid is of exogenous, dietary orign. There is no evidence of any endogenous synthesis. It is consumed by humans in considerable quantities in vegetable and animal products. Although phytol can be metabolized by humans to phytanic acid, most phytol in the diet is bound to chlorophyll and little is absorbed. Hence, the contribution of phytol to the phytanic acid concentration in humans is negligible. In view of the large intake and the presence of only trace amounts in human tissue, the catabolic pathway that disposes of phytanic acid must be very efficient. The accumulation of large amounts of this unusual fatty acid in various tissues and lipid classes is probably the cause of a series of symptoms, both acute and chronic. The experience with treatment resulting in a reduction of phytanic acid levels in the body and the experience with loading experiments indicate that there is indeed a causal relationship between phytanic acid and symptomatology in RD. It is probable that the incorporation of phytanic acid into myelin sheaths leads to a less stable myelin structure. The methyl branching of phytanic acid probably disrupts the packing of the hydrocarbon tails in the bimolecular lipid leaflet due to steric hindrance, and in this way destabilizes the myelin. Once phytanic acid levels reach a critical point, myelin dissolution occurs. The phytanic acid levels are higher

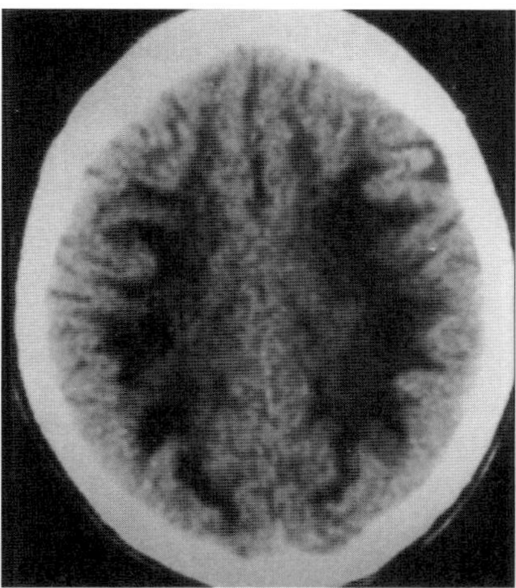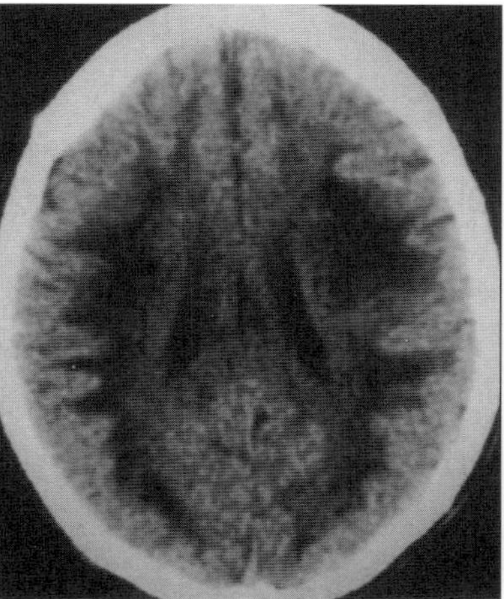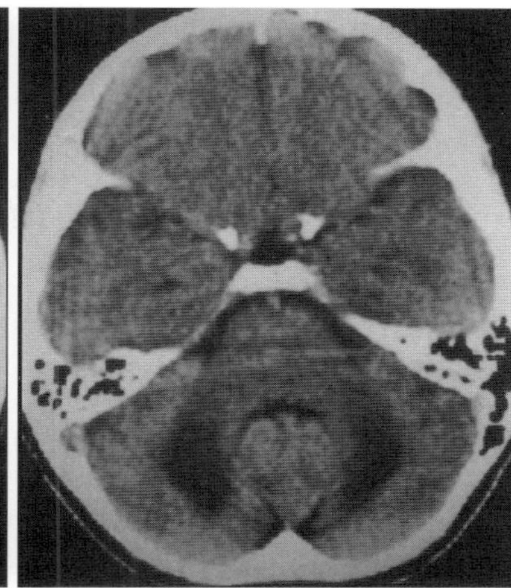

Fig. 25.1. CT scan in this case of RD shows extensive symmetrical low density in the cerebellar and cerebral white matter. Courtesy of Kendall (1992), with permission

in peripheral nerve myelin than in CNS myelin and demyelination starts earlier and is more severe in the PNS than in the CNS.

The higher concentration of phytanic acid in myelin of the PNS than in myelin of the CNS requires explanation. There are indications that the turnover rate of myelin is higher in peripheral nerves than in brain and spinal cord. Phytanic acid may, therefore, accumulate more easily in the peripheral nerves. Another possibility is that the blood-nerve barrier in the PNS is less restrictive than the blood-brain barrier in the CNS, allowing a more rapid increase in phytanic acid content of peripheral nerves.

The distribution of demyelination in the CNS, with preferential involvement of brain stem and cerebellum, has not been explained.

25.5 Therapy

As the origin of phytanic acid is exclusively exogenous, further accumulation of the substance can be prevented by a strict diet, low in phytanic acid. The need to restrict phytol is questionable. Furthermore, the diet should contain an adequate amount of energy to prevent considerable weight loss. An appreciable quantity of phytanic acid is present in body fat stores. During conditions of increased mobilization of body fat, phytanic acid is liberated from body stores, and serum concentration increases even with low intake of phytanic acid. During periods of important weight loss serious worsening of neurological or myocardial pathology may occur, even resulting in death.

Strict diet and supply of sufficient energy to maintain a near-constant body weight lead to a gradual drop in serum phytanic acid levels to normal or slightly increased levels. The treated RD patients show definite clinical improvement. They no longer have apparently spontaneous relapses. The improvement in particular concerns the signs and symptoms that change rapidly: neuropathy, cerebellar ataxia, cardiomyopathy and ichthyosis. Problems such as visual disturbances, anosmia and deafness usually stabilize and do not deteriorate any further. Some neurological problems are due to irreversible damage and are not influenced favorably by lowering phytanic acid levels. Early diagnosis and treatment is important to prevent irreversible handicaps. The advice to furnish sufficient energy applies particularly at the start of treatment, when the serum phytanic acid levels are still very high. Later, when the phytanic acid content of the serum has been reduced to safer levels, a gradual weight reduction is acceptable.

Plasmapheresis provides the means to lower serum phytanic levels rapidly. Very high serum levels are toxic and may precipitate life-threatening symptoms. In these circumstances, plasmapheresis can be used as an emergency measure. Furthermore, plasmapheresis has been shown to be an excellent supplement to dietary treatment. When applied with a low frequency, it can compensate for a less strict dietary regimen.

25.6 Magnetic Resonance Imaging

There are few reports on imaging findings in RD, probably because of the rarity of the disease and the fact that the site of major involvement is the PNS rather than the CNS. Considering histopathological findings, MR signs of demyelination can be expected to occur mainly in brain stem tracts, cerebellar peduncles and the cerebellar white matter. One case has been described with CT findings (Fig. 25.1). In addition to hypodensity of the cerebellar white matter, diffuse, symmetrical, cerebral hemispheral white matter hypodensity was also found (Fig. 25.1).

The nucleus of the cell contains the structural information for all proteins present in the cell, and is responsible directly or indirectly for the synthesis of all molecules in the cell. The information is coded in deoxyribonucleic acid (DNA) by the sequence of four nitrogenous bases: the purines adenine and guanine (A and G), and the pyrimidines cytosine and thymine (C and T). The information is carried in the form of a three letter code, the letters being A, G, C and T. Different arrangements of three consecutive bases code for different amino acids in the peptides to be synthesized. Such coding triplets are called codons. The segment of DNA that codes for one peptide chain is called a gene. Peptides are strings of amino acids that form the building blocks of enzymes and other proteins. There are 20 naturally occurring amino acids.

DNA has a helical structure with two chains of nucleotides twisted together to form a double helix. Nucleotides are base-deoxyribose-phosphate complexes. The backbone of DNA, which is constant throughout the molecule, consists of deoxyribose molecules linked by phosphates. The bases are on the inside of the helix, whereas the deoxyribose phosphate backbone is on the outside. In the two chains of the helix, adenine always appears opposite thymine and guanine opposite cytosine. This makes the chains complementary; that is, the sequence of bases in one chain dictates the sequence of bases in the other chain. The stability of the double helix is accounted for by the enormous number of hydrogen bonds that connect the complementary bases along the entire length of the double helix.

In the nucleus the long molecules of DNA are squeezed into tightly compacted, discrete lengths, the chromosomes. DNA varies in both length and base composition from chromosome to chromosome. In human cells, each of the 23 different chromosomes has a characteristic length and a distinctive sequence of genes. The specific sites on chromosomes where genes are situated are called loci. Chromosomes exist in homologous pairs, and so do the genes. As a result of an alteration of the structure of a gene, individual genes may exist in different forms, called alleles, only two of which can be present in one individual. An allele can be either dominant or recessive. Both chromosomes of a homologous pair may carry identical alleles (homozygosity for that allele) or different alleles (heterozygosity). The complete set of DNA sequences carried on all the 46 chromosomes, is the genome. Total nuclear DNA contains 3×10^9 base pairs and 10000 to 40000 genes in duplo.

The process of synthesis of peptides based on information coded in DNA is divided into a transcription step and a translation step. Both steps depend on the presence of different ribonucleic acid (RNA) molecules. Chemically, RNA is similar to DNA except for the presence of ribose instead of deoxyribose. DNA is transcribed into messenger RNA (mRNA) by the action of an enzyme called RNA polymerase. Because of the rules of base pairing, mRNA is a mirror image of the DNA from which it is copied, but uracil is used instead of thymine. Most genes consist of alternating coding and noncoding segments of DNA. The coding segments are called exons. The noncoding segments are called introns. Both introns and exons are transcribed into mRNA, but before mRNA is transported from the nucleus to the cytoplasm, introns are removed by the process of so-called RNA splicing. After various processing steps, mRNA moves from the nucleus to the cytoplasm of the cell where it acts in the process of translation as a template for protein synthesis. Protein synthesis takes place on ribosomes, located free in the cytoplasm or on the surface of the endoplasmic reticulum. The ribosomes become attached to mRNA and carry the growing peptide chains. Ribosomes contain ribosomal RNA (rRNA), which does not contain genetic information to be translated into proteins, but has both a structural and a functional role in ribosomes and is required for protein synthesis. Amino acids do not bind directly to mRNA, but first become attached to transfer RNA (tRNA). Each tRNA molecule is specific for both a particular amino acid and for an appropriate mRNA codon. A tRNA molecule binds to a particular codon on mRNA by carrying an anticodon, a group of three nucleotides with a sequence complementary to the mRNA codon. Successive tRNAs carry their amino acids to the mRNA template and hence a peptide chain is built up with the correct sequence of amino acids. After releasing the amino acid at the ribosome, the tRNA is released and is free to attach to another amino acid of the same kind.

Ribosomes are either located free in the cellular cytoplasm or are bound to the membranes of the rough endoplasmic reticulum. These locations are related to the final destination of the newly synthesized proteins. Proteins synthesized on free polyribosomes are liberated into the cytoplasm from which they can be transported to another location, such as the nucleus, mitochondria or peroxisomes. The proteins formed on membrane-bound polyribosomes are directly transported through the membrane into the lumen of the rough endoplasmic reticulum. The routing of proteins is conducted by the first part of the forming proteins that contains a signal peptide. Proteins synthesized on the rough endoplasmic reticulum can have different destinations, including secretory vesicles, lysosomes, plasma membrane, rough endoplasmic reticulum and the Golgi complex. Proteins can be modified in the rough endoplasmic reticulum by means of glycosylation. All proteins with destinations other than the rough endoplasmic reticulum are transported to the cis Golgi complex, from where they are transported to the trans Golgi complex while undergoing further modifications. Proteins are sorted in the Golgi complex according to their site of destination.

DNA molecules contain endless stretches of information. In order to transcribe a particular gene or group of genes, RNA polymerase must recognize where to begin transcription of DNA and where to terminate it. At the beginning of a gene or group of genes is a site consisting of a short sequence of bases, called a promotor, that serves as a start signal. At the end of the gene or genes another sequence of bases, the terminator site, signals the RNA polymerase to stop.

The nucleus plays a central role in two essential biosynthetic processes of the cell: transcription (RNA synthesis) and replication (DNA synthesis). DNA synthesis is in human cells a discontinuous process and occurs only during the synthetic phase (so-called S-phase) of the cell cycle. The DNA helix is opened, so that both DNA chains can be copied with help of the enzyme DNA polymerase. Each strand is used as a template for constructing new complementary strands. At the end of the DNA replication the cell has two copies of its genome, each of them consisting of an old and a newly synthesized strand of DNA. This is a very precise process.

Every cell in the human body contains the complete complement of genes necessary to make an entire human being. Since most organs are made up of cells with very special functions, it follows that only a small proportion of their genes must be active and come to expression. The basis of cellular differentiation is regulation of expression of genes. Many genes are required to function only at specific phases of development and they must be activated and switched off at the appropriate times. All individual genes must be so regulated that they produce just the right quantity of product for the physiological requirement of the cell. This is determined by the rate of gene transcription.

In differentiated cells, DNA synthesis occurs first in DNA of active genes and last in DNA of genes that are not expressed in these cells.

The extraordinary fidelity of DNA replication is crucial for the accurate transfer of genetic information. Errors in this process are a common source of deleterious mutations, which are inherited in successive cell cycles. Considering the magnitude of the job (about 3×10^9 base pairs per haploid human genome), it is a tribute to the precision of the DNA replication machinery that more errors do not accumulate during the multitude of cell divisions that occur during a lifetime. The accuracy of the overal DNA replication process is assured by several mechanisms, including nucleotide selection by DNA polymerase, exonuclease proof-reading activity associated with the DNA polymerases, and post-replicative mismatch repair system. These mechanisms assure a final mutation rate of 10^{-10} to 10^{-12} errors per base pair per generation, which is still acceptable for individual and species.

Despite the high accuracy of the DNA replication process some errors arise during DNA replication, most often due to the incorporation of noncomplementary bases by DNA polymerase. Furthermore, chemical and physical hits to DNA cause a variety of structural and chemical lesions to the genome. The chemical compounds damaging DNA can be of endogenous or exogenous origin. DNA changes may result from attacks by endogenous reactive chemicals produced during cell metabolism, such as oxygen radicals. Cells are rich in enzymatic and nonenzymatic radical scavenging systems and the most dangerous chemical reactions are confined to specialized organelles, such as mitochondria and peroxisomes, to prevent injury. Other chemical compounds which react with nucleic acids range from metals, alkylating agents, polycyclic hydrocarbons, aromatic amines, azo dyes, mitomycin C, aflatoxin B1, and urethane. Among the physical agents damaging DNA most common are ultraviolet and ionizing radiation. Damage that is not repaired before DNA replication may become fixed by copying in subsequent replication cycles or may result in breakdown of DNA replication and cell death.

There is a variety of DNA repair systems which are able to remove the damage and restore the normal nucleotide sequence. They can be divided into several categories. The first category includes repair systems characterized by the direct reversal of DNA damage in which a single enzymatic step is able to restore the normal state of DNA. The second category includes the base excision repair and the nucleotide excision repair. In the excision repair system the unusual or modified base or nucleotide is removed, and a new DNA chain a few nucleotides long is synthesized which is then joined to the adjacent preexisting nucleotides by the action of DNA ligase. The third category includes DNA repair systems that come into action when bulky lesions are left in the DNA template and stop the DNA replication machinery. The synthesis of one strand is interrupted in front of the lesion and reinitiated at some points in the undamaged region beyond the lesion. The deriving gap cannot be handled by excision repair which requires an intact complementary strand. The gap in front of the damage is repaired by recombination, and the damage is subsequently repaired by a process that is called "daughter strand gap repair".

DNA repair systems do not repair the entire genome homogeneously. Repair in inactive genes is slow. Repair in active genes is fast. Repair in the transcribed strand of active genes is also accelerated. Hence, poorly expressed DNA regions can be repaired slowly, and consequently DNA lesions may accumulate in these sequences of the genome. There is evidence that nondividing, post-mitotic cells (such as neurons) contain lower levels of DNA repair enzymes and repair DNA slower than proliferating cells. This could render nerve cells prone to an accumulation of DNA damage during their life span.

In many ways, DNA and DNA alterations are related to myelin disorders.

1. Defects in DNA repair may lead to abnormalities in myelin synthesis and myelin maintenance.

2. Defects concerning genes coding for myelin proteins may lead to disturbances of myelin build-up, maturation and maintenance.

3. Genetic defects concerning enzymes involved in the metabolism of myelin components may result in disturbances of myelin build-up, maturation and maintenance.

4. Genetic defects may have indirect implications for processes of myelination and myelin maintenance; for instance, by toxic influences of metabolic derangements.

5. In many aspects, the genetic make-up influences the vulnerability to the occurrence of myelin disorders; for instance, by influence on immunological reactions.

The following chapters discuss myelin disorders caused by defects in DNA repair or by defects concerning genes coding for myelin proteins.

27 Cockayne's Disease

27.1 Clinical Features and Laboratory Investigations

Cockayne's Disease (CoD) is a rare, inherited disorder characterized by cachectic dwarfism, cutaneous photosensitivity and progressive neurological dysfunction. The mode of inheritance is autosomal recessive. Two types of the disease are distinguished: classical CoD or CoD type I and severe CoD or CoD type II.

In CoD type I, the children seem normal at birth. Their weight, length and head circumference are normal. Growth failure generally begins within the first year of life and is profound. Weight is affected to a greater extent than length, leading to cachectic dwarfism. Subcutaneous fat is lost diffusely and almost completely, giving the patients a starved appearance. A thin, prominent nose, narrow mouth and chin, sunken eyes and loss of adipose tissue from the face result in the characteristic facies of an old man or woman. This appearance becomes more and more evident in the course of a few years. Within the first 2 years almost all patients have become microcephalic. A thin and dry skin, fine hair and large and sometimes malformed ears contribute to the characteristic facies of CoD patients. Dermal photosensitivity is present in 75% of the patients and can appear as acute sun sensitivity that results in desquamation, scarring and atrophy of exposed areas. Pigmentary abnormalities with hypopigmentation and hyperpigmentation have occasionally been described. Anhidrosis may occur. Dental problems are common with moderate to severe caries.

The posture of CoD patients is typical. Even at an early age there is an abnormal flexion of hips and knees while standing. In older patients the posture is stooped due to kyphosis combined with progressive hip, knee and ankle contractures. The trunk is small, the arms and legs are disproportionately long and hands and feet are large.

The earliest commonly noticed neurological abnormality is delayed psychomotor development which usually becomes apparent at the time when sitting, walking and speech should develop. The delay in the acquisition of functions becomes progressively greater as the patient grows older. All patients with CoD type I are mentally retarded, but mental capacities vary from mildly to profoundly deficient. Among the higher functioning patients, intellectual deterioration usually becomes evident in the teenage years. Behavioral problems are rare and the patients are usually described as happy, and social. In the course of the years progressive neurological abnormalities become apparent. Cerebellar signs are present with tremor, lack of coordination, dysarthric speech and gait ataxia. Pyramidal signs are usually present with hypertonia and hyperreflexia. The gait disorder in patients who become ambulatory is striking and progressive, due to a combination of spasticity, ataxia and contractures of the hips, knees and ankles. Sensorineural hearing loss occurs in over half the patients. Myoclonus, and involuntary choreiform and athetoid movements are rare. Overt signs of peripheral neuropathy are rare until late stages of the disease, when there is a progressive, diffuse muscular atrophy, muscle weakness and areflexia. Some patients have diminished lacrimation, decreased sweating, miotic pupils, and cool and acrocyanotic limbs. This could be due to autonomic dysfunction, but formal assessment of autonomic function has not been documented. Seizures occur late and in a minority of the patients.

Pigmentary degeneration of the retina of the salt and pepper type is found in the majority of the patients. The retina changes are progressive and during the first few years of life normal findings do not exclude the diagnosis of CoD. Other common ophthalmological abnormalities are cataract and optic atrophy. Miotic pupils which are poorly responsive to mydriatics, corneal dystrophy and decreased or absent lacrimation may be found. Despite the extensive ocular abnormalities some visual acuity usually remains, although blindness may occur.

Renal problems develop in about 10% of the CoD patients with decreased renal function, and very rarely renal failure. Hypertension may occur.

Undescended or small testes are seen in about 30% of the male CoD patients. In female patients breasts are often small and menstrual cycles irregular.

The neurological abnormalities in CoD type I become gradually more severe and mental failure is progressive. Death by inanition and infection, most commonly respiratory infections, usually occurs in the fourth decade of life.

A growing number of patients of CoD type II has been described with an earlier onset of symptoms and a more severe course than in CoD type I patients. CoD type II patients often have a low birth weight and little postnatal increase in height, weight and head circumference, although some patients have a normal birth weight and a normal gain in weight during the first few months of life. The infants develop an emaciated appearance characteristic of CoD with little subcutaneous fat, deep-set eyes and a prominent, beaked nose. In the neonatal period the children are hypotonic, but develop spastic quadriplegia. Few or no developmental milestones are reached which are subsequently lost in the process of neurological deterioration. Congenital cataract is often present. Other reported ocular abnormalities include hypoplastic optic nerves, microphthalmus, iris hypoplasia, microcornea and reduced lacrimal secretion. Kyphosis and progressive contractures of hips and knees occur. Photosensitivity has been reported. Generally, dental, auditory and cutaneous complications are less commonly described in these patients, probably because of the severe neurological problems and early age at death. Death usually occurs by the age of 6 or 7 years, but may also occur during the first few years of life.

The clinical pictures of CoD type II, cerebro-oculo-facio-skeletal syndrome (so-called COFS syndrome) and cataracts-microcephaly-failure to thrive-kyphoscoliosis syndrome (so-called CAMFAK syndrome) overlap. Which of these disorders are genetically related and which are distinct genetic entities will remain open to discussion until the underlying biochemical and genetic defects are discovered.

Laboratory investigations of blood and CSF reveal no consistent and no diagnostic abnormalities. In CSF an elevated protein content may be found. Few patients have biochemical evidence of a decreased renal function with decreased creatinine clearance. In incidental patients elevated serum cholesterol or lipoprotein levels have been noted. Nerve conduction velocities are markedly slowed, consistent with a demyelinating polyneuropathy, in the majority of the patients. In skeletal muscle, denervation changes can be found. EEG is normal in some patients, but may show slowing and sometimes epileptic discharges. Evoked potentials are often abnormally delayed. Radiological investigations of the skeleton in CoD show microcephaly, with a thick cranial vault and sometimes intracranial calcifications. General skeletal maturation may be within normal limits, advanced or delayed. Less common findings include shortness and broadness of the metacarpals and phalanges, whose epiphyses sometimes have an ivory-dense appearance, and flattening of the vertebral bodies, lipping of their upper and lower anterior margins, and osteoporosis.

The clinical suspicion of CoD can be confirmed by ultraviolet irradiation of cultured skin fibroblasts of the patients. Cell lines from CoD patients show failure of DNA and RNA synthesis to recover to normal rates after irradiation. The failure of RNA synthesis to recover in CoD cells after ultraviolet irradiation can be used in prenatal diagnosis. Carrier detection is as yet not possible.

27.2 Pathology

The leptomeninges in classical CoD appear thickened and fibrotic. The brain is usually small and has an atrophied appearance. Cerebellar atrophy is most severe. On sectioning, the lateral ventricles appear to be enlarged and the corpus callosum is thin. The white matter is decreased in volume and has a mottled appearance. Calcium depositions are present bilaterally in the basal ganglia and dentate nuclei and may also be found in the white matter and cerebral and cerebellar cortices. The dura may be focally calcified.

Microscopic examination of the leptomeninges reveals increased collagenous connective tissue without any inflammatory changes. The principal finding in classical CoD is tigroid demyelination with patchy loss of myelin sheaths, relative preservation of axons, and numerous islands of preserved myelin sheaths. A relationship between blood vessels and myelin loss or presence has not been demonstrated. All levels of the brain are involved, including cerebral hemispheral white matter, cerebellar white matter and brain stem. The U fibers are not spared. In the spinal cord the descending tracts are focally demyelinated, whereas the ascending tracts are relatively spared. The demyelinated areas contain fewer oligodendrocytes than the areas of myelin preservation. Sudanophilic lipids are scanty, but sometimes seen in the walls of vessels and in microglial cells in the brain parenchyma. No inflammatory infiltration is found. Astrogliosis is seen in the demyelinated areas. The cerebral cortex is generally intact, but sometimes there is a slight diffuse loss of neurons. The cerebellar cortex is less well preserved and the number of Purkinje cells and granule cells is reduced. Calcium deposits are present perivascularly and within the neuropil. The typical locations of calcium deposits include the basal ganglia and dentate nucleus, and may also involve cerebral and cerebellar cortex and the white matter. The small deposits may coalesce into larger calculi. In some cases of CoD nuclear abnormalities have been found in astrocytes and neurons. In these cases many of these cells have a single, large, hyperchromatic, atypical nucleus. Some cells are multinucleated. Similar nuclear abnormalities have been described in cells from patients with ataxia telangiectasia and in mammalian fibroblasts, supralethally irradiated in vitro with ionizing radiation. In incidental cases neurofibrillary tangles have been found in the nucleus basalis, substantia nigra, locus coeruleus and the cerebral cortex. Their presence may be considered to be a premature senile change of the brain or a nonspecific finding occurring in chronic neurological conditions.

Sural nerve biopsies demonstrate chronic segmental demyelination and remyelination with onion bulb formation. Onion bulbs are nonspecific signs of repeated demyelination and remyelination. They are more pronounced in older than in younger patients. In some cases of CoD, electron-dense, membrane-bound, finely granular or lamellated inclusions have been reported in Schwann cells. The nature and role of these inclusions is unknown.

Renal pathology may include thickening of the glomerular basement membrane.

In early-onset cases of CoD, neuropathological findings are very similar to those of classical CoD. The leptomeninges are thickened. The brain is small and atrophic and the ventricles are enlarged. The white matter is reduced in volume. In the CNS severe but discontinuous demyelination in a tigroid fashion is found with concomitant gliosis. The cerebrum, cerebellum, brain stem and spinal cord are affected. Calcium depositions, present perivascularly and in the neuropil, may be found in basal ganglia, thalamus, dentate nucleus, cerebral and cerebellar cortex and meninges. Cerebral cortex is intact; in the cerebellar cortex loss of Purkinje cells and granule cells is found. Bizarre astrocytes with large and multiple nuclei may occur.

27.3 Chemical Pathology

In CoD the white matter shows a marked loss of myelin lipids and some increase in cholesterol esters. Besides this usual picture of demyelination, no specific abnormalities are found.

27.4 Pathogenetic Considerations

A defect in DNA repair is the cause of a number of human genetic disorders, including xeroderma pigmentosum, ataxia telangiectasia, and CoD.

Despite the high accuracy of the DNA replication process some errors arise during DNA replication. Furthermore, chemical and physical hits to DNA cause a variety of structural and chemical lesions. The chemical compounds which react with nucleic acids range from oxygen radicals, alkylating agents, polycyclic hydrocarbons, aromatic amines to aflatoxin, whereas the most common physical agents are ultraviolet and ionizing radiation. If not repaired, DNA damage leads to defects in subsequent replication cycles and to abnormalities in transcription and translation of the information coded in DNA. The variety of DNA damage is reflected by a variety of DNA repair systems which are able to remove the damage and restore the normal nucleotide sequence.

In CoD, both the classical and the severe form, there is a defect in DNA repair. Cultured fibroblasts from CoD patients are more sensitive than normal to killing by ultraviolet irradiation. In CoD cells there is a marked, prolonged inhibition of synthesis of DNA and RNA after ultraviolet irradiation. Damage produced by ultraviolet light in DNA in normal cells depresses rates of both DNA and RNA synthesis, but these rates soon become normal. In CoD cells this recovery does not occur. The rapid recovery of DNA and RNA synthesis in normal cells can be attributed to preferential rapid repair of DNA damage in regions of DNA which are actively transcribed, in contrast to a much slower repair in the bulk of DNA. In CoD cells, this preferential repair of transcriptionally active DNA does not take place, damage in these regions being repaired at the same (slow) rate as in the bulk of DNA. This failure to effect the rapid repair of crucial regions of DNA is the cause of the hypersensitivity of the cells to the lethal effects of ultraviolet light. In CoD cells, global DNA repair is normal and there is no increase in chromosomal breakage, as seen in xeroderma pigmentosum. The molecular basis of the inability to repair transcriptionally active DNA in CoD has not yet been elucidated. The chromosomal location of the CoD gene has not yet been established.

There is evidence of genetic heterogeneity: in classical CoD, cell fusion studies have shown the presence of more than one complementation group. Several patients have signs of CoD and xeroderma pigmentosum, both clinically and in cell culture studies. In several patients in whom the clinical diagnosis CoD was made, no defect in recovery of DNA and RNA synthesis after ultraviolet irradiation of fibroblasts could be shown. Several patients have been described with an unusually mild clinical presentation, and in at least one of them, the abnormalities in DNA and RNA metabolism typical of CoD were found. Until now the clinical finding of enhanced photosensitivity has proven the best correlation with a positive cellular diagnosis.

The photosensitivity of CoD patients is due to the damaging effects of ultraviolet radiation in sunlight. It is hypothesized that the death of photoreceptor cells (resulting in retinitis pigmentosa), myelin producing oligodendrocytes and Schwann cells (resulting in demyelination in the CNS and PNS), and fat cells (resulting in extreme cachexia) is due to the inability of these normally long-lived, nondividing cells to repair their

DNA which has been damaged by certain intracellular metabolites. Nuclear atypia of neurons and astrocytes may also result from the accumulation of unrepaired DNA damage.

27.5 Therapy

To date no effective mode of therapy has been found in CoD and the management of the disease is purely symptomatic. Patients should be monitored for treatable complications, such as hypertension, hearing loss and dental caries. Physical therapy can be helpful to avoid contractures. Emollients for dry skin, avoidance of excessive sun exposure and use of sun-screens are helpful in diminishing skin problems. Genetic counseling is important.

27.6 Magnetic Resonance Imaging

CT scan may demonstrate bilateral calcifications of the basal ganglia, dentate nucleus and other areas of the brain (Fig. 27.1). Cerebral, cerebellar and brain stem atrophy with prominence of sulci and ventricular enlargement is usually seen.

MRI confirms the presence of variable atrophy, most pronounced in brain stem and cerebellum. There is a loss of white matter volume and ventricles are mildly enlarged. However, atrophy is not reported in all patients. MRI is less sensitive than CT in showing the presence of calcium depositions (Fig. 27.2), but is more accurate in delineating the locations. The globus pallidus is most often involved, followed in frequency by the dentate nucleus. In addition calcium depositions may be seen in the putamen, caudate nucleus and as irregular, not necessarily symmetrical areas in the cortex and white matter of cerebrum and cerebellum. In addition, there are symmetrical white matter abnormalities (Figs. 27.1, 27.2). On T_2-weighted images the signal intensity of the cerebral white matter is abnormally high, but not so high as in completely unmyelinated white matter in neonates. The white matter often seems to have a finely irregular, mottled aspect, probably reflecting the tigroid pattern of myelin presence. In many of the reported patients the moderately high signal intensity is seen throughout the hemispheral white matter, including periventricular white matter and U fibers, sometimes also the internal capsule. The corpus callosum has a better state of myelination. The images resemble those of Pelizaeus-Merzbacher disease, apart from the calcium deposits. In other patients the white matter is better myelinated in the subcortical areas and the white matter hyperintensity is most marked in the periventricular area. Apparently delayed and disturbed myelination (dysmyelination) as well as demyelination play a role in CoD. Images in type I and type II CoD are essentially the same.

The MRI pattern as described is highly suggestive of CoD, in particular in combination with the clinical findings. Apart from the calcifications the images may resemble those of Pelizaeus-Merzbacher disease, CAM-FAK syndrome (cataracts-microcephaly-failure to thrive-kyphoscoliosis) and COFS (cerebro-oculo-facio-skeletal) syndrome (Fig. 27.3). A similar MRI pattern can be seen in mitochondrial disorders, but these can easily be differentiated from CoD on the basis of clinical and biochemical findings.

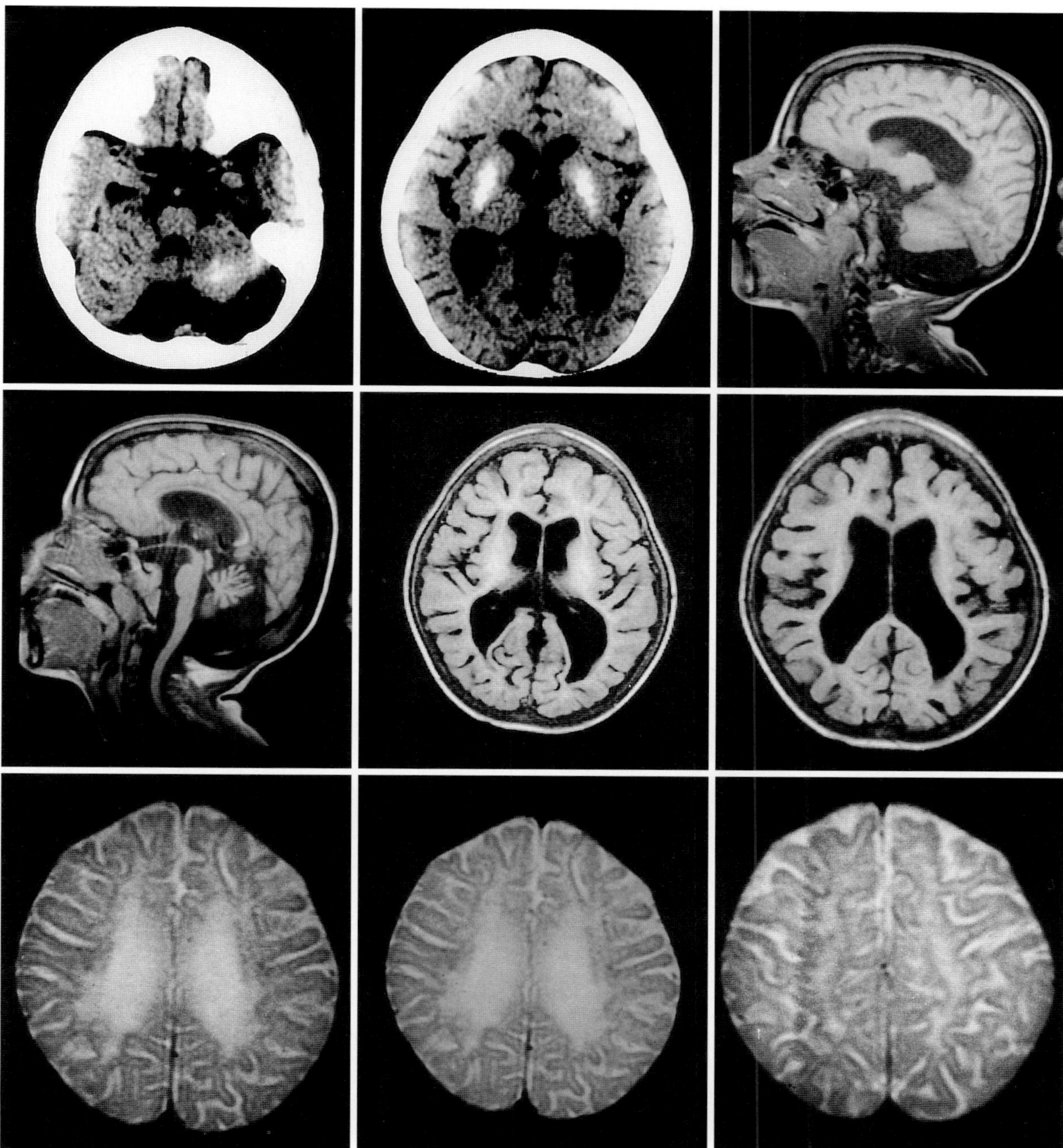

Fig. 27.1. 6-year-old girl with CoD. CT scans (*left upper row*) through the posterior fossa and the lateral ventricles show calcifications in the dentate nucleus and the basal ganglia, with ventricular and sulcal widening and cerebellar atrophy. The T_1-weighted sagittal images show the atrophy of cerebellar vermis and hemispheres, especially on the left side. Calcifications are less conspicuous on MRI. The T_2-weighted images (*lower row*) show the poor state of myelination of the white matter. Courtesy of I.N. Snoek, Eindhoven, the Netherlands, with permission

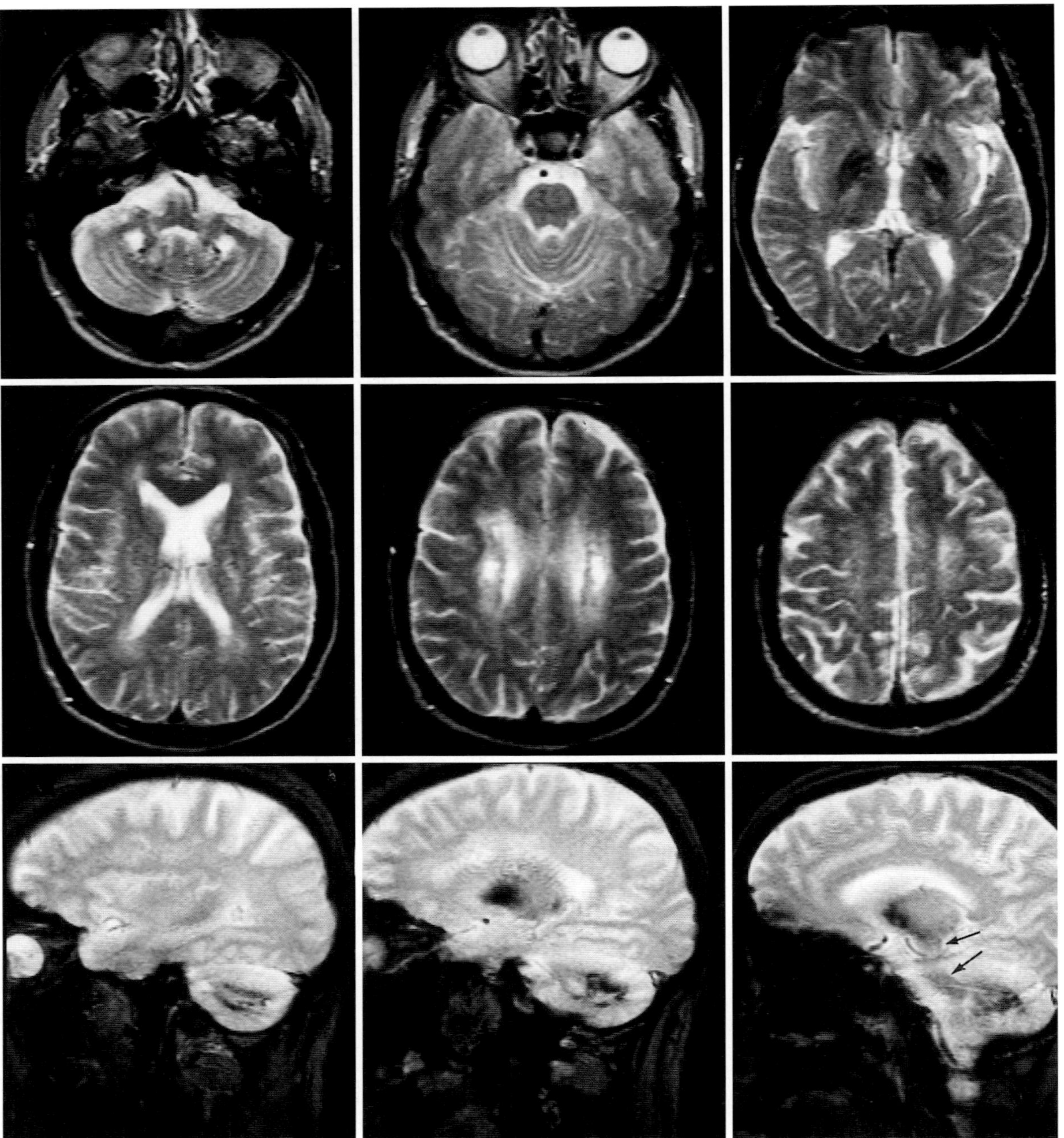

Fig. 27.2. 34-year-old male with CoD. The T_2-weighted transverse series (*upper two rows*) show the involvement of the cerebellar white matter and the cerebral periventricular white matter, and the widening of the cerebral sulci. Note the low signal intensity of the globus pallidus (at 0.6 Tesla). Also the dentate nucleus contains areas of low signal intensity. Gradient echo images (*lower row*) are helpful in identifying the calcifications in the basal ganglia, the superior cerebellar peduncle (*arrows*), the dentate nucleus and cerebellar white matter

Fig. 27.3. A baby-boy at the ages of 3.5 months (*upper two rows*) and 6 months (*lower two rows*), in whom the diagnosis COFS syndrome was made. The images, showing an arrest of myelination in combination with some atrophy, are indistinguishable from those of Pelizaeus-Merzbacher disease. There is no evidence of calcium deposits

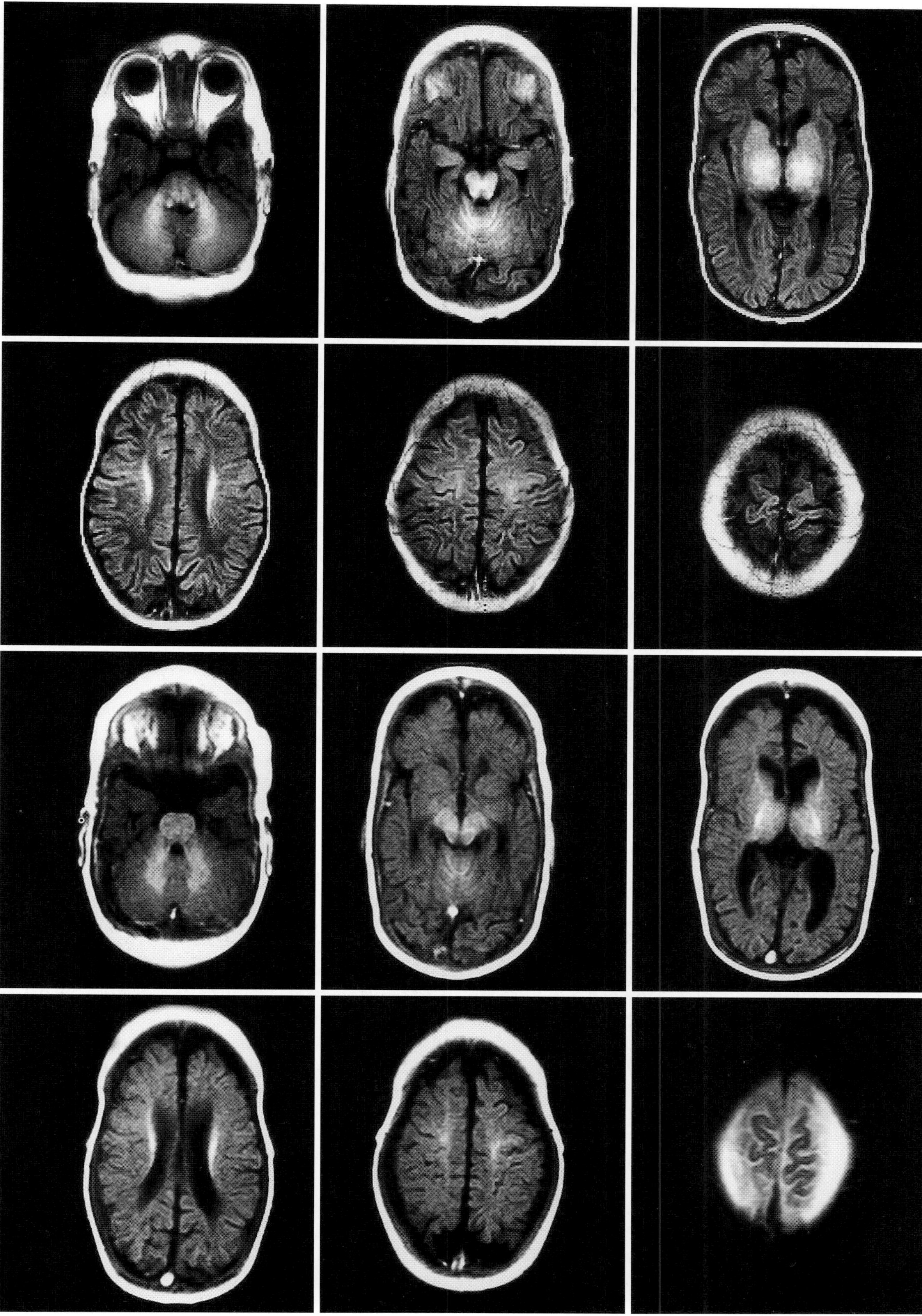

28 Pelizaeus-Merzbacher Disease

28.1 Clinical Features and Laboratory Investigations

Pelizaeus-Merzbacher disease (PMD) is a rare neurological disorder affecting the myelination of the CNS in children. The disease is usually subdivided into three types: the classical type (type I), the connatal type (type II) and the transitional type (type III).

The classical type has its onset in the infantile or late-infantile period. The disease has an X-linked recessive mode of inheritance. It manifests initially by irregular nystagmoid eye movements referred to as "dancing", "trembling", or "roving". In some children stridor occurs, either caused by laryngeal abductor paralysis or laryngomalacia. There is a variable but always marked or severe developmental delay with only very slow developmental progression. Growth is also retarded and the head size is small, in the low normal or microcephalic range. Seizures occur early in the course of the disease. Characteristically there is a tremor or bobbing, nodding or shaking movement of the head. Signs of tetraspasticity, cerebellar ataxia and extrapyramidal movement disturbances with hyperkinesia, dystonia and choreoathetosis become manifest as the patient matures. The sensory system is usually well preserved. Optic atrophy with visual failure is common. Nystagmus disappears in the course of a few years. Skeletal abnormalities, such as osteoporosis, kyphoscoliosis result from the chronic motor disease and they invariably occur after the disease has been manifest for many years. The course of the disease is chronic. After the age of 5 or 6 years a very slow progression of the neurological signs and a decline of mental level can usually be noted, but in the presence of severe developmental delay and motor handicap, signs of regression can be difficult to detect. Death occurs in most patients in late adolescence or young adulthood and is usually due to malnutrition and intercurrent illnesses.

The connatal type, also called Seitelberger type, is a rarer and more severe form of PMD. The disease is already manifest in the neonatal or early infantile period. Both males and females can be affected. The disease has an X-linked transmission in some families, an autosomal recessive transmission in others. The neonatal period may be characterized by hypotonia, absent primitive reflexes and sometimes stridor. Abnormal, nystagmoid eye movements and extrapyramidal hyperkinesia occur early, followed by the development of epilepsy, spasticity, cerebellar ataxia and optic atrophy. From birth onwards there is a complete failure of psychomotor development or an early loss of attained milestones. Microcephaly and growth retardation develop in the subsequent years. Progression is rapid, with death occurring in the first decade, usually in early childhood.

The transitional form between the classical and connatal types resembles the latter, but its course is less rapid. The onset of disease is neonatal or in early infancy, and average age at death is about 8 years. The disease is sporadic or possibly autosomal recessive.

The nosology of PMD is quite unclear. In the first place the distinction between the classical and connatal forms of PMD is ill-defined. The age of onset does not appear to be a valuable discriminating factor between the types of PMD. The rate of progression is the most useful and earliest reliable means of differentiating the connatal from the classical type. Age at death is another distinguishing factor. Secondly, three further classes of PMD have been suggested: the adult or Löwenberg-Hill type with autosomal dominant inheritance (type IV), variants with patchy demyelination (type V), and Cockayne syndrome with an autosomal recessive mode of inheritance (type VI). Cockayne syndrome, however, is evidently a separate disease and it is doubtful whether types IV and V are variants of PMD. Finally, the variable mode of inheritance of PMD is a problem. Some authors only include those patients in whom an X-linked mode of inheritance is evident. Other authors also include affected females. In particular in connatal PMD, female patients can be found, but mothers of boys suffering from classical PMD can also have some neurological problems. Incidentally female patients in sibships with classical PMD show identical clinical and postmortem neuropathological findings. The so-called Lyon hypothesis is invoked to explain these female cases. This hypothesis explains the female cases by preferential inactivation of the X-chromosome without the PMD mutation. Sporadic male cases can be explained as new mutations.

Laboratory investigations are of no help in establishing the diagnosis. Skeletal X-ray survey may reveal abnormalities which are secondary and not diagnostic for PMD. Nerve conduction velocities and electromyography are normal. Evoked potential studies may be of some help. In BAEP studies usually only wave I or waves I and II are present and later components are absent. ERG is normal. VEP and SSEP are absent or abnormal with increased latency, abnormal shape and decreased amplitude. Definite diagnosis is established by postmortem examination of the CNS and in some patients by establishing a defect in the proteolipid protein gene with DNA-based tests.

Prenatal diagnosis and carrier detection is possible in some of the families using DNA techniques.

28.2 Pathology

In PMD, the brain is too light for the patient's age and shows signs of diffuse atrophy, involving cerebral hemispheres and in particular brain stem and cerebellum. On sectioning the white matter appears reduced in volume to a variable extent and the corpus callosum is markedly reduced in width. Microscopic examination shows lack of myelin in all parts of the CNS. The pathological picture is basically the same in all PMD patients irrespective of subtype, but with variable severity.

In connatal PMD, the pathological picture varies from a marked lack of myelin to a complete absence of myelin in all parts of the brain and spinal cord. The myelin present is usually found in the deeper parts of the brain: the diencephalon (globus pallidus, posterior limb of the internal capsule, thalamus), the brain stem (tegmentum of pons and mesencephalon, mesencephalic pyramidal tracts) and the central part of the cerebellum. The myelin present is usually found in perivascular islets. Also, residual myelin islets are sometimes present in the subcortical white matter, especially in the pre- and postcentral gyri. There are no signs of active demyelination. There are no or little sudanophilic breakdown products in the white matter. Oligodendrocytes with normal size, shape, number, and distribution may be found, but they may also be reduced in number or be completely absent, or they may show morphological abnormalities. The axons are relatively well preserved. A certain amount of axonal loss may be seen in completely demyelinated areas. The severity of the concomitant fibrillary gliosis varies from slight to dense. The gray matter is also affected; the intracortical myelin is completely or almost completely absent. However, the normal cytoarchitecture is preserved. The cerebellar cortex shows loss of Purkinje cells and granular cells. Myelin is present in normal amounts for age in the PNS, including the spinal roots and cranial nerves but with the exception of optic nerves and chiasm.

At the other end of the spectrum the abnormalities in classical PMD are less pronounced and myelin deficiency is less severe. There is a patchy absence of myelin with preservation of numerous myelin islets giving the white matter a so-called tigroid pattern. Most of the myelin islets surround small blood vessels. The myelin sheaths in these islets are thin and composed of only a few myelin lamellae. Microscopically some remaining myelin sheaths are also seen in the areas which are otherwise devoid of myelin. At most, small amounts of sudanophilic lipid products are found. Oligodendrocytes are often numerically reduced, especially in the areas lacking myelin. All parts of the CNS are affected in the same way, but the spinal cord, brain stem, cerebellum, diencephalic structures, and subcortical white matter show a relatively good state of myelin preservation. In all areas of the CNS axons are relatively well preserved. Where myelin is absent, the remaining white matter is mainly composed of naked axons. Fibrillary gliosis varies from slight to intense. The astrocytes are sometimes hypertrophied. The gray matter is also involved in the process. Myelin sheaths are reduced in number or are absent, but the cortical cytoarchitecture as well as the individual nerve cells are normal, although a certain loss of and damage to nerve cells may be seen. In particular in the cerebellar cortex, loss of Purkinje cells and granule cells may be evident. Within the cortex a diffuse proliferation of astrocytes may be present. No myelin deficiency is seen in the PNS, including spinal roots and cranial nerves with the exception of the optic nerve.

The transitional type shows abnormalities intermediate in severity between the connatal and the classical types.

In all types of PMD, ultrastructural examination of oligodendrocytes often reveals abnormalities. Oligodendroglial cells are described with scanty cytoplasm and commensurately fewer organelles, and a reduction in the number of cytoplasmic processes, in their diameter and extent. Their nuclei display large aggregations of condensed chromatin granules in the periphery and focally throughout the center. On the other hand, oligodendrocytes are also described that are larger than normal with voluminous cytoplasm and abundant organelles. Their nuclei are enlarged, and the chromatin is fairly evenly dispersed. The nucleolus is prominent. The oligodendrocytes may contain spherical, lamellated cytoplasmic inclusions and may also have numerous myelin balls at their periphery, appearing in association with myelinated fibers. Nonspecific crystalloid inclusions or lipid droplets may be found in astrocytes.

28.3   Chemical Pathology

Chemical analysis of the remaining myelin in PMD reveals that its lipid content is greatly reduced and its protein content, conversely, relatively increased. The cerebrosides are reduced in quantity and the sulfatides are greatly reduced in quantity. The remaining glycolipids contain an abnormally high proportion of glucose with a proportional reduction of galactose. The myelin ganglioside content and cholesterol content are near normal. Phospholipids are increased, mainly at the level of sphingomyelin, choline phosphoglycerides and inositol phosphoglycerides, whereas ethanolamine phosphoglycerides and plasmalogens are reduced. Protein analysis shows that proteolipid protein is absent, myelin basic protein is decreased, whereas so-called Wolfgram proteins are increased.

The chemical composition of whole white matter depends on the amount of myelin that is present. The water content is abnormally high. Those lipids that are generally recognized as myelin lipids, are either absent or markedly reduced. No or very little sulfatide is present. A marked reduction is seen in cerebroside, cholesterol and phospholipids. The cholesterol: pholpholipid: cerebroside ratio is similar to the ratio in brain prior to myelination. Gangliosides are found in normal concentrations. No or only a very small amount of cholesterol esters are present. The protein composition of white matter is also altered with absence of proteolipid protein and reduction of other myelin proteins.

In contrast to white matter, the chemical composition of gray matter is much closer to normal. The concentration of sulfatides and cerebrosides is decreased, but the concentration of phospholipids, cholesterol and gangliosides is normal or close to normal.

28.4   Pathogenetic Considerations

For many decades the pathogenesis of the lack of myelin in the CNS in PMD has been a matter of debate. The original contention of Merzbacher was that the lack of myelin sheaths was due to faulty or absent myelination. Subsequently, many authors have classified PMD among the leukodystrophies and described the histopathological findings as tigroid demyelination. However, several histological and chemical findings are not consistent with demyelination, but are consistent with a defect in myelin deposition. Histological examination fails to reveal signs of active demyelination. The small amounts of myelin degradation products are in conformity with at best a very slow breakdown of myelin. Usually the oligodendrocytes are found to be decreased in number, showed morphological abnormalities and appeared inactive. The chemical findings of no or at most a low level of cholesterol esters in the white matter is not in agreement with active demyelination. The cholesterol: phospholipid: cerebroside ratio in PMD corresponds with the ratio in the brain prior to myelination. The low ratio of ethanolamine phosphoglycerides: choline phosphoglycerides in PMD is an indication of a poor state of maturation of the brain, as the ratio increases with maturation. The high glucose content of glycolipids is also an indication of the immature state of the brain; as maturation proceeds, glucolipids are replaced by galactolipids.

The basic defect in at least a proportion of the PMD families is a defect in the gene coding for proteolipid protein. The proteolipid protein gene is localized on the long arm of the X-chromosome and has been assigned to Xq21.2–Xq22. The gene has been cloned and sequenced. This gene encodes for proteolipid protein as its major gene product, and additionally for DM20, another myelin protein that is identical to proteolipid protein but approximately 35 amino acids shorter. DM20 is also absent in PMD.

Proteolipid protein is a major myelin membrane protein. Myelin basic protein and proteolipid protein normally constitute more than 80% of the total myelin proteins and they are present in myelin in approximately equal amounts. They are considered to be myelin-specific. Proteolipid protein is confined to the CNS and is absent from the PNS. The compact lamellar structure of myelin is organized and stabilized by these two main proteins, myelin basic protein as a peripheral membrane protein, and proteolipid protein as a strongly hydrophobic integral membrane protein. Myelin basic protein contributes to the compaction of the major dense lines and proteolipid protein to the tight apposition of the intraperiod lines in the myelin sheath. The spatial structure of proteolipid protein, and with this its function, is easily perturbed. Even minor changes in proteolipid protein compromise the functional integrity of this myelin protein.

The mode of action of changes in or absence of proteolipid protein has not yet been elucidated. The defect may result in a change in the compaction of the myelin sheath, in a failure to form myelin sheaths, it may interfere with the metabolism of oligodendrocytes, lead to disturbance of normal oligodendroglial maturation, or may lead to early oligodendroglial cell death. There is some evidence for all of these possibilities. The presence of a normal or increased number of oligodendrocytes in the absence of myelin may point to failure of myelin deposition. The lack of typical oligodendrocytes in some other cases may be a result of a defect in cellular differentiation or of early oligodendroglial cell death.

The severity of the disease may be related to the degree of deficiency of normal proteolipid protein. A complete or nearly complete absence may lead to connatal PMD, and a relative deficiency may lead to later-onset PMD. The topography of the myelin present is in conformity with an inhibition of myelination, which apparently sets in before birth (connatal form) or within the first year of life (classical and transitional form). Apparently the developmental age at which further myelination is inhibited, determines the amount of myelin present. It is possible that the myelin present is unstable leading to a very slow breakdown. It is not clear whether the rather slow deterioration of PMD patients is due to progressive degradation of the defective myelin sheath or decay of unmyelinated axons.

A number of PMD families has been investigated. Several different point mutations in the proteolipid protein gene, a complex rearrangement of the gene and a complete deletion of the whole gene have been described. It is evident that defects in the proteolipid protein gene may account for many cases of X-linked PMD. However, sequencing of the entire coding region of the gene has failed to reveal mutations in several other PMD patients who showed X-linked inheritance of the disease. This observation suggests that defects in the noncoding regions of the gene may also be responsible for PMD or that another X-linked gene may be involved. As there is evidence for autosomal recessive inheritance in some families, particularly in the connatal form of the disease, autosomal genes may also be related to PMD. It is obvious that PMD is a genetically heterogeneous disease and that only part of its genetic basis has been elucidated.

28.5 Therapy

At present no therapy is known for PMD. Antenatal diagnosis is possible in some families.

28.6 Magnetic Resonance Imaging

CT scanning is of no help in the diagnosis of PMD, showing only atrophy.

In contrast, the MRI pattern in PMD is usually highly suggestive of the disorder. In most cases, MRI shows an arrest of myelination in a stage that is in itself normal. In some cases no myelin at all is present (Fig. 28.1). The T_2-weighted images show a high signal intensity of all unmyelinated white matter structures, whereas these structures have a low signal intensity on T_1-weighted images. In fact, no high signal intensity areas are seen on T_1-weighted images in these cases. In other cases myelin is present in (parts of) the brain stem, (parts of) the cerebellar white matter, the posterior limb of the internal capsule, the thalamus and the

globus pallidus (Fig. 28.2). In some cases additional myelin is present in the directly periventricular part of the corona radiata, in the subcortical white matter and cortex of the pre- and postcentral gyri and in the directly periventricular part of the radiatio optica. The myelinated structures have a low signal intensity on T_2-weighted images and a high signal intensity on T_1-weighted images. The pattern described is a normal stage of myelination for a neonate or an infant in the first few months of life, although not normal for the age of the patient. Apart from this, the brain has an abnormal appearance. The white matter is variably but usually markedly reduced in volume with a mild enlargement of the ventricular system, a thin corpus callosum, folding of the cortex in thin, deep gyri and enlargement of the subarachnoid spaces. The aspect of the white matter is not completely identical to normal unmyelinated white matter, but is somewhat speckled, possibly reflecting the presence of some myelin in a tigroid pattern. Atrophy of brain stem and cerebellum may be striking. If MRI is performed during the first few months of life, the images are not diagnostic as they merely show atrophy and delay of myelination or may even be near normal in appearance, but repeated MRI confirms the absence of progress of myelination. Seeing the described pattern in a boy who is a few years old is highly suggestive of PMD. Arrest of myelination may be seen in other conditions, such as severe asphyxia or late congenital infections, but in these conditions usually additional focal brain lesions are present, which are lacking in PMD. Most conditions other than PMD, having an adverse effect on myelination, lead to a delayed but slowly progressive myelination with advancement of the degree of myelination on each repeat MRI if made after a sufficiently long interval. Hence, repeated MRI is of help in establishing the diagnosis of PMD. We saw MR images very similar to those of PMD in a patient with the cerebro-oculo-facio-skeletal (COFS) syndrome (see Chap. 27). However, the clinical picture in this syndrome differs from PMD.

Evidence has been found that, as expected from histopathological findings, the stage of myelination, as shown on MR images, correlates with the type of PMD. In connatal PMD, either no myelin at all is seen, or some myelin consistent with a prenatal arrest of myelination. In transitional and classical PMD, more myelin is present.

In some incidental cases, reported in the literature, more myelin is present in the cerebral hemispheres. The pattern of myelination is patchy and myelination may involve the subcortical areas in particular. The images are different from those described above although the clinical picture may be quite typical for PMD. Considering the genetic heterogeneity and the fact that most cases reported in the MR literature were not tested for the presence of an abnormality in the

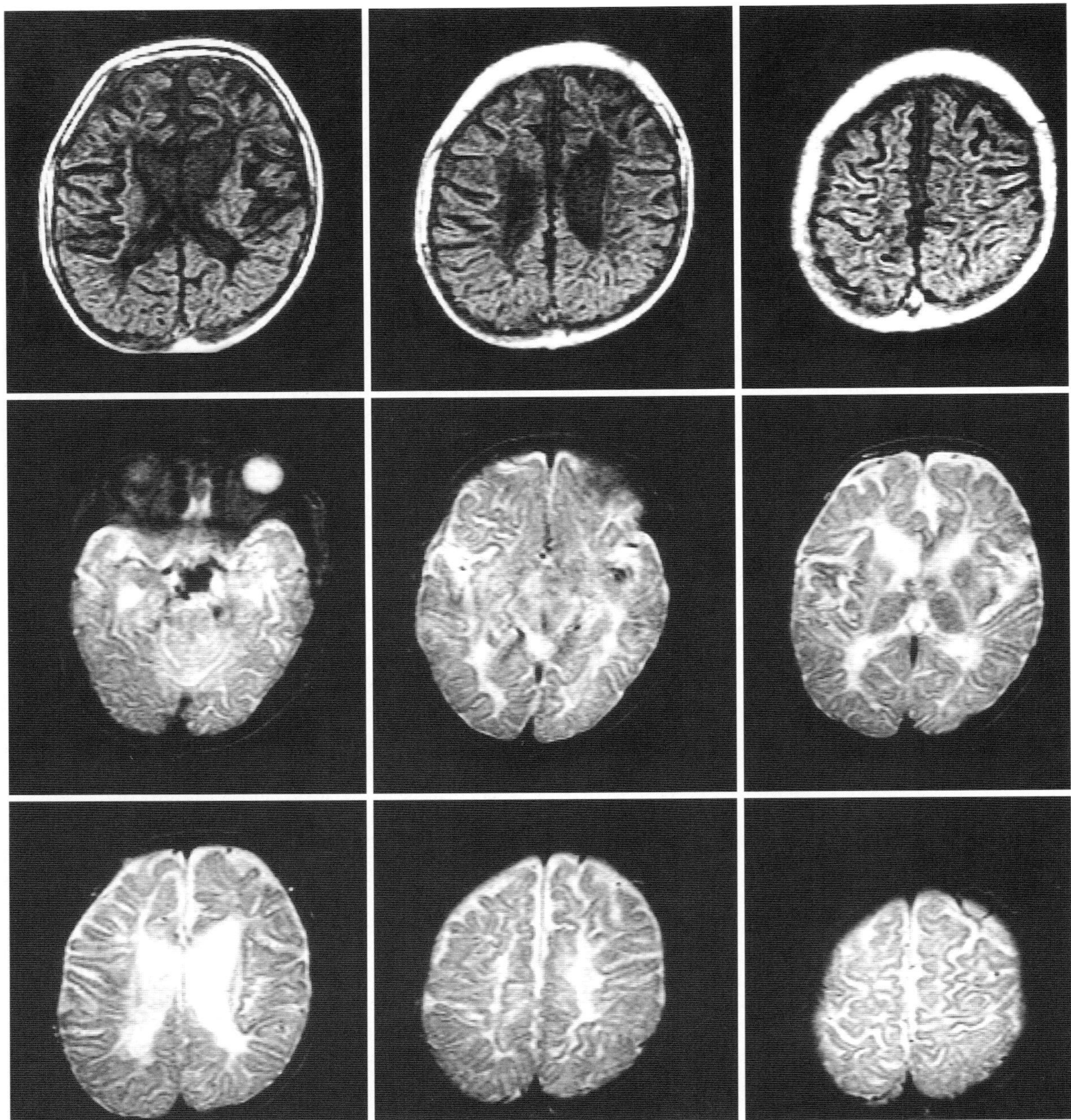

Fig. 28.1. Boy, 10 years old, with the diagnosis connatal form of PMD. The T_1-weighted (*upper row*) and T_2-weighted transverse images do not show any myelin formation. There is considerable atrophy. The pattern is consistent with amyelination of the brain

proteolipid protein gene, some heterogeneity is also expected in observed MRI patterns.

Some female carriers of the disease have been shown to have multiple foci of increased signal intensity in the cerebral white matter, but others have not. MRI is not suitable as a tool for carrier identification.

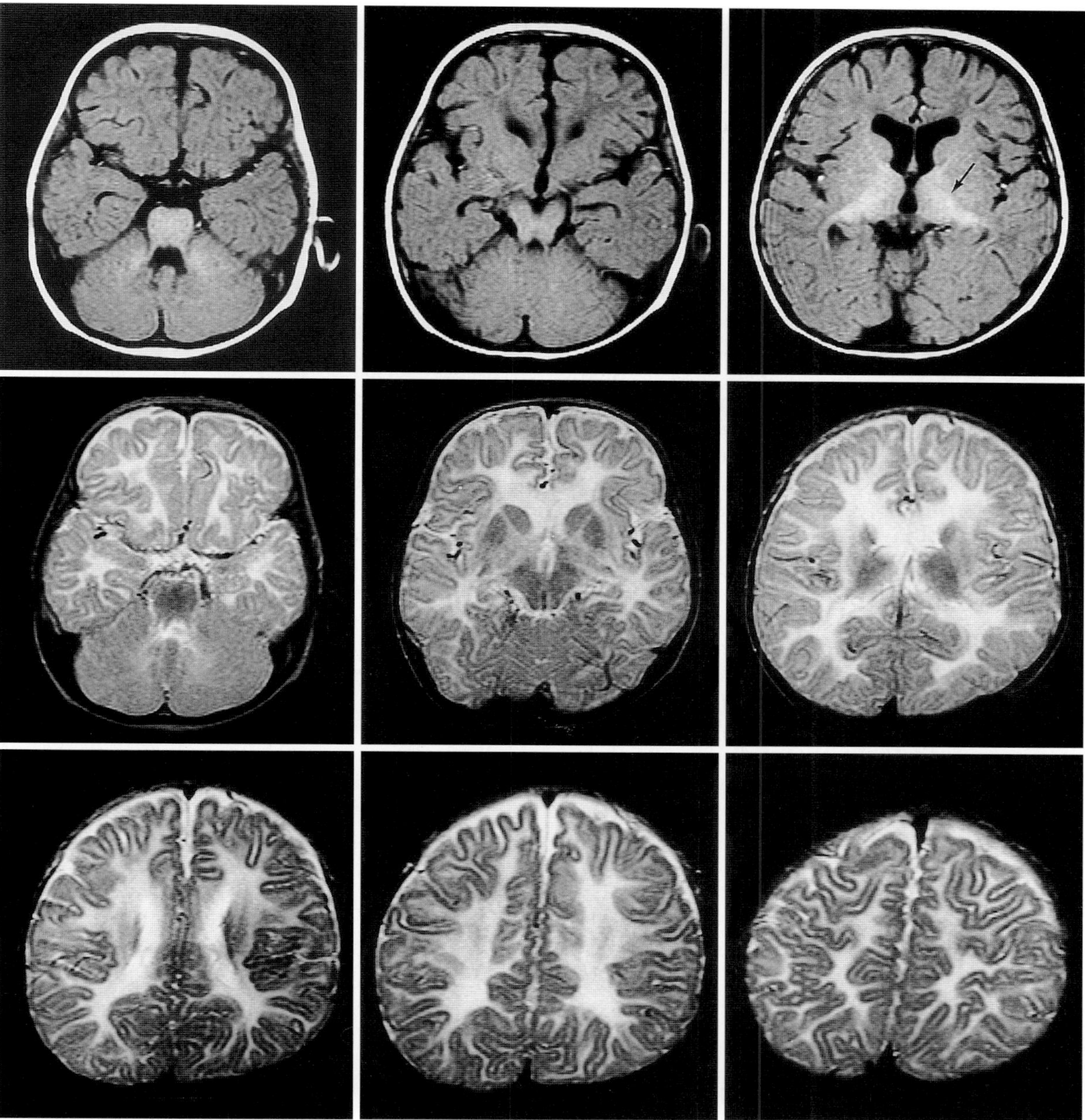

Fig. 28.2. Boy, nearly 2 years old. Clinical diagnosis: classical type of PMD. The MRI shows presence of myelin in the central areas (*arrow, right upper row*). Also in the T$_2$-weighted images (*lower two rows*) some myelin is seen in the cerebellum and brain stem. The pattern of myelin presence is consistent with an arrest of myelination soon after birth. There is some atrophy. Courtesy of J.J.M. van Collenburg, Zwolle, the Netherlands, with permission

29　18q⁻ Syndrome

29.1　Clinical Features and Laboratory Investigations

The 18q⁻ syndrome is an autosomal deletion disorder with variable phenotype. Most patients have a de novo deletion, but in some patients it is inherited. The most frequent disease characteristics include mental retardation, short stature, microcephaly, midface hypoplasia, hypertelorism, epicanthus, carp-shaped mouth, high or cleft palate, preauricular skin tags, narrow or atretic ear canals, conductive hearing deficit, short neck, tapering fingers, clinodactyly, proximal thumbs, prominent finger whorls, widely spaced nipples, congenital heart disease, genital abnormalities, and foot deformities. Mental capacities vary from borderline to severely deficient. Apart from mental retardation, neurological abnormalities include hypotonia, seizures, nystagmus, poor coordination and increasing choreoathetosis.

Routine and metabolic laboratory investigations reveal no abnormalities. IgA deficiency is relatively frequently found. Peripheral nerve conduction is normal. Study of evoked potentials may reveal prolonged central conduction. Chromosomal analysis reveals a partial deletion of the long arm of chromosome 18, including the bands q22.3 → qter.

29.2　Pathology

Reduction of cerebral white matter and delay of myelination are the main histopathological findings. Ventricles and subarachnoid spaces may be mildly enlarged.

29.3　Pathogenetic Considerations

The deletion of the 18q22.3 → qter region includes the locus for the myelin basic protein gene (18q22–23). It is possible that the impairment in myelination of the CNS is related to heterozygosity for the absence of the myelin basic protein gene. The two most important proteins of CNS myelin are proteolipid protein and myelin basic protein. Myelin basic protein accounts for 30%–40% of the total myelin protein, proteolipid protein for 40%–50%. The 18q⁻ syndrome is considered to be the autosomal counterpart of X-linked Pelizaeus-Merzbacher disease, which is caused by mutations of the proteolipid protein gene. However, an important difference is that one normal myelin basic protein gene is present in the 18q⁻ syndrome, whereas no normal proteolipid protein gene at all is present in males suffering from Pelizaeus-Merzbacher disease. Pelizaeus-Merzbacher disease is characterized by a severe impairment of myelination of the CNS. The extent of impairment of myelin deposition is probably more variable in the 18q⁻ syndrome.

The so-called shiverer mouse has an autosomal recessive disease related to a mutation of the myelin basic protein gene. In this mouse a defect in CNS myelination is found. Clinical disease is characterized by generalized action tremor, increasingly frequent convulsions and premature death. Histopathological examination reveals that CNS myelin is largely absent and when present, appears as abnormal whorls of cytoplasm-filled membranes, tightly compacted at the intraperiod line, but uncompacted at the major dense line. The so-called myelin-deficient mouse has a duplication of the myelin basic protein gene and a low level of myelin basic protein mRNA. The phenotype of the myelin deficient mouse is similar to that of the shiverer mouse, but less severe.

Myelin basic protein is also a component of PNS myelin. A curious feature is that absence or mutation of the gene has little effect on PNS myelin. PNS is only subtly altered and functionally normal. It is suggested that some component specific to peripheral myelin is functionally equivalent to myelin basic protein and capable of substituting for this protein in its absence.

In the 18q⁻ syndrome, more genes are missing than the myelin basic protein gene, explaining other features of the clinical picture. The variability of the clinical picture may be related to the site and size of the deletion.

29.4　Therapy

Supportive care is the only therapeutic option.

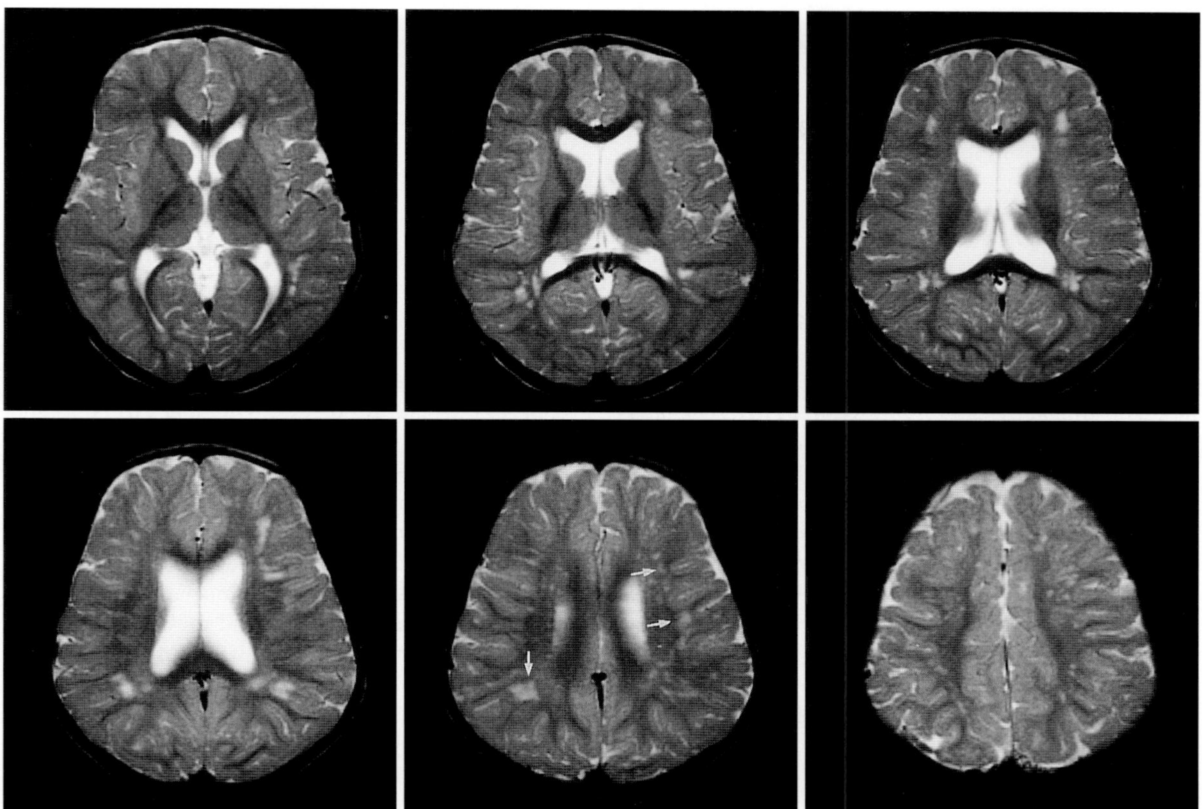

Fig. 29.1. The transverse T_2-weighted MR series of this 3-year-old boy shows wide-spread patches of hypomyelination (*arrows*). The appearance of the lesions would also be consistent with patchy demyelination. Similar images have been observed in other patients with the 18q⁻ syndrome. Courtesy of Prof.Dr. U. Stephani, Kiel and Prof.Dr. B. Terwey, Bremen, Germany, with permission

29.5 Magnetic Resonance Imaging

The few MR images published show a variable myelin deficit. In a follow-up study of a child up to the age of 3 years, a delay in myelination was found, but myelination was further advanced at every repeat MRI. In a 16-month-old boy, a near-total absence of myelin in cerebral and cerebellar white matter, internal capsule and corticospinal tracts was seen with relatively normal myelination of the corpus callosum. The cortical gyri were relatively thin and the sulci relatively deep due to reduction in white matter volume. His mother, who also had the 18q⁻ syndrome, had a better state of myelination and hypomyelination was restricted to the corticospinal tracts in the brain stem, posterior limb of the internal capsule, centrum semiovale, optic radiations and external capsule. The corpus callosum, frontal and temporal lobes were better myelinated. Focal white matter lesions have also been reported (Fig. 29.1).

30 Phenylketonuria

30.1 Clinical Features and Laboratory Investigations

Phenylketonuria (PKU) represents a heterogeneous group of disorders with autosomal recessive inheritance. PKU, or hyperphenylalaninemia, is caused by a deficiency of the phenylalanine hydroxylating system. The phenylalanine hydroxylating system consists of two essential components: phenylalanine hydroxylase and coenzyme tetrahydrobiopterin (Fig. 30.1). PKU is in most patients caused by deficiency of phenylalanine hydroxylase, and in a minority of patients by deficiency of tetrahydrobiopterin.

Classical PKU due to severe phenylalanine hydroxylase deficiency. Infants with this disease are normal at birth. In the course of the first year of life psychomotor retardation becomes obvious. Eczema is present in a considerable number of patients, usually from infancy to late childhood. The patients often have blond hair, fair skin and blue eyes, but this is not necessarily the case. They often have a mousy, musty odor. Seizures may occur, taking the form of tonic-clonic seizures, myoclonic seizures, but also typical infantile spasms. Irritability, frequent vomiting and insufficient growth are part of the clinical picture. The final mental level of PKU children is deficient, but the children are trainable. Verbal IQ is lower than performal IQ. The children are small and often microcephalic. Pyramidal signs are present with hypertonia, gait disturbances, hyperreflexia and extensor plantar reflexes. Frequently a rapid, fine and irregular tremor of the hands is present. Abnormal choreoathetoid movements may be present with twisting movements, continuous repetitious finger movements and rhythmical swinging body movements. Psychiatric disturbances with severe hyperactivity, destructiveness, self-mutilation and uncontrollable attacks of rage or excitement are common.

World-wide neonatal screening programs have led to early detection of almost all PKU patients. Early dietary treatment prevents most of the described abnormalities, which are now rarely seen. Intelligence is usually within the normal range, although mean intelli-

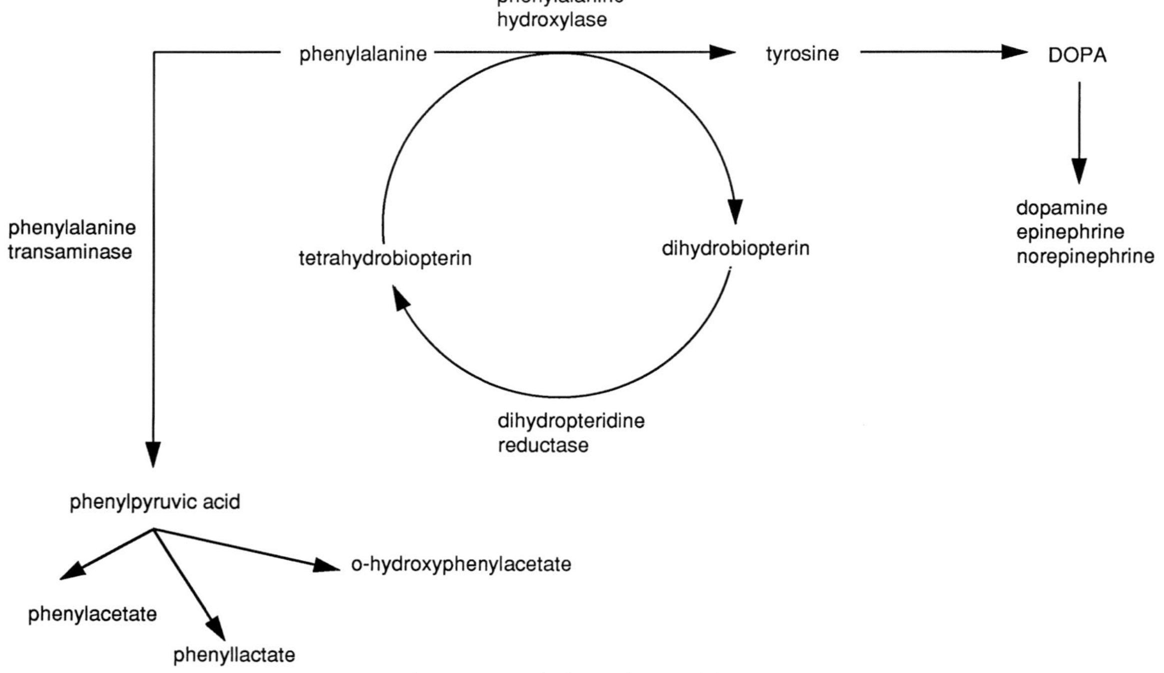

Fig. 30.1. Metabolism of phenylalanine

gence in patients with classical PKU who are treated early is roughly half a standard deviation lower than the IQ of unaffected siblings and population norms. Treated PKU patients are generally slower to acquire language, have a higher frequency of learning difficulties and behavioral disturbances with hyperactivity, anxiety and poor concentration. Strict dietary treatment was formerly thought to be important only during the period of major cerebral maturation and used to be ameliorated or stopped in mid to late childhood. However, there is now evidence that with discontinuation of strict diet and rise in phenylalanine levels, some cognitive deterioration and emotional problems develop in many patients, together with an increase in motor problems consisting of tremor and signs of spasticity of the legs. Reinstitution of strict diet may result in these problems disappearing.

Maternal PKU appears to have detrimental effects on embryogenesis and fetal development. The offspring of females with classical PKU, who are no longer being treated, show a high frequency of microcephaly, mental handicap and impaired growth, occasionally accompanied by malformations of the heart or other organs. The incidence of these aberrations appears to be correlated with the maternal concentration of serum phenylalanine. Reinstigation of dietary treatment prior to conception has a favorable effect on outcome.

Mild variants of classical PKU lead to less severe mental retardation if untreated. Patients tolerate a larger intake of phenylalanine and successful treatment requires a less rigid diet than in the case of severe classical PKU.

In so-called persistent hyperphenylalaninemia mildly elevated serum phenylalanine levels are found, but there are no clinical symptoms and treatment is not necessary.

Patients with deficiency of tetrahydrobiopterin have so-called malignant PKU. In these patients progressive neurological dysfunction occurs despite dietary treatment with phenylalanine restriction. Patients present early in life with microcephaly, disturbed psychomotor development and the other neurological problems associated with hyperphenylalaninemia. In addition, signs of extrapyramidal dysfunction are prominently present and consist of parkinsonism, chorea, dystonia, oculogyric spasms, or myoclonus. Typical signs of parkinsonism are hypokinesia, bradykinesia, rigidity and mask-like facies. In addition, sweating, hyperpyrexia without infection, drooling, swallowing difficulties, pin-point pupils, truncal hypotonia, limb hypertonia and hyperreflexia, infantile spasms and tonic-clonic seizures often form part of the clinical picture. Symptoms may be less marked and consist mainly of extrapyramidal dysfunction and/or slow development. In a subclass of tetrahydrobiopterin deficient patients, caused by dihydropteridine reductase deficiency,

rapidly progressive demyelination of the CNS may occur additionally and cause spasticity, pseudobulbar palsy, long tract sensory loss and cognitive deterioration.

Neonatal screening is performed between 6 and 14 days after birth. Increased blood phenylalanine concentration indicates a positive test. In phenylalanine hydroxylase deficiency, phenylpyruvic acid and o-hydroxyphenylacetic acid are excreted in the urine (Fig. 30.1). The blood level of tyrosine is normal or lower than normal excluding hyperphenylalaninemia secondary to disorders of tyrosine metabolism. Apart from tyrosinemia hyperphenylalaninemia secondary to prematurity, hepatic insufficiency, chronic renal insufficiency and trimethoprim medication should be considered. An oral phenylalanine loading test is performed when the child is several months old and leads to elevated serum levels of phenylalanine without elevation of tyrosine. Severe and mild variants of phenylalanine hydroxylase deficiency are distinguished by the level of serum phenylalanine before treatment, the level of serum phenylalanine and the duration of the increase after phenylalanine loading, and the tolerance of phenylalanine in the diet. Residual phenylalanine hydroxylase activity can be determined in liver biopsy material. Prenatal diagnosis and carrier detection can be performed with the help of DNA techniques.

If elevated serum phenylalanine concentrations are found on neonatal screening, total biopterin concentrations and dihydropteridine reductase are measured to exclude dihydropteridine reductase deficiency and disorders in the synthesis of tetrahydrobiopterin (Fig. 30.2). Assessment of the ratio between total biopterin and neopterin in urine is helpful in differentiating between the various enzyme defects. In dihydropteridine reductase deficiency, the total biopterin level is very high, whereas neopterin level is normal or moderately increased; in 6-pyruvoyl tetrahydropterin synthetase deficiency, the neopterin level is elevated and the biopterin level is very low; and in case of guanosine triphosphate cyclohydrolase deficiency both neopterin and biopterin levels are extremely low. Examination of urine pteridine profiles makes it possible to make a tentative diagnosis of the basic defect. In cases of tetrahydrobiopterin deficiency, CSF and urine levels of homovanillic acid (HVA), 5-hydroxyindoleacetic acid (5HIAA), vanillyl mandelic acid (VMA), and 3-methoxy-4-hydroxyphenylglycol (MH-PG), the major metabolites of dopamine, serotonin and (nor)epinephrine in the human CNS, are reduced. The levels of these metabolites may also be reduced, although less markedly, in classical PKU. However, in classical PKU the levels normalize with a phenylalanine restricted diet, which is not the case in disorders characterized by tetrahydrobiopterin deficiency. In dihydropteridine reductase deficiency, serum folate lev-

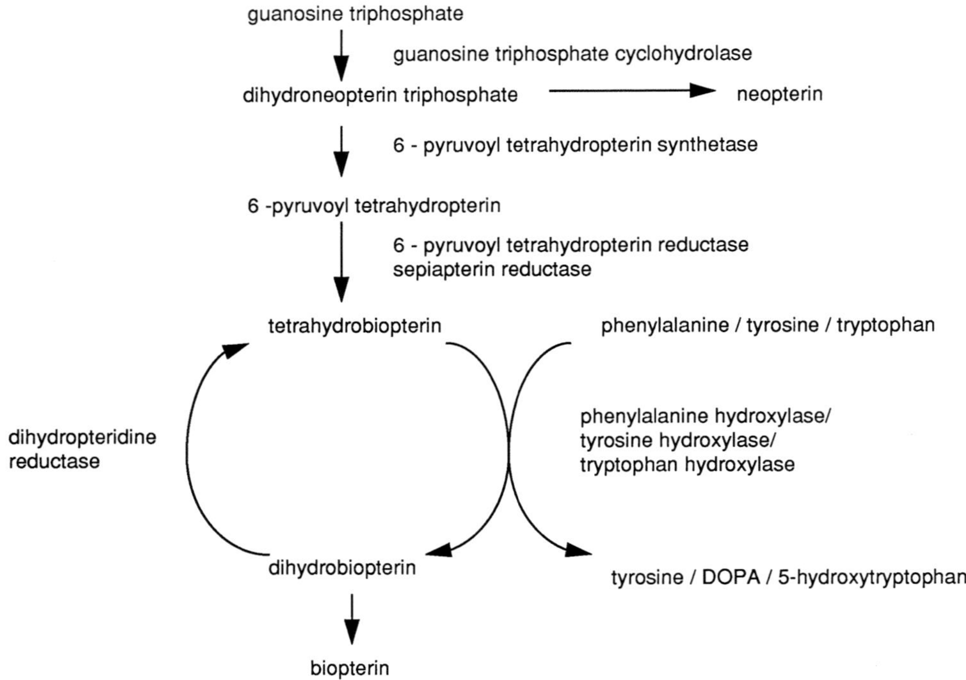

Fig. 30.2. Synthesis of tetrahydrobiopterin

els may be low. The diagnosis should be confirmed by enzyme studies in erythrocytes (dihydropteridine reductase, 6-pyruvoyl tetrahydropterin synthetase), lymphocytes (guanosine triphosphate cyclohydrolase) or liver biopsy (6-pyruvoyl tetrahydropterin synthetase, guanosine triphosphate cyclohydrolase). Prenatal diagnosis can be performed by assessing pterin levels in amniotic fluid or enzyme activity in fetal erythrocytes, amniocytes or chorionic villi, depending on the different enzyme defects.

30.2   Pathology

In untreated classical PKU, the weight of the brain is below normal. The reduction in volume is greater in the white than in the gray matter. The ventricles are enlarged. The cortical pattern of gyri and sulci is normal.

Microscopic examination of the cortex reveals evidence of a general developmental delay with reduction in number and size of cortical neurons, paucity of dendritic arborization and reduced synaptic density. In addition, glial scars or defects attributable to post-convulsive necrosis may be seen.

The white matter shows a lack of myelination in untreated PKU children. Apart from hypomyelination a status spongiosus of the white matter may be seen. The status spongiosus is most marked in the optic tracts, the periventricular white matter, the centrum semiovale and in the central part of the cerebellar white matter, although at times spongy lesions are also seen in the subcortical white matter. Apart from occasional sudanophilic fat droplets in perivascular spaces, no signs of active myelin loss are seen. There is little gliosis.

In older untreated children and adults, areas of demyelination are seen in the periventricular and lobar white matter, sparing the subcortical U fibers. In some cases the areas are sharply defined; in others the borders of the lesions are indistinct. In the areas of demyelination an intense gliosis and deposition of sudanophilic material is seen. Oligodendrocytes are reduced in number. The axis cylinders are relatively better preserved than the myelin sheaths. The cerebellar white matter may also be involved. Spongy lesions, similar to those observed in children, may be noted immediately adjacent to the demyelinating areas. With advancing age white matter changes tend to become more pronounced and diffuse, although not in all cases.

30.3   Chemical Pathology

Analysis of cerebral lipids reveals a deficiency of myelin lipids, particularly involving cerebroside and cholesterol. In the few studies performed, the deficiency of myelin lipids is more severe in older patients. Cholesterol esters are absent or present in only small amounts.

30.4 Pathogenetic Considerations

Phenylalanine is an essential amino acid, ubiquitous in dietary protein. It is normally transformed into tyrosine, which is in turn used for protein synthesis and is the immediate amino acid precursor for melanin, dopamine, norepinephrine and epinephrine. The conversion of phenylalanine to tyrosine requires the presence of phenylalanine hydroxylase and tetrahydrobiopterin as a proton donor (Fig. 30.1). Tetrahydrobiopterin is reconverted from dihydrobiopterin by dihydropteridine reductase. In the majority of cases, PKU is caused by a deficiency of the hepatic enzyme phenylalanine hydroxylase, and in a minority ($\pm$ 2%) by dihydropteridine reductase deficiency or a defect in the synthesis of tetrahydrobiopterin (Fig. 30.2). At present three different enzymopathies are known to affect tetrahydrobiopterin synthesis: a defect in guanosine triphosphate cyclohydrolase, 6-pyruvoyl tetrahydropterin synthetase, and pterin-4a-dehydratase activity.

The phenylalanine hydroxylase gene has been mapped to the long arm of chromosome 12, position q22-24.1. The gene has been sequenced and a large number of different mutations (more than 80 at present) have been reported. There is evidence that the phenotypic heterogeneity of the disorder reflects underlying genetic heterogeneity. Some of the mutations lead to absence of residual hydroxylase activity, whereas others result in the presence of some variable residual activity. Most patients are compound heterozygotes leading to a range of residual activities. A good correlation has been found between the residual level of activity of mutant phenylalanine hydroxylase enzymes and clinical severity of the disease. The residual enzyme activity also correlates with the pretreatment serum level of phenylalanine, serum phenylalanine levels measured in standardized loading tests, and phenylalanine tolerance. Severe classical PKU is caused by mutations with zero residual enzyme activity (so-called null phenotype). Higher enzyme activity is associated with a milder phenotype. In persistent benign hyperphenylalaninemia without clinical manifestations residual enzyme activity is relatively high.

Deficiency of phenylalanine hydroxylase results in the accumulation of phenylalanine, which is transaminated to phenylpyruvate, phenyllactate, phenylacetate and o-hydroxyphenylacetate (Fig. 30.1). The metabolites derived from phenylalanine contribute little to the cerebral damage in PKU. Probably the most important effects are related to direct toxic influences of phenyl-

alanine itself. In theory, deficiency of phenylalanine hydroxylase activity could lead to systemic tyrosine deficiency. However, no consistent or significant reduction in plasma tyrosine has ever been demonstrated in untreated PKU patients and postnatal tyrosine supplementation does not prevent occurrence of neurological abnormalities. Hyperphenylalaninemia has a number of adverse effects. Owing to the competitive nature of amino acid transport across the blood-brain barrier, the brain in patients with PKU is exposed to both high phenylalanine levels and low concentrations of other large neutral amino acids, including histidine, tyrosine, arginine, tryptophan, and ornithine. A number of studies have provided evidence that hyperphenylalaninemia interferes with protein synthesis, which may be related to the inhibition of transport of amino acids across the blood-brain barrier. High levels of phenylalanine have a double effect on tyrosine and tryptophan metabolism. Not only is the transport across the blood-brain barrier inhibited, but high phenylalanine levels also lead to competitive inhibition of the enzymes tyrosine hydroxylase and tryptophan hydroxylase, enzymes involved in the synthesis of dopamine, (nor)epinephrine (from tyrosine) and serotonin (from tryptophan). As a result of both enzyme inhibition and deficiency of the amino acid substrates for these enzymes, the neurotransmitters dopamine, (nor)epinephrine and serotonin are decreased in untreated patients with phenylalanine hydroxylase deficiency.

It is important to distinguish permanent from reversible effects of hyperphenylalaninemia. Reversible neuronal dysfunction, which disappears on treatment, is probably related to neurotransmitter dysfunction. If left untreated, reversible dysfunction may become irreparable damage consisting of a reduction in number and growth of neuronal cells and synapses. The defect in protein synthesis may contribute to this damage. Reversible white matter damage consists of delay in myelination and white matter sponginess, probably related to a combination of phenylalanine toxicity on cells and disturbed protein synthesis. Long standing, severely disturbed myelination and demyelination may only be partially repairable. The vulnerability of the brain for hyperphenylalaninemia is lifelong. Discontinuation of diet may again lead to neuronal dysfunction with epilepsy, enhanced occurrence of EEG abnormalities and cognitive decline, and to white matter damage as evident from MRI.

The tetrahydrobiopterin deficiency states can be divided into defects in synthesis and defects in recycling. Dihydropteridine reductase deficiency is the only defect in recycling. The gene encoding this enzyme is located on chromosome 4 region p15.1–p16.1. Deficiency of the enzyme, which may be partial or complete, leads to tetrahydrobiopterin deficiency, which is not only a cofactor (proton donor) in the hydroxylation of phenylalanine to tyrosine, but also in the hydroxylation of tryptophan to 5-hydroxytryptophan and in the hydroxylation of tyrosine to L-DOPA (Fig. 30.2). 5-Hydroxytryptophan is the precursor of serotonin and melatonin, L-DOPA is the precursor of dopamine, epinephrine and norepinephrine. In addition, hyperphenylalaninemia has a competitive inhibitory effect on tyrosine hydroxylase and tryptophan hydroxylase. So, deficiency of dihydropteridine reductase has a profound effect on multiple neurotransmitter systems, which explains many of the neurological features of the disorder. This effect cannot be improved by lowering phenylalanine intake only. The defects of tetrahydrobiopterin synthesis have similar effects on these neurotransmitter systems. A special aspect of dihydropteridine reductase deficiency is related to folate metabolism. The enzyme also reduces dihydrofolate to tetrahydrofolate. Defective folate metabolism is important in dihydropteridine reductase deficiency. Megaloblastic changes of blood cells are unusual, even in very low folate concentration. However, progressive neurological damage is frequent. Histological changes in the brain are similar to congenital folate malabsorption and 5,10-methylene tetrahydrofolate reductase deficiency and consist of multifocal, perivascular demyelination, accompanied by perivascular microcalcification in the basal ganglia.

30.5 Therapy

Classical PKU is treated with a low-phenylalanine diet. Such a diet depends on the use of manufactured substitutes for many natural foods (meat, fish, eggs, nuts, dairy products, bread), making the diet difficult to sustain over long periods. Treatment should be monitored regularly with assessment of serum phenylalanine levels. Both early onset of dietary treatment and strict compliance to the diet contribute to a favorable intellectual outcome. IQ is clearly correlated with the quality of dietary control. Current treatment of PKU patients is not perfect and cognitive level is, on average, lower than expected. For many years it has been customary to stop dietary treatment in mid to late childhood or in adolescence in the asumption that hyperphenylalaninemia is only harmful in the immature brain. However, discontinuation of diet leads to some cognitive deterioration in many of the PKU patients. There is a lack of concentration, and sometimes agitation and emotional instability. Hypertonia of the legs, hyperreflexia and extensor plantar responses are frequently present and may lead to difficulty in walking. Epilepsy, slowness of speech, dysarthria and tremor, in particular intention tremor, may occur. With high levels of phenylalanine EEG shows background slowing. The complaints may be reversible if phenylalanine restriction is resumed, but may become permanent if longstanding. Life-long continuation of dietary treatment is advisable. In particular, restriction of phenylalanine intake during pregnancy is important for the benefit of the offspring.

In PKU related to tetrahydrobiopterin deficiency deterioration continues under conventional dietary treatment. In these patients the therapeutic goal is two-fold: not only to control the blood level of phenylalanine but also to normalize monoamine neurotransmission. The administration of tetrahydrobiopterin is insufficient to achieve this latter purpose. The introduction of oral administration of a combination of tetrahydrobiopterin, L-DOPA, carbidopa and 5-hydroxytryptophan, given to bypass the impaired activity of tyrosine hydroxylase and tryptophan hydroxylases, is followed by some (and sometimes a dramatic) degree of clinical and biochemical improvement. Carbidopa is a peripheral decarboxylase inhibitor to prevent peripheral conversion of L-DOPA to dopamine and so prevent systemic adverse effects and enhance central beneficial effects. The treatment should not only be monitored by evaluation of serum phenylalanine levels, but also by assessment of CSF neurotransmitter metabolites. In the case of dihydropteridine reductase deficiency the folate disturbance also requires treatment. Tetrahydrofolate should be administered in sufficient amounts to keep CSF concentrations in the high-normal range. This level of tetrahydrofolate prevents the occurrence of demyelinating disease.

30.6 Magnetic Resonance Imaging

During the last few years it has become clear that white matter abnormalities occur with high frequency in patients with classical PKU. The earliest and most frequent abnormalities consist of high signal intensity lesions on T_2-weighted images in the parieto-occipital periventricular white matter (peri-atrial and peritrigonal region) (Fig. 30.3). In more severe cases, the frontal periventricular white matter is also involved and the white matter abnormalities may extend into the subcortical area. The corpus callosum is relatively, but not always completely spared. The internal capsule, brain stem and cerebellar white matter are preserved. The white matter lesions are symmetrical and either bandlike or patchy and partly confluent in an irregular fashion. Additional isolated white matter spots may occasionally be present. Frequently the frontal, and less often the occipital white matter changes have a peculiar configuration extending like little "flames" from the ventricular border in line with the ventricles. In few patients some generalized cerebral atrophy is seen.

These white matter changes have been reported in older children, adolescents and adults. At present there

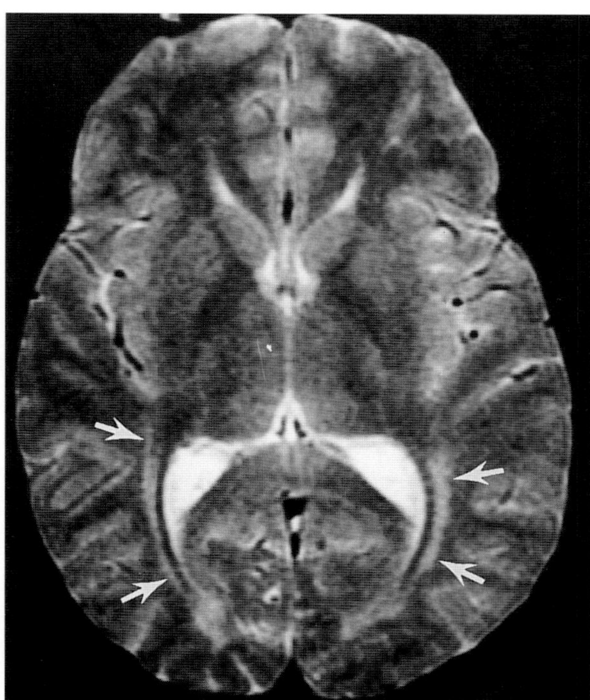

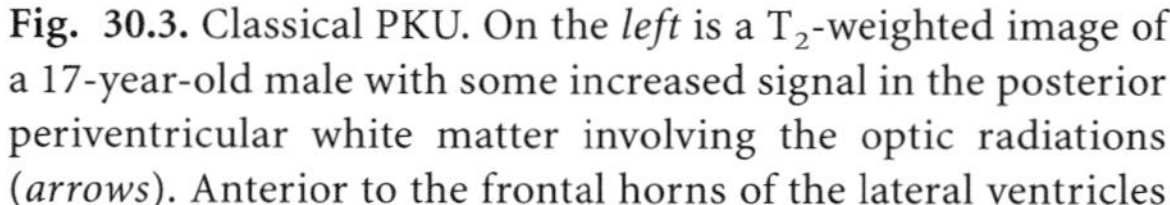

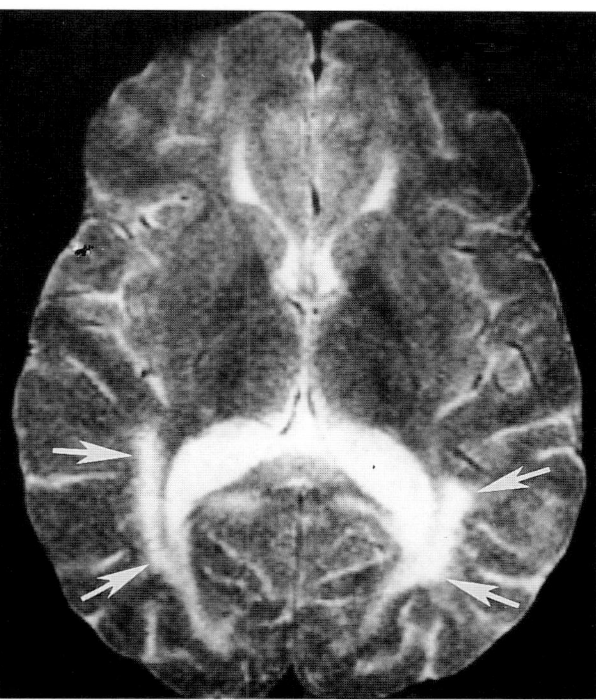

Fig. 30.3. Classical PKU. On the *left* is a T$_2$-weighted image of a 17-year-old male with some increased signal in the posterior periventricular white matter involving the optic radiations (*arrows*). Anterior to the frontal horns of the lateral ventricles less severe changes are seen. On the *right* is a T$_2$-weighted image of a 21-year-old man with a similar but more severe pattern. Courtesy of Shaw et al. (1991), with permission

is no systematic MRI study involving infants and young children. From the studies performed it is apparent that white matter abnormalities are less likely to be present in children under dietary control and in patients with milder variants of PKU. The white matter changes are predominantly present in patients after stopping the phenylalanine restricted diet. There is a positive correlation between the presence and severity of the white matter abnormalities and both the degree of recent exposure to high phenylalanine levels and the number of years after stopping the low phenylalanine diet. The presence of white matter changes is not correlated with the age of onset of diet (early versus late treatment) or the quality of dietary control during the first years of life or subsequent years. These data suggest that recently sustained exposure to high phenylalanine concentrations rather than the quality of long-term control is the major determinant of white matter signal abnormalities as detected by MRI. A few patients developing neurological abnormalities several months or years after stopping or relaxing the phenylalanine restricted diet underwent sequential MRI studies. Whereas initial MRI investigations showed symmetrical periventricular white matter changes, follow-up scans after resumption of a strict diet showed resolution of the abnormalities within a few months in some but not all patients.

The nature of the white matter changes is still a matter of conjecture as there are no direct correlative studies comparing MRI and histopathological findings in the same patients. Considering the rapid reversal of MRI changes that may be produced by effective dietary intervention, white matter edema may be assumed. Considering the fact that reversibility of MRI changes was not confirmed in all cases and considering the known histopathological sequence of events in untreated PKU patients (hypomyelination → white matter (myelin) vacuolation and edema → demyelination), an attractive hypothesis is that the early MRI changes observed represent white matter edema with intramyelinic vacuole formation and that the late changes represent permanent myelin damage and loss. The initial stage is reversible, the later stage is not.

The white matter changes are clinically correlated with motor problems, in particular spasticity of the legs, processing of visual information, and changes in mood and personality. No relationship between MRI changes and IQ has been found.

The imaging changes observed in patients with PKU due to a deficiency of tetrahydrobiopterin are different from those in classical PKU. There are only a few reports on imaging findings, and so their incidence and extent are not fully known. In one report (Brismar et al. 1989) the basic enzyme defect is not specified. In

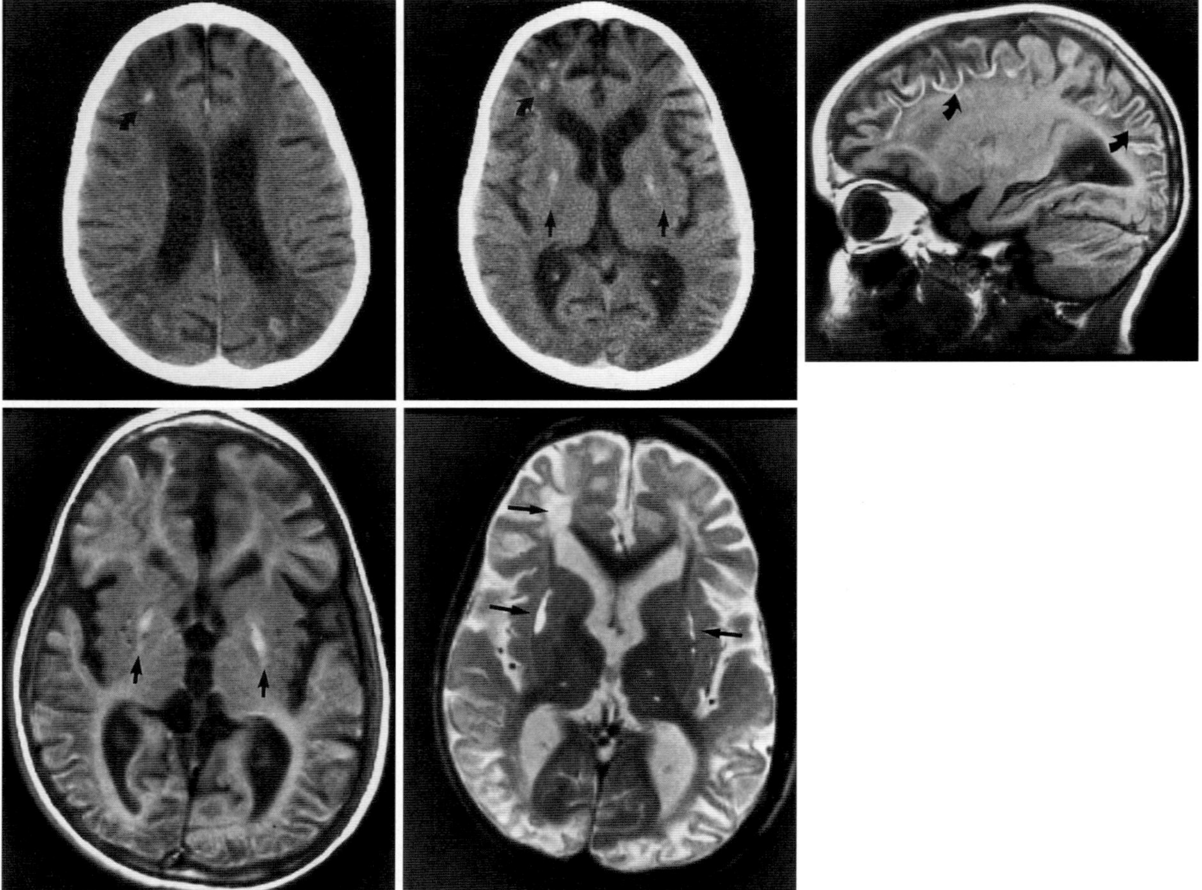

Fig. 30.4. In a girl with malignant PKU due to dihydropteridine reductase deficiency, aged 2 years and 8 months, CT scans (*upper row left*) show dilated ventricles with cortical atrophy and calcifications in the striatum and in the frontal and occipital gray and white matter junction. The white matter is hypodense in these areas. The transverse T_1 and T_2-weighted MR images at the age of 4.5 years (*lower row*) show basal ganglia tesious (*arrows*). There is a high signal intensity in the calcified spots in the basal ganglia on T_1-weighted images (*arrows*). The subcortical white matter has too low a signal intensity on the T_1-weighted images, too high a signal intensity on the T_2-weighted images. The parasagittal T_1-weighted MR image (*upper row right*) shows a gyriform band of high signal intensity in the cortex and corticomedullary junction, probably due to calcification (*arrows*). Courtesy of Gudinchet et al. (1992), with permission

this study CT is reported to be normal in the youngest patients up to the age of about one year. In older children CT shows atrophy with enlargement of the ventricular system and subarachnoid spaces. In some of the patients, diffuse hemispheral white matter hypodensity is reported. MRI shows diffuse hemispheral white matter hyperintensity on T_2-weighted images in these patients. In other studies, a combination of gray and white matter changes has been reported in dihydropteridine reductase deficiency (Figs. 30.4–30.6). CT scan shows atrophy with enlargement of the ventricular system and subarachnoid spaces. In addition, calcium depositions develop and are seen bilaterally in the basal nuclei (globus pallidus, possibly also putamen), and frontal subcortical region. Variable white matter hypodensity is seen. MRI shows some evidence of calcium deposition in the areas mentioned, with mottled hyperintensity on T_1-weighted images and heterogeneous signal loss, sometimes in combination with high signal intensity areas on T_2-weighted images. In one case the T_1-weighted images are reported to show diffuse cortical hyperintensity, probably representing diffuse cortical calcification (Fig. 30.4). The MR images show white matter abnormalities, either focal and partly cystic, involving the occipital region bilaterally, or diffuse and involving all hemispheral white matter. In the latter case differentiation between severely disturbed myelination and demyelination may not be possible.

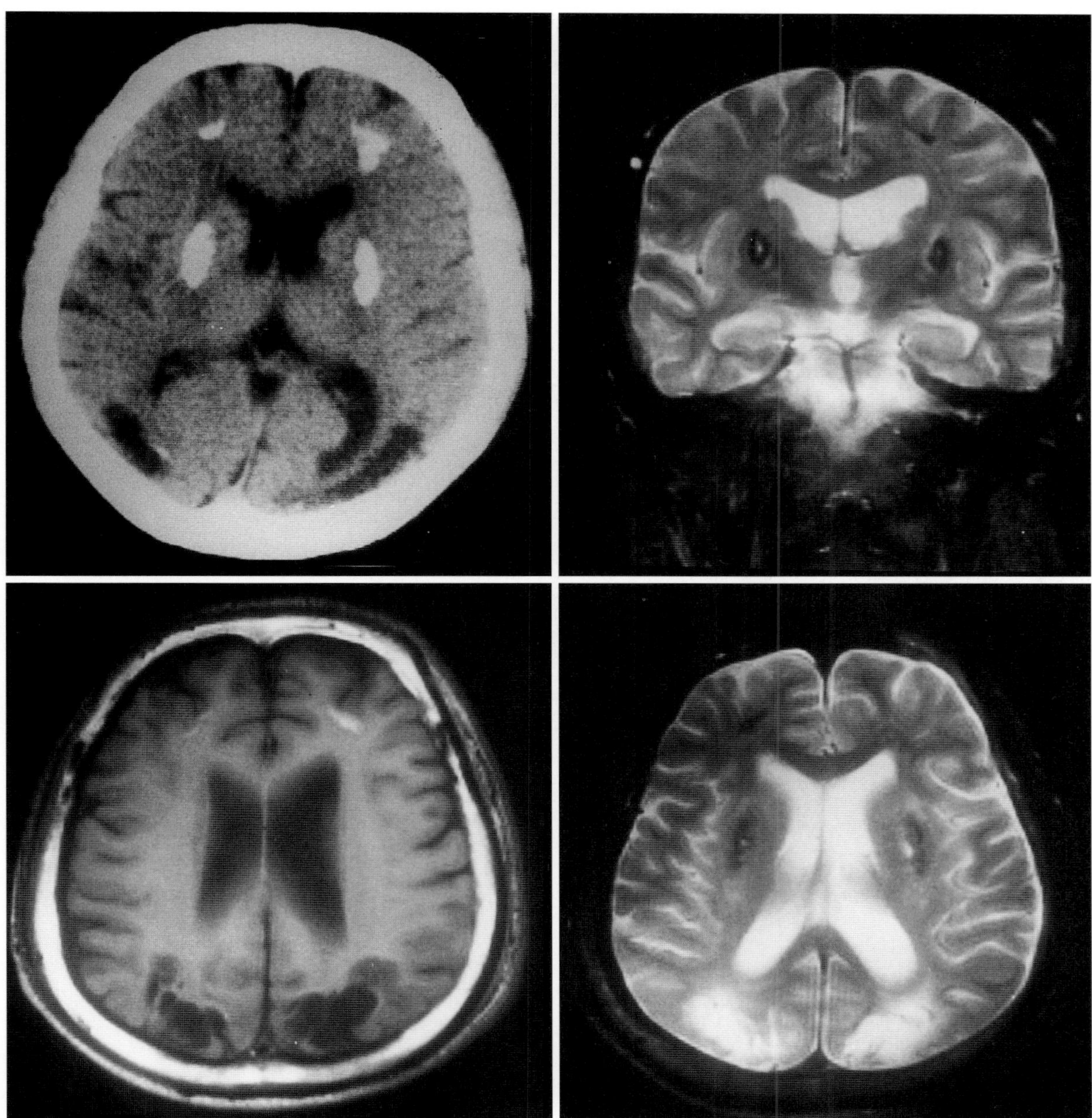

Fig. 30.5. A 26-year-old male with hyperphenylalaninemia due to dihydropteridine reductase deficiency. CT (*upper left*) shows extensive calcification in the basal ganglia and in the frontal cortico-medullary junction. Coronal T$_2$-weighted MRI shows enlarged ventricles (*upper right*). The basal nuclei have a low signal intensity with a central area of high signal intensity, similar to the eye-of-the-tiger phenomenon of Hallervorden Spatz disease. The transverse T$_1$- and T$_2$-weighted images (*lower row*) show, like the CT scan, cyst formation in the occipital lobes. Note the high signal intensity on the T$_1$-weighted image in a calcified subcortical lesion (*lower left*), and the low and high signal intensity in the basal ganglia on the T$_2$-weighted transverse MR image (*lower right*). Courtesy of Sugita et al. (1990), with permission

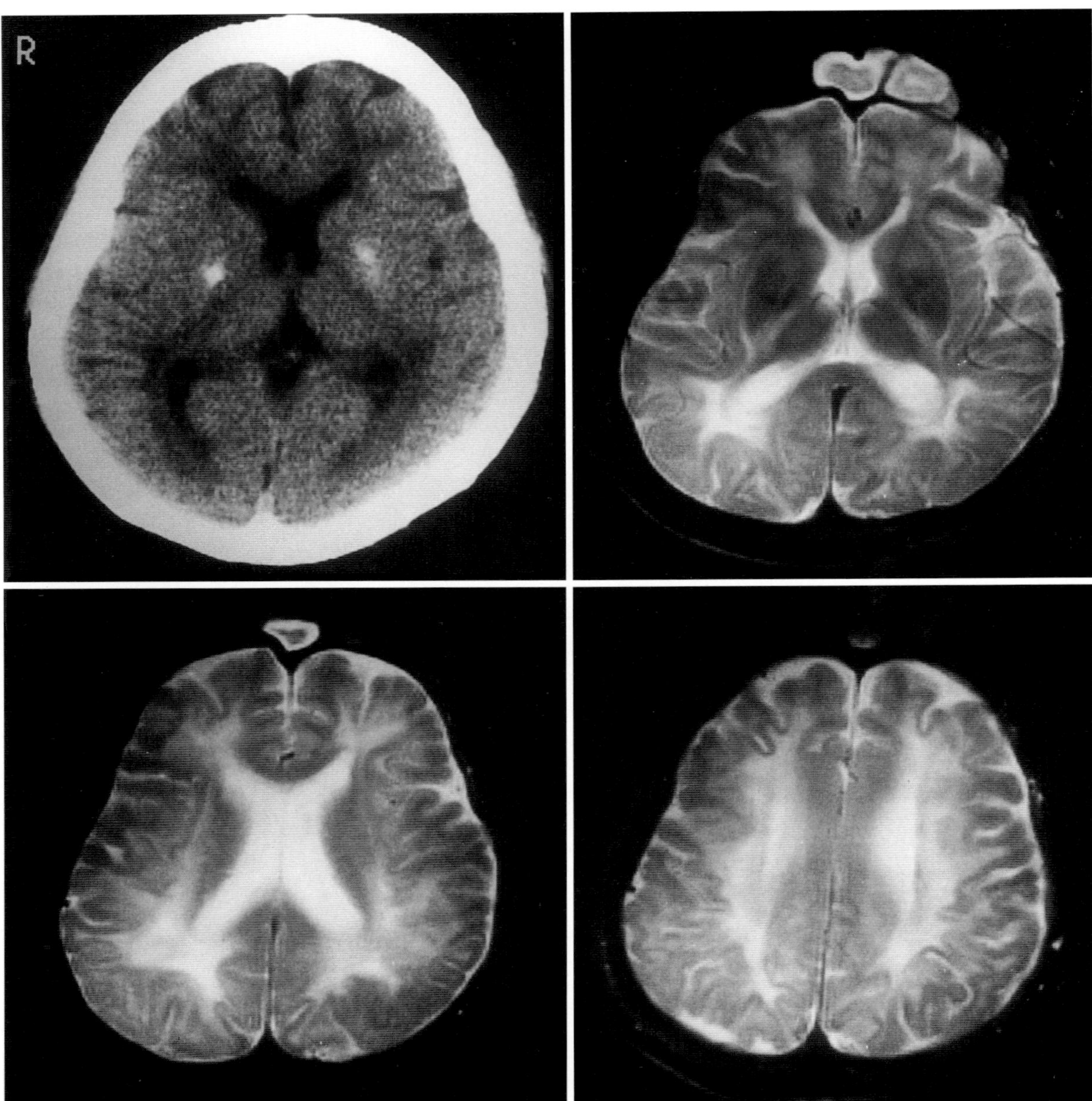

Fig. 30.6. A 20-year-old male with dihydropteridine reductase deficiency. CT (*upper left*) shows some calcification of the basal ganglia. In this patient, MR shows diffuse involvement of the white matter in the centrum semiovale, reaching the U fibers, and involving the peritrigonal white matter and external and internal capsule. The frontal white matter is less severely affected. Courtesy of Sugita et al. (1990), with permission

31 Glutaric Aciduria Type 1

31.1 Clinical Features and Laboratory Investigations

Glutaric aciduria type 1 is a rare autosomal recessive metabolic disorder with highly variable clinical symptomatology.

The disease usually presents with an acute encephalitis-like encephalopathy in infancy or childhood after normal initial development. The first episode occurs in most cases during the second half of the first year of life. Frequently, the only abnormality preceding the first episode is a developing macrocephaly. The encephalopathic episode is usually triggered by an infectious illness. The episode is characterized by seizures, lowering of consciousness, coma, opisthotonic posturing, hypotonia, loss of head control, spasticity, dystonia, orofacial dyskinesia, grimacing and rigidity. Recovery is slow and often incomplete. After onset, the course of disease is usually slowly progressive with episodes of acute deterioration, often associated with an infection. Patients frequently have a tendency to sweat profusely. There may be episodes of unexplained fever. Death usually occurs in the first decade, in the course of an episode of acute deterioration during an infection or in the course of a Reye syndrome-like episode. In other patients the course of disease is more chronically progressive with retarded development during the first year of life. Subsequently, hypotonia, dystonia, athetoid involuntary movements and spasticity develop gradually over the years with loss of motor skills. Progressive dystonia is invalidating and leads to a loss of walking and writing abilities. Also, articulate speech may become progressively difficult and may be lost altogether. Mental capabilities are relatively preserved. Some patients remain asymptomatic and asymptomatic adults have occasionally been found while screening families known to be affected. With early treatment the prognosis of the patients improves and most or all of the neurological damage can be prevented.

In glutaric aciduria type 1, excessive urinary excretion of glutaric acid, glutaconic acid and 3-hydroxyglutaric acid suggests the diagnosis. The defect in metabolization of glutaryl-CoA leads to accumulation of this substance in body fluids, partly esterified with carnitine and excreted as glutaryl-carnitine. Carnitine deficiency can be the result of this excessive carnitine use. Lysine, hydroxylysine and tryptophan, precursors of glutaryl-CoA, are not elevated in urine or body fluids. During episodes of clinical decompensation a metabolic acidosis, ketosis, hyperammonemia and elevation of serum transaminases may be found. Occasionally hypoglycemia occurs in an acute episode. The diagnosis of glutaric aciduria type 1 may be difficult to establish. Enhanced urinary excretion of the mentioned metabolites may be intermittent and only detectable during episodes of metabolic derangement. In some cases the urine concentration of glutaric acid, glutaconic acid and 3-hydroxyglutaric acid may even remain normal during episodes of clinical decompensation. In most (but not all) of these patients a decrease in plasma carnitine levels and an increase in urinary glutarylcarnitine levels can be found indicative of glutaric aciduria. In some patients only elevated levels of glutaric acid can be found in CSF. Definite diagnosis can be established by assay of glutaryl-CoA dehydrogenase in leukocytes and fibroblasts. Prenatal diagnosis can be performed by enzyme assessment in chorion villi or cultured amniotic cells.

31.2 Pathology

Most commonly noted abnormalities involve the putamen and head of the caudate nucleus, less often the globus pallidus. Changes tend to be more marked in patients who die after several years than in infants. The lesions are characterized by loss of neurons associated with gliosis. The cortex is well preserved. Ventricular enlargement is often noted.

Marked spongiform changes are seen in the hemispheral white matter in some patients. It is the periventricular white matter which is particularly involved, whereas the subcortical arcuate fibers are spared. In addition, optic nerves, corpus callosum, anterior limb of the internal capsule, deep cerebellar white matter and long tracts of the upper brain stem are involved. The posterior limb of the internal capsule, cerebral peduncles and superior cerebellar peduncles are not involved. Vacuolation is caused by myelin splitting and intramyelinic vacuole formation. In electron microscopy splitting is seen to occur along the intraperiod line. Mild spongiform changes due to myelin splitting may be seen in subcortical gray matter structures rich in myelin, such as the thalamus, globus pallidus and brain stem reticular formation.

31.3 Pathogenetic Considerations

Glutaric aciduria type 1 is caused by deficiency of glutaryl-CoA dehydrogenase. Glutaryl-CoA, a catabolite of lysine, hydroxylysine and tryptophan, is dehydrogenated to glutaconyl-CoA and subsequently decarboxylated to crotonyl-CoA, both steps being catalysed by a single enzyme, glutaryl-CoA dehydrogenase. The enzyme is present in both mitochondria and peroxisomes. In glutaric aciduria type I the mitochondrial enzyme is lacking. An incidental case of peroxisomal glutaryl-CoA dehydrogenase deficiency has been described. Mitochondrial glutaryl-CoA dehydrogenase is a flavin adenine dinucleotide (FAD) requiring enzyme. Deficiency of this enzyme activity has been reported in glutaric aciduria type I and in multiple acyl-CoA dehydrogenase deficiency, also called glutaric aciduria type II.

The cause of striatal dysfunction and necrosis in glutaric aciduria is not known. A number of factors may contribute to the damage. It has been shown that glutarate is toxic to striatal cells in culture and some suggest that the striatal lesions are due to the direct effects of glutarate. Glutaric acid, glutaconic acid and 3-hydroxyglutaric acid are competitive inhibitors of glutamic acid decarboxylase, the enzyme involved in biosynthesis of γ-aminobutyric acid (GABA), an inhibitory neurotransmitter. Biochemical analysis of the brains of a few patients demonstrated elevated levels of glutaric acid in the frontal cortex and basal ganglia, very low glutamic acid decarboxylase activity and very low concentrations of GABA in the caudate nucleus and putamen. Also, low CSF GABA levels have been found. The low GABA is not necessarily related to inhibition of glutamic acid decarboxylase, but may also be the result of destruction or dysfunction of GABA-ergic neurons. Another theory is that quinolinic acid, an intermediate in the metabolism of tryptophan and lysine, and a potent neurotoxin, contributes to the neuronal damage in glutaric aciduria. Another possible pathogenetic mechanism involves N-methyl-D-aspartate (NMDA) receptors, of which glutamate is the normal activator. Glutaric acid may interfere with the reuptake of glutamate, resulting in its accumulation in the synapse, or it could activate glutamine receptors, resulting in enhanced activation of NMDA receptors with deleterious results.

Still less is known about the pathogenesis of myelin splitting and vacuolation. Myelin splitting is probably caused by toxic effects of accumulating substances.

The cause of the macrocephaly has not been adequately explained. Contributing factors may be presence of extracerebral fluid collections, hydrocephalus and myelin splitting with intramyelinic accumulation of fluid.

There is marked clinical variability among homozygous individuals with identical biochemical profiles within the same kindred with consanguineous parents. This excludes allelic heterogeneity and suggests the existence of unrelated, genetically polymorphic protective mechanisms. Clinical variability may also be related to the flexibility of associated enzyme systems like those involved in GABA or glutamate metabolism.

31.4 Therapy

A diet low in protein, in particular low in tryptophan and lysine, is recommended, supplemented with riboflavin and carnitine. Riboflavin is a coenzyme for glutaryl-CoA dehydrogenase and large doses have been shown to decrease the excretion of glutaric acid, presumably by increasing its metabolism. Carnitine is used to stimulate the formation and excretion of glutarylcarnitine. After onset of neurological problems this treatment protocol leads to no or only modest improvement, but in most cases further deterioration is halted and no further episodes of acute encephalopathy occur. Early treatment has been shown to be effective in preventing the occurrence of most or all problems. Some patients, however, still show some deterioration, and an encephalopathic episode may even occur. With early treatment, improvement or resolution of neuroimaging abnormalities can be observed.

There are some additional therapeutic options. In view of the decreased GABA levels, treatment with a GABA analog, baclofen, is logical and has produced some symptomatic improvement with a decrease in dystonia. Gamma-vinyl GABA (vigabatrin) causes an irreversible inhibition of GABA transaminase, the first step of GABA catabolism, and in this way leads to increased GABA levels. Decreased dystonia has been noted with vigabatrin therapy. Valproate has been recommended because of its inhibitory action on GABA transaminase. However, valproate is partly excreted as valproylcarnitine and may cause further stress to the already compromised carnitine system.

Whether subdural fluid collections should be evacuated, and whether shunt implantation should be performed in cases of ventricular enlargement and progressive macrocephaly, is questionable. Spontaneous resolution of these abnormalities has been documented, as well as ongoing deterioration despite neurosurgical intervention.

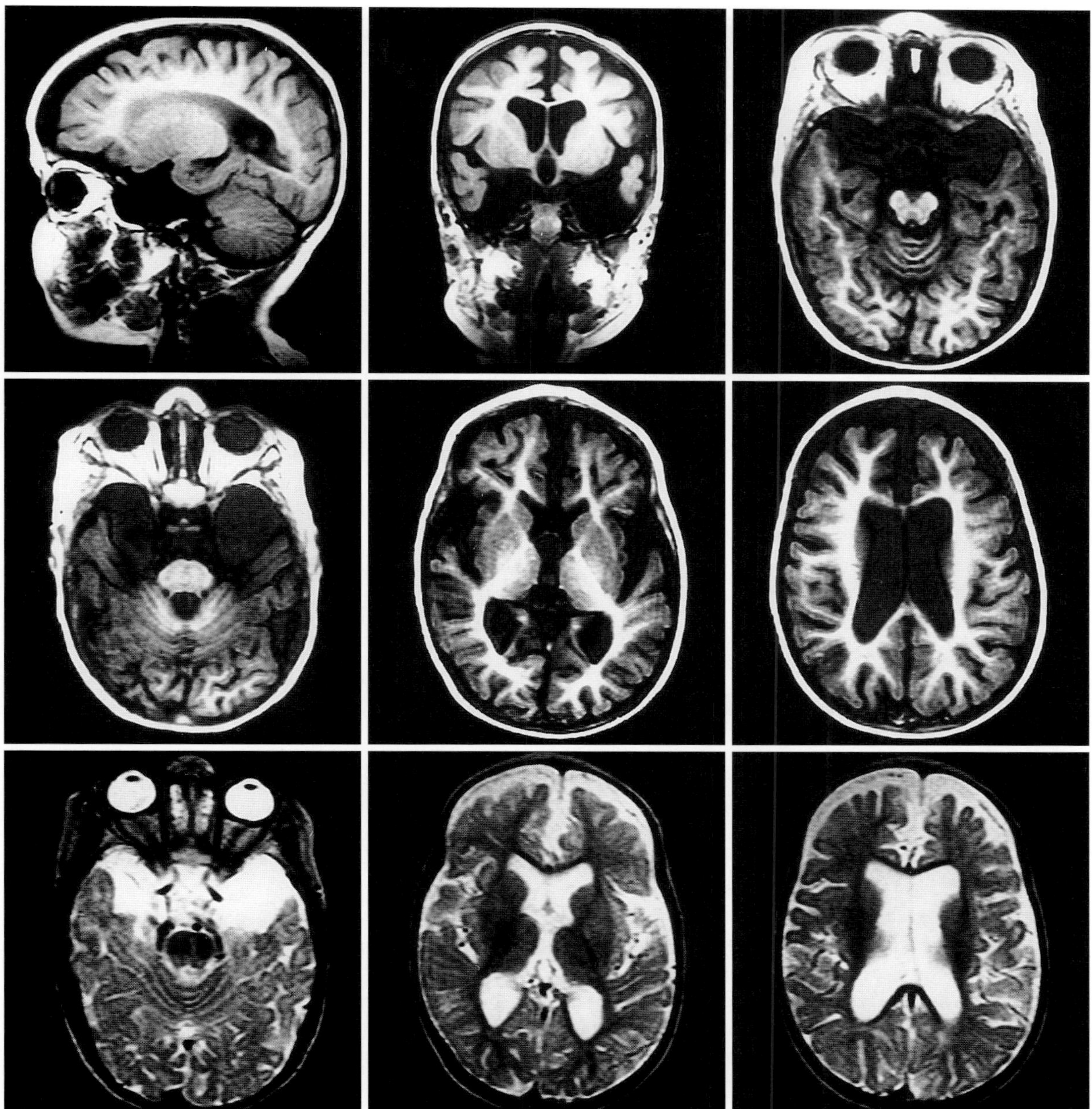

Fig. 31.1. A 2-year-old boy with glutaric aciduria type 1. The MR images show some of the typical features: large insular and temporal fluid collections, with underdevelopment of the temporal lobes. Over the hemispheres there are subdural fluid collections and enlargement of the arachnoid space. The dura in between is visible on the T_2-weighted images (*lower right*). The ventricles are mildly enlarged. In this case the T_2-weighted images (*lower row*) do not show high signal intensity in the putamen. Myelination is delayed, the subcortical white matter still having a relatively high signal intensity

31.5 Magnetic Resonance Imaging

CT scan of the brain discloses enlarged CSF spaces in most patients with glutaric aciduria type 1, even if asymptomatic without treatment. The most often noted are fluid collections over the convexities in the frontoparietal and frontotemporal areas. In some cases the frontoparietal fluid collections have the appearance of subdural hygromas, usually bilateral, occasionally unilateral. In most cases the fluid collections consist of enlarged subarachnoid spaces, frequently ascribed to cerebral atrophy, sometimes to communicating hydrocephalus. Considering the presence of absolute or relative macrocephaly, mild enlargement of the ventricular system and absence of significant cortical damage at autopsy, communicating hydrocephalus may be the

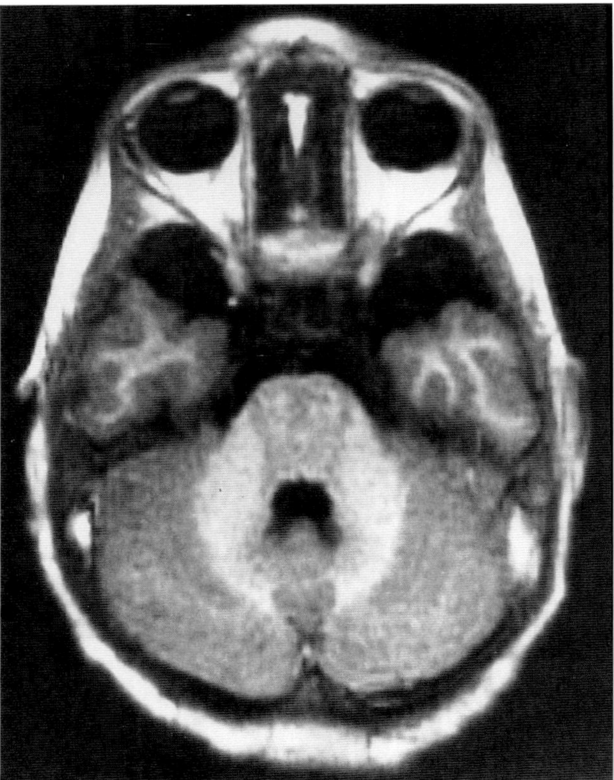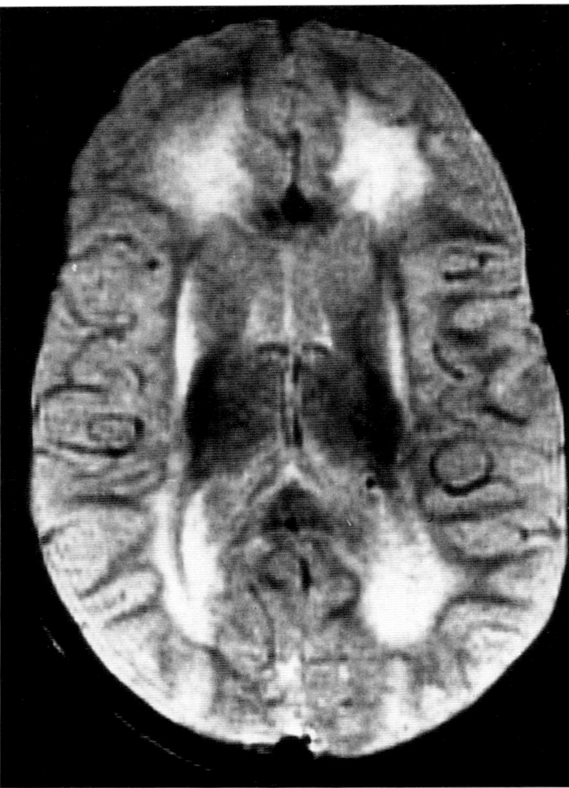

Fig. 31.2. A 5-year-old boy with glutaric aciduria type 1. T$_1$-weighted image through the level of the 4th ventricle shows bilateral pretemporal enlarged CSF spaces (*left*). The T$_2$-weighted image at the level of the basal ganglia shows high signal intensity of the putamen and symmetrical white matter involvement in the frontal and occipital region, sparing the arcuate fibers (*right*). Courtesy of Altman et al. (1991), with permission

most probable explanation. In many glutaric aciduria type I patients, the Sylvian fissure is widely open forming a large CSF space anterior to the temporal lobes. Some authors ascribe these CSF collections to the presence of bitemporal arachnoid cysts, but this is rarely in conformity with the configuration of the CSF collections. Usually they are ascribed to either frontal and temporal atrophy or failure of opercularisation. The aspect of the incompletely formed frontal and temporal operculum is most consistent with a failure of opercularisation. However, in incidental patients a normal Sylvian fissure has been noted soon after birth, whereas widely opened Sylvian fissures are seen several months later, forming an argument for atrophy. Decrease of enlarged CSF spaces has been noted to occur spontaneously and with treatment. In some patients hemispheral white matter hypodensity has been found.

MRI also depicts the fluid collections (Figs. 31.1, 31.2). In most cases the aspect of the widely opened Sylvian fissures is not consistent with arachnoid cysts but more probably with hypoplasia of the frontal and temporal operculum. The enlarged peripheral fluid spaces are the result of enlarged subarachnoid spaces, subdural spaces or a combination of the two (Fig. 31.1). In addition, bilateral lesions are often seen in the head of the caudate nucleus and in the putamen with abnormal signal intensity and/or atrophy (Fig. 31.2) In some of the patients white matter changes are seen. Delay in myelination has been reported (Fig. 31.1). Symmetrical, diffuse hemispheral white matter involvement has been observed in older patients. The white matter abnormalities are most marked in the frontal and occipital periventricular white matter and in the centrum semiovale with sparing of the arcuate fibers (Fig. 31.2).

On the whole, the imaging findings are highly variable. In some patients no abnormalities are noted at all (own observation), whereas in others only or mainly enlarged CSF spaces are seen; other cases show a predominance of striatal lesions, while others have a combination of striatal and white matter abnormalities.

It is probable that most cerebral abnormalities can be prevented by early treatment.

32 Propionic Acidemia

32.1 Clinical Features and Laboratory Investigations

Propinonic acidemia, also called ketotic hyperglycinemia, is a disorder of organic acid metabolism with autosomal recessive inheritance. Two forms of the disease can be distinguished: the severe neonatal onset form and the late onset form.

Many patients with propionic acidemia present in the neonatal period with a progressive encephalopathy. They are normal at birth, but after a few hours or days deterioration sets in with lethargy, poor feeding, vomiting, tachypnea and unexplained coma. Abnormalities in tone and movement occur. Limb hypertonia and opisthotonic posturing or axial hypotonia are often present. Abnormal pedaling movements, myoclonic jerks and tremors may be present. Convulsions may occur. In the more advanced stage, there are signs of respiratory distress and bradycardia. Mortality is high, and survivors frequently have severe lasting neurological impairment, in particular characterized by mental retardation and extrapyramidal movements.

In the late onset form, the patients are older when they present with an acute encephalopathy. Most patients are older than 1 year at presentation and some may even present in adulthood. The acute metabolic decompensations are precipitated by enhanced protein catabolism of exogenous origin (high protein intake) or endogenous origin (catabolic states, such as in fasting, infections or other forms of stress), but sometimes no cause is found. The encephalopathic episodes are characterized by ataxia, lethargy and coma, sometimes with focal neurological abnormalities like hemiplegia. Often the children already had chronic problems before the first episode, including chronic feeding problems, persistent vomiting, failure to thrive, hypotonia, osteoporosis and developmental retardation. These chronic problems can be present for a long time without acute metabolic decompensation and without correct diagnosis. Mortality rate of the encephalopathic episodes with delayed onset is lower than that of the neonatal onset form, and the prognosis with respect to intelligence is better. Some patients with the later onset form of propionic acidemia are mildly retarded, but some patients have a normal intelligence. Some patients have a lasting extrapyramidal movement disorder, usually chorea.

During episodes of acute metabolic decompensation, laboratory investigations reveal signs of dehydration, metabolic acidosis with ketonuria, elevated ammonia levels and decreased carnitine levels. Lactate may be elevated and hypoglycemia may be present. Neutropenia and thrombopenia are consistent findings. Specific laboratory findings suggesting the diagnosis are elevated plasma and urine levels of propionate, glycine, hydroxypropionate, propionylglycine, and methylcitrate. CSF glycine is not elevated as is the case in nonketotic hyperglycinemia. The diagnosis is confirmed by assessment of the enzyme propionyl-CoA carboxylase in leukocytes or fibroblasts. Prenatal diagnosis can be performed by enzyme assessment in cultured amniocytes and chorionic villi.

32.2 Pathology

Few data are present on histopathological findings in propionic acidemia. In the neonatal form, myelin splitting and myelin vacuolation have been reported, affecting the structures that contain myelin in a term neonate: posterior limb of the internal capsule, globus pallidus, thalamus, brain stem tegmentum, cerebellar white matter and spinal cord. The progress of myelination is normal for a neonate. The cortical cytoarchitecture is normal.

In older children, post-mortem reveals atrophy and in some children a status spongiosus affecting the cerebral hemispheres. In others the white matter was reported to be normal. Atrophy, nerve cell loss and gliosis may be found in the caudate nucleus and putamen, to a lesser extent in the globus pallidus and thalamus. Hypermyelination may occur in the affected basal nuclei.

32.3 Pathogenetic Considerations

The basic defect in isolated propionic acidemia is a deficient activity of the mitochondrial enzyme propionyl-CoA carboxylase. This enzyme has biotin as its cofactor and consists of two nonidentical subunits (α and β). Both α-subunit deficiency and β-subunit deficiency have been described. The genes encoding the α and β-subunits have been mapped to chromosomes 13 and 3, respectively. Mutations have been described.

Propionyl-CoA carboxylase converts propionyl-CoA into methylmalonyl-CoA, which is subsequently converted into succinyl-CoA, which enters the Krebs cycle. Isoleucine, valine, threonine and methionine are precursors of propionic acid, explaining the observed protein and amino acid intolerance.

The myelinopathy with splitting and vacuole formation is seen in a number of inborn errors of metabolism, including Canavan disease, maple syrup urine disease and nonketotic hyperglycinemia, and a number of intoxications, including hexachlorophene, cuprizone and triethyltin intoxication. The myelinopathy is probably a toxic phenomenon.

32.4   Therapy

In episodes of acute metabolic decompensation, treatment consists of removal of toxic products by dialysis or exchange transfusions. At the same time further catabolism of proteins should be prevented and an anabolic situation should be achieved to prevent the production of more toxic products. This can be achieved by continuous parenteral nutrition with a protein-free product and continuous intravenous infusion of insulin. Insulin has the capacity to stimulate protein synthesis. Biotin can be added to stimulate residual enzyme activity. Carnitine is administered to stimulate excretion of propionylcarnitine in urine.

Long-term treatment consists of dietary protein restriction while maintaining normal development and nutrition status and preventing catabolism. Chronic treatment with biotin and carnitine can be considered.

32.5   Magnetic Resonance Imaging

Neuroimaging reports on propionic acidemia are scarce. CT findings have been reported as being normal, or showing cerebral atrophy. In some cases hypodensities are seen in the basal nuclei. White matter hypodensities have been reported. Both hypodensities of white matter and basal nuclei may disappear at follow-up (Surtees et al. 1992).

MRI findings are also scarce. Cerebral atrophy, delayed myelination and abnormalities in the caudate nuclei, globus pallidus, and putamen have been reported. In one patient with a hemiplegia during an acute metabolic decompensation, MRI revealed no corresponding contralateral cerebral lesion, apart from slight local cortical atrophy. We found a delay in myelination and some cerebral atrophy in two patients. In another patient more extensive abnormalities were found, consisting of delayed and disturbed myelination in addition to persisting lesions in caudate nucleus and putamen (Fig. 32.1).

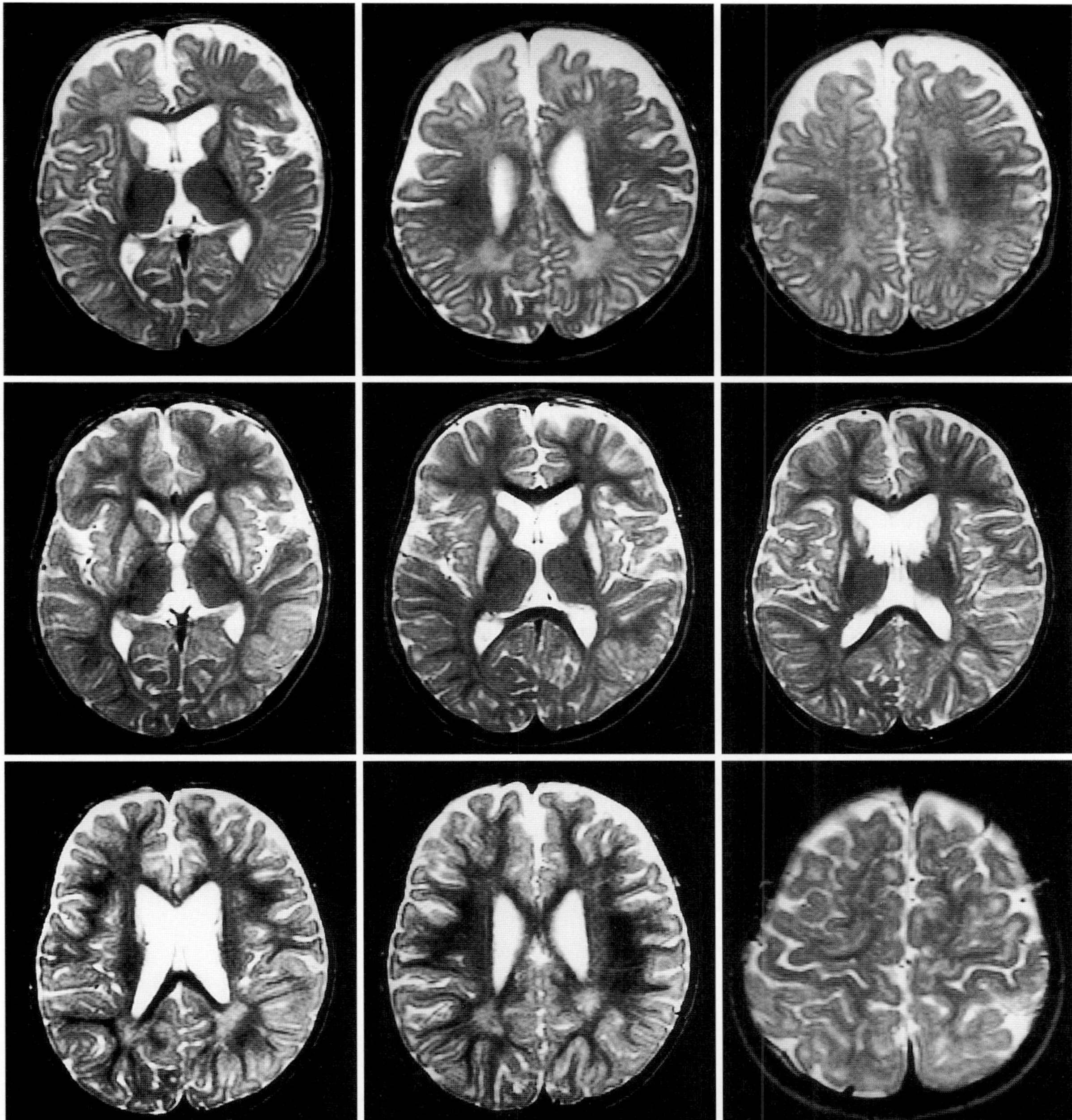

Fig. 32.1. T$_2$-weighted images in a boy with propionic acidemia at the ages of 10 months (*upper row*) and 2 years (*two lower rows*). At the age of 10 months, myelination is delayed and irregular. At the age of 2 years, myelination is more advanced, but still incomplete in the periventricular occipital area and in the subcortical area. In addition, there are lesions in the caudate nucleus and putamen and there are signs of some cerebral atrophy. The globus pallidus contains minor abnormalities

Two types of hyperprolinemia can be distinguished: type I related to deficiency of proline dehydrogenase and type II related to deficiency of Δ^1-pyrroline-5-carboxylic acid dehydrogenase. Both forms have an autosomal recessive mode of inheritance. There is doubt about the relationship with clinical symptomatology for both types of hyperprolinemia. Mental retardation, epilepsy and renal dysfunction have been reported in both type I and type II hyperprolinemia, but the metabolic disturbances can also be free of any associated clinical manifestations.

In hyperprolinemia type I, plasma proline levels are usually elevated up to 5-fold, whereas they are increased 10- to 15-fold in type II. Urine proline levels are also elevated. In addition, in type II, plasma and urine levels of Δ^1-pyroline-5-carboxylate are elevated.

Neuropathological observations are very scarce. Woody et al. (1969) found vacuolation of cerebral and cerebellar white matter in a boy of 3 months. Myelin was present in the cerebellum, but deficient in the cerebral hemispheres, consistent with a disturbance of myelination. Ventricles were dilated.

The second mention of white matter disease came from CT and MRI (Steinlin et al. 1989). In a 10-year-old boy with hyperprolinemia type I and neurological problems in the form of mental retardation, cerebral palsy, epilepsy and nystagmus, CT showed diffuse cerebral white matter hypodensity and moderate dilation of ventricles and subarachnoid spaces. MRI confirmed the presence of diffuse cerebral hemispheral white matter abnormalities with high signal intensity on T_2-weighted images. The condition of the cerebellar white matter, brain stem, internal capsule and corpus callosum was not described.

34 Nonketotic Hyperglycinemia

34.1 Clinical Features and Laboratory Investigations

Nonketotic hyperglycinemia (NKH) is an autosomal recessive disorder of which two types are distinguished: the neonatal type and the late-onset type.

Patients with neonatal NKH are normal at birth. Within a few days there are progressive neurological abnormalities, including lethargy, hypotonia, convulsions and apneic spells. Most patients die within a few weeks. The few patients who survive, show signs of spasticity, opisthotonus, absence of any development, severe seizures and microcephaly. Most children who survive the neonatal period, die within the first year of life but some survive into childhood in a severely disabled condition.

In the late-onset variant, patients are normal throughout the neonatal period. Development is retarded.

During the first weeks of life a characteristic EEG pattern is seen with short bursts of high complex waves alternated with hypoactivity. This burst-suppression pattern changes into hypsarrhythmia in the course of a few weeks.

Laboratory abnormalities include elevated levels of glycine in plasma and urine in the absence of ketoacidosis. The CSF level of glycine is elevated, as is the ratio of CSF to plasma glycine. Elevation of CSF glycine is most unusual and essential for the diagnosis.

NKH is caused by a defect in the glycine cleavage system. This system is specifically expressed in liver, kidney and brain, but not in fibroblasts and leukocytes. Liver biopsy was therefore necessary for enzymatic diagnosis of NKH. Recently, however, it was shown that the glycine cleavage system can be induced in lymphocytes which are transformed into lymphoblasts by Epstein-Barr virus infection. This procedure proves reliable and makes enzymatic diagnosis of NKH feasible using peripheral blood. Carrier detection is also possible with this test. Prenatal diagnosis using cultured amniotic cells is not possible, because the glycine cleavage system is not manifest in these cells. However, prenatal diagnosis using chorionic villi cells is feasible. DNA diagnosis is also possible when the mutation of the family is known.

34.2 Pathology

The external configuration of the brain in patients who died from NKH in the neonatal period is normal with a normal gyral pattern. The quantity of myelin found by microscopic examination of the brain is normal, but all myelinated areas have a striking spongy appearance imparted by the presence of numerous vacuoles. In conformity with the neonatal state of myelination, the spinal cord, brain stem (in particular brain stem tegmentum), cerebellar white matter, posterior limb of the internal capsule and optic nerves, tracts and chiasm are prominently involved, whereas cerebral hemispheral white matter devoid of myelin is free of vacuoles. There is usually a good correlation between myelin density and density of vacuoles. There are no sudanophilic deposits and there is a paucity of phagocytic and astroglial reactions. In children beyond the neonatal period variable delay in myelination has been reported.

In electron microscopy, the vacuoles are shown to be located within myelin sheaths and formed by splitting of myelin lamellae along the intraperiod lines.

Additional neuropathological changes can be found related to the serious condition of the child and occurrence of complications: neuronal incrustation with calcium in the cortex and thalamus, more acute anoxic neuronal changes in the cerebral cortex, and ischemic and/or hemorrhagic white matter changes in the periventricular area.

Neuropathological findings have also been described in a boy, who had a neonatal presentation of NKH and survived until 17 years of age (Agamanolis et al. 1993). A mild diffuse decrease in white matter mass was found with some ventricular enlargement. The white matter of the CNS showed diffuse vacuolation, contrasting with the more limited vacuolation in neonates in whom unmyelinated white matter is not vacuolated. The amount of myelin was normal in this boy. There was no evidence of a progressive myelin disease and no myelin loss. Also, cortical architecture was normal. The cerebellum was diffusely atrophic with a severe loss of Purkinje cells and granule cells. Numerous crystals were present in perivascular spaces and vessel walls of cerebellar tissue, probably calcium oxalate crystals. Oxalate is a product of glycine metabolism via glyoxylate.

34.3 Pathogenetic Considerations

The basic defect in NKH is in the glycine cleavage system. The glycine cleavage system is composed of four proteins: P-protein (a pyridoxal phosphate dependent glycine decarboxylase), H-protein (a lipoic acid containing protein), T-protein (a tetrahydrofolate requiring enzyme), and L-protein (lipoamide dehydrogenase). The glycine cleavage activity is undetectable or extremely low in the neonatal type, whereas in the late-onset type there is still some residual activity. The majority of the NKH patients have a defect in the P-protein and the remaining patients a defect in the T-protein. The gene coding for P-protein has been sequenced and a number of mutations have been described.

In NKH, the brain and CSF have an elevated concentration of glycine which is held responsible for the neurological impairment. Glycine is a major inhibitory neurotransmitter in spinal cord and brain stem, acting on strychnine-sensitive receptors. However, recent evidence indicates that glycine is also active in the cerebral cortex and that it has not only inhibitory but also excitatory properties. It is a positive modulator of the N-methyl-D-aspartate (NMDA) receptor of glutamate which plays an important role in glutamate-induced neurotoxicity. NMDA receptors are located throughout the brain. Glycine increases the frequency of NMDA receptor channel opening by accelerating recovery of the receptor following glutamate-induced desensitization. In this way, glycine potentiates the excitotoxic action of glutamate. In animal experiments it has been shown that glycine administration enhanced NMDA-induced seizures in mice whose classic glycine receptors located in spinal cord and brain stem had been blocked with strychnine. This experiment indicates that glycine is a harmful enhancer of the NMDA-response in vivo. It has been shown that the developing brain has heightened susceptibility to NMDA-mediated injury and high levels of glycine may be particularly devastating to the CNS of the neonate. This is in accordance with the clinical observation that most acute neurological problems are present in the neonatal period, and that stabilization is seen in patients surviving this period, albeit with a severe neurological handicap.

The relationships between high glycine levels and myelin vacuolation and between myelin vacuolation and clinical symptomatology is unclear. A myelin disorder does not as a rule lead to severe epilepsy, but rather to spasticity and other forms of loss of neurological function. The myelin disorder may explain at least part of the clinical impairment in the chronic stage of the disease. Myelin vacuolation is seen in inborn errors of metabolism (Canavan disease, maple syrup urine disease) and in intoxications (hexachlorophene, triethyltin, cuprizone). The pathogenetic mechanisms of myelin vacuolation are unclear in all these conditions, but are probably toxic in nature.

34.4 Therapy

Many therapeutic approaches have been attempted to lower glycine concentrations in patients with the neonatal-onset form of NHK. Dietary restriction of glycine and serine or of all protein, administration of drugs to stimulate excretion of glycine in urine or bile, peritoneal dialysis, hemodialysis and exchange transfusions have failed to achieve much success. The seizure activity may decrease under such regimens and the sensorium may improve. Strychnine blocks glycinergic inhibitory effects, but strychnine is only effective on the classic glycine receptors present in brain stem and spinal cord. Strychnine treatment is clinically not effective. Diazepam is a competitor of glycine receptors. The drug has a favorable anticonvulsant effect.

Since gaining insight into the importance of NMDA receptors in NKH, treatment with NMDA receptor antagonists has been attempted. Ketamine, an NMDA receptor antagonist, has been reported to lead to a decrease in irritability, improvement of gross motor movements, decrease in epilepsy, and improvement of sucking. Dextromethorphan, another NMDA receptor antagonist, has been reported to lead to cessation of seizures, improved alertness and social interest and initiation of some motor development with grasping. During temporary cessation of treatment and during febrile infections, severe but reversible neurological deterioration can occur. Until now, the results of dextromethorphan treatment are the most promising, but the neurological handicap of the treated children remains serious and there is only minor development. Possibly, if treatment is initiated very early on in the neonatal period, prognosis may improve.

34.5 Magnetic Resonance Imaging

Very few imaging data are available on NKH. Progressive cerebral and cerebellar atrophy has been described with ventricular enlargement, enlargement of the subarachnoid spaces and thinning of the corpus callosum. Delay in myelination has been reported after the neonatal period.

In the neonatal phase, MR images similar to those of maple syrup urine disease would have been expected, with abnormalities in the signal intensity of the myelinated areas due to myelin vacuolation (brain stem, in particular brain stem tegmentum, cerebellar white matter and posterior limb of the internal capsule), but these have not been reported.

35 Maple Syrup Urine Disease

35.1 Clinical Features and Laboratory Investigations

Maple syrup urine disease (MSUD) is a heterogeneous disorder. Classification is based on clinical presentation and outcome. Clinically, four phenotypes can be distinguished: classical, intermediate, intermittent and thiamine-responsive forms of MSUD. All forms have an autosomal recessive mode of inheritance.

In classical MSUD, the infants appear normal at birth. By the end of the first week symptoms emerge with lethargy, poor feeding (but rarely vomiting), alternating periods of hypertonia and hypotonia, opisthotonus, convulsions, bulging fontanelle, irregular respiration and apnea. An odor of maple syrup is frequently noted, but may not initially be present. If the disease is not treated, rapidly progressive neurological deterioration occurs with cerebral edema, coma and death usually within the first month of life. If an untreated patient survives the first few weeks of life, signs of severe brain damage remain, with profound psychomotor retardation, generalized dystonia, bilateral ptosis, ophthalmoplegia and facial diplegia.

Early diagnosis and treatment may avert or reverse the neurological abnormalities, but mental and neurological residua are common in treated patients. It has been shown that the length of time after birth that the metabolic derangement is not adequately treated, and the quality of long-term metabolic control both have important influences on eventual intellectual capacities. If the disease is identified and treated within a few days after birth, IQ scores are higher and may be normal. A problem is that intercurrent illnesses, even minor illnesses, may lead to severe metabolic derangement, cerebral edema and possibly death.

In the intermediate variant of MSUD, progressive mental retardation is the major clinical feature, usually becoming apparent during the first year of life. Generalized hypotonia and an odor of maple syrup are present.

In the intermittent form of MSUD, clinical signs are first seen between the ages of 2 months and 40 years, triggered by infection, vaccination, operation or sudden increase in dietary protein. The episodic deterioration is characterized by maple syrup odor, cerebellar ataxia, irritability and progressive lethargy. With sup-portive care the patient recovers, but will experience repeated similar episodes until the correct diagnosis is established and specific dietary treatment started.

In thiamine-responsive MSUD, clinical course of disease tends to be relatively mild, even if untreated, although thiamine responders may also be found among patients with the classical, severe form of the disease. The clinical course of the disease is greatly ameliorated by simultaneous thiamine administration and dietary treatment. Outcome is favorable.

Laboratory investigations reveal a ketoacidosis in episodes of metabolic decompensation. Concentrations of branched-chain amino acids (leucine, valine and isoleucine) and related keto acids (α-ketoisocaproic acid, α-ketoisovaleric acid and α-keto-β-methylvaleric acid) are elevated in blood, urine and CSF. Smaller amounts of the respective 2-hydroxy acids are formed by reduction of the keto acids. An unusual isomer of isoleucine, alloisoleucine, is also found. Diagnosis is confirmed by demonstration of a deficiency of branched-chain keto acid dehydrogenase in leukocytes or cultured fibroblasts.

In the early stages of untreated classical MSUD, EEG shows characteristic abnormalities, variously called a "comb-like", "picket fence" rhythm or "central theta spindle". The pattern consists of bursts and runs of 5–7 Hz primarily monophasic, negative, mu-like activity in the central and central-parasagittal regions during wakefulness and sleep with the most abundant bursts occurring during quiet, non-REM sleep. The background pattern shows diffuse slowing, loss of reactivity to auditory stimuli, suppression-burst patterns, and spike and sharp wave patterns. The abnormalities disappear on treatment. Motor and sensory peripheral nerve conduction velocity is normal.

Prenatal diagnosis can be performed by assessing branched-chain keto acid dehydrogenase in cultured amniocytes or chorionic villus cells. In families with known genomic mutations, DNA analysis can replace the enzyme assay. Heterozygote testing is possible in families with a known mutation.

35.2 Pathology

In young infants, dying in the acute stage of the disease, the brain is enlarged due to generalized edema.

Brain weight is increased. Gyri may be broadened and flattened. Microscopic examination reveals a status spongiosus of myelinated areas. Regions are spared if myelination has not yet started. And so in neonates, the areas involved are the spinal cord, medulla oblongata, dorsal part of pons, mesencephalon, cerebellum, cerebellar pedunculi, and posterior limb of the internal capsule. Sponginess may also be present in the basal nuclei, in particular in the globus pallidus due to its density of myelinated fibers. The sponginess is caused by myelin splitting and vacuolation. No signs of active myelin breakdown are seen and no sudanophilic breakdown products. In the spongy white matter marked astrocytic gliosis is present.

In older, untreated infants neuropathological findings consist of a delay in myelination and, again, a status spongiosus and astrogliosis of the myelinated white matter. Myelin stains reveal myelin paucity, but there is no evidence of active myelin breakdown. There are no phagocytic cells and no or little depositions of sudanophilic breakdown products. The myelin abnormalities occur in all regions and no areas are spared. Gray matter is essentially normal.

In treated infants and children myelination is normal and white matter sponginess is minimal.

35.3 Chemical Pathology

In neonates the lipid composition of the brain is normal or near-normal. In older, untreated infants the findings of chemical analysis of the brain are in conformity with delayed myelination without active myelin breakdown. Major myelin components, including sulfatide, cerebroside and proteolipid protein are significantly reduced. Cholesterol esters are not elevated. Free amino acids in the brain are not altered with the exception of the branched-chain amino acids which are markedly increased. Glutamine, glutamate and GABA are significantly reduced. In older, treated patients, the lipid composition of the brain is normal.

35.4 Pathogenetic Considerations

MSUD is caused by a deficiency of branched-chain α-keto acid dehydrogenase. This is a mitochondrial multi-enzyme complex catalysing the oxidative decarboxylation of branched-chain α-keto acids derived from transamination of branched-chain amino acids such as valine, leucine and isoleucine. The multi-enzyme complex consists of three catalytic components: branched chain α-keto acid decarboxylase (E_1), dihydrolipoyl transacylase (E_2), and dihydrolipoamide dehydrogenase (E_3). E_1 is further composed of two α and two β subunits. The complex also contains two specific regulatory enzymes, a kinase and a phosphatase, compounds that are responsible for regulating the catalytic activity through phosphorylation and dephosphorylation. $E_1\alpha$ is the catalytic subunit which is phosphorylated at two serine residues and hence responsible for regulation of the catalytic activity of the complex. Phosphorylation inactivates and dephosphorylation activates the complex. $E_1\alpha$ binds thiamine pyrophosphate to create the active site for decarboxylation of the keto acid substrate. E_2 forms the structural core of the enzyme complex to which E_1, E_3, kinase and phosphatase are bound. E_3 is identical to the dehydrogenases associated with pyruvate dehydrogenase and α-ketoglutarate dehydrogenase complexes.

The enzyme complex has six components. Thus, there are at least six genetic loci encoding this multienzyme complex and a mutation in any of these loci can result in dysfunction of the branched chain α-keto acid dehydrogenase complex. $E_1\alpha$ has been mapped to chromosome 19 at position q13.1–13.3; $E_1 \beta$ has been mapped to chromosome 6 at position p21–22; E_2 has been mapped to chromosome 1 at position p21–31 and E_3 has been mapped to chromosome 7 at position q31–32. In classical MSUD, mutations in the $E_1\alpha$, $E_1 \beta$ and E_2 genes have been found; most mutations identified so far affect the E_2 subunit. Compound heterozygotes having two different mutations within a subunit have also been reported. Patients with a deficiency of E_3 activity have combined lactic aciduria and branched-chain keto aciduria.

The process of understanding the molecular genetic basis of MSUD has started, but no clear relationship between genotype and phenotype has yet emerged. There is some relationship between clinical phenotype and residual enzyme activity. In classical MSUD, the ability to decarboxylate leucine by intact cells is less than 2% of normal. In intermittent MSUD, leucine decarboxylation ability is between 2% and 40% of normal.

All patients with thiamine-responsive MSUD have some residual enzyme activity. Administration of pharmacological doses of thiamine leads to enhanced tolerance to intake of branched-chain amino acids, but patients still need a continued, moderate restriction of these amino acids. Pharmacological doses of thiamine alone will not restore normal enzyme function. The biochemical mechanisms for thiamine responsiveness probably consist of a stabilizing effect of thiamine on the mutant enzyme complex.

Mechanisms for toxic effects of increased branched-chain amino acids and keto acids remain largely unelucidated. The toxic effects may be related to disturbance of neurotransmission, energy depletion and direct myelin damage. Branched-chain keto acids and their hydroxyderivatives compete with glutamate for decarboxylation and so reduce GABA production. Excess leucine may reduce cerebral serotonin. Ketoisocaproic acid inhibits pyruvate dehydrogenase and α-ketoglutarate dehydrogenase, two important enzymes in mitochondrial energy production.

Hexachlorophene and triethyltin are toxins which also lead to myelin vacuolation. These substances are inhibitors of mitochondrial oxidative phosphorylation. From experimental studies it is known that lasting effects only follow chronic exposure and that early discontinuation of exposure is followed by repair. This course of events is similar to that observed in MSUD: early treatment leads to resolution of abnormalities. Only in untreated cases are lasting effects seen. The precise pathophysiological mechanisms of myelin splitting are unknown, either in exogenous intoxications or in MSUD.

35.5 Therapy

In cases of acute metabolic decompensation with very high blood and tissue levels of branched chain amino acids and keto acids, emergency treatment is necessary. Exchange transfusions, peritoneal dialysis and hemodialysis are effective in acutely ill patients. These therapeutic measures should be supplemented by high energy intake to reverse the catabolic condition caused by infection or fasting. For this purpose intravenous glucose, intravenous lipids or a special formula containing a mixture of complete nutrients, lacking only branched-chain amino acids, can be used. Concomitant administration of insulin is very effective in achieving an anabolic situation. In acutely ill but not comatose patients, the nutritional therapy may be sufficient. During the course of therapy, isoleucine and valine should be added to the regimen to prevent depletion of these essential amino acids and thus ensure effective protein synthesis.

Minor illnesses may lead to catabolic conditions with release of amino acids from body tissues. Toxic levels of branched-chain amino acids may be reached within a few hours with onset of as yet mild clinical symptoms. Immediate high energy intake and temporary removal of all natural protein from the diet may prevent a full-blown metabolic decompensation. Catabolic conditions after surgery can be prevented by administration of insulin and a branched-chain amino acid-free parenteral nutrition regimen.

All patients with classical MSUD require life-long dietary treatment. The long-term treatment aims at maintaining the whole-body content of branched-chain amino acids close to the minimum requirement for normal body function. The amount of branched-chain amino acids necessary for adequate protein synthesis is given in the form of natural proteins in a protein-restricted diet. A branched-chain amino acid-free mixture of amino acids is used to supplement the diet. The levels of branched-chain amino acids in blood are measured regularly to monitor treatment. Deficiency of branch-chain amino acids leads to growth failure, skin rash and exfoliative dermatitis.

If onset of dietary treatment leads to lowering of blood levels of branched chain amino acids within a few days after birth and if adequate dietary control is maintained over the years prognosis is excellent and intellectual capacities may be normal. Later onset of treatment or poor dietary control contribute to mental deficiency.

With adequate dietary treatment and careful monitoring, female MSUD patients may enjoy successful pregnancies.

Patients with milder forms of MSUD tolerate a higher protein intake.

In thiamine-responsive MSUD, use of thiamine increases protein tolerance. However, a protein restricted diet should be used and the plasma levels of branched-chain amino acids monitored.

35.6 Magnetic Resonance Imaging

In MSUD with neonatal presentation, CT shows a very characteristic pattern with hypodensity and swelling of the cerebellar hemispheres, dorsal part of pons, mesencephalon, posterior limb of the internal capsule, the globus pallidus, and often the thalamus (Fig. 35.1). In addition, a mild, generalized, cerebral white matter hypodensity is seen.

MRI confirms the pattern. On T_2-weighted images swelling and high signal intensity is seen in the posterior part of the pons, in the mesencephalon, the cerebellar white matter, posterior limb of the internal capsule, lateral thalamus and globus pallidus (Fig. 35.1). Besides, mild diffuse edema is present. Without treatment edema gradually decreases and atrophy ensues. Edema is most pronounced between the third week and the end of the second month. With treatment edema resolves more rapidly. Remaining abnormalities are variable, depending on the severity and duration of the initial episode of metabolic derangement. In some cases MRI becomes normal. In others delay in myelination and some signs of atrophy are found.

Milder variants of MSUD usually come to medical attention in the second year of life because of retarded development. CT and MRI at that time show diffuse abnormality of the white matter of both the cerebellum and the cerebral hemispheres (Fig. 35.2). The internal and external capsules and the brain stem are involved. Both the thalamus and globus pallidus are affected, whereas putamen and caudate nucleus are normal. Also the cortex is normal. Improvement after treatment

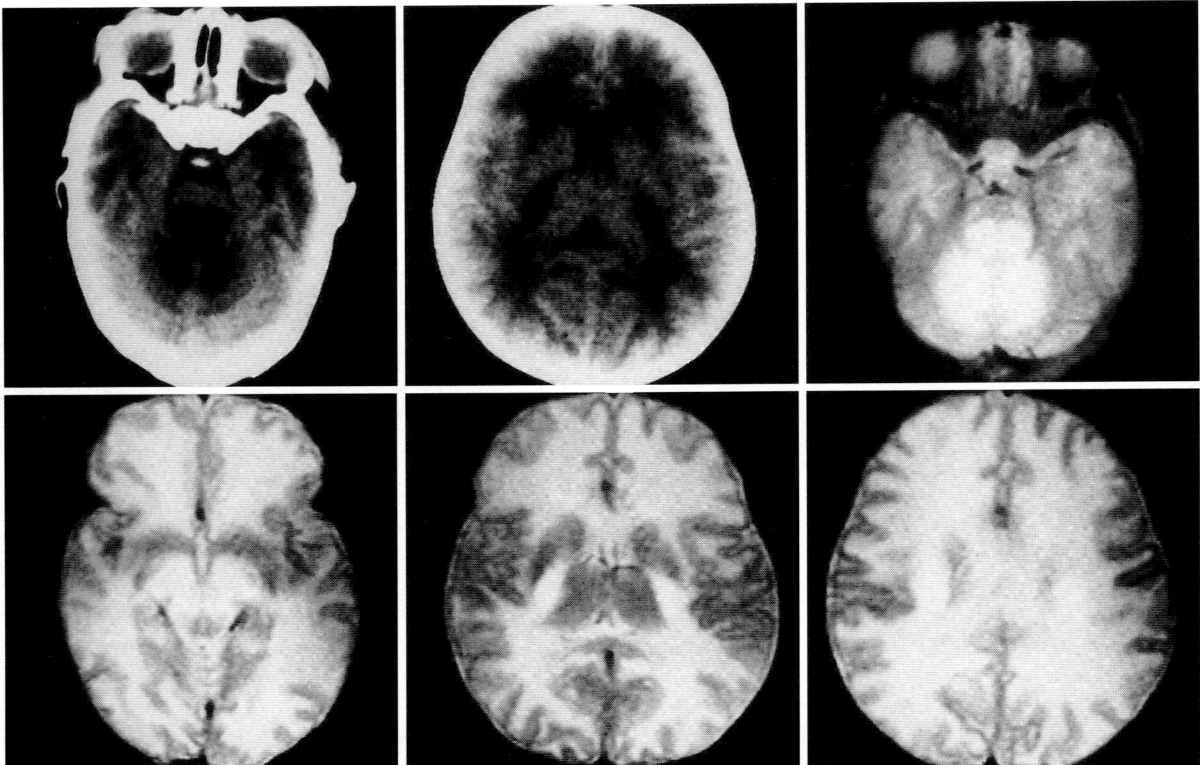

Fig. 35.1. MSUD in a neonate. On CT (*upper row, left and middle*) low density of the white matter is seen, particularly conspicuous in the cerebellum, dorsal part of the pons and internal capsule. MRI (*upper row, right; lower row*) shows very high signal intensity and swelling in the cerebellar white mat- ter, the dorsal part of the pons, the mesencephalon and the posterior limb of the internal capsule. The remainder of the cerebral white matter shows some increase in signal intensity and some swelling, but less severe. Courtesy of Brismar et al. (1990), with permission

has been reported. In earlier treated variant cases CT and MRI may be normal.

If MRI is performed during an episode of metabolic decompensation in adequately treated and normally developing children with classical MSUD, it has been reported to show diffuse brain swelling and abnormally increased signal intensity on T_2-weighted images in the subcortical U fibers, periventricular white matter, posterior limb of the internal capsule, brain stem, putamen and caudate nucleus. If adequate treatment is initiated immediately, most or all abnormalities disappear.

The images of patients with classical MSUD during the neonatal period are diagnostic. All areas which are normally myelinated at that age have an abnormal signal intensity and are swollen. This pattern is exclusively seen in vacuolating myelinopathies of neonatal onset. The images of patients with milder variants of MSUD during the second year of life are very similar to those of Canavan's disease. However, clinical history and laboratory findings differentiate between the two.

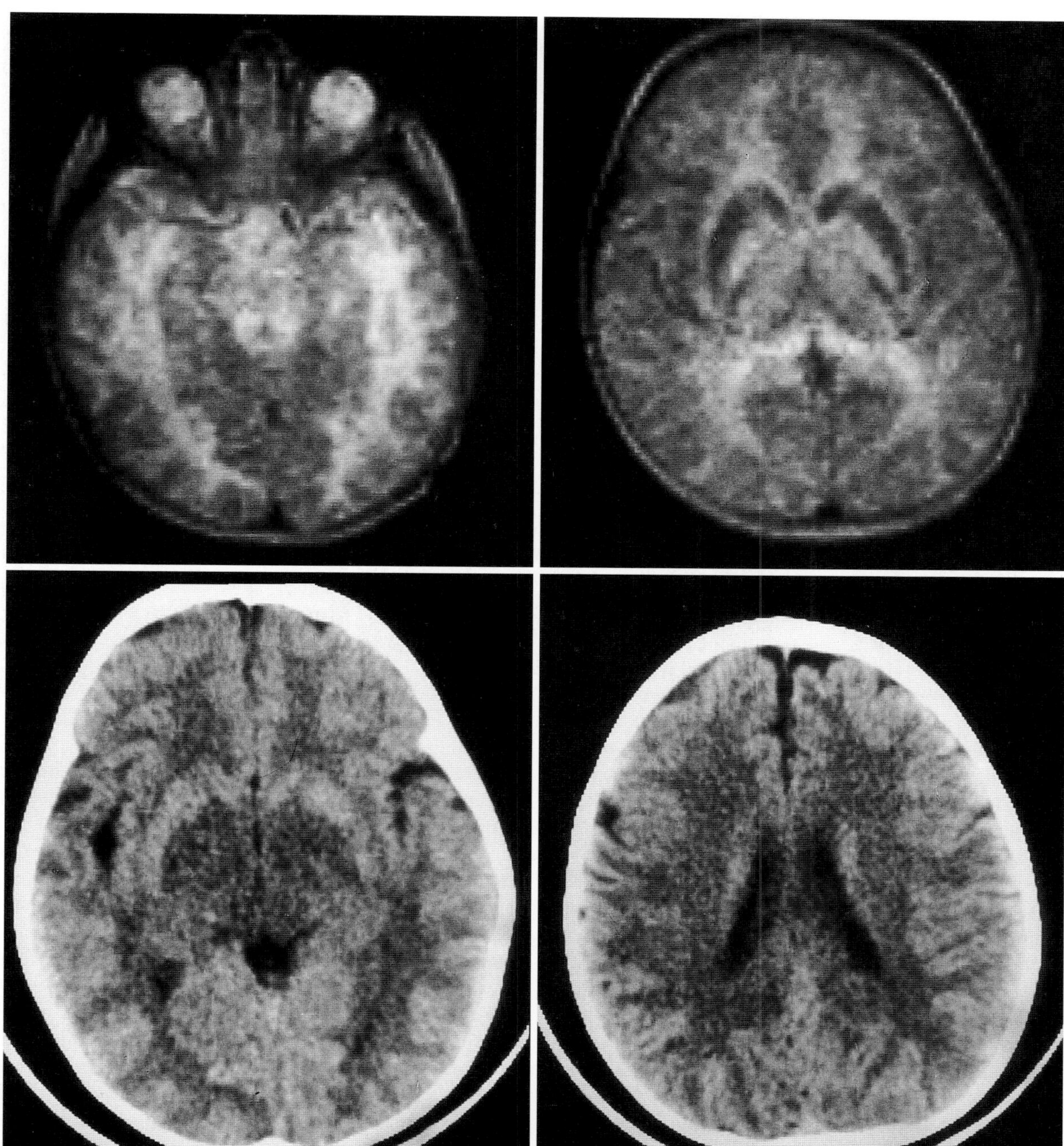

Fig. 35.2. Late form of MSUD in a baby boy of 18 months. In this MSUD of later onset CT scans (*lower row*) show low density in the cerebral hemispheres, the globus pallidus and thalamus. The MR images (*upper row*) show a hyperintense signal in the white matter, with involvement of the brain stem and relative sparing of the posterior limb of the internal capsule. Thalami and globus pallidi have an abnormally high signal; the nucleus caudatus and putamen are normal. The MR image has many features in common with Canavan's disease. Courtesy of Uziel et al. (1988), with permission

36 Canavan's Disease

36.1 Clinical Features and Laboratory Investigations

Canavan's disease (CD) is a rare hereditary neurological disorder affecting infants and children. The disease is also called spongy degeneration of the CNS of the Van Bogaert-Bertrand type. CD has an autosomal recessive mode of inheritance. It is most frequently found in children of Jewish Ashkenazi or Saudi Arabian origin.

The infantile form of CD is the most common. The patients appear normal at birth and the initial stages of development are normal. The disease usually becomes apparent within the first 6 months of life. Early signs include hypotonia with poor head control, decreased motor activity, irritability, visual loss, poor sucking ability and accelerated skull growth. The abnormal increase in skull growth results in macrocephaly. Failure of developmental progress and regression occur. Gradually, hypotonia of arms and legs is replaced by spasticity and tonic extensor spasms may occur. Axial hypotonia persists. Blindness with coarse nystagmoid eye movements and pale optic discs at funduscopy become evident. Occasionally deafness is noted. Choreoathetosis, dystonia and tonic or myoclonic seizures occur in some patients. Eventually a chronic vegetative state with decerebrate or decorticate rigidity appears. Autonomic crises may occur with episodically increased vasomotor responses, disturbed temperature regulation and vomiting. The patients generally die before the age of 4 years. However, a considerable number of patients has a more protracted course with a life-expectancy beyond 10 years.

In the congenital variety children may appear normal at birth or may be in a poor condition. During the first few days after birth, inactivity and lethargy become manifest. The children cry frequently and exhibit difficulties in sucking and swallowing. They are hypotonic. They die within a few days or weeks.

A few case reports of juvenile variants of CD have appeared in the literature, but in these cases the diagnosis has not been verified biochemically, since they date from a period before definitive metabolic diagnosis was possible. No biochemically proven case with juvenile phenotype has been reported.

Laboratory investigations in CD are diagnostic. An increased amount of N-acetylaspartic acid is found in urine and plasma. CSF protein is sometimes raised. EEG is diffusely slow with paroxysmal features. Evoked potentials are delayed or absent. Nerve conduction velocity is normal. Decreased activity of the enzyme aspartoacylase is found in cultured fibroblasts. Carrier detection is possible. Prenatal diagnosis can be performed by assessment of enzyme activity in amniocytes and chorionic cells, but these techniques are unreliable owing to the low levels of aspartoacylase in these cells. Assessment of the level of N-acetylaspartate in amniotic fluid is more reliable. DNA techniques are being developed.

36.2 Pathology

The brain is abnormally enlarged in CD. Otherwise the external appearance of the cerebral gyri, cerebellum, and brain stem are normal. On sectioning, an ill-defined demarcation between cortex and white matter is seen in all parts of the cerebral and cerebellar hemispheres. The deeper cortex and subcortical white matter are edematous and soft. There is no tendency towards cavitation. During the first few years, the ventricles are slightly narrowed. Thereafter, they gradually increase in size as a result of loss of tissue.

Histological examination shows vacuolation with presence of innumerable minor cavities, most striking in the subcortical cerebral white matter and in the deep layers of the cortex, giving the affected areas a spongy appearance. No substances can be demonstrated within the vacuoles. Myelin degeneration is present in a pattern that closely follows the status spongiosus. In the subcortical area moderate to severe loss of myelin is seen, but axons and oligodendrocytes are largely intact. The periventricular white matter, corpus callosum, internal capsule and fornix are less severely vacuolated and their myelin content is better preserved. Myelin vacuolation and loss is accompanied by astrogliosis. Myelin breakdown products are scarce; some sudanophilic lipids may be present in macrophages. Cortical neurons are normal in number and appearance, while intracortical myelin is lost.

Within the cortex, there is a marked proliferation of astroglia. Their nuclei are abnormally large, variably shaped with unevenly dispersed nuclear chromatin which tends to accumulate near the nuclear membrane. These cells are also seen in the subcortical white matter, but they do not prevail in other areas of vacuolated white matter. They are so-called Alzheimer type II cells.

On electron microscopy, the vacuoles observed in the white matter appear to be formed as a result of separation of myelin lamellae with intramyelinic vacuole formation. Splitting of the myelin lamellae occurs at the intraperiod lines, where external surfaces of the original oligodendroglial membrane were closely apposed in the formation of the myelin sheath. The swollen astrocytes with enlarged nuclei and watery cytoplasm contribute to the vacuolated aspect, in particular within the cortex. On electron microscopy these cells are shown to contain abnormal, enormously elongated mitochrondria.

Sponginess is also present in the globus pallidus and thalamus, whereas caudate nucleus and in particular putamen tend to be better preserved. Alzheimer type II cells are present in the basal ganglia.

Within the cerebellum the most severe vacuolation is seen in the Purkinje cell layer, the deeper areas of the granule cell layer and the subcortical white matter. Purkinje cells and granule cells are well preserved. Myelin loss is accompanied by astrocytosis, but axons are spared. The deep white matter of the cerebellum is better preserved. Vacuolation is present in the dentate nucleus, but nerve cells are intact.

Vacuolation, demyelination and astrocytosis are present in midbrain, pons, medulla and spinal cord, both in descending and ascending tracts. Cranial nerve nuclei, other brain stem nuclei and spinal cord gray matter show a variable degree of vacuolation. However, involvement of brain stem and spinal cord is more variable and severe. The optic nerve, containing CNS myelin, is involved in the process. The other cranial nerves, the spinal roots and the peripheral nerves are normal.

In protracted infantile patients, who survive for a relatively long time, the lateral ventricles are markedly dilated as a result of severe loss of white matter tissue. Myelin is now also lost in the deep white matter. In addition, neuronal loss is severe, and vacuolation is seen in all layers of the cortex.

In the congenital variant the sponginess is most severe in the cerebellum and brain stem, which are the parts with the highest myelin content at that time.

36.3 Chemical Pathology

In CD, chemical abnormalities in the brain are limited to the white matter; the chemical composition of the gray matter is near normal. The most prominent white matter abnormality is its increased water content. There is a drastic decrease in myelin lipids and protein as manifestations of the severe myelin loss. There is a marked decrease of galactolipids and a relatively smaller decrease in cholesterol and total phospholipids. No cholesterol esters are detected in the white matter.

The composition of myelin is altered. Cholesterol is increased, and phospholipids are decreased, especially ethanolamine phosphyglycerides. Galactolipids are severely diminished, cerebroside more so than sulfatide. The total ganglioside concentration is normal.

This abnormal pattern of white matter and myelin composition is also seen in several other diseases and is probably a result of nonspecific destruction of myelin.

Electrolyte analyses show that the composition of the excess fluid in the brain of a CD patient is similar to that of plasma ultrafiltrate.

36.4 Pathogenetic Considerations

Kvittingen et al. (1986) reported on a patient with macrocephaly, leukodystrophy, progressive cerebral atrophy and massive N-acetylaspartic aciduria. The first patient with a leukodystrophy and N-acetylaspartic aciduria, in whom a deficiency of aspartoacylase was demonstrated, was reported by Hagenfeldt et al. (1987). Matalon et al. (1988) correlated aspartoacylase deficiency with CD by demonstrating the characteristic spongy degeneration at brain biopsy in children with N-acetylaspartic aciduria. The gene for aspartoacylase has been identified and mutations have been described in CD families.

N-acetylaspartate is synthesized from acetyl-CoA and aspartate by L-aspartate-N-acetyl transferase exclusively in the CNS. It is metabolized to aspartate and acetate by aspartoacylase. In deficiency of aspartoacylase N-acetylaspartate concentrations in the brain are elevated and the substance is excreted in large amounts in the urine.

The brain is the only organ in which the biosynthesis of N-acetylaspartate has been demonstrated. Its concentration in the brain is very high and higher in gray than in white matter. It has been shown that N-acetylaspartate is mainly or exclusively localized in neurons. To date, the functional role of this compound has not been elucidated. Some suggest it is an inert metabolite. Others suggest it is involved in neurotransmission. N-acetylaspartate is converted to aspartate and has been implicated in the formation of glutamate. Both aspartate and glutamate are excitatory neurotransmitters. The high concentration of N-acetylaspartate in neurons may be a form of chemical compartmentation serving neurotransmission. It has been proposed that N-acetylaspartate is an acetyl group donor in the synthesis of brain lipids, including myelin lipids. In particular, the substance would be important in the formation of cerebronic acid, which is a precursor of ceramide, which in turn is a constituent of sulfatide and cerebroside. Some others suggest N-acetylaspartate is important in protein synthesis.

The relationship between accumulation of N-acetylaspartate and myelin vacuolation and formation of abnormal astrocytes has not been elucidated. Those who suggest that the substance is essential for the normal synthesis of myelin lipids, explain the myelin abnormality by faulty formation of one of its constituents. However, the chemical composition of myelin in CD shows merely nonspecific abnormalities related to the myelin breakdown process and no specific deficiencies of some of its components. Others suggest that accumulation of N-acetylaspartate may have toxic effects leading to myelin splitting. In this respect, the comparison to hexachlorophene intoxication and triethyltin intoxication is important, as both conditions are characterized by myelin splitting, vacuolation and loss, and presence of Alzheimer type II cells with abnormal mitochondria, as is the case in CD. Hexachlorophene and triethyltin both interfere with mitochondrial oxidative phosphorylation. N-acetylaspartate is synthesized in mitochondria and if this substance accumulates, its toxic effects may well be mainly exerted in these organelles. However, the relationship between possible mitochondrial dysfunction and myelin vacuolation is unclear. In a recent study no signs of mitochondrial dysfunction could be found (De Coo et al. 1991), in contrast to earlier studies in which abnormalities in mitochondrial Na^+/K^+-ATPase were reported (Adachi et al. 1966, 1972).

Recently, two highly unusual cases of aspartoacylase deficiency were reported by Toft et al. (1993). The clinical disease was much milder than in the usual form of CD, with normocephaly, epilepsy and mild psychomotor retardation without regression at any time up to the age of 6 years. MR images did not show white matter changes but abnormal signal intensity in globus pallidus, putamen and caudate nucleus. The nature of this condition awaits further elucidation. It is important to recognize that the assessment of aspartoacylase activity is difficult and not always reliable. One should, therefore, hesitate before establishing a diagnosis of "atypical CD" without confirmation by DNA techniques.

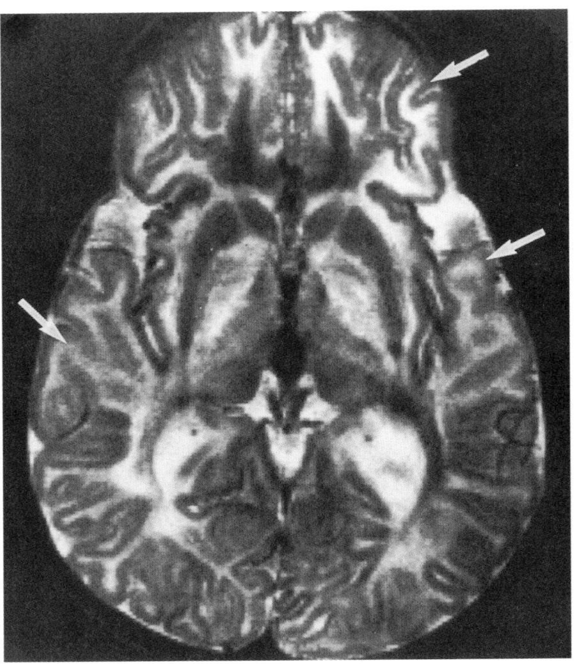

Fig. 36.1. Patient with CD. The subcortical white matter is extensively involved (*arrows*), whereas the periventricular white matter is partially spared. Note the involvement of the globus pallidus, contrasting with the sparing of putamen and caudate nucleus. Courtesy of Runge et al. (1988), with permission

36.5 Therapy

At present, no specific therapy is available for CD patients.

36.6 Magnetic Resonance Imaging

CT shows diffuse hypodensity of the white matter of cerebral hemispheres and cerebellum. Involvement of the globus pallidus with sparing of caudate nucleus and putamen is usually seen.

In all stages of the disease, MRI shows the most severe abnormalities in the subcortical white matter of cerebrum and cerebellum (Figs. 36.1–36.3). Central white matter structures, such as the periventricular rim of white matter, internal capsule, corpus callosum and brain stem are preserved longer (Figs. 36.1, 36.2). As the disease progresses, the central white matter also becomes involved (Fig. 36.3). Thus, the spread of the white matter changes is centripetal. The subcortical white matter has a mildly swollen aspect, broadening the gyri. In contrast to pachygyria the thickness of the cortex is normal. The white matter abnormalities are always confluent and are symmetrical in distribution.

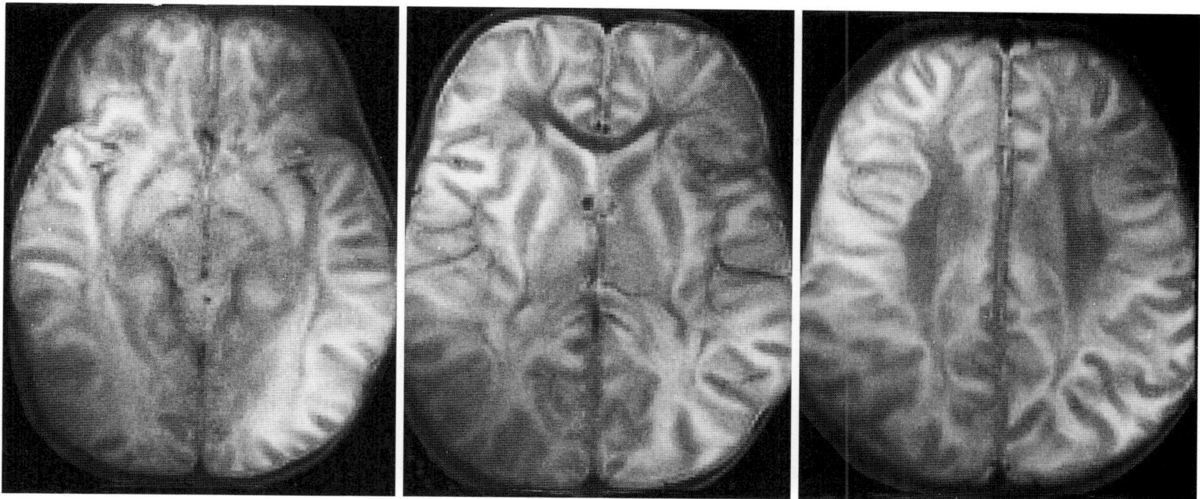

Fig. 36.2. A 21-month-old boy with CD. These mildly T_2-weighted images show the involvement of the subcortical white matter, globus pallidus, and, to a lesser extent, of the thalamus. The corpus callosum, periventricular white matter and posterior limb of the internal capsule are spared. Courtesy of Meyding-Lamadé and Sartor (1993), with permission

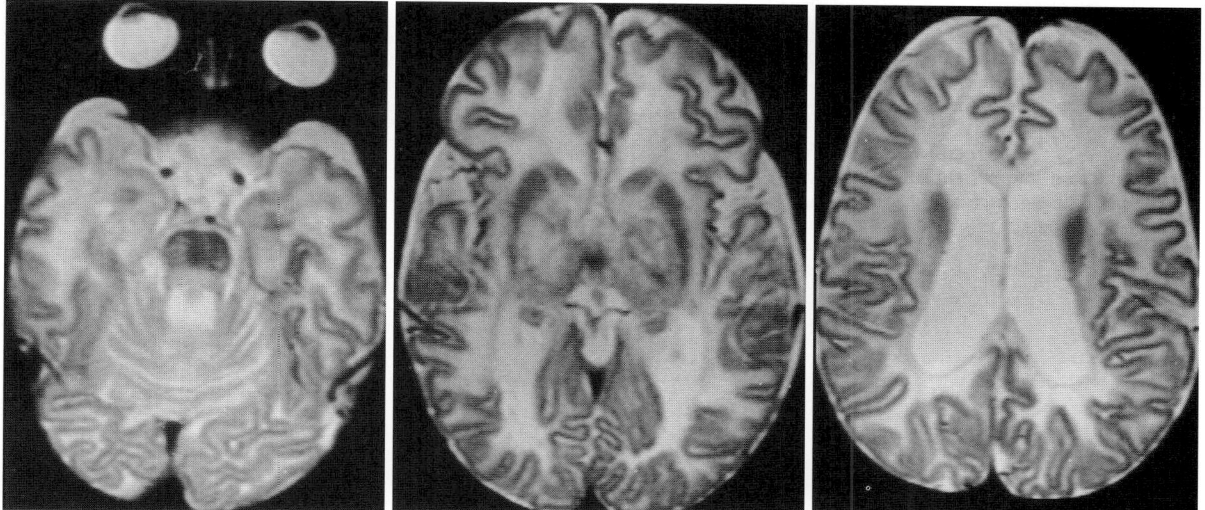

Fig. 36.3. A 32-month-old child with CD. These T_2-weighted images show there is now involvement of all white matter structures, including corpus callosum and periventricular white matter. The globus pallidus and thalamus are involved bilaterally. The brain stem is relatively, but not completely spared. There are signs of diffuse atrophy. Courtesy of Kendall (1992), with permission

Bilateral involvement of the globus pallidus is always seen (Fig. 36.1–36.3), involvement of the thalamus regularly (Fig. 36.3). The resulting image with sparing of putamen and caudate nucleus is very typical for CD.

After several years cerebral atrophy ensues with enlargement of the ventricular system and subarachnoid spaces (Fig. 36.3). Cerebellar atrophy is also evident.

The differential diagnosis of diffusely swollen white matter changes includes mainly late onset variants of maple syrup urine disease, Alexander's disease, congenital muscular dystrophy and the disease described as infantile-onset spongiform leukoencephalopathy with a discrepantly mild clinical course. In the presence of lesions of the globus pallidus with preservation of the caudate nucleus and putamen, the images are highly suggestive of CD, but maple syrup urine disease should be excluded by biochemical tests.

37 L-2-Hydroxyglutaric Aciduria

37.1 Clinical Features and Laboratory Investigations

L-2-Hydroxyglutaric aciduria is a rare neurometabolic disorder with autosomal recessive inheritance. The children are initially normal. In the second year of life a delay in unsupported walking, abnormal gait, speech delay or febrile convulsions form the presenting symptoms in most cases. In other patients no abnormalities are noted until learning disabilities become apparent during early school years. Over the years slowly progressive neurological dysfunction is noted, characterized predominantly by cerebellar ataxia with nystagmus, dysarthria, head titubation, trunk ataxia, dysmetria and intention tremor. Slow intellectual decline is noted in all patients. Frequently noted abnormalities are extrapyramidal signs such as dystonia and choreoathetosis, pyramidal signs, pseudobulbar signs, myoclonus, and macrocephaly. Seizures occur in the majority of the patients.

Laboratory investigations reveal elevated urinary excretion of L-2-hydroxyglutaric acid; plasma and CSF levels are also increased. Lysine levels in urine, plasma and CSF may also be elevated.

37.2 Pathology

Only few descriptions of brain pathology are available. In one case histological findings were described as polycystic white matter degeneration (Kaabachi et al. 1993); in another as patchy loss of myelin with reactive astrocytes and enlarged perivascular spaces in the white matter (Wilcken et al. 1993). In 1994, Larnaout et al. described diffuse demyelination, spongiosis and cystic cavitation of the cerebral white matter in a patient who died at the age of 30 years. The abnormalities were most pronounced in the subcortical region, in the axis of cerebral convolutions. In the cerebellum, loss of granule cells and Purkinje cells and moderate pallor of the white matter were noted. The dentate nucleus and globus pallidus showed marked cell loss and severe spongiosis. The putamen and caudate nucleus were less severely affected. Myelin was normal in the corpus callosum, genu of the internal capsule, optic tracts and optic radiations. Cerebral cortex, thalamus, brain stem and spinal cord were normal.

37.3 Pathogenetic Considerations

The basic defect in L-2-hydroxyglutaric aciduria is not known. The disease has only recently been defined (Barth et al. 1992, 1993). It has been shown that L-2-hydroxyglutaric acid is degraded in a dehydrogenase reaction. Possibly, a deficiency of L-2-hydroxyglutarate dehydrogenase is responsible for the disease. The elevations of lysine may be secondary rather than primary, as lysine loading appears to have no effect on the level of L-2-hydroxyglutaric acid.

37.4 Therapy

As yet no treatment is available.

37.5 Magnetic Resonance Imaging

MRI in patients with L-2-hydroxyglutaric aciduria shows a highly characteristic and consistent pattern. The abnormalities begin within the subcortical white matter with multiple foci of high signal intensity on T_2-weighted images (Fig. 37.1). The lesions have a tendency to become confluent, first in the frontoparietal region (Fig. 37.2), later involving all subcortical white matter in a confluent manner. The white matter abnormalities are mildly swollen with some broadening of the gyri (Fig. 37.2). The aspect of swollen white matter changes suggests that the basic histopathological abnormality may be a spongiform leukoencephalopathy. Centrally located white matter structures, such as periventricular white matter, corpus callosum, internal capsule, and brain stem are spared. The caudate nucleus is atrophic and the lateral ventricles are slightly enlarged. Changes in signal intensity are seen in the caudate nucleus and globus pallidus in some patients (Fig. 37.1).

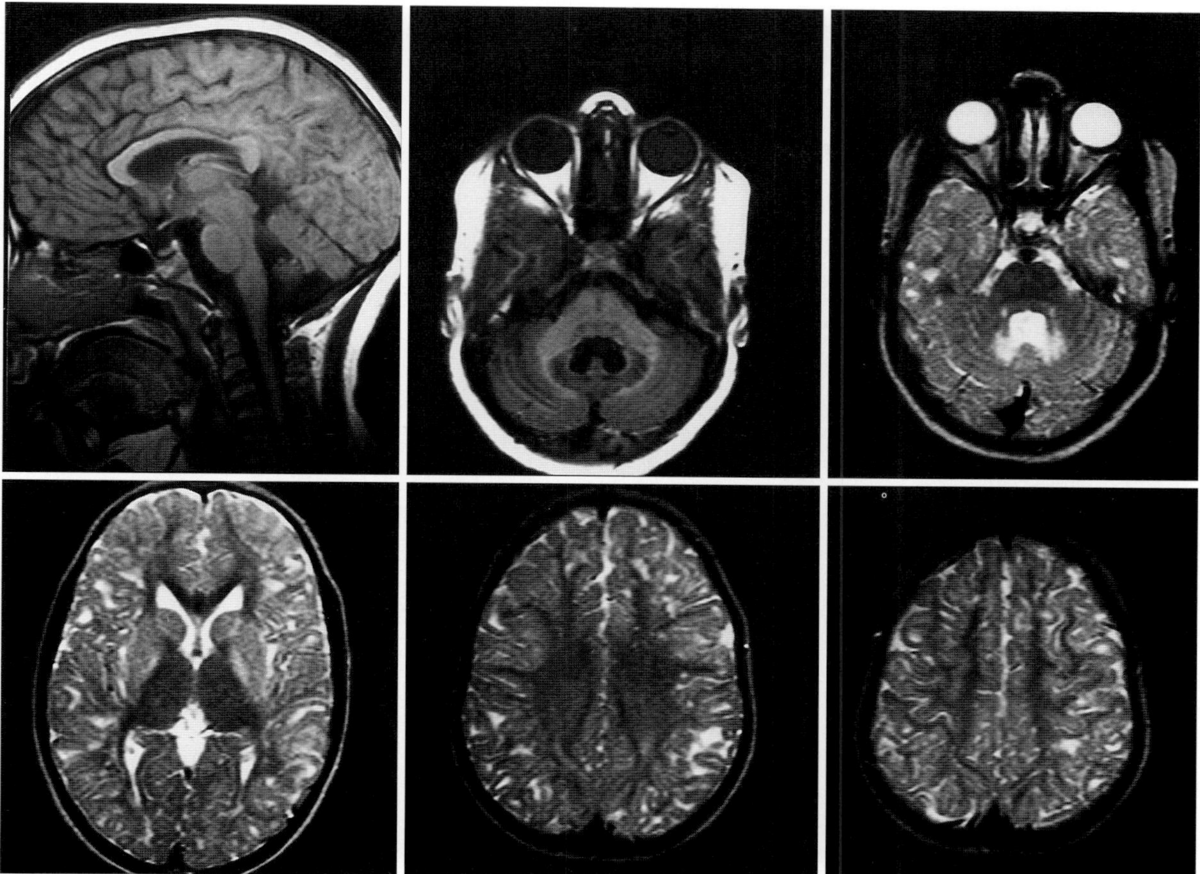

Fig. 37.1. A 10-year-old boy, who has L-2-hydroxyglutaric aciduria, showing the involvement of subcortical white matter and the sparing of the central white matter including the corpus callosum. Lesions are also present in the nucleus dentatus and globus pallidus; part of the vermis inferior is absent

The cerebellar vermis is highly atrophic in all patients. The cerebellar hemispheres are also atrophic, but less severely. In the dentate nucleus a change in signal intensity is present (Figs. 37.1, 37.2). The cerebellar white matter is normal.

The pattern of symmetrical abnormalities with supratentorial subcortical white matter lesions, infratentorial atrophy of the cerebellum (vermis more than hemispheres) and lesions in both dentate nuclei has never been described in any other disorder. As far as is presently known, it is pathognomonic.

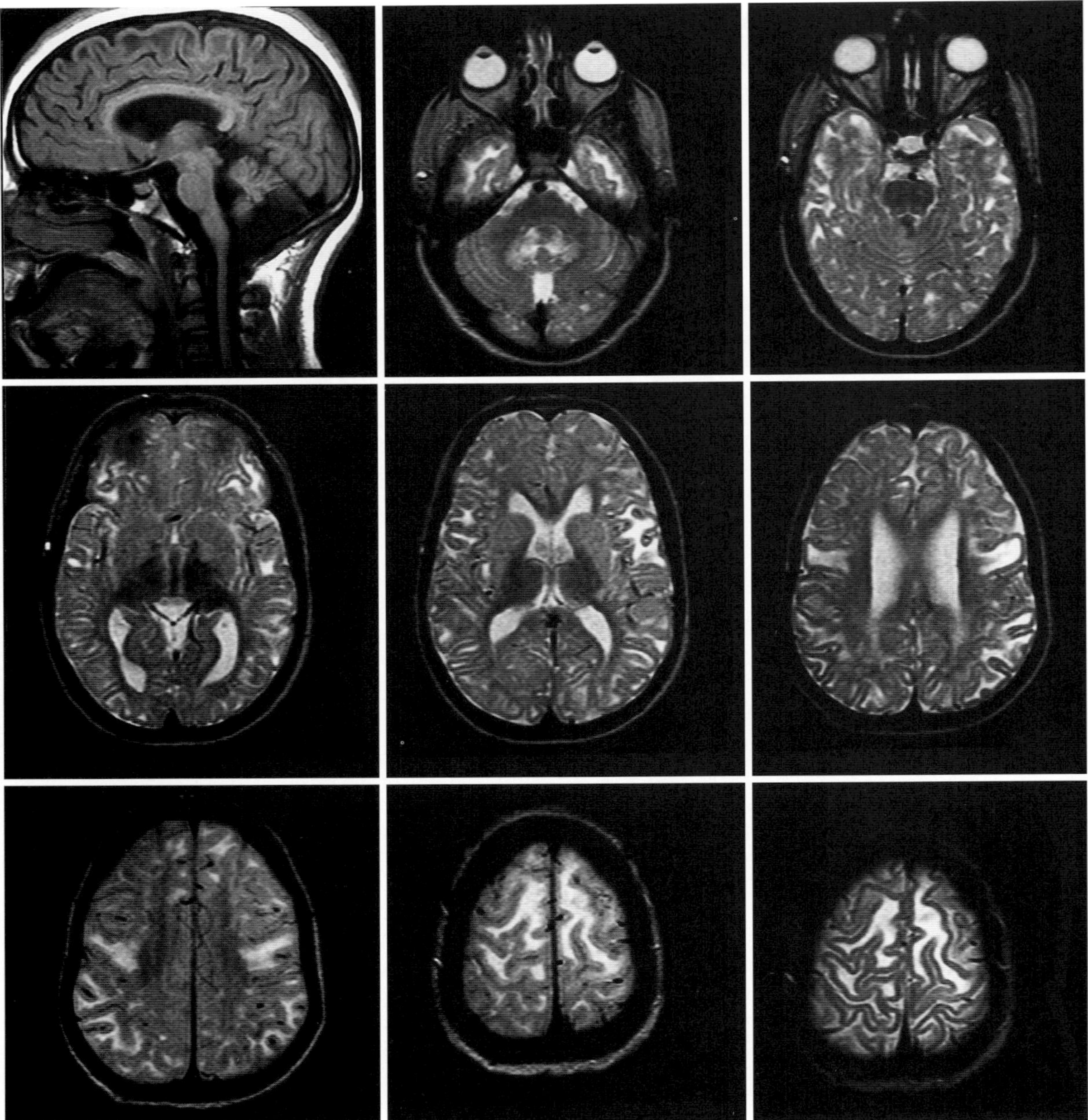

Fig. 37.2. MR images of the 16-year-old brother of the patient described in Fig. 37.1, showing the typical features of L-2-hydroxyglutaric aciduria: atrophy of the cerebellar vermis, and irregular involvement of the subcortical white matter with focal signs of some white matter swelling. The nucleus dentatus is also affected

38 Hyperhomocysteinemias

38.1 Introduction

Hyperhomocysteinemias are associated with a diversity of neurological problems, ranging from mental retardation to signs of subacute combined degeneration of cord and brain, and to cerebral infarctions.

Homocysteine lies at an important branch point of sulfur amino acid metabolism. It is formed from methionine by demethylation. It may either be converted to cysteine through the transsulfuration reaction or remethylated to form methionine. Remethylation to methionine requires methyl donors such as betaine or 5-methyltetrahydrofolate. The metabolism of homocysteine requires folate and cobalamin (vitamin B_{12}) (Fig. 38.1). Consequently, a number of defects may underly hyperhomocysteinemia: a defect in the transsulfuration pathway, a defect in cobalamin metabolism and a defect in folate metabolism.

The most common defect of the transulfuration pathway and the most frequent cause of severe hyperhomocysteinemia is a deficiency of cystathionine β-synthetase. This enzyme normally catalyzes the conversion of homocysteine to cystathionine, which is converted to cysteine.

5,10-Methylenetetrahydrofolate reductase deficiency is the most common defect of folate metabolism. This enzyme deficiency leads to a lack of 5-methyltetrahydrofolate, a cosubstrate for the methionine synthetase reaction, which in turn leads to an impairment of the remethylation of homocysteine to methionine.

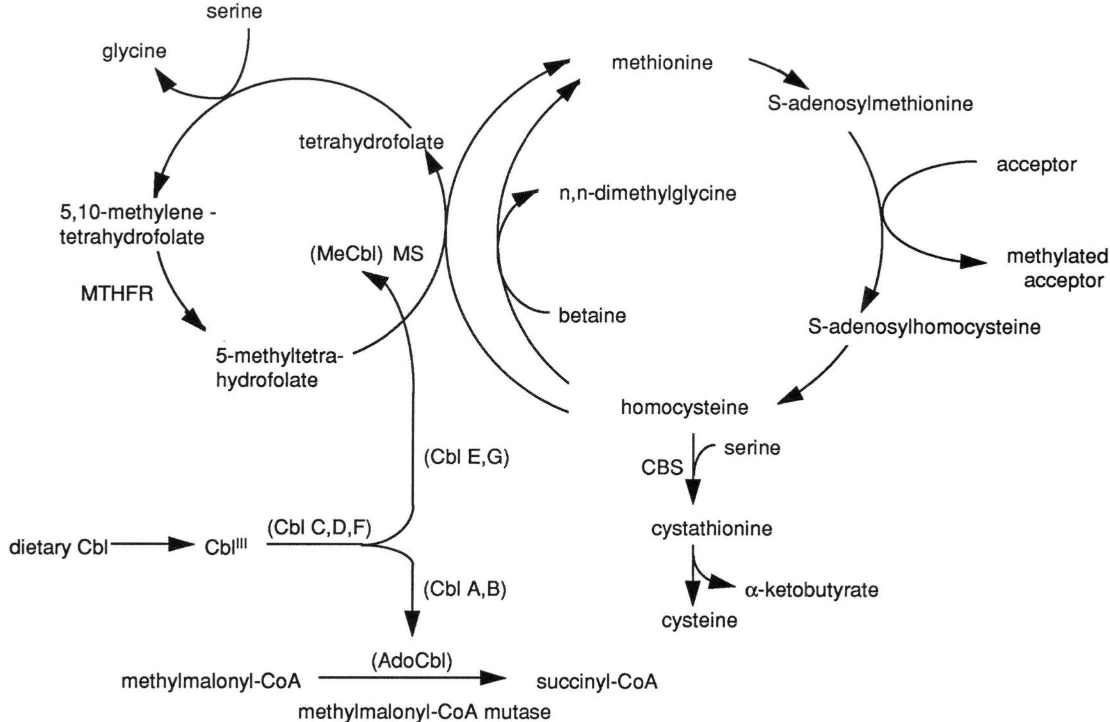

Fig. 38.1. Homocysteine metabolism

Deficiency of methionine synthetase, also known as methyltetrahydrofolate: homocysteine methyltransferase, is not known in human patients.

Folic acid deficiency leads to a disturbance of the folate cycle and, as a consequence, to hyperhomocysteinemia.

Inborn errors affecting intracellular cobalamin metabolism lead to a deficiency of methylcobalamin and/or adenosylcobalamin. Methylcobalamin is an essential cofactor for methionine synthetase, the enzyme catalyzing the conversion of homocysteine to methionine. Adenosylcobalamin is a cofactor for methylmalonyl-CoA mutase. The inborn errors of cobalamin metabolism can be divided into three main groups: isolated defects in methylcobalamin synthesis, isolated defects in adenosylcobalamin synthesis and defects in the synthesis of both methylcobalamin and adenosylcobalamin. The patients with isolated defects in methylcobalamin synthesis can be divided into two complementation groups (CblE and CblG), which are very similar clinically and biochemically with the presence of hyperhomocysteinemia. The patients with isolated defects in adenosylcobalamin synthesis can be divided into two complementation groups, designated CblA and CblB. Biochemically they are characterized by methylmalonic aciduria without hyperhomocysteinemia. As hyperhomocysteinemia is not present in these diseases, they are not discussed in this chapter. Among the patients with a defect in the synthesis of methylcobalamin and adenosylcobalamin three complementation groups can be distinguished (CblC, CblD, and CblF). Biochemically they are characterized by presence of both hyperhomocysteinemia and methylmalonic aciduria.

Cobalamin cannot be synthesized by the body and is dietary in origin. Deficiency leads to a disturbance of function of both methionine synthetase and methylmalonyl-CoA mutase and consequently to a combination of hyperhomocysteinemia and methylmalonic aciduria.

So-called mild hyperhomocysteinemia, both in the fasting state and after methionine loading, can be the consequence of heterozygosity for cystathionine β-synthetase deficiency. Heterozygosity for 5,10-methylenetetrahydrofolate reductase deficiency does not lead to hyperhomocysteinemia. However, homozygosity for a mutant form of 5,10-methylenetetrahydrofolate reductase, characterized by thermolability, can lead to mild hyperhomocysteinemia, although not necessarily. Heterozygosity for this mutation does not lead to hyperhomocysteinemia. Compound heterozygotes for the classical and thermolabile mutation of 5,10-methylenetetrahydrofolate reductase may also be mildy hyperhomocysteinemic.

38.2 Clinical Features and Laboratory Investigations

Cystathionine β-synthetase deficiency leads to the classical clinical picture commonly associated with the term "homocystinuria". The disease has an autosomal recessive inheritance. There is a considerable clinical variability, even within the same family. Psychomotor retardation is often a feature of the disease and becomes evident during the first or second year of life. In the course of time, the optic lenses become dislocated in most patients. Other ophthalmological abnormalities include myopia, and less frequently glaucoma, optic atrophy, retinal abnormalities and cataract. There are often skeletal abnormalities including osteoporosis, scoliosis, arachnodactyly, thinning and lengthening of the long bones and other abnormalities in configuration and maturation of the skeleton. The combination of ectopic lenses and tall and thin habitus may give the patient a Marfanoid appearance. Patients often present with signs of premature arteriosclerosis and thromboembolism. Vascular occlusion can occur in any vessel at any age. Fifty percent of the untreated patients suffer a cardiovascular incident before the age of 30 years, and cerebral infarction accounts for more than 60% of these incidents. Related neurological problems include hemiparesis and other focal neurological signs. In addition, generalized dystonia, other extrapyramidal movement disturbances, and epilepsy, usually with grand mal convulsions, may occur. Behavioral disturbances and personality problems occur in a considerable number of patients. There are no signs of bone marrow dysfunction.

The clinical severity of 5,10-methylenetetrahydrofolate reductase deficiency varies greatly from case to case, even within the same family. The disease has an autosomal recessive mode of inheritance. Onset of clinical manifestations varies from early infancy to adulthood. More than half of the patients become symptomatic during the first year of life. Among the most common early clinical manifestations are lethargy, epilepsy, hypotonia and severe developmental delay, often in combination with microcephaly. In early onset disease, early death is not rare and can occur during an episode of apnea or may follow respiratory problems. In older children, a disturbance of gait is a common finding. Neurological examination reveals a combination of spasticity and sensory disturbances of the legs, consistent with combined dysfunction of the dorsal columns and pyramidal tracts of the spinal cord (combined degeneration of the cord), variably mixed with signs of a peripheral polyneuropathy with weakness and sensory disturbances with a glove-and-stocking distribution. The disturbances of postural sense lead to loss of coordination. Seizures, psychiatric manifestations, athetosis and parkinsonism may occur. There are no signs of megaloblastic anemia. Vascular complications are not common in patients with 5,10-methylenetetrahydrofolate reductase deficiency, but recurrent cerebral infarction and superior sagittal sinus thrombosis have been reported.

Folate deficiency is one of the most common vitamin deficiencies. The major causes are poor dietary intake; conditions leading to malabsorption, such as steatorrhea and sprue; and treatment with anticonvulsants such as phenytoin or with antifolate drugs including methotrexate, trimethoprim and triamterene. In an advanced stage, the deficiency can cause macrocytic anemia, neutropenia, thrombopenia or pancytopenia with macrocytosis. Neurological complications are exceptional. However, there is convincing evidence that folate deficiency without cobalamin deficiency can cause subacute combined degeneration of the cord and brain. Hereditary congenital folate malabsorption has been described in a small number of patients. These patients present at the age of 2–5 months with severe megaloblastic anemia, diarrhea, mouth ulcers and failure to thrive. Most patients show progressive neurological deterioration, with mild to severe mental retardation, seizures, peripheral neuropathy, ataxia and athetosis.

Inborn errors of cobalamin metabolism are autosomal recessive disorders with a variable clinical picture. Most patients become manifest in infancy, but delay in onset of clinical manifestations to adolescence or adulthood has been described. In infancy, the patients present with gastrointestinal (feeding problems, vomiting, atrophic stomatitis, glossitis, alternating diarrhea and constipation and failure to thrive), hematological (macrocytic anemia, less often thrombocytopenia), and neurological problems compatible with subacute combined degeneration of the cord and brain and a polyneuropathy. In older children the gastrointestinal problems are less prominent and hematological and neurological problems dominate. In young patients neurological manifestations include psychomotor retardation or regression, lethargy, hypokinesis, hypotonia, brisk reflexes, ataxia, optic atrophy and seizures. In older children the syndrome of subacute combined degeneration of the cord and brain is easier to diagnose with signs of a myelopathy, peripheral neuropathy, optic atrophy, dementia and behavioral problems.

Cobalamin deficiency can be observed in a number of conditions. Deficiency due to insufficient dietary intake is rare, but can be observed in strict vegetarians (vegans) and in breast-fed babies of mothers who are cobalamin deficient. Cobalamin in the diet is released from protein in the acid environment of the stomach. Here it binds to R proteins of gastric and salivary origin. Pancreatic proteases digest the R proteins and liberate cobalamin in the upper small intestine, where it forms a complex with intrinsic factor, synthesized by gastric parietal cells. The newly formed complex binds with specific receptors in the terminal ileum and is transported into the enterocyte. The complex is dissociated and cobalamin is transported into the portal blood bound to transcobalamin II. Transcobalamin II is the transport protein for cobalamin and also facilitates cobalamin uptake by tissues. Disturbances of cobalamin uptake and transport can arise at all levels. R protein deficiency as an inherited defect has been described in a small number of patients. Intrinsic factor deficiency can be caused by deficient synthesis, synthesis of a mutant protein with decreased activity, autoimmune gastritis with antibodies against parietal cells and intrinsic factor, or a gastrectomy. Cobalamin malabsorption may be due to defective receptor on the enterocyte, defective receptor internalization, surgical resection of the terminal ileum, inflammatory diseases of the ileum (sprue, colitis ulcerosa, Crohn's disease) and transcobalamin II deficiency. Nitrous oxide (N_2O) is a very special cause of deficient cobalamin activity. It oxidizes active cobalamin to an inert form. Long-term exposure to this anesthetic substance, formerly used in the artificial ventilation of tetanic patients, leads to megaloblastic and aplastic bone marrow changes and combined degeneration of the spinal cord. Patients with latent cobalamin deficiency are exceedingly sensitive to neurological deterioration following nitrous oxide anesthesia.

The clinical signs and symptoms of cobalamin deficiency usually follow a chronic course and have a delayed onset because of the large cobalamin stores in the body. In infants fed on breast milk with a low cobalamin content, symptoms are delayed by several months. The signs and symptoms are hematological (macrocytic anemia, usually mild thrombocytopenia, hypersegmentation of neutrophils, aplastic anemia), gastrointestinal (atrophic glossitis, stomatitis, constipation, diarrhea) and neurological. The neurological signs and symptoms usually follow a chronic course, but a more or less acute spinal cross-section syndrome does occur. Neurological abnormalities consist of a progressive spastic paraparesis with ataxia due to impairment of postural sense. The arms are usually affected later and to a lesser extent than the legs. Peripheral neuropathy occurs with progressive weakness, loss of reflexes (but plantar reflexes usually remain extensor) and distal sensory disturbances. Visual problems may occur caused by optic atrophy. Mental signs are frequent and range from disturbed development in infants to regression and dementia, lability, depression, irritability, confusion, psychosis and lethargy in older patients. Affected infants are often microcephalic. Epileptic seizures may occur.

Longstanding mild hyperhomocysteinemia related to heterozygosity for cystathionine β-synthetase deficiency and probably also to thermolability of 5,10-methylenetetrahydrofolate reductase deficiency con-

Table 38.1. Laboratory findings in the hyperhomocysteinemias

	Homocysteine	Methionine	Methylmalonic acid	Macrocytosis
Cystathionine β-synthetase deficiency	↑	↑	–	–
5,10 methylene-tetrahydrofolate reductase deficiency	↑	–	–	–
cbl C, D, F	↑	–	↑	+
cbl E, G	↑	–	–	+
Folate deficiency	↑	–	–	+
Cobalamin deficiency	↑	–	↑	+

tributes to premature arteriosclerosis of small and large vessels, which may become manifest with transient ischemic attacks, lacunar infarctions and cerebral infarcts in large arterial territories. The clinical symptomatology of stroke in these patients does not differ from that in cerebrovascular disease of any other origin.

Most important laboratory investigations include assessment of the levels of homocysteine, methionine, and methylmalonic acid in plasma and urine and assessment of hematological abnormalities, in particular megaloblastic anemia (see Table 38.1). It is important to note that there may be no hematological abnormalities, even in the presence of overt neurological abnormalities. In cystathionine β-synthetase deficiency, low levels of cystathionine and cystine are additional findings. The homocysteine levels are highest in cystathionine β-synthetase deficiency, lowest in the socalled mild hyperhomocysteinemias. Mild hyperhomocysteinemia can be detected by performing a methionine loading test or by assessment of serum homocysteine levels in fasting condition. The assessment of the CSF level of S-adenosylmethionine is of value as a decrease is associated with present or imminent demyelination.

Direct enzyme assessment confirms the diagnosis in cystathionine β-synthetase deficiency and 5,10-methylenetetrahydrofolate reductase deficiency. The enzyme assessment can be performed in liver biopsy specimens, cultured fibroblasts and lymphocytes. Serum folate is low in folate deficiency. In case of dietary cobalamin deficiency or deficiency due to gastrintestinal absorption problems, serum cobalamin levels may only be slightly or moderately low, despite other clinical evidence of important deficiency. Total serum cobalamin is normal in transcobalamin II deficiency, and in CblC, CblD, CblF and CblE and CblG. Disturbances of cobalamin absorption can be investigated with the Schilling test. This test measures urinary excretion of radioactively labeled cobalamin after oral administration. If the urinary level is below normal, the test is combined with addition of intrinsic factor to distinguish between cobalamin deficiency caused by lack of intrinsic factor and other causes of disturbances of the vitamin absorption. Differentiation of CblC,

CblD, CblF, CblE and CblG is possible by biochemical and complementation studies on cultured fibroblasts. Cystathionine β-synthetase activity and 5,10-methylenetetrahydrofolate reductase activity can be assessed in chorionic villi and cultured amniocytes, facilitating prenatal diagnosis. Prenatal diagnosis in disorders of intracellular cobalamin metabolism can be performed on amniocytes or chorionic villus samples.

In case of subacute combined degeneration of the spinal cord, CSF protein is usually slightly elevated. SSEPs show normal or moderately slowed peripheral conduction, normal conduction or mild slowing across the cervical portion of the median SSEP and absence or severe slowing of impulse propagation along the spinal cord with the peroneal SSEP. The conduction velocity of peripheral nerves is normal or mildly to more markedly reduced. There may be signs of denervation.

38.3 Pathology

Two types of cerebral pathology are consistently seen in severe hyperhomocysteinemias: subacute combined degeneration of the spinal cord and brain and the cerebral consequences of premature arteriosclerosis.

Subacute combined degeneration of the spinal cord is a demyelinating disorder, principally affecting the CNS. The form the disorder takes, both clinically and histopathologically, is strongly influenced by the age of the patient, or rather, the progress of myelination at the time of onset of disease. In early infantile onset the disease may take the form of delayed and disturbed myelination rather than demyelination, whereas after completion of myelination the classical picture of subacute combined degeneration of the cord and brain arises.

Degeneration and demyelination of the spinal cord, in particular the dorsal and lateral columns, lent the disease its name: subacute combined degeneration of the cord. The midthoracic segments of the cord are mainly involved where a zone of white matter destruction may affect the whole cord and not only the long tracts. In the upper cervical segments the posterior columns are predominantly affected and at the lower lumbar levels predominantly the pyramidal tracts. As pathological changes predominate in the midthoracic segments, subsequent Wallerian degeneration may play a role in the affection of the ascending tracts in the cervical segments and of the descending tracts in the lumbar segments. The first changes consist of swelling and splitting of myelin sheaths, followed by spongiform white matter degeneration and demyelination. At electron microscopy it is shown that the myelin splitting occurs at the intraperiod line. A variable astrocytic reaction is present, but sometimes it is considerable.

In the cerebral white matter variable demyelination is present. In many cases the demyelinating lesions are small, ill defined and located perivascularly. Their number is variable. They may be scanty or disseminated over wide areas. Sometimes the cerebral white matter changes become extensive and diffuse, but internal capsule and brain stem remain relatively spared. In incidental cases a predominance of subcortical white matter involvement has been mentioned, with the brunt of abnormalities in the white matter at the junction of the cortex. The histology of the cerebral lesions is similar to that of the spinal cord. There is first a fusiform swelling of myelin sheaths, myelin splitting, formation of intramyelinic vacuoles, followed by demyelination and finally also axonal degeneration. The optic nerves are often involved in the demyelinating process. The basal nuclei including the thalamus may also become involved in the process of myelin vacuolation. In more extensive white matter disease loss of white matter volume occurs with enlargement of ventricles and subarachnoid spaces.

Peripheral nerves show signs of a combination of segmental demyelination and axonal degeneration.

In cystathionine β-synthetase deficiency main pathological findings are arteriosclerosis, arterial thromboembolism and venous thrombosis in children and young adults. Resulting lesions consist of arterial and venous infarcts. Most often multiple small infarcts of different ages are seen, spread over the brain. In cystathionine β-synthetase deficiency demyelination is rare. In one patient (Chou and Waisman 1965), a vacuolating white matter disease was documented, predominantly involving the subcortical white cerebral and cerebellar white matter, relatively sparing the corpus callosum, internal capsule, and brain stem. Spinal cord was also involved. In one patient a combination of demyelination and extensive vascular abnormalities with multiple small infarcts was found (Dunn et al. 1966).

In 5,10-methylenetetrahydrofolate reductase deficiency vascular pathology is present but less severe than in cystathionine β-synthetase deficiency and cerebral infarcts are rare. Demyelination of brain and spinal cord as described in subacute combined degeneration of cord and brain is the most common type of pathology. The findings in folate deficiency are similar.

In the inherited defects in cobalamin metabolism and in cobalamin deficiency, spongy demyelination in the pattern of subacute combined degeneration of cord and brain is the predominant finding. Additional changes are present in arterioles and capillaries with thickening, fibrosis and hyalination, but cerebral infarctions have not been reported.

Until now, cerebral infarction is the only type of pathology observed in mild hyperhomocysteinemia, in most cases related to heterozygosity for cystathionine β-synthetase deficiency. This observation may be biased as children and young adults with cerebrovascular accidents are screened for the presence of mild hyperhomocysteinemia. Systematic data on neuropathological findings in unselected patients are not available.

38.4 Pathogenetic Considerations

Two types of pathology dominate in the hyperhomocysteinemias: vascular pathology and myelinopathy. The relative contribution to the clinical symptomatology varies per disease. In cystathionine β-synthetase deficiency, but also in mild hyperhomocysteinemia, vascular pathology dominates, whereas in 5,10-methylenetetrahydrofolate reductase deficiency, disturbances of cobalamin metabolism (CblC, CblD, CblF, CblE and CblG), exogenous folate deficiency and cobalamin deficiency, the myelinopathy dominates.

The pathogenesis of the vascular pathology is only partially understood. There is evidence from experimental animal work and from in vitro research that homocysteine damages the vascular endothelium. Injury of arterial and venous vessel walls predisposes to early arteriosclerosis and thrombosis. It has been found that micromolar amounts of copper, as present in ceruloplasmin, catalyze oxidation of homocysteine. During the course of this process hydrogen peroxide is produced, which may play a role in the endothelial damage. Platelet abnormalities and abnormalities in soluble factors involved in blood coagulation may contribute to the thrombotic diathesis.

Plasma homocysteine levels are highest in cystathionine β-synthetase deficiency, explaining the high incidence of vascular accidents in this disorder. It is remarkable, however, that vascular abnormalities and vascular accidents occur relatively frequently in the mild hyperhomocysteinemias, which have a lower level of homocysteine than for instance the inherited cobalamin disorders, whereas vascular pathology is rare in the latter conditions. The chronicity of elevated homocysteine levels before detection and treatment, in view of the absence of other clinical problems in heterozygosity for cystathionine β-synthetase deficiency, may form part of the explanation.

Most current evidence points to deficiency of S-adenosylmethionine being critical to the development of demyelination. In the human brain S-adenosylmethionine is the universal methyl group donor, acting in a wide variety of biological methylations, that modify proteins, nucleic acids, fatty acids, phospholipids and polysaccharides. S-adenosylmethionine is necessary for the inactivation of catecholamines and other biogenic amines. The methyl transfer pathway provides precursors for polyamine synthesis. A relationship has been found between the presence of demyelination and deficiency of S-adenosylmethionine in the CSF, whereas remyelination under treatment is associated with a return of the S-adenosylmethionine level to normal. Additional evidence comes from animal experimental work, in which cycloleucine is used to elicit subacute combined degeneration of the spinal cord. Cycloleucine causes deficiency of S-adenosylmethionine by inhibition of methionine adenosyltransferase. The precise mechanism of a deficiency of S-adenosylmethionine leading to demyelination is not known. The failure of methylation of arginine$_{107}$-myelin basic protein may be important in this respect. In addition, methyl groups are necessary for synthesis of choline from ethanolamine, and these methyl groups are provided by S-adenosylmethionine. Deficient synthesis of choline may contribute to the myelinopathy.

Administration of folic acid in patients with cobalamin deficiency may precipitate or exacerbate demyelination. Folic acid is not active and requires conversion to active tetrahydrofolate. This reaction is very slow. Folic acid competes with the transport of active tetrahydrofolate in the CNS. The resulting decreased availability of tetrahydrofolate for nervous tissue is probably the cause of enhanced demyelination.

The folate cycle is not only involved in the remethylation of homocysteine to methionine, a reaction that is crucial to the synthesis of S-adenosylmethionine, it is also involved in the transfer of methyl groups necessary for the synthesis of purines and pyrimidines, major constituents of DNA. There is general agreement that megaloblastic anemia or pancytopenia and the defective proliferation of rapidly dividing cells with sequelae as glossitis, intestinal problems and hypospermia, are related to impairment of DNA synthesis due to interference with folate metabolism. The main problem with folate metabolism in the cobalamin disorders (CblC, CblD, CblF, CblE and CblG) and cobalamin deficiency is that 5-methyltetrahydrofolate is not converted to tetrahydrofolate, whereas the conversion of 5,10-methylenetetrahydrofolate to 5-methyltetrahydrofolate is irreversible. This is called the methyl-folate trap. The trap leads to deficiency of folate coenzymes derived from tetrahydrofolate, necessary in the production of purines and pyrimidines.

In cases of deficiency of folate or cobalamin, or in inborn errors of folate or cobalamin metabolism, CSF levels of 5-hydroxyindolacetic acid (5-HIAA) and homovanillic acid (HVA), metabolites of serotonin and dopamine, respectively, are found to be decreased. The decrease is independent of the level of S-adenosylmethionine. Why these metabolites are reduced is not known. Neurotransmitter disturbances may be responsible for the frequently observed extrapyramidal movement abnormalities, epilepsy and changes in mood and personality.

The gene encoding cystathionine β-synthetase has been mapped to chromosome 21q22.3. The gene has been sequenced and several mutations have been described. Cystathionine β-synthetase requires pyridoxal phosphate (vitamin B$_6$) as a cofactor. In case of a mutation, there is either no residual enzyme activity, a reduced activity and normal affinity for the cofactor, or reduced activity and reduced affinity for pyridoxal phosphate. The vitamin B$_6$ responsive patients do better in all aspects of the disease than non-responsive patients, even if both groups are untreated. They have a higher IQ and all other manifestations of the disease occur later.

38.5 Therapy

About half the patients with cysthationine β-synthetase deficiency respond to large oral doses of vitamin B$_6$ (pyridoxine). After a variable period, up to a few weeks, homocysteine levels become normal, hypermethioninemia decreases and hypocysteinemia increases to normal values. In some patients the response is only partial and very large doses of vitamin B$_6$ are needed. If this is not enough to correct the biochemical abnormalities, a diet low in methionine and high in cystine should be initiated. A mildly methionine restricted diet may be advisable for vitamin B$_6$-responsive patients too. Extra supplementation of betaine has been proposed to promote remethylation of homocysteine to methionine, but has not been effective. Folate utilization may be increased in patients with cystathionine β-synthetase deficiency, since it is required in methylation of homocysteine to methionine. Folate deficiency can mask vitamin B$_6$-responsiveness and simultaneous administration of folate is necessary in some patients to achieve biochemical normalization. Aspirin has been used to reduce the tendency to develop thromboses, but has not proven to be beneficial. With early installment of treatment, most of the clinical manifestations of the disease can be prevented or delayed.

Also, in mild hyperhomocysteinemia due to heterozygosity for cystathionine β-synthetase deficiency, vitamin B_6 combined with folate can normalize plasma homocysteine levels. The long-term effects of this treatment have not been fully assessed.

5,10-Methylenetetrahydrofolate reductase deficiency has proven very resistant to treatment and only limited success has been achieved. Therapeutic options include (1) use of folates such as folic acid or folinic acid in an attempt to maximize any residual enzyme activity; (2) use of methyltetrahydrofolate to replace the missing product; (3) use of methionine to correct the cellular methionine deficiency; (4) use of pyridoxine to lower homocysteine levels because of its role as a cofactor for cystathionine β-synthetase; (5) cobalamin because of its role as a cofactor for methionine synthetase; (6) carnitine; and (7) betaine in order to lower homocysteine levels and supplement methionine levels. In most patients several agents are used in combination.

Folate deficiency can be corrected by supplementation of the deficient substance.

All inborn errors of intracellular cobalamin metabolism are treated with intramuscular hydroxycobalamin. After induction, the hydroxycobalamin can be given orally because cobalamin absorption and transport are normal. The biochemical and hematological response to the therapy is usually rapid. Plasma levels of methionine and homocysteine can be used to monitor treatment. In CblE and CblG the use of hydroxycobalamin is usually sufficient, although supplementation with methionine has been shown to have additional beneficial effects. In CblC of infantile onset, hydroxycobalamin cannot always fully reverse the biochemical abnormalities. Betaine can be used as additive. A synergistic action of betaine and hydroxycobalamin has been shown in CblC. The long-term outcome of treatment depends to a great extent on the swiftness of installment of treatment after onset of symptoms, or, in other words, on the extent of irreversible neurological damage.

In all causes of cobalamin deficiency, hydroxycobalamin can be administered. In transcobalamin II deficiency large doses of hydroxycobalamin are required to correct cellular cobalamin deficiency. The effect of treatment depends on the presence and extent of irreversible neurological damage.

38.6 **Magnetic Resonance Imaging**

The cerebral infarctions occurring in cystathionine β-synthetase deficiency, both lacunar and large infarctions, can be visualized by MRI. The images as such are not specific, only the age category of the patient is unusual. MRI of a small number of patients has been reported and changes suggestive of single or multiple small infarcts are most commonly observed. When the lesions are scattered over the brain with a predilection for the periventricular area, the picture may resemble that of multiple sclerosis.

So far, no systematic study of MRI findings of the brain has been reported in mild hyperhomocysteinemia. An enhanced frequency of (silent) infarcts can be expected. One case of severe cerebrovascular occlusive disease in mild hyperhomocysteinemia has been reported (Van Diemen-Steenvoorde et al. 1990).

MRI may reveal spinal cord abnormalities in subacute combined degeneration with an increased signal intensity of the posterior part of the cervical spinal cord on T_2-weighted images in sagittal or transverse direction. The abnormality in signal intensity may also be more extensive and not limited to the posterior columns. With treatment, disappearance of the lesion can be followed.

MRI of cerebral white matter abnormalities has been documented in a limited number of patients with 5,10-methylenetetrahydrofolate reductase deficiency, disorders of intracellular cobalamin metabolism (Surtees et al. 1991; Walk et al. 1994) and dietary cobalamin deficiency (Fig. 38.2). One of the patients of Surtees et al. (1991) was still young, and MRI only showed a delay in myelination with improvement after therapy. Two other, older children had a slightly increased signal intensity of all deep white matter, sparing brain stem, internal capsule and subcortical white matter, consistent with a slight degree of demyelination or still insufficient myelination. Improvement was noted after therapy. The patient of Walk et al. (1994) showed symmetrical periventricular white matter abnormalities, most prominent in the occipital region, but extending along the border of the lateral ventricles. In a case of generalized dystonia, low signal intensity of the globus pallidus on both sides was found, consistent with disturbed function. In our cobalamin deficient patient, aged 1 year and 7 months, a severe cerebral hemispheral white matter abnormality was found, whereas corpus callosum, internal capsule and brain stem were spared (Fig. 38.2). The white matter abnormalities were most severe in the parietal area, extending through the corona radiata into the arcuate fibers. In addition, the hemispheral white matter had too high a signal intensity on T_2-weighted images with a patchy distribution, most pronounced in the subcortical white matter, probably related to delayed and disturbed myelination.

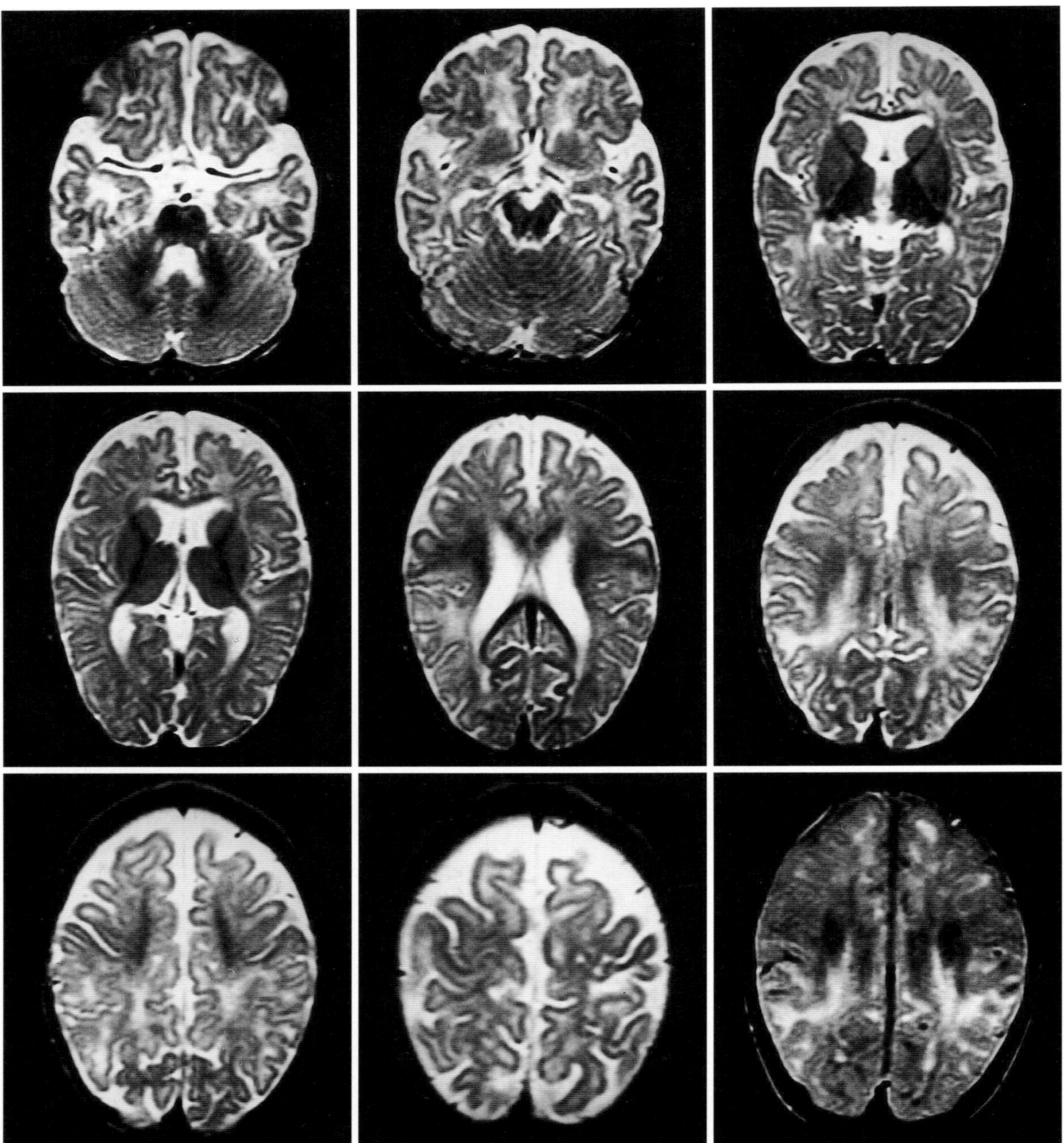

Fig. 38.2. Girl, 1 year and 7 months of age, with cobalamin deficiency. She was breast-fed and her mother had been a strict vegetarian for years. These T_2-weighted MR images suggest a combination of delayed and disturbed myelination of the cerebral hemispheres, and of demyelination and gliosis in the parietal area. Corpus callosum, internal capsule and brain stem are spared. The proton density image (*right lower image*) shows the extent of the demyelination and gliosis. In addition there is some cerebral atrophy with enlargement of ventricular system and subarachnoid spaces

39 Urea Cycle Defects

39.1 Clinical Features and Laboratory Investigations

There are five well-documented urea cycle defects:
- Carbamyl phosphate synthetase deficiency (CPSD)
- Ornithine transcarbamylase deficiency (OTCD)
- Argininosuccinate synthetase deficiency (ASSD), also called citrullinemia
- Argininosuccinate lyase deficiency (ASLD), also called argininosuccinic aciduria
- Arginase deficiency, also called hyperargininemia.

These disorders have an autosomal recessive mode of inheritance, with the exception of OTCD, which has an X-linked recessive inheritance.

Clinical signs of metabolic derangement may appear at any time, but peak periods include the neonatal period, change to a diet with high protein content (replacement of milk feeding by a higher protein content diet, parenteral nutrition) and episodes of infectious diseases. Valproate may also induce an episode of metabolic derangement.

In the case of neonatal presentation, a normal baby is born after normal pregnancy and delivery. After 1 or a few days the child becomes lethargic and hypotonic. Vomiting, seizures, hypothermia and hyperventilation occur. Lethargy increases and coma follows. There are signs of elevated intracranial pressure with bulging fontanelle and increasing head size. In most cases the disease progresses rapidly to death within a few days. Survivors almost always have severe neurological sequelae.

In the case of later onset, the disease is episodic. Occurrence of symptoms may be related to protein intake or infections, but not infrequently, an episode occurs without any obvious cause. The episodes are characterized by headache, lethargy, irritability, agitation, confusion, hallucinations, vomiting, hypotonia, ataxia, dysarthria, and coma. In the children with later onset of clinical symptoms mortality rate is still high, and highest during the initial presenting illness.

Apart from the episodic worsening, the clinical course of the disease is characterized by variable psychomotor retardation, ataxia, seizures, growth retardation and hepatomegaly. However, normal development and neurological function have been reported in rare cases. In ASLD, coarse and friable hair (trichorhexis nodosa) is a special characteristic.

The clinical features and course of disease are indistinguishable in CPSD, OTCD, ASSD and ASLD. It is only in hyperargininemia that the clinical manifestations differ. The clinical symptoms are slowly progressive and include growth failure, psychomotor retardation, spastic tetraplegia, the legs being more severely involved than the arms, tremor, ataxia, choreoathetosis, epilepsy, and hyperactivity. In addition, episodes with lethargy, vomiting and coma may occur. There is some variability in onset and rate of progression of the disease. Life span is usually longer than in the other urea cycle defects.

Females heterozygous for OTCD are usally free of symptoms, but approximately 10% become symptomatic and have a milder and more variable course of disease than affected males. Symptoms are episodic and include headaches, vomiting, irritability, bizarre behavior, lethargy, ataxia, tremors, seizures and coma. A high-protein diet, infection, surgery and the postpartum state may precipitate attacks. Deterioration following use of valproate has been described repeatedly.

Laboratory investigations reveal hyperammonemia in all urea cycle disorders with the exception of hyperargininemia in which blood ammonium levels may be normal. Respiratory alkalosis is often present. Urinary orotic acid is increased because of the shunting of nitrogen waste from the urea cycle. In CPSD and OTCD citrulline is decreased in plasma. In ASSD plasma citrulline is elevated, whereas in ASLD argininosuccinate is elevated and citrulline is moderately increased. In these four disorders, plasma levels of glutamine and alanine are frequently raised, wherease arginine and ornithine are decreased. In hyperargininemia, ariginine is elevated in plasma. In urine, elevation of arginine, lysine, cystine, ornithine, citrulline, glutamine and orotic acid is found.

Definite diagnosis can be established by enzyme assessment in liver cells. In hyperargininemia and ASLD enzyme assessment is also possible in erythrocytes.

All five urea cycle defects can be diagnosed antenatally. The techniques necessary for prenatal diagnosis vary from measurement of abnormal metabolites in amniotic fluid, analysis of DNA from chorionic villi or amniocytes, to measurement of enzyme activity in cultured amniocytes or in utero liver biopsy samples. Protein loading, alanine loading and allopurinol challenge to induce orotic aciduria can be used for carrier detection in OTCD. However, a negative test does not rule out the carrier status. DNA techniques can be used for carrier detection if DNA is available from an affected patient.

39.2 Pathology

Neuropathological findings are variable and depend on the age of the patient and on the relative effects of present and past acute and chronic metabolic derangements. Neuropathological findings are similar in the various urea cycle disorders.

Actual high elevations of ammonium levels lead to brain swelling. On light and electron microscopy, astrocyte swelling is found. Hyperammonemia induces the so-called Alzheimer type II change in astrocytes. This change consists of an increase in the number and size of astrocytic nuclei, which may become nearly twice their normal size. These nuclei are vesicular with a prominent nuclear membrane and an optically empty nucleoplasm with sparse chromatin particles. The cytoplasm is not discernible with the light microscope. Alzheimer type II astrocytes are mainly present in cerebral cortex, basal nuclei, cerebellar cortex and nuclei and brain stem nuclei. The presence of Alzheimer type II cells depends on the presence of hyperammonemia. In adequately treated cases with normal ammonia levels Alzheimer type II cells are absent.

Chronic hyperammonemia leads predominantly to neuronal damage.

In neonates dying in the acute phase of metabolic decompensation diffuse brain swelling is found. Alzheimer type II astrocytes are present in gray matter structures. There is no or little neuronal damage. Myelination is normal for age. In some neonates a status spongiosus of cortex and/or white matter has been described.

In older children, variable, focal and multifocal cortico-subcortical necrosis may be seen with a tendency to microcavitation. Acute lesions are swollen; old lesions are atrophic with presence of ulegyria. On microscopic examination, cortical findings vary from normal to pseudolaminar neuronal necrosis to complete depopulation of the cortex. The cortical damage may have a spongiform aspect. Spongy changes may also be seen in basal nuclei and brain stem. White matter changes are variable. Myelination may be normal or mildly to severely delayed. Signs of active myelin breakdown may be absent or present. The white matter changes may be spongiform with presence of myelin splitting and vacuolation.

In female carriers of OTCD, neuropathological findings are different and apparently mainly related to chronic hyperammonemia. Variable, sometimes extreme cerebral atrophy is the predominant finding. The hemispheric walls are thin and the lateral ventricles are dilated. The cerebral cortex shows signs of neuronal loss and gliosis. There is also loss of neurons in the basal nuclei and thalamus. Alzheimer type II astrocytes are present in the cerebral cortex, basal nuclei, dentate nuclei and brain stem nuclei. The white matter becomes rarefied and gliotic with a reduced number of myelinated fibers.

39.3 Pathogenetic Considerations

The urea cycle serves two purposes: it contains, in part, the biochemical reactions required for the de novo biosynthesis and degradation of arginine, and it incorporates the surplus of nitrogen into urea, which serves as a waste nitrogen product. The enzymes involved in urea synthesis are partly located within the mitochondria (carbamyl phosphate synthetase, ornithine transcarbamylase), whereas the other enzymes are located within the cytosol (argininosuccinate synthetase, argininosuccinate lyase, arginase).

A urea cycle defect has two consequences: arginine becomes an essential amino acid (except in hyperargininemia) and nitrogen accumulates in a variety of molecules, in particular ammonia. Ammonia is highly toxic to the brain where it interferes with energy production and normal metabolism of neurotransmitters. Ammonia influences the glutamine-glutamate-GABA balance. Glutamate is the most important excitatory neurotransmitter, whereas γ-amino butyric acid (GABA), formed by decarboxylation from glutamate, is the most important inhibitory neurotransmitter. In the presynaptic neuron, glutamate is formed from glutamine by glutaminase. After release by the presynaptic neuron, glutamate is taken up by the astrocyte in which it is processed by glutamine synthetase into glutamine. Glutamine is transported to the presynaptic neuron where glutaminase catalyzes the formation of glutamate available for neurotransmission. Hyperammonemia has a great impact on this cycle by stimulating synthesis of glutamine from ammonia and glutamate with consumption of ATP. The disturbance of the balance between excitatory and inhibitory neurotransmitters may contribute to the cerebral dysfunction. Glutamine synthetase is mainly located in astrocytes and high plasma levels of ammonia lead to accumulation of glutamine within astrocytes. During hyperammonemia, the concentration of glutamine in the brain becomes highly elevated. It has been proposed that the consequent osmotic effect causes astrocytes to swell with subsequent cerebral edema.

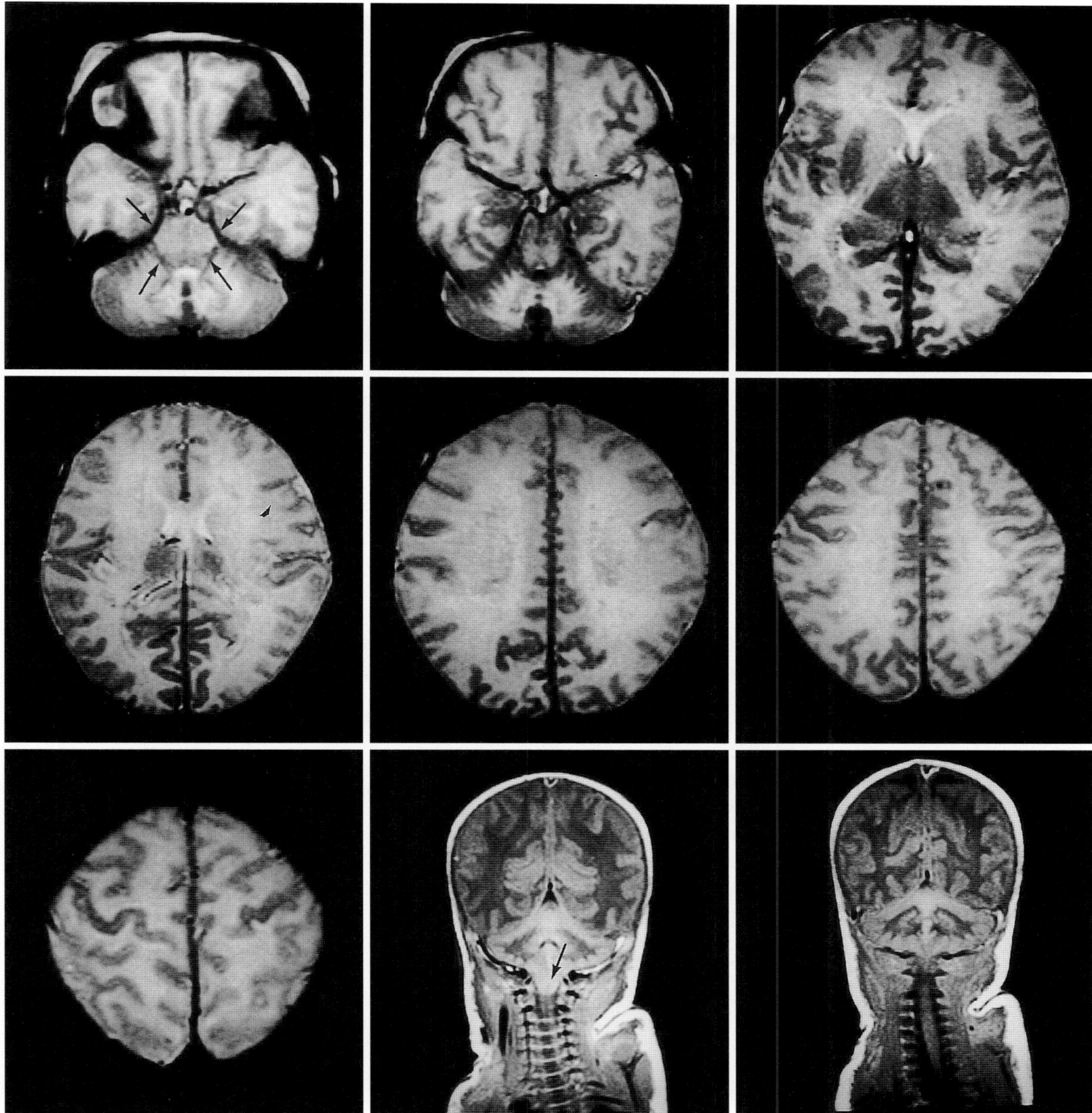

Fig. 39.1. MRI series of a baby boy, 1 week of age, with ASLD. The T$_2$-weighted transverse images show generalized edema with, in particular, severe swelling of the brain stem (*arrows, upper left*). The T$_1$-weighted coronal slices show tonsillar herniation (*arrow, bottom middle view*) and also the generalized edema. MR spectra of this patient are shown in Chap. 71

Recently, the excitotoxin quinolinic acid has been advanced to explain aspects of neuronal injury. Quinolinic acid accumulates under hyperammonemic conditions and derives from tryptophan metabolism. Under such conditions there is an increased transport of tryptophan across the blood-brain barrier. Tryptophan oxidation leads to the formation of quinolinic acid, which acts as an excitotoxin at the N-methyl-D-aspartate (NMDA) receptors. Moderate elevations of CSF levels of quinolinic acid have been found in patients with a urea cycle defect.

Unlike patients with liver failure, where ammonia is only one of several toxins, ammonia appears to be the only cause of the acute encephalopathy seen in urea cycle defects, with the exception of hyperargininemia, where an increase in arginine may also play a role. In hyperammonemia due to liver failure, MRI of the brain shows, as expected in generalized disorders, a symmetrical pattern. There are changes in signal intensity in the basal nuclei, in particular due to T$_1$ shortening. In contrast, brain pathology in urea cycle disorders is often characterized by focal, usually asymmetrical lesions. It remains to be explained why cerebral abnormalities related to hyperammonemia in urea cycle disorders are so different from those observed in liver failure, and why the lesions tend to be asymmetrical.

In all urea cycle disorders apart from hyperargininemia, arginine is deficient unless externally supplied. Chronic arginine deficiency is characterized by dermatological features with erythematous scaling. A dramatic improvement of this cutaneous eruption occurs with dietary arginine supplementation. High levels of citrulline or argininosuccinate are probably not toxic. The similarity in presentation among the different urea cycle defects is related to hyperammonemia. The variability is principally a function of the different mutations (and hence different levels of residual enzyme activity) responsible for them. Some of the variability may also be related to the metabolic consequences of the various enzyme deficiencies, which have some differences. In females carrying an OTC mutant allele on one chromosome, variability in expression is related to the proportion of hepatocytes in which the normal or mutant allele is active (lyonization).

The gene locations in urea cycle defects have been largely identified. The gene of carbamyl phosphate synthetase has been sequenced and located on the short arm of chromosome 2. That for ornithine transcarbamylase is located on the short arm of the X-chromosome; it has been sequenced and a number of mutations have been identified. In OTCD, one-third of the new patients appear to be new mutations. The gene for argininosuccinate synthetase is located on chromosome 9. The gene for argininosuccinate lyase is located on chromosome 7; it has been sequenced and mutations have been described. The gene for arginase is located on chromosome 6; it has been sequenced and mutations have been described.

39.4 Therapy

Urea cycle defects can be treated by a protein restricted diet, a sufficient caloric intake to avoid catabolic situations with breakdown of endogenous protein and supplementation of absent substances. Protein restricted diets have to be supplemented with essential amino acid mixtures to avoid deficiencies. In all urea cycle disorders apart from hyperargininemia, arginine cannot be synthesized endogenously; it has become an essential amino acid and has to be supplied. If an essential amino acid is lacking, protein breakdown cannot be remedied. Long term treatment with restriction of high protein food, including milk and meat, leads to deficiency of minerals, trace elements and vitamins, which have to be supplemented. Enzyme replacement therapy through liver transplantation has been attempted recently. The future prospects of gene therapy look promising.

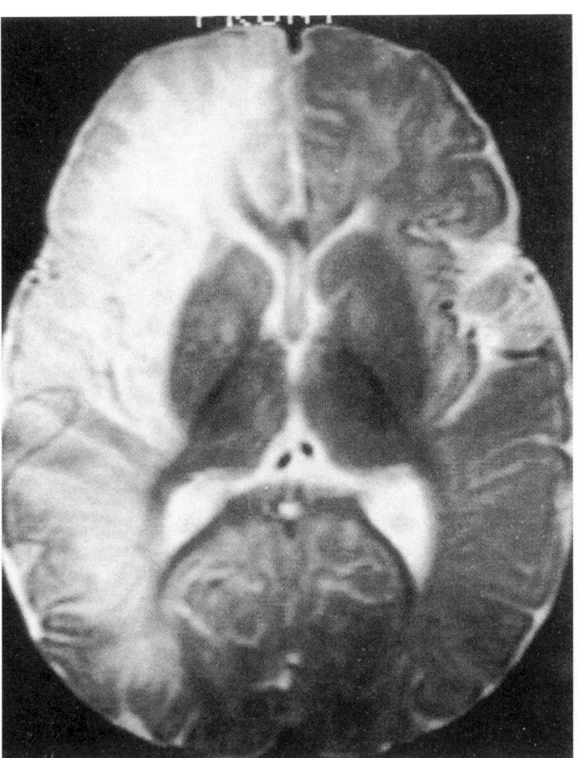

Fig. 39.2. A 12-year-old girl, carrier of OTCD, with an acute episode of convulsions and hemiplegia. The T_2-weighted transverse image shows an extensive area of high signal intensity in the right frontal and parietal white matter and an area of slightly increased signal intensity in the left frontal white matter. The cortex is involved, too. Especially in the right frontal region there is blurring of the corticomedullary junction. Courtesy of Kendall (1992), with permission

Infections and insufficient caloric intake due to anorexia carry the risk of triggering an episode of severe hyperammonemia. Therefore, such conditions have to be treated vigorously. In acute episodes of hyperammonemia, measures are necessary to augment nitrogen disposal. Benzoate, supplied orally or intravenously, can be used as a substrate for an alternate route of nitrogen disposal. Lactulose binds ammonia in the intestinal tract and can enhance ammonia disposal in faeces. Hemodialysis can be used in acute, life threatening situations.

The use of valproic acid as antiepileptic drug should be avoided. Valproic acid may accelerate the appearance of hyperammonemia.

The overall long-term prognosis has improved with treatment, in particular in patients presenting after the neonatal period. However, a high percentage of treated patients is still mentally retarded. The mortality rate in neonatal presentation is still very high and most (or all) surviving patients are severely handicapped.

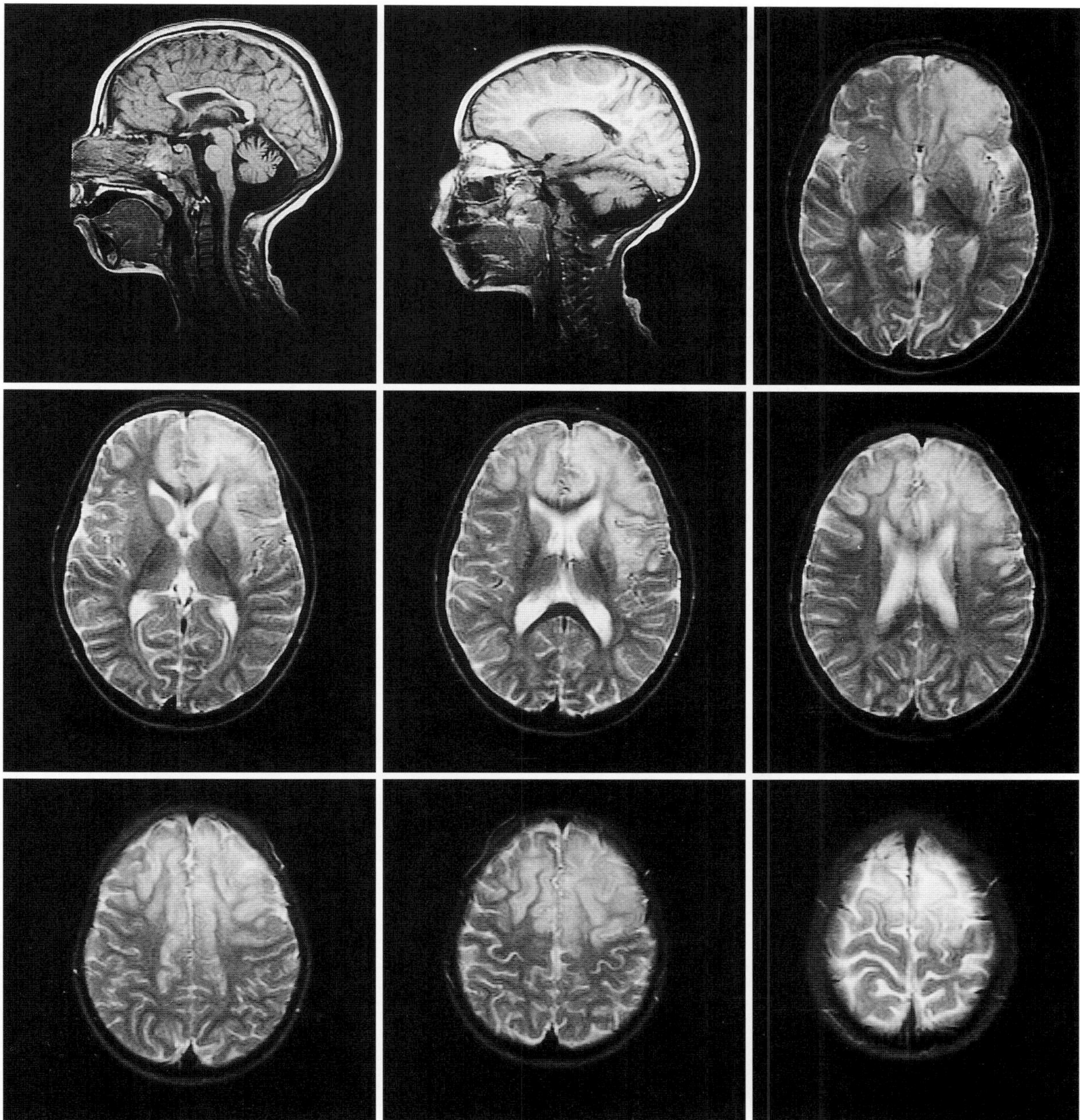

Fig. 39.3. Boy, 6 years of age, with hyperargininemia. The MR images were made during an episode of acute metabolic decompensation following protein-rich gavage feeding. The sagittal images, T_1-weighted, show cerebellar atrophy. The transverse T_2-weighted images show the signal changes bilaterally in the frontal lobes, accentuated on the left side, with involvement of both gray and white matter, typically blurring the gray-white matter junction. The corpus callosum is not involved, nor are the basal ganglia. With treatment, all changes in signal intensity disappeared; some atrophy remained

39.5 Magnetic Resonance Imaging

In urea cycle defects, cerebral abnormalities change, depending on the stage of disease. In acute episodes of metabolic derangement, lesions appear, which may improve under treatment and leave their traces. Chronic hyperammonemia also has its deleterious effects. MRI has the advantage over neuropathological examinations of being able to depict the dynamics of cerebral lesions in urea cycle disorders.

In neonates, neuroimaging shows severe brain swelling (Fig. 39.1). The images carry little diagnostic value apart from showing cerebral edema. MR spectroscopy may contribute by showing highly elevated glutamine levels. See also Chap. 71.

In acute metabolic derangement in older infants and children, large areas of abnormal signal intensity are seen in the brain involving both cortex and underlying white matter, giving them an infarct-like aspect (Figs. 39.2, 39.3). These areas are moderately swollen. Often multiple lesions are seen. The distribution of the lesions is as a rule asymmetrical or even unilateral. In some cases one hemisphere is totally involved. A combination of high plasma ammonia levels and an MRI picture with one or more large, moderately swollen areas involving cortex and white matter is highly suggestive of a urea cycle defect. This pattern is present in all urea cycle defects when an episode of acute metabolic derangement is present, including those in female carriers of OTCD (Fig. 39.2). In the chronic stage, swelling resolves and atrophy with patchy changes in signal intensity of cortex and subcortical white matter remain.

In chronic hyperammonemia, defective myelination and progressive cerebral atrophy are seen.

40 Galactosemia

40.1 Clinical Features and Laboratory Investigations

Three major types of galactosemia can be distinguished based on three different enzyme deficiencies. The most commonly detected type, classical galactosemia or galactosemia type 1, is caused by a deficiency of galactose-1-phosphate uridyltransferase. Galactosemia type 2 is caused by galactokinase deficiency. Galactosemia type 3 is the result of a deficiency of uridine diphosphate galactose-4-epimerase. All three types have an autosomal recessive mode of inheritance.

Galactosemia type 1 has an incidence of 1:40000 to 1:60000. Affected infants are normal at birth. Clinical manifestations develop a few days after the baby has started to have milk feeds. Symptomatology includes a failure to thrive, refusal to feed, vomiting, diarrhea and hypotonia. Signs of a deranged liver function with jaundice and hepatomegaly usually become apparent after the first week of life. Hemolysis occurs in some patients contributing to the jaundice. There is an enhanced susceptibility to infections, in particular Escherichia coli infections. Sepsis often develops within the first 2 weeks of life. Ascites may occur and is a serious prognostic sign with an associated mortality of about 20%. Cataracts appear within days or weeks and become irreversible within a matter of weeks. There may be signs of elevated intracranial pressure with lethargy and diffuse cerebral edema on neuroimaging. If milk is not withdrawn, neonatal death may follow.

There are less severe variants of the disease. Clinical presentation may be later and less life-threatening. Some patients are seen later in the first year of life because of retarded psychomotor development, cataracts and hepatomegaly. In rare cases, a child who is several years of age is presented with psychomotor retardation and cataracts. These children often have a history of reduced milk intake because of recurrent vomiting after drinking milk.

If galactose is not eliminated from the diet, cataracts, progressive liver failure, and mental deficiency develop in patients surviving the neonatal period. A galactose-free diet causes a striking regression of all present signs and symptoms. Nausea and vomiting cease, lethargy disappears, weight gain ensues, liver problems clear,

and cataracts regress. However, the long-term outcome is less optimistic. Over the years, verbal and performal IQ slowly decline and a substantial number of patients has a subnormal intelligence. School achievements are often worse than those of healthy sibs. At the end of the first decade of life, many children develop a tremor, resting and postural. Other neurological signs that may develop over the years include a cerebellar ataxia with clumsiness, intention tremor and dysdiadochokinesis; hyperreflexia, apraxia, seizures and choreoathetosis. Some children are microcephalic. Many children have speech abnormalities, varying from dysarthria, verbal dyspraxia, dysgrammatism to stuttering. A high incidence of ovarian failure with hypergonadotropic hypogonadism has been documented in female patients. Amenorrhea may be primary or secondary and can also occur after pregnancy. Successful pregnancies in female patients are rare, but have been described. No correlation between onset and strictness of diet and development of late complications has ever been established. A relationship between development of cataract and dietary control is present. With introduction of tighter dietary control lens opacities usually gradually resolve. The patients with milder variants of galactosemia type 1 have a better outlook with normal physical, motor and mental development when treated.

In patients with signs of CNS problems, EEG often shows nonspecific abnormalities. SSEPs show prolonged central conduction times.

Galactosemia type 2 is much rarer than galactosemia type 1, and much milder. Cataracts are the only consistent manifestation of the untreated disorder. They develop insidiously within weeks of birth. In exceptional cases, mild hepatomegaly, mental retardation or pseudotumor cerebri have been described.

Galactosemia type 3 exists in two forms. Infants with the mild form appear healthy and remain so. The severe form is similar to galactosemia type 1. Presentation is neonatal with jaundice, vomiting, weight loss, hypotonia, and hepatomegaly. Despite treatment, motor and intellectual development are retarded and neural deafness is present.

Whenever the diagnosis galactosemia is considered in neonates, it is essential to stop milk feeding immediately. In galactosemia type 1, a positive reduction test in urine may be the first diagnostic lead. Apart from galactosuria, there may be evidence of a renal tubular defect with some proteinuria, glucosuria, amino aciduria, phosphaturia and renal tubular acidosis. Galactitol in urine is elevated. The intermittent nature of the galactosuria makes its detection difficult, in particular when milk feeds are withheld from very ill infants. The diagnosis is confirmed by the finding of high levels of galactose-1-phosphate in red blood cells and the demonstration of a deficiency of galactose-1-phosphate uridyltransferase in red or white blood cells. The assay on red blood cells may, of course, be falsely negative after exchange blood transfusion. When a child has received exchange transfusion, assays in blood must be postponed for 3 to 4 months. Enzyme activity can also be determined in cultured skin fibroblasts. Patients with some residual enzyme activity appear to follow milder clinical courses (mild variants) than patients with no demonstrable activity.

In galactosemia type 2, elevated galactose is found in blood and urine. Galactose-1-phosphate is not elevated. Final diagnosis is established by demonstrating of a deficiency of galactokinase in red blood cells or fibroblasts.

In galactosemia type 3, elevated galactose is present in blood and urine. The diagnosis may be suspected when galactose-1-phosphate in erythrocytes is elevated and the activity of galactose-1-phosphate uridyltransferase is normal. The diagnosis can be confirmed by demonstrating a deficiency of epimerase activity in red blood cells and leukocytes. In the mild form of galactosemia type 3, the enzyme deficiency is limited to blood cells and normal activity is found in fibroblasts and liver cells. In the severe form generalized deficiency of epimerase is present.

In several countries, mass newborn screening is performed. Diagnostic difficulties arise in cases of partial galactose-1-phosphate uridyltransferase deficiency. A mutation at the transferase locus, called the Duarte variant, causes diminished red cell transferase activity but usually no clinical disorder. The gene frequency of the Duarte variant is high and compound heterozygotes with one Duarte allele and one classical galactosemia allele are the most common biochemical phenotype detected by screening newborn infants. This condition is usually benign, but neonates may have symptoms of galactose toxicity. Several other benign mutations of the galactose-1-phosphate uriyltransferase gene have been described.

Prenatal diagnosis can be performed by analysis of galactitol in amniotic fluid and by enzyme analysis in chorionic villus cells or amniotic fluid cells. Prenatal diagnosis, however, is only rarely performed with a view to terminating the affected pregnancy.

40.2 Pathology

Only few neuropathological descriptions are present and they only concern patients with classical galactosemia (type 1). Most prominent findings concern the cerebral white matter and cerebellar cortex. The cerebral white matter is diffusely gliotic. On myelin staining, patchy pallor is found, but no signs of active demyelination. The white matter changes are most pronounced in the periventricular area. The white matter may be reduced in volume with some enlargement of the lateral ventricles and subarachnoid spaces. The cerebral cortex has either been described as normal or as exhibiting some neuronal loss. Gliosis and pigmentary degeneration of the globus pallidus and reticular zone of the substantia nigra have been described. There is a loss of Purkinje cells within the cerebellar cortex.

40.3 Pathogenetic Considerations

Galactose is metabolized in 3 sequential enzymatic steps. The first step comprises the phosphorylation of galactose by galactokinase to form galactose-1-phosphate. The second step is mediated by galactose-1-phosphate uridyltransferase and results in an exchange of galactose-1-phosphate for the glucose-1-phosphate moiety of uridine diphosphate glucose to form uridine diphosphate galactose and free glucose-1-phosphate. In the third step, uridine diphosphate galactose is transformed to uridine diphosphate glucose by the enzyme epimerase. In this step galactose is converted to glucose. This step can be reversed leading to endogenous synthesis of galactose from glucose.

The most common type of galactosemia, type 1, is related to a deficiency of galactose-1-phosphate uridyltransferase. The gene encoding this enzyme has been mapped to chromosome 9. It has been sequenced and a growing number of mutations have been described. Furthermore, gene polymorphism has been found leading to enzyme polymorphism. The most common variants are the Duarte variants (D_1 and D_2), but other benign variants have also been described. There is evidence that the molecular heterogeneity forms the explanation for the variable clinical outcome.

The human galactokinase gene has been previously mapped to chromosome 17 (GK_1). It is not known whether GK_1 is altered in patients with galactokinase deficiency. Recently another galactokinase gene has been cloned and mapped to chromosome 15 (GK_2). It is possible that humans have two galactokinase genes.

The epimerase gene has been mapped to chromosome 1.

The pathogenetic mechanisms of tissue damage in galactosemia are understood to only a very limited extent. The mechanisms may be organ-specific.

Galacticol toxicity is probably responsible for the development of cataracts. In the presence of high galactose levels, the enzyme aldose reductase irreversibly reduces galactose to galactitol. Very little galactitol leaves the intracellular compartment and no further metabolism is possible beyond the galactitol step. The intracellular concentration of galactitol increases and alters the cell osmotic environment. Water is drawn into the cell and results in lens swelling, with denaturation and precipitation of proteins and disruption of lens architecture.

There is evidence that galactose-1-phosphate is responsible for many of the acute toxic effects in galactosemia, including liver and brain damage. Galactose-1-phosphate may trap high energy phosphate bonds or may directly interrupt energy production at cellular level. High galactose and galactose-1-phosphate levels may inhibit the normal entry of glucose into the brain with resulting curtailment of glycolytic flux, sufficient to disrupt the cerebral energy state. Aldose reductase activity is also present in the brain, where galactitol may accumulate intracellularly and contribute to cellular swelling and death.

The observation that a galactose-free diet cannot be realized and that galactose and galactose-1-phosphate can also be made from endogenous sources, make it probable that galactose-1-phosphate and galactitol also contribute to the occurrence of late complications.

In particular, the late complications of classical galactosemia have been ascribed to a depletion of uridine diphosphate galactose, one of the products of galactose-1-phosphate uridyltransferase activity. Uridine diphosphate galactose is the donor of the galactosyl moiety in the biosynthesis of glycoproteins and glycolipids, including gangliosides, cerebroside and sulfatide. A deficiency of uridine diphosphate galactose could limit the synthesis of these macromolecules, which include major myelin lipids. However, recent studies have cast doubt on this hypothesis, as the presence of decreased uridine diphosphate galactose levels could not be confirmed. The theory is also difficult to reconcile with the metabolic pathways which enable synthesis of uridine diphosphate galactose from glucose-1-phosphate by pyrophosphorylase and epimerase.

Depletion of myo-inositol and inositol phospholipids has been found in the brain of galactosemia patients. Myo-inositol is essential for the synthesis of inositol phospholipids, which are membrane components. An important surface signal transduction system relies on induction of hydrolysis of plasma membrane phosphoinositides to generate intracellular second messenger molecules which induce the cell to respond to various extracellular agonists, such as neurotransmitters and peptide hormones. Insufficient levels of these membrane phosphoinositides may lead to impaired cell function. Myo-inositol is synthesized from glucose-6-phosphate. Aldose reductase is activated by high levels of galactose, and activation of this pathway leads to myo-inositol depletion.

The cause of ovarian failure is not known. Prenatal and postnatal factors probably play a role.

40.4 Therapy

The predominant source of galactose is lactose, present in mammalian milk or artificial milk formulae. Patients with galactosemia type 1 are treated with a galactose-free diet, causing all symptoms of acute galactose toxicity to disappear, including vomiting, diarrhea, jaundice, hepatomegaly, cerebral edema and cataracts. Levels of galactose-1-phosphate in red blood cells and galactitol in urine drop. Monitoring of treatment by assessing galactose-1-phosphate in red blood cells or galactitol in urine is of limited value. Even with strict adherence to diet, the values remain elevated. After increased galactose intake, it takes several weeks before galactitol in urine rise and even longer before galactose-1-phosphate rises. On the whole, changes in galactose intake have relatively little effect on metabolite levels. Perfect treatment is not attainable, probably because food products may still contain some galactose and, possibly more important, because of endogenous production of galactose from glucose. There is no evidence that the occurrence of late complications depends on strictness of compliance to the diet, which is also an argument in favor of endogenous galactose production. In addition, an abnormal prenatal intrauterine biochemical environment may be responsible for part of the cerebral and ovary dysfunction, which cannot be reversed by postnatal treatment. Experimental therapeutic strategies include replacement of depleted metabolites, such as inositol or uridine to increase uridine diphosphate galactose.

There is no evidence that dietary treatment of heterozygous mothers pregnant with a galactosemic fetus has beneficial effects. Lactation in galactosemic mothers may cause a significant rise in galactose-1-phosphate in red blood cells and galactitol in urine. Considering these biochemical signs of self-intoxication, breast feeding is discouraged. Hormonal replacement therapy is given to female patients with ovary dysfunction.

Treatment of galactosemia type 2 may be limited to the elimination of milk from the diet. It is not necessary to apply a strict galactose-free diet.

Treatment of the mild form of galactosemia type 3 is not necessary. Treatment of the severe form is similar to treatment of galactosemia type 1, but more difficult. Galactosemia type 3 patients are unable to synthesize galactose from glucose and are therefore dependent

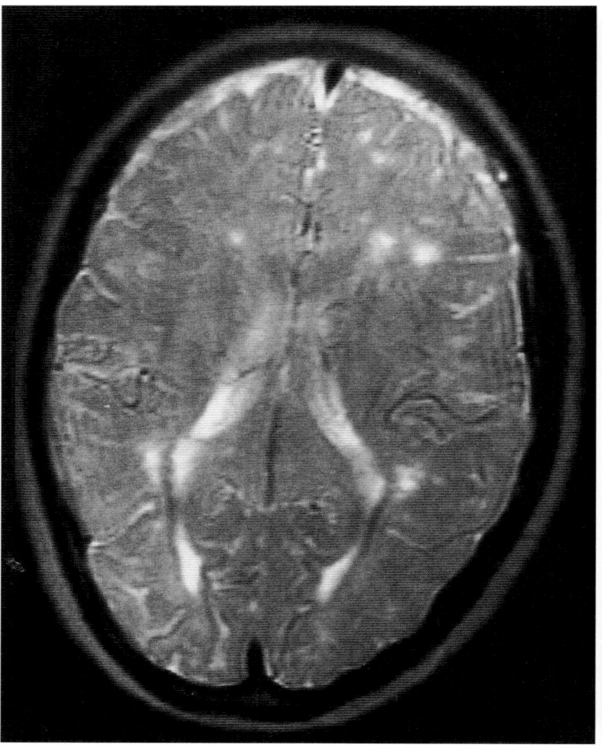 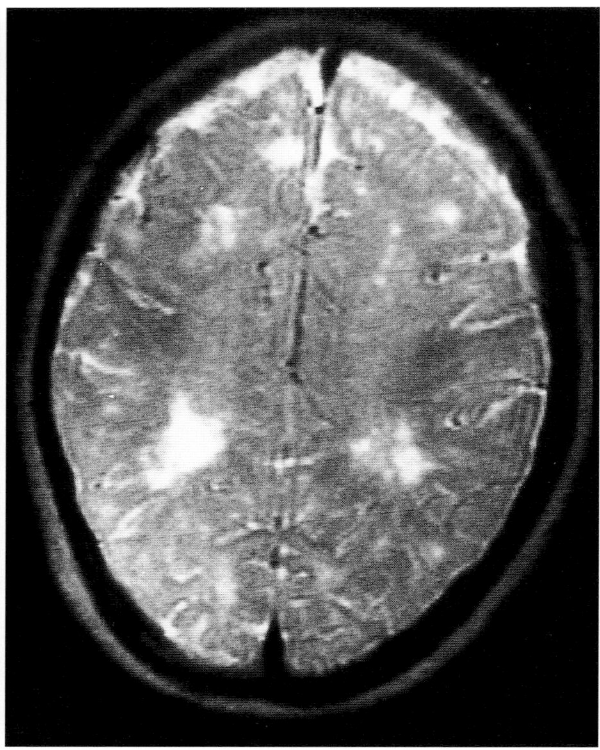

Fig. 40.1. Girl, 14 years of age, with galactosemia type 1. The T$_2$-weighted images show a combination of hypomyelination and patchy high signal intensity white matter abnormalities, consistent with gliosis. There is some widening of the arachnoid spaces

upon exogenous sources for galactose. When too small amounts of galactose are ingested, synthesis of galactosylated compounds, such as galactoproteins and galactolipids (myelin lipids!), is impaired. Unfortunately, there is no easily available chemical parameter for monitoring galactose allowance.

40.5   Magnetic Resonance Imaging

Neuroimaging reports all concern galactosemia type 1. CT scan of the brain has been reported to show signs of generalized atrophy in patients with neurological abnormalities. The ventricular system is enlarged and the cerebellum is atrophic.

The first abnormality noted by MRI is that after normal initial myelination the directly subcortical white matter does not become as hypointense on T$_2$-weighted images as in normal children older than 1 year, indicative of hypomyelination (Fig. 40.1). This can still be seen in adult patients. In addition, multiple foci of high signal intensity are seen in many patients, spread over the hemispheral white matter (Fig. 40.1). The foci are bilateral and more or less symmetrical in distribution, although not perfectly symmetrical. The white matter abnormalities are most pronounced in the periventricular area, round the frontal and occipital horns.

In many patients the ventricular system is slightly enlarged. Cerebellar foliae are prominently visible in some patients.

In none of the patients with mild variants of galactosemia type 1 are abnormalities noted on MRI.

41 Sjögren-Larsson Syndrome

41.1 Clinical Features and Laboratory Investigations

Sjögren-Larsson syndrome (SLS) is a rare disorder with an autosomal recessive mode of inheritance. The three cardinal clinical signs are mental retardation, congenital ichthyosis and spastic diplegia or tetraplegia. The ichthyosis is seen at birth and initial presentation may be as a collodion baby. The ichthyosis tends to worsen with time, and usually presents after infancy as a brownish verrucous, lichenified hyperkeratosis. The signs of spasticity usually become manifest at 4–30 months of age. Many of the patients are never able to walk without assistance and a considerable number are wheelchair-dependent. Those able to walk have a typical spastic gait. Tendon reflexes are high and bilateral Babinski signs are often present. Short stature and thoracolumbar kyphoscoliosis may be present. Mental deficiency varies from moderate to severe. Speech defect is usually present and can be attributed to a combination of mental deficiency and pseudobulbar palsy. Occasionally epilepsy is present. Some SLS patients have ocular abnormalities, including a pathognomonic circular pattern of glistening white dots in the macular region of the retina. Defective development of tooth enamel is a minor feature of the syndrome.

Clinical diagnosis of SLS is confirmed by finding deficient fatty alcohol-NAD$^+$ oxidoreductase activity in leukocytes and cultured fibroblasts. Carrier detection can be performed by enzyme assessment in cultured fibroblasts. Prenatal diagnosis is possible with the help of enzyme assessment in cultured amniocytes and fetal skin biopsy tissue.

41.2 Pathology

External appearance of the brain is normal. A considerable loss of myelin is seen in the hemispheral white matter, the area involved extending from frontal to occipital. Ballooning of myelin sheaths is a notable feature within the areas of myelin loss. Lipid-laden macrophages and histiocytes are present. Small lipid droplets are contained in the cytoplasm of microglia, scattered diffusely through the white matter. In the area of myelin loss, degeneration and loss of axis cylinders and astrocytosis are found. The corpus callosum is well myelinated. Within the brain stem the pyramidal tracts show depletion of myelin and loss of axis cylinders. Myelin loss is also demonstrated in some of the descending tracts of the spinal cord, including the lateral corticospinal tracts, but the ascending tracts are normal. Cerebellar white matter is normal.

Microscopy of the cerebral cortex reveals diffuse cell loss in all areas with an increase in astrocytes and accumulation of sudanophilic droplets of fat. Within the cerebellar cortex some loss of Purkinje cells is seen. Some neuronal cell loss is also seen in the basal nuclei, in particular in putamen and substantia nigra.

41.3 Pathogenetic Considerations

The basic defect of SLS is an impairment in fatty alcohol oxidation due to deficient activity of fatty alcohol-NAD$^+$ oxidoreductase. This enzyme consists of two proteins that sequentially catalyze the oxidation of fatty alcohol to fatty aldehyde and fatty acid, reactions that are catalyzed by fatty alcohol dehydrogenase and fatty aldehyde dehydrogenase, respectively. SLS patients are specifically deficient in the fatty aldehyde dehydrogenase component. As a consequence of this enzyme deficiency, long-chain alcohols accumulate in SLS patients. The finding that SLS patients are deficient in fatty aldehyde dehydrogenase and not in fatty alcohol dehydrogenase raises the possibility that the SLS phenotype results partly from fatty aldehyde accumulation. Accumulation of this substance could, however, not be confirmed in studies with intact SLS fibroblasts.

The biological consequences of either long-chain fatty alcohol or fatty aldehyde accumulation are unknown. Long-chain alcohols have been shown to partition into artificial lipid bilayers and synaptic vesicles. If fatty alcohols accumulate in the skin of SLS patients, it could alter the epidermal water barrier, which is critically dependent on the lipid composition of the stratum corneum, and lead to increased transepidermal water loss and ichthyosis. Partition of long-chain fatty alcohols or fatty aldehydes into membranes could alter the myelin membrane and lead to myelin instability and loss.

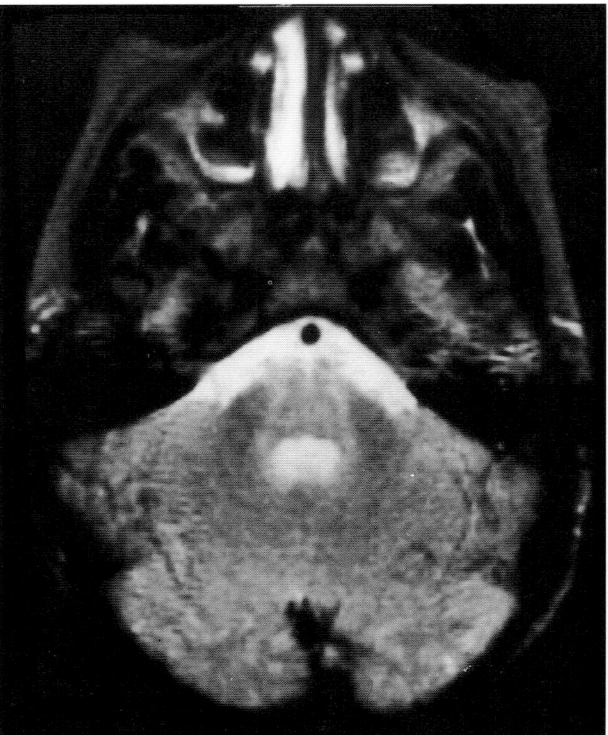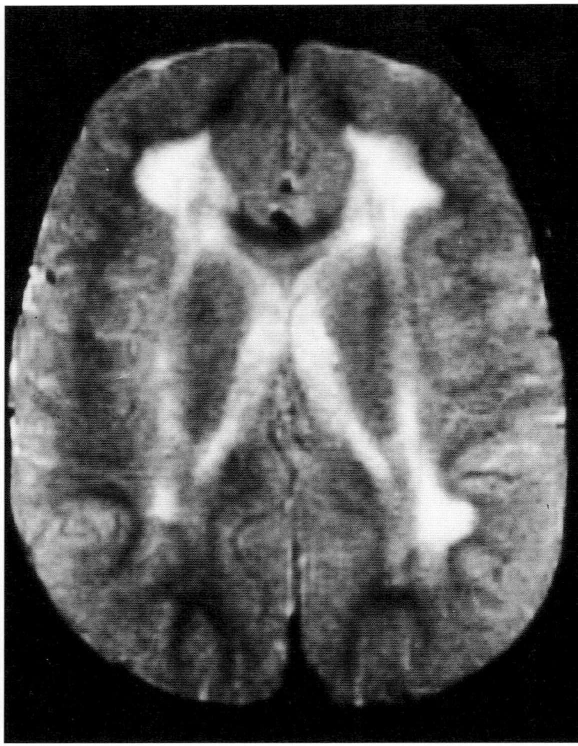

Fig. 41.1. MR images of a 4-year-old patient with SLS. Note the diffuse hemispheral white matter changes with sparing of the arcuate fibers, internal capsule, corpus callosum, and cere- bellum. Pontine tracts are also involved. Courtesy of DiRocco et al. (1994), with permission

41.4 Therapy

At present there is no causal treatment. Symptomatic treatment, including care of the dermatological problems, and supportive care are the only options.

41.5 Magnetic Resonance Imaging

Only very few imaging data are available. In several CT studies diffuse or more patchy hemispheral white matter hypodensity has been reported, most marked in the frontal area. No enhancement is present after contrast administration.

MRI confirms the presence of diffuse hemispheral white matter abnormality with sparing of the arcuate fibers, corpus callosum and cerebellar white matter, and involvement of corticospinal tracts in the brain stem (Fig. 41.1).

42 Lowe Syndrome

42.1 Clinical Features and Laboratory Investigations

Lowe syndrome (LS), or oculocerebrorenal syndrome, is a rare, X-linked hereditary disease. It is present in all races, with a predominance in those with Caucasian and Asian ancestries.

Affected males present themselves with congenital ocular manifestations including congenital cataract, often associated with glaucoma and miotic pupils. Buphthalmos may be present. Sight is poor and eye movements are nystagmoid. Additional early features include muscle hypotonia and hyporeflexia or areflexia. During the first year of life psychomotor developmental delay becomes obvious. The infants have excessive crying with a high-pitched scream. Asymptomatic amino aciduria and proteinuria are usually found during this stage.

During early childhood the symptoms of renal tubular dysfunction develop with metabolic acidosis and losses of calcium and phosphate. Severe demineralization and rickets may develop and lead to frequent fractures, pain, and delay of normal physical development. Linear growth decreases after one year of age and between 1 and 3 years of age height falls below the third percentile. Head circumference is either normal or borderline microcephalic. Noninflammatory arthropathy of unknown pathogenesis with pain, contractures and joint swelling may occur, affecting both large and small joints. Mental retardation is usually moderate, but intelligence varies between normal and profoundly decreased. Some patients have epilepsy. Unusual stereotypic movements are often seen. Maladaptive behavior is frequently present and consists of temper tantrums, high-pitched scream, and stubbornness.

Patients with LS continue to grow in early adulthood. Final height, however, remains below the third percentile of normal values. Severe bone disease leads to orthopedic disability. Renal dysfunction is slowly progressive. Terminal renal failure occurs in the mid-thirties. Death may occur between the first and the fourth decade, secondary to inanition pneumonia or uremia.

Laboratory findings show renal tubular dysfunction similar to Fanconi syndrome. The tubular dysfunction leads to urinary loss of bicarbonate, calcium, phosphorus, protein, and amino acids. The results are metabolic acidosis, hypophosphatemia, secondary hyperparathryoidism, and rickets. Urinary excretion of carnitine is increases with decreased serum carnitine. The serum muscle enzymes creatine kinase, aspartate aminotransferase and lactate dehydrogenase, have been reported to be elevated in some cases. Over the years progressive glomerular dysfunction develops with uremia. A linear relation between reciprocal serum creatine level and age reflects the progressive renal failure. Abnormalities of blood chemistry values are mitigated by replacement therapy for renal tubular losses.

Skeletal X-ray examinations reveal rachitic changes. EEG often shows nonspecific abnormalities, sometimes epileptic activity.

Detection of female carriers is possible. Progressive lenticular opacities are present in LS carriers and even young carriers can be identified reliably in this way. Lack of opacities cannot be considered as proof of not being a carrier, but is highly suggestive. DNA techniques are becoming available for carrier detection and prenatal diagnosis.

42.2 Pathology

In LS, data on neuropathological findings are limited. The brain weight is usually below normal. Moderate, diffuse atrophy may be seen with cortical atrophy, some ventricular enlargement and thinning of the corpus callosum. The meninges are diffusely fibrotic without inflammatory changes.

Variable cortical changes have been described ranging from pachygyria and polymicrogyria to neuronal loss in combination with gliosis. The cortex may also be found to be normal.

The white matter changes described are also variable. The most frequent finding is gliosis. Myelination has been described as normal in some patients, whereas myelin paucity was described in others. Myelin paucity is usually ascribed to dysmyelination. White matter abnormalities are most pronounced in the centrum semiovale and periventricular white matter. Active myelin breakdown has never been reported. In rare cases, there are no white matter abnormalities.

Cerebellum may be atrophic or normal. Gliosis of the cortex and white matter have been observed.

Variable and inconsistent abnormalities of the peripheral nervous system has been reported. Nerve biopsy has been found to exhibit signs of an axonal neuropathy in several, but not all patients. Muscle biopsy has indicated selective type 1 fiber atrophy with type 1 fiber predominance, considered to be consistent with congenital fiber type disproportion myopathy or, alternatively, to abnormal neuronal influence upon muscle. In other patients, muscle biopsy revealed no abnormalities.

Renal pathology demonstrates dilated tubules with atrophy of tubular epithelium. Many tubules contain eosinophilic, granular protein casts. Interstitial fibrosis is present. Glomerular changes have also been observed, in particular on ultrastructural examination. Glomerular endothelal cells have been found to be swollen with a reduction in the number of endothelial slit pores, fusion of endothelial foot processes and thickening of the glomerular basement membrane.

42.3 Pathogenetic Considerations

LS is an X-linked disorder. The LS locus has been mapped to region Xq25–q26. Recent evidence suggests that the gene product is involved in the inositol phosphate metabolism. Inositoltriphosphate is involved in signal transduction and phosphatidylinositol participates in anchoring membrane proteins, but the function of many inositol phosphates, either free or esterified in phospholipids, is unclear.

In highly exceptional cases, the LS phenotype has been observed in female patients. Possible explanations for this observation include the simultaneous presence of mutations on both X-chromosomes, and the presence of a mutation or a translocation within one LS locus together with a preferential inactivation of the normal X-chromosome.

The relationship between the genetic defect and the clinical symptomatology is unclear in LS. The lenticu-lar opacities are already present at birth in affected males and are not the result of the metabolic changes. The cause of the hypotonia is a matter of debate. Some ascribe it to muscular involvement, others to an axonal neuropathy.

42.4 Therapy

In renal tubular acidosis and rickets a combination of sodium-potassium citrate, phosphorus and vitamin D therapy has a beneficial effect. Ocular surgery is essential for establishing some visual acuity. The retina in patients with LS is usually well-formed and capable of receiving a light stimulus.

42.5 Magnetic Resonance Imaging

MRI in LS shows a much more consistent pattern than suggested by neuropathology. In patients with an advanced degree of myelination patchy, partially confluent white matter changes are seen suggestive of gliosis (Fig. 42.1). During the first months of life these white matter abnormalities may not be noticeable due to the still unmyelinated aspect of the white matter. The changes are most pronounced in the periventricular area and centrum semiovale. The distribution of the white matter changes is globally symmetrical, but not in detail. Often small cystic lesions are seen within the abnormal white matter. Arcuate fibers, corpus callosum, internal capsule, brain stem and cerebellum are spared. Mild ventriculomegaly may be present. No major cortical abnormalities have been reported. Some evidence of polymicrogyria has been reported incidentally.

The images with somewhat irregular, patchy white matter abnormalities and small cysts are reminiscent of those of congenital infections, in particular cytomegalovirus infections. Cortical gyrational abnormalities are also seen in early prenatal cytomegalovirus infections.

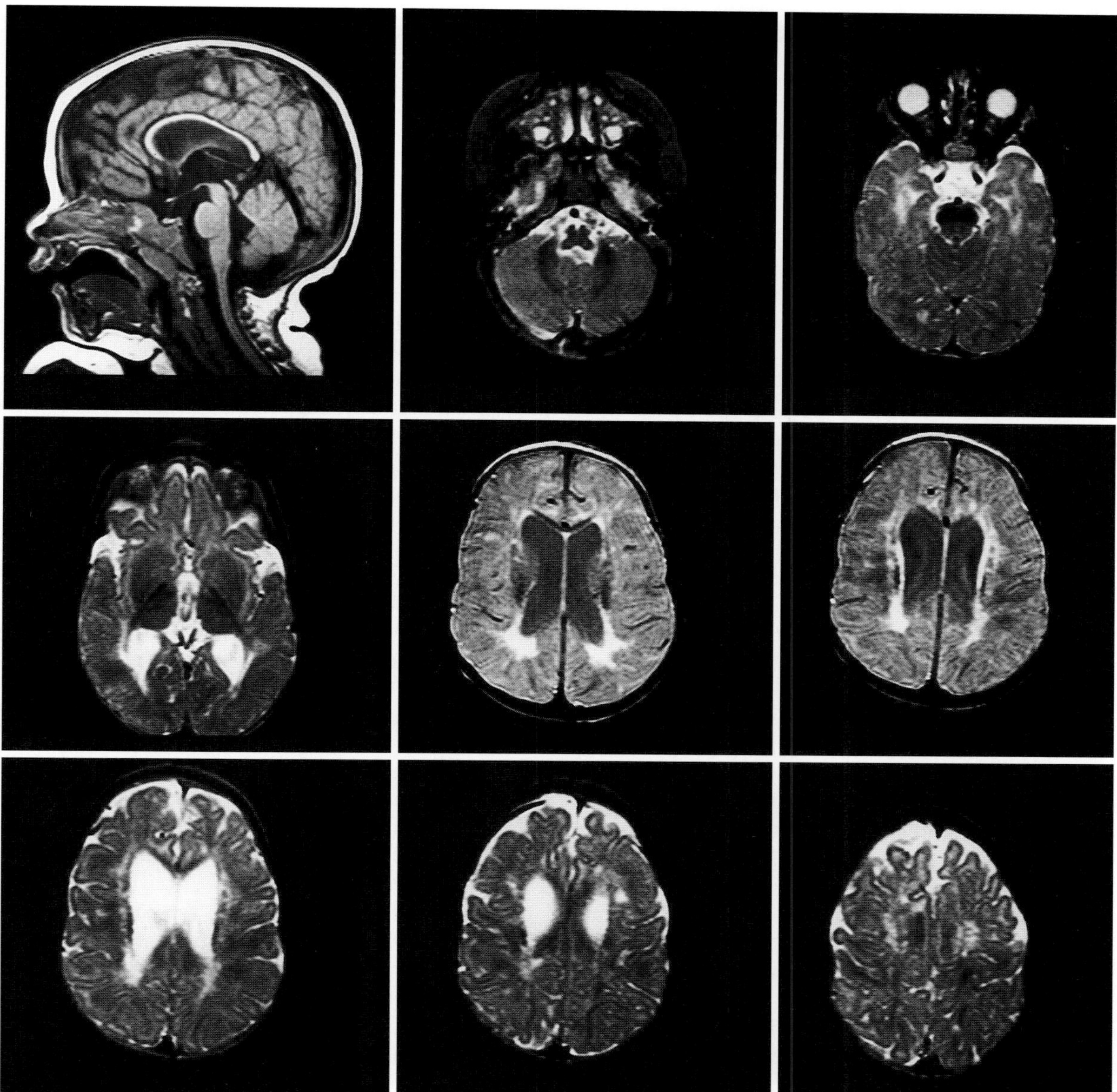

Fig. 42.1. MR study of a 14-month-old boy with LS. The ventricles are dilated and there is a rather symmetrical rim of patchy hyperintensity around the ventricles, interrupted by some areas of low signal intensity. The corpus callosum is thin. In the frontal areas the U fibers are not yet myelinated

43 Wilson Disease

43.1 Clinical Features and Laboratory Investigations

Hepatolenticular degeneration was first described by Kinear Wilson in 1912 and has been named after him. Wilson disease (WD) is a genetically determined, autosomal recessive disease with a prevalence of 20–30 per million. The clinical picture is extremely variable, also depending on the age of presentation. Patients present with hepatic, neurological or psychiatric symptomatology in roughly equal proportions, with some overlap. In children, hepatic manifestations predominate, whereas in adolescents and adults neuropsychiatric manifestations are more frequent. Symptoms rarely occur before the age of 6, and half of the patients are symptomatic by the age of 15. Onset after the age of 40 is rare, but patients presenting in the fifth and sixth decades have been described.

Hepatic manifestations in WD encompass a spectrum of acute and chronic liver diseases. Some patients, usually younger patients, present with fulminant hepatic failure, leading to jaundice, hypoalbuminemia, ascites, coagulation defects, hyperammonemia and hepatic encephalopathy. Massive liver failure in WD is often accompanied by hemolytic anemia. However, if the liver failure is less massive, only certain features of this syndrome may be present. In older patients liver failure tends to be chronic and is associated with portal hypertension, hypoalbuminemia, edema and ascites. Some patients present with a clinical picture of hepatitis and/or cirrhosis without elements of liver failure. They may be jaundiced, reflecting a period of hemolysis. Most patients with WD, whatever their clinical presentation or presymptomatic status, have some degree of liver disease. They often have evidence of portal hypertension, including gastric or esophageal varices, and/or hypersplenism with thrombopenia or leukopenia.

The patient with WD who presents with neurological disease is typically in his/her late teens or twenties. The signs and symptoms are usually chronic, but occasionally acute in presentation. Frequent early symptoms include tremor, speech problems, clumsiness and personality changes. Kayser-Fleischer rings are almost invariably present in patients with neurological manifestations of WD. The rings are typically 1 to 3 mm in diameter, green, yellow or brown, and located at the periphery of the cornea. They begin as crescents in the superior quadrant and subsequently extend to the inferior, lateral and medial regions until they become circumferential and broader, spreading centrally from the limbus. Kayser-Fleischer rings may be seen with the unaided eye, but a slit-lamp examination is often necessary to detect these. Adolescents may present with a deterioration of performance at school and in athletics, difficulties with handwriting and loss of dexterity. Without treatment, neurological deterioration continues. The full-blown neurological picture of WD encompasses a variable combination of the following signs: dysarthria, drooling, dysphagia, grimacing, abnormal eye movements, dystonia, rigidity, bradykinesia, athetosis, wing beating, spasticity with increased tendon reflexes and Babinski signs, cerebellar ataxia, and tremor (resting, intention, or postural), but cognitive and sensory functions are typically preserved. Seizures may occur. Because of increasing difficulty in controling movement, the patient becomes unable to feed him- or herself, and becomes bedridden. Flexion contractures develop. Ultimately, the patient becomes helpless, is usually alert, but unable to talk.

Psychiatric and behavioral symptoms are variable and include reduced performance at school or at work, inability to cope, depression, very labile moods ranging from mania to depression, sexual exhibitionism, and frank psychosis. Personality changes, particularly irritability, emotionality and increased anger are the most commonly noted problems.

Ophthalmological abnormalities include, in the first place, the Kayser-Fleischer rings, and, less frequently, sunflower cataracts consisting of green, golden-brown, or gray granular deposits in the lens of the eye, appearing as discoid opacities in the anterior lens capsule with petal-like fronds that radiate toward the lens periphery like a sunflower. Neither Kayser-Fleischer rings nor sunflower cataracts affect vision significantly.

Hematological presentation is rare, but WD should be considered in young patients with nonspherocytic, Coombs-negative intravascular hemolysis of unclear etiology. Severe hemolysis frequently occurs in the setting of fulminant hepatic failure.

Patients may have abnormalities of renal tubular function with amino acduria, proteinuria, uricosuria, hypercalciuria, hyperphosphaturia, or defective urine acidification. Occasionally, full-blown Fanconi syndrome is present. Renal stones are not uncommon.

Osteomalacia, rickets, osteoporosis, osteoarthritis, polyarthritis, localized bone demineralization, spontaneous fractures, peri- and intra-articular calcifications, and joint hypermobility may occur in WD. However, musculoskeletal symptoms are rarely the presenting complaints. Hyperpigmentation of the skin may occur. Congestive heart failure and cardiac dysrhythmias have been reported. The most frequent endocrinological disturbances are gynaecomastia and delayed puberty due to hepatic dysfunction. Primary or secondary amenorrhea due to liver disease is common. Successful pregnancy is exceptional in untreated female WD patients and spontaneous abortions occur frequently.

There is often an unacceptable delay in establishing a diagnosis of WD. Whenever the diagnosis is suspected, Kayser-Fleischer rings should be sought by an experienced ophthalmologist, using a slit lamp. Kayser-Fleischer rings are almost always present in WD patients with neurological problems, but their absence does not mean the diagnosis is wrong. Kayser-Fleischer rings are also not pathognomonic for WD and may be seen in some other hepatobiliary diseases or as a result of topical ocular application of copper-containing solutions. In most patients suspected of WD, the presence of both Kayser-Fleischer rings and at least one, if not all three, biochemical markers confirm the diagnosis: low serum level of ceruloplasmin, elevated serum copper concentration and an increased urinary copper excretion. However, one should recognize the limited value of these tests. Ceruloplasmin is low in about 90% of WD patients, but some patients have levels in the low-normal range due to hepatic inflammation, pregnancy or use of estrogen. A low serum ceruloplasmin can also be found in heterozygotes for WD, in other hepatic disorders, normal neonates and in patients with malabsorption, malnutrition or nephrosis. Free serum copper and urinary copper concentrations can be elevated in other hepatobiliary diseases. In case of doubt, in particular if the ceruloplasmin level is normal and/or Kayser-Fleischer rings are absent, conditions most often seen in patients with hepatic presentation, liver biopsy for copper analysis and microscopic examination are essential. Hepatic copper concentrations are always elevated in untreated WD patients and also higher in patients than in heterozygotes. Histological abnormalities in WD range from steatosis to cirrhosis. Normal liver histology is seen in heterozygotes. However, in patients with chronic cholestatic liver disease, elevations of liver copper concentrations may be similar to those in WD patients. In selected patients a test of incorporation of a copper isotope into serum ceruloplasmin is informative. Because the biochemical copper profile of a normal neonate mimics that seen in WD and clinical manifestations of WD are rarely seen before the age of 6, conventional screening of potentially affected children should begin no earlier than 3 years of age. Since the WD gene has been sequenced recently, DNA techniques are becoming available for definite diagnosis in patients suspected of WD and for distinction between presymptomatic patients and heterozygotes in families with WD. Prenatal diagnosis is possible using DNA techniques.

Evoked potential studies do not contribute to the diagnosis in WD, but they may be used in monitoring treatment. SSEPs and BAEPs are frequently prolonged in neurologically symptomatic patients, more so than VEPs.

43.2 Pathology

External examination of the brain usually reveals no abnormalities except for some shrinkage of the insular cortex.

Within the brain parenchyma, lesions are invariably present in the corpus striatum, which appears shrunken. Cavitation is often present in the putamen, sometimes also in the caudate nucleus, rarely in the globus pallidus, thalamus and red nucleus. On microscopic examination, neuronal loss is found in the putamen and caudate nucleus. Astrocytic proliferation is present. Some astrocytes have the appearance of Alzheimer type II cells; few resemble Alzheimer type I cells. When cavities are present, variable numbers of lipophages and siderophages are seen in relation to the cavities; old and recent hemorrhages can be found. Depositions of copper have been described by some, in particular in the putamen. Less constantly and less severely involved nuclei are the globus pallidus, the subthalamic nucleus, the thalamus, dentate nucleus, substantia nigra and other brain stem nuclei. Opalski cells are typically present in the thalamus, globus pallidus and zona reticularis of the substantia nigra, but less often in the caudate nucleus and putamen. Opalski cells are large cells with voluminous cytoplasm and small nuclei. Their origin is uncertain, but they are typically present in WD.

In some patients destructive lesions are present in the cerebral cortex and white matter. The distribution of the cortical involvement corresponds with that of the white matter involvement. These lesions may be very impressive and exceed the lesions in the basal nuclei. The lesions are typically located in the superior and middle frontal gyri; widespread involvement posterior to the frontal lobes is uncommon. The changes are usually symmetrical, but may also be asymmetrical. Cavitation of the white matter lesions may occur. The outer layers of the cortex always retain sufficient structural integrity to form a continuous shell. In microscopic examination of the affected cortex, the deep cortical layers appear to be affected predominantly, whereas the more superficial cortical layers are relatively intact. The cortical abnormalities may have a spongiform appearance. The white matter abnormalities vary from myelin paucity to clear-cut necrosis with presence of sudanophilic breakdown products.

The cerebellum is relatively spared. Some loss of cortical neurons may be seen and some myelin pallor. The dentate nucleus is most frequently involved. White matter degeneration in the region of the dentate nucleus has been described.

43.3 Pathogenetic Considerations

WD is characterized by failure to incorporate copper into ceruloplasmin in the liver, and failure to excrete copper from the liver into bile. The gene responsible for WD has been identified and assigned to band q14.3 on chromosome 13. The gene has been cloned and sequenced and a number of disease-specific mutations have been detected. The gene product is a cation transporting P-type ATPase protein, probably involved in copper transport. This protein is present predominantly in liver, kidney and placenta.

Copper is an essential trace element, being an integral component of a variety of important enzymes, including superoxide dismutase, cytochrome oxidase and other electron transport proteins. In excess, copper is also a very toxic ion, because it can oxidize proteins and lipids in membranes, bind to proteins and nucleic acids and enhance generation of free radicals. Dietary intake of copper generally far exceeds the trace amounts required. Consequently, efficient and appropriate mechanisms must exist to ensure copper homeostasis and to transport copper to the sites where it is required without allowing toxic accumulation of free ions. Various proteins have been recognized to be involved in copper homeostasis and transport: albumin for copper transport in the blood, ceruloplasmin as a possible copper donor to tissues and enzymes, metallothionein for intracellular copper storage. The newly detected copper transporting ATPase probably plays a role in copper export out of the liver. Deficiency of this protein leads to failure to excrete copper from the liver into bile and to incorporate copper into ceruloplasmin during ceruloplasmin biosynthesis in the liver. This results in toxic accumulation of copper in the liver, with subsequent overflow to the kidney, brain and cornea. Accumulation of copper leads to liver cirrhosis, progressive neurological damage and/or renal problems. Very high free serum copper levels, in particular caused by sudden massive release of copper from the liver, may result in hemolytic crises.

The cause of pathology in WD is copper toxicity. Organs affected by the disease contain elevated copper levels, and lowering of copper leads to cessation of progression, some repair and clinical improvement. Excess copper causes cell injury, inflammation and cell death. Copper has damaging effects on mitochondria and peroxisomes. Effects on microtubules, on crosslinking of DNA and on plasma membranes, as well as inhibition of a large number of enzymes, have also been shown. The state of copper is important. Copper bound to ceruloplasmin, metallothionein or albumin is nontoxic. It is ionic copper or copper that is easily dissociable, that is toxic. Copper toxicity probably occurs because of the generation of oxidant radicals. In this respect it is important to note that the pattern of preferential involvement of gray matter structures in WD shows some striking similarities to the patterns observed in respiratory chain defects and in hypoxia. Caudate nucleus and putamen are preferentially affected. Other frequently involved gray matter structures are thalamus, globus pallidus, subthalamic nucleus and periaqueductal gray matter.

43.4 Therapy

Therapeutic strategies in WD can focus on inhibition of the intestinal uptake of copper, induction of metallothionein to detoxify copper, and chelation.

Penicillamine is the drug of first choice in WD. It acts by reductive chelation, reducing the copper bound to protein, thereby decreasing the affinity of the protein for copper and allowing penicillamine to bind copper. Reductive chelation is much more effective than chelators with a high affinity for copper, such as EDTA. The copper mobilized by penicillamine is excreted in urine. Penicillamine probably also induces hepatic metallothionein, thereby holding potentially toxic copper in a nontoxic form. Some patients improve clinically soon after therapy begins, whereas some may require several months of therapy before improvement occurs. In about 10%–20% of WD patients with neurological complaints, temporary exacerbation of symptoms is seen with institution of therapy. However, some patients never recover to their pretherapy baseline. Penicillamine therapy should be continued for life in WD patients, whether asymptomatic or symptomatic. With treatment, asymptomatic patients remain asymptomatic. Inadvertent discontinuation of penicillamine therapy may lead to catastrophic clinical deterioration and death. Adverse effects of penicillamine are, unfortunately, common. A considerable number of the patients develop an early hypersensitivity reaction to penicillamine mandating its discontinuation. Treatment is restarted in conjunction with corticosteroids until tolerance develops. Long-term use of penicillamine can result in serious side-effects forcing discontinuation of its use. These side-effects include induction of a variety of autoimmune-like disorders and induction of a skin problem due to alterations of dermal collagen and elastin.

Triethylene tetramine dihydrochloride (trientine or trien) is both a chelator, acting primarily by enhancing urinary excretion of copper, and an inhibitor of copper absorption in the intestine. Far less clinical experience has been gained with this drug than with penicillamine, but it can be used in WD patients who do not tolerate penicillamine. Tolerance of triethylene tetramine dihydrochloride is generally excellent.

Oral zinc as zinc acetate or zinc sulfate, inhibits intestinal copper absorption and promotes fecal copper excretion. There is also evidence that zinc may induce the synthesis of metallothionein in enterocytes and possibly hepatocytes. Although zinc appears to be a more potent stimulus to metallothionein synthesis than copper, copper is more avid in binding to metallothionein. Complexed copper may then either be transferred into the portal circulation or remain complexed within the cytosolic fraction of the enterocyte and be excreted in the feces with sloughed cells. Zinc therapy is usually well tolerated, but the therapy acts slowly producing a modestly negative copper balance.

Because of the ubiquity of copper in our diet, a negative copper balance cannot be achieved by dietary modification alone. It seems prudent, however, to recommend that WD patients avoid food with a high copper content.

Despite the effectivenes of medication in most WD patients, occasional patients require liver transplantation because of hepatic failure. This procedure corrects the metabolic defect localized in the liver and transplanted patients no longer need specific medication for WD.

The prognosis of WD patients has generally improved greatly with the advent of treatment. In particular, when treatment is started in a presymptomatic stage, patients never become symptomatic. Also, the vast majority of symptomatic patients improve considerably or recover completely. The patients with hepatic presentation have the least optimistic prognosis. Assuming they survive the initial episode, the greatest risks are variceal bleeding and hepatic insufficiency. The patients with neurological or psychiatric presentation have a better prognosis, although their quality of life can be problematic if the residual deficit is considerable. It is therefore important to start treatment as early as possible, before irreparable damage has occurred. Under adequate treatment, successful pregnancy is possible. Anti-copper therapy should be continued during pregnancy. Zinc is probably safest as both penicillamine and triethylene tetramine dihydrochloride are possibly teratogenic.

43.5 Magnetic Resonance Imaging

CT scan of the brain in WD may reveal a number of different abnormalities including mild ventricular dilatation, cortical atrophy, brain stem atrophy, hypodense areas in the region of the putamen and globus pallidus and dentate nucleus, and white matter hypodensities, in particular in the frontal subcortical area.

MRI most often shows lesions in the thalamus, putamen and caudate nucleus. Gray matter structures which are also regularly involved are the globus pallidus and claustrum. The lesions are usually bilateral and symmetrical, and asymmetry is rare. The lesions most often have a high signal intensity on T_2-weighted images and a low signal intensity on T_1-weighted images. These changes in signal intensity are thought to reflect edema, necrosis and gliosis. In some patients, areas of low signal intensity are seen in the putamen, head of the caudate nucleus and globus pallidus on T_2-weighted images. The nuclei either have a generalized low signal intensity, or there are small areas of low signal intensity within the high signal intensity. Some assume that the low signal intensity on T_2-weighted images is related to iron deposition, as phagocytes containing iron pigment after small hemorrhages are seen in histology. Others assume that the low signal intensity is related to the paramagnetic effect of copper. It is well established that copper ions in vitro have a pronounced effect on both T_1 and T_2. An increased concentration of copper ions causes a decrease in T_1 and T_2. However, the effects of T_1 shortening with a high signal intensity of the basal nuclei on T_1-weighted images has never been reported. Sometimes multiple small cavities are seen within the basal nuclei with a signal intensity similar to that of CSF on all sequences. No contrast enhancement is seen.

Atrophy is a frequent finding. It may be focal, most frequently involving the caudate nuclei or brain stem. The atrophy may also be generalized with enlargement of subarachnoid spaces and ventricular system.

Subcortical white matter lesions are not rare in WD, in contrast to what was formerly thought (Fig. 43.1). The white matter lesions are most often found in the frontal lobes, sometimes with extensions into the parietal area. White matter lesions in other areas are rare. Their location is largely subcortical, and they may not reach the ventricular wall. The white matter lesions are usually large and confluent, but multiple, small, isolated lesions can also be found. In exceptional cases the white matter lesions are cystic. The white matter changes are often asymmetrical, which contrasts with the symmetry of the gray matter lesions. No contrast enhancement is present.

Cerebellar lesions are less frequent in WD, but do occur. Bilateral lesions in the dentate nuclei are most

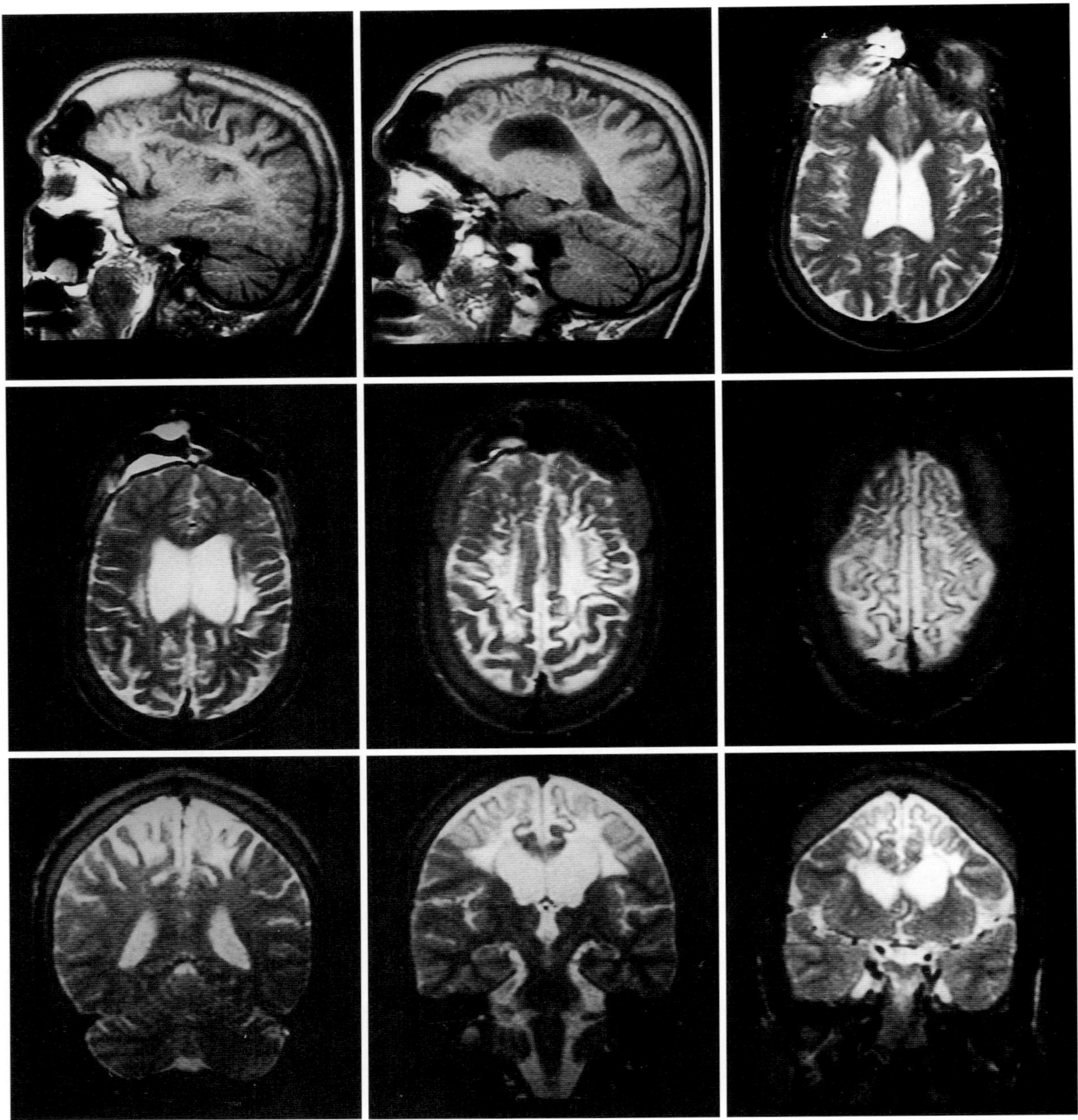

Fig. 43.1. A 48-year-old male patient with WD. The sagittal T_1- and transverse and coronal T_2-weighted MR images show frontoparietal involvement of the white matter, extending into the arcuate fibers. There is atrophy in the area of white matter involvement. In this case there are no abnormal signals from the basal ganglia, but the caudate nucleus is atrophic

often seen. In the white matter round the dentate nucleus, abnormal signal intensity may be present.

Brain stem lesions are by no means rare. The areas most frequently involved are the tectum and tegmentum of the midbrain, red nucleus, substantia nigra, central part of the base of the pons, and pontine tegmentum. Atrophy of midbrain and pons may be seen. A T_2-weighted image through the midbrain may reveal the so-called "face of the giant panda" appearance, with a low signal intensity of the superior colliculus, loss of the normal, characteristic low signal intensity of the lateral portion of the substantia nigra, presence of the normal low signal intensity of the red nucleus and high signal intensity of the tegmentum of the midbrain and the thalamus.

MRI is of value in WD, both for diagnostic and monitoring purposes. The diagnosis of WD may be difficult, and MRI may suggest this possibility. The most important differential diagnostic options are respiratory chain defects and extrapontine myelinolysis, in particular if a central lesion is present in the basis of the pons. However, clinical history and laboratory tests differentiate between these disorders.

MRI is abnormal in almost all patients with neurological complaints and in some neurologically normal patients. In exceptional cases normal MRI has been reported despite the presence of neurological abnormalities. With successful treatment, MRI abnormalities have been shown to improve or disappear.

Some correlations have been found between cerebral lesions and clinical symptomatology. Dystonia is related to putamen lesions; dysarthria correlates with lesions in both putamen and caudate nucleus. Both lesions in the substantia nigra and in the putamen and caudate nucleus are associated with parkinsonism. Abnormalities in efferent cerebellar pathways, including superior cerebellar pedunculus, red nucleus an thalamus, are associated with clinical cerebellar signs. Lesions in the dentate nucleus are associated with a kinetic tremor and dysmetria. Lesions in the red nucleus are associated with proximal kinetic tremor. Generalized atrophy and subcortical white matter lesions are associated with cognitive decline.

44 Neuronal Ceroid Lipofuscinoses

44.1 Clinical Features and Laboratory Investigations

The neuronal ceroid lipofuscinoses (NCL), often called Batten disease, constitute a group of progressive neurodegenerative disorders either with an autosomal recessive mode of inheritance in infants, children and adults or, in rare instances, with an autosomal dominant mode of inheritance in adults. Usually four types are distinguished: infantile NCL (INCL, NCL1 or Santavuori disease), late-infantile NCL (LINCL, NCL2 or Jansky-Bielschowsky disease), juvenile NCL, (JNCL, NCL3, Spielmeyer-Vogt disease or Batten disease) and adult NCL (ANCL, NCL4 or Kufs' disease). The classification of NCL is based on the age of onset, clinical course of the disease, and neurological, ophthalmological, neuropsychological and ultrastructural findings. About 10% of all NCL patients represent variant or atypical forms, which are difficult to classify into the main groups.

INCL is the earliest and most severe major form of NCL. The disease occurs most frequently in Finland, the incidence being there 7:100 000. The early psychomotor development is normal until 6–18 months. Many children manage to stand up and to speak single words, but few learn to walk alone. Then rapid psychomotor deterioration sets in. Head growth slows down. The children develop muscular hypotonia, microcephaly, ataxia, choreoathetosis, stereotyped hand movements, myoclonic jerks, epilepsy, irritability and visual failure. The stereotyped hand movements are similar to those observed in Rett syndrome. Visual failure becomes apparent between 12 and 20 months. Most patients are blind before the age of 2. Slow or absent pupillary responses, optic atrophy and macular and retinal degeneration without pigment aggregations can be found on ophthalmological examination. Partial and generalized seizures and, occasionally, a Lennox-Gastaut-like epileptic syndrome are seen. Between 24 and 36 months most children are bed-ridden. They are grossly mentally retarded and do not perform voluntary movements. Opisthotonus, decorticate posturing and hyperexcitability to any kind of stimulation increasing the myoclonic jerks are characteristically present. Flexion contractures are common. After a number of years the hyperexcitability ceases. The final vegetative state is dominated by extensor posturing, unresponsiveness, blindness, gross microcephaly, stimulus-sensitive myoclonus and seizures. Death ensues before the age of 15, usually between 8 and 11 years.

LINCL has its onset between 2 and 4 years of age. Usually epilepsy is the first symptom. Often several types of seizures occur, including generalized tonic-clonic seizures, myoclonic jerks, absences and drop attacks. As disease progresses, myoclonia becomes the most predominant type. Onset of epilepsy is soon followed by mental and motor deterioration. Ataxia, especially truncal ataxia, hypotonia and slurring of speech occur. Speech diminishes and disappears within a year. Typically, visual failure appears after the neurological symptoms and progression is slow. Blindness usually occurs at the age of 6 years. Funduscopic examination may initially be normal, but within 2 years after onset macular degeneration and retinal pigmentation are seen. Progression of disease is otherwise rapid with precipitous regression of mental and motor faculties. The initial hypotonia gives way to spasticity, painful flexor spasms and severe flexion contractures. Excessive drooling and difficulty with swallowing occur. The final stage of the disease is one of unresponsiveness, myoclonic hyperexcitability and blindness. Death occurs between 10 and 15 years.

JNCL is the most common type of NCL in the world with the highest incidence in North European countries (0.5:100 000), in particular in Finland (5:100 000). The first clinical symptom is visual failure starting at the age of 4–8 years. Subsequently, mental slowing, epilepsy and motor disturbances occur. The disease progresses at a slow pace and long periods of ostensible arrest, sometimes even improvement, are common. Ophthalmological examination reveals macular degeneration and pigmentary retina degeneration. Blindness is present by the age of 6–14 years. Seizures increase in frequency and severity and are usually of a generalized and complex partial nature. Mental deterioration with widening gap between JNCL patients and classmates become obvious after the age of 12 years. Patients are unable to follow a regular school program and begin to lose acquired cognitive skills. Speech impediment becomes noticeable in that the tone is monotonous. Patients also demonstrate echolalia and perseveration. Motor skills are lost. Rigidity, hypokinesia and dystonia are frequently observed and movements are slow. Intention tremor, tremor at rest and myoclonias are often noted. Spasticity does not set in until a late stage and is never severe. Many teenagers become depressed. Some manifest restlessness, rage, physical violence, insomnia, and visual and auditory hallucinations with paranoid delusions. Chewing and swollowing become more difficult, eventually necessitating nasal tube feeding. Myoclonia may become severe. Life expectancy is 18–40 years.

ANCL usually starts around the age of 25–30 years. Two main clinical subtypes are usually distinguished, although there is considerable overlap. Clinical phenotype A is characterized by behavioral changes, dementia, progressive myoclonus epilepsy, cerebellar ataxia and dysarthria. Vision is normal and there are no signs of optic atrophy, macular degeneration or pigmentary retinal degeneration. In the course of the disease seizures become intractable. Signs of involvement of the pyramidal, extrapyramidal and lower motor neuron systems are absent or only seen terminally. Clinical phenotype B is characterized by behavioral changes, dementia and motor abnormalities. Cerebellar or extrapyramidal features are prominent, the latter most frequently taking the form of a hyperkinetic movement disorder, rarely parkinsonism. Tic-like facial dyskinesias may be present. Pyramidal signs are rarely prominent. Visual failure and retinal abnormalities are not present. Seizures are rare and may only occur late in the course of the disease. Death in both phenotypes usually occurs about 12 years after the onset of the disease, ranging from a few years to over 4 decades.

There are several variant forms of NCL. The congenital form of NCL with onset at birth is very rare. Death usually occurs within hours, days or weeks. However, more prolonged survival for several years has also been described (chronic congenital form of NCL). Another variant form is either called LINCL-variant or early JNCL. The onset (4–5 years) and course of the disease are between those of classical LINCL and JNCL.

Findings of repeated neurophysiological examinations are very important in establishing the diagnosis. In INCL, EEG shows characteristic disappearance of sleep spindles from the age of 1.3 years onwards and sleep spindles are certainly absent by 2.0 years at the latest. When the patient is 1.5–2 years old, the EEG slows and begins to attenuate to become iso-electric at the age of 3–4 years. There is no abnormal photic response. ERG abnormalities, especially a marked loss in amplitude, are early findings and may precede impairment of vision. ERG is usually negative at 12 months of age. VEP is markedly reduced in amplitude and becomes negative. It has been demonstrated that the SSEP becomes negative at an early stage, even before the ERG and VEP become negative. In LINCL, EEG already shows typical large polyspikes after low rate photic stimulation or single flashes at an early stage of the disease. ERG is negative by the age of 3–4 years. Other very typical findings are giant VEPs and SSEPs. In variant-LINCL/early JNCL, these giant VEPs and SSEPs are also found and ERG is negative by the age of 4–5 years. In JNCL, EEG findings are progressively abnormal, but not specific. There is no abnormal photic response. ERG becomes absent by the age of 5–7 years. The amplitudes of the VEP and SSEP are reduced. In ANCL, the resting EEG is abnormal, but nonspecifically so. An intense photoparoxysmal response and an unusual sensitivity to low frequency photic stimulation is of more diagnostic significance. ERG and VEP are normal. Giant short-latency SSEPs can be observed. They are common to many forms of progressive myoclonus epilepsy, and are of limited value in the differential diagnosis.

Ultrastructural findings are essential for the diagnosis of NCL. Skin biopsy and rectum biopsy are mostly used for this purpose. Peripheral lymphocytes can also be examined, in particular in JNCL. In this disorder peripheral lymphocytes can already be shown to contain vacuoles by means of light microscopy. Vacuolated lymphocytes on light microscopy are not a feature of the other NCL forms. A general rule is that the older the patient the less easy it is to find characteristic inclusions, which is true for ANCL. In ANCL, a brain biopsy containing full thickness cortex may be necessary to demonstrate the disease. The biopsied tissues examined by electron microscopy show characteristic, membrane-bound deposits in vascular endothelium, sweat gland epithelium, smooth muscle cells, neurons and in lymphocytes. In INCL, granular osmiophilic deposits (GROD) are the predominant type of inclusions. In LINCL, variant LINCL/early JNCL, and JNCL curvilinear bodies and fingerprint bodies are seen. Fingerprint bodies are more numerous in JNCL, while curvilinear bodies are more common in LINCL. In ANCL both GROD and fingerprint structures are seen.

Urinary sediment levels of dolichols are elevated in all forms of NCL. False negative results occur in 7%–15% of the cases, but usually become positive on repeat testing. False positive results are seen in about 15% of age-matched normal children and children with other neurological diseases. Known causes of false positive results include strenuous exercise, urinary tract infection, menstrual fluid contamination, I cell disease and Niemann-Pick disease type II.

Prenatal diagnosis is possible for INCL, LINCL and JNCL using electron microscopy of chorionic villus specimens and amniotic fluid cells, searching for the characteristic inclusions in affected fetuses. Quantitation of subunit c of mitochondrial ATP synthetase in chorionic villus samples can be used in LINCL and JNCL. Since the DNA locus of INCL and JNCL is known, DNA-based prenatal diagnosis is possible in the majority of the families. At present, the different techniques are used in combination. The DNA techniques make carrier detection possible in selected cases.

44.2 Pathology

The hallmark of neuropathological findings in NCL consists of neuronal lipofuscin storage. The storage leads to displacement of the nuclei and distention of the proximal axon segment, but usually not to ballooning of the cells. On light microscopy the storage material is pale yellow with hematoxylin-eosin stains, slightly pigmented and granular. It is strongly PAS-positive, stains with Sudan dyes and with many other stains for lipofuscin. Examination with ultraviolet light reveals bright yellow autofluorescence. The deposits are readily shown by an acid phosphatase reaction, indicative of their lysosomal location. The ultrastructural appearance of the storage material is different, depending on the form of NCL.

In INCL atrophy of the brain is exceedingly severe, affecting cerebral hemispheres and cerebellum. The brain stem and spinal cord are relatively spared. Microscopic findings change with age. Up to the age of about 2.5 years, neuronal storage is observed with slight to moderate cortical neuronal loss, intense fibrillary astrocytosis and presence of macrophages. The white matter shows only slight changes. From about 2.5 to 4 years of age, neurons become grossly depleted, with the exception of the giant cells of Betz in the motor cortex. There is a massive cortical macrophagocytosis and astrocytosis. The white matter shows moderate to severe loss of myelin. Above the age of about 4 years, the atrophic cortex is entirely depleted of nerve cells and consists of a spongy network of fibrillary astrocytes and capillaries with some macrophages. The white matter shows a complete loss of myelin, also in the subcortical U fibers. Only a few large myelinated nerve fibers apparently derived from the preserved Betz cells are still present. At this stage also the cerebellar cortx shows complete atrophy. Most subcortical nuclei show florid neuronal storage, destruction, macrophagocytosis and astrocytosis, although the primary motor and sensory nuclei of brain stem and spinal cord are remarkably resistant. The stored material in INCL has a similar ultrastructural appearance, wherever found. The substance is osmiophilic and consists of globules with a granular matrix, present either singly or as aggregates of globules. The single globules and the aggregates are stored in larger vesicles surrounded by a unit membrane of lysosomal origin. The deposits have been designated as GROD and can be found in neurons, ependymal cells, choroid plexus epithelium, macrophages, Schwann cells, smooth muscle cells, renal glomerular endothelium, renal distal tubular epithelium, Kupffer cells, vascular endothelium, germinal epithelium of the testis, sweat gland epithelium, thyroid follicle cells, cells of the exocrine and endocrine pancreas, fibroblasts and about 10% of lymphocytes.

In LINCL, neuropathological changes are less severe. The external atrophy is variable and sometimes more pronounced in the cerebellum than in the cerebral hemispheres. Neuronal storage, neuronal loss and mild to moderate cortical astrocytosis are found, but neurons remain present, even in older patients. There may be some loss of myelin in the white matter, but this is not marked. In electron microscopy the stored material mostly has the appearance of curvilinear profiles, but may also take the form of fingerprint profiles. Curvilinear profiles consist of stacks of curved lamellae forming little arcs or semicircles. Accumulations of these are membrane-bound. These curvilinear bodies are also widespread outside the nervous system, similar to in INCL. Although no vacuoles containing lymphocytes are seen on light microscopy, curvilinear bodies may be shown in lymphocytes on electron microscopy.

Also in JNCL diffuse cerebral and cerebellar atrophy is seen, the degree being proportional to the duration of the disease. The cortical neurons show signs of storage and degeneration. Astrogliosis is usually mild. The white matter shows little evidence of myelin loss. In electron microscopy of stored material, the fingerprint pattern predominates, but may be admixed with curvilinear profiles. Fingerprint profiles are formed by groups of parallel paired lines, each pair of lines separated by a lucent space. The lines tend to be equidistant, straight or curved. Groups of lines form whorl-like patterns of fingerprints. The deposits are membrane-bound. Also in JNCL the storage bodies are widespread in other tissues than the nervous system. A small proportion of the lymphocytic vacuoles, seen on light microscopy, are shown to contain fragments of fingerprint profiles in electron microscopy.

In ANCL, variable cerebral atrophy is found. Neuronal storage and neuronal loss is found in the cerebral cortex (sometimes confined to layers III and V), the cerebellar cortex and central nuclei. On electron microscopy fingerprint profiles and GROD are found. These storage bodies can also be found in several non-neural tissues.

All infantile and childhood forms of NCL have a severe, progressive retinopathy. Ganglion cells show signs of lipofuscin pigment storage, similar to neurons in the brain. The same pigment is present in the cells of the bipolar layer. Most conspicuous is the degeneration and loss of photoreceptor cells, spreading from the macula outwards. A severe atrophy of all retinal layers develops with narrowing of small retinal vessels and displacement of melanin-containing pigmented cells into the atrophic retina through the external limiting membrane. These displaced melanin-containing cells may also harbor NCL type-specific lipopigments. On electron microscopy the storage materal has the appearance specific for the form of NCL.

44.3 Chemical Pathology

Analysis of brain biopsy tissue from INCL cases shows some lipid disturbance in the cerebral cortex, but a more severe reduction in myelin lipids in the cerebral white matter. At autopsy, when the end-stage of the disease is reached, the cerebral and cerebellar tissues are extremely lipid-poor. The concentrations of cholesterol and phospholipids in cerebral gray matter are reduced to about 40% of those in age-matched controls. In cerebral white matter the lipid changes are still more pronounced. The concentration of cholesterol is reduced to about 10% of the control value, that of phospholipids to about 20%, and the concentrations of cerebrosides and sulfatides to values of often less than 1%. These results demonstrate an extreme reduction of myelin lipids, and in the terminal stage of INCL all attempts to isolate myelin from cerebral hemispheres and cerebellum fail. The ganglioside concentration and pattern of individual gangliosides are the same in gray and white cerebral matter, which means a more severe reduction in gangliosides for gray matter (to about 15% of control value) than for white matter (about 40% of control value). Lipid changes are much less pronounced in brain stem and spinal cord.

The other forms of NCL show only minor lipid alterations.

Protein is the major component of intralysosomal storage material which accumulates in all forms of NCL. Over 40%–60% of the dry weight of isolated storage material is protein. In INCL the saposins A and B constitute a major proportion of the accumulated protein. Saposins are sphingolipid activator proteins essential for the hydrolysis of sphingolipids in lysosomes. In LINCL, JNCL and ANCL subunit c of the mitochondrial ATP synthetase constitues a considerable proportion (up to 85% in LINCL, about 20% in JNCL) of the accumulated protein. The protein molecules are intact and there is no evidence of any abnormality in amino acid sequences. Dolichols, which are unesterified alcohols, represent up to 2% of the dry weight of storage bodies.

44.4 Pathogenetic Considerations

The term lipopigment is a general one given to yellow-brown pigments that stain with lipid stains and fluoresce under ultraviolet light. The prototype pigment is lipofuscin (age pigment), ubiquously present in cells of aged individuals. The term ceroid has been used to describe any pathological lipopigment, including the lipopigment of NCL. The nature of the fluorophores in the NCL-specific ceroid has been studied but is still not clear.

In storage disorders, the primary goal of most biochemical studies has been to discover unique biochemical markers which will give some clue about the nature of the basic defect. In all forms of NCL, there is lysosomal storage of ceroid, which could be isolated and analyzed. In contrast to other lysosomal storage disorders, the chemical analysis of ceroid has not led to the elucidation of the unique biochemical defect of NCL.

The initial hypothesis was that lipid peroxidation was the cause of NCL. It was generally accepted that autofluorescent lipopigments represented cross-linked products of lipid peroxidation. Autofluorescent lipopigments were also found in disorders of impaired vitamin E metabolism and in vitamin E deficiency. In addition, tissue analysis indicated losses of polyunsaturated fatty acids in patients and carriers, and the presence of a secondary product of lipid peroxidation, 4-hydroxynonenal. The significance of the biochemical findings has not been elucidated. The discovery of elevated dolichols in urine and brain tissue of NCL patients led to another hypothesis, namely that the basic biochemical defect in NCL involved the metabolism of dolichols and retinoids. However, dolichol concentrations in the aging brain are even higher and dolichols are enriched in lipofuscin. The more recent view is that the dolichol accumulation is a nonspecific secondary alteration. Also the accumulation of dolichol-linked oligosaccharides is probably a secondary phenomenon. A possible role of deficient proteases or protease inhibitors in NCL was considered after studies showed that inhibition of lysosomal thiol proteases would induce formation of autofluorescent lipopigments in brains of animals. This hypothesis could, however, not be confirmed. A wide variety of other hypotheses has been advanced including disturbances in fatty acid metabolism, disturbances in very low density lipoprotein synthesis, defective processing of amyloid precursor protein, and abnormal protein methionine S-methylation. None of these has been substantiated. The abnormal storage of normal subunit c of mitochondrial ATP synthetase has more recently been reported in LINCL, JNCL and ANCL. The reasons for the storage of this protein are not apparent. There are two subunit c genes, both of which encode identical mature polypeptides but with different targeting sequences. Both targeting sequences lead to mitochondrial uptake. Abnormalities in sequence or expression of one of the subunit c genes have, however, not been found. The finding that the mature form of subunit c accumulates within lysosomes implies that the polypeptide has entered the lysosome via the mitochondrion. Little is known about the normal catabolism of mitochondrial proteins, and at present it is not known what causes the accumulation of subunit c and whether this accumulation has primary pathogenetic significance. It has recently been found that a major proportion of the protein component of the storage bodies in INCL consists of saposins A and B. The cause and significance are not known.

The gene of INCL has been mapped to chromosome 1p32; the gene of JNCL to chromosome 16p12.1–11.2. The genes of the other forms of NCL have still to be mapped. There is evidence that LINCL is not allelic to either JNCL or INCL. It is not known whether ANCL is allelic to any of the other NCL variants. The results of these genetic studies imply that NCL represents a group of nonrelated disorders, which share a number of clinical, biochemical and histopathological characteristics.

Atrophy of the brain and retina is a feature of NCL, in particular of INCL, not shared to the same degree by other neuronal storage diseases. It is unlikely that neuronal necrosis is due to overloading of cells by storage material. It is more likely that there is something inherently toxic in the disease process. The severe loss of myelin in INCL is striking. The myelin loss is more severe than can by explained by the neuronal loss.

44.5 Therapy

Treatment continues to be mainly supportive. Anticonvulsants are important and need to be tailored to patient, seizure type and side-effects. Tegretol is often quite helpful in the setting of behavioral disturbances. In the management of INCL, irritability, sleeping disorders, choreoathetosis and late pains have responded best to baclofen, tizanidine, levomepromazine and benzodiazepines. Only a few children with LINCL show important irritability and sleeping disturbances. Behavioral problems, depression and psychosis are often present in JNCL. Meaningful hobbies and individual, not too demanding teaching are of basic importance in the management of these problems. Medication is necessary periodically. Valproate and benzodiazepines can be of help in coping with the sleeping problems. Severe behavioral problems and psychotic symptoms can be treated with haloperidol, levomepromazine and benzodiazepines. In the bedridden stage, motor restlessness or panic attacks can be alleviated with baclofen and tizanidine. Antiepileptics, neuroleptics, antidepressants and anxiolytics have been used to try to suppress involuntary movements, but with no clear effect. Nasogastic tube or, preferable, gastrostomy tube feeding is important in the later stages of the disease and has prolonged and improved the quality of life.

Causal treatment trials have been without effect. Antioxidant therapy with vitamin E, vitamin C, vitamin B_6 and selenium was without success. The results of dietary supplementation with polyunsaturated fatty acids are equivocal.

44.6 Magnetic Resonance Imaging

In INCL, CT scan of the brain shows severe atrophy, more severe in the cerebral hemispheres than in the cerebellum. Some atrophy of the brain stem can also be seen. The ventricles and subarachnoid spaces are enlarged. The entire white matter is hypodense and reduced in volume. The cortex is abnormally thin, whereas the volume of the basal ganglia is not reduced, except in the oldest patients. The calvarian bone is thickened in patients over 2 years of age. MRI is already abnormal in an early stage of disease in INCL, before

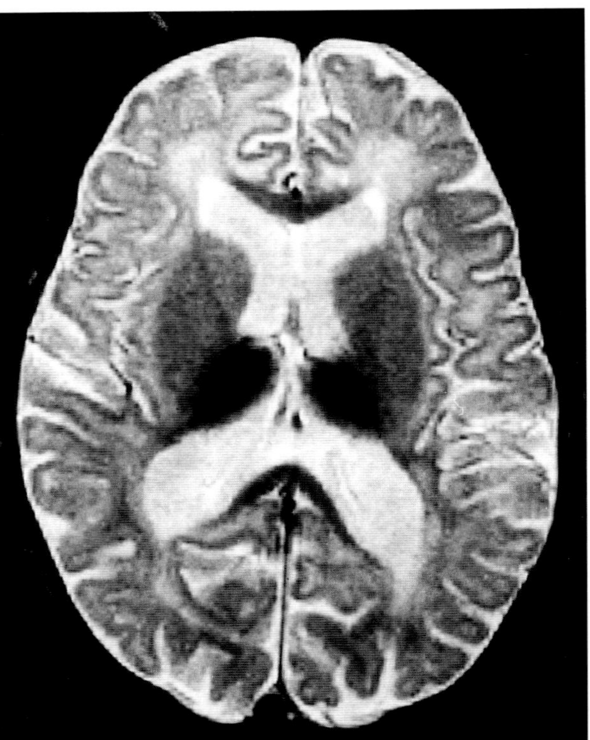

Fig. 44.1. An 18-month-old child with INCL. Note the cerebral atrophy with enlarged ventricles and subarachnoid spaces. The white matter has a higher signal intensity than gray matter in most areas, consistent with disturbed and delayed myelination. Low signal intensity consistent with myelin deposition is seen in the occipital area and the corpus callosum. In the periventricular region, including the occipital area, the white matter has a more pronounced high signal intensity, consistent with myelin loss. The thalami have a low signal intensity. Courtesy of Santavuori et al. (1992), with permission

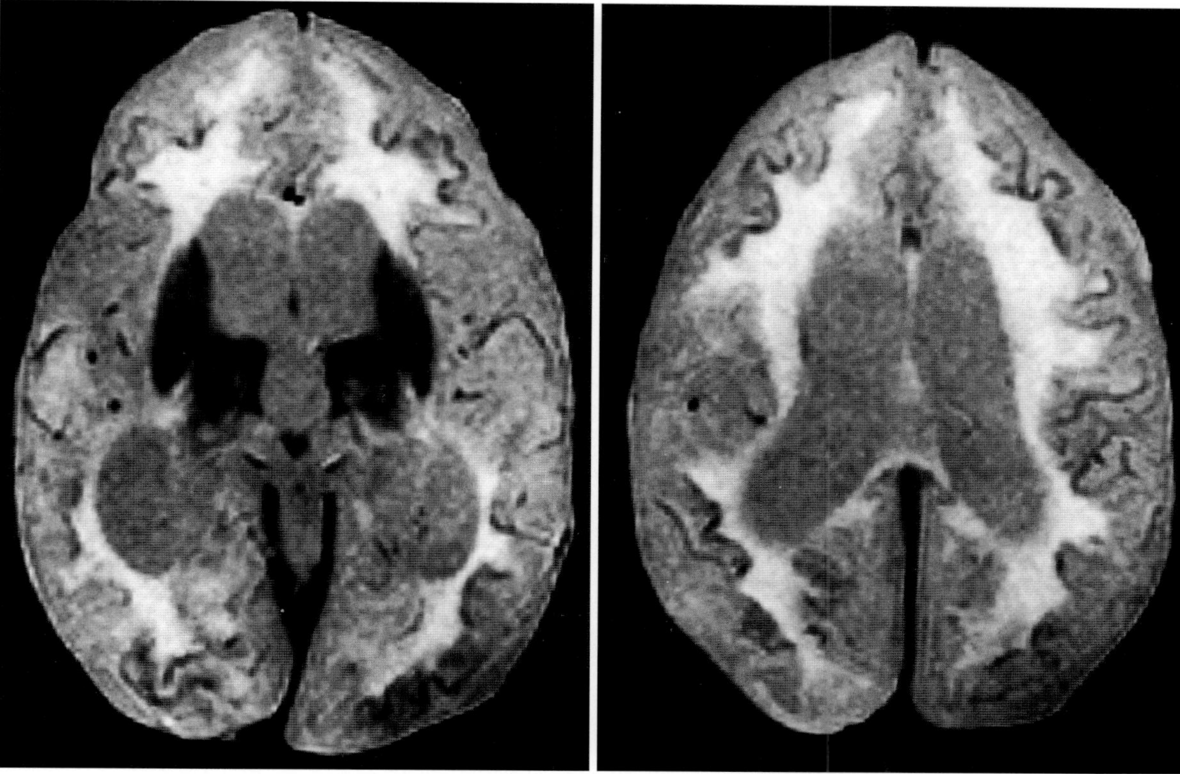

Fig. 44.2. A 6-year-old child with INCL. Note the severe generalized atrophy and the low signal intensity of the thalami and basal ganglia on these mildly T_2-weighted images. The white matter has a high signal intensity throughout, consistent with absence of myelin and presence of gliosis. Courtesy of P. Santavuori and S.L. Vanhanen, Helsinki, Finland, with permission

the appearance of clinical symptoms. With increasing age there is increasing atrophy. The white matter has a high signal intensity on T_2-weighted images in all stages of the disease (Figs. 44.1, 44.2). The signal intensity is highest in the periventricular area (Fig. 44.1). The corpus callosum and internal capsule are myelinated normally. The appearance of the white matter abnormalities suggests a combination of delayed and disturbed myelination (subcortical area) and myelin loss with gliosis (periventricular area). With increasing age the loss in white matter volume becomes extreme. In the end only a thin cerebral mantle is left with highly abnormal signal intensity of the white matter throughout, compatible with complete absence of myelin and severe gliosis (Fig. 44.2). The cortex becomes increasingly thin. The basal ganglia and in particular the thalamus have a low signal intensity on T_2-weighted images. Initially, their volume is relatively normal, but subsequently also the central nuclei become severely atrophic.

In the NCL variants of later onset, CT shows progressive atrophy, involving cerebral hemispheres and cerebellum. The atrophy involves both gray and white matter. In LINCL cerebellar atrophy is more severe than cerebral atrophy. MRI in LINCL has been reported to show a rim of mildly increased signal intensity around the lateral ventricles and, additionally, a decrease in signal intensity in thalami and/or basal ganglia. In JNCL abnormalities appear later and initial MRI may be normal. Apart from progressive atrophy, most severe in the cerebellum, the rim of mildly increased signal intensity in the periventricular white matter may also be seen in JNCL (Fig. 44.3). In ANCL, CT and MRI show atrophy. White matter abnormalities have not been reported.

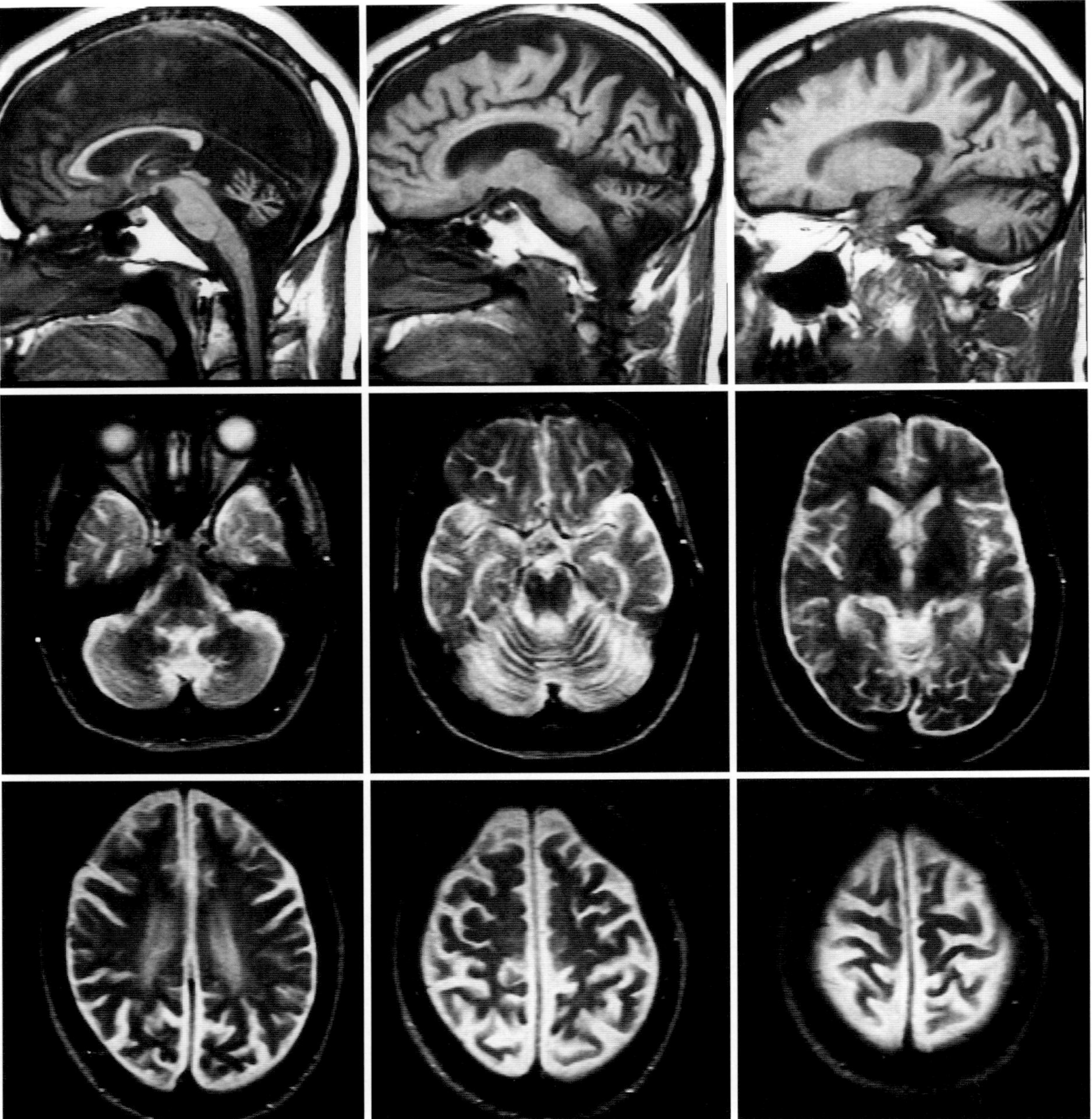

Fig. 44.3. A 23-year-old patient with JNCL. The cerebellum is more severely atrophic than the cerebellar hemispheres. Around the lateral ventricles a small rim of slightly increased signal intensity is seen

45 Alexander's Disease

45.1 Clinical Features and Laboratory Investigations

Alexander's disease (AD) is a rare, nonfamilial disorder of the CNS which is also called dysmyelinogenetic leukodystrophy. The disease occurs sporadically without clear familial incidence. Three clinical subgroups of AD can be distinguished: infantile, juvenile and adult.

In infantile AD, the onset of symptoms varies from birth to early childhood. The average age of onset is 6 months. There is an increasing megalencephaly together with signs of neurological deterioration. Retarded motor and mental development, loss of acquired developmental milestones, spastic quadriparesis and seizures are usually present. In some of the patients there are clinical signs of elevated intracranial pressure with bulging fontanelle, vomiting and papilledema at funduscopy. Usually funduscopic findings are normal. Pupillary reactions are intact. Nystagmus may occur. Choreoathetosis has been observed. The average duration of the illness is 2–3 years, ranging from a few months to 8 years.

In juvenile AD, the onset of symptoms varies from 7 to 14 years with an average age at onset of 9 years. Initial development is normal. The patients suffer from progressive bulbar and pseudobulbar symptoms and spasticity. Nystagmus and ataxia may also occur. Seizures, behavioral changes and cognitive deterioration may occur but are less prominent. The average duration of illness is 8 years.

In adult AD, the onset of symptoms is highly variable, occurring between the second and seventh decades. The clinical features reported are highly variable. The disease may resemble multiple sclerosis with intermittent neurological manifestations. A chronic progressive course with dementia, spastic tetraplegia and ataxia has also been reported. Sometimes the disease remains asymptomatic. Considering the fact that there is no diagnostic laboratory test for AD, that the disease is defined by the presence of Rosenthal fibers in brain tissue and that Rosenthal fibers are also known to occur in conditions other than AD, it is questionable whether this entire range of clinical syndromes represents adult AD.

Laboratory investigations are not helpful in establishing the diagnosis of AD. CSF is normal or shows a nonspecific increase in protein level. High-voltage slow-wave activity and focal discharges are recorded on the EEG in most cases with predominance of abnormalities over the frontal area.

45.2 Pathology

In AD the brain is abnormally enlarged. External examination may reveal macrogyria. In many patients the lateral ventricles are enlarged. In most cases the hydrocephalus is caused by narrowing of the aqueduct. Incidental cases have been reported with a greatly expanded cavum septi pellucidi, bulging into the lateral ventricles and compressing the foramina of Monro. Subependymal cysts may be seen beneath the inferior surfaces of both frontal horns.

On microscopic examination the most distinctive feature of AD is the presence of innumerable Rosenthal fibers throughout the CNS. Rosenthal fibers are irregularly shaped, elongated or round hyaline eosinophilic bodies up to 50 mm in length with a diameter of 1–25 mm. They are arranged radially around blood vessels and perpendicularly to the surface of the cerebral hemispheres, brain stem, cerebellum and spinal cord in the subependymal and subpial regions. In addition, they are scattered throughout the white matter in all areas of the CNS. Rosenthal fibers are most prominent in the frontal white matter, the basal ganglia, thalamus and hypothalamus. The neurons of the cortex and basal ganglia are relatively well preserved regardless of the degree of Rosenthal fiber deposition. In the brain stem the subependymal accumulation of Rosenthal fibers may lead to narrowing of the lumen of the aqueduct resulting in hydrocephalus.

Throughout the CNS there are focal accumulations of hypertrophic fibrillary astrocytes, most marked in the subpial, subependymal and periventricular regions. Their distribution corresponds to the greatest concentration of Rosenthal fibers. The astrocytes are often large and may contain bizarre nuclei. They have large amounts of cytoplasm and in their perikaryon hyaline droplets which show the staining characteristics of Rosenthal fibers. On electron microscopy it is evident that the Rosenthal fibers are abundant in astrocytic processes and present in smaller amounts in the astrocytic perikarya. On electron microscopy Rosenthal fibers appear as granular osmiophilic deposits closely associated with intermediate glial filaments. The granular deposits are non-membrane-bound.

Another distinctive histological feature is paucity of myelin. The lack of myelin sheaths is generally speaking most pronounced in the frontal white matter, temporal white matter, centrum semiovale, tegmentum of the brain stem and ventral and lateral columns of the spinal cord. There is little or no sparing of the arcuate fibers. The internal capsule, optic radiations and cerebellum are relatively better myelinated. However, in some cases the cerebellar white matter is also extensively involved. As a rule the frontal white matter is most severely involved. Cavitation occurs relatively frequently in AD, is usually present in the deep white matter of the frontal lobes and is sometimes seen in the parietal lobes adjacent to the lateral ventricles. In these areas the white matter may be severely reduced in thickness. In the areas of myelin paucity most axons are intact. The affected white matter is markedly cellular due to abundance of abnormal, hypertrophied astrocytes. No inflammatory reaction is present. Oligodendroglia do not show any pathological changes, but may be reduced in number.

In most cases there is a discrepancy between the lack of myelin and the scarcity of sudanophilic material. Some authors suggest that the absence of typical features of active breakdown of myelin sheaths points to dysmyelination rather than demyelination. However, in other cases presence of sudanophilia and macrophages accumulating neutral fat have been reported. Possibly, myelin paucity can be explained by a variable combination of dysmyelination and demyelination, dysmyelination being most pronounced in the patients with early onset of disease.

45.3 Chemical Pathology

Chemical analysis of brain tissue in AD reveals signs of immature myelin with a relatively high content of glucolipids instead of galactolipids and with a relatively low cerebroside content. All myelin constituents are present in a lower than normal concentration as a consequence of the myelin paucity. Cholesterol esters are not elevated. A major constituent of the Rosenthal fibers is αB-crystallin.

45.4 Pathogenetic Considerations

The hallmark of pathological findings in AD is detected in the Rosenthal fibers. It is known that the formation of Rosenthal fibers is a nonspecific process. They have been reported as a focal phenomenon in different types of glial tumors, in glial scar tissue and areas of longstanding reactive gliosis, in multiple sclerosis, encephalomalacia, and syringomyelia. More widespread formation has been described in diffuse gliomatosis, central pontine and extrapontine myelinolysis, vincristine therapy, radiation and chronic inflammatory processes. Rosenthal fiber formation appears to reflect chronic pathological processes affecting astrocytes.

It has been established that αB-crystallin is a major component of Rosenthal fibers. α Cristallin is a major water-soluble lens protein of enormous size. It is a heterogeneous aggregate produced by the products of two genes, αA and αB. The αA-crystallin appears to be confined to the lens. In contrast, αB-crystallin is found in many extralenticular tissues, including heart, muscle, kidney, and brain. Both αA- and αB-crystallin are members of the so-called small heat shock protein (HSP) family. In addition to αB-crystallin another small heat shock protein, HSP27, has been noted as a component of Rosenthal fibers. Both αB-crystallin and HSP27 are normally present in the brain in small amounts and are water-soluble. The expression of these proteins is enhanced by various stress conditions. They accumulate in reactive and neoplastic astrocytes in a variety of pathological conditions, and this accumulation is associated with translocation of the proteins from the soluble fraction to the insoluble or cytoskeleton-related fraction. In the Rosenthal fibers, αB-crystallin and HSP27 are present as insoluble aggregates bound to the intermediate glial filaments. The association of αB-crystallin and HSP27 with intermediate filaments is probably critical in the formation of Rosenthal fibers. Ubiquitin is another component of the Rosenthal fibers. It has been shown that Rosenthal fibers contain mono- and polyubiquitinated conjugates of αB-crystallin. Conjugation with ubiquitin is the first step in a series of reactions that lead to intracellular nonlysosomal degradation of proteins, but probably proteolysis is not the only function of ubiquitin. Ubiquitin is present in various neuronal inclusions, such as the neurofibrillary tangles of Alzheimer disease, Lewy bodies of Parkinson disease and Pick bodies in Pick disease. The presence of ubiquitin in these inclusions may represent an abortive or only partially successful attempt to degrade proteins that accumulate in the pathological states mentioned.

In conclusion, Rosenthal fibers are stress protein inclusions. It is possible that the formation of Rosenthal fibers is the result of overexpression of stress protein genes and as such an important pathogenetic mechanism in AD, but it is probably not the primary abnormality that underlies AD. The astrocytes in AD are probably responding to some as yet unknown stimulus. The primary defect in AD is not known; it may be astrocytic in origin. Recently, the gene for crystallins has been located on chromosome 11. In this context, it is of importance that a child has been described with a partial deletion of the long arm of chromosome 11 and, apart from the usual clinical features, abnormality of the cerebral white matter. However, direct sequencing of the promoter and coding regions of the crystallin gene has revealed a normal sequence in several AD patients investigated.

The relationship between astrocytic abnormalities and myelin paucity, whether due to dysmyelination, demyelination or both, is unknown. However, astrocytes have multiple important functions and astrocytic dysfunction may have pathological consequences. Astrocytes provide structural support for the nervous system, and they play a central role in regenerative repair. Astrocytic foot processes provide physical and electrical insulation for synapses, thus preventing activity at one synapse from influencing the excitability of neighboring synapses. Furthermore, they have an important role in potassium distribution, preventing the accumulation of potassium in the extracellular space during neuronal activity. They are involved in the metabolism of various neurotransmitters, and probably have a reservoir function for nutrients. It is likely that astrocytes and their interaction with oligodendrocytes are a prerequisite for the deposition and maintenance of myelin sheaths. There are junctions between astrocytes and oligodendrocytes providing a means of interaction. Astrocytes are the "third factor" allowing oligodendrocytes to myelinate axons and to maintain the myelin sheaths already deposited around axons. These data indicate clearly that astrocytic dysfunction in the immature brain of infants, in which myelin must still be laid down, may have an adverse effect on the process of myelination and myelin maturation, resulting in dysmyelination. In older patients astrocytic dysfunction may lead to disturbance of myelin maintenance resulting in demyelination.

As already indicated, there is evidence that myelin paucity is explained at least in part by disturbed myelination. In truly demyelinating disorders, a macro- and microglial reaction of variable intensity is always found with evidence of phagocytic activity and presence of products of myelin breakdown. In AD, no phagycotic transformation of macroglia and microglia is seen, despite a conspicuous absence of myelin sheaths. There is a lack of histological and histochemical evidence for the presence of lipoid products of myelin breakdown. There is chemical evidence of a disturbance of myelin maturation. Finally, in analogy with Pelizaens-Merzbacher disease the areas that myelinate relatively early, such as the dorsal columns of the spinal cord, the internal capsule, the cerebellar white matter and the optic radiations, are relatively better myelinated, whereas myelin paucity is most pronounced in those areas that myelinate relatively late, such as the frontal and temporal white matter, and the ventral columns of

the spinal cord. This latter argument is not completely convincing, as the lateral columns of the spinal cord and brain stem tegmentum myelinate relatively early, but usually contain little myelin; in some cases the cerebellar white matter also shows a profound lack of myelin. To stress the differences between AD and the regular "myelinoclastic leukodystrophies," the disease has been called a "dysmyelinogenic leukodystrophy."

The megalencephaly in AD is caused by a combination of astrocytic proliferation and massive deposition of Rosenthal fibers. The subsequent atrophy and cyst formation would be secondary to progressive astrocytic cell death in association with loss of other nervous tissue components. The contrast enhancement, seen in neuro-imaging in the frontal periventricular white matter, caudate nucleus, thalamus and hypothalamus is probably related to a defect in the blood-brain barrier related to impaired function to astrocytic foot plates. The Rosenthal fibers are in particular present in astrocytic cell processes and foot plates. These foot plates form an integral part of the blood-brain barrier. The areas that show contrast enhancement are the areas that have the highest density of Rosenthal fibers. Another reason for blood-brain barrier disruption, in particular inflammation, is not found in these areas.

There is some doubt about the adult cases of AD. The clinical picture often resembles multiple sclerosis and it is known that Rosenthal fibers may be present in multiple sclerosis plaques. These patients may in reality be suffering from multiple sclerosis with unusually extensive Rosenthal fiber formation. Only a handful of patients have been described with adult AD in the neurologically normal subgroup. The striking clinical feature common to all of these cases is that all had severe complicated medical illnesses that resulted in their death. These illnesses may have induced reactive Rosenthal fiber formation in the CNS.

45.5 Therapy

No definitive therapy is available.

45.6 Magnetic Resonance Imaging

CT scan findings have been reported in many cases of infantile AD, several cases of juvenile AD, but not in any case of adult AD.

In infantile AD, CT discloses bilateral, usually symmetrical, moderately well demarcated areas of reduced density in the frontal lobes with extensions to the temporal and parietal lobes and the external and extreme capsules. The internal capsule is usually spared, but the anterior limb may be involved. The subcortical arcuate fibers are involved in the process. Temporarily, the

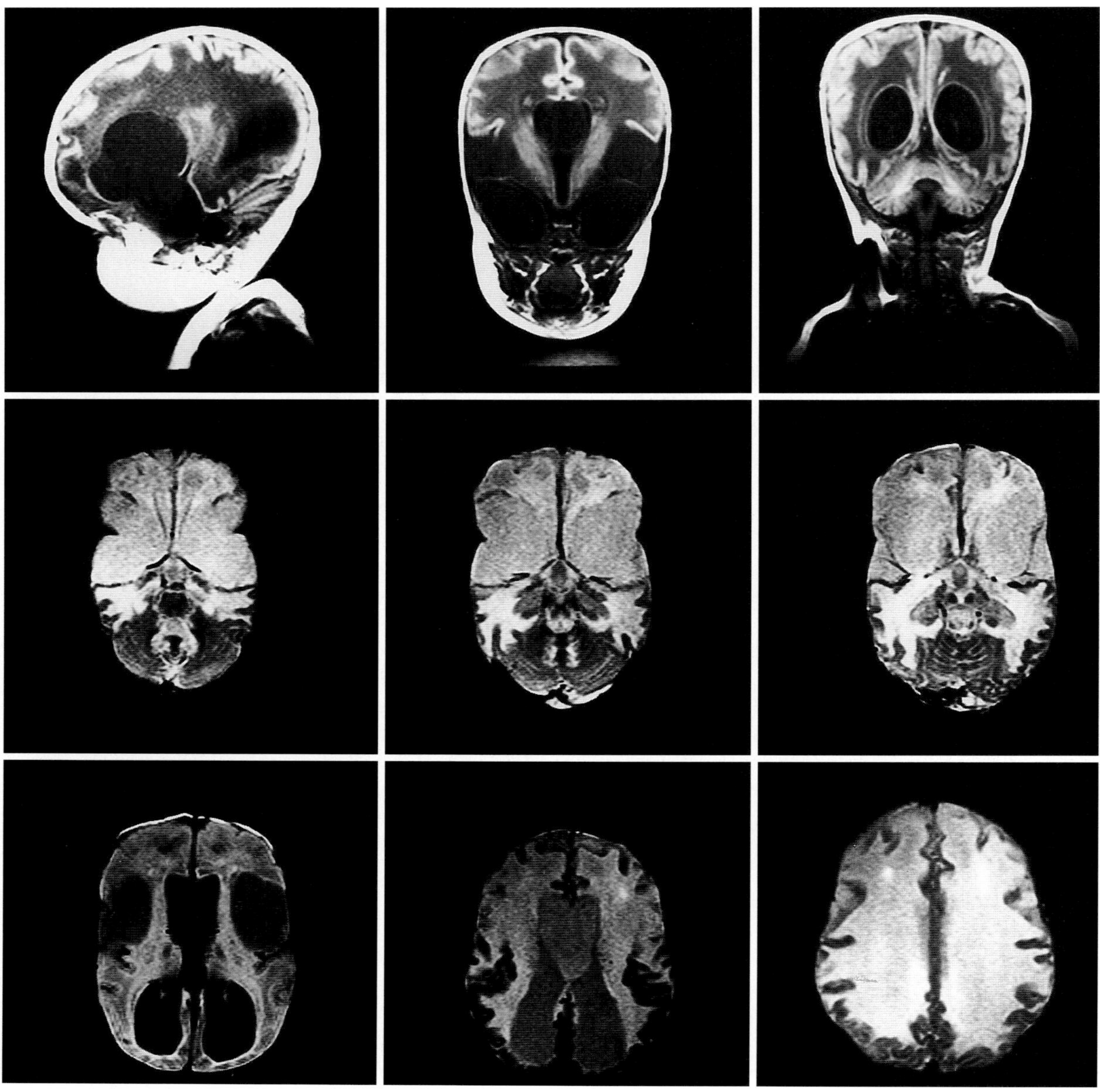

Fig. 45.1. A 3-month-old baby girl with infantile AD. The *upper row* of T_1-weighted coronal images shows large fronto-temporal cystic areas. The third ventricle is wide; the cavum septi pellucidi is grossly dilated. The T_2-weighted transverse series shows white matter involvement, which has already progressed towards the occipital lobe. There are a large cystic cavum septi pellucidi and cavum Vergae. The lateral ventricles are enlarged with rounded occipital horns. Initial involvement of the cerebellar white matter in the hilus of the dentate nucleus is apparent

white matter abnormalities may show mass effect with compression of the ventricles, but there is usually a mild to moderate enlargement of the lateral and third ventricles, either caused by atrophy or by aqueduct stenosis. The frontal white matter may be cystic. In many cases normal or increased density is seen in a rim in the subependymal region, including frontal periventricular white matter, caudate nucleus, thalamus, hypothalamus, fornix and the occipital periventricular white matter. In some cases increased density has also been reported in the subpial layers with a more patchy appearance. In the majority of the patients, contrast enhancement is seen in the areas of increased density. Contrast enhancement has also been reported in the dorsal part of the brain stem. However, some patients show no contrast enhancement, possibly

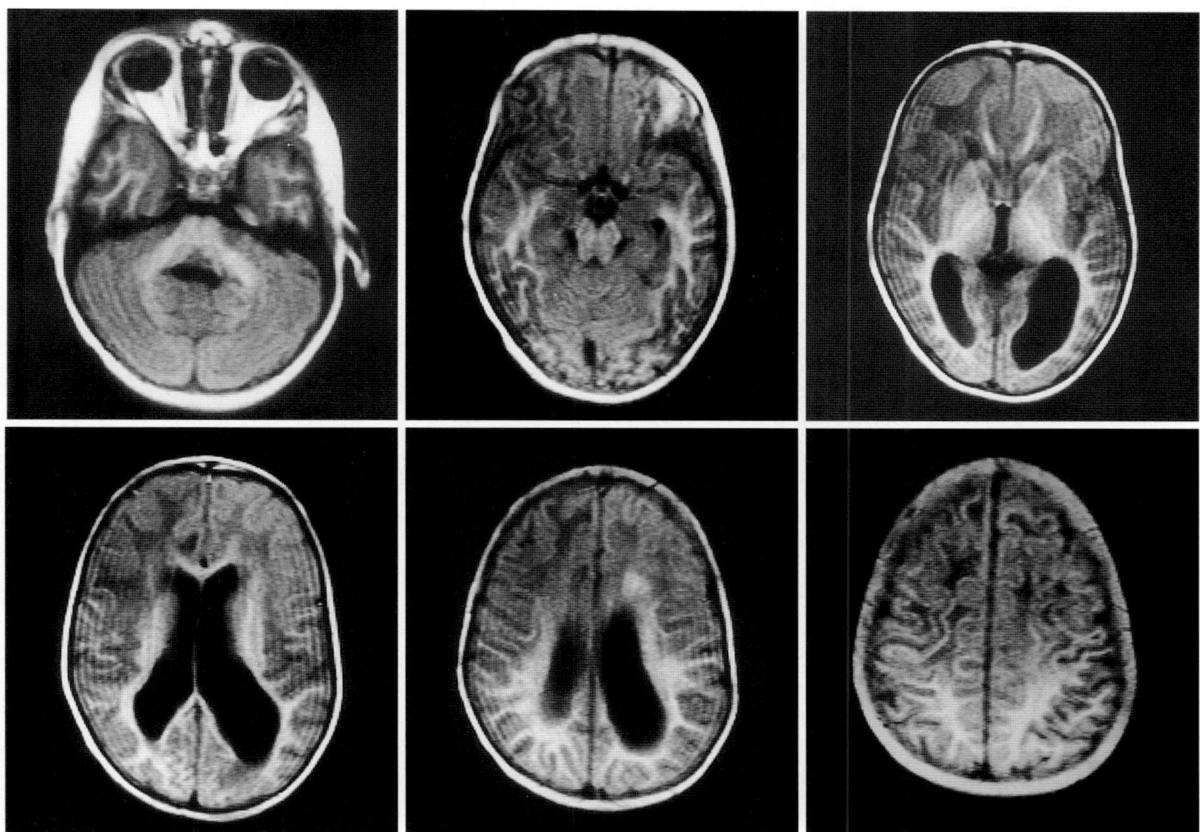

Fig. 45.2. Series of T_1-weighted images in a 9-year-old girl with juvenile AD. From these images the ventro-dorsal gradient in white matter disease is evident. The ventricles are widened in this case

depending on the time of examination, because the higher density enhancing regions decrease as the disease progresses.

In all cases reported, the frontal white matter abnormalities are most severe and occipital white matter and cerebellum are completely or relatively spared. However, cerebellar white matter may become involved extensively and cerebellar involvement should not exclude the diagnosis AD.

In the course of the disease, the white matter abnormality increases in extent, cysts arise and atrophy ensues. Contrast enhancement is absent in later stages of the disease.

In juvenile AD, CT findings include frontal white matter hypodensity which expands in the course of time. Details about areas of increased density and contrast enhancement are less well known.

MRI shows abnormal signal intensity of the white matter in a symmetrical distribution with frontal predominance and relative sparing of the occipital white matter (Figs. 45.2, 45.3). The arcuate fibers are involved in the process. The abnormal white matter has a swollen aspect with broadening of gyri and stretching

of the overlying cortex (Fig. 45.1). The external and extreme capsules are involved. The anterior limb of the internal capsule and the anterior part of the corpus callosum are often affected, but spared in some patients. Cavitation of the frontal white matter may be shown in the course of the disease (Fig. 45.3). Contrast enhancement has not been reported but will be similar to that observed in CT scanning. Abnormal signal intensity may also be seen in basal nuclei, cerebellar white matter and brain stem.

The ventricles may be enlarged and MRI can easily differentiate between obstruction of the foramen of Monro due to an enormously enlarged cavum septi pellucidi (Fig. 45.1), narrowing of the aqueduct and atrophy. Subependymal cysts may be seen at the level of the head of the caudate nucleus.

Although brain biopsy is necessary to establish a definite diagnosis, MRI is capable of suggesting the diagnosis with a high probability of accuracy. The characteristic MRI features are the frontal predominance of the white matter abnormalities, the swollen aspect of the abnormal white matter, the prominent involvement of arcuate fibers, the tendency to form

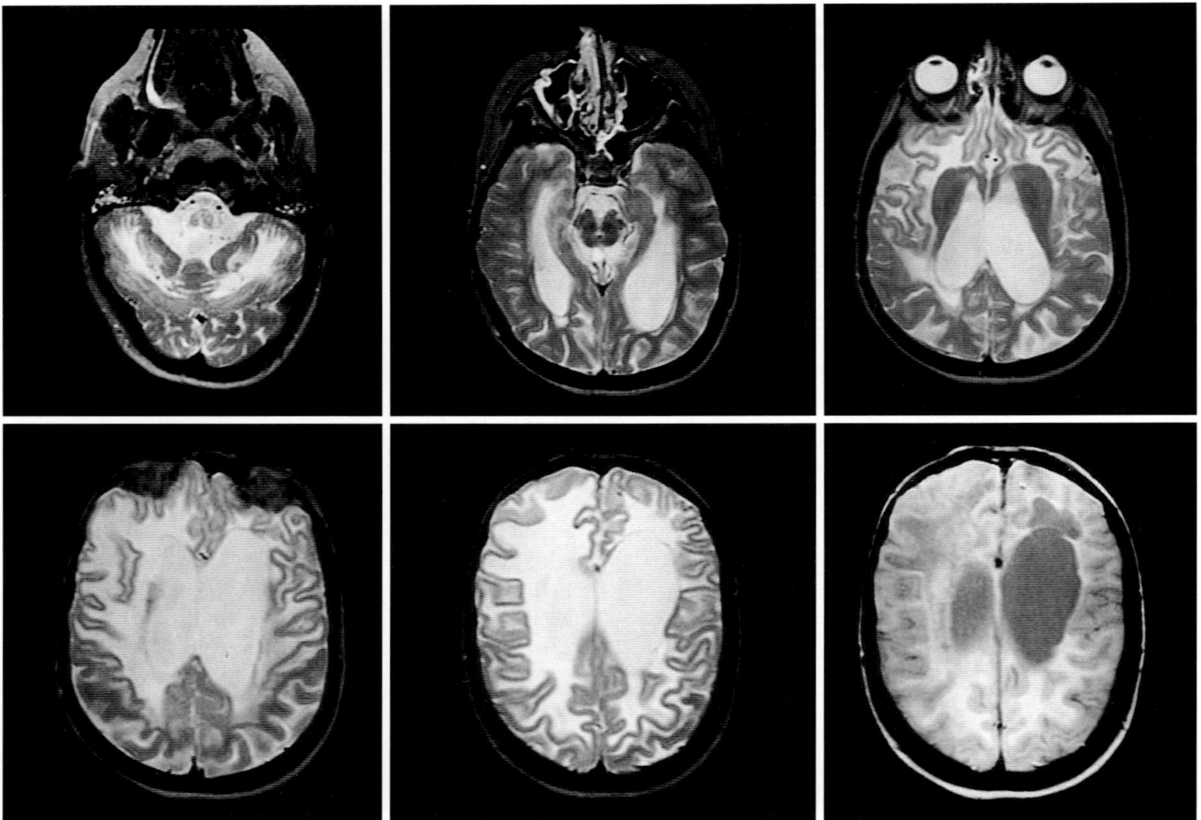

Fig. 45.3. At the age of 14 years (same girl as in Fig. 45.2, but now in a vegetative state), the disease has spread over the entire brain, with the exception of the occipital and temporal subcortical white matter, which are still preserved. The cere-bellar white matter is now also affected. In the frontal periventricular white matter, cysts have appeared. The affected white matter appears swollen

cysts and the peculiar pattern of contrast enhancement. Variants of metachromatic leukodystrophy, globoid cell leukodystrophy and X-linked adrenoleukodystrophy may exhibit frontal predominance, but in these disorders the arcuate fibers are relatively preserved, the white matter abnormalities are not swollen, the tendency to cystic degeneration is less prominent and the typical contrast enhancement is lacking. In Canavan's disease, the white matter also appears swollen, but in this condition the occipital white matter is not spared and the thalamus and globus pallidus are typically involved.

46 Myotonic Dystrophy

46.1 Clinical Features and Laboratory Investigations

Myotonic dystrophy (MD) of Curschmann-Steinert is a dominantly inherited degenerative myopathy. Symptoms of the disease usually become apparent between the ages of 15 and 40 years, but may be found in childhood. Major symptoms include myotonia and progressive muscle weakness and atrophy. In particular the face, jaw, neck and distal muscles are affected. Myotonia leads to a prolonged after-contraction of the affected muscles which persists after the voluntary muscle contraction has ceased. Myotonia is increased by fatigue, emotion and cold. Other features of the disease inclue cataract, early frontal baldness (more conspicuous in males than in females) and gonadal atrophy leading to impotence and infertility. The myocardium is often affected and heart block may occur. Smooth muscles, particularly those of the pharynx, esophagus and gastrointestinal tract are also involved. Diabetes mellitus occurs with enhanced frequency. Low intelligence and mental subnormality are frequently present. Hypersomnia may occur.

MD has a congenital variant, with variable hypotonia and weakness present at birth. This variant is present in 10%–15% of the patients. In congenital MD respiratory problems and feeding difficulties are common. Joint deformities may be present. Myotonia is not usually present in neonates and seldom develops until later in childhood. Cataracts and endocrine abnormalities usually develop even later. Mental subnormality is present in nearly all patients with congenital MD. The disease has a gradual downhill course.

A characteristic feature of MD is the tendency of the symptomatology to worsen with transmission to subsequent generations, a phenomenon that has been termed anticipation. In early generations, cataract was often the only abnormality; in a subsequent generation adult myotonia and weakness would occur, while in the next generation congenital MD would be seen. The disease is transmitted as an autosomal dominant trait, but the mother is the affected parent in over 90% of the cases of congenital MD.

Diagnosis is established by clinical examination and EMG. On EMG prolonged trains of high-frequency discharges arising from single fibers or groups of muscle fibers occur in response to electrode insertion or movement. EMG can be negative in young patients. DNA techniques are available to establish final diagnosis and prenatal diagnosis.

46.2 Pathogenetic Considerations

MD is caused by an increased number of cytosine-thymidine-guanine (CTG) trinucleotide repeats in the untranslated region of a protein kinase gene located in the q13.3 band of chromosome 19. The normal gene has between 5 and 40 CTG trinucleotide repeats, whereas MD alleles have from approximately 90 to several thousands such repeats. The longer the CTG repeat sequence, the more severe the clinical symptomatology. The phenomenon of anticipation is associated with an increase in the length of the CTG repeat sequence with transmission to subsequent generations. Rare cases of reverse mutations have been reported, in which the prolonged CTG repeat sequence in the parent is decreased in size to a normal length in the offspring. The primarily maternal transmission of congenital MD may be the result of genomic imprinting leading to a differential expression of maternally and paternally inherited DNA.

The deduced amino acid sequence of the MD gene forms a protein homologous to a protein kinase. In MD the excitability of the muscle membrane is altered, presumably as a result of altered phosphorylation of skeletal muscle ion channels. Altered phosphorylation of other proteins may give rise to the extramuscular manifestations, including signs of cerebral dysfunction.

46.3 Therapy

Symptomatic relief of the myotonia can, if necessary, be obtained by using drugs such as procainamide and diphenylhyantoine. The effect of these drugs lies in the stabilization of the muscle membrane; they have no effect on muscle weakness. Physiotherapy may be necessary. Cataract extraction can be important in order to preserve visual acuity.

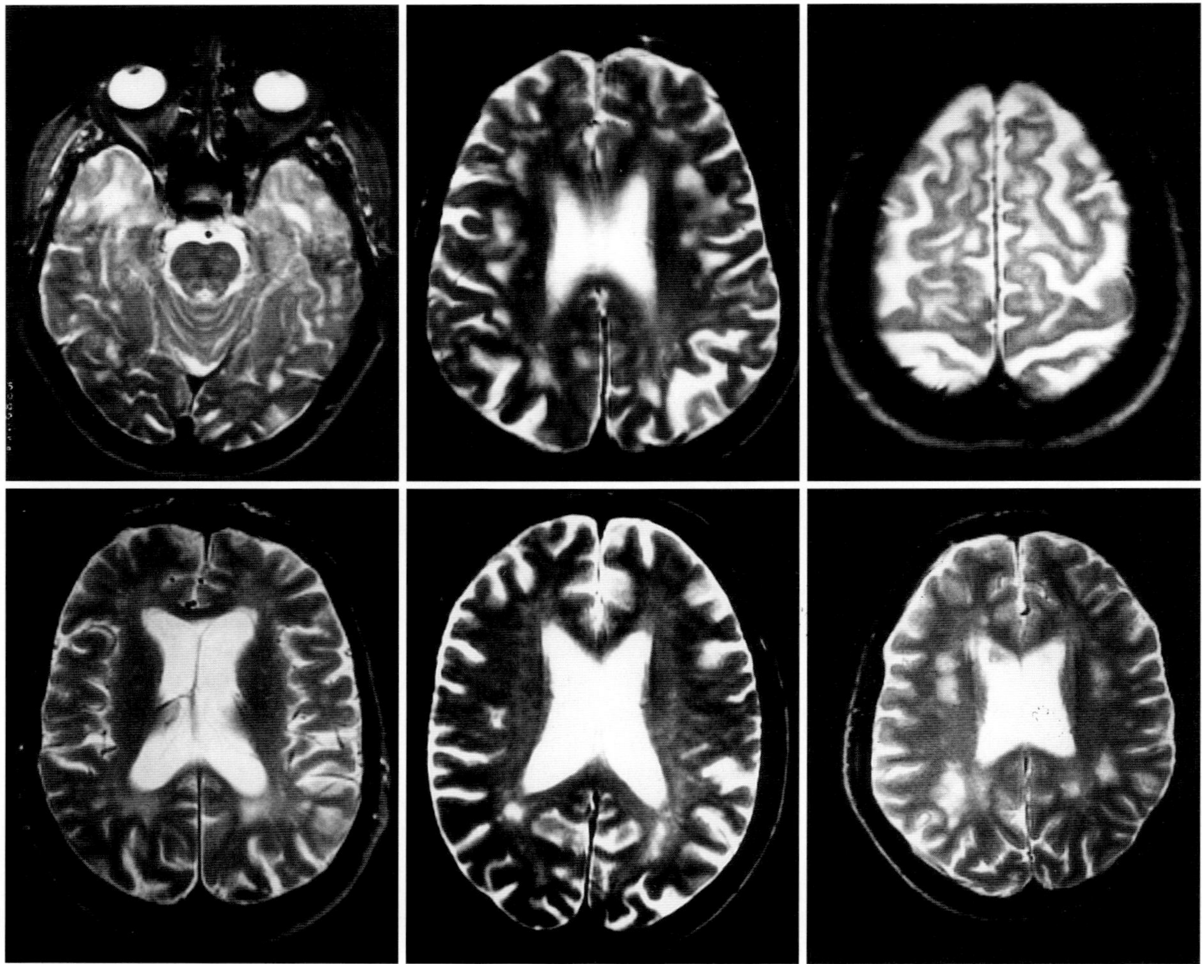

Fig. 46.1. The *upper row* of T$_2$-weighted MR images shows the white matter changes in a 60-year-old female MD patient. The white matter abnormalities are patchy and predominantly located in the subcortical area. There is some atrophy with enlargement of the subarachnoid spaces. The *lower row* of T$_2$-weighted MR images show the variability of white matter involvement in three different MD patients. Courtesy of Damain et al. (1992), with permission

46.4 Magnetic Resonance Imaging

It was already known from CT, that mild ventricular enlargement and white matter hypodensity are not rare in MD.

MRI confirms the frequent presence of mild ventriculomegaly and enlargement of subarachnoid spaces. In the majority of the patients MRI also shows white matter abnormalities in the cerebral hemispheres. The distribution of the white matter lesions is variable, ranging in location from predominantly in the periventricular region to predominantly in the lobar white matter or predominantly in the subcortical areas (Fig. 46.1).

Involvement of the anterior part of the temporal lobes has been found repeatedly. The white matter changes are often patchy with partly isolated and partly irregularly confluent lesions of variable size (Fig. 46.1). The lesions tend to be bilateral but are often not symmetrical in detail. The extent of the white matter changes varies from minor, with some small white matter lesions, to more extensive and more confluent lesions.

The white matter changes occur both in congenital MD and later onset forms and have the same imaging characteristics in both conditions.

The histopathological correlate of these white matter changes has not been described.

47 Congenital Muscular Dystrophy

47.1 Clinical Features and Laboratory Investigations

Congenital muscular dystrophies (CMD) are a heterogeneous group of congenital myopathies that are hereditary and often progressive. They can be subdivided according to the associated CNS abnormalities:

I. CMD with major disturbances of neuronal migration and gyration and with delayed myelination:
    a. Fukuyama type
    b. Santavuori type
    c. Walker-Warburg type
    d. Fowler type
II. CMD with prominent white matter abnormalities and minor abnormalities in neuronal migration and gyration
III. CMD with macrocephaly and severe white matter changes and no abnormalities in neuronal migration and gyration
IV. CMD with cerebellar ataxia
V. CMD without associated CNS abnormalities

In Japan, the *Fukuyama type of CMD* is the second most frequent of the muscular dystrophies, Duchenne muscular dystrophy being the most frequent. The disease is almost exclusively reported in Japan and one should hesitate to suggest this diagnosis in a non-Japanese patient. Inheritance is autosomal recessive. Onset of clinical symptoms is in the neonatal or early infantile period with obvious hypotonia and hypokinesia. Motor development is delayed to a variable degree. In most patients motor functions are acquired gradually, and the maximum motor development has been reached by the age of 2–8 years. The majority of patients never manage to stand or walk, the highest developmental level is usually crawling on hands and knees. The distribution of affected muscles is generalized, but proximal muscles are slightly more severely affected than distal muscles. The facial muscles are also affected, resulting in a hypotonic facial expression. Muscular atrophy is prominent. Pseudohypertrophy of the calves is found in some patients. After the age of about 8 years, motor functions gradually deteriorate. Joint contractures are not usually found in the neonatal period, but flexion contractures of hips, knees, and elbow joints, limited anteflexion of the cervical spine, and contractures of the joints of the hands develop

consecutively during the first few years of life. There is invariable involvement of the CNS often with microcephaly, and always with severe mental retardation, which is not progressive. Convulsions occur in more than half the patients, usually in the form of generalized tonic-clonic convulsions. In a minority, infantile spasms are found. Ophthalmological abnormalities include optic nerve pallor, severe myopia, and less often chorioretinal degeneration and retinal vascular abnormalities. The average life span in Fukuyama type CMD is estimated to be about 12 years; patients rarely live beyond the age of 20. Acute respiratory failure due to pneumonia is the most frequent cause of death.

Santavuori type of CMD is also called muscle-eye-brain (MEB) disease. Most reports come from Finland, but the total number of patients reported is small. The disease has an autosomal recessive mode of inheritance. Clinical symptoms are very similar to the Walker-Warburg syndrome, but tend to be milder. Muscle hypotonia and poor visual contact are noted in the neonatal or early infantile period. Typical facial appearance is characterized by a relatively large head with a high and prominent forehead, wide fontanelle, flat midfacies and short nose and philtrum. In about half of the patients there are some signs of hydrocephalus during the first year of life with a mildly increased skull growth rate, but shunt implantation is only required in a minority. Motor development is variably, but generally severely retarded. Some of the patients show hardly any developmental progress, whereas others achieve sitting without support at the age of 10 years and walking with support after more than 10 years of life. Muscle weakness is generalized, but in the extremities weakness is slightly more prominent in the proximal muscles. Facial muscles are not involved. Contractures develop gradually and not in every patient. There is always involvement of the CNS with marked mental retardation. However, some patients do acquire the ability to speak. Most patients develop seizures, incidentally infantile spasms. Ophthalmological examination typically reveals severe visual failure with severe myopia. Additional ocular signs include glaucoma, retinal dystrophy, choroidal hypoplasia, optic nerve pallor and cataract. Between the ages of 5 and 25 years progress of psychomotor development ceases in many patients and deterioration sets in with loss of mental and motor abilities and development of signs of spasticity, particularly in the legs. The age at death is highly variable: some patients die at the age of 6 years, whereas others survive until their fifties.

Walker-Warburg syndrome has many alternative names, including Walker's lissencephaly, Warburg syndrome, cerebro-oculo-muscular syndrome, cerebro-ocular dysplasia-muscular dystrophy syndrome and HARD±E syndrome (hydrocephalus, agyria and retinal dysplasia with or without encephalocele). The disease has an autosomal recessive mode of inheritance. Severe neurological dysfunction is evident from birth onwards. Hypotonia is profound and neonatal reflexes are often poor or absent. In about 40% of the patients congenital contractures are present. The affected neonates are immobile and unreactive. In many patients progressive hydrocephalus is evident from birth onwards with macrocephaly and bulging fontanelle. In other patients hydrocephalus is not evident at birth but develops soon afterwards. Microcephaly is present in a minority. About 30% of the patients have an occipital meningocele or encephalocele. Epileptic seizures occur frequently. Ophthalmological abnormalities are multiple and diverse and include defects of the anterior and posterior chambers: corneal opacities, iris atrophy, iridolental synechiae, narrow iridocorneal angle with or without glaucoma and buphthalmos, persistent hyperplastic primary vitreous, retinal dysplasia, retinal detachment, optic disc hypoplasia, optic disc coloboma and unilateral or bilateral microphthalmia. Some patients have cleft palate and cleft lip. Genital abnormalities including small penis and undescended testes are common in males. In the months following birth, the infants show profound mental and motor retardation with rarely any development beyond the newborn level. However, the clinical picture varies considerably, even within the same sibship. Survival varies from the neonatal period to 3 years, but most children die within the first year of life.

Fowler syndrome, also called proliferative vasculopathy with hydranencephaly-hydrocephaly, is characterized by prenatal or perinatal death, limb contractures with joint webs and severe hydrocephalus. Eye pathology has not been reported.

CMD with white matter abnormalities and minor cortical dysplasia represents a milder disease. It is also called the occidental type of cerebromuscular dystrophy. Considering the variability in clinical and neuroimaging findings it is possible that more than one disease entity is represented in this condition. Inheritance is autosomal recessive. Diffuse hypotonia and generalized weakness are evident from birth or early infancy and lead to a delay in motor development. Some children never acquire the ability to stand or walk, whereas others achieve this ability within a few years. The majority of patients have contractures of the joints, sometimes already present at birth. Muscle atrophy is prominent. The facial muscles are involved and the children often have long, thin faces. In some cases external ophthalmoplegia is found. Some of the patients have normal intelligence, whereas some have mental impairment, varying from mild to severe. A minority of patients have seizures. Most patients remain stable, but in others a slowly progressive weakness is noted after several years. The development of pyramidal signs with Babinski reflexes and presence of ataxia are sometimes seen in later years. Little is known about the precise life expectancy but most patients live for decades.

CMD with macrocephaly and white matter abnormalities without cortical dysplasia a better defined disease. Inheritance is autosomal recessive. Generalized hypotonia is noted in infancy with a delay in motor development. Some children acquire the ability to walk, others do not. Generalized muscle weakness is noted with atrophy. Facial weakness is also present. Contractures are usually present, either at birth or later in life. In most children intelligence is normal, some have a mild intellectual impairment, but none are severely retarded. Some children develop generalized seizures. Considering the limited number of patients described, the outlook is uncertain. In some patients progression of weakness is noted at the end of the first decade with death between 10 and 20 years. However, survival beyond 20 years has been described.

Recently, one family has been described by Van Engelen et al. (1992) with adult onset of clinically evident muscular dystrophy and in the oldest patient (29 years old) progressive signs of CNS dysfunction with development of seizures, pyramidal and cerebellar signs. MRI findings consisted of severe white matter abnormalities similar to those observed in the congenital variant of the disease.

CMD in combination with cerebellar atrophy has been reported. Cerebral cortex and CNS white matter are intact.

In *pure CMD* no clinical and paraclinical signs of CNS dysfunction are found.

In laboratory investigations a variably elevated creatine kinase (CK) level is found, which is never as high as in Duchenne muscular dystrophy. After 6 years of age the CK level tends to fall gradually, but usually does not reach normal values. EMG examination reveals myopathic discharges of low amplitude and short duration. EEG often shows paroxysmal discharges and abnormal background rhythms. Diagnosis of CMD is established by finding dystrophic changes in muscle biopsy tissue.

47.2 Pathology

In *Fukuyama type CMD* extensive cortical dysplasia of cerebrum and cerebellum is present. The pattern of the cortical dysplasia may vary from site to site and from case to case. The pattern is, however, symmetrical. The primary sulci (central, calcarine, parieto-occipital and cingulate) are present, secondary sulci are shallow and the gyral surfaces have an irregular appearance. The cortical dysplasia may take the form of unlayered polymicrogyria or smooth, four-layered pachygyria or verrucose dysplasia with superficial cellular nodules within a normally stratified 6-layer cortex. The polymicrogyria is also called pachygyric polymicrogyria, because the microgyri are fused, the external appearance of the brain is pachygyric, and unlayered polymicrogyria is only found on microscopic examination. In most patients the 3 mentioned types of cortical dysplasia are present to a variable extent. The border between cerebral cortex and white matter is irregular. Ectopic nerve cells are found in the subcortical white matter, near the ventricles and disseminated within the white matter. The ventricles are often mildly dilated. Overt hydrocephalus is not present. Occasionally the frontal cortex shows focal interhemispheric fusions. The pyramidal tracts in the brain stem are hypoplastic and dysplastic. Within the cerebellar cortex, areas of polymicrogyria are present. Superficial glio-mesenchymal proliferation is present on the surface of the brain and spinal cord, leading to thickened leptomeninges adherent to the surface of the CNS. The white matter changes vary in severity. Myelin paucity and gliosis are seen, but without signs of breakdown, particularly in the younger children, whereas normal myelination is seen in older children. In a case in which brain tissue was investigated at two different points of time, myelination was very poor and astrogliosis marked in brain biopsy material, whereas at autopsy 4 years later, myelination proved to be only slightly less than normal and astrocytosis was mild. Myelin paucity in younger children is caused by severe delay of myelination.

The number of patients reported with the *Santavuori type of CMD* is limited and there are few data about histopathological findings (Santavuori et al. 1989). The hallmark of abnormalities is the cortical dysplasia, in particular polymicrogyria. The ventricles are dilated to a variable extent. Septum pellucidum may be absent. There are no data on the condition of the white matter.

Much more is known about *Walker-Warburg type of CMD*. On external examination the brain surface may be smooth with only an interhemispheric fissure present and a markedly foreshortened sylvian fissure due to incomplete development of the opercula. The brain surface may also have an irregular verrucous appearance with areas of pachygyria and polymicrogyria.

The leptomeninges are thick and may obliterate the subarachnoid space with fibrous and heterotopic glial tissue. On sectioning, the lateral ventricles are markedly to severely enlarged; only in exceptional cases are ventricles normal. The corpus callosum and septum pellucidum are often absent or hypoplastic. The aqueduct is small and stenotic. The cerebellar vermis, especially the posterior vermis, and the cerebellar hemispheres are hypoplastic, often associated with an enlarged fourth ventricle and a retrocerebellar cyst, constituting a Dandy-Walker malformation. In about 25% of the patients a posterior encephalocele or meningocele is present, containing either an extension of a retrocerebellar cyst, cerebellar tissue or, rarely, tissue of supratentorial origin. Factors contributing to ventricular enlargement are aqueduct stenosis, disturbed fluid dynamics associated with the Dandy-Walker malformation, and blockage of the arachnoid granulations by fibroglial tissue. The cerebral cortex is abnormally thick with absent white matter interdigitations or with irregular, shallow indentations in the otherwise smooth cortical ribbon. On microscopic examination the cortex is severely disorganized with no recognizable lamination and widespread disruption by gliofibrillary bundles accompanying vessels from the pial surface. Agyria with severe disorganization of the cortex and absence of lamination is called lissencephaly type II. The observation of widespread pachygyria and polymicrogyria rather than agyria in some of the patients with otherwise typical pathological changes of type II lissencephaly confirms that the pachygyria and polymicrogyria are lissencephalic variants. Neuronal heterotopias are present scattered in the white matter and in the subependymal region. The white matter is reduced in volume, poorly myelinated and gliotic. Myelination is virtually absent in some cases. In the brain stem corticospinal tracts are grossly absent. Within the smooth, afoliar cerebellar cortex microscopic changes are found reminiscent of those in the cerebral cortex. Cerebellar white matter is better myelinated.

Very little information is available on histopathological findings in the *Fowler type of CMD* (Norman and McGillivray 1988). Changes are similar to those described in Walker-Warburg syndrome. Hydrocephalus is severe and the cerebral mantle is narrow. Cortical dysplasia is present and there is an unusual proliferation of cerebral cortical arteries.

There have been only a few histopathological reports of *CMD with prominent white matter abnormalities and subtle cortical dysplasia*. Jervis (1955) described neuronal heterotopias in the subcortical white matter in combination with a widespread, symmetrical demyelinating process involving the cerebral hemispheres with sparing of the arcuate fibers. There were small areas of demyelination in the cerebellum. No signs of active myelin loss with presence of myelin breakdown products were noted. Egger et al. (1983) and Trevisan et al. (1991) described the variable presence of focal areas of some polymicrogyria, pachygyria and small hetertopias, but no generalized, severe cortical dysplasia. Both described widespread, patchy or more confluent areas of demyelination in the cerebral white matter. Myelin sheaths in those areas showed moderately severe degeneration, but no myelin breakdown products were demonstrated. The white matter changes were consistent with a slow demyelinating process, or a focal disturbance of myelination.

In *CMD with severe white matter abnormalities and macrocephaly* only one histopathological report has been published (Echenne et al. 1984). External appearance of the brain was normal. Furthermore, no abnormalities of cerebral and cerebellar cortex were found on microscopic examination and there were no neuronal heterotopias within the white matter. Extensive absence of myelin was found bilaterally with sparing of the arcuate fibers. Abnormalities were most severe in the frontoparietal white matter, whereas the occipital white matter was less extensively involved. On microscopic examination the white matter appeared spongy. Moderate astrocytic proliferation was found. No changes were found in basal ganglia, brain stem or cerebellum, including cerebellar white matter.

In CMD, dystrophic changes are seen in muscle tissue. These include marked variation in fiber size with presence of atrophic and hypertrophic fibers, fiber necrosis with presence of phagocytes, increased number of fibers with internal nuclei, increased interstitial fibrosis and replacement by adipose tissue. No inflammatory infiltration is found. There are no significant differences between the subdivided groups of CMD. Little attention is paid to cardiac muscle involvement. In the Fukuyama type of CMD, degeneration and loss of myocardial fibers as well as myocardial fibrosis may be found at autopsy.

47.3   Pathogenetic Considerations

All types of CMD discussed have an autosomal recessive mode of inheritance. The basic defect and the location of the related gene(s) have not yet been identified in most types. An exception is Fukuyama type CMD, the gene for which has recently been localized to chromosome 9q31–33. There is recent evidence that the Walker-Warburg syndrome is linked to the same chromosomal locus, but Santavuori type of CMD is not. CMD with prominent white matter abnormalities, macrocephaly and no cortical dysplasia is linked to chromosome 6q3, the merosin gene. This type of CMD is now also called merosin-negative CMD.

The nature of the relationship between CMD and derangement of neuronal migration and organization is not known.

The white matter abnormalities reported in CMD are variable. In the Fukuyama type of CMD there is convincing evidence that the white matter abnormalities, so often reported in neuroimaging, are caused by retarded but ongoing myelination. In repeated neuroimaging, improvement of the white matter abnormality has been reported and progression of myelination has been described in one child in whom brain biopsy and autopsy findings were compared. Retarded myelination is probably also present in the other types of CMD with major disturbances of neuronal cortical organization.

In CMD with mild cortical dysplasia the white matter abnormalities are described as demyelinating, although no signs of active demyelination were found. The abnormalities are often focal with normal myelination in other areas. In incidental cases progression of the abnormalities is documented with repeated neuroimaging, confirming that the lesions are probably demyelinating. However, stationary white matter changes were found in other patients.

In merosin-negative CMD the white matter abnormalities are diffuse and spongiform. The precise nature of the sponginess is not known and the location of the vacuoles remains to be established: intramyelinic, intracellular, or interstitial.

The role of the white matter abnormalities in determining the clinical picture of the patients seems to be minor in all CMD variants. The disease is mostly explained by the severity of the cortical dysplasia and the muscular dystrophy. Probably the white matter changes play a role in those patients who show signs of progressive cerebral dysfunction.

47.4   Treatment

No definitive treatment is possible, only supportive care. Physiotherapy is of major importance. In some patients a slight improvement in strength and a fall in CK activity have been noted on administration of corticosteroids. However, in other patients no improvement was found. Considering the major adverse effects of chronic use of corticosteroids, this mode of therapy remains controversial.

47.5   Magnetic Resonance Imaging

CT scan in *Fukuyama type of CMD* shows some evidence of cortical dysplasia with broad, smooth gyri and incomplete opercularization. In younger children

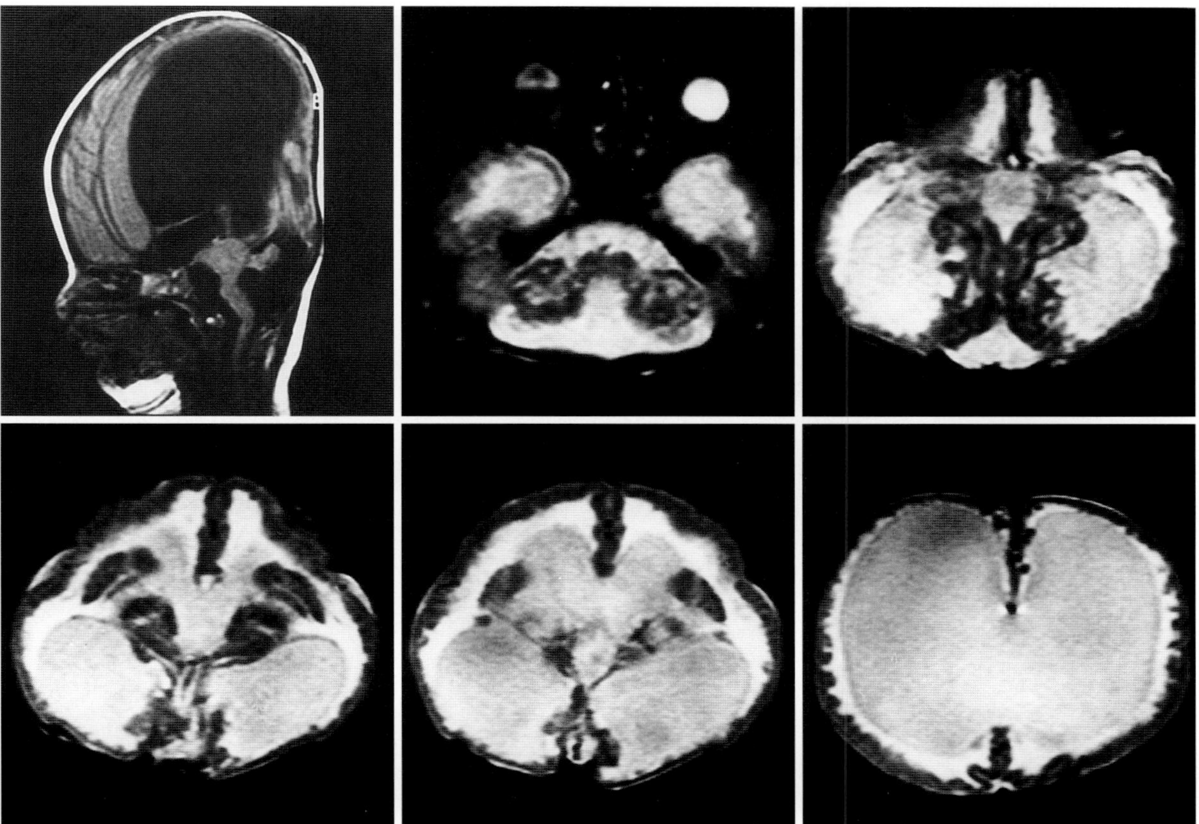

Fig. 47.1. Walker-Warburg type of CMD in a 4-month-old boy. Note the enlarged ventricles, absent septum pellucidum, hypoplastic pons, and cerebellum with characteristics of a Dandy-Walker malformation, hypoplastic corpus callosum, and cortical irregularities of lissencephaly type II. The brain stem and possibly the cerebellum contain some myelin. Cerebral hemispheres and internal capsule contain no myelin at all

the white matter diffusely has a low density, which improves on repeated CT. MRI is able to depict the cerebral cortical dysplasia in greater detail. The images show too few, too broad gyri and incomplete opercularization. In most areas the cortex has an irregular aspect with little dots, reflecting polymicrogyria and verrucose cortical dysplasia. MRI also shows cerebellar cortical dysplasia, with irregularly distorted folia. The ventricular system is mildly enlarged and often has a colpocephalic aspect. In young children very little myelin is seen. For instance, in children at the age of 12 months myelin is only present in cerebellum, brain stem, internal capsule, corpus callosum and in occipital and pericentral parietal white matter. On repeated MRI, after an interval of at least 6 months, progress of myelination is seen, the rate being variable. Cases have been reported in which hardly any myelin was seen after several years.

In the *Santavuori type of CMD*, CT scan shows a markedly dilated ventricular system. The gyri are few and broad. Opercularization is incomplete. The cortex

cannot be depicted in detail by CT, but some images suggest irregularities, consistent with polymicrogyria, constituting the so-called pachygyric polymicrogyria. Septum pellucidum and corpus callosum are absent or incomplete in some patients. In some cases hypoplasia of the inferior vermis is reported. The white matter is hypodense, in particular in the frontal area. MRI has been reported to show a variable ventricular enlargement, ranging from normal to markedly dilated. Cortical gyri and sulci are distinctly visible, but are abnormal, in particular in the frontal, temporal and parietal areas. Neuronal heterotopias may be seen in the white matter. Pons and cerebellum are hypoplastic. Variable, but generally subtle white matter abnormalities are seen without typical appearance or distribution.

In the *Walker-Warburg type of CMD*, CT and MRI almost invariably show severe hydrocephalus (Fig. 47.1). A normal ventricular size is highly unusual and may suggest the presence of the Sanatvuori type of CMD. Corpus callosum and septum pellucidum are of-

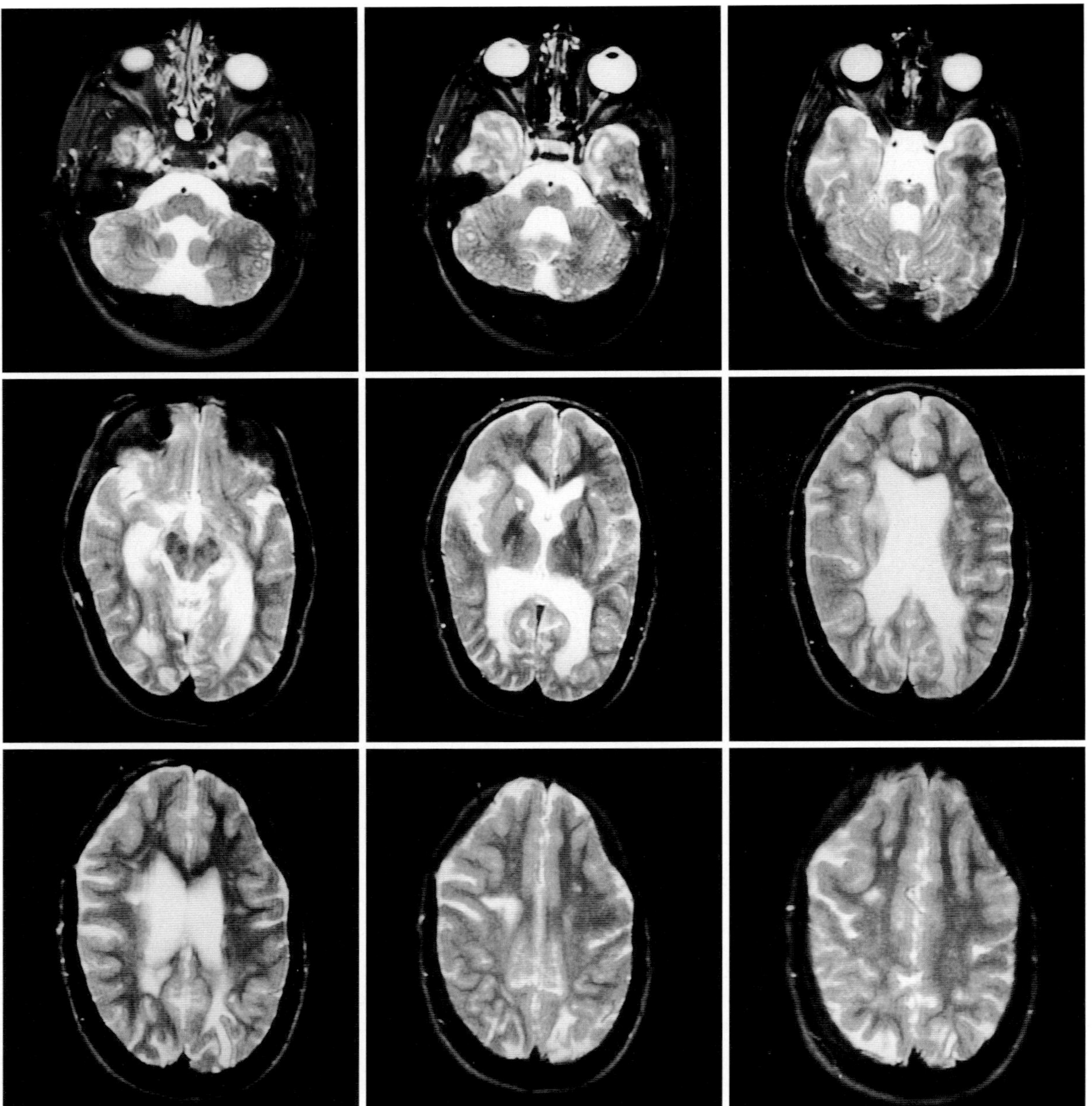

Fig. 47.2. A 13-year-old girl with CMD. In this case MR shows ventricular enlargement, vermis hypoplasia, disseminated focal white matter abnormalities, and mild cortical dysplasia. Courtesy of R. le Coultre and J.H. Begeer, Groningen, The Netherlands, with permission

ten absent or hypoplastic. The third ventricle is also enlarged, the aqueduct is narrow. The cerebellum is very hypoplastic in all its elements, in particular in the vermis. The cerebellar surface is smooth, without foliae. The fourth ventricle is enlarged and is in open communication with an enlarged retrocerebellar space, forming either the full-blown Dandy-Walker malformation or the less severe Dandy-Walker variant. A posterior meningocele or encephalocele is often present.

Because of the severe hydrocephalus and very thin cerebral mantle, the quality of white and gray matter may be difficult to assess. The cortex is smooth on the external side. The border with the white matter is often irregular, reflecting the polymicrogyria or disruption of the cortex by gliofibrillary bundles. In some cases extensive subcortical and subependymal heterotopic neuronal nodules are seen. Fusion of the frontal cortex in the interhemispheral area can be visualized. In ex-

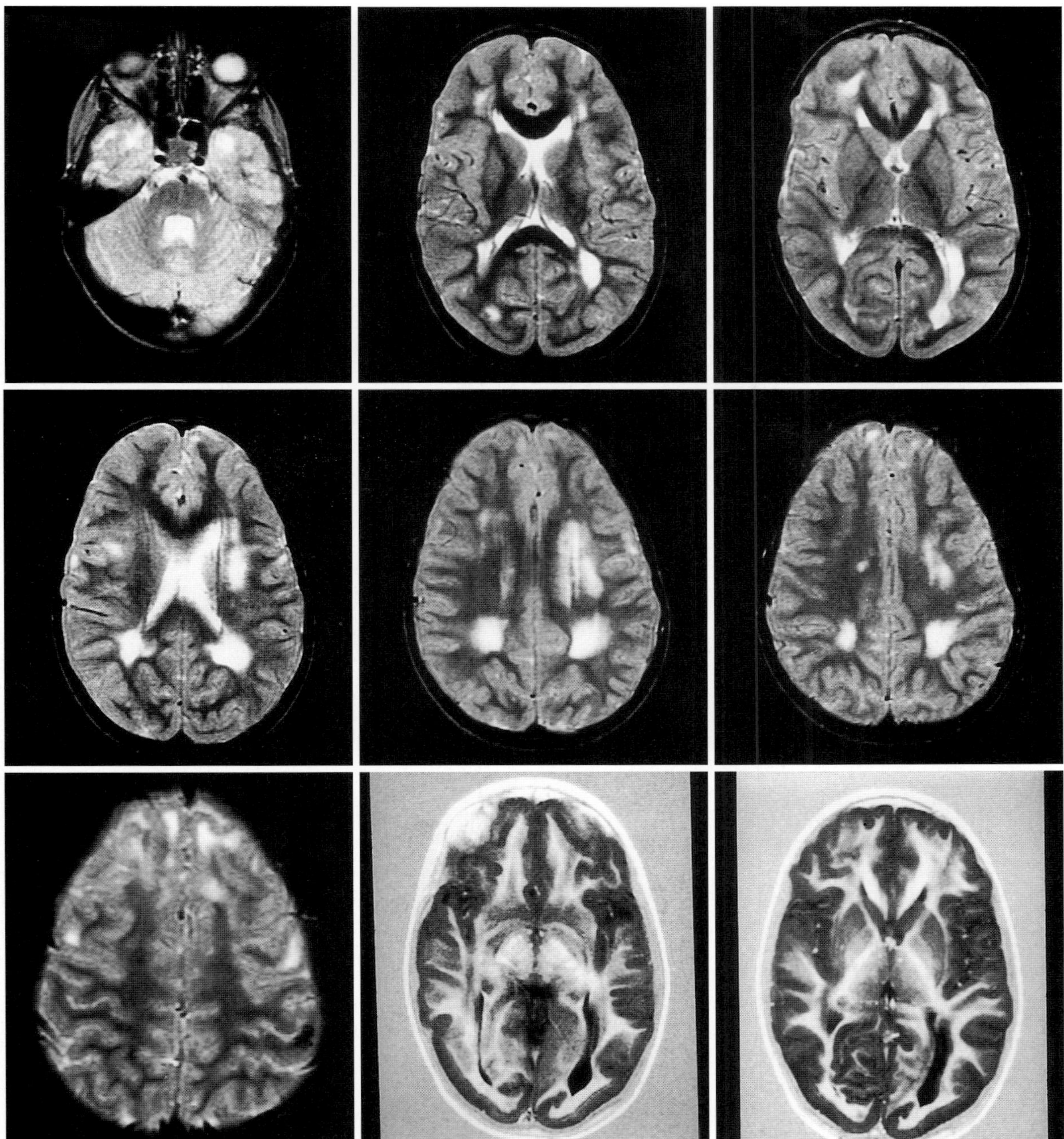

Fig. 47.3. A 7-year-old boy with CMD. The T$_2$-weighted images show widespread involvement of the white matter, confluent and isolated, periventricular and subcortical, with normal-sized ventricles. The T$_1$-weighted (IR) images (*lower row, right*) show the cortical dysplasia in the occipital lobe. Courtesy of H. Stroink and C.E. Catsman-Berrevoets, Rotterdam, The Netherlands, with permission

ceptional cases, broad but somewhat better formed gyri have been described. The white matter is poorly myelinated (Fig. 47.1).

In *CMD with mild cortical dysplasia and marked white matter abnormalities* only CT scan findings have been reported so far. CT fails to show the rather subtle cortical dysplasia. In most cases there is enlargement of the subarachnoid spaces and in some cases the ventricles are somewhat enlarged. A marked low density of the white matter of the cerebral hemispheres is found,

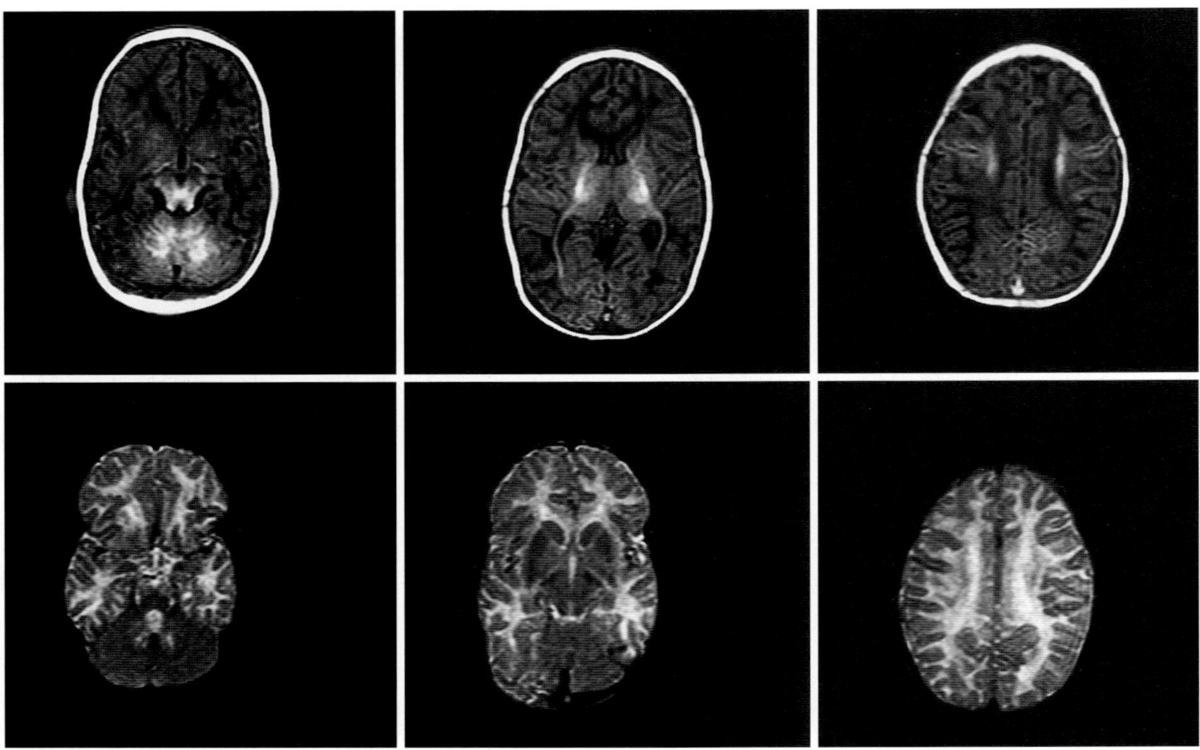

Fig. 47.4. A 3-month-old baby girl with merosin-negative CMD. The T_1- (*upper row*) and T_2- (*lower row*) weighted images are normal for this age (see also Fig. 47.5)

which is unchanged on repeated CT scanning. Increasing areas of white matter hypodensity were only found in one patient. In the two cases we saw with MRI, the localized cortical dysplasia was easily seen (Figs. 47.2, 47.3). The white matter changes remained unchanged in one patient (Fig. 47.3).

In *merosin-negative CMD with white matter changes and macrocephaly*, CT and, to a greater extent, MRI show prominent white matter changes. The white matter appears swollen, leading to stretching of the overlying cortex which is folded in gyri broader than normal. On CT it is hardly possible to distinguish between primary cortical dysplasia and secondary broadening of the gyri as a consequence of white matter swelling. MRI shows the normal aspect of the cortex, which is not thicker than normal and does not have the irregular aspect of pachygyric polymicrogyria (see Fig. 47.5). In our experience the white matter is near-normal in the first few months of life (Fig. 47.4). From the second year of life onwards MRI shows swollen white matter with a high signal on T_2-weighted images, low on T_1-weighted images (Fig. 47.5). The abnormalities have a frontal predominance and the occipital white matter is better preserved. The corpus callosum, internal capsule, brain stem and cerebellum are preserved and well myelinated. In some cases some myelin

is present in the subcortical areas. The white matter changes appear to be nonprogressive over the years.

In the two patients with adult onset signs of muscular dystrophy and cerebral dysfunction, reported by Van Engelen et al. (1992), the white matter abnormalities are identical to those of the merosin-negative CMD patients (Fig. 47.6). A special finding is that the oldest patient, 29 years of age, has cysts in the subcortical area in the tips of the temporal lobes and the parietal area (Fig. 47.6). With these cysts the MR pattern becomes identical to the pattern of the spongiform leukoencephalopathy described in Chap. 48.

The CMD patients described by Cook et al. (1992) have a marginal microcephaly with a head circumference at or just above the second percentile. The MR pattern in these patients shows diffuse white matter disease, but is slightly different in that the subcortical white matter is more extensively preserved and the white matter swelling is not evident. The corpus callosum and internal capsule are also preserved. The white matter abnormalities did not change over the years.

It is clear that MRI plays an important role in the classification of CMD patients during life. The cortical dysplasia, cerebellar malformation and different types of white matter involvement are depicted in detail. MRI is highly sensitive in demonstrating white matter lesions, their location and extent and up to now MRI has

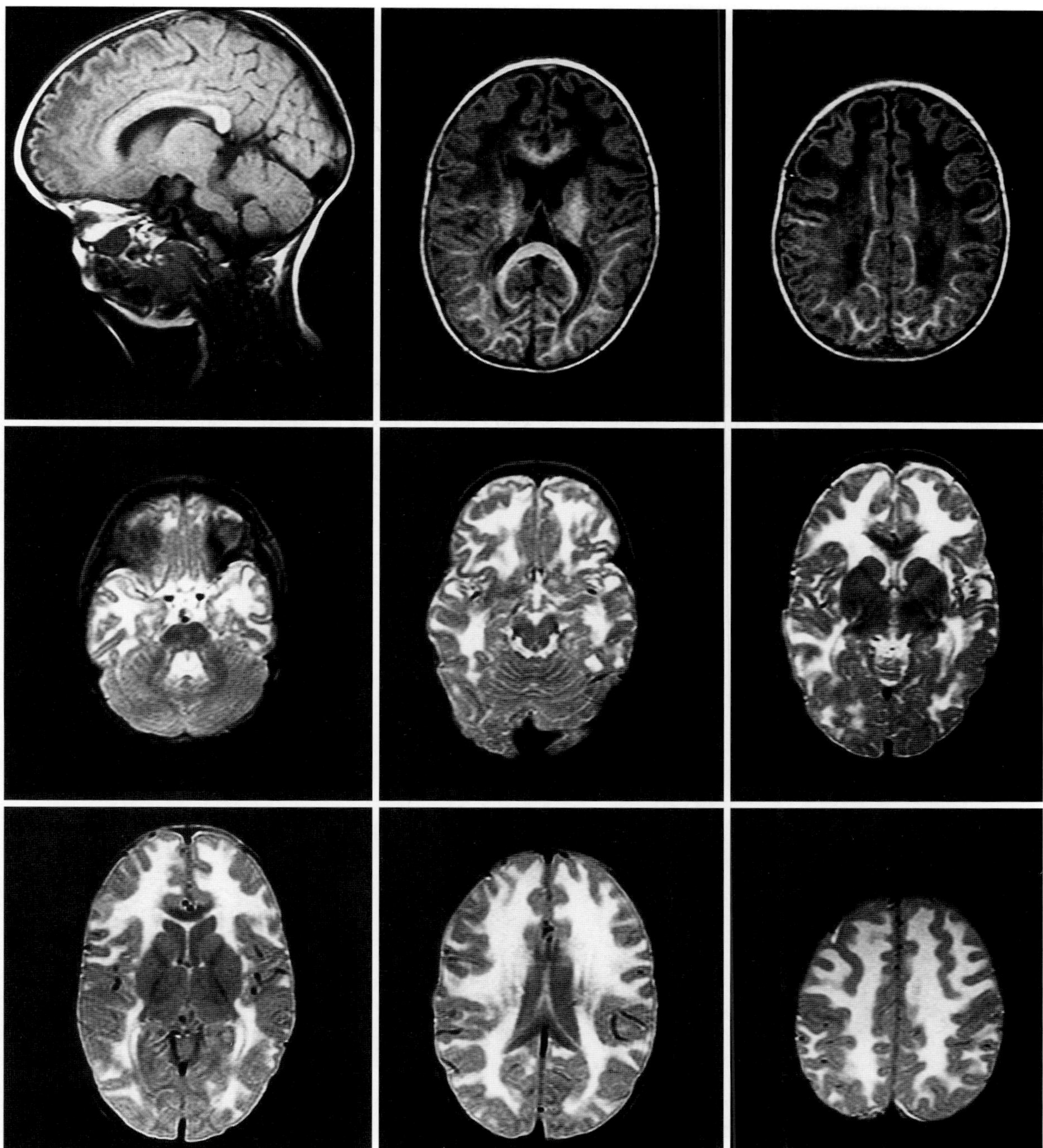

Fig. 47.5. Same patient as in Fig. 47.4, now 2 years of age. Extensive white matter abnormalities are seen. There is some swelling of the white matter suggesting spongiform white matter pathology. The corpus callosum and some subcortical white matter fibers, particularly in the occipital area, contain myelin. No cysts are seen in this patient

not shown progressive white matter disease, in contrast to some CT reports. Considering MRI findings, white matter changes may be (entirely or largely) caused by delayed myelination, focally or more generally disturbed myelination and white matter sponginess.

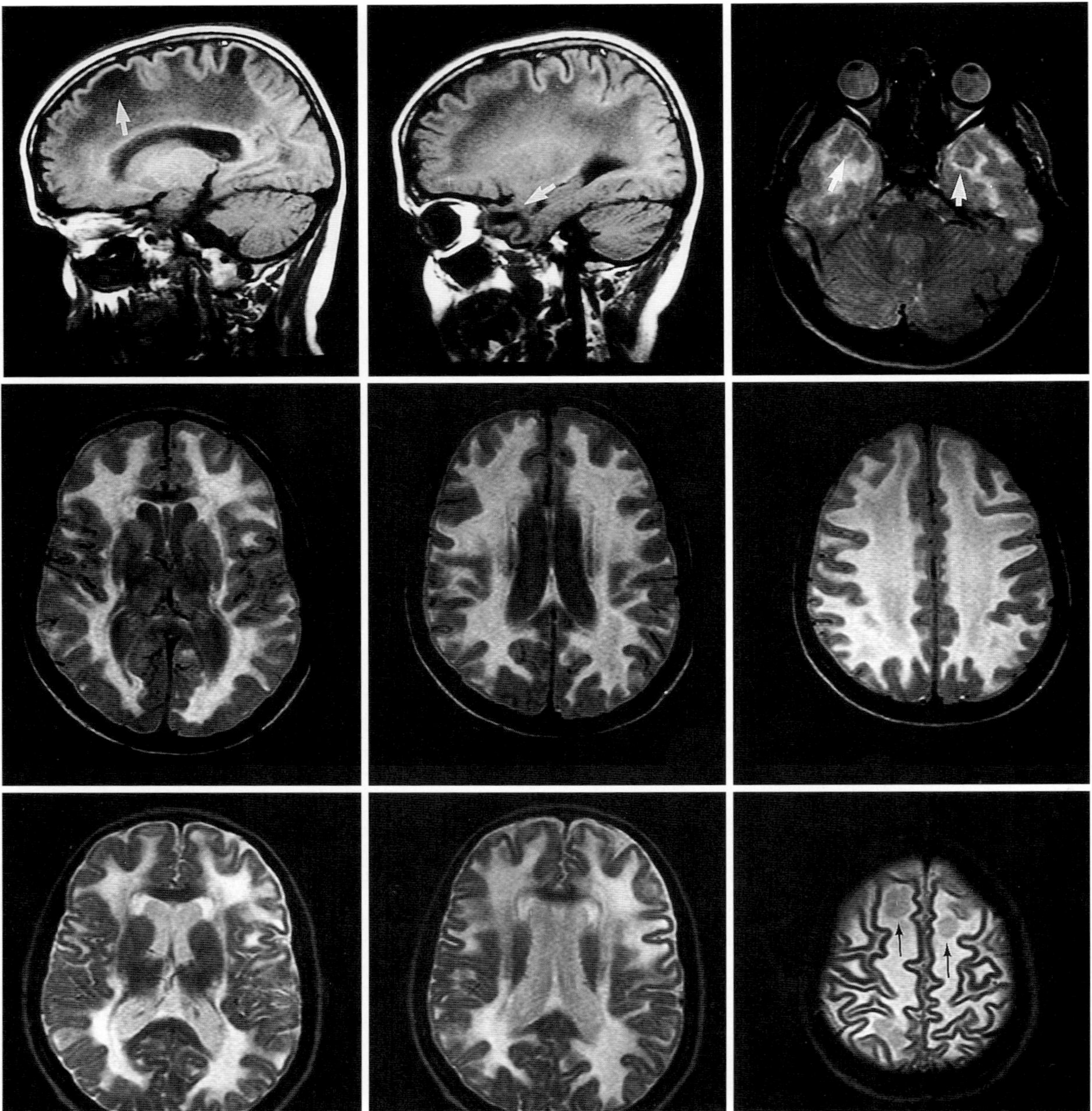

Fig. 47.6. A 29-year-old woman with later-onset signs of muscular dystrophy. The images have about the same features as in Fig. 47.5 with widespread involvement of white matter, suggestive of spongiform white matter pathology. Now, however, cysts have also been formed (*arrows*) in the frontal, fronto-parietal and temporal regions (see also images in Chap. 48)

48 Infantile-Onset Leukoencephalopathy with Swelling and a Discrepantly Mild Clinical Course

48.1 Clinical Features and Laboratory Investigations

Recently, an as yet unidentified disease, characterized by cerebral leukoencephalopathy and megalencephaly with infantile onset, was discovered (Van der Knaap et al. 1993, 1994a,b,c, 1995a,b). Considering the high rate of consanguinity among the parents and the presence of two affected sibs in one family, an autosomal recessive mode of inheritance can be assumed.

Macrocephaly is present at birth or, more frequently, develops during the first year of life. Initial mental and motor development is normal in most cases, mildly delayed in the minority of the patients. Apart from progressive macrocephaly, the first clinical sign is usually a delay in walking. Walking is unstable and the child often falls. Subsequently a slow deterioration of motor function is noted over the years with development of axial ataxia and limb ataxia. Signs of pyramidal dysfunction are late and minor, and are always dominated by the signs of cerebellar ataxia. Muscle tone tends to be low, apart from some ankle hypertonia. Reflexes become high and Babinski signs become apparent. Gradually the ability to walk independently is lost and the children become completely wheelchair-dependent at the end of the first decade or in the second decade of life. Mental deterioration is late and mild. Decreasing school performance becomes evident during the later years of primary school. In a minority of patients, intellectual capacities are mildly decreased from the beginning. A relatively late and slow decrease in intelligence is also noted in these patients. The majority of the patients have mild epilepsy, easily controled with medication.

The oldest known patient is 22 years of age. At present the final course of the disease is not known.

In laboratory investigations no abnormalities are found. There is no evidence of a lysosomal dysfunction (in particular no evidence of sphingolipidoses) a peroxisomal dysfunction or mitochondrial disorder. No abnormalities of amino acid and organic acid metabolism are found. CSF GABA, amino acids and amines are normal. There is no evidence of muscular dystrophy. Peripheral motor and sensory nerve conduction velocity is normal. Evoked potentials are initially normal in most patients. BAEPs remain normal, but VEPs and SSEPs deteriorate over the years with prolongation of latencies and abnormal cortical responses. EEG is initially normal. Subsequently, background slowing occurs and abnormalities are seen like sharp waves, spikes and spike-wave complexes with variable location. No abnormal photic responses are seen.

48.2 Pathology

Brain biopsy was performed in one patient. The cortex was normal. A status spongiosus of the white matter was found with presence of innumerable vacuoles. The precise location and nature of the vacuoles has not yet been identified. Most myelin sheaths have a normal appearance and there are only minor signs of myelin breakdown.

48.3 Pathogenetic Considerations

Among the progressive cerebral disorders characterized by megalencephaly and leukoencephalopathy, the present disorder can be defined on the basis of clinical and MRI findings.

It is apparent that the disease has an early onset with progressive macrocephaly during the first year of life. From about the end of the first year of life, head growth rate becomes normal and growth follows a line parallel to the 98th percentile, though far above it. The most important change in the brain in the first year of life is myelination, from an almost complete absence of myelin in the cerebral hemispheres in the neonatal period to a state of near-completion of myelination at the end of the first year of life. The simultaneous occurrence of the normal process of myelination and the onset of the white matter disease in these patients may suggest a connection.

The white matter has a very abnormal aspect on MRI at an early age (youngest child was 2 years when imaging was performed), when neurological examination is still normal or near-normal and evoked responses are normal. Consequently, despite its highly abnormal appearance, the white matter is functionally intact or largely intact during these early years.

Over the years, MRI shows some decrease in white matter swelling and some enlargement of lateral ventricles and subarachnoid spaces. Clinically, the patients show very slow deterioration: initially mostly motor deterioration, later also mental deterioration. Evoked responses deteriorate with progressive slowing and abnormal cortical responses.

The cause of the disease is unknown. Considering the usual clinical course and paraclinical findings of demyelinating disorders or vacuolating myelinopathies (e.g., Canavan's disease), it is highly improbable that these types of pathology underly the disease. Not only is the basic pathology unknown, but also the cause of the clinical deterioration is unknown. Probably the large number of sometimes microscopically enormous vacuoles eventually compromises the white matter in its normal structure and function.

48.4   Magnetic Resonance Imaging

In all patients supratentorial hemispheral white matter is diffusely abnormal and swollen. The swelling is most marked during the first years of life, with obliteration of peripheral CSF spaces and narrowing of ventricles (Fig. 48.1). In older children the hemispheral white matter swelling is less severe, peripheral CSF spaces are more prominently visible and the ventricular system becomes slightly enlarged (Figs. 48.2, 48.3). There are subcortical cysts with a typical location: anterior temporal and/or frontoparietal area. The cysts are bilateral; they tend to become larger with age and in a few patients they have been shown to increase in number. The signal intensity of the contents of the cysts is always similar to that of CSF. In accordance with this, T_1 and T_2 of cyst contents and CSF are also similar. A patent cavum septi pellucidi and cavum Vergae are often present.

In contrast with the diffuse abnormality of the hemisperhal white matter there is a characteristic sparing of central white matter structures, including corpus callosum, anterior limb of the internal capsule, (partially) posterior limb of the internal capsule and a periventricular rim of occipital white matter. The posterior limb of the internal capsule either shows a line-shaped abnormality in signal intensity over its whole length (Fig. 48.2), or an abnormality in its distal part only (Fig. 48.3). In addition, some sparing of subcortical fibers is seen most often in the occipital area. In the majority of patients, the cerebellar white matter shows only a slight abnormality in signal intensity and no swelling. In some patients minor abnormalities are seen in the pyramidal tracts of the brain stem. Cortical gray matter structures and basal nuclei are always normal.

Similar white matter changes with swelling have been reported in Canavan's disease, Alexander disease, L-2-hydroxyglutaric aciduria and one variant of congenital muscular dystrophy. However, in Canavan's disease, as a rule, MRI demonstrates additional involvement of the thalamus and globus pallidus, not found in our patients. Special MRI findings in Alexander disease are contrast enhancement in the periventricular region, caudate nuclei and thalami, the frequent presence of hydrocephalus and the often prominent cavitation starting in the frontal periventricular white matter. None of these are present in the disease described in this chapter. In L-2-hydroxyglutaric aciduria MRI shows additional involvement of caudate nuclei, putamen, dentate nuclei and severe atrophy of the cerebellar vermis, not observed in the present disease. The MRI abnormalities observed in one variant of congenital muscular dystrophy are very similar to those observed in the disease described here. The typical cysts were observed in one patient with a later onset variant of muscular dystrophy with leukoencephalopathy and swelling. The nature of the leukoencephalopathy in congenital or later onset muscular dystrophy has not been elucidated (see also Chap. 47 on congenital muscular dystrophy).

Incidental reports mention similar cases of megalencephaly and leukoencephalopathy of infantile onset and unknown origin. These cases are usually presented under the heading of atypical variants of Alexander disease. In 1990, Harbord et al described two sibs, aged 3.5 and 4.5, with onset of macrocephaly during the first year of life. After normal initial development ataxia, spasticity and epilepsy occurred. One sib was never able to walk unaided, and the other only managed for a few months in the third year of life. Mental capacities were intact. CT scan of the brain showed severe white matter hypodensity and swelling, but cysts were not reported. It is possible that these two sibs suffered from a severe variant of the disease described here.

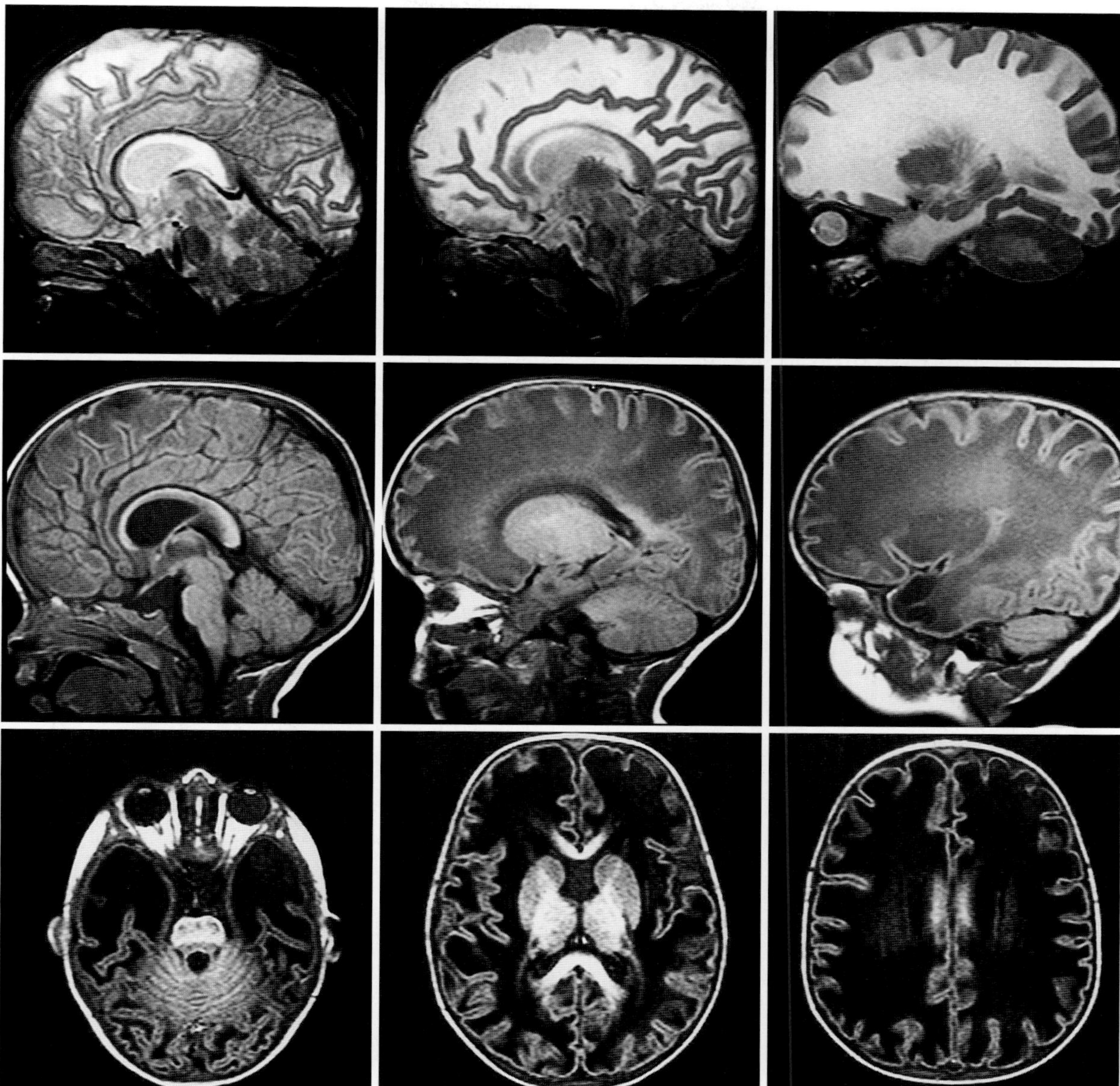

Fig. 48.1. MRI series of a 2-year-old girl with the disease entity described in this chapter. The *upper row* of T$_2$-weighted sagittal images show the macrocephaly, the swollen white matter, and the cysts in the frontal and temporal region. The *middle row* shows these features in a T$_1$-weighted sagittal direction. The *lower row* presents transverse T$_1$-weighted (IR) images, making it obvious that corpus callosum, basal ganglia, capsula interna, and pons are spared

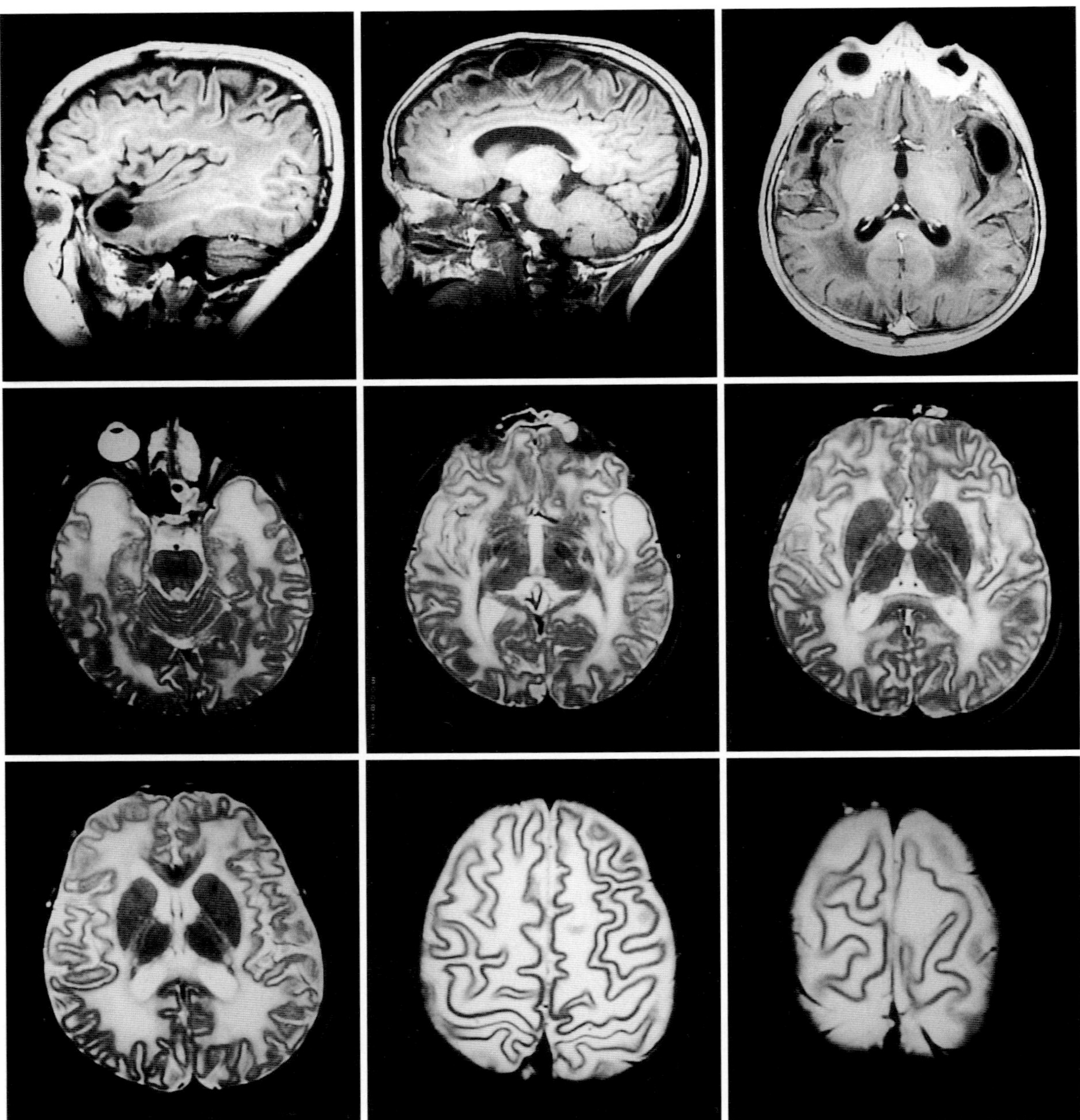

Fig. 48.2. Another example of the MRI features of the disease in a 12-year-old boy. Note again the swelling of the white matter and the sparing of the corpus callosum and basal ganglia, this time with a line-shaped high signal from the posteri- or limb of the internal capsule. The white matter swelling is somewhat less severe than in the 2-year-old patient. The cystic lesions are present in their usual spots

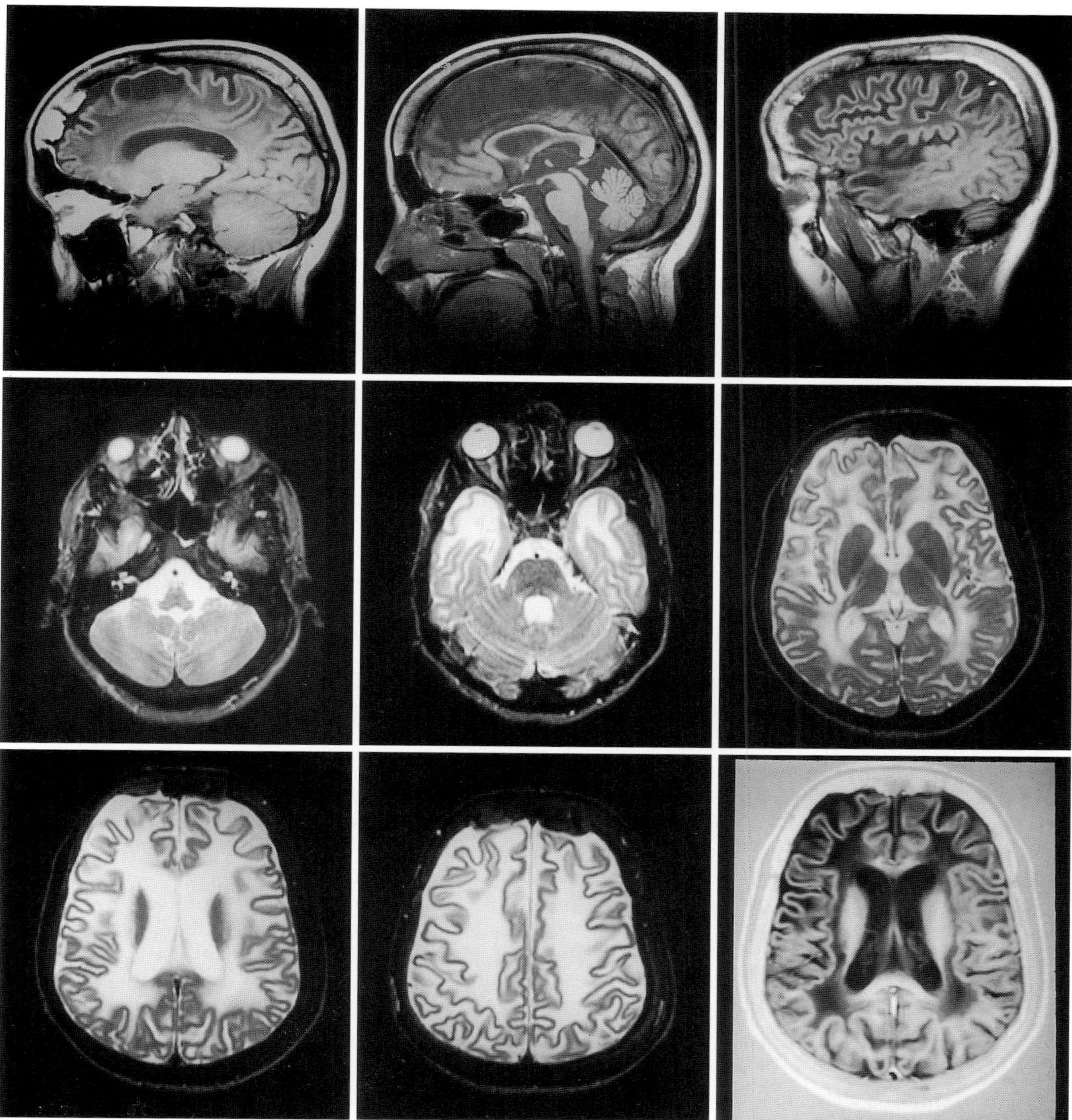

Fig. 48.3. A 20-year-old woman, showing that some atrophy has now developed. The cysts have become larger

49 Childhood Ataxia with Diffuse Cerebral Hypomyelination

49.1 Introduction

Recently, a disorder characterized by childhood ataxia and diffuse cerebral white matter abnormalities has been described in detail by Hanefeld et al. (1993) and Schiffmann et al. (1992, 1994). Apart from progressive cerebellar ataxia, seizures and optic atrophy were noted. Cognitive functions were relatively preserved. MRI showed diffuse high signal intensity of the hemispheral white matter on T_2-weighted images.

Reviewing the literature, it is probable that in the past several similar cases have been presented under the heading of Behr syndrome. Behr syndrome is defined as an autosomal recessive disorder characterized by optic atrophy, cerebellar ataxia, variable pyramidal tract dysfunction and variable mental deficiency. Considering the great variation in course of disease, presence of additional abnormalities, and cerebral pathology (presence or absence of abnormality in myelin content), it is evident that Behr syndrome is not a genetically homogeneous entity but harbors a number of different degenerative disorders. One of them is defined by diffuse abnormalities of the cerebral white matter (Hanefeld et al. 1993; Schiffmann et al. 1994; Marzan and Barron 1994).

49.2 Clinical Features and Laboratory Investigations

Initial development is normal. Age at onset of deterioration lies in early childhood, but onset in infancy may also occur. Presenting signs are clumsiness and progressive ataxia with dysmetria and intention tremor of the extremities. Truncal ataxia and head titubation occur. The disease is progressive over the years, often with episodic deterioration following infections and minor head traumas. The capability to walk independently and sit without support is lost. Progressive dysarthria is noted. Progressive optic atrophy leads to visual failure. Variable spasticity develops and becomes particularly pronounced in the legs. Reflexes are markedly increased and plantar responses are extensor. Head growth continues at a normal rate. Initial cognitive development is normal or mildly delayed and re-mains relatively preserved. Epileptic seizures may occur but only incidentally.

No abnormalities are found in laboratory investigations. CSF is normal. Extensive screening for inborn errors of metabolism reveals no abnormalities. Peripheral nerve conduction and EMG are normal.

49.3 Pathology

On brain biopsy, the cortex appears to be unremarkable, except for some mild gliosis. White matter pathology is characterized by hypomyelination, presence of thin myelin sheaths with normal periodicity, occasional myelin splitting and intramyelinic vacuole formation, and a component of later demyelination, astrogliosis and microglial activation (Schiffmann et al. 1994).

49.4 Pathogenetic Considerations

The basic defect is unknown, but the disease is probably inheritable with an autosomal recessive mode of inheritance. We observed the condition in five patients from two families.

It has been noted repeatedly (Schiffmann et al. 1994; Marzan and Barron 1994; own observation) that MRI shows diffuse hemispheral white matter abnormalities from the onset of clinical symptoms and remains unchanged over the years despite evident clinical deterioration. Surprisingly, the MRI abnormalities are already extensive whereas clinical symptomatology is mild, and MRI does not change much in contrast to the clinical downhill course. The histopathological basis of the clinical deterioration is unknown. The pattern of MRI abnormalities and the histopathological findings suggest a combination of hypomyelination and demyelination.

49.5 Therapy

No causal treatment is possible. Prenatal diagnosis cannot be performed.

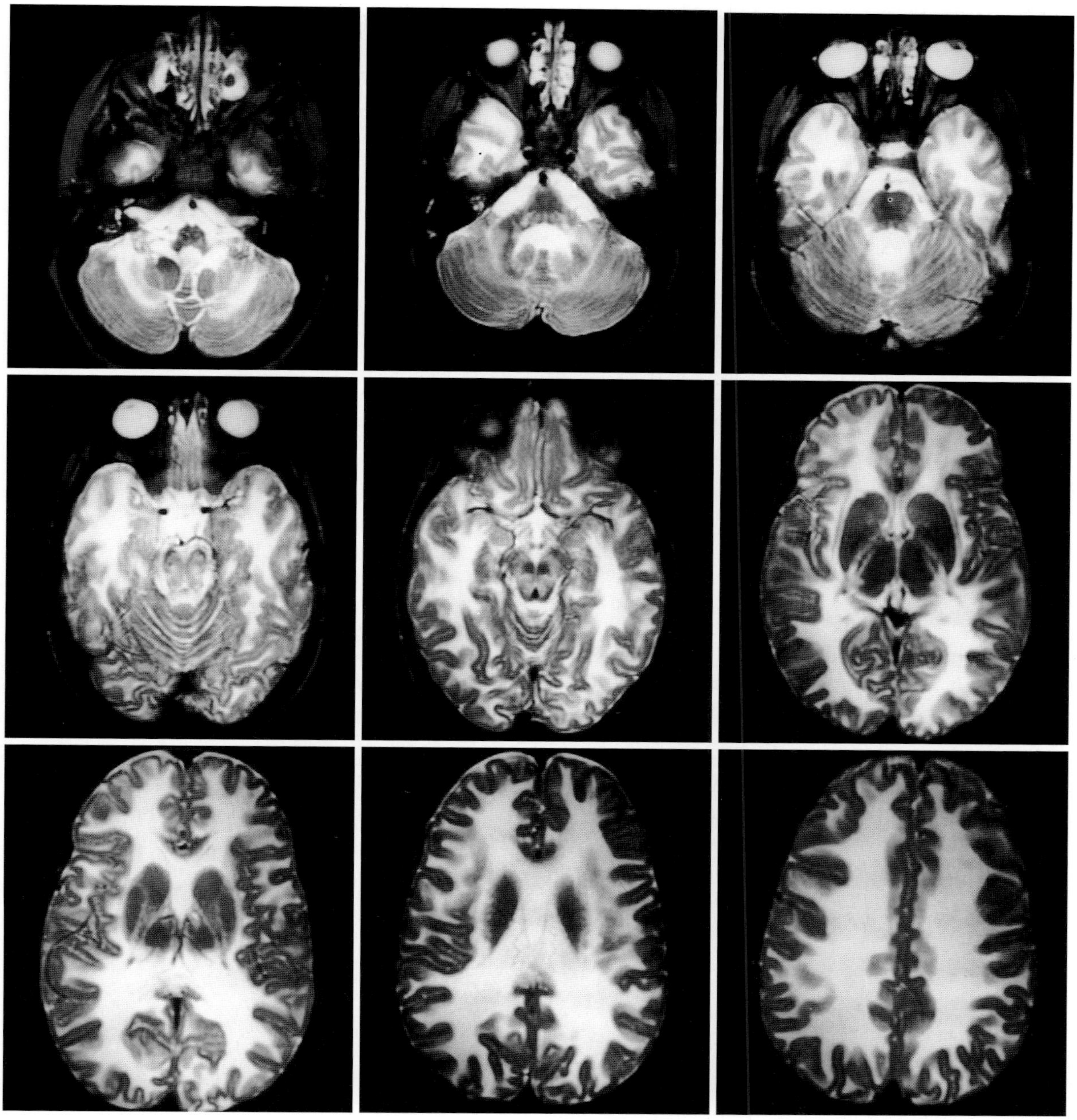

Fig. 49.1. T_2-weighted transverse series through the brain of a 5-year-old girl showing the extent of white matter changes in the brain. Clearly, the white matter in the cerebellum and cerebral hemispheres is affected. The U fibers are also involved in this case. The genu of the corpus callosum and the basal ganglia are spared. The posterior limb of the internal capsule is partially affected; a streak of myelin remains

49.6 Magnetic Resonance Imaging

CT scan shows diffuse white matter hypodensity.

MRI depicts the white matter abnormalities in more detail. The hemispheral white matter is severely abnormal. In our patients, the white matter abnormalities are diffuse and homogeneous (Figs. 49.1, 49.2). The subcortical U fibers may be extensively involved (Fig. 49.1) or partly preserved (Fig. 49.2). The corpus callosum is partially preserved. The external capsule and extreme capsule are affected, while the internal capsule is variably involved. The ventricles may be mildly enlarged, but severe atrophy has not been observed. The brain stem is better, although not completely preserved. The

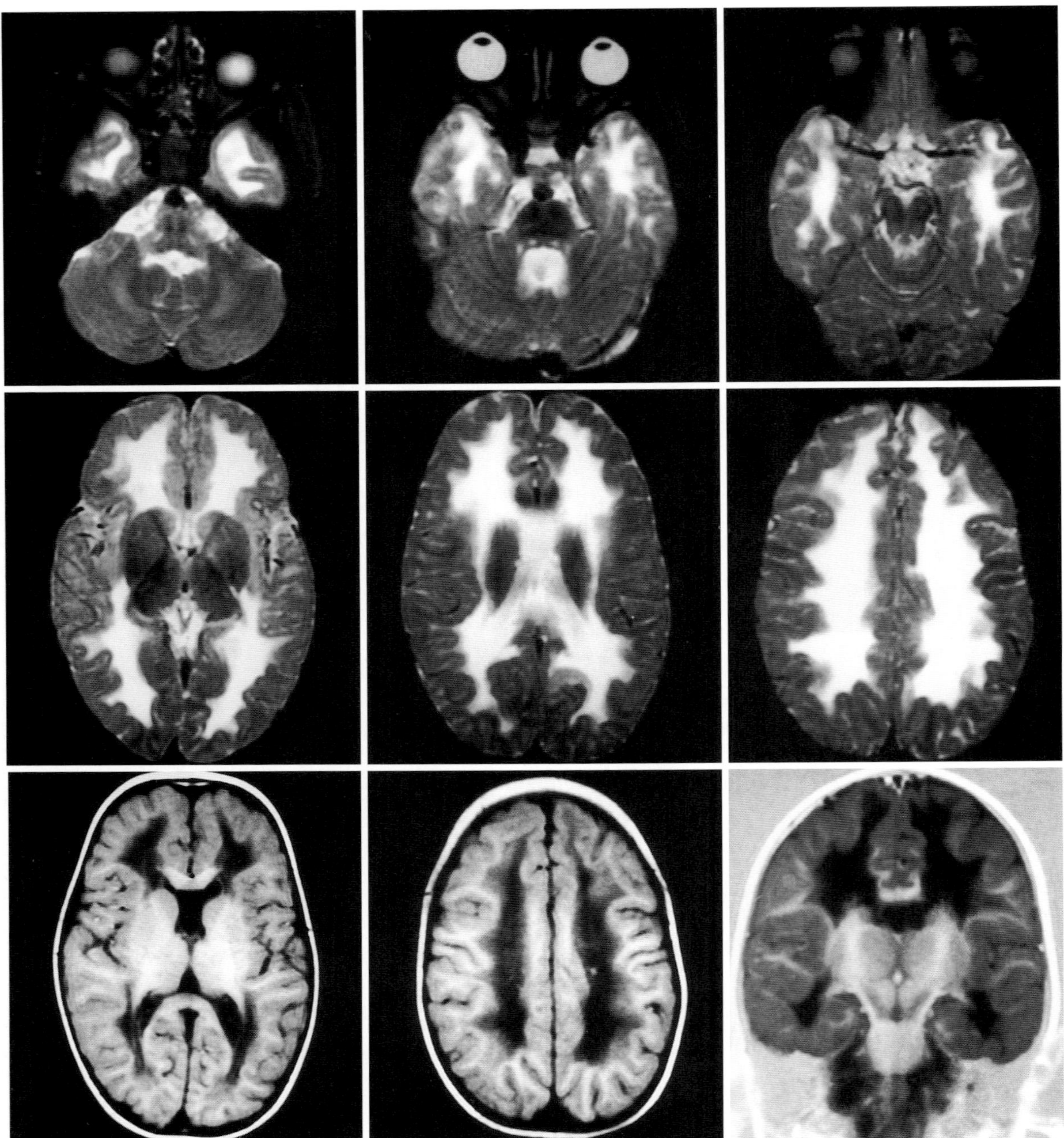

Fig. 49.2. T$_2$-weighted transverse series (*upper two rows*) of the 3-year-old sister of previous patient, also suffering from the same disease. The changes in the posterior fossa are less conspicuous and the U fibers are partially preserved. There is sparing of the genu and splenium of the corpus callosum and the internal capsule

cerebellar white matter is, at most, partially affected.

The pattern of myelin presence (brain stem, cerebellar white matter, internal capsule) is consistent with an early stage of myelination. However, the presence of some myelin in the corpus callosum and subcortical white matter is not. MR images are compatible with a combination of disturbed myelination and demyelination.

MRS findings are discussed in chapter 70.

50 Leukoencephalopathy, Cerebral Calcifications, and Chronic Cerebrospinal Fluid Lymphocytosis (Aicardi-Goutières Syndrome)

50.1 Introduction

In 1984, Aicardi and Goutières described eight infants with progressive microcephaly, spasticity, dystonia, persistent lymphocytic pleiocytosis and elevated CSF protein; neuroimaging revealed a combination of white matter abnormalities and calcium depositions, most prominent in the basal nuclei. The course of disease was fatal over a period of months or years. Some patients were sibs, and autosomal recessive inheritance was suggested. Among the eight infants some variability was noted. The CSF lymphocyte count varied from only slightly elevated to over 100 cells/mm^3; protein level varied from normal to more than 1 g/l. A variation in CSF composition was found in the same patient at different occasions and between patients. In two patients, CT showed no calcifications, whereas their sibs had calcifications of the basal nuclei. In two patients calcium depositions were not only seen in the basal nuclei, but punctate calcifications were also present in the white matter alongside the ventricle wall.

In the past a number of similar patients have been described with a combination of severe neurological dysfunction, white matter disease and calcium deposits in the basal nuclei. However, several patients have additional characteristics suggesting they may belong to another diagnostic category. For instance, in some patients degenerative retinitis is observed (Neill and Dingwall 1950; Lyon et al. 1968; patients 1 and 3 of Melchior et al. 1960; patients 1–4 of Billard et al. 1989); some are normocephalic (Boltshauser et al. 1991); occasionally, additional cortical calcifications are seen at autopsy (Hallervorden 1950; Jervis 1954; case 1 of Koussef 1980; Troost et al. 1984), while in many cases no information is present about CSF composition. Reviewing the literature it is evident that we are probably dealing with a heterogeneous group of patients, but that one better-defined disease entity can be pointed out, which is characterized by severe, early onset and often early fatal neurological abnormalities, microcephaly, CSF lymphocytosis with or without elevated protein, and, on neuroimaging or post-mortem examination, a combination of white matter changes and calcium depositions with variable location but mainly in the basal nuclei (Babbit et al. 1969; Troost et al. 1984; Aicardi and Goutières 1984; Mehta et al. 1986; Razavi-Encha et al. 1988).

50.2 Clinical Features and Laboratory Investigations

The disease presents itself at birth or within the first few months of life. Early signs are irritability, jitteriness, feeding problems and failure to thrive. Often a high-pitched cry is noted. Generalized hypertonia and spasticity are present from the beginning, or develop in the course of the first months. Truncal hypotonia, poor head control or opisthotonic posturing are noted. Head growth is poor with progressive microcephaly. Gain in height and weight is below normal. Some but not all patients have convulsions. Vision is poor. Some patients have pale optic discs, whereas others have normal fundi. Pupillary reactions are normal. There is a severe developmental delay. No, or at most few, developmental milestones are reached. The disease is usually considered to be progressive, although because of its severity and early onset, it is difficult to determine whether this is the case. Most children die early, either within weeks or within a few years of birth. The majority die in a vegetative state from pneumonia. Incidentally, survival for more than 6 years has been reported.

On repeated occasions, more than one affected patient has been observed within the same family, suggesting autosomal recessive inheritance.

Laboratory investigations have revealed no abnormalities apart from an obligatory, chronic, lympocytic pleocytosis in the CSF, with or without an elevation of the protein content, without evidence of intrathecal immunoglobulin synthesis. There is no evidence of congenital infections. Extensive screening for inborn errors of metabolism has never revealed abnormalities.

50.3 Pathology

Post-mortem investigations demonstrate micrencephaly. On sectioning, reduction in white matter volume and some enlargement of the ventricles may be noted. Calcium depositions are consistently present.

Most dense calcium deposits are seen in the globus pallidus, putamen, caudate nucleus and dentate nucleus. Less dense calcium deposits are variably noted in the cerebral cortex, cerebral white matter, and cerebellar white matter. The calcium deposits are usually punctate, but large concrements may also be seen. On microscopy the calcium deposits are shown to be vascular and perivascular as well as axonal. Within the cortex and basal nuclei some neuronal loss is found.

The state of myelination in the cerebral and cerebellar white matter is poor, with little myelin present. Some ascribe this to hypomyelination, and others to myelin loss. No sudanophilic material is present. The white matter shows enhanced fibrillary gliosis.

50.4 Pathogenetic Considerations

The disease is probably hereditary with an autosomal recessive mode of inheritance. The basic defect is unknown. An alternative explanation includes a maternally transmitted congenital infection, but this could never be shown, either in the child or in the mother.

50.5 Therapy

At present, there is no therapy apart from supportive care. Prenatal diagnosis is as yet not possible.

50.6 Magnetic Resonance Imaging

CT is very important in the diagnosis of this disease, easily demonstrating the presence of calcium deposisions (Fig. 50.1). The calcium deposits are most often reported in the globus pallidus, putamen, caudate nucleus and dentate nuclei. Additionally, calcium deposits have been reported in the white matter, in particular in the periventricular area alongside the ventricle wall. The deposits are often punctate, but may also form larger concrements. However, in several affected sibs of typical cases of leukoencephalopathy with cerebral calcifications and chronic CSF lymphocytosis, CT did not reveal any calcification. Apparently the calcifications are a characteristic, but not obligatory part of the disease. On CT, variable white matter hypodensity has been reported, in contrast to the invariable lack of myelin found on post-mortem examination. Calcifications are less easily seen on MRI, but MRI more easily shows the abnormality of the white matter (Fig. 50.1).

CT and MRI may show only some of the characteristic abnormalities, despite the presence of the typical clinical picture. A female patient became symptomatic 3 weeks after birth with inconsolable, high-pitched crying, severe feeding problems necessitating gavage feeding, spastic tetraplegia, opisthotonic posturing, poor vision, progressive microcephaly and a poor gain in weight and height. The only laboratory abnormality that could be found, was a chronic lymphocytosis in the CSF in combination with some elevation of the total protein level and no elevation of CSF immunoglobulins. Extensive and repeated investigations for congenital infections were negative. CT scan of the brain (Fig. 50.2) was performed at 4 and 10 months, and on both occasions revealed an identical pattern of punctate calcium deposits alongside the ventricle wall, probably including the caudate nucleus. No calcium deposits were seen in the putamen, globus pallidus or dentate nucleus. The cerebral white matter was hypodense. MRI was performed at 6 and 10 months and on both occasions revealed an identical pattern of a severe white matter abnormality of the cerebral hemispheres with cystic degeneration in the anterior temporal and parieto-occipital subcortical areas. Myelin was shown to be present in the brain stem, cerebellar white matter, basal nuclei, a rim of the optic radiation and the tracts of the corona radiata which are in contact with the primary motor and sensory cortices. Outside these areas no myelin was seen. This pattern was identical at 6 and 10 months, consistent with an arrest of myelination at a very early stage. These MRI findings form an argument for a disturbance of myelination, rather than demyelination as a cause of the white matter abnormalities. However, the appearance of the white matter is different from normal unmyelinated white matter, being slightly and homogeneously swollen and partly cystic.

The MRI pattern shows similarities to other diseases characterized by disturbed myelination and presence of calcium deposits, including Cockayne's disease, CAMFAK syndrome (cataracts, microcephaly, failure to thrive, kyphoscoliosis) and COFS (cerebro-oculo-facio-skeletal) syndrome (see Chap. 27 on Cockayne's disease). In these cases CSF may reveal an elevated protein level, but not a chronic lymphocytic pleocytosis.

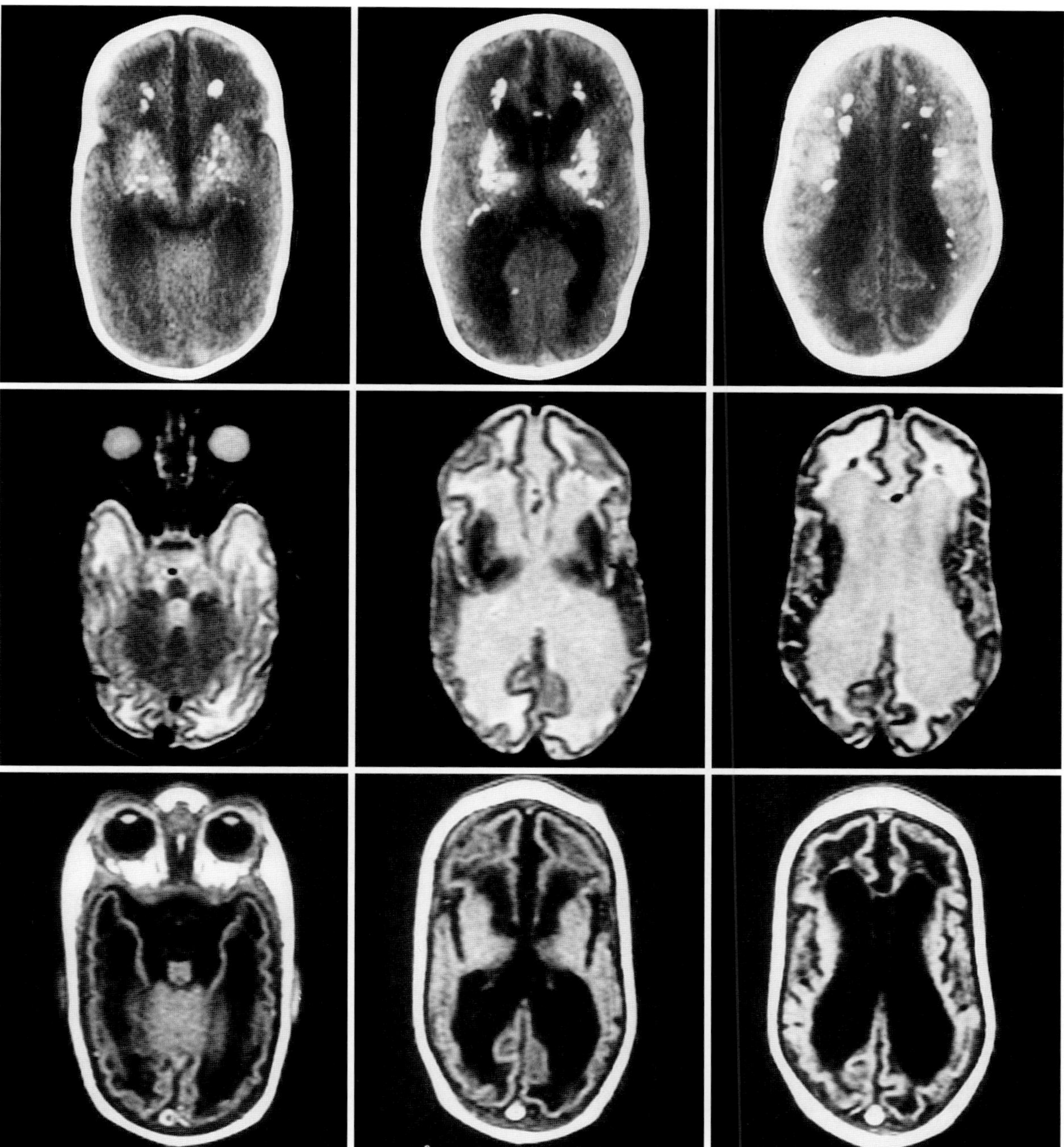

Fig. 50.1. CT (*upper row*) and MRI (*lower two rows*) in a 7-month-old patient with Aicardi-Goutières syndrome. There are calcium deposits in the thalamus, basal ganglia, and periventricular white matter. The calcium deposits in the white matter have the typical punctate appearance. The MRI scans show an abnormal signal intensity of the hemispheral white matter throughout. Note the presence of cystic degeneration in the anterior temporal area. Courtesy of P.G. Barth, Amsterdam, The Netherlands, with permission

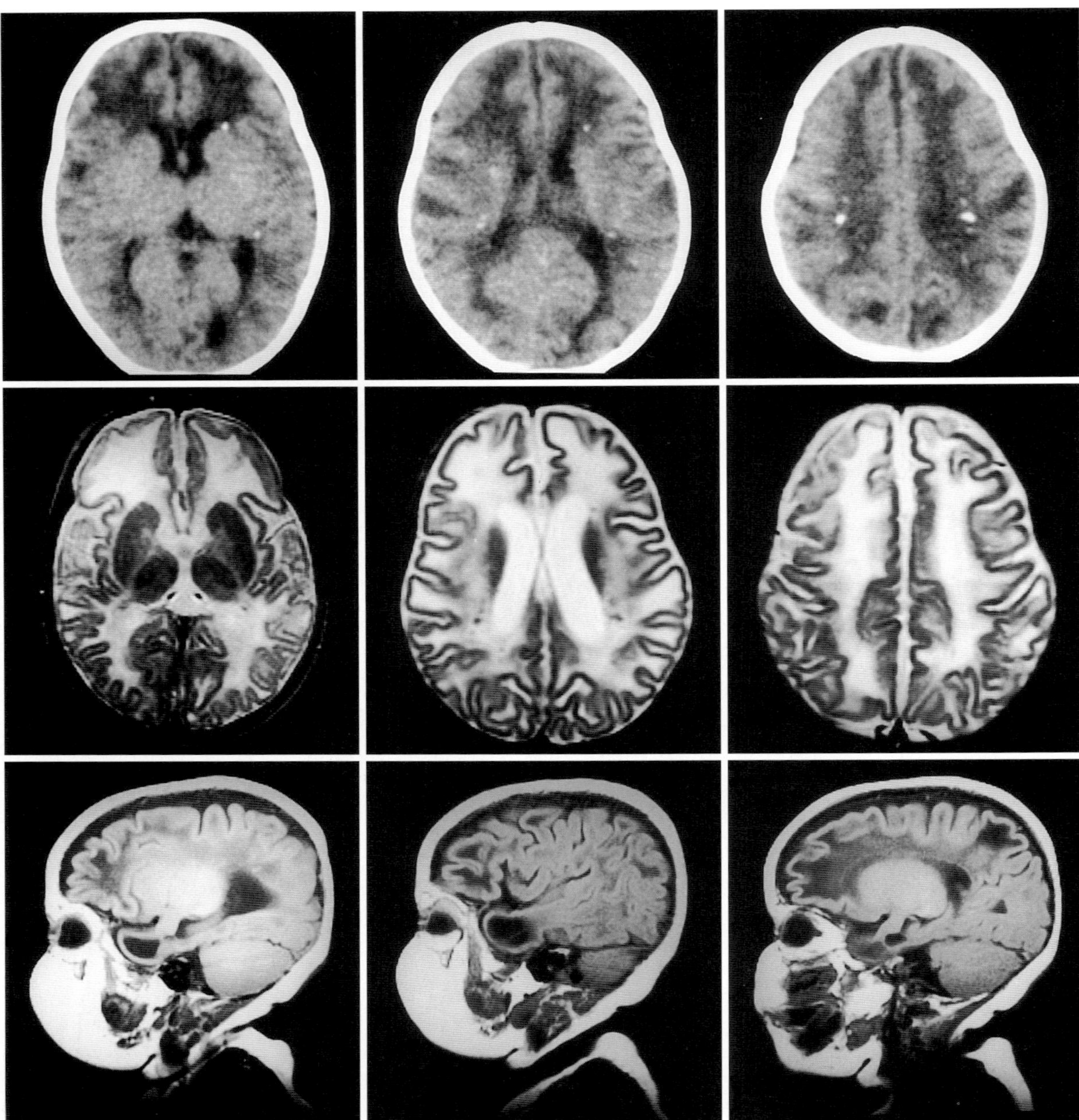

Fig. 50.2. Female patient, described in the text. Note the punctate calcium depositions in the white matter alongside the ventricle wall and probably in the head and tail of the caudate nucleus. Myelination is severely delayed and the unmyelinated white matter is abnormal in appearance. Note on the sagittal images the cysts in the temporal and parieto-occipital white matter

Although apparently different with respect to the underlying cause, inflammatory and infectious diseases have much in common. In both conditions the human defense system plays an active role, counteracting the cause of the disturbance, killing the intruder and repairing the tissue damage.

Inflammation has principally a protective role. Paradoxically, in a large number of human diseases inflammatory reactions are part of the pathogenetic mechanisms causing tissue damage. Inflammatory reactions can be both protective and histotoxic. This histotoxicity has prompted a huge effort of the pharmaceutical industry to develop effective antagonists and inhibitors of the molecules involved in these reactions, the inflammatory mediators. The inflammatory process is characterized by a complex interplay between blood cells, blood vessels and tissue. These responses are complex, but relatively stereotyped.

Many components of the defense system have to come into action to destroy the invading micro-organism or counteract adverse interactions. The defense system depends largely on the immune system, which can be subdivided into an *innate (nonadaptive)* and an *acquired (adaptive)* part. Repeated infections do not improve the innate system, whereas the adaptive immune system has a "memory-bank" with improved resistance after repeated insults. In both systems a *molecular* (solvable, humoral) component can be distinguished from a *cellular* component.

In the *innate system* the *soluble factors* are lysozyme, complement, acute phase proteins, and interferon.

The enzyme lysozyme is a soluble bactericidal substance, abundantly present in body fluids. It is capable of splitting the exposed peptidoglycan wall of susceptible bacteria.

Complement consists of a complex series of some twenty proteins, and forms one of the enzyme systems in plasma triggered during inflammation. Once activated, the complement system produces a rapid, highly amplified response to a trigger stimulus, mediated by a cascade phenomenon in which the product of one reaction is the enzyme catalyst of the next reaction. Components of complement are designated by the letter "C" followed by a number, related to the chronology of its discovery. Unfortunately, the sequence in which the complement components come into action is not completely identical to the sequence of their discovery. The actions of activated complement range from increasing vascular permeability to mast cell degranulation, opsonization and phagocytosis of bacteria, neutrophil activation and chemotaxis, and lysis of bacteria and foreign cells. Two ways of activating complement are distinguished. One is the so-called alternative pathway, which is activated by a microbial polysaccharide. This pathway belongs to the innate, nonspecific immune system. The other, the classical pathway, is a specific response triggered by antibody-antigen complexes. Both systems work closely together.

Acute phase proteins are plasma proteins which undergo a dramatic increase in concentration in response to infection or injury. A number of factors belong to this group, including C-reactive protein (CRP) and fibrinogen. CRP has the ability to bind to a number of micro-organisms which contain phosphorylcholine on their membranes. The complex formed is able to activate complement by the classical pathway, resulting in opsonization of the microbe for adherence to phagocytes.

Interferons (IFN) are broad-spectrum anti-viral agents. Different molecular forms of interferon have been identified. There are at least 14 different IFN-α, produced by leukocytes, while fibroblasts and other cells produce IFN-β, IFN-γ and macrophage activating factors, which switch on the microbicidal mechanisms of the macrophage. A subpopulation of T lymphocytes, T-helper cells, will produce lymphokines, amongst which IFN-γ, if bound to an antigen in association with a major histocompatibility complex class II molecule on a macrophage surface. IFN-γ is also produced by cytotoxic T lymphocytes which recognize antigen in association with MHC class I molecules.

The major histocompatibility complex (MHC) is the name of the genome which is of predominant importance in the transplant rejection process. In man the MHC is the human leukocyte antigen (HLA) cluster encoded for by chromosome 6. It has been recognized that proteins encoded in this particular region of chromosome 6 are involved in many aspects of immunological recognition, including both interaction between lymphoid cells, and interaction between lymphocytes and antigen presenting cells. Three classes of MHC molecules are distinguished. Class I molecules associate with antigen on the surface of virally infected cells to signal cytotoxic T lymphocytes. Class II molecules signal T-helper cells for activating B cells and macrophages. T-helper cells are only activated when both antigen and MHC class II molecules are presented on the antigen presenting cell. Class III genes encode complement components.

The *cellular* part of the *innate immune system* is formed by phagocytes, natural killer cells and mast cells.

The phagocytes can be distinguished in monocytes and polymorphonuclear granulocytes. The latter can be differentiated into neutrophils, eosinophils and basophils, according to the histological staining of their granules. Granulocytes do not show any specificity for antigens, but together with antibodies and complement, they play an important role in protection against micro-organisms. Their predominant role is phagocytosis. In the process of phagocytosis both oxygen-dependent and oxygen-independent mechanisms play a role. The oxygen-burst is the process in phagocytosis by which oxygen is converted to free radicals.

Oxygen radicals and their metabolites constitute an important class of inflammatory mediators. Free radicals are atoms or molecules containing an unpaired electron in the outer orbit. Phagocytic cells, when activated, exhibit a sharp increase in molecular oxygen consumption, the so-called respiratory burst, and produce a battery of biologically active oxygen radicals and derived metabolites. The stimuli for phagocyte derived oxygen radical production are multiple, including endotoxins, γ-immunoglobulins and cytokines. Reduction of molecular oxygen by addition of a single electron results in formation of the superoxide anion ($O_2\cdot$). In aqueous environments $O_2\cdot$ exists in equilibrium with its protonated form, $H_2O\cdot$ (perhydroxyl radical). In the presence of superoxide dismutase $O_2\cdot$ can undergo dismutation, resulting in H_2O_2 formation. Hydrogen peroxide has the capacity to oxidize directly a wide spectrum of biological molecules. Phagocyte derived oxygen radicals and their metabolites are important mediators of tissue damage in inflammatory disorders. The concurrent rise in pH due to free radical formation allows cationic proteins to function optimally, damaging the bacterial membrane. The process of phagocytosis is adequately supported by the complement system, that can prepare micro-organisms for phagocytosis by opsonization.

Natural killer cells are large granular lymphocytes with a characteristic morphology, capable of recognizing structures on high molecular weight glycoproteins which appear on the surface of virally infected cells and which allow them to be differentiated from noninfected cells. At the binding site, pores are forced in the infected cell and the cell is then killed by nuclear fragmentation through calcium-dependent endonuclease. The

various interferons produced by virally infected cells augment natural killer cytotoxicity and form an integrated feed-back defense system.

Mast cell have a central role in the acute inflammation process. They are loaded with granules containing preformed mediators, which are released upon triggering. This triggering occurs by components of the complement system. Mast cell activation follows two major pathways. The first pathway involves the release of the preformed mediators from the granules, such as histamine, causing vasodilatation, increased capillary permeability and chemokinesis; neutral proteases, which activate complement; eosinophil and neutrophil chemotactic factor; and platelet activating factor which induces mediator release, including interleukins and tumor necrosis factor with multiple actions such as macrophage activation and triggering of acute phase proteins. The second pathway results in the release of newly synthesized mediators via the phospholipase A_2 pathway. This enzyme initiates arachidonic acid degradation. Breakdown of arachidonic acid is achieved by different enzymes. Lipoxygenase leads to the promotion of leukotrienes which influence the microcirculation and enhance chemotaxis. Cyclo-oxygenase leads to the formation of prostaglandins and thromboxanes, which affect bronchial muscle, platelet aggregation and vasodilatation.

Complex and efficient as the innate immune system appears, many micro-organisms find ways to circumvent these attacks. Therefore the *adaptive immune system* was developed with also humoral and cellular components. The *humoral adaptive immune system* leads to the formation of antibodies, which form specific answers to specific antigens. Antibodies form a highly specific answer to those micro-organisms which escape the innate immune system. Antibodies are capable of binding specifically to the attacking microbe, of activating the complement system, and of stimulating phagocytic cells. The antibody molecule therefore has three main regions, two regions concerned in communicating with complement and phagocytes, and one region for binding to an individual micro-organism. The latter region carries the external recognition function. The first two functions are constant. The recognition function, however, demands numerous adaptations of recognition sites. Antibodies, when bound to a microbe, will link to the first molecule in the classical complement sequence.

The *cells* involved in the *adaptive immune system* are mainly lymphocytes. All the cells of the immune system are derived from pluripotent stem cells through two main lines of differentiation: the lymphoid lineage, producing lymphocytes and the myeloid lineage producing phagocytes and mast cells. There are three kinds of lymphocytes with different functions: T cells and B cells and the so-called third population cells. T cells differentiate initially in the thymus; B cells in fetal liver, spleen, and in adult bone marrow. Morphologically, T and B cells are identical; functionally they can be distinguished. B cells are classically defined by the production of immunoglobulins (antibodies) which are presented on the cell surface. The T cells can be subdivided into T-helper cells, T-suppressor cells and T-killer cells. Their function is to recognize foreign intruders, to activate B cells, and to kill invading micro-organisms. The third population cells do not consistently carry markers of either T or B cells. They possess specific receptors for g-immunoglobulins and form the greater part of natural killer and antibody-dependent cellular cytotoxic effectors. In another classification system, dependent on the surface proteins reacting to clusters of antigens (CD= cluster determinants), lymphocytes can be subdivided in terms of different cell types. The T-helper cells are classified as CD4+ cells, formerly T4 cells; the T-suppressor/killer cells as CD8+ cells, formerly T8 cells.

To orchestrate the actions of all the cells involved in the inflammatory process, a great variety of solvable mediators are used for communication between the cells. Also on the effector side many solvable factors play an important role in the inflammatory reaction. An important group of such mediators has been given the name cytokines. Cytokines can be distinguished into monokines, produced by monocytes and macrophages, and lymphokines, produced by lymphocytes. Cytokines are hormone-like substances and are the most important mediators of the action of T lymphocytes. The immunofunctions of T lymphocytes are reflected by a specific set of cytokines, the lymphokines, produced by these cells after activation. Subpopulations of T cells, such as T1 and T2 helper cells, can be distinguished by the specific lymphokines they produce. Important lymphokines, some of which have been referred to before, are interleukins, interferons, lymphotoxin, growth factors and tumor necrosis factor. CD4+ cell has the cytokine profile of the T1 helper cell. The T1 helper cell activates the B lymphocytes to produce antibodies and it causes eosinophilia and mast cell hyperplasia. The CD8+ lymphocyte has T2 cell characteristics and is responsible for cytotoxicity, complement fixation, and macrophage activation. The CD8+ lymphocyte profile, therefore, protects against viruses, tumors and infections. It is also responsible for transplant rejection, inflammation and auto-immune reaction. Cytokines form a functional network. The various factors, messengers and effectors, act in a subtle interaction. These interactions may be synergistic, additive or antagonistic and function in order to maintain a balance of optimal efficacy in the protection of the host.

The cooperative cellular and mediator activity in *inflammatory* (either *infectious* or *noninfectious*) *disorders* of the CNS can be briefly sumarized as follows:

Circulating T cells recognize the concerned antigen in combination with the major histocompability complex class II on antigen presenting cells and start to proliferate. The antigen presenting cells in the CNS may be perivascular macrophages, the gate keepers of the CNS. Microglial cells may also act as antigen presenting cells within the CNS. Sensitized or activated T cells start to release substances such as IFN-γ, which activate local cells such as microglia, astrocytes and perivascular macrophages. This local activation results in upregulation of adhesion molecules on endothelial cells, enhanced expression of major histocompability complex, and release of chemo-attractive substances, which attract and facilitate the entrance of more T cells, macrophages and B lymphocytes. B cells are triggered to become plasma cells and produce antibodies. Macrophages, microcytes, astrocytes and mast cells start to produce inflammatory mediators such as tumor necrosis factors, reactive oxygen species, interleukins, vasoactive amines, leukotrienes, complement and hydrolytic enzymes. The result is, eventually, vascular dilatation, increased capillary permeability, exsudation of fluid in tissue and extravasation of numerous cells, leading subsequently to disruption of the blood-brain barrier, perivascular inflammation, formation of edema and demyelination. Phagocytosis of myelin by macrophages may be initiated by antimyelin antibodies, or by opsonization via their receptor for complement component.

Knowledge of the factors mediating inflammation has stimulated attempts to undo undesired reactions by counteracting or blocking the involved pathways. IFN-γ, for example, proved to have a negative influence on the course of secondary progressive multiple sclerosis. IFN-β, known to counteract the action of IFN-γ, seems to have a beneficial effect on the course of this disease.

In *infectious disorders* several pathogenetic factors play a role in evoking the host response. Exotoxins, for example, are produced by micro-organisms during their growth. They have a proteinaceous nature and therefore act as antigens. They evoke an antibody response and in this way give rise to neutralizing antitoxins. Endotoxins are membrane molecules, lipopolysaccharides, present in the outer cell membrane of gramnegative bacteria. The polysaccharide chain is variable and determines the antigenic structure of the bacteria. The lipid fraction anchors the lipopolysaccharide in the outer bacterial membrane, is less variable and is responsible for the toxic effects. After liberation of the lipopolysaccharides from the bacterial membrane they adsorb on the lipid membrane of many cells, especially neutrophils. This triggers a whole cascade of immune reactions. Another way to evoke immune reactions is

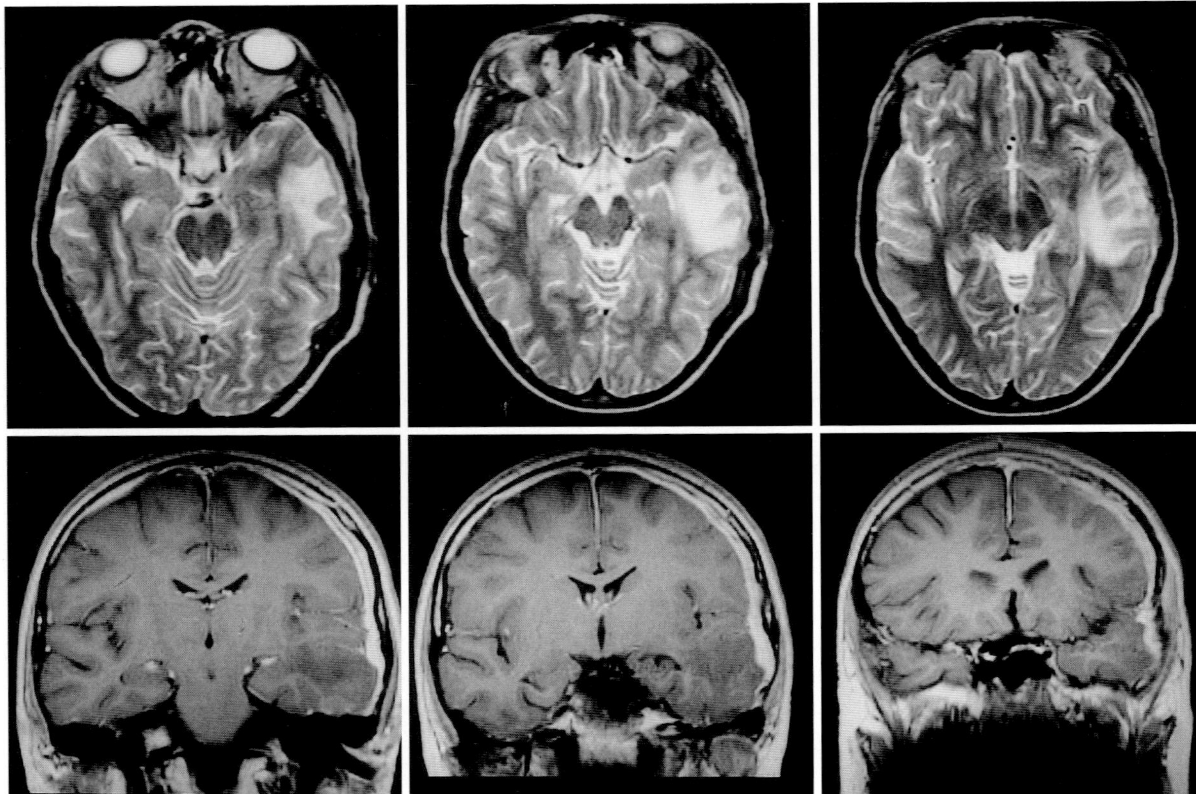

Fig. 51.1. A 13-year-old male with herpes simplex encephalitis. Involvement of the left temporal area is shown on the transverse T_2-weighted MR series. Both white and gray matter are involved. The coronal T_1-weighted MR images show slight swelling and loss of contrast between gray and white matter in the same area and meningeal thickening and enhancement over the left hemisphere. The cortex in the left frontal area is also slightly thickened

by presentation of antigens by specialized cells, also called antigen presenting cells, such as the Langerhans and dendritic cells. These cells recognize the foreign intruders probably by lack of identifying cell surface membrane MHC class I compounds. Viruses use the replication system of host cells and bring their antigens to expression on the surface of the host cells, activating natural killer cells.

The presence and multiplication of the original micro-organism sustains the disease or expands it. The micro-organisms produce a gamut of products to assist in their spread, including streptokinase, hyaluronidase, and neuraminidase. In many cases it is difficult to distinguish the direct influence of the micro-organisms on the tissue from the immunological reaction the attack provokes. A demonstration of this is found in subacute sclerosing panencephalitis, caused by the measles virus. In subacute sclerosing panencephalitis, as in other persistent viral infections, deposits of immune complexes can be demonstrated in the wall of small cerebral blood vessels. The presence of immune complexes and the histological findings of perivascular edema, inflammation and demyelination provide strong evidence that, in addition to the actual invasion by the virus, there is a contemporaneous immune-mediated response to this virus, responsible for most of the tissue damage. The same could be true for progressive rubella panencephalitis, subacute AIDS encephalitis and tropical spastic paraparesis due to HTLV-1 infection.

Selective neuronal and/or glial damage in infectious disorders and the predilection for particular areas (topistic areas) is in most cases difficult to understand. Experience has taught that herpes simplex virus has affinity for the frontal and temporal lobes (Fig. 51.1); fungal infections attack primarily gray matter structures; Hemophilus influenzae has preference for cortical-subcortical areas (Fig. 51.2); cytomegalovirus (CMV) and AIDS encephalopathy in adults is predominantly located in the cerebral white matter and spares the U fibers. There is often a considerable difference between the course of a disease and the predilection sites between congenital infections and infections acquired later, after birth. A good example is the differ-

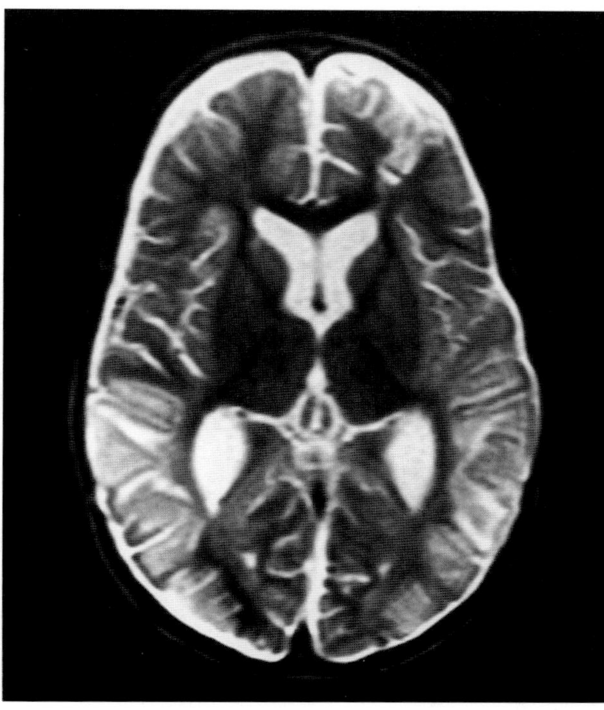 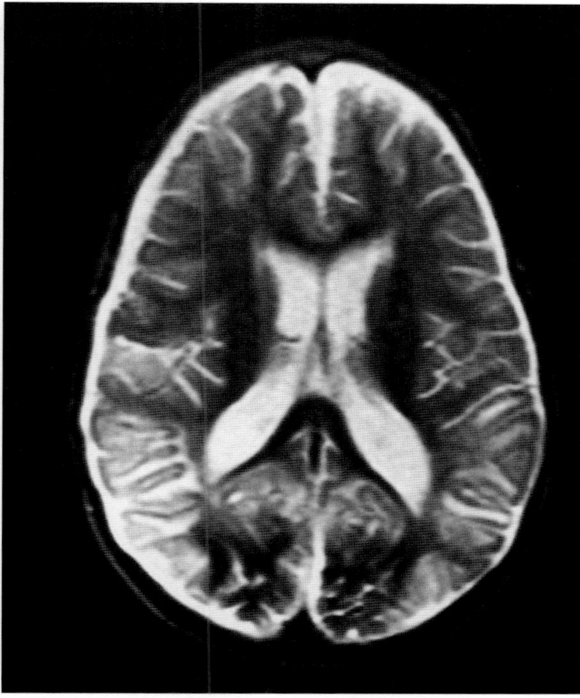

Fig. 51.2. A 5-year-old boy with Hemophilus influenzae meningoencephalitis. The T_2-weighted images show the pericerebral fluid collection and the cortical/subcortical involvement in the right and left occipital and left frontal region. This kind of involvement of cerebral structures was seen by us several times in Hemophilus influenzae meningoencephalitis

ence between congenital, connatal and adult CMV infection (Figs. 51.3, 51.4), and between congenital and postnatal toxoplasmosis.

In some infections the preferential location is simply related to the porte d'entrée. For example, infections that involve the leptomeninges will enter the brain via the Virchow-Robin spaces and are located predominantly in the cortex (Hemophilus influenzae) and in the basal ganglia (Cryptococcus neoformans) or both. In herpes simplex virus, a primary infection in the throat or mouth is followed by the persistent presence of latent virus in sensory ganglia and possibly also in the brain, after entry via the olfactory route. Following activation of the latent virus, direct spread may explain the frontotemporal predominance. Within the affected area, herpes simplex virus infects all types of cells.

For many viruses a necessary condition for the entry into cells is the availability of specific receptor molecules at the surface of such cells. The distribution of these receptor molecules will largely determine the specific regions of the brain preferentially attacked by the virus and the population of cells in the affected regions that are injured or destroyed. Some viruses like JC papovavirus, responsible for progressive multifocal leukoencephalitis, infect oligodendrocytes with sparing of the neurons. This explains the affinity of this virus for white matter. Rabies virus has great affinity for the cerebellum and limbic system, whereas poliomyelitis affects the motor nuclei in the cortex, brain stem and anterior horns of the spinal cord. Creutzfeldt-Jakob disease, caused by prions, has recently been shown by MRI to affect in particular the basal ganglia. These differences in topographical distribution are considered to be the result of specific receptor interactions.

Viruses enter the cells of the host either by fusing with the plasma membrane, and discharging their contents directly in the cytosol, or by being internalized through the endocytotic pathway. The first way is used by Herpes simplex and corona viruses. Internalization does not have special requirements in these cases. Other viruses do not have this option and have to follow the other path, involving binding to a receptor and collection of receptor-ligand complexes at the cell membrane. The viruses are then transported within endocytotic vesicles. After penetration of the cell membrane, the replicative machinery of the virus itself comes into play. Using the host cell system of nucleic acid (DNA/RNA) replication and transcription, viruses can replicate and transcribe their DNA or RNA and in so doing multiply themselves; the new virus particles leave the cell in search of new host cells. Ultimately the

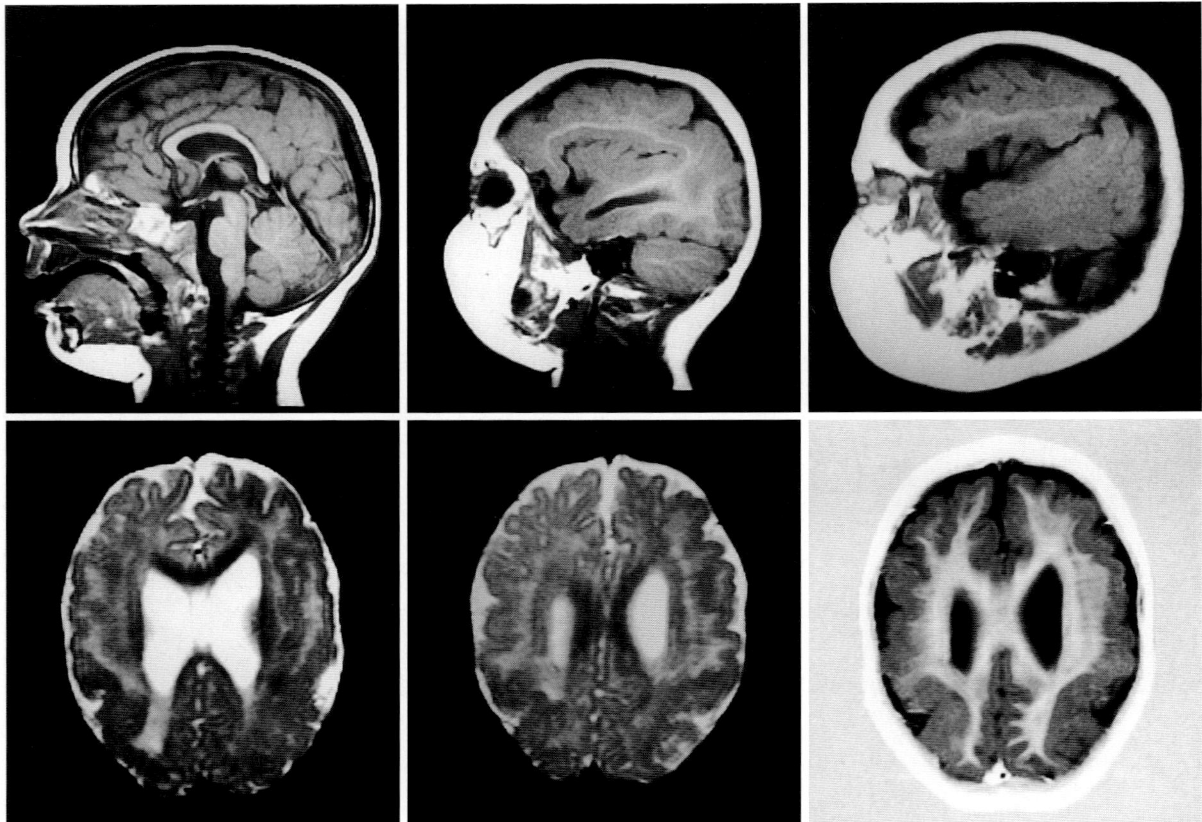

Fig. 51.3. A 1-year-old boy with history of maternal cytomegalovirus infection in the first trimester of pregnancy. The sagittal T_1 series (*upper row*) shows the gyral abnormalities, especially in the peri-insular and occipital regions. The two T_2-weighted transverse images (*left and middle, lower row*) show enlarged ventricles with persistent cavum septi pellucidi and cavum Vergae, and disfigured posterior horns. There is a linear pattern radiating from the ependymal lining of the ventricles towards the surface, representing neurons arrested during the process of migration. The T_1-weighted IR image (*right, lower row*) shows the thick cortical layer most pronounced in the occipital lobe and the radiating pattern of arrested migrating neurons

balance between the viral machinery and the host immune system will determine the outcome of the infection.

In the *noninfectious inflammatory disorders* other mechanisms play a role in invoking the host response, not all of which are well understood. The inflammatory reactions may be triggered by "primary" auto-immune reactions in which auto-antibodies are primarily directed against auto-antigens, as is the case in vasculitis of the CNS in systemic lupus erythematosus, Behçet's disease, giant cell arteritis and rheumatoid vasculitis. The hypothesis is that these primary autoimmune disorders are the result of a dysfunction of T-cell regulation. The inflammatory response in the CNS may also be secondary to an infectious disease elsewhere in the body or a vaccination. Mycoplasma infections of the lung, for example, may lead to an acute disseminated encephalomyelitis, caused by the formation of antibodies that cross-react with CNS antigens on myelin membranes or surface molecules of CNS cells. This reaction resembles in many aspects the experimental allergic encephalomyelitis provoked by immunization with components of the myelin membrane (basic myelin protein for example). Such a secondary auto-immune response probably also forms the basis of several paraneoplastic syndromes of the CNS, such as limbic encephalitis, and Purkinje cell degeneration. Here too, the hypothesis is that antibodies formed against tumor antigens cross-react with structural components of the CNS.

As far as the involvement of myelin in inflammatory and infectious disorders is concerned, several biomechanisms can be distinguished:
— Immune reaction against one of the components of myelin. This occurs in acute disseminated encephalomyelitis. This condition can be simulated in an animal model: experimental allergic encephalomyelitis. In the latter condition the animal has been sensitized against basic myelin protein.

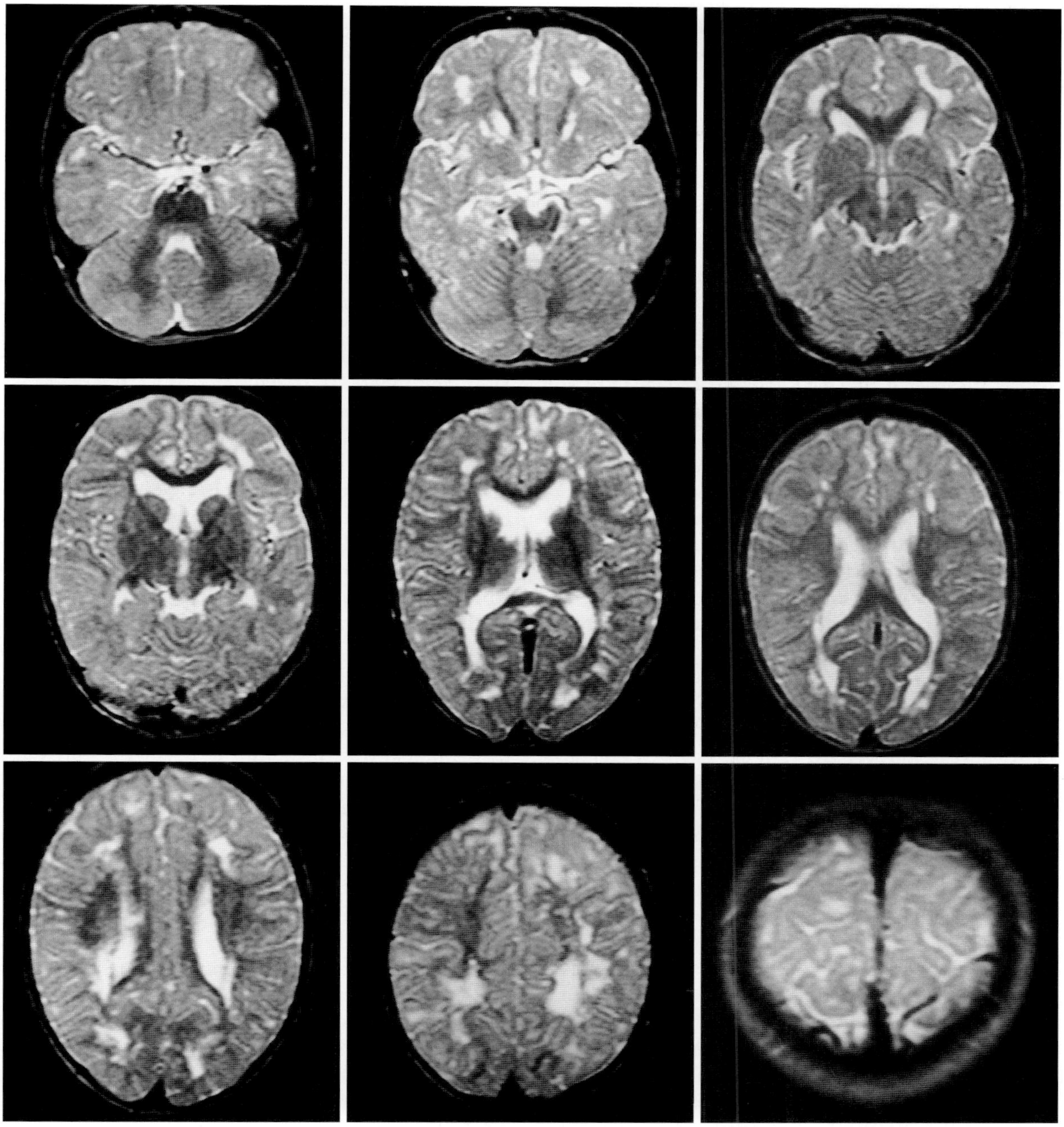

Fig. 51.4. An 18-month-old girl with an early neonatal cytomegalovirus infection. Compared to the image in Fig. 51.3, this observation makes clear that age is also a pathoplastic factor in infections. This set of T_2-weighted transverse images shows irregular myelination and areas of high signal intensity in both hemispheres, with a tendency towards symmetry. There is no evidence of a disturbed neuronal migration or gyration

— Specific infection of oligodendrocytes leading to cell death and subsequent loss of the myelin sheath extension of the oligodendrocytes. This is the case in progressive multifocal leukoencephalitis.

— Myelin can also be an innocent bystander and become a victim in a process that hits all white matter components and possibly gray matter as well. This occurs in a multitude of infections, such as Hemophilus influenzae, herpes simplex and toxoplasmosis.

— Finally, dysmyelination may be the consequence of infectious or inflammatory changes to unmyelinated white matter, damaging the white matter matrix. Most of the congenital infections can have this effect, often in addition to other visible structural lesions.

52 Multiple Sclerosis

52.1 Clinical Features and Laboratory Investigations

Multiple sclerosis (MS) is the most common demyelinating disorder of the CNS. The peak incidence is at 30 years of age. MS rarely commences in childhood or over the age of 50 years. Females are affected twice as frequently as males. MS shows a characteristic geographical distribution. It is rare in tropical areas and increases in frequency at higher latitudes. It has been estimated, for example, that the prevalence rate in the United States varies from 6–14 per 100 000 inhabitants in the southern states to about 40–60 per 100 000 inhabitants in the northern states. No definite relationship has been established with the climatic characteristics of the latitude. Within this overal latitudinal distribution a rather large range of incidences of MS has been observed at the same latitudes. Incidental clusters of MS have been reported. In these instances a remarkable number of patients acquire MS within a short period of time (a few months), and they share a common exposure in their history. Etiological factors for these MS pockets are as yet unknown. Sometimes such clusters of MS assume the proportions of an epidemic, the incidence of MS rising over a period of several years in a larger area. In these cases the nature of the introduced environmental factor or factors still remains to be elucidated. The importance of environmental factors is stressed by the findings of migrational studies. A decrease in the risk of developing MS has been noted in young individuals migrating from high-risk to low-risk areas and an increase in risk after migration from low-risk to high-risk areas. Such changes in risk have not been found in older individuals, and the data suggest that the risk of acquiring MS is largely established around the age of 15. There is also increasing evidence of a genetically influenced susceptibility to MS. In general, first-degree relatives of probands have a risk that is 30–50 times greater than the risk for the general population.

A number of variants of MS can be distinguished: classical MS (also called Charcot's disease), neuromyelitis optica (NMO, or Devic's disease), concentric sclerosis (CS, or Baló's disease), and diffuse sclerosis (DS, or Schilder's disease).

The clinical presentation of classical or Charcot's type of MS is extremely variable. The extreme acute progressive form of Marburg is rare. For the more slowly developing forms it has become usual to distinguish four types: The initial course is usually *relapsing-remitting*, followed in two of three patients by a *secondary progressive* course with increasing disability as measured on a disability scale over a period of 12 months. One-third of the patients with a relapsing-remitting course have a *benign form* of MS with little remaining disability after 10 years or more. Finally there is a *primary progressive form* in a minority of the patients, with progressive disability from the onset.

Clinical symptoms are related to lesions in various tracts of the CNS. Sometimes symptoms of extremely short duration occur, lasting for seconds to hours. Common features in MS are fatigue, impairment of vision due to optic neuritis, motor disturbances caused by pyramidal tract involvement, sensory disturbances including Lhermitte's symptom, cerebellar ataxia and dysarthria, diplopia, micturition problems, sexual disturbances, hearing loss, vertigo and balance abnormalities. Less common are epileptic seizures, signs of peripheral neuropathy, trigeminal neuralgia, hemifacial spasms, and dementia, although some degree of cognitive impairment is present in up to half of MS patients. There is almost always a tendency for the frequency of episodes to decrease as time passes, or for the progression of the progressive variety to slow down. The extent of the resulting disability is extremely variable. In general, it appears that the average life expectancy in young patients after the onset of MS is about 35 years. About 60%–70% of patients remain ambulant. Long-term prognosis is not influenced by pregnancy, illness, or anesthesia.

Before discussing the diagnostic problems in MS, the clinical picture of the less frequently occurring variants of MS are described briefly.

NMO (Devic's disease) is a clinical syndrome, consisting of optic neuritis, often bilateral with total blindness, in combination with transverse myelitis, which usually has a thoracic localization. The optic neuritis and transverse myelitis occur either simultaneously or are separated by a brief interval of several days to several weeks. Men and women are affected more or less equally. The age of patients ranges from 5 to 65 years, but patients are rarely older than 50 years. The group most commonly affected are young adults. This disease occurs most frequently in the Asian population, where the overall incidence of MS is low. The prognosis is rather poor. Until recently, about 15%–20% of patients died in the acute stage due to an ascending spinal disorder with respiratory paralysis; another 30% died with complications after many nonths. A poor neurological outcome with severe disability is reported in another 15% of patients. Complete or nearly complete recovery is found in about 35%. Improved supportive care has reduced mortality and residual disability. About half of surviving patients experience no recurrence of neurological disease; about one-third of the remainder suffer a relapse of optic neuritis, one-third a relapse of optic neuritis and transverse myelitis, and one-third develop a multifocal white matter disease.

CS (Balo's encephalitis periaxialis concentrica) is a very rare MS variant which usually affects young adults. For unknown demographic reasons there is a much higher incidence in the Philippines. Both sexes are affected more or less equally. Compared to classical MS, CS runs a more rapidly progressive, usually monophasic course. The initial symptoms are often suggestive of a stroke; less frequently psychiatric symptoms predominate. The neurological symptoms are sometimes associated with fever and headache and then resemble the clinical picture of an infection or tumor. The disease is progressive and can be fatal, usually as a consequence of respiratory problems and infection. A more prolonged survival for several years has also been reported.

DS (Schilder's encephalitis periaxialis diffusa) is a demyelinating disease related to MS which primarily affects children. Clinical features are intellectual impairment, epileptic seizures, signs of pyramidal tract involvement, occasionally unilaterally with hemiplegia, cerebellar ataxia, visual impairment caused by retrobulbar neuritis or demyelination of the occipital lobes, pseudobulbar palsy with disturbances of swallowing, deafness, diplopia, extrapyramidal movement abnormalities, and incontinence. A predominatly psychiatric symptomatology is relatively frequent. In most cases there is a rather rapid progression of neurological signs over the course of 1–2 years. In a minority the demyelinating process is fulminant and accompanied by cerebral edema. Rarely, the course of disease is characterized by exacerbations. In exceptional cases significant and prolonged improvement occurs; an arrest of the disease is observed in exceptional cases.

Definite diagnosis has always been a problem in MS. The clinical features may mimic many other neurological disorders, including tumors, metastases, vasculitic disorders, granulomatous disease and infections.

Specific diagnostic tests are lacking. This diagnostic uncertainty has led to the definition of diagnostic criteria. In 1965, Schumacher was the first to draw up clinical criteria for the diagnosis of definite MS (Schumacher et al. 1965). The basic idea behind these criteria is that there must be symptoms and objective signs of multifocal white matter disease with dissemination in space and time, for which there is no better neurological explanation. These criteria have been repeatedly modified, and clinical criteria for possible and probable MS added (McAlpine, Rose). In 1983, Poser was the first to draw up new diagnostic criteria that were not completely clinical but incorporated supportive laboratory data (CSF abnormalities) and paraclinical evidence of multifocal white matter lesions (CT and evoked responses) (Poser et al. 1983). Since that time, MRI has become more generally used and has acquired a prominent role as a paraclinical test.

Valuable laboratory findings supporting the diagnosis of MS are oligoclonal bands in the CSF and an increased IgG index as a sign of increased intra blood-brain barrier synthesis of IgG. The sensitivity of assessment of the IgG index in MS is about 80% and that of oligoclonal banding about 90%. The specificity and predictive value of these CSF investigations are highly dependent on the so-called pretest probability of MS. The problem is that a number of diseases mimicking MS, such as infections, acute disseminated encephalomyelitis, and vasculitis, are apt to lead to an increased production of IgG in the CSF with oligoclonal banding. It should be noted that some patients with clinically definite MS have a normal CSF IgG index and lack oligoclonal bands. Levels of CSF IgM and IgA may also be elevated in MS. The CSF protein content may be slightly raised, but very rarely exceeds the level of 1 g/l. The white cell count may also be increased, but only in exceptional cases is it higher than 20 cells/ml. Another CSF abnormality may be an elevation of myelin basic protein in active MS. Its level is normal in stable MS. The finding of increased amounts of myelin basic protein is indicative of active demyelination and as such not specific for MS. Increased CSF free light chains of immunoglobulins and an increased CSF $\kappa{:}\lambda$ light chain ratio have been described. Increased CSF free κ chains appear to be relatively specific for MS. Abnormally high levels have been found in 85% of patients with clinically definite MS, in 20% of patients with CNS infections, and only exceptionally in noninfectious controls.

A number of changes in the subset distribution of T cells has been reported in the peripheral blood of MS patients. CD4+ T (helper) cells can be subdivided in two mutually exclusive subsets: „naive" cells that have not yet been stimulated, and „memory" cells that have been stimulated before. These subsets can be recognized by differences in CD antigens. Memory cells can produce large amounts of cytokines after activation and show increased expression of a set of adhesion molecules. In the peripheral blood of patients with active MS, decreased numbers of naive cells have been found. In inactive MS this fraction is normal. In the peripheral blood of active MS patients, lymphocytes have been found with increased expression of the activation marker CD26 compared to patients with inactive MS and healthy controls. In CSF of active MS patients CD4+ cells are relatively over-represented compared to CD4+ cells in peripheral blood. Among CD4+ T cells memory cells are increased whereas naive cells are almost absent in CSF. Subset changes, therefore, may reflect disease activity and can be used for monitoring purposes. Further examinations are required to reveal the true significance of these findings.

Other tests often used in the diagnostic assessment of MS are the evoked potentials VEP, SSEP and BAEP. These tests are helpful in detecting silent white matter lesions, in this way providing evidence of a multifocal white matter affection in cases of clinically indefinite MS. VEPs and SSEPs appear to give a higher diagnostic yield than BAEPs. However, abnormalities are nonspecific and must be interpreted with care in the context of the clinical picture.

In NMO, CSF abnormalities are similar to those in MS, with the exception of a more common occurrence of lymphocytic pleocytosis. Nonspecific slowing of the EEG pattern is often observed; epileptic changes do not occur.

Laboratory examinations in CS rarely yield much information. CSF usually reveals no pleocytosis, sometimes an increased amount of red blood cells. Total protein is only occasionally elevated.

In DS the CSF is often normal, but slight lymphocytosis is occasionally found. The protein level is not infrequently elevated, as is the IgG index. Oligoclonal bands have been reported. EEG abnormalities are nonspecific and reflect only the location and extent of the cerebral lesion.

52.2   Pathology

Usually the external appearance of the brain is normal in MS. In chronic cases slight atrophy may be present with widening of sulci and slight enlargement of the ventricular system. Occasionally firm, depressed lesions are seen on the surface of the brain stem, spinal cord and in the optic nerves. On sectioning, numerous lesions of varying size become apparent in the white matter of CNS, and even more are revealed by microscopic examination. The distribution of plaques varies greatly among MS patients, but the following are recognized as preferential localizations: the periventricular white matter, in particular the lateral angles of the lateral ventricles, the floor of the aqueduct, floor of the fourth ventricle, cerebellar peduncles, cervical part of the spinal cord, and the optic nerves. In severe, longstanding cases, numerous lesions are found in most parts of the CNS. Although the distribution of lesions is not precisely symmetrical, predominant involvement of one hemisphere is rare. A significant proportion of the plaques is found in the border zone between gray and white matter; a smaller number of plaques involves only gray matter.

Microscopically, the earliest stage of the MS plaque consists of perivenular lymphocytic infiltration. The subsequent stage is characterized by a more diffuse tissue infiltration by inflammatory cells and macrophages associated with edema, demyelination, proliferation and hyperplasia of astrocytes, and appearance of increased numbers of lipid-laden macrophages and demyelinated axons. Loss of myelin and oligodendrocytes eventually becomes complete. As plaques enlarge and coalesce, the perivenular distribution becomes less apparent. The axons are relatively spared, but some axonal loss occurs in all lesions. In the course of time, axonal loss can become very substantial, but the extent of axonal loss in the demyelinated areas is highly variable. The myelin is also predominantly affected in plaques in the gray matter, and neuronal cell bodies are largely preserved. In lesions of several months duration, inflammation is far less pronounced, fewer lipid-laden macrophages are seen, and fibrillary gliosis becomes increasingly prominent. Chronic-inactive MS plaques have a sharply demarcated border, and are hypocellular, demyelinated and gliosed with almost total oligodendrocyte loss. Inflammatory cells and lipid-laden macrophages are no longer present. The remaining elements are axons and astrocytic processes. Axonal damage has led to Wallerian degeneration, which is most evident in the long tracts. Rarely is the damage sufficiently severe to produce a cyst. In the same patient lesions of different ages are present.

In MS, plaque-like areas are observed in which myelin has not completely disappeared, and which do not have the appearance of the typical plaque. These lesions are called shadow plaques. The myelin sheaths in these plaques are abnormally thin and are of relatively uniform thickness. The internodes are short. The number of oligodendrocytes is increased in the lesion. These features are characteristic of remyelination, and so the shadow plaques probably represent areas of remyelination and not areas of partial demyelination, as has been suggested.

The description as given fits the relapsing-remitting form of MS. Histological description of the clinically distinguishable subentities of classical MS faces difficulties. Histological examination is usually performed in patients who have been suffering from the disease for a long time, with the exception of the acute form of MS (Marburg type) in which the lesions are days to weeks old and show acute inflammatory and demyelinating changes. As a consequence of the lack of this histological information, there is no parallel description of histology in clinical MS subtypes, such as primary progressive and benign MS. A known histological pattern shows more diffuse demyelination with more diffuse and less intense inflammation. Whereas multiple lesions are more often seen in young patients, the latter diffuse pattern is more common in older patients. A mixture of the two patterns is seen in patients in whom the disease was initially relapsing-remitting, but secondarily became progressive in its course.

Immunocytochemical studies have demonstrated that the inflammatory cells of acute MS plaques are mostly macrophages and lymphocytes with few plasma cells. Macrophages stain positive for the major histocompatibility complex (MHC) class II, which implies a role for these cells in local antigen presentation to T cells. The T cells present are a mixture of CD4+ (helper-inducer) and CD8+ (suppressor-cytotoxic) T lymphocytes. Initially these T lymphocytes are predominantly present in the center of the plaque, but as the lesion enlarges T cells move to the peripheral part of the lesion. The CD4+ cells invade the normal white matter. The majority of the inflammatory T cells in MS are memory phenotype cells. The margins of the plaque contain predominantly CD8+ cells and increased numbers of oligodendrocytes and astrocytes. With increasing age of the plaque, myelin and macrophages disappear from the central part; the plaque margins contain lymphocytes, oligodendrocytes, lipid-laden macrophages, and astrocytes, suggestive of low-grade activity at these margins. In chronic-active MS, small numbers of inflammatory cells are scattered throughout the normal-appearing white matter, suggestive of a diffuse, slow, demyelinating process. Chronic-inactive MS lesions contain few inflammatory cells. In chronically affected tissue another interesting recent finding is the presence of so-called "γ δ" T cells in MS plaques and their association with heat shock proteins expressed on oligodendrocytes. These cells have previously been implicated in the pathogenesis of rheumatoid arthritis, but the presence of these cells with still unclear function now seems to be a more general finding in autoimmunity. They may either play a role in tissue repair or in perpetuating the inflammatory process.

Apart from demyelination, electron-microscopic examination reveals accumulation of dense bodies and myelin figures in oligodendroglia and astrocytes. No unequivocal virus particles are present.

The correlation between pathological findings and clinical signs and symptoms is rather poor. The most striking example is the recognition of subclinical MS at autopsy, which is estimated to comprise about 5%–20% of all MS cases.

In NMO the spinal cord, optic nerves, and chiasm appear swollen and congested externally if the patient has died relatively early in the course of disease. Demyelination and inflammation with perivascular lymphocytic infiltration and fat granules are seen at microscopy. In severe cases necrosis of gray and white matter occurs, leading to cavitation. However, at the periphery of such lesions the relative sparing of axons is evident. Acute lesions may be hemorrhagic. The spinal cord lesion is often large and extends over many segments, usually in the low cervical and high thoracic areas. Lesions in the conus may also occur. In the optic nerves and chiasm extensive loss of myelin, gliosis and some loss of axons occurs. As a rule, additional areas of demyelination are found in the predilectional regions of classical MS, such as periventricular areas and the brain stem.

The characteristic lesions in CS are areas of alternating zones of myelinated and demyelinated tissue, either with a concentric pattern or with a more irregular arrangement. The size of lesions varies from tiny to about 4–5 cm in diameter. The location and number of lesions vary widely. Sometimes larger areas are almost completely involved. The lesions may occur anywhere in the CNS; only the spinal cord is rarely affected. The rings of the lesion terminate abruptly where they contact gray matter. The central core is the starting point of the lesion and consists of a venule with a cuff of inflammatory cells. In the course of time, the central core becomes intensely gliotic. The core is surrounded by zones of demyelination in which axons are preserved, and myelin is replaced by gliosis. With increasing distance from the core, the stage of myelin breakdown in the affected zones becomes less advanced, and the gliosis is less severe. Acute lesions are surrounded by edema. In chronic lesions the involved area becomes scarred and atrophic. The concentric lesion may become so disintegrated that it is difficult to recognize. Ultrastructural examination of the myelinated zones reveals that they are largely composed of thinly myelinated fibers. A few normally myelinated and some demyelinated axons are also present. These bands contain many cells, including oligodendrocytes, lymphocytes, and astrocytes. These changes are reminiscent of those seen at the edge of a chronic-active MS plaque and are interpreted by some as zones of remyelination. Throughout the white matter, numerous venules show cuffs of inflammatory cells. Very often there are also lesions characteristic of classical MS.

In pure DS widespread demyelination is found, with variable axonal damage in the centrum semiovale of both cerebral hemispheres, most often involving the occipital lobes. Usually the corpus callosum is also affected and interconnects the lesions of the two sides.

The lesions are not completely symmetrical. They have a sharp edge. A rim of subcortical white matter is commonly preserved, but a lesion may also spread into the gray matter. In the acute stage demyelination is associated with dense perivascular infiltrates of lymphocytes, plasma cells, and lipid-filled macrophages. The myelin disintegration leads to the formation of sudanophilic material. Areas may be become frankly necrotic, and cavitation may occur. Glial reaction is present, with giant multinucleated and hypertrophied astrocytes. In cases of long duration, inflammatory cells and macrophages containing sudanophilic material disappear. Evidence of Wallerian degeneration is common. There are not only naked axons but also axons partially covered with thin layers of myelin as signs of abortive remyelination. Histologically DS cannot be differentiated from X-linked adrenoleukodystrophy.

Transitional sclerosis is a pathological variant of DS in which the described histological changes are accompanied by scattered smaller plaques in other parts of the CNS, more typical of MS. The pathological pattern of transitional sclerosis is usually found in young adults, i.e., a slightly older age group than in pure DS. It is not usually possible to establish a definite clinical diagnosis of transitional sclerosis. The clinical signs and symptoms are dominated by the large demyelinated areas, but a more episodic occurrence with remissions has been reported.

52.3 Chemical Pathology

Chemical analysis of the composition of MS plaques reveals a number of alterations: increase of water, decrease of total lipid, in particular of cholesterol, cerebrosides, sulfatides, ethanolamine plasmalogens, and serine phosphoglycerides. Cholesterol esters are increased. In the lesion the major myelin proteins – myelin basic protein, proteolipid protein, myelin-associated glycoprotein, and Wolfgram proteins – are reduced. Myelin basic protein is in fact virtually absent from the center of most plaques, and the decrease in concentration of myelin-associated glycoprotein extends into the normal-appearing white matter around the plaque, suggesting that this protein disappears or is altered before myelin breakdown starts. The protein losses in the plaque are accompanied by an increase in proteins of a lower molecular weight, which may be proteolytic breakdown products. In and around the MS lesion proteinases and other hydrolytic enzymes are increased. The observed chemical changes in the MS plaques are variable and depend on the extent of demyelination. As is demonstrated histologically, old plaques have no or little myelin left and lack sudanophilic material. An early MS lesion contains more

myelin and more sudanophilic material, which is biochemically defined as cholesterol esters.

Myelin isolated from the plaque has a composition typical of abnormal myelin during aspecific degradation. No myelin abnormalities specific for MS have been demonstrated.

Much effort has been devoted to the study of the chemical composition of normal-appearing white matter in MS in the hope of finding an underlying biochemical defect. In the first place, the myelin yield of the normal-appearing white matter is strikingly low. There is a decrease in total lipid, in phospholipids (particularly ethanolamine plasmalogens), in both galactolipids (cerebroside, and sulfatide), and in myelin proteins. Frequently, cholesterol esters are found. Minor alterations of fatty acids have been repeatedly demonstrated but without a consistent pattern. Several investigators found an elevation of hydrolytic enzymes in normal-appearing white matter. These findings are qualitatively similar to those observed in MS plaques, but are considerably smaller in magnitude. Furthermore, the chemical composition of many white matter samples is completely normal. All these data together provide strong evidence for the presence of minor microscopic abnormalities of the MS type in the white matter that appears macroscopically normal. This suggestion has been confirmed by microscopic examination of samples of normal-appearing white matter. It is clear that the disease process is widespread and not simply restricted to plaques. There is a general myelin deficit throughout the white matter.

Compositional abnormalities have been reported in myelin isolated from normal-appearing white matter, but the reported changes are minor, variable, and contradictory. Most investigators agree that the myelin is chemically normal. An explanation for the observed abnormalities is found in the assumption that normal-appearing white matter contains normal myelin together with myelin in various stages of degradation.

52.4 Pathogenetic Considerations

The search for the cause of MS has engaged many investigators for many years, but it has still not been successful. Two main lines can be distinguished in theories about the etiology of MS: one line pointing to the evidence for genetic factors, the second line advocating environmental factors.

The evidence for a genetic factor or factors comes from reports of familial cases and unusually high risk families and from studies which consistently show higher concordance rates for MS in monozygotic twins than in dyzygotic twins. The concordance rate in monozygotic twins reported in the literature varies from 10% to 70% and in dizygotic twins from 2.3% to

20%. Selection bias probably leads to overestimation of the rate of concordance among twins. On the other hand, however, a twin sample collected at one point in time probably underestimates the concordance rate, as more individuals will develop MS in the course of time, and the concordance rate will increase with increased duration of follow-up. The prevalence of MS among relatives of MS patients is increased, and the increase becomes more pronounced the closer the degree of kinship to the propositus. This observation is consistent with a genetic hypothesis, but common environmental experiences with relatives, and especially twins, may also play a role. The low overall twin concordance rate (a concordance rate of 100% would be expected among monozygotic twins if MS were exclusively genetically determined), and the increased prevalence of MS in dizygotic twins compared to siblings (1%–6% of the siblings of MS patients are also affected) strongly suggests the involvement of environmental as well as genetic factors.

Further evidence for a genetic component in the etiology of MS comes from the observation of associations between MS and specific human leukocyte antigen (HLA) alleles. The HLA genes encoding for these antigens, which are expressed on cell surfaces of lymphocytes, are found on the short arm of chromosome 6. The HLA system consists of five loci – A,B, C, D, and DR – and each of the HLA loci has a large number of alleles. The HLA region can be used as an excellent genetic marker with known chromosomal location. There is a highly significant association between HLA-DR2 and MS and a less strong association between HLA-A3 and B7 in Caucasians. However, there are great differences in observed HLA associations in populations of different racial background, and it is clear that the mentioned HLA alleles in themselves are neither necessary nor sufficient to lead to the development of MS. The meaning of the HLA associations is not entirely clear. A likely explanation is that the MS-related gene or genes lie on the same chromosome as the HLA genes and are in linkage disequilibrium with specific HLA alleles. This means that certain combinations of alleles occur significantly more frequently than would be expected by chance. It is also possible that specific HLA alleles are directly involved in the etiology of MS. The HLA system is part of the immune response system. In MS a number of immunological abnormalities have been observed, and it is possible that the HLA system is in this way related to MS.

It is obvious that MS is not a genetically determined disease with a Mendelian mode of inheritance. It is more probable that a susceptibility gene (or genes) for MS exists, and that the expression of this gene (or these genes) depends on environmental factors. The chromosomal localization of the genetic material determining susceptibility to MS is probably in or near the HLA region, or its expression depends on the action of certain HLA alleles.

Epidemiological studies of migrants suggest that environmental factors, particularly before the age of 15 years, are involved in the etiology of MS. One of the most important theories about the nature of the environmental factors consists of speculation on a viral etiology, in particular a measles infection. However, a causative virus has never been reproducibly isolated from the CNS of MS patients, nor has viral antigen been demonstrated in a consistent fashion. Ultrastructural examination of brain tissue has never unequivocally revealed virus particles. Not only are antibodies to measles elevated in the CSF, but also antibodies to other viruses. It is probable that these antibodies result from a nonspecific immunostimulation. Nevertheless, the viral hypothesis cannot be completely dismissed and finds some support in many experimental viral models of demyelination.

Another major theory proposes that MS results from alterations in the immune system. A suggestion in this direction came from the observation of some similarity between MS and experimental allergic encephalomyelitis in animals, an autoimmune demyelinating disease induced by sensitization against myelin antigens. Abnormalities of immunoregulation and of humoral and cellular immunity seem to be an important part of the disease process in MS. Inflammatory cells – lymphocytes, plasma cells, and macrophages – are present in perivascular areas in the CNS in active disease and take part in the disease process. In nearly all MS patients evidence is found for an increased synthesis of immunoglobulins within the blood-brain barrier. It has been repeatedly observed that a low T suppressor cell activity and a high ratio of T helper to T suppressor cells is present in the blood during exacerbations of MS, and also chronically progressive MS patients have identical abnormalities of peripheral blood T lymphocyte subsets. The high levels of antiviral antibodies, indicative of hyperactive B lymphocytes, and the deficiency of suppressor T lymphocyte function may be signs of a fundamental defect in immunoregulation. The cause of the immunological alterations in MS and their role in the pathogenesis of MS have, however, not yet been elucidated. The antibody response in the CSF may be an expression of an autoimmune process against normal or altered brain constituents. This autoimmune process might be idiopathic, or triggered by a viral infection or other exogenous or endogenous antigens that cross-react with brain constituents. Low concentrations of antibodies have been demonstrated in the CSF reacting with myelin proteins, oligodendroglia, glycolipids, and nuclear antigens, but no single MS-specific antigen that reacts with most of the IgG has ever been identified. It is not excluded that the observed antibodies are epiphenomena without pathogenetic importance. Another explanation may be that T helper-inducer lymphocytes in MS are activated and autoreactive. Many other changes in immune-related factors have been observed, such as circulating immune complexes, altered levels of cytokines and complement components, and prostaglandin synthesis, but the significance of these findings is not known. A very convincing observation about the role of immune responses in MS has been the decrease in MS activated lesions in pregnant women. We have seen a sharp decrease in lesions in all cases, with a return to the pre-pregnant status in the subsequent months. In another study, the beneficial effect of pregnancy was indicated by the finding that the mean disease duration before becoming wheelchair dependent was 50% longer in patients who became pregnant after the first symptoms of MS.

It is clear that immunological abnormalities, either primary or secondary, play a role in the disease process of MS, but no coherent theory of the etiology and pathogenesis can as yet be formulated. The best formulation at the moment seems to be that MS is a disease produced by an environmental agent in genetically susceptible individuals in whom there is an abnormality of immune mechanisms.

The correlation between neuropathological lesions and clinical signs and symptoms is rather poor in MS. There are many silent lesions. Clinically silent lesions probably occur when demyelination affects some but not all fibers of a pathway. A conduction block occurs in demyelinated fibers, but conduction remains intact in unaffected fibers. The very transient symptoms in MS are probably related to a reduction of the functional reserve of a fiber tract for the conduction of nerve impulses by demyelination. Slight alterations of conduction capabilities, for instance, those due to a rise in body temperature, may result in the appearance of symptoms from a fiber tract in which a plaque has reduced the functional reserve but not to less than the minimum number of fibers necessary for normal function. Improvement occurs as soon as conduction of electrical impulses is restored. Recovery after a relapse is probably largely related to remyelination, which leads to abolition of the conduction block.

The precise nature of the relationship between MS, CS, NMO, and DS is not known. The frequent occurrence of histopathologically typical MS lesions in CS, NMO, and DS provides evidence for some essential similarities in etiology and pathogenesis. In NMO, it is important to distinguish the MS-related disease from acute disseminated encephalomyelitis and a vasculitic process, especially lupus erythematosus, both of which may produce an identical clinical picture and a rather similar pathological picture. As NMO is relatively frequent in Asian populations, it has been suggested that racial-genetic factors lead to a modified appearance of MS.

In CS, some consider the concentric lesion to be a variant of an MS plaque in which the center of the lesion represents the initial small focus of acute demyelination, and in which the concentric lesion is formed by a centrifugal progression of episodes of demyelination and remyelination. They suggest that the zones of preserved myelin with the concentric lesions are episodically formed by remyelination at the borders of demyelinating foci, which is followed by further centrifugal spread of demyelination. The observation of a lamellar configuration alongside common MS lesions leads others to the assumption of a local physicochemical cause of concentric features, for instance, edema. A remarkable difference with MS is that the concentric lesion never invades gray matter structures contrary to MS plaques. There is, as yet, no explanation for the higher incidence of CS in the Philippines.

Loose and indiscriminate use of the term DS has led to a great deal of confusion in nomenclature. Schilder was the first to describe the disease in three cases of what he called encephalitis periaxialis diffusa. However, on closer inspection of clinical data and neuropathological findings one of these patients probably had X-linked adrenoleukodystrophy and another acute disseminated encephalomyelitis. Only one patient is now considered to be an example of DS. After Schilder many authors used the name DS for a wide range of unrelated demyelinating disorders. It is true that in a number of diseases, especially in X-linked adrenoleukodystrophy, it is extremely difficult to differentiate from DS only on clinical and pathological grounds. In these cases, ultrastructural examination and assessment of various enzyme activities are indispensible in establishing the correct diagnosis. In the course of time, an increasing number of diseases could be distinguished from DS, and some have suggested abandoning the term Schilder's DS. However, we and others are of the opinion that designation as Schilder's DS should be reserved for myelinoclastic DS as a variant of MS. The pathology of DS does not differ substantially in its light- or electron-microscopic appearances from the classical disseminated form of MS. The only difference involves the dimension of the demyelinating lesions and the rapid progression of the process. In 1985, Poser offered the following definition of DS: the disease is a subacute or chronic myelinoclastic disorder resulting in the formation of one or more, commonly two, roughly symmetrical plaques measuring at least 2×3 cm in two of the three dimensions, involving the centrum semiovale of the cerebral hemispheres. Other diseases that can lead to a similar picture should be excluded. The pathogenesis of DS is largely identical in this case to that of MS, and the question is which factor is responsible for the difference. It has been suggested, that the large areas of demyelination may be due to the fact that the child's nervous system, being still immature, is more susceptible to an injurious agent. It is improbable, however, that the immaturity of the brain alone accounts for the difference compared to classical MS, as classical MS can also occur during childhood. So far, the problem has not been solved.

52.5 Therapy

There are many palliative measures to ease the problems of MS patients: physiotherapy is helpful in keeping the patient mobile as long as possible, spasmolytic drugs have a place in combatting spasticity and bladder dysfunction, and antibiotics are necessary in intercurrent infections. But as long as the etiology of MS is unknown, a causal treatment cannot be developed. During the past few years, theories about an immunological basis for MS have received much attention, and at the same time a variety of treatments have been advocated, designed to alter or suppress the immune response. One of the first studies about immunotherapy in MS was that of Rose in 1976 on the use of adrenocorticotropic hormone (ACTH) in acute exacerbations. It was demonstrated that ACTH shortens the recovery time but does not affect the eventual level of recovery. More recent studies indicate that high-dose intravenous corticosteroids also hasten recovery. Intrathecal corticosteroids did not prove to be any more helpful than orally administered corticosteroids. More aggressive immunosuppressive agents have also been used, such as azathioprine and cyclophosphamide. There is some suggestion that azathioprine may have a slightly favorable influence in relapsing-remitting MS with some slowing of progression. It has no influence in chronic-progressive disease. There is evidence that cyclophosphamide is of some help in chronic-progressive MS, especially when the patient is relatively young, the disease duration relatively short, and the progression relatively rapid. However, the beneficial influence does not last long, and renewed progression starts as a rule within one to several years. This indicates that repeated treatment courses or maintenance treatment is necessary. Cyclophosphamide is not well tolerated because of its side effects. Plasma exchange has been used in limited studies. As this mode of treatment is almost always used in conjunction with immunosuppressive agents, its merits cannot be clearly defined. The invasiveness of this mode of treatment limits its use. Total lymphoid irradiation is an experimental treatment with major immunosuppresive effects. It has been reported to benefit patients with chronic-progressive MS.

Levamisol, another immunopotentiating agent, may be of some benefit in chronic-progressive MS. Cyclosporin A has also been tested in MS patients but has the disadvantage of serious side effects. In a comparative study between azathioprin and cyclosporin A therapy in MS patients, it was observed that a strong rebound phenomenon occurred after completing the cyclosporin A therapy and that the annual number of exacerbations increased three-fold. Recently the intravenous administration of immunoglobulins has received new interest. Clinical trials are underway. Copolymer 1 has been reported to reduce the number of relapses with possible improvement of abilities. Following initial optimistic reports, large scale clinical trials must be carried out to prove the efficacy of this mixture of polypeptides, that acts as an immunological agent and appears to simulate myelin basic protein. Its greatest advantage is the low toxicity. New treatment modalities are based upon the recent knowledge of T cell activation and cytokine production in autoimmune diseases. From a therapeutic point of view there are several ways in which excessive effector functions of activated T cells can be counteracted, for instance by injection of monoclonal antibodies against T cell membrane molecules. The excessive intrathecal presence of immunoglobulins in MS might be related to the activation of CD4+ T lymphocytes also inducing B lymphocyte production. A large multicenter anti-CD4 antibody trial is currently underway. With this kind of therapy one must always consider the systemic effects on other organs or organsystems, also dependent on T cell activition for their protection. It does not make sense to cure the autoimmune response in the MS plaque, and by so doing induce a life-threatening pneumonia or sepsis. As monoclonal antibodies act more selectively, they may be more effective in suppressing disease activity.

Recently, success has been reported in a multicenter trial with interferon-β (IFN-β) in relapsing-remitting MS. There were highly significant favorable effects on exacerbation rates, times between first and second excacerbations, severity of exacerbations, and MS activity and lesion load as determined by MRI. It has also become clear that IFN-β is only partially effective at the tested doses: patients in the high dose group continued to have exacerbations, albeit at a reduced rate and of milder clinical severity. The effect is probably due to the ability of IFN-β to inhibit IFN-γ synthesis, to improve defective suppressor activity in MS patients and to inhibit class II MHC antigen expression induced by IFN-γ on the surfaces of antigen presenting cells. IFN-β has antiviral activity. Although there is little support for the proposition that MS results from direct viral infection, IFN-β might modify the response to viral infections, which most often form the trigger of exacerbations in MS.

Far fewer therapeutic trials have been performed in CD, NMO, and DS. In CD a beneficial effect of prednisone therapy has been described, but not consistently. In NMO remarkable improvement has been reported under treatment with corticosteroids, immunosuppressants, and lymphocytoplasmapheresis. However, due to the very low incidence of NMO, no controlled trial has provided proof of such favorable effects. In DS a good clinical reaction to corticosteroids, ACTH, and immunosuppressants is generally observed.

52.6   Magnetic Resonance Imaging

CT is now rarely used in the diagnosis and follow-up of MS. With CT it was possible to visualize lesions in about 35% of the MS patients. Areas of hypodensity were seen in the white matter, particularly in the periventricular region. New MS lesions might show enhancement after contrast injection. In long-standing and severe cases ventricular dilatation and cortical atrophy were observed. In NMO CT was usually normal. In CS CT showed usually round, hypodense lesions sometimes enhancing after contrast injection. In DS CT revealed large hypodense areas bilaterally in the centrum semiovale. After contrast injection there was ring-like enhancement.

Very early in the development of MR systems it became apparent that the unsurpassed tissue contrast of MRI was of importance in the diagnosis of MS. The first publication by Young et al. (1981) appeared in the Lancet (November 14, 1981) and already made clear that MRI was far superior to CT in detecting lesions in patients who were suspected of suffering from MS. This has since been confirmed many times, and the general policy today is that, if an imaging modality is used in the search for MS, it should be MRI. Also, however, in the Lancet (December 1984) one finds a warning against overenthusiasm by Ormerod et al. (1984) stating that MRI provides a sensitive means of demonstrating both vascular and demyelinating lesions, and that "with the sequences presently in use it is not possible to distinguish them." Since then more and more conditions have been identified that lead to isolated or confluent white matter lesions with prolonged T_1 and T_2. This, naturally, prompted questions concerning the role of MRI in MS. Through the years many centers have contributed to this discussion and identified the role of MRI in diagnosis, therapy-monitoring and research.

Most of the research has concentrated on relapsing-remitting and secondary progressive forms of MS. This is because there is no necessity to examine benign forms of MS repeatedly, and because in the primary progressive group, despite the progressive neurological symptoms, one finds only a few lesions on MRI. In the follow-up studies in the relapsing-remitting and secondary progressive groups it became clear that lesions as seen on T_2-weighted images may come and go without evident clinical changes. Although the findings are not specific, it is possible to describe the most common MRI appearance of the relapsing-remitting and secondary progressive forms of MS. There are multiple lesions with intermediate signal intensity on T_1-weighted images, high signal intensity on T_2-weighted images, isolated or confluent or both, with a bilateral but asymmetrical distribution, and preferentially located along the lateral angles of the ventricles in the efferent and afferent tracts of the corpus callosum (Fig. 52.1). The corpus callosum is thinner than usual and has an irregular border. Parasagittal T_2-weighted images show this relationship with the corpus callosum to best advantage (Fig. 52.2). There are few or no lesions in the basal ganglia. Lesions may occur in the mesencephalon (8%), the pons (12%), the cerebellar hemispheres (4%) and the medulla oblongata (1%–2%). Lesions are spread through the frontal, parietal and occipital lobes and, less frequently, the temporal lobe. However, many cases of definite MS do not fit this description. Nearly anything goes with MS. Lesions may show mass-effect or become cystic. Some of the lesions may enhance after intravenous administration of gadolinium. Enhancement of the lesion may be global, irregular or only affect the rim of the lesions (Fig. 52.3). Enhancement indicates disruption of the blood-brain barrier, pathophysiologically probably the first local change of a developing MS plaque. Inflammation and edema will follow. The enhancement lasts between 2 and 6 weeks. MRI provides the possibility to identify acute, new or reactivated, lesions. However, it has become obvious that activity of the disease as measured by gadolinium-enhancing lesions does not correspond with clinical exacerbations or worsening of the disability of the patient (mostly quantitated via the Expanded Disability Status Scale of Kurtzke, EDSS). The relationship between the lesions demonstrated on MRI and clinical findings is generally speaking poor. In cases with advanced disease of the secondary progressive type, the correspondence between the developing atrophy and the number of white matter lesions and the EDSS is better (Figs. 52.4, 52.5).

In NMO, one does not necessarily expect lesions in the cerebral white matter as the clinical condition mainly consists of problems of vision (optic neuritis) and paraplegia (transverse myelitis). In the cases we have seen, however, we have always found serious white matter lesions of the cerebral hemispheres. These MRI findings are in accordance with histology.

In DS the lesions are large, at least 32 cm in size, mostly localized in the parietal region on both sides and, in accordance with the original drawings of Schilder, connected via the corpus callosum. From the

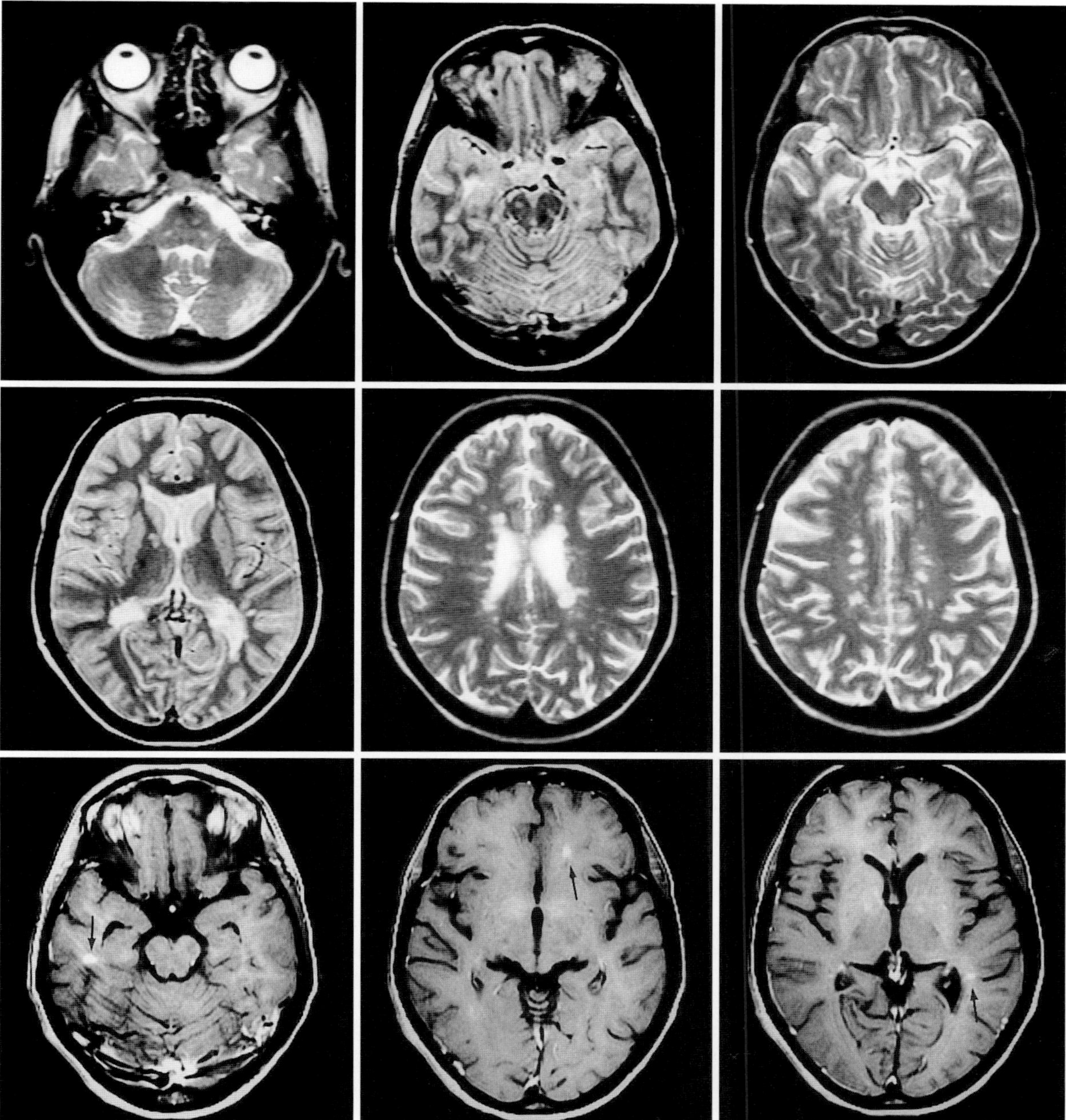

Fig. 52.1. A 32-year-old woman with clinically definite, classical MS. Typical lesions are seen on the transverse T_2-weighted series of MR images. Lesions are present in the mesencephalon, in the right genu of the internal capsule, near the trigonum on both sides, abutting the lateral wall of the ventricles and along the tracts of the corpus callosum. After injection of gadolinium (*lower row*) some of the lesions take up contrast (*arrows*)

drawings of Schilder's original publication (Fig. 52.6), one can also conclude that the lesions will appear symmetrical in some transverse sections but not in all. These lesions spare the arcuate fibers, unless the case is very advanced. After injection of gadolinium there is enhancement of the peripheral active rim (Fig. 52.7). It may be difficult to distinguish DS from X-linked adrenoleukodystrophy on the basis of imaging findings. Bilateral, confluent white matter lesions connected via the corpus callosum and showing rim enhancement are also seen as a rule in X-linked adrenoleukodystrophy. However, in X-linked adrenoleukodystrophy the localization of the lesions is preferentially occipital and the lesions are symmetrical. It is in the

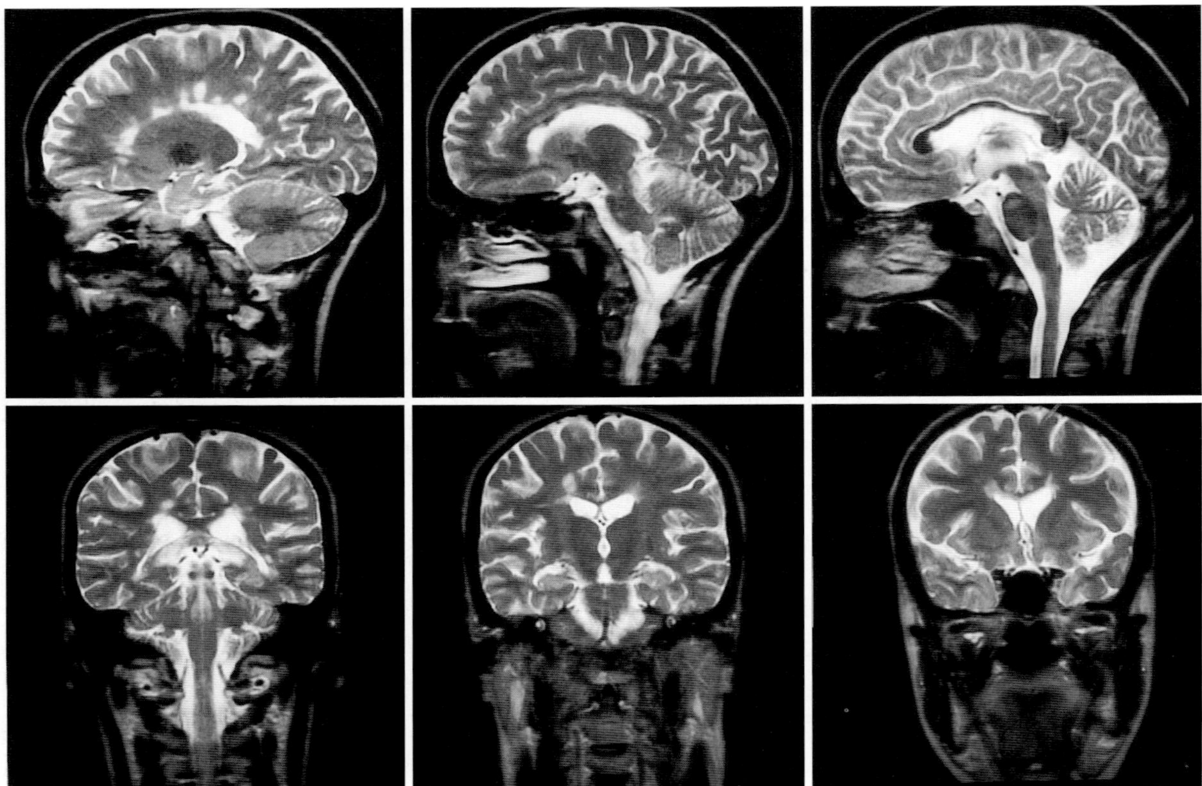

Fig. 52.2. Suggestions have been made to improve the specificity of MR images with respect to MS. Adding other imaging planes is considered to be helpful (as are other pulse sequences). The sagittal T_2-weighted series shows the typical lesions extending upward from the borders of the lateral ventricles. The corpus callosum is extremely thin, lesions as a rule undermining the ventral surface. The coronal images do not add much to the specificity but show nicely the lesions around the temporal horns

atypical cases of X-linked adrenoleukodystrophy with frontal or pariental, asymmetrical lesions that confusion with DS may exist. However, with laboratory investigations it is easy to distinguish X-linked adrenoleukodystrophy from DS. DS is very rare, but it should be borne in mind when diagnosing cases of severe white matter affection occurring in the first two decades of life.

CS is easily recognizable on MRI and shows alternating layers of myelinated and unmyelinated fibers, leading to a striking appearance (Fig. 52.8). In CS the MR images show the ring-like lesions, often already visible on the proton density and T_2-weighted images, with an enhancing rim after contrast injection.

It is evident that MRI plays a role in the diagnosis of MS. The clinical classifications of MS, according to Schumacher, Rose and Poser, have had a great impact on research into MS. On the Schumacher-Rose scale, the diagnosis of definite, probable, or possible MS is made on clinical grounds only, with dissemination in time and space of the clinical presentation of the lesions as the main criterion. Poser added to this the laboratory (CSF) and paraclinical (evoked responses, CT, MRI) findings. In his classification one finds clinically definite MS and laboratory-supported definite MS. This has led to considerable controversy because now at least two forms of definite MS seem to exist. Poser's concept has made the relative contributions of the various laboratory and paraclinical tests in the diagnosis of MS a subject of further research. A study by Paty et al. (1988) compares the diagnostic capabilities of MRI, CT, evoked potentials, and CSF oligoclonal banding in 200 patients with clinically probable and possible MS. MRI appeared to be the most sensitive paraclinical test, being very successful in identifying MS-like lesions in patients who fulfilled the criteria of Poser's classification for laboratory-supported definite MS. In follow-up its predictive value with respect to the development of clinically definite MS appeared to be very high, surpassing all other paraclinical tests. The examiners were struck, however, by the lack of specificity of the "strongly suggestive MRI pattern," due to the fact that this can be produced by other

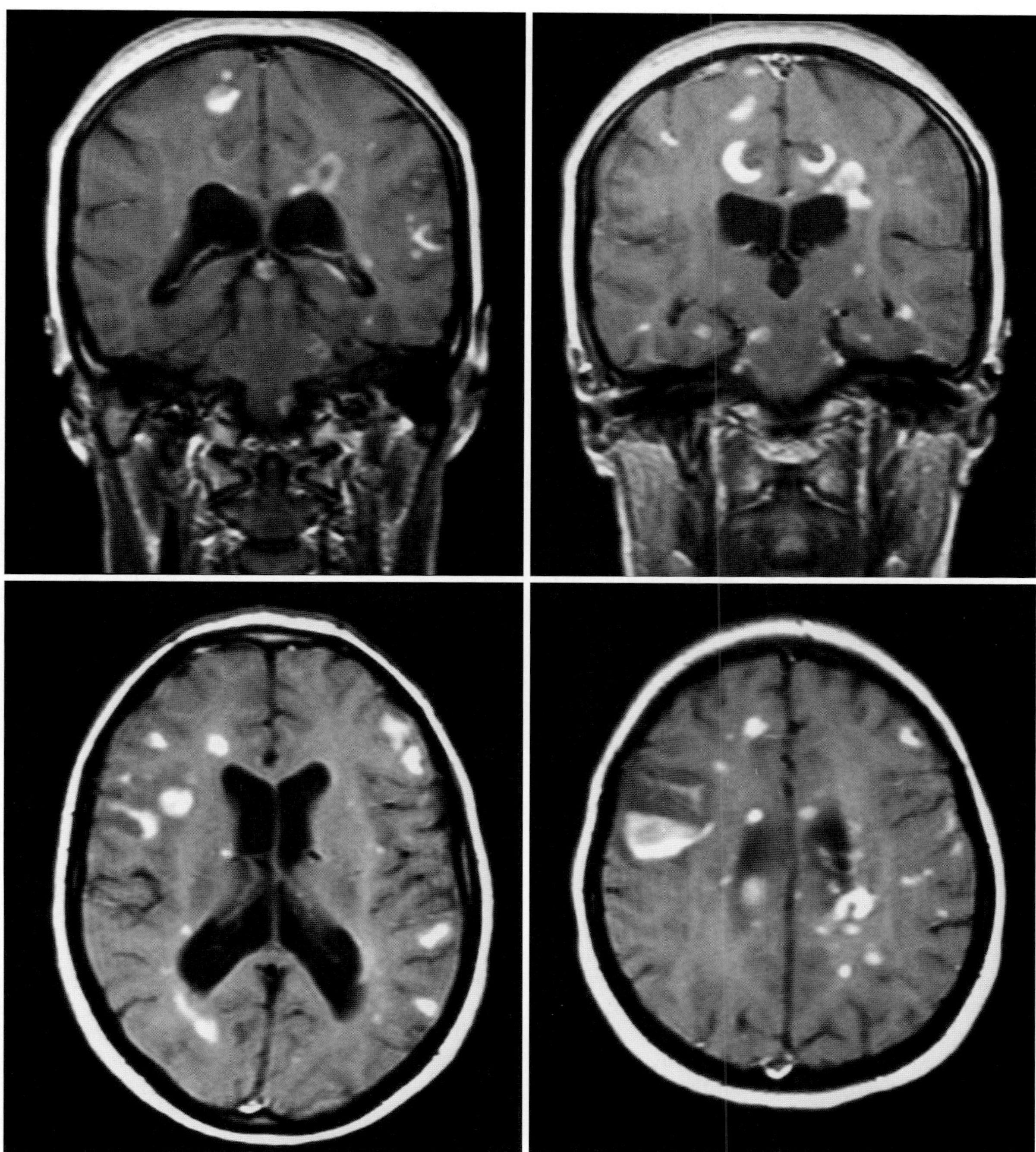

Fig. 52.3. Occasionally the enhancement of lesions is quite striking, as in this 38-year-old woman with definite MS. Note that the trigeminal nerve is also enhanced

disease states. They believe that clinical judgement remains the most important in making the distinction between MS and other diseases. In a reaction to this article, Kurtzke (1988) presented a further analysis of the results of Paty et al. He looked particularly at the patients in whom there was a reliance on paraclinical evidence for demonstration of multiplicity of lesions.

He presented an analysis of the sensitivity (ratio of all patients with MS with positive test to all patients with MS), the specificity (ratio of all patients without MS with negative test to all patients without MS), and the positive predictive value of the MRI (ratio of all patients with MS and positive test to the sum of patients with and without MS with a positive test). It becomes

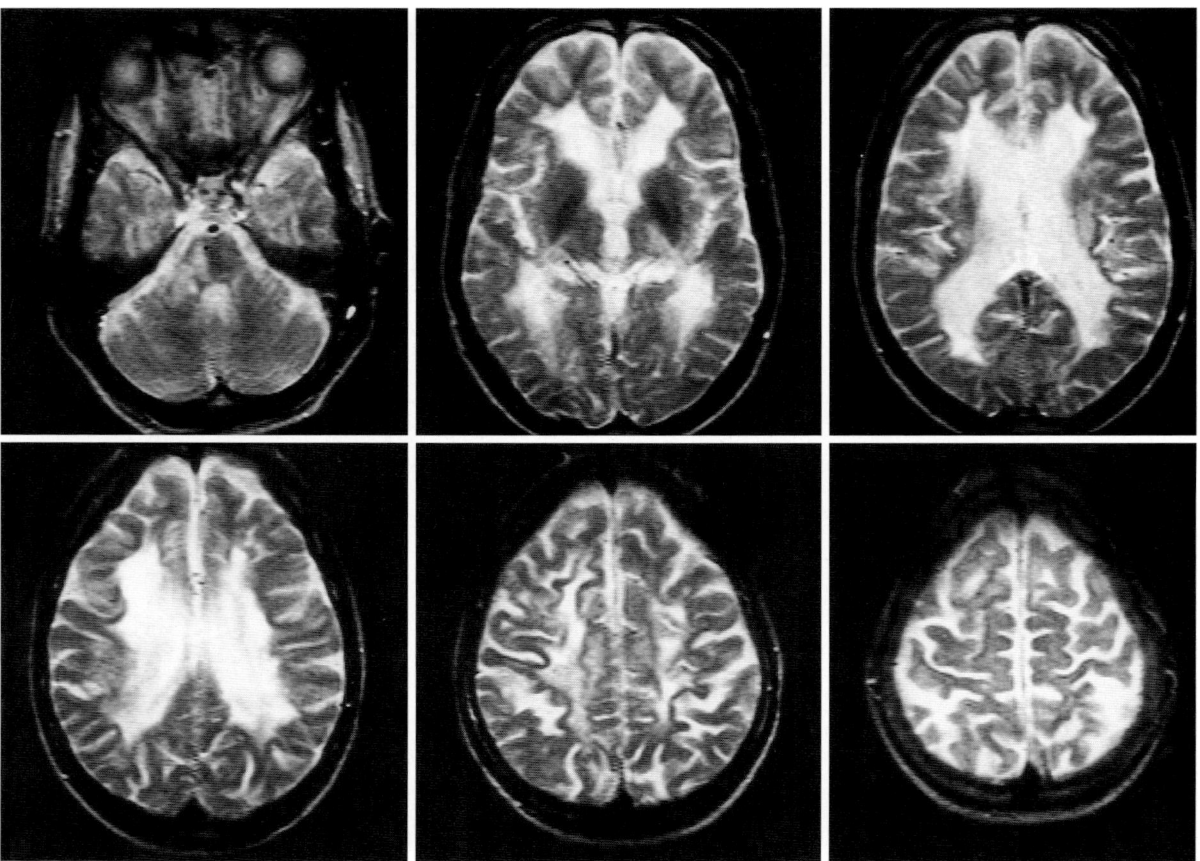

Fig. 52.4. A 36-year-old man who had been suffering from secondary progressive MS since the age of 20. The T_2-weighted MR series shows extensive confluent involvement of the white matter in the centrum semiovale, involving the U fibers. There are also lesions in the pons and middle cerebellar peduncle and generalized atrophy. In long-standing cases of progressive MS this pattern of confluent lesions may be seen

clear that if the pretest probability of MS is in the order of 90%, sensitivity, specificity, and positive predictive value of the MRI would all be in the order of 90%. If, however, the prevalence of MS in an examined population were only 1 per 100, there would be a positive predictive value of only 10%, or, one true positive would lead to nearly ten false positives. As the prevalence of MS in the general population is even lower, it is evident that MRI cannot be used as a screening method for MS. The same reasoning, of course, applies to all screening tests. What remains is that in patients with a clinical classification of possible or probable MS, MRI (and oligoclonal banding) can in individual cases certainly add to the probability of the diagnosis. This view has recently been confirmed in a study by Morrissey et al. (1993). In a 5-year follow-up study of patients who initially presented with isolated neurological symptoms suggestive of MS they found that MRI was a powerful predictor of the later diagnosis of definite MS, better than the presence of HLA-DR2 antigen or CSF oligoclonal bands.

Various other diseases can be excluded by MRI. Caution is essential, however, in all cases. Many other conditions can lead to multifocal lesions located chiefly in the white matter with prolonged T_1 and T_2. They are found in arteriosclerotic disorders, head trauma, migrainous headache, vasculitis (systemic lupus erythematosus, Behçet), early metastatic lesions, leukemic deposits in the brain, Lyme's disease, neurosarcoidosis, toxoplasmosis and as age-related white matter changes in the elderly. Without further information, MRI cannot reliably differentiate between these conditions. However, MRI is not the only tool which can be used to reach the diagnosis. Clinical evidence, patient's history, age, and laboratory findings may suggest a diagnosis other than MS. The fact that some of the above-mentioned causes for "MS-like" white matter lesions are often seen in the fifth and sixth decades of life, and that the incidence of MS is low in this age group, argues for the reservation of MRI as a tool in the classification of MS for research mainly in the under-50 age group.

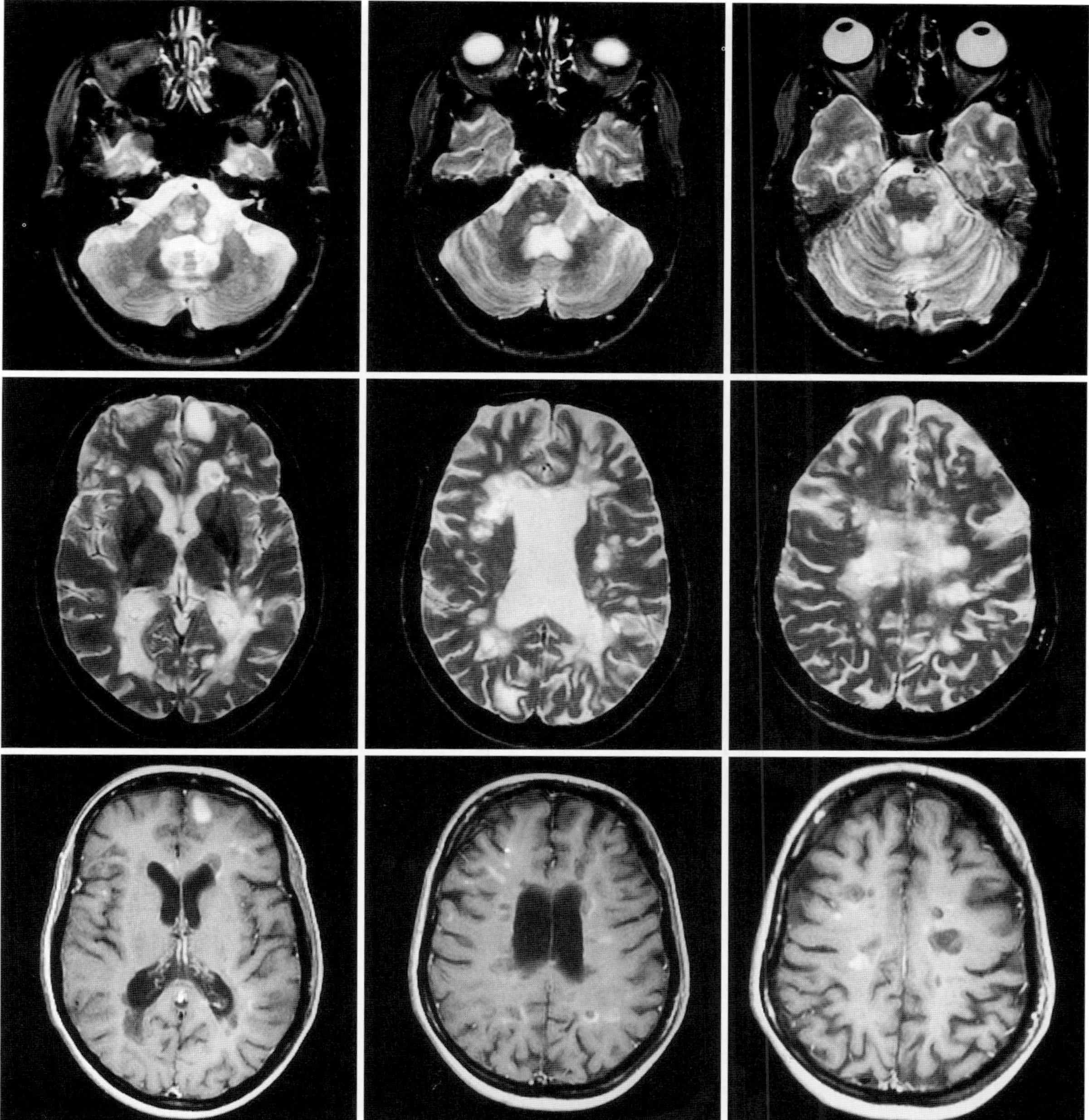

Fig. 52.5. A 34-year-old woman with long-standing, secondary progressive MS. The *upper three T_2-weighted images* show an abundance of lesions in the pons, cerebellum, and cerebellar peduncles. Supratentorially the lesions are partly isolated, partly confluent. The T_1-weighted image after contrast injection (*right lower row*) shows the enhancement of some lesions, but also another phenomenon, the so-called black holes, which are nonenhancing lesions with low signal intensity. In these areas axons are probably also lost. The presence of black holes correlates with a poor neurological outcome

The role of MRI in the diagnosis of MS can be described as being of little extra value in cases with clinically definite MS, of considerable help in individual cases with clinically probable and possible MS, and of dubious help in those cases which clinically provide only a minimal suspicion of MS. The value of MRI with respect to the diagnosis of MS in patients over the age of 50 is low.

The use of intravenous gadolinium-DTPA as a paramagnetic contrast agent has added to the value of MRI

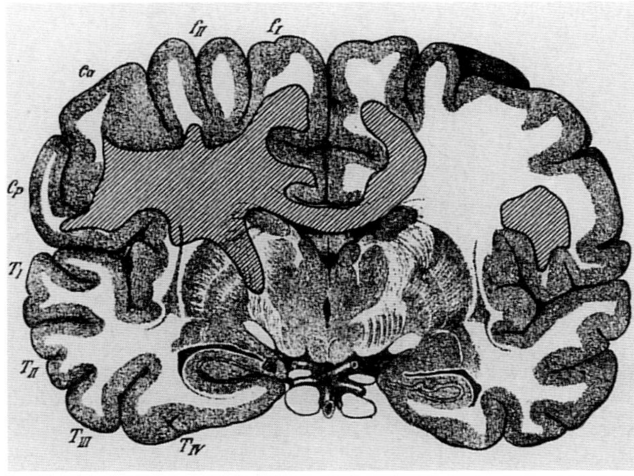

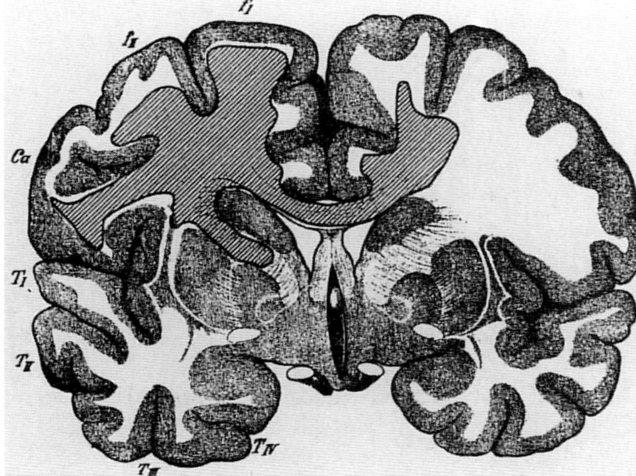

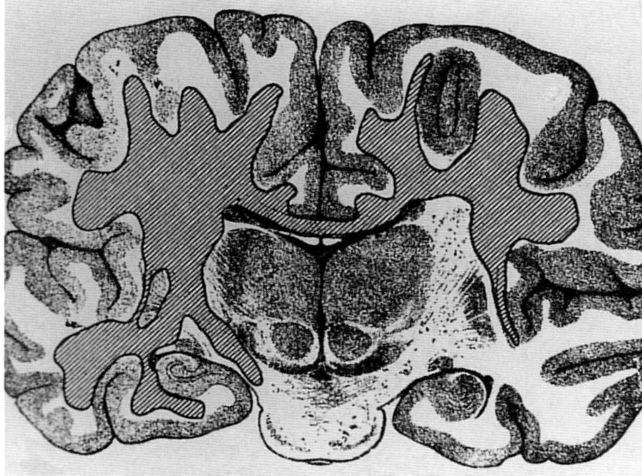

Fig. 52.6. Illustrations from the original paper of Schilder (1912) on DS. The drawings show the extensive, asymmetrical involvement of the frontal and parietal lobes, connected via lesions in the corpus callosum

in MS. In cases with a clinical suspicion of MS, MRI cannot only help to demonstrate "dissemination in space" with the presence of more than one lesion in the CNS at different locations, but gadolinium-enhanced MRI can also demonstrate "dissemination in time," by

showing older nonenhancing or no longer enhancing lesions together with new or reactivated lesions with blood-brain barrier disruption. The most important role of gadolinium-enhanced MRI has emerged as monitoring the efficacy of drug treatment. Longterm follow-up studies have shown that newly appearing gadolinium-enhancing lesions are far more frequent in relapsing-remitting and secondary progressive forms of MS than clinical exacerbations. If one accepts gadolinium-enhancement as a sign of new disease activity, then one has a means of monitoring the therapeutic response of the disease to new drugs. It has been shown by Barkhof et al. (1992) that changes in the number of gadolinium-enhancing lesions during the course of the disease correspond far better to changes in the EDSS than changes in lesion load on T_2-weighted images. The apparent advantage for therapeutic trials is the gain in time and the smaller population one has to examine to obtain statistical significance of results. The eventual clinical trial based on clinical results can thus be limited to the most promising compounds.

Lately there has been a growing interest in remyelination, part of the healing process of MS. Some lesions disappear from MRI in MS patients with follow-up MRI, whereas others do not. The question is whether the disappearing lesions remyelinate and therefore become invisible or shrink and turn into little gliotic scars. New MR methods may be helpful in answering this question, for example by changes in the magnetization transfer contrast ratio or changes in the diffusion constant. Other techniques may also be considered, such as functional MRI or MR spectroscopy.

One has to be aware that MS can occur in very young children. Actually MS has been diagnosed in children aged 2 years. As in adults the diagnosis has to be considered when multifocal white matter abnormalities are seen, some of which may take up contrast after injection. The lesions in young children may be larger, and have less affinity for the lateral borders of the ventricles. Although the numbers reported are small, the incidence of brain stem lesions may be somewhat higher in children than in adults. As in adult MS, the contrast uptake disappears after several weeks and the lesions become less conspicuous on T_2-weighted images.

Two manifestions of MS outside the brain deserve special mention: optic neuritis and spinal cord lesions, because they both require special MRI techniques. Both can occur in all other forms of MS with the possible exception of DS. In some cases of optic neuritis, it has been possible, using special techniques, to demonstrate a lesion within the optic nerve (Fig. 52.9). Especially the STIR sequence has been recommended for this purpose. Other fat suppression techniques have a better signal to noise ratio and are also applied successfully. Fat saturation techniques can be very well com-

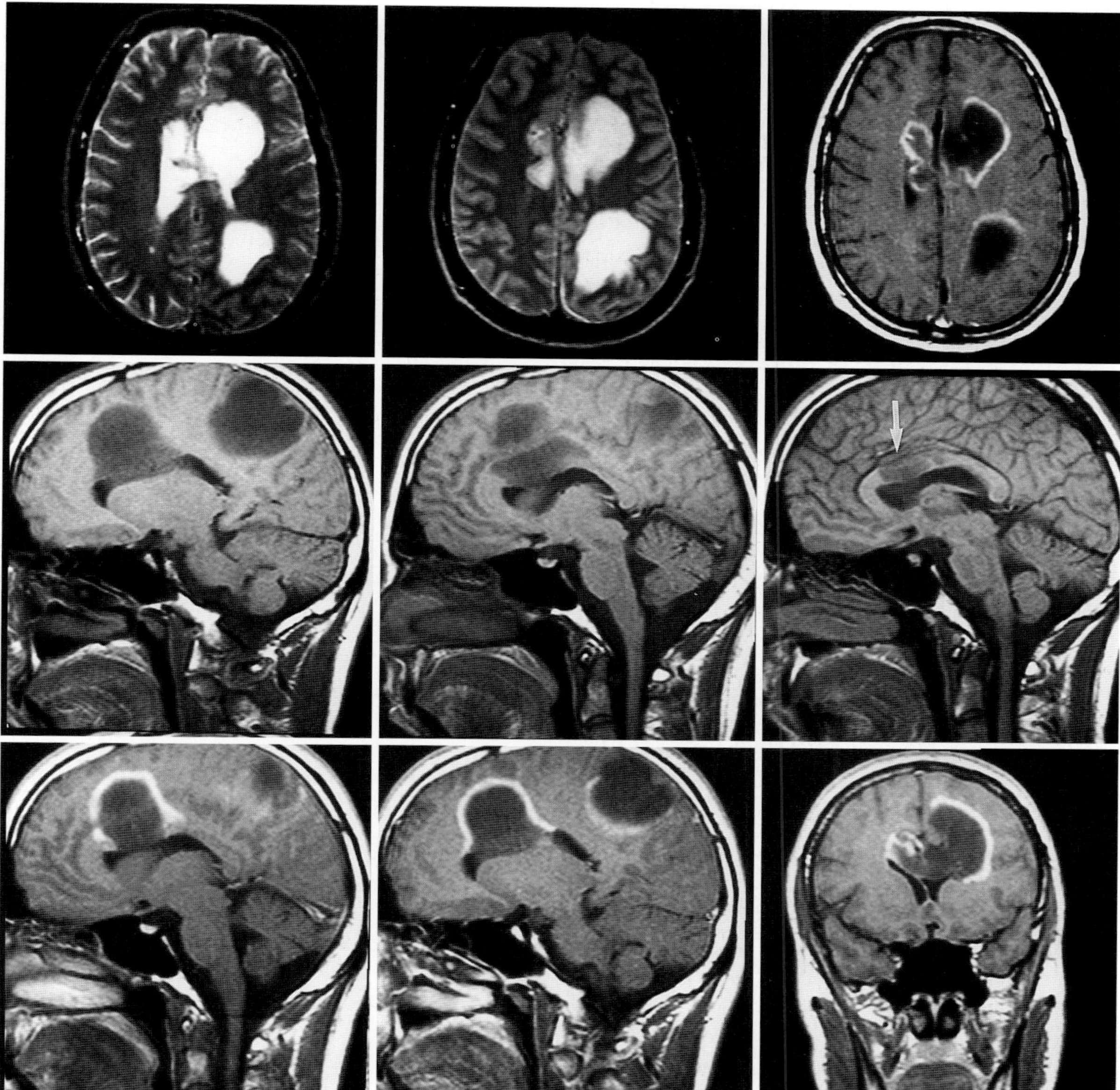

Fig. 52.7. A 27-year-old man with a recent acute excacerbation of neurological signs and symptoms, including hemiplegia, aphasia, headache, and drowsiness. The MR tableau is a collage of T_2-weighted images (*upper left*) and T_1-weighted images with and without contrast in three planes. Compare especially the coronal image with Schilder's diagrams (Fig. 52.6). Large lesions are seen on both sides in the frontal and parietal regions, with an asymmetrical distribution, preponderance to the left, and involvement of the corpus callosum (*arrow*) connecting the lesions on the left and right sides. There is a ring-like enhancement in the zone of acute inflammatory response. There was a considerable improvement after 6 weeks of treatment with corticosteroids

bined with gadolinium-enhancement. The majority of MS lesions of the spinal cord occur in the cervical and conal region. They appear mostly as high signal intensity lesions on T_2-weighted images and may enhance after contrast injection (Fig. 52.10). There is, as a rule, no or very little mass effect. Mass effect can incidentally be considerable and mimic an intramedullary tumor. It is, of course, very important to perform this study in patients presenting with spinal cord symptoms to confirm the diagnosis and to rule out other disorders. If a lesion indicative of MS is found, an MR study of the head should be considered to look for corroborative evidence of lesions in the brain to support the diagnosis of MS. The greatest technical problems in detecting MS lesions are encountered in the thoracic region. Phased array coils have increased the signal to noise

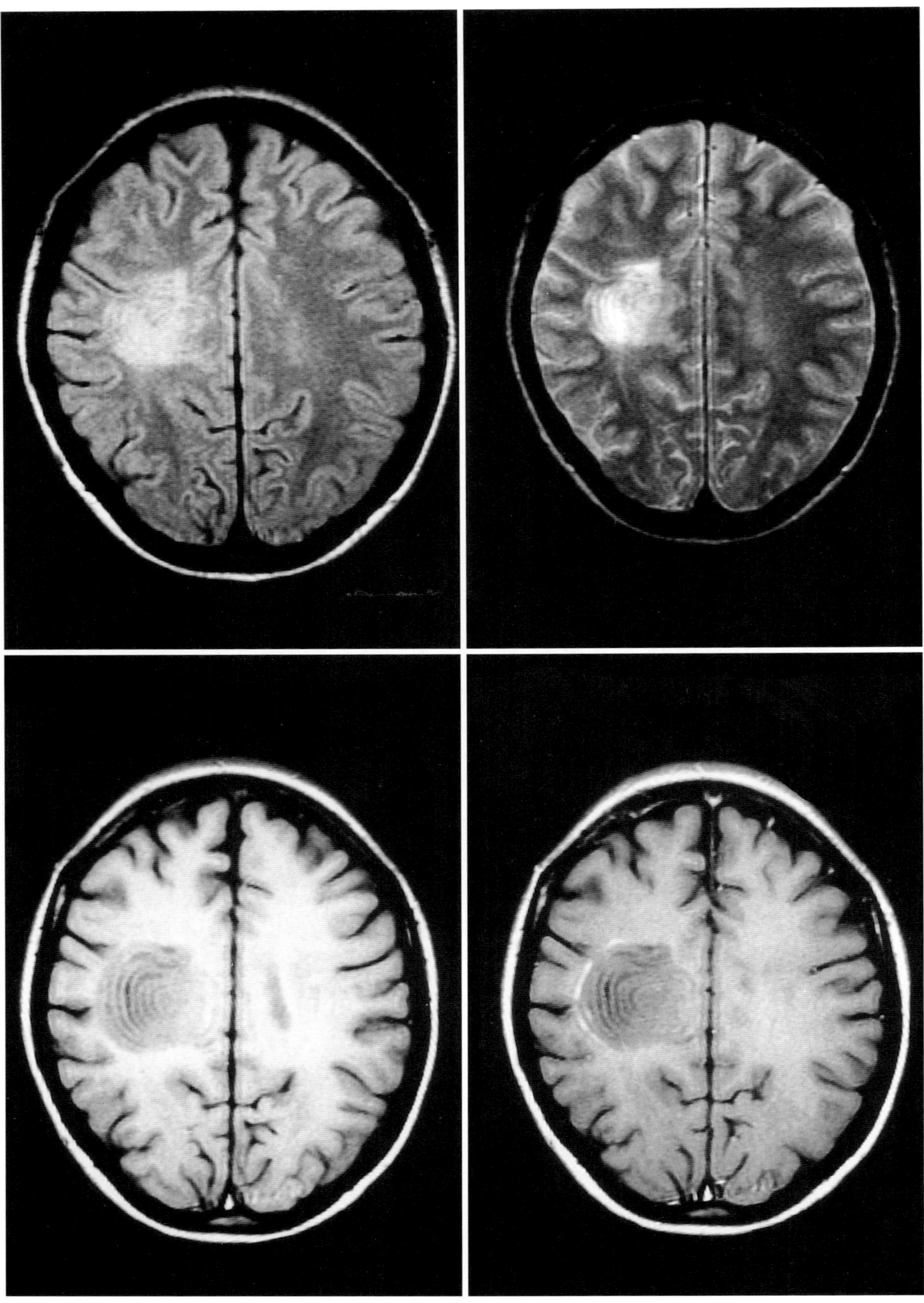

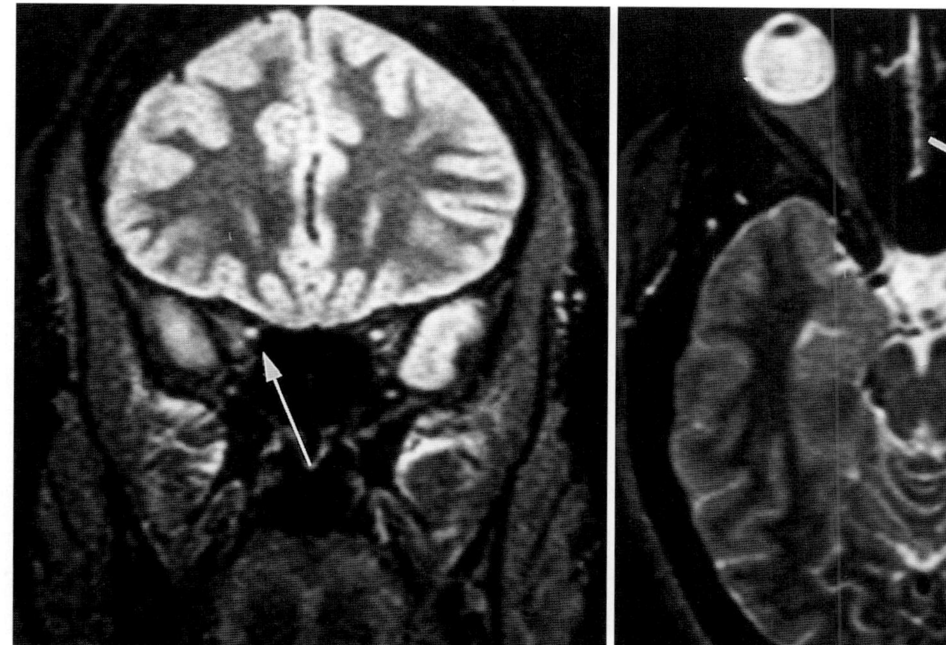

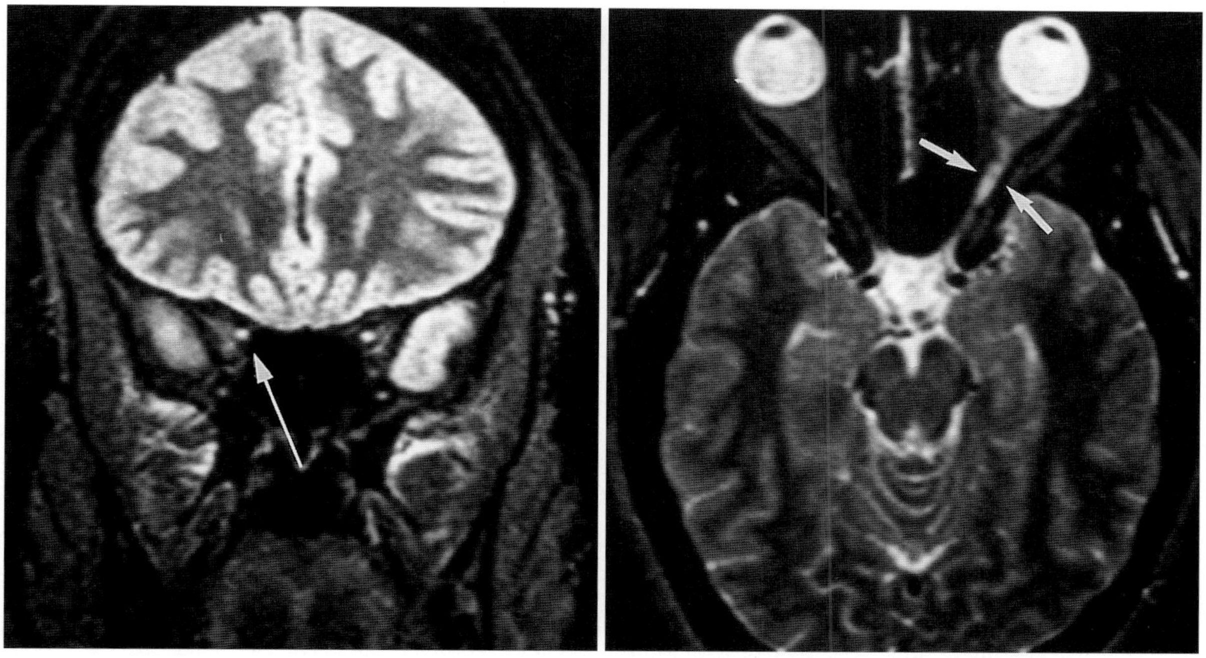

Fig. 52.9. The STIR technique is shown in a patient with NMO (*left*). Bilaterally the optic nerve has too high a signal intensity, consistent with the diagnosis. On the *right* a T_2-weighted image is shown with TR 4000, TE 150. Also with T_2 weighting the fat signal is reduced. The lesion in the optic nerve can be clearly seen (*arrows*)

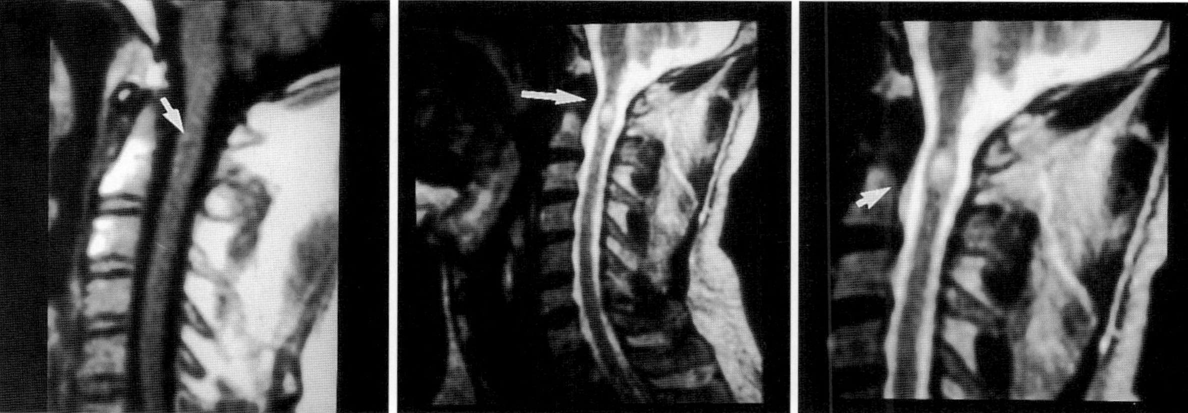

Fig. 52.10. Spinal lesions in MS usually present as shown here in a 42-year-old man who had clinical signs of transverse myelitis. The T_1-weighted image shows a slight irregularity in the upper cervical cord (*left, arrow*). The T_2-weighted image (*middle*) shows the lesion much more clearly (*arrow*). On the *right view* this is shown in more detail (*arrow*)

ratio and detail in studies of the spinal cord. This will improve thoracic cord studies. There is some evidence emerging that the findings of spinal cord plaques correspond better with the degree of disability and symptoms of the patient than lesion load, localization or number of events in the brain, perhaps with the exception of brain stem lesions.

Fig. 52.8. A 25-year-old woman with CS. MRI shows a large lesion with a concentric pattern in the white matter on the right side. An abrupt termination of the concentric rings is present where the lesion abuts on the gray matter. After contrast administration only the outer rings enhance. Courtesy of Korte et al. (1994), with permission

53.1   Introduction

MR images showing multiple white matter lesions, isolated or confluent, bordering the edges of the lateral ventricles, located in the corpus callosum, sometimes the mesencephalon, basis pontis, middle cerebellar peduncles, in any number and size, partly enhancing with gadolinium contrast, are by no means specific for multiple sclerosis (MS). Of course many of the conditions mentioned below will not be confused with MS if the clinical side of the illness is also taken into consideration. However, the finding of MS-like lesions in patients suffering from one of these conditions might lead to confusion, and the presence of two disorders might be considered. Then it is important to know that MS-like lesions may form part of the disease.

A short survey will be given of the most frequent conditions that may mimic MS on MRI, and that have not been discussed in separate chapters (see the chapters on acute disseminated encephalomyelitis, progressive multifocal leukoencephalopathy, vasculitis, vascular white matter lesions in elderly, and Leber's hereditary optic atrophy).

53.2   Lyme's Disease or Borreliosis

Neurosyphylis and neuroborreliosis are currently the most important spirochetal diseases that can affect the human nervous system. An increasing number of cases of Lyme's disease have recently been reported, probably due to the increasing deer population. The disease is now second to AIDS as an infectious disorder problem. Lyme's disease is a worldwide zoonosis and the most common vector-borne illness in the United States and Europe. It is caused by Borrelia burgdorferi, carried by the hard-shelled ticks, Ixodes domini, Ixodes pacificus and Ixodes ricinus. After intradermal inoculation, the spirochetes proliferate within the dermis and cause a spirochetemia, followed by invasion of the CNS and possibly also the PNS. Within a few weeks after infection, the disease manifests itself by nonspecific neurological complaints such as myalgias and headaches. Often there is a characteristic rash: erythema chronicum migrans. Positive polymerase chain reaction (PCR) tests have been obtained in the CSF of patients with

erythema migrans. This contradicts the conviction that the spirochetes do not enter the CNS until approximately 1 month after infection. Clinical manifestations of the CNS are generally explainable by a chronic basal meningitis, with cranial neuropathies, most frequently facial nerve weakness, often bilateral. Encephalopathy and peripheral neuropathy, heralding the third stage of the infection, tend to occur many months after the initial infection. The CNS involvement can be mild, with mood and mild memory disturbances, or present as a severe encephalomyelitis. The diagnosis is made by a consistent history, clinical signs and symptoms, CSF pleiocytosis and raised anti-Borrelia burgdorferi antibody levels in serum and CSF. Techniques like enzyme-linked immunosorbent assay (ELISA) and the indirect fluorescent antibody tests are used. Also, nowadays, the PCR test is available to amplify specific spirochetal DNA. The diagnosis is very important because the disorder can be treated well by antibiotics with or without corticosteroids.

The MR images of Lyme's disease may look very similar to MS (Fig. 53.1). In some of the reported cases the widespread lesions tend to be larger, with all lesions showing ring-like enhancement, whereas meningeal enhancement is also present. Lesions are often located in the frontal subcortical white matter, but lesions may also be disseminated through the brain. Not all cases with CNS symptoms have positive MRI findings (in one series 7/14). Because of the lesion characteristics, Lyme's disease should be on the list when differentiating multifocal white matter disease.

53.3   Sarcoidosis of the CNS

Neurosarcoidosis is always mentioned in textbooks and reviews as a condition that may mimic MS. In most cases, however, sarcoidosis of the CNS has some characteristics that will rule out the diagnosis MS.

Sarcoidosis is a chronic disease of unknown cause, involving multiple organ sytems. The typical pathology is a noncaseating granuloma. The pulmonary manifestations are the best known, such as bilateral hilar lymphadenopathy. Increased angiotensin-converting enzyme levels, or defects in cell-mediated immunity help in establishing the diagnosis. Gallium scanning

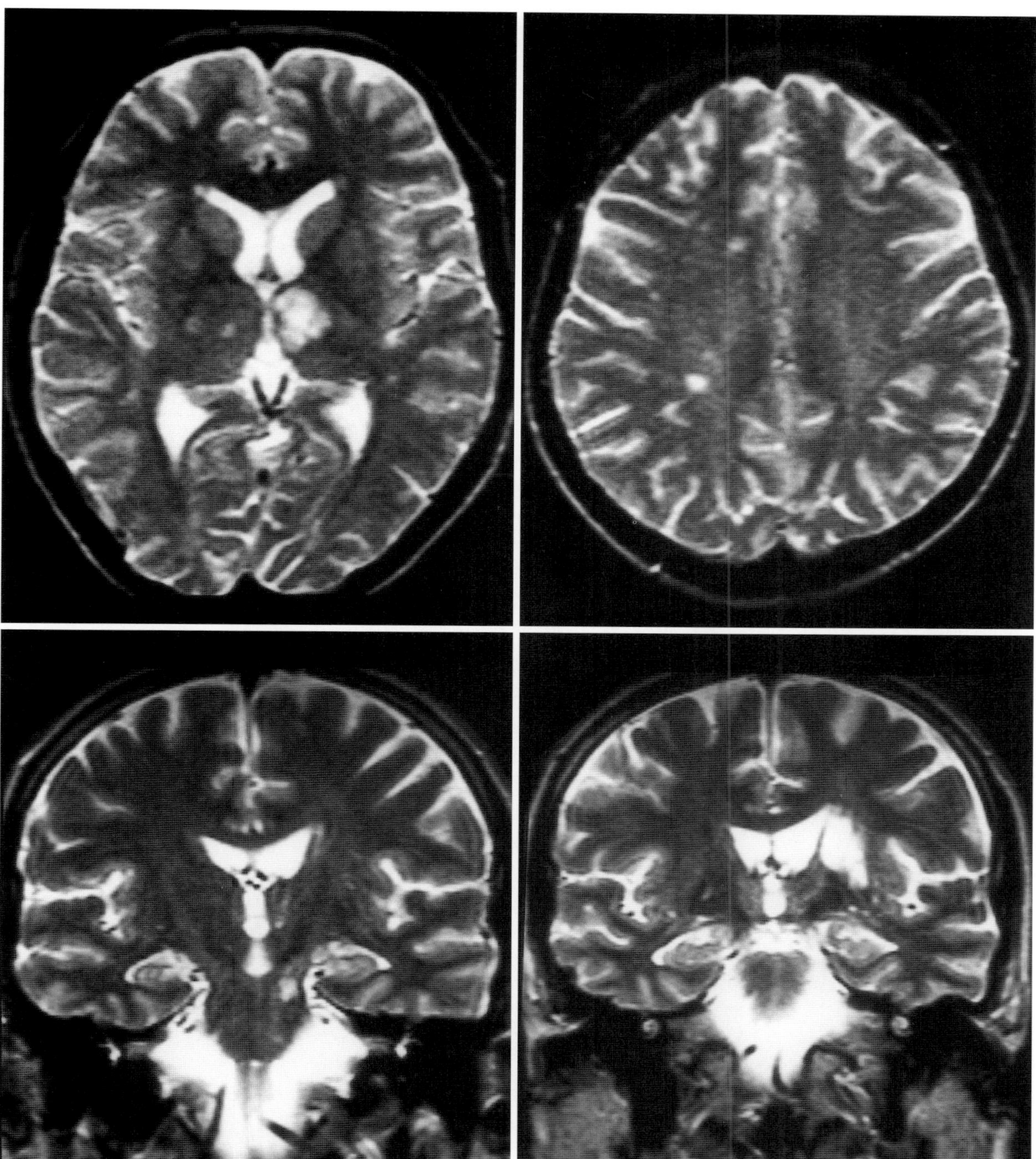

Fig. 53.1. A 48-year-old man with Lyme's disease. The small white matter lesions scattered over the centrum semiovale and brain stem are indistinguishable from MS lesions. Only the large lesion in the thalamus on the left suggests a diagnosis other than MS

may identify disease of the lung or salivary glands. Typical findings of neurosarcoidosis are hypothalamic or pituitary dysfunction (in particular diabetes insipidus), myelopathy, cranial neuropathy, and symptoms of an intracranial mass lesion. In the CSF the findings may cause confusion with MS: mild lymphocytic pleiocytosis, increased protein and sometimes oligoclonal bands. Neurosarcoidosis has been reported without systemic involvement. There is usually a good response to steroids, expecially in the active forms.

MRI of neurosarcoidosis may have the same appearance as is usually found in MS. This, however, is not the rule. In neurosarcoidosis the lesions often involve the

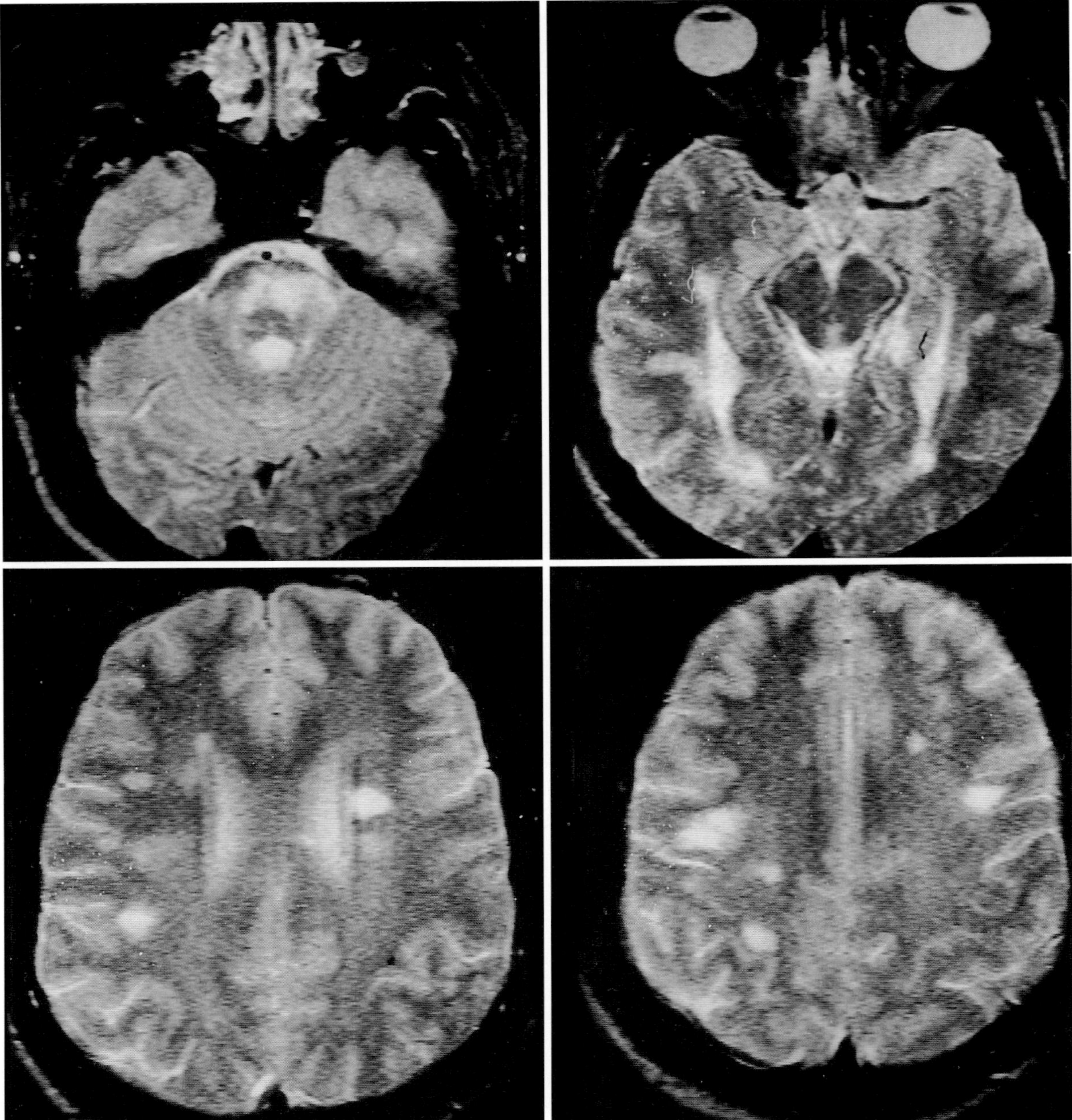

Fig. 53.2. A 36-year-old woman with tropical spastic para-paresis. There are multiple white matter lesions in the pons and the hemispheral white matter, in both the periventricular and subcortical areas, potentially compatible with a diagnosis of MS

hypothalamus and the pituitary stalk. After contrast injection these lesions usually enhance and there is often meningeal enhancement as well. Lesions may also be located at the surface of the brain and show enhancement, including meningeal enhancement.

53.4 Tropical Spastic Paraparesis

Tropical spastic paraparesis is a neurological disorder, mainly of the Caribbean areas. It presents as a progressive spastic paraparesis and urinary dysfunction. This is caused by an infection with human T-cell lympho-tropic virus type I (HTLV-1). The lesions are usually restricted to the spinal cord and optic nerve (as in Devic's disease), but on MRI, lesions have been found

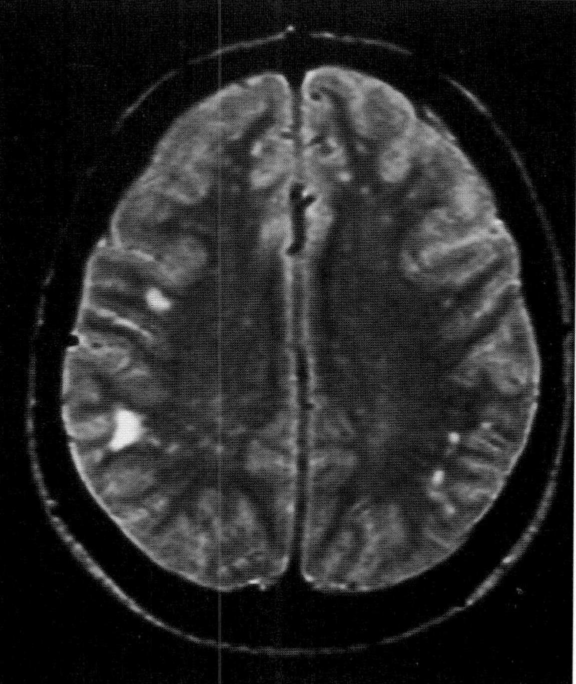

Fig. 53.3. A 38-year-old woman with long history of „migraine accompagnée." Aspecific lesions are seen on the T_2-weighted images, dispersed through both hemispheres, some located in the arcuate fibers, especially the larger ones, the smaller ones in the centrum semiovale and the periventricular white matter without particular preference for the periventricular region. These lesions are probably vascular in origin, either caused by the migraine or by the vasoactive medication

in the brain which are indistinguishable from lesions seen in MS, with discrete white matter lesions disseminated in the centrum semiovale and along the lateral borders of the ventricles (Fig. 53.2). Some lesions enhance after gadolinium injection. Usually no lesions are found in the basal ganglia, brain stem and cerebellum. Especially in the West Indian population, tropical spastic paraparesis is common and MS is rare. Shift of large parts of West Indian populations to regions where MS is common and tropical spastic paraparesis is not, may lead to confusion. In two cases in our experience, the disease manifested with subacute symptomatology of the medulla oblongata and upper cervical spine. MRI showed lesions with clear mass effect and enhancement in those areas.

53.5 Chronic Inflammatory Demyelinating Polyneuropathy

Chronic inflammatory demyelinating polyneuropathy bears a close clinical and pathological resemblance to the Guillain-Barré syndrome. The course, however, is chronic progressive or chronic relapsing. In a number of patients a multifocal CNS disorder has been reported, with combined clinical features of MS and chronic inflammatory demyelinating polyneuropathy. The lesions, as seen on MRI, are strikingly similar to what can be found in MS patients, indicative of a chronic multifocal demyelination. It is not well understood why combinations of the two diseases are relatively rare. Chronic inflammatory demyelinating polyneuropathy can be treated with high doses of corticosteroids, immunosuppressive drugs, plasmapheresis and with high doses of intravenous gammaglobulin.

53.6 Migrainous Headache

In cases of migrainous headache, white matter lesions have been described, that cannot readily be distinguished from MS (Fig. 53.3). The medical history, of course, is helpful. The nature of the lesions is not clear. Vascular spasms may play a role in local disturbance of cerebral blood flow. A relationship with anti-migrainous medication, for example, ergotamine-like preparations, has to be considered.

53.7 Eclampsia and Pre-eclampsia

In patients with eclampsia and pre-eclampsia, cerebral white matter lesions can usually be found and may become quite extensive. They are usually transient. Hy-

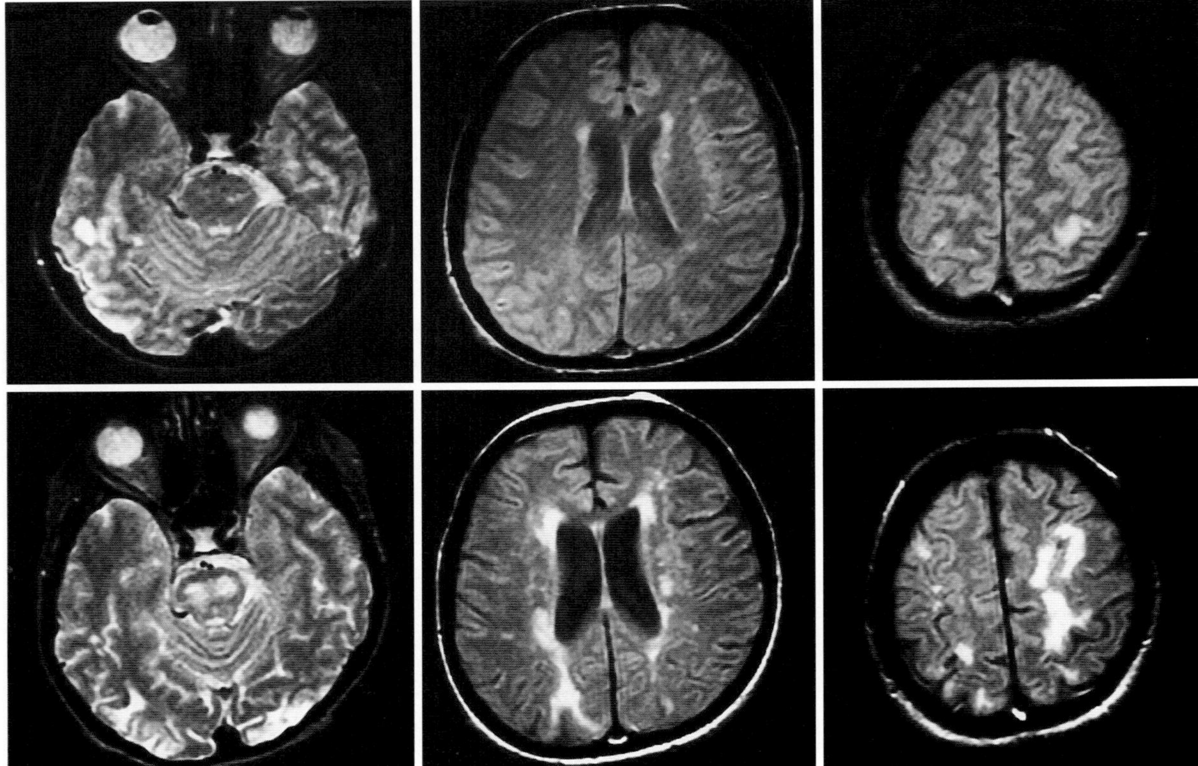

Fig. 53.4. A 48-year-old woman with eosinophilia-myalgia syndrome presented with neurological symptoms, including extremity weakness, dysarthria, and ataxia. She also complained of diffuse muscle and joint pains, skin rash, edema, and headaches. The *upper row* of T_2-weighted MR images was made shortly after first presentation; the *lower row* 22 months later, shortly after the diagnosis was established. The images show lesions of the white matter in the brain stem, in the periventricular region, and in the centrum semiovale which were worse at the second examination. The lesions are partly patchy and isolated, partly confluent. The gray matter is not completely spared. Courtesy of Lynn (1992), with permission

pertension and hypertensive vascular changes obviously play a role. The lesions may involve the basal ganglia, thalamus and the parieto-occipital subcortical white matter. Being large and multifocal, they may mimic progressive multifocal leukoencephalopathy rather than MS.

53.8 Multiple Metastases

Multiple metastasis, for example in melanoma, can present as multiple high signal lesions on T_2-weighted MR images. Usually additional information on the images, such as hemorrhage and uptake of contrast in all lesions, or in the case of melanoma the paramagnetic effect of melanin with T_1 shortening, may be helpful, as are the medical history and laboratory data. But MS can also produce hemorrhagic and expanding lesions and incidentally all MS lesions enhance after contrast injection.

53.9 Eosinophilia-Myalgia Syndrome

The eosinophilia-myalgia syndrome is a multi-system disease first recognized in 1989. The disease is defined by generalized debilitating myalgias, peripheral eosinophilia, and the absence of any infection or neoplasm. The condition is associated with the ingestion of L-tryptophan-containing products. The symptom complex includes myalgias, arthalgias, rash, cough or dyspnea, fever, fatigue and peripheral edema. Peripheral neuropathy has been reported in the condition. Recently also multiple white matter lesions have been seen in a patient with additional signs of cerebral dysfunction. The clinical story of the patient is different from MS patients (Fig. 53.4).

53.10 Waldenström's Macroglobulinemia

Leukoencephalopathy has been described in Waldenström's macroglobulinemia, a chronic illness of insidious onset characterized by a proliferation of plasmacytoid lymphocytes. The disease primarily affects males aged between 50 and 70 years and usually results in death within 2–5 years. Physical findings include painless lymphadenopathy and hepatosplenomegaly. Unlike multiple myeloma, bone lesions other than marrow infiltration are unusual. The cell product is a high molecular weight gammaglobulin, whose presence in the blood results in hyperviscosity, retinal hemorrhages and mucosal bleeding. Bence-Jones proteinuria is found in 10%–15% of cases. The clinical association with CNS disease is referred to as Bing-Neel syndrome. The neurological manifestations include encephalopathies of a multifocal nature, peripheral or cranial neuropathies, cerebrovascular accidents and subarachnoid hemorrhage. Clinically the disease cannot be confused with MS. Small infarctions disseminated through the brain may mimic the MRI appearance of MS.

54.1 Clinical Symptoms and Laboratory Investigations

Acute disseminated encephalomyelitis (ADEM) is an uncommon inflammatory disorder within the CNS, predominantly within the white matter of the brain and spinal cord. Postinfectious-postvaccination encephalopathy is a frequently used synonym. Poser used the term disseminated vasculomyelinopathy indicating the probably causative small vessel vasculopathy (Poser 1969). Many other synonyms exists.

ADEM and acute hemorrhagic encephalomyelitis (AHEM) represent two clinical variants of a single pathological process. They occur following a viral infection or vaccination or without recognized antecedent. Implicated viral infections are measles, chickenpox, rubella, smallpox, infectious mononucleosis, herpes simplex, herpes zoster, mumps, influenza and Mycoplasma pneumoniae. They rarely occur following a bacterial infection. A nonspecific upper respiratory tract infection is the most common antecedent. The latent period varies from several days to several weeks, the mean being 4–6 days. Onset of the neurological symptoms is usually abrupt, with convulsions and progression to somnolence and coma. Illness may also commence subacutely with symptoms of headache, fever, irritability, drowsiness, and vomiting. Nuchal rigidity is often present. The neurological signs are quite polymorphic and consist of hemiplegia, diplegia or tetraplegia, cerebellar ataxia, cranial nerve palsies, optic neuritis, nystagmus, sensory loss, and bladder dysfunction. Subcortical blindness is rare. Extrapyramidal motor abnormalities such as chorea, athetosis, and ballismus may be found. The progression of the disease is variable. Patients with AHEM progress more rapidly into delirium and coma. The highest mortality is seen during the first week of the illness, and in fact most patients who survive the first week eventually recover, with varying degrees of disability. Prolonged disturbances in level of consciousness entail a poor prognosis both for morbidity and mortality. Neurological sequelae include epilepsy, spastic paresis, ataxia, decreased vision and cognitive and psychiatric disturbances. Most of the neurological syndromes have a monophasic course lasting several weeks. Recurrent attacks of ADEM/AHEM have been described. The occurrence of the neurological abnormalities is apparently independent of the nature and severity of the antecedent infection or immunization.

There is a close relationship with the Guillain-Barré syndrome and in fact a combination of ADEM and Guillain-Barré syndrome has been described. Clinically, ADEM can usually be distinguished from multiple sclerosis because it presents with signs of severe multifocal involvement of the CNS at the same time. If initially monosymptomatic with optic neuritis, the optic neuritis tends to be bilateral. No clinical feature, however, is exclusive to one or the other disorder.

Laboratory investigations reveal a peripheral leukocytosis. The CSF shows pleocytosis. The cellular exsudate is mainly lymphocytic and rarely exceeds 100 cells/ml in ADEM. In AHEM the initial cells are granulocytic, and erythrocytes are also often seen. Glucose concentration is normal. There is usually a mild elevation of the CSF proteins, with an oligoclonal banding pattern and a heightened IgG index as signs of intrathecal IgG synthesis. An elevated level of myelin basic protein is shown, indicating myelin destruction. CSF abnormalities may persist for a long time after clinical recovery. Rarely, the CSF is completely normal throughout the course of the illness. The EEG often shows bilateral slow activity, suggesting either widespread diffuse disease of both hemispheres or disease in the diencephalic projection system. These abnormalities are nonspecific and add little to the diagnosis.

54.2 Pathology

Edema is often the most conspicuous gross finding in ADEM, but the external appearance of the brain may also be completely normal. Microscopic examination demonstrates a diffuse inflammatory process in the brain, brain stem, and spinal cord with inflammatory cells around veins and venules. Sometimes the perivascular infiltrates are associated with signs of a vasculitis, showing inflammatory cells in vessel walls with or without frank necrosis. The cerebral hemispheres are usually more or less symmetrically involved. Both the white and gray matter are affected, but the white matter shows more severe changes. The most distinctive histological change is perivascular demyelination. Within the lesions myelin sheaths are lost, but the axons are relatively unaffected. Occasionally the demyelinating lesions are confluent and form large demyelinated areas. At later stages of the disease, the inflammatory exsudate is replaced by fibrous gliosis.

In AHEM, necropsy reveals the brain to be swollen and soft in consistency. On sectioning, numerous small hemorrhages are seen, mainly in the white matter. The cerebral cortex and basal ganglia are often spared. The hemorrhagic lesions are often but not always symmetrical. Confluence of many small lesions leads to large hemorrhagic lesions. On microscopic examination the abnormalities are seen to be related to blood vessels, predominantly small veins but also small arteries. There is necrosis of vessel walls, with fibrinous exsudation, perivascular edema, hemorrhages, neutrophilic granulocytes in the vessel walls, perivascular spaces and adjacent brain tissue and perivascular demyelination. The demyelination is usually associated with necrosis and at least some loss of axons. In severely necrotic areas all axons may disappear. Perivascular demyelination is also seen surrounding apparently normal vessels.

Both in ADEM and in AHEM the severity, type, and localization of the pathological changes are unrelated to the type of preceding disease. In both syndromes the parenchymal pathology is often associated with meningeal lymphocytic infiltrates.

54.3 Pathogenetic Considerations

The early theories on ADEM and AHEM speculated that these syndromes might represent a delayed but direct invasion of the CNS by a virus or reactivation of a latent virus. There has, however, been a considerable amount of evidence against these theories. The pathological changes are fairly uniform and quite unlike those of the viral encephalitides, the demonstration of viral antigens or viral particles in the brain or the CSF being an exception.

Some observations led to the theory that ADEM and AHEM represent an autoimmune response to myelin constituents. First of all, the same neurological syndrome was found in patients vaccinated with rabies vaccine grown in rabbit spinal cord. Secondly, a comparable neurological syndrome was reported in animals after the repeated injection of CNS homogenate in combination with Freund's adjuvant. This syndrome is known as experimental allergic encephalomyelitis. Pathologically, the lesions of ADEM and experimental allergic encephalomyelitis have marked similarities. The white matter shows perivascular cuffing by inflammatory cells and demyelination. The cerebral hemispheres, cerebellum, brain stem and spinal cord are involved. A hyperacute form of allergic encephalomyelitis has been induced in animals with alteration of the immunization regimen. Pathologically, more hemorrhagic features are present, similar to AHEM. Sensitization of lymphocytes to nervous tissue antigen and especially to myelin basic protein has been shown in a variety of postinfectious neurological disorders, including ADEM and AHEM. Experimental allergic encephalomyelitis results from T cell sensitization to myelin basic protein. The delayed hypersensitivity to myelin basic protein leads to an attack on myelin sheaths with subsequent demyelination. The demyelination is predominantly perivascular as the responsible T cells originate from the blood. ADEM and AHEM may represent the human counterparts of experimental allergic encephalomyelitis with breakdown of tolerance to myelin antigens. It is possible that the viral proteins serve as an antigen that cross-reacts with myelin antigens. It is also possible that during the initial phase of viral invasion there is subclinical involvement of the CNS, with release or exposure of sequestered neural antigens and subsequent sensitization to them. These theories, however, do not explain the rarity of ADEM and AHEM following a viral infection of the CNS, such as herpes virus or cytomegalovirus, nor its low incidence in general. How a wide variety of infections and vaccinations can induce similar sensitization to myelin antigens has also not been explained satisfactorily.

An alternative theory stresses the importance of the vascular changes, which are almost invariably present, and has coined the term disseminated vasculomyelinopathy. The detection of circulating antigen-antibody complexes in the serum of patients with a variety of postinfectious neurological disorders led to the assumption of a vascular lesion due to the entrapment of immune complexes in vessel walls and the subsequent inflammatory response. Because perivascular demyelination can result from vascular injury alone, the participation of delayed hypersensitivity would not be necessary. The presence or absence of immune complexes, the size and the number of the complexes, and not the antecedent illness would thus be the major factor in the development of ADEM and AHEM, and the development of delayed hypersensitivity to myelin antigens would be merely an epiphenomenon resulting from nervous tissue damage. However, it is not clear why the nervous system should be preferentially involved in immune complex mediated vasculitis. Only some indirect evidence supports this theory: the detection of circulating complexes in some patients with various postinfectious neurological disorders, the presence of systemic features compatible with immune complex disease in occasional patients, and the occurrence of similar nervous system abnormalities in other human disorders caused by immune complexes. Immune complexes have, however, not been found at sites of vessel injury, and it is not impossible that the complexes themselves only represent an epiphenomenon.

The two hypotheses explained here are not mutually exclusive. Immune complex vasculitis results in increased vascular permeability. Changes in vascular permeability and perivascular inflammation can either alter the antigenicity of myelin or release an antigen previously sequestered by a competent blood-brain barrier. The cell-mediated immune response could then perpetuate the damage and lead to demyelination. In some patients perivascular demyelination is seen, whereas in others the pathological picture is dominated by perivascular necrosis. It is hypothesized that pure demyelination may be caused by hypersensitivity to myelin antigens alone and that necrosis associated with inflammatory infiltration occurs when there is production of antibodies directed against several components of the brain parenchyma.

54.4 Therapy

Corticosteroids have frequently been used in the management of ADEM and AHEM. Occasionally, dramatic clinical improvement is seen. Relapses have occurred when steroids were withdrawn, and improvement recurred when steroids were reinstituted. The fact that the improvement is sometimes absent or only slight may be explained by the presence of irreversible structural damage prior to institution of the steroid therapy. It is recommended that corticosteroid therapy be initiated as soon as possible in the treatment of these syndromes.

54.5 Magnetic Resonance Imaging

In ADEM, CT scan of the brain shows multifocal or diffuse white matter damage, but it may be normal in the acute stage, or may remain normal throughout. In addition to nonenhancing lesions, enhancement may be seen. There is a limited correlation between clinical signs and the radiological distribution of the lesions. CT can seldom explain the full extent of clinical disability, and, conversely, several lesions may be seen for which no correlative clinical signs are observed. Clinical improvement is accompanied by disappearance of contrast enhancement and complete or partial resolution of low-density lesions.

In AHEM the white matter lesions are characterized on CT by extensive edema with prominent mass effect.

MRI in ADEM shows multiple, usually large white matter lesions with an asymmetrical distribution (Figs. 54.1, 54.2). In very extensive cases, in which almost all white matter is involved, the asymmetrical distribution becomes less clear. Symmetry of lesions is exceptional. Smaller, multiple sclerosis-like lesions may also occur. The lesions have a preference for the occipital and parietal area. The white matter lesion may "spill into" the cortex with some focal cortical involvement. Mass effect is rare. Spinal lesions have been visualized by MRI. After contrast injection some of the white matter lesions may enhance. The enhancement is sometimes patchy, while sometimes filling the lesion. Ring-enhancement has also been reported. The presence of both enhancing and nonenhancing lesions argues in favor of the lesions being in different stages of development. Repeated MRI during the course of the disease may show disappearance of some lesions and concurrent appearance of others. These observations modify the view that ADEM is always simply monophasic. Improvement of white matter lesions may take a long time, as much as 18 months, and part of the white matter damage may be permanent (Figs. 54.2, 54.3). New lesions may appear despite clinical improvement.

Apart from the difference in preferential involvement of brain structures, it may be difficult to distinguish ADEM from multiple sclerosis. If the clinical story is not indicative of a preceding infection or vaccination, or when the disease presents with a single symptom such as optic neuritis, it is impossible to differentiate between acute multiple sclerosis and ADEM on the basis of an MR image. Extensive lesions with parietal and occipital lesions are indicative of ADEM. Repeated MRI examinations over a long period of time may be helpful, in particular in combination with follow-up of the clinical course. Stationary lasting lesions are indicative of ADEM while newly appearing lesions dispute this diagnosis, but this is by no means an absolute rule.

In exceptional cases, one may find a clinical picture suggestive of ADEM while MRI shows predominantly or exclusively gray matter lesions. These gray matter lesions may disappear. Probably the "gray matter-ADEM" is the counterpart of the "regular" ADEM, just like Guillain-Barré syndrome is usually a demyelinating polyneuropathy, but sometimes axonal.

In AHEM the hemorrhagic component can be identified with confidence by MRI. The hemorrhagic aspect which is unusual in multiple sclerosis and its variants, may help to establish the correct diagnosis (Fig. 54.4).

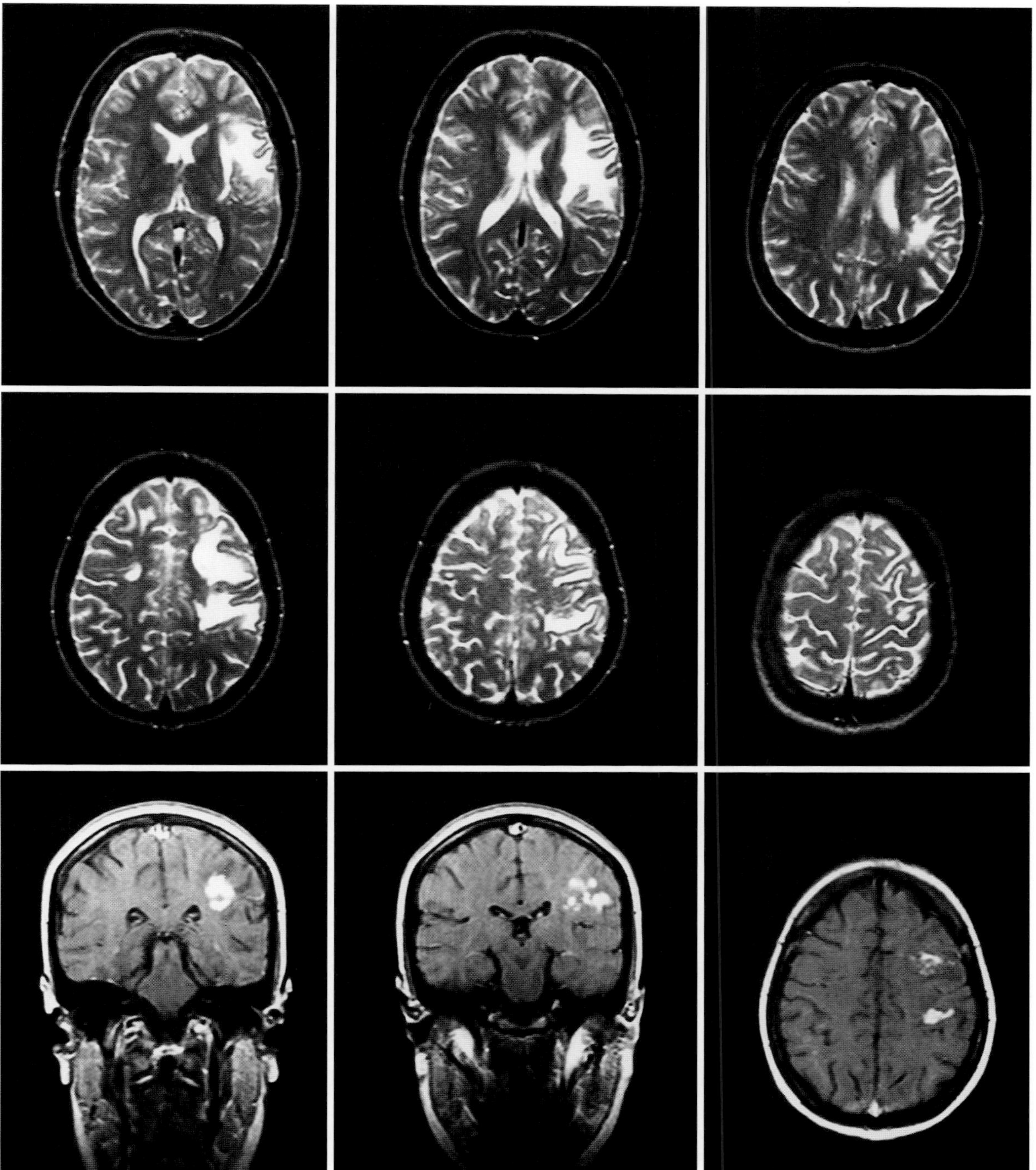

Fig. 54.1. A 14-year-old girl with acute onset of hemiplegia, fever, drowsiness, and disorientation. The chest X-ray showed pneumonia, which proved to be caused by Mycoplasma pneumoniae. The T_2-weighted transverse series shows involvement of white matter in the left peri-insular region, the left fronto-parietal region, extending into the arcuate fibers and several smaller foci in the right hemisphere. After injection of gadolinium, some of the lesions enhance. This image can also be seen in children with multiple sclerosis or infections of the brain

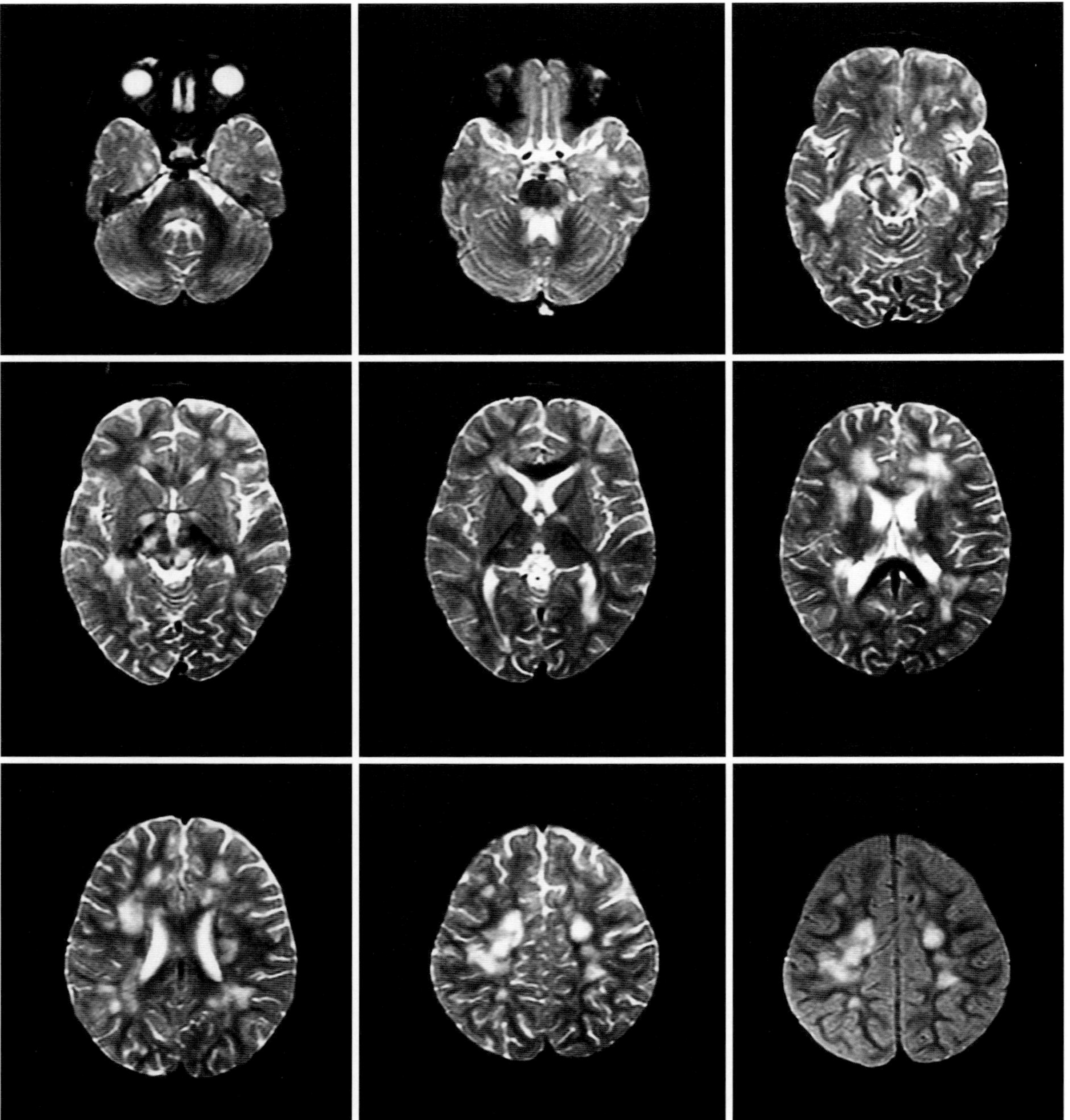

Fig. 54.2. A 3-year-old girl who had suffered a viral infection 3 weeks previously. She then became acutely ill with lowered consciousness. The T_2-weighted MR series shows the involvement of the pons, mesencephalon, and basal ganglia and an irregular pattern of focal areas of high signal intensity with an asymmetrical distribution, and relative sparing of the occipital lobe

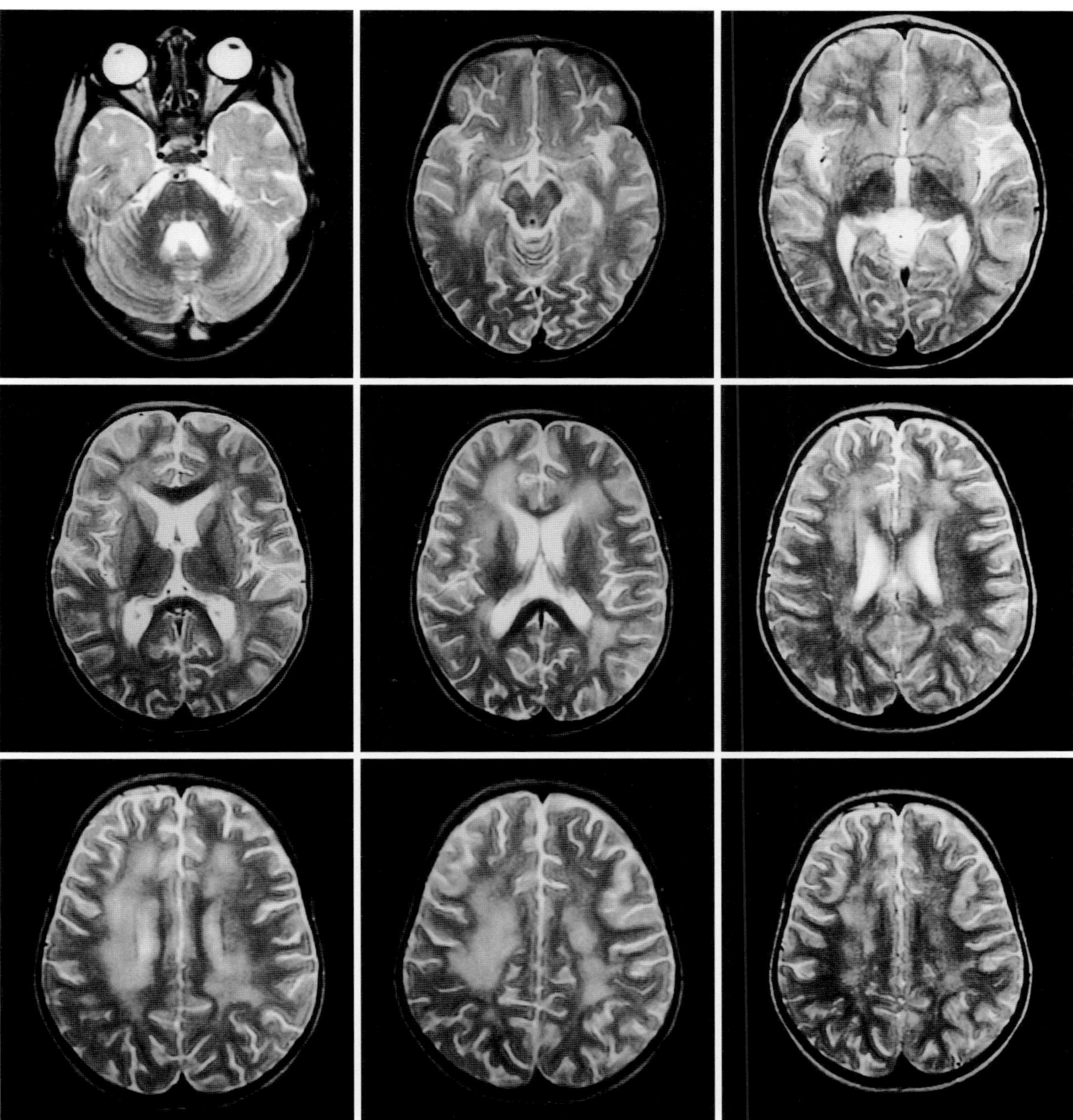

Fig. 54.3. Same patient as in Fig. 54.2. With corticosteroid treatment, this patient showed gradual clinical improvement. In the MR images, the abnormal areas show a less high signal intensity and blurring of the borders. In a matter of weeks the lesions resolved almost completely

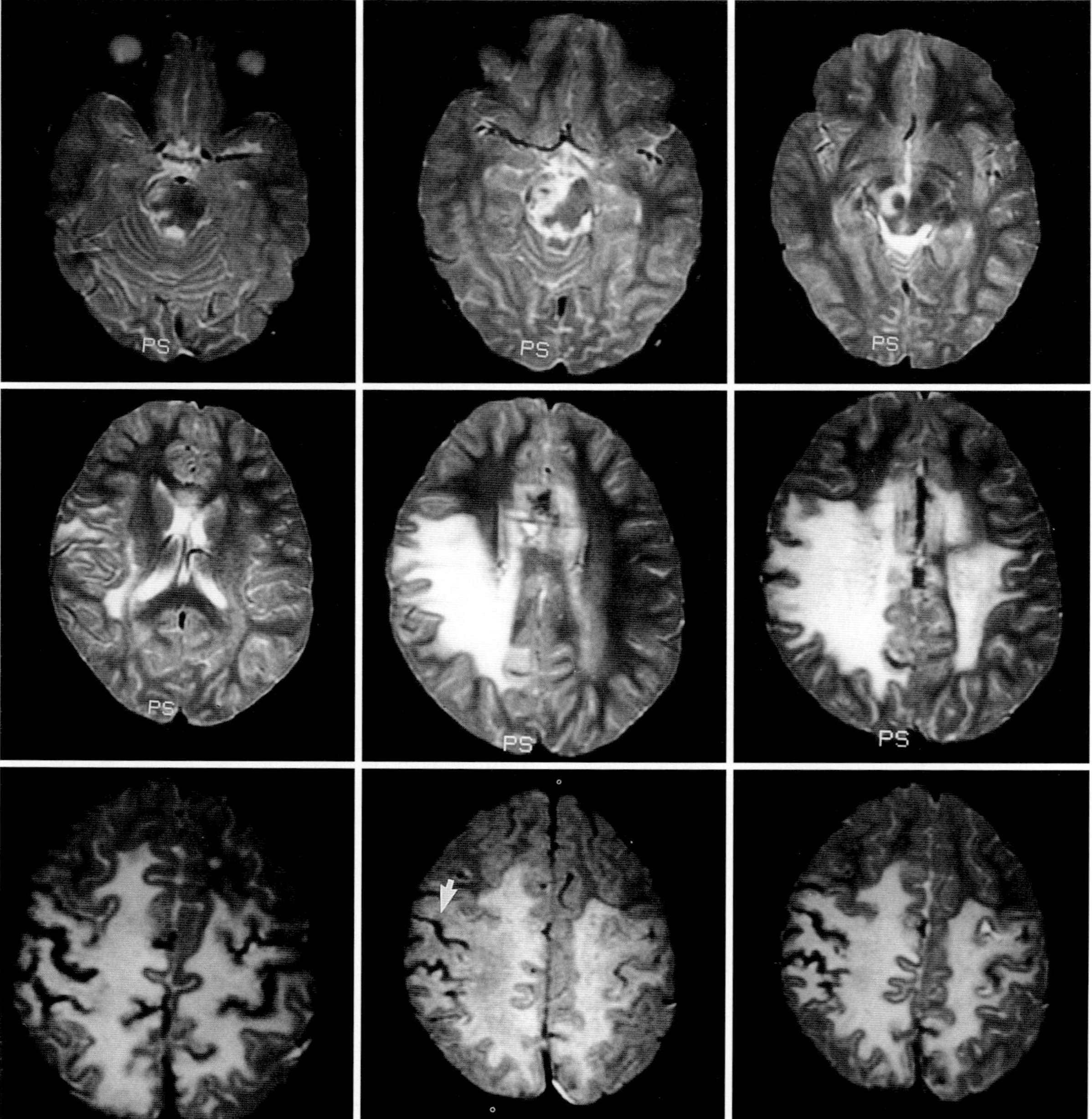

Fig. 54.4. Acutely ill boy, 8 years of age, following a minor infection a few weeks prior to admission. The T$_2$-weighted MR images show involvement of pons and mesencephalon, especially on the right side, and supratentorially large confluent areas of abnormal white matter. The abnormalities extend into the U fibers. The gyral pattern is marked by a very low signal intensity (*arrow*), caused by the presence of breakdown products of hemoglobin. The presence of a considerable degree of hemorrhage classifies this patient as a case of AHEM. (Courtesy of A. Goulao, Lisbon, Portugal)

55 Acquired Immunodeficiency Syndrome

55.1 Clinical Features and Laboratory Investigations

The acquired immunodeficiency syndrome (AIDS), as defined according to the criteria from the Centers of Disease Control, is a state characterized by one or more opportunistic diseases indicative of underlying cellular immunodeficiency in the absence of underlying causes of cellular immunodeficiency other than human immunodeficiency virus type 1 (HIV-1) infection and in the absence of all other causes of reduced resistance reported to be associated with opportunistic diseases. The opportunistic diseases in AIDS include opportunistic infections and neoplasms that can result from immunodeficiency. AIDS is caused by the retrovirus HIV-1. This virus has previously been designated human T-cell lymphotropic virus type III (HTLV-III), lymphadenopathy-associated virus (LAV), and AIDS-related virus (ARV). High-risk groups in non-Third World countries have been defined as homosexual or bisexual males, intravenous drug abusers, immigrants from Haiti and Central Africa, blood transfusion recipients, heterosexual partners of AIDS patients, children of mothers with AIDS, and hemophiliacs who have received factor VIII concentrate. About 72% of the AIDS patients originate from the first mentioned risk group, 17% from the second risk group. The other risk groups constitute only minor percentages of the total AIDS patient population.

AIDS can manifest itself in many different ways. Most patients present with malignant tumors and/or infections that are infrequently seen in immunocompetent individuals. The most common tumors in AIDS are Kaposi's sarcoma, primary CNS lymphoma, systemic non-Hodgkin lymphoma, and plasmocytoma. The opportunistic infections most frequently include Pneumocystis carinii pneumonia, toxoplasmosis, cryptococcal meningitis, candidiasis of the upper gastrointestinal tract, and many other viruses, fungi, mycobacteria, and parasites. Nonspecific signs and symptoms of the disease are weight loss, fatigue, malaise, night sweats, fever, and generalized lymphadenopathy. Neurological signs and symptoms are frequent and are reported in 30%–75% of patients. Malignant lymphoma and metastatic Kaposi's sarcoma may affect the CNS. Opportunistic infections of the CNS include her-

pes simplex encephalitis, herpes zoster encephalitis and radiculitis, cytomegalovirus encephalitis, papovavirus infection with progressive multifocal leukoencephalitis, infection with Aspergillus fumigatus, Candida albicans, and Cryptococcus neoformans, nocardiosis, coccidioidomycosis, Mycobacterium tuberculosis, and atypical mycobacterial infections, toxoplasmosis, and neurosyphilis. However, only a minority (about 30%) of the CNS affections can be attributed to opportunistic infections. A primary HIV-1 infection is the most common cause of neurological dysfunction. Acute diffuse leukoencephalitis, subacute encephalitis, aseptic meningitis, vacuolar myelopathy, and inflammatory demyelinating peripheral neuropathy are generally assumed to be probably caused by direct HIV-1 infection. Subacute HIV-1 encephalitis, also called AIDS encephalopathy or AIDS dementia complex, is the most frequent neurological manifestation of AIDS and eventually afflicts many AIDS patients. Subacute HIV-1 encephalitis usually develops after other complications of AIDS have appeared, but it may also be the first major or even the sole clinical manifestation of HIV-1 infection. Acute diffuse leukoencephalitis, with severe neurological symptoms and often fatal outcome has been described in a limited number of cases. Other neurological complications include cerebral hemorrhage and cerebral infarction. Thrombocytopenia predisposes AIDS patients to cerebral hemorrhage, while nonbacterial thrombotic endocarditis may lead to cerebral infarction.

Demyelinating white matter lesions are a major neuropathological finding in HIV-1 infections of the CNS, and the remainder of this chapter focuses on acute and subacute HIV encephalitis and vacuolar myelopathy.

In subacute HIV encephalitis, cognitive, motor, and behavioral abnormalities are usually early features. Early cognitive abnormalities are impaired memory, loss of concentration, confusion, and slowing of mentation and movement. The onset of dementia is usually insidious, but a rapid onset over a period of a few days and accelerations are not rare. Behavioral abnormalities include apathy, social withdrawal, dysphoric mood, organic psychosis, and regressive behavior. Early motor symptoms are lack of balance, weakness of the legs, tremor, and loss of coordination. Neurological examination often reveals ataxia and pyramidal tract signs. The majority of patients develop a severe and global dementia within 2 months after the onset of symptoms, but sometimes the initial course is more protracted, and a mild or moderate impairment of intellectual functions is present for several months prior to the subsequent onset of a more severe global dementia. The dementia of subacute HIV-1 encephalitis has been described as subcortical because of the relative absence in many patients of seizures and other signs of focal cortical involvement. The affected patients usually remain alert. Neurological symptoms in the end stages are variable and include aphasia, ataxia, hypertonia, motor weakness with paraparesis, quadriparesis or hemiparesis, pseudobulbar palsy with dysphagia and dysarthria, tremor, blindness, extrapyramidal signs with rigidity, incontinence, myoclonus, epileptic seizures, and sometimes organic psychosis. Retinopathy is found in about one-third of the patients with subacute HIV-1 encephalitis. Cotton wool spots are the most frequently observed retinal abnormalities; less frequently a hemorrhagic retinitis is seen. Optic neuritis is a rare finding. Death usually occurs within 1 year after the first signs of encephalopathy are noted.

Acute diffuse leukoencephalitis is a much rarer condition, described in a small number of patients. Clinically the disease is characterized by a rapid mental deterioration, progressive tetraparesis and in some cases death within a few days. A relapsing-remitting course of disease has also been described, indistinguishable from multiple sclerosis.

The majority of children with AIDS are born to women who have AIDS or pre-AIDS themselves and who are intravenous drug abusers, sexual partners of male members of high-risk groups, or of Haitian origin. In a smaller percentage of the affected children, transfusion-associated AIDS has been implicated. Clinical characteristics of AIDS in children include failure to thrive, generalized lymphadenopathy, hepatosplenomegaly, recurrent bacterial infections, and infections with opportunistic agents. Neurological abnormalities are variable. The most consistent findings are acquired microcephaly and moderate to severe mental retardation. Motor deficits ranging in severity include pyramidal tract signs with spastic paraparesis or tetraparesis and pseudobulbar palsy. Hypotonia with hyperreflexia is frequent in affected children, especially early in the course of disease. In some children, psychomotor retardation is stationary. In others progressive mental and motor deterioration occurs with a remitting course. Subacute HIV-1 encephalitis can be found in this latter group of patients.

Vacuolar myelopathy is a common neurological complication in AIDS. It is frequently difficult to correlate spinal cord abnormalities with clinical symptoms and signs in individual patients since many patients have coexistent encephalopathy or peripheral neuropathy. Clinical features may be a spastic monoparesis, paraparesis, or tetraparesis with hyperreflexia and extensor plantar reflexes, but sometimes reflexes are absent. Incontinence and sexual disturbances are frequent as well as sensory abnormalities with sensory ataxia. Neuropathologically, grades I, II and III myelopathy can be distinguished. A steadily progressive spastic-ataxic paraparesis which usually evolves over several weeks to months is most characteristic of patients with grade III, severe myelopathy. Signs and symptoms are similar but less severe in patients with grade II myelopathy. Clear myelopathic signs are infrequent in patients with grade I myelopathy.

Patients with AIDS are susceptible to a number of PNS complications. Peripheral nerve affections occur in about half of the patients with subacute encephalitis. Cranial nerve signs are less prominent. Apart from herpes zoster radiculitis, a distal symmetrical peripheral polyneuropathy, chronic inflammaotry demyelinating polyradiculoneuropathy, and mononeuritis multiplex have been described. Distal symmetrical peripheral neuropathy manifests itself by distal sensory disturbances and a mild degree of weakness in the distal muscles of the lower extremities. The symptoms are predominantly sensory with burning, painful paresthesias, and numbness. In more advanced stages the muscular weakness may become more marked and spread to the arms. Chronic inflammatory demyelinating polyradiculoneuropathy resembles the Guillain-Barré syndrome but the course is subacute or chronic more often. Weakness is most severe in distal muscles but also affects proximal muscles. Sensory abnormalities are usually less marked. In severe cases weakness becomes generalized, and facial diplegia, bulbar weakness, and respiratory difficulties result. In mononeuritis multiplex, nerve dysfunction is relatively abrupt in onset. In the course of time, multiple nerves become involved, resulting in patchy weakness and sensory loss.

The evaluation of a patient suspected of AIDS includes investigations of the immune system and diagnostic studies to determine whether localized or disseminated infection or malignancy exists. Serological studies for a number of infections are frequently positive, such as hepatitis A and B, herpes group viruses, and toxoplasmosis. If indicated, cultures of body fluids for bacteria, mycobacteria, viruses, and fungi may be performed. Immunological investigations may include tests demonstrating cutaneous anergy to recall antigens, depressed response in lymphocyte transformation assays, and usually a decreased natural killer cell activity. Studies of T lymphocyte subpopulations in AIDS reveal a depletion of CD4+ T helper cells with an inversion of the CD4+ helper to CD8+ suppressor cell ratio. Lymphopenia may be present. These immunological abnormalities may be absent early in the disease. Abnormalities in B cell function and humoral immunity have been reported. Immunoglobulin levels may be high due to nonspecific polyclonal B cell activation. Circulating immune complexes may be present. The most specific diagnosis of HIV infection is by direct identification of the virus in tissue or blood of suspected patients or indirectly by demonstrating the presence of antibodies to the virus. Longitudinal studies have shown that in serum, HIV-1 antigens appear early and transiently in primary HIV-1 infection. Antibody production follows, after which HIV antigens may disappear. Symptomless carries have serum anti-HIV antibodies, but rarely serum HIV antigens. Most AIDS patients, on the other hand, have serum HIV antigens as well as antibodies. Persistence or reappearance of HIV antigens seems to correlate with the development of full-blown AIDS.

The CSF of patients with HIV infection of the CNS usually has a slightly raised protein content and less often a mononuclear pleocytosis with cell counts of up to 50 cells/mm^3. The CSF of children with AIDS encephalopathy shows these abnormalities less often. The CSF of patients with AIDS encephalopathy often contains oligoclonal immunoglobulin bands which have anti-HIV activity. CSF anti-HIV antibodies are present in most AIDS patients, irrespective of the presence of neurological complications. These antibodies occur early in the course of the disease, indicative of an early seeding of HIV to the CNS. A longitudinal study showed that HIV-1 antigen is present transiently in CSF before the occurrence of antibody. HIV-1 antigen continues to be present in children and adults with progressive AIDS encephalopathy. As a rule, it is not found in the CSF of symptomless seropositive controls, some of whom have anti-HIV antibodies in the CSF. Persistence of HIV-1 antigens in the CSF most probably reflects ongoing CNS involvement. HIV-1 antigens in the CSF are not a result of leakage of viral proteins through the blood-brain barrier, as in some patients the quantity of HIV-1 antigens is larger in CSF than in serum, whereas other patients have extremely high serum levels and no HIV-1 antigens in the CSF. The same arguments apply to anti-HIV antibodies, proving that the synthesis of these CSF antibodies occurs within the blood-brain barrier.

The EEG often shows moderate, generalized slowing of the background pattern in subacute HIV-1 encephalitis, occasionally with nonperiodic high-voltage spiking. Even in patients with seizures or myoclonic jerks, paroxysomal discharges are not usually seen.

In patients with distal symmetrical peripheral neuropathy the nerve conduction velocity is normal or slightly reduced. EMG shows some signs of denervation in distal muscles. In chronic inflammatory demyelinating polyneuropathy a marked slowing of nerve conduction is the rule. The abnormalities are frequently patchy. F responses are prolonged or absent, which is in conformity with a component of radiculopathy. Conduction block is a common finding. EMG is either normal or shows signs of denervation and reinnervation.

55.2 Pathology

It has been estimated that approximately 40% of patients with AIDS have clinically apparent CNS dysfunction. At autopsy, neuropathological abnormalities are found in about 80% of patients, and 20% of patients have multiple coexisting CNS disease processes. Neuropathological signs of subacute HIV-1 encephalitis are found in about 50% of patients with AIDS, and it is accordingly the most common CNS illness associated with AIDS.

The brains of patients with subacute HIV-1 encephalitis usually show some degree of atrophy at postmortem examination. Mild to moderate ventricular dilatation is associated with an apparent reduction of cerebral white matter and shrunken cortical gyri. The most prominent microscopic abnormalities in the brain involve the white matter and deep-seated gray matter. Subacute HIV-1 encephalitis, also called giant cell encephalitis or microglial nodule encephalitis, is characterized by intraparenchymal and perivascular infiltrations of lymphocytes and macrophages, located both in gray and white matter. The perivascular infiltrations occur typically around capillaries and venules and are most frequently detected in the centrum semiovale, basal ganglia, and pons. In mild cases the infiltrates are lymphocytic and scanty. In more severe cases, inflammatory infiltrates are composed mainly of foamy macrophages, in some instances intermixed with multinucleated giant cells. These multinucleated cells are thought to be derived from macrophages as they display macrophage markers, and are considered to be a histopathological hallmark.

The most common white matter abnormality is diffuse pallor, demonstrated by myelin staining. The borders of these large areas of pallor are ill defined. The subcortical white matter is relatively spared. There is some variability in the regional intensity of the pallor, which is most prominent in the centrum semiovale. The myelin loss is accompanied by a loss of axons, but the axons are relatively better preserved. Diffuse reactive astrocytosis occurs and generally parallels the inflammatory and parenchymal changes. In addition, most patients have small, poorly defined foci of more complete demyelination. These usually have a perivascular distribution. The lesions are associated with inflammatory infiltrates, which are composed of lymphocytes, lipid-laden foamy macrophages, reactive astrocytes, microglia, and sometimes multinucleated cells. Another common finding is vacuolation of the white matter, most frequently observed in the centrum semiovale and less commonly in the internal capsule, brain stem, and cerebellum. Electron-microscopic examination shows intramyelin vacuoles.

The cerebral cortex is relatively normal. Astrocytosis is usually only found in the deep cortical layers. Considerable neuronal damage and loss is seen only in cases of severe white matter changes. Inflammatory infiltrations with presence of macrophages, lymphocytes, multinucleated cells, and reactive astrocytes are present in the basal ganglia and brain stem. Sometimes focal areas of coagulation necrosis with cavitation are seen, principally in the basal ganglia.

Microglial nodules with multinucleated giant cells are found in both gray and white matter, in the latter case often accompanied by demyelinating lesions. HIV-1 virus has been identified in these nodules. In a number of cases, however, the microglial nodules contain cells with the intranuclear and intracytoplasmic inclusion material typical of cytomegalovirus infection. Microglial nodules may be the consequence of either HIV-1 infection or cytomegalovirus infection. Cytomegalovirus-associated nodules are usually distinguished by their predominant localization within the cortical gray matter and by the presence of characteristic intranuclear inclusion bodies within or near the nodules.

Ultrastructural studies of the brain in subacute HIV-1 encephalitis reveals many virus-like particles in the cytoplasm of most macrophages and multinucleated giant cells and, less often, in astrocytes, but not in neurons and oligodendrocytes. These particles are double-membraned structures which contain cylindrical nucleoids characteristic of the lentivirus subfamily of the retrovirus group. These structures have been identified as HIV-1. In addition to complete infectious HIV-1 virions, HIV-1 RNA, HIV-1 DNA, and HIV-1 core proteins have been identified in the brains, but also in the CSF, of patients with subacute HIV-1 encephalitis. Macrophages and multinucleated cells of macrophage origin appear to be infected, but there is evidence that some other cells are also infected to a lesser extent.

Histological examination of acute diffuse leukoencephalitis reveals demyelination, most pronounced in the centrum semiovale. There is also axonal loss, but axons are relatively better preserved than myelin. Microglial nodules and multinucleated giant cells may be present but have also been reported as absent. Inflammatory reaction is variable. The demyelinating lesion may extend into the frontal, occipital and temporal area. The basal nuclei, thalamus, and brain stem may also be involved in the process. The lesions may be large and multifocal or highly confluent, symmetrical or asymmetrical. Presence of HIV-1 genome in the brain has been shown. Tests for all other infections, in particular cytomegalovirus, were negative.

In multiple sclerosis-like leukoencephalopathy, multiple, large, well-defined areas of demyelination can be shown, which may involve hemispheral white matter, internal capsule, basal nuclei, optic tracts, corpus callosum, brain stem and cerebellum. These lesions are characterized by myelin loss with presence of lipid-laden macrophages and preservation of axons and nerve cell bodies, associated with marked gliosis and presence of perivascular inflammatory infiltrates. Multinucleated giant cells and microglial nodules are reported as absent. Direct evidence of HIV-1 infection has not (yet) been provided, although in one case, increase in CSF HIV-1 antigen during exacerbations has been demonstrated.

In children with progressive HIV-1 encephalopathy, brain weight is below normal for age, and sometimes there is obvious atrophy. Most of the brains show evidence of white matter disease, including pallor, diffuse lack of myelin, and astrocytosis. Probably both hypomyelination and demyelination are responsible for the diffuse lack of myelin. The axons are relatively better preserved than in adults. Calcification often occurs within or adjacent to the walls of small vessels in the basal ganglia and central white matter of the cerebral hemispheres, especially in the frontal lobes. Inflammatory cell infiltrates which resemble classic microglial nodules but which are larger are commonly observed. They consist of microglia, astrocytes, lymphocytes, a few plasma cells, and often multinucleated cells, which in part have the proportions of multinucleated giant cells. The inflammatory infiltrates are most often located in basal ganglia and pons but also in other gray and white matter structures of brain and spinal cord. In addition, vascular or perivascular inflammation may be present, involving small or medium-sized arteries or veins. The inflammation of intraparenchymal vessels is accompanied by intimal fibrosis of medium-sized vessels and endarteritis obliterans with focal thrombosis of small vessels.

Spinal cord disease afflicts approximately 25% of AIDS patients. Pathological changes are most prominent in the lateral and posterior columns at the thoracic level, less severe in the anterolateral and anterior columns. White matter changes are often asymmetrical and are not confined to specific anatomic tracts. Microscopically, the disease is characterized by intramyelin vacuoles, similar to those seen in cerebral and cerbellar white matter. Axons are intact except in the most severely affected areas. The white matter vacuolation is associated with few lipid-laden macrophages, usually located within the vacuoles. Reactive astrocytes are rare, and inflammation is not present as a rule.

55.3 **Pathogenetic Considerations**

HIV-1 has been clearly identified as the primary cause of AIDS. HIV-1 is the prototypical member of the Lentivirinae subfamily of retroviruses affecting humans. Lentiviruses characteristically cause indolent infections in their host. These infections are notable for involvement of the nervous system, long periods of clinical latency and weak humoral immune responses complicated by persistent virus presence. One feature that distinguishes the lentiviruses from other retroviruses is the remarkable complexity of their viral genomes. Most retroviruses capable of replication contain only three genes. HIV-1, however, contains in its RNA genome at least six additional genes. It is probable that the distinct but concerted actions of these additional genes underlie the profound pathogenicity of HIV-1. From a therapeutic standpoint, this same genomic complexity may also be the Achilles heel of the virus. A broad-based search for antagonists specific for these HIV-1 gene products has started. High-resolution electron microscopy has revealed the HIV-1 virion as an icosahedral structure containing 72 external spikes. These spikes are formed by the two major viral-envelope proteins, gp120 and gp41. The HIV-1 lipid bilayer is also studded with various host proteins, including class I and class II major histocompatibility (MHC) antigens, acquired during virion budding. Details about the core of the virion are now also known. HIV-1 has a selective tropism of CD4+ T helper-inducer lymphocytes. The human CD4+ T lymphocyte and monocyte are the major cellular targets for HIV-1 infection, because the CD4 membrane antigen represents the principal, if not sole, high affinity receptor for this retrovirus. After entry of the CD4+ T lymphocyte, the viral RNA is transcribed into DNA and subsequently integrated into the CD4+ T lymphocyte DNA during cell divison. In inactive CD4+ T cells much of the viral DNA remains unintegrated in the cytoplasm. The HIV replication cycle is restricted until the CD4+ T cell is activated by other pathogens (for instance, hepatitis B virus, herpes simplex virus, cytomegalovirus) or by allogeneic stimulation (for instance, exposure to allogeneic semen, blood, or allografts). After activation transcription occurs in RNA, followed by protein synthesis. Viral proteins and viral RNA assemble. Mature viruses are formed by budding from the cytoplasmic membrane. In the process of HIV replication the CD4+ T cell is killed. The mechanism of cell death is unclear. The killing of CD4+ T-cell lymphocytes leads to depletion of this type of cells. Faster depletion of CD4+ T cells may result from enhanced susceptibility to superinfection by other pathogens, for example, by cytomegalovirus. CD4+ T lymphocytes play a central role in the immune response, and their depletion leads to many immunological abnormalities. The cellular (T-cell) immune system essentially ceases to function, but there are also marked abnormalities in B cell activation (humoral immune system) and immunoregulation. There is a state of polyclonal B cell activation with high immunoglobulin levels and a poor antibody response to new antigens. The deficiency of cellular immunity leads to an extreme susceptibility to viruses, fungi, mycobacteria, and parasites – agents that require cell-mediated immunity for containment. Neoplasms arising in a cellular immunodeficiency state include primarily lymphomas and Kaposi's sarcoma. The B cell dysregulation may explain the frequent occurrence of severe pyogenic infections, in particular with Streptococcus pneumoniae and Haemophilus influenzae. The elevated production of nonspecific immunoglobulins may lead to autoimmune processes, such as immune thrombocytopenia. In addition, CD4+ T antigens are also present on the cell surface of certain types of macrophages and monocytes, which may therefore also be infected by HIV-1. The infection of these cells results in additional immunological deficits, especially in chemotaxis.

HIV-1 leads to a persisting infection. The viral genetic information is integrated in the DNA of the host cell, and the virus can only be destroyed by killing the infected cells. It has been demonstrated that a small percentage of infected cells may survive and contribute to virus persistence. Infected monocytes and macrophages may contribute to the persistence of HIV-1 as they appear to be relatively resistent to the cytolytic effect of HIV-1.

HIV-1 appears to be transmitted predominantly by contact with infected blood or semen. However, the virus has also been isolated from cervicovaginal secretions, tears, urine, saliva, breast milk, and CSF. Although there is no proof that these fluids are involved in the transmission of AIDS, the possibility cannot be excluded. HIV may be transmitted to a child in utero, during birth, or postnatally through infected breast milk.

The clinical picture of patients with HIV-1 infections can range from asymptomatic (carrier with viremia or antibody or both) through chronic generalized lymphadenopathy to a variable degree of clinically manifest immunodeficiency. Currently, there is no specific test to predict which patients are likely to have the full-blown disease. The latency period between infection and full-blown AIDS ranges between several months and several years.

Substantial evidence supports a direct etiological role for HIV-1 in subacute encephalitis, aseptic meningitis, vacuolar myelopathy, and peripheral neuropathy. The intra-blood-brain barrier synthesis of HIV-1-specific antibodies has been demonstrated in the majority of AIDS patients with neurological symptoms but also in patients without these. The oligoclonal IgG bands in the CSF of AIDS patients have been demonstrated to contain anti-HIV activity. The presence of HIV-1 antigens in CSF appears to be strongly associated with CNS involvement. HIV-1 has been isolated from CSF in patients with subacute encephalitis and aseptic meningitis. The fact that virus has been isolated from CSF cannot be attributed solely to the presence of infected lymphocytes since many samples are free of cells. HIV DNA and RNA sequences have been demonstrated in CNS tissue of patients with subacute encephalitis. HIV-1 has been isolated from brain in subacute encephalitis, from the spinal cord in vacuolar myelopathy, and from the sural nerve in a patient with peripheral neuropathy. The multinucleated giant cells, seen in subacute encephalitis, show a striking similarity to the multinucleated cells that develop from the fusion of T lymphocytes infected by HIV-1 in vitro. Ultrastructural examination has identified intact retroviral particles within the multinucleated giant cells in some cases. The multinucleated cells are probably of macrophage origin, as they share morphological features and macrophage markers. Very similar multinucleated giant cells have been reported in lymph nodes in AIDS patients. There is evidence that the multinucleated giant cells are of hematogenous origin. It is possible that the virus penetrates the CNS by migration of infected mononuclear cells from the blood, but a direct viral invasion of the CNS is not excluded. Immunohistochemical identification of HIV antigen has shown that the most frequently infected cells include macrophages, microglia, and multinucleated giant cells; less frequently capillary endothelial cells, astrocytes, and oligodendroglia are infected, and also neurons, but only rarely. The virus is concentrated in, although not limited to the white matter.

The precise mechanisms underlying the structural cerebral damage remains to be determined. The low-level infection, sometimes seen in a few neurons, astrocytes, and oligodendrocytes cannot be held responsible for the severe CNS damage that is often present. The functional and structural damage of the CNS is therefore probably related indirectly to the HIV-1 infection, which primarily affects monocytes and macrophages and to a lesser degree endothelial cells. Data indicate that the extent of endothelial and macrophage infection is more commensurate with the clinical findings than the extent of neuronal and glial infection. This observation led to the suggestion that the CNS dysfunction reflects an infection of the endothelial cells that impairs the blood-brain barrier and leads to fluctuations in fluid and electrolyte levels and to structural damage. Another possibility is that activated macrophages secrete a variety of materials, such as tumor necrosis factor, interleukin, and proteolytic enzymes, that cause brain tissue damage and impairment of neurological function. An alternative is that the release of HIV-1 envelope glycoproteins from infected macrophages may interfere directly with neuronal function as these HIV-1 proteins may directly suppress neuronal responses to neurotrophic factors and cause shortened neuronal survival.

The frequent involvement of the CNS in AIDS is probably related to a number of factors. The brain is an immunologically privileged organ. HIV-1 within brain tissue may be hidden and protected from immune surveillance. In addition, the damage to the immune system caused by HIV infection promotes the persistence of viral infection. In infants the known susceptibility of the immature CNS to viral invasion plays a role and may explain the high incidence of AIDS encephalopathy in young children infected with HIV.

55.4 Therapy

From the discussion so far it is obvious that there are at least four entries to the therapeutic approach to HIV-1 infection, based upon the specific characteristics of the HIV-1 infection.

The first approach is based upon the complexity of the HIV-1 genome, which contains at least six genes in addition to the three essential genes of other retroviruses. A search is in progress to find antagonists for these HIV-1 gene products.

The second approach is based upon the dominant role played in HIV-1 infection by CD4+ T cells. An attempt has been made to use soluble forms of CD4 protein as receptor decoys; however, with little success so far. Also, primary viral isolates seem to be quite resistant to soluble CD4 analogs.

The third approach is based upon the inhibition of the viral reverse transcriptase. Several products have been tested and the best results so far have been obtained with these drugs. Three products have been used to date: $3'$asido-$2',3'$-dideoxythymidine (zidovudine), $2',3'$-dideoxycytidine (ddC), and $2',3'$-dideoxy-inosine (ddI). It has been proven in clinical trials that these products have had the best effect until now in counteracting the HIV-1 infection. Each is phosphorylated to an active triphosphate after entry into the cell and then acts either as a chain terminator of the nascent DNA strand produced by the reverse transcriptase or as a simple competitor blocking the incorporation of the respective normal nucleosides. The viral reverse transcriptase appears to incorporate these dideoxynucleoside analogs preferentially, which probably accounts for their therapeutic effectiveness. Zidovudine has been shown to prolong survival and to reduce the frequency and severity of opportunistic infections in patients with AIDS. Probably the drug also delays the progression of the disease in asymptomatic but seropositive persons. In one case of acute diffuse leukoencephalitis white matter disease was reversed with Zidovudine therapy. The principal toxic effect of zidovudine is bone marrow suppression, which frequently manifests as anemia and macrocytosis. Zidovudine and the other two compounds can be taken orally, have good CSF penetration and have toxicity patterns that do not overlap: peripheral neuropathy with ddC and ddI, pancreatitis with ddI and bone marrow suppression with Zidovudine. Alternating regimens are therefore possible.

The fourth approach is the development of an HIV-1 vaccine. The development of such a vaccine has been complicated by the remarkable sequence heterogeneity of the HIV-1 envelop proteins. Hyperimmunization of chimpansees with HIV-1 envelop protein was insufficient following injection with small quantities of the same strain of HIV-1. Recent vaccination studies (in Asian monkeys) with a simian virus (SIV-1) infection which causes an AIDS-like disease have generated exciting results and suggest that an effective HIV-1 vaccine may be an achievable goal. Given the complexity of the problem, it is not reasonable to expect such a vaccine, whole virus or subunit HIV-1, within the next 2–5 years.

Preventive measures still prevail in the battle against AIDS, the universally propagated "safe sex" being the major public prevention factor. Other preventive measures are directed towards the avoidance of contact with infected blood, screening of blood donors for AIDS, inactivation of virus in blood products such as factor VIII concentrate.

Specific measures have also been advocated in the management of HIV-1 positive pregnant women, in order to reduce the risk of neonates acquiring the disease in the peri- or postnatal period.

It is obvious that in opportunistic infections and CNS tumors appropriate therapeutic measures have to be taken. Identifying the causative agent in infections or the nature of the tumor is, therefore, important and the major role of MRI. Recently, Thallium-201 SPECT has changed the imaging algorithm of neurologically symptomatic HIV-1 patients, as it has resulted in the differentiation of CNS lymphomas from infections, making earlier and more adequate treatment possible.

55.5 Magnetic Resonance Imaging

Neuroimaging studies are essential in the evaluation of AIDS patients with neurological symptoms. A high percentage of the patients infected with HIV-1 has CNS complications, including the AIDS dementia complex, opportunistic infections and brain tumors. The primary purpose of brain imaging is to detect potentially treatable opportunistic lesions.

Most patients with advanced HIV-1 encephalitis have CT evidence of cerebral atrophy with enlargement of subarachnoid spaces and ventricles. CT evidence of atrophy may precede clinical signs of encephalitis, whereas in other cases initial CT scans may be normal and the atrophy becomes evident on later scans. Marked hypodensities in the white matter of both cerebral hemispheres are sometimes noted. An additional abnormality shown by CT scan in some children with HIV-1 infection of the CNS and less frequently in adults is calcification of basal ganglia and, less often, of the periventricular white matter and the frontal subcortical white matter. CT scans may, of course, also reveal abnormalities which are a consequence of opportunistic infections, tumors, and vascular lesions of the brain. The presence of more than one kind of lesion within one patient frequently complicates the interpretation of CT findings.

MRI has greater sensitivity than CT to identify CNS lesions in this patient population, with the exception of calcifications in basal ganglia and subcortical areas as reported in the pediatric population with AIDS. HIV-1 infection of the brain leads to a number of patterns identifiable on MRI. The most common finding in AIDS dementia complex is generalized atrophy with widened ventricles and enlarged cortical sulci with loss of cortical tissue. Probably, however, atrophy is a relatively late finding. It has been suggested that MR spectroscopy is more sensitive, already showing a decrease of the N-acetylaspartate (considered to be a neuronal marker) concentration, whereas images are still normal.

The second pattern represents the subacute HIV-1 encephalitis and reflects the histological findings of diffuse, mild myelin pallor or demyelination with preference for the frontal and parietal lobes. MRI shows symmetrical periventricular areas of mildly increased signal intensity of the white matter, not involving the U fibers, with the mentioned topological preference (Figs. 55.1–55.4). There is no enhancement after gadolinium injection. The brain stem and cerebellum are not involved. In the course of the disease the white matter abnormalities progress, eventually resulting in severe hemispheric involvement.

In acute diffuse leukencephalitis, large multifocal or more diffuse and extensive white matter abnormalities have been reported. In the case of multifocal lesions, these are not necessarily symmetrical. Hemispheral white matter, internal capsule, thalamus and brain stem may be involved. In cases in which the disease course resembles multiple sclerosis, multifocal white matter involvement is seen. Enhancement of the lesions has not been reported.

The frequency of superimposed infections is relatively low but double and multi-infections occur. Of the opportunistic infections, cerebral toxoplasmosis is the

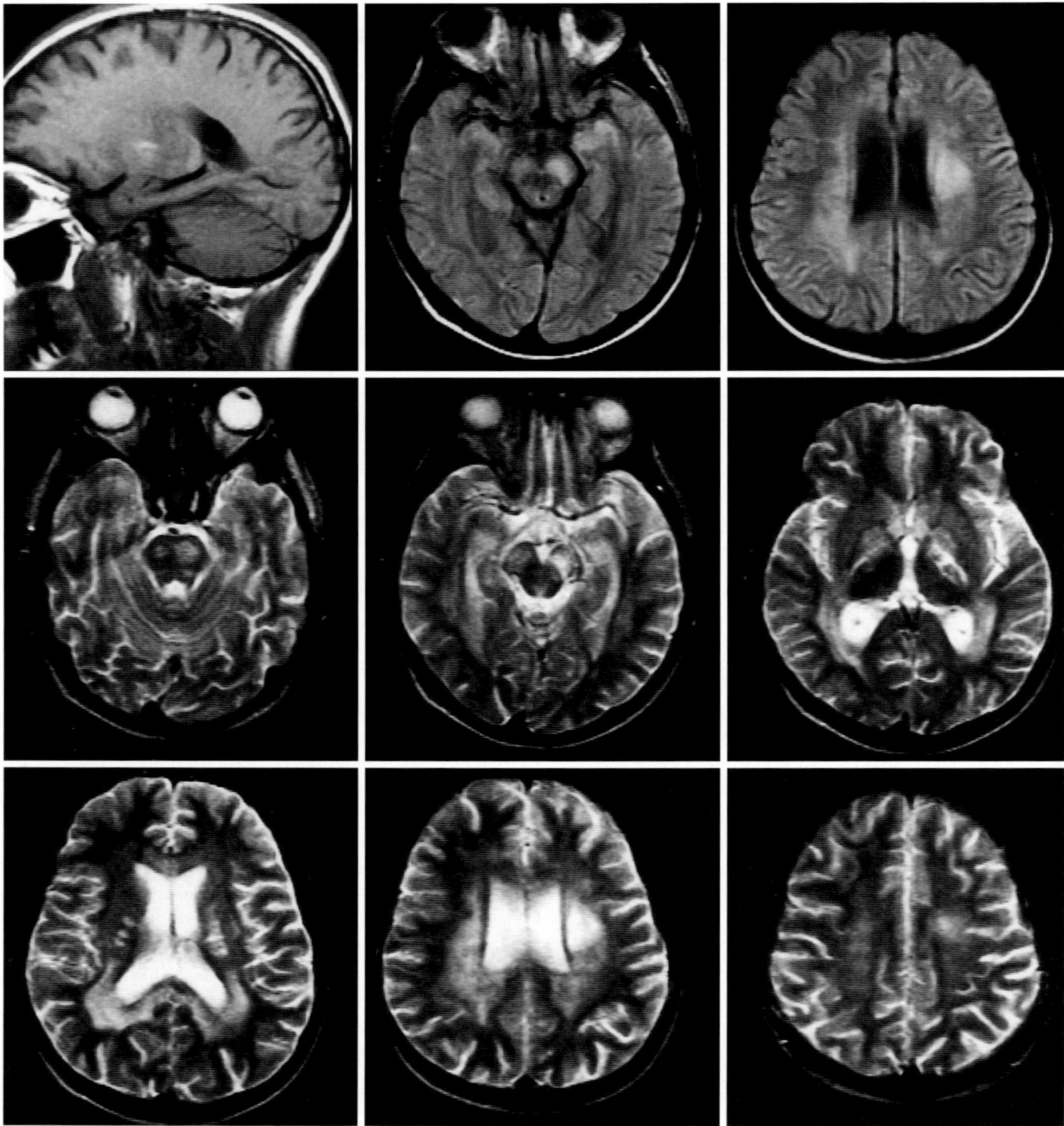

Fig. 55.1. A 24-year-old man, suffering from AIDS, with a progressive neurological syndrome and mental and emotional deterioration. The T_1-weighted sagittal image shows a mixed signal intensity lesion in the basal ganglia on the left side, probably an old hemorrhage. The transverse proton density (*upper row*) and T_2-weighted (*lower two rows*) images show lesions consistent with subacute HIV encephalitis. There is a mildly increased signal intensity in the centrum semiovale and around the ventricles, also involving the posterior limb of the internal capsule and the white matter tracts in the pons. The lesions are not perfectly symmetrical at the level of pons, mesencephalon, and periventricular area. This asymmetry is unusual for subacute HIV encephalitis, and one cannot exclude a second, superimposed type of pathology

most common. It is the presenting opportunistic infection in at least 5% of the AIDS patient population. The lesions of toxoplasmosis are multifocal, unequal in size (Fig. 55.2). Sometimes the lesions show the so-called "target" sign, with a rim of high signal intensity on T_2-weighted images and a core that is isointense with normal white matter. Lesions occur in all areas including the subcortical region, basal ganglia, brain stem and less frequently the cerebellar hemispheres. The lesions can be very large, have contact with the ventricles

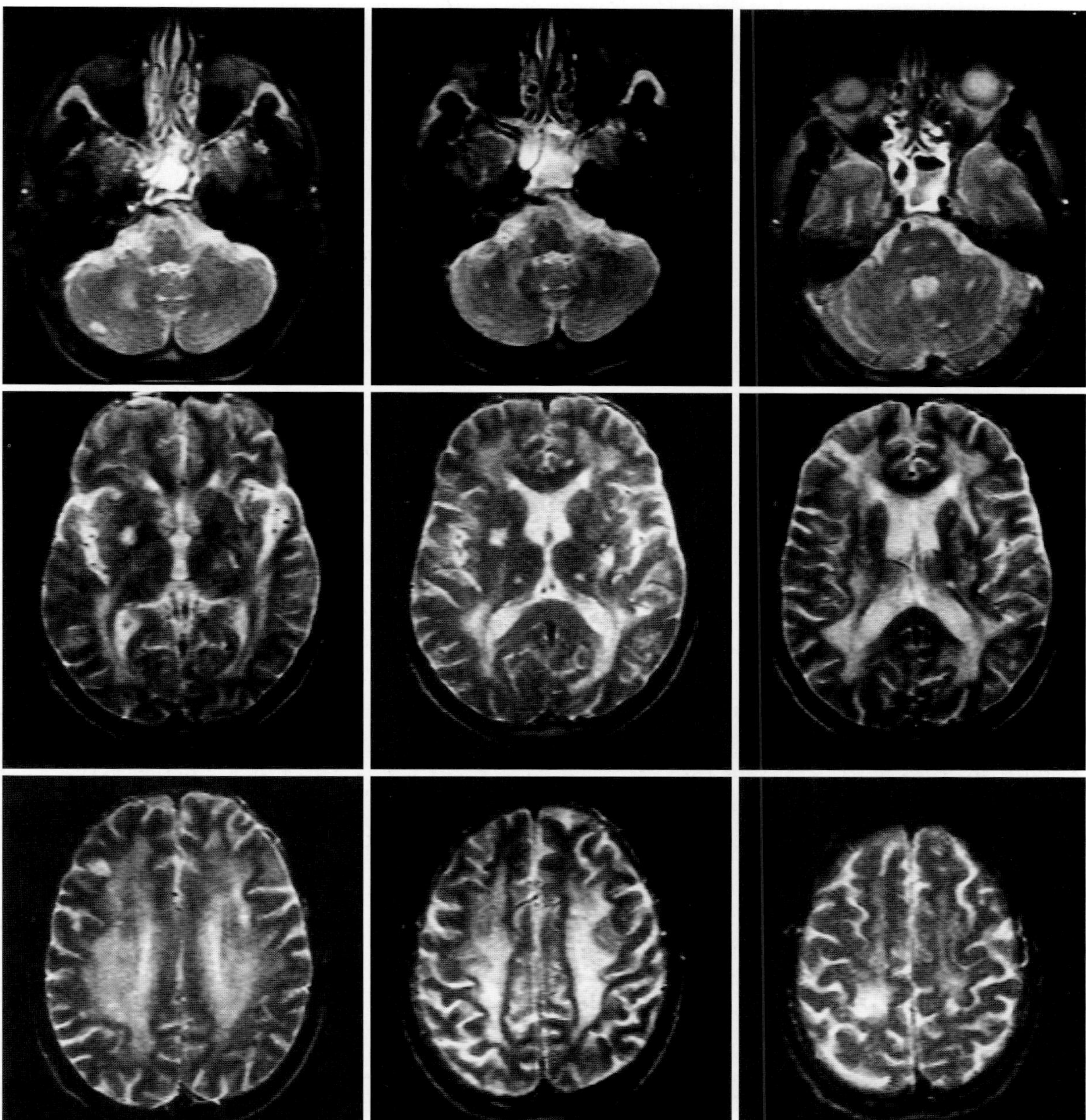

Fig. 55.2. A 48-year-old male AIDS patient admitted to the hospital with general malaise and neurological symptoms consisting of left-sided hemiparesis, cerebellar ataxia and diplopia. He also showed intellectual deterioration. The MR images show two types of lesions. The first type consists of multiple smaller, isolated lesions in the cerebellum, pons, and basal ganglia. The second type of lesion consists of a more symmetrical involvement of the centrum semiovale, abutting the lateral edges of the ventricles, and some faint involvement of the cerebellar white matter. The latter lesion represents the subacute HIV encephalitis; the dispersed, smaller lesions were proven to be toxoplasmosis

and mimic lymphoma. After contrast injection the lesions usually enhance. In about 5% of the cases, however, no or only slight enhancement is seen. This may be due to the absence of inflammation as a consequence of the defective immune system of the patient, resulting in little or no capsule formation around the toxoplasmosis abscess. Possibly, this finding could predict a poor prognosis. Pragmatically one could consider anti-toxoplasmosis treatment when multiple focal lesions with ring enhancement are seen. If toxoplasmosis is present, the lesions will improve within 2 weeks of therapy. Progressive multifocal leukoencephalitis is discussed in a separate chapter. In this disease, the lesions are confined to the white matter and extend

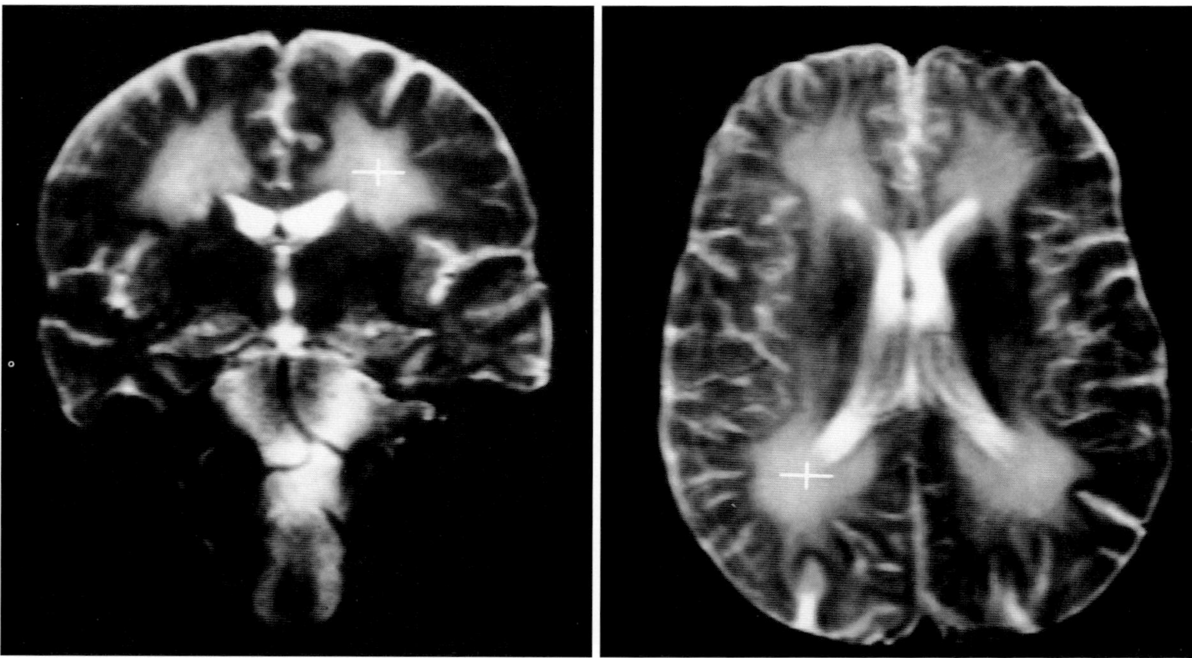

Fig. 55.3. A 40-year-old male AIDS patient with gradual intellectual deterioration. The MR images show symmetrical involvement of centrum semiovale, sparing the U fibers, abutting the lateral upper edges of the ventricles, a pattern as seen in subacute HIV encephalitis

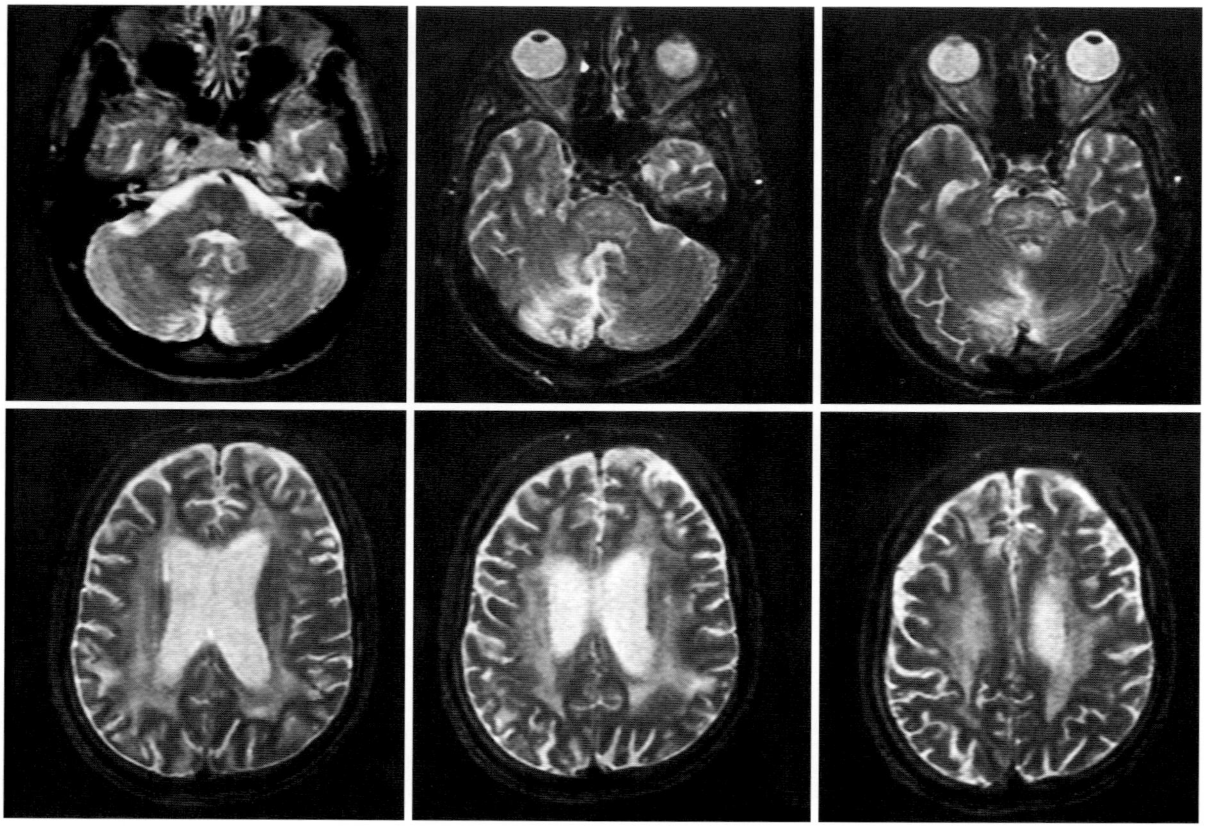

Fig. 55.4. A 45-year-old male AIDS patient with intellectual deterioration, behavioral disturbances, and recent cerebellar symptoms. The T_2-weighted images show general atrophy of the brain and a pattern of white matter involvement that is characteristic for HIV encephalitis. The lesion in the right cerebellar hemisphere is an infarction, also seen regularly in combination with HIV encephalitis, sometimes together with tuberculosis

into the arcuate fibers. There is a typically sharp border between gray matter and demyelinated white matter, leading to a characteristic pattern. Cryptococcus neoformans infection is the most frequent intracranial fungus infection (2%–7.5% of AIDS patients). The infection is preferentially located in the basal ganglia spreading along the Virchow-Robin spaces. This pattern of spread may produce a very typical appearance, suggestive of this type of infection. Cytomegalovirus encephalitis resembles in many aspects the subacute AIDS encephalitis and may present clinically with the same symptoms. Patients may also be asymptomatic. On MRI, diffuse, symmetrical, periventricular high signal intensity changes are seen on T_2-weighted images. This aspect is indistinguishable from subacute HIV encephalitis. In some cases a ventriculitis will develop. After contrast injection this appears as an enhanced subependymal rim around the ventricles.

Of the CNS tumors complicating AIDS, the primary lymphoma is the most frequently observed (about 5% of AIDS). In AIDS, lymphomas may be multifocal, which is rare in other patients. Also the enhancement of lymphoma in AIDS patients may be less homogeneous. Differentiation from toxoplasmosis on MRI may be very difficult. Both can present as single or multifocal lesions with mass effect, both can be connected with the ventricular wall and enhance after contrast administration. Thallium-201 SPECT may offer a solution in the distinction between infection and lymphoma. Leptomeningeal lymphoma can be diagnosed by presence of pericerebral tissue, enhancing with contrast. Metastases of Kaposi's sarcoma have been described in the CNS and in the skull base, but are extremely rare.

In HIV-1 encephalitis in children, apart from the ventriculomegaly and atrophy also found in adults, there is often a symmetrical bilateral calcification of the basal ganglia and the white matter adjacent to the frontal horns. Contrast enhancement of the basal ganglia has also been described, sometimes starting unilaterally, becoming bilateral later on. In some cases the calcifications are supposed to be due to a concurrent cytomegalovirus infection. White matter disease is not a prominent feature of HIV-1 encephalitis in children, although white matter changes may be present. Opportunistic infections are more rare in children than in adults. Central mass lesions are usually caused by primary lymphoma.

In the spinal cord lesions have been described in AIDS patients. On MRI these lesions are not distinguishable from lesions as seen in transverse myelitis in multiple sclerosis. Swelling of the cord is seen initially with moderate enhancement, eventually followed by atrophy.

56.1   Clinical Features and Laboratory Investigations

Progressive multifocal leukoencephalitis (PML) is a rare demyelinating infection of the CNS caused by a polyoma virus, the JC virus. It usually occurs in immunodeficient patients. Its association with such underlying diseases as lymphoma, multiple myeloma, leukemia, sarcoidosis, tuberculosis, Whipple's disease, lupus erythematosus, systemic carcinomas, renal transplantation and bone marrow transplantation, AIDS, and immunosuppressed states is well documented, although the disease has also been reported in patients without evidence of an immunological deficit. During the last few years, most PML cases were AIDS patients. The prevalence of PML in AIDS patients is estimated to be in the range of 4%–7%, which is probably an underestimation. In most cases, PML is a late complication of such preexisting chronic systemic disease which has typically been present for a long time before the neurological abnormalities appear. This underlying disease does not differ appreciably either in its clinical or pathological aspects from the same disease in other patients in which PML does not occur. There is no way of predicting the occurrence of PML. PML occurs predominantly in adults. There is a male preponderance of about 5:3.

The clinical signs and symptoms of PML are those expected from the presence of multiple CNS lesions of varying size, mainly affecting the white matter of the cerebral hemispheres but indiscriminate in their localization. In the early stages the most frequently observed signs are monoparesis, hemiparesis, personality change, mental impairment, ataxia, dysarthria, dysphasia, and cerebral visual impairment. Quadriparesis, severe dementia, and coma characterize the more advanced stages. Headaches and seizures are unusual, and there is no evidence of increased intracranial pressure. Rarely, involuntary movements indicative of an extrapyramidal disorder are observed, such as choreiform movements, dystonia, athetosis, or parkinsonism. Once the disease appears, it generally progresses until the patient dies. Usually, as with many incapacitating cerebral diseases, death results from terminal bronchopneumonia. In most cases a period of about 2–6 months elapses between the first appearance of neuro-logical symptoms and death. In a few patients the illness is extremely brief, lasting only a few days. At the other end of the scale, it can last for 1 year or more. Exceptional patients showing spontaneous improvement have been described.

It is clear that a wide range of clinical neurological abnormalities may be encountered in PML, and no syndrome is especially distinctive for the disease. The combination of a coexisting chronic systemic disease with a fairly rapidly progressive multifocal or diffuse cerebral disease should suggest the presence of PML.

Routine laboratory investigations are usually negative or show nonspecific abnormalities. The CSF is generally normal. In some patients a mild elevation of protein or mild increase in lymphocytes is observed. EEG reveals abnormalities in most PML patients, but is nonspecific. Definite diagnosis requires brain biopsy, but new and promising diagnostic tests are becoming available. New tests include an anti-JC virus IgM antibody assay and a PCR (polymerase chain reaction) technique. Although the IgM assay may help in the investigation of disease associated with primary or reactivated infection, a potential problem is that antibody detection methods are unlikely to be informative in patients with diminished immune responses. The PCR technique has the advantage of being able to detect low concentrations of viral genome in sites other than the brain, e.g., in CSF cells, obviating the need for invasive brain biopsies. Several PCR studies have also shown subclinical JC viral infection of circulating B lymphocytes and CNS tissue of HIV-infected individuals. However, since many of the JC virus studies were performed on postmortem CNS material, the value of the tests in the clinical situation, in particular with respect to detection of subclinical infection, is not yet known.

56.2   Pathology

In PML the brain shows no external abnormalities. On sectioning, multiple grayish granular-appearing lesions are seen in the white matter, often associated with a loss of the distinct border between the cortex and subcortical white matter. Asymmetrical involvement is the rule. Although the lesions are often found bilaterally, they are usually more extensive in one cerebral hemisphere than in the other.

Microscopically the lesions vary from small foci of demyelination to extensive areas of myelin loss, occupying the major portion of a cerebral lobe or hemisphere. The small foci tend to be rounded or oval, but the larger areas of demyelination are irregularly outlined, probably resulting from coalescence of smaller lesions. The lesions may occur anywhere in the white matter of the CNS, no part of the CNS being entirely spared. However, the lesions tend to be less frequent in the brain stem and the cerebellum, and involvement of the spinal cord and peripheral nerves is uncommon. Localization of lesions in the corticomedullary junction and subcortical white matter is very typical. The deep cortical layers often also show loss of myelin sheaths, but the cortical cytoarchitecture remains intact.

The lesions are characterized by loss of myelin with relative sparing of the axons. Sometimes the axons are destroyed along with the myelin, leaving nothing but a meshwork of astrocytic processes and glial fibrils or actual cavities. In the center of the lesion, where myelin sheaths have been destroyed, oligodendrocytes are absent. At the periphery of the lesions the oligodendrocytes are markedly altered, with enlargement of their nuclei and effacement of the normal chromatin pattern. These abnormal nuclei often contain basophilic or eosinophilic inclusion bodies. Another cellular change is a conspicuous alteration of astrocytes. Some of the astrocytes in and around the lesion are enlarged into gigantic forms, and their nuclear structure is profoundly altered. Hyperchromatism, occasionally bizarre lobulation of the nucleus, multinucleation, or mitotic figures are characteristic abnormalities. The change in individual cells is at times so severe that they become indistinguishable from the neoplastic cells that typify malignant astrocytomas. The relative absence of a cellular inflammatory reaction is striking. In many cases inflammatory cells are absent altogether, and in other cases they are few. Numerous lipid-laden macrophages can be identified within the area of demyelination.

PML does little damage to nerve cell bodies. Lesions may be situated in gray matter structures, especially the deep cortical layers. Within these lesions the myelin sheaths are destroyed, and the astrocytes and oligodendrocytes show the characteristic changes, whereas most of the nerve cells appear to be intact.

Electron microscopic studies show virus-like particles within the abnormal oligodendrocytic nuclei and, to some extent, also in altered astrocytes. These particles are seen in isolation, in irregular groups, in a crystal-like pattern or in the form of filaments. The size, shape, surface details, and arrangement of these particles are characteristic of the polyoma virus subgroup of papovaviruses. This observation is confirmed by immunofluorescent studies with the use of specific antibodies against polyomavirus. Using the in situ hybridization techniques with a polyomavirus DNA probe, the infection of oligodendrocytes and astrocytes with this virus can also be shown.

56.3 Pathogenetic Considerations

PML is a demyelinating disease associated with a polyomavirus, which belongs to the Papovaviridae. The family Papovaviridae consists of two genera, papillomavirus and polyomavirus. These are small DNA-containing viruses. A human polyomavirus, designated JC virus after the individual from whom it was first isolated, has been implicated as the etiological agent in nearly all cases of PML. In a minority of the cases a related polyomavirus, simian virus 40, has been held responsible for the disease. Although the disease PML is rare, infection with the JC virus is quite common. Antibodies to JC virus have been found in up to 80% of the population, and the prevalence of antibodies rises with increasing age. Infection is usually acquired early in life: by the age of 15, 65% of children have anti-JC virus antibodies. The virus is distributed throughout the world. The route of infection is unknown. In a given PML patient there is no information about whether these antibodies were present before the onset of the disease. It has been postulated that the disease results from activation of latent virus in the brain or other tissue when the immune response has become impaired. For instance, JC virus has been found in mononuclear cells of bone marrow and spleen in PML patients and in the Virchow-Robin spaces in the brain. These findings suggest that JC virus can be present in mononuclear cells in bone marrow during latency, and that virus-infected lymphocytes enter the perivascular space of the brain, which may result in PML. Another hypothesis is that PML may occur as a primary infection in a person who has not acquired immunity to the virus during childhood, and who later becomes immunologically impaired in adult life. Simian virus 40 is of minor importance in PML. In general, infection with this virus is rare in humans, only 5% showing antibodies. The source of the virus is unknown.

Various polyomaviruses are known to induce cell transformation in vitro and are oncogenic in hamsters. Papovaviruses, their antigens, or viral DNA sequences have been detected in some human tumor cells, but the evidence that these viruses play any significant role in human cancer has yet to be determined. Pathologically, two cell types in the brain are infected by the polyomavirus. Oligodendrocytes are lytically infected, and virus particles fill the nucleus to give it a characteristic appearance. Oligodendroglial cell death causes de-

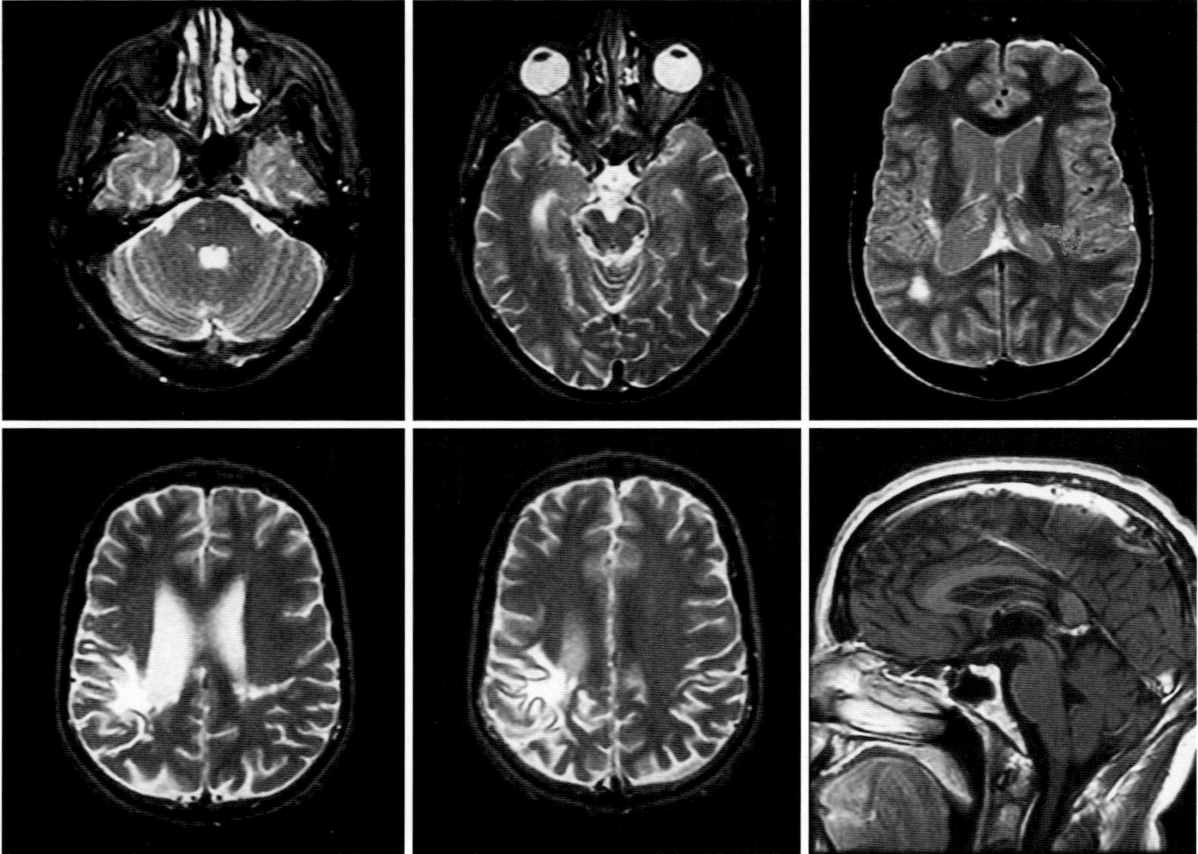

Fig. 56.1. A 46-year-old man, with AIDS and subsequent neurological symptoms due to PML. The T_2-weighted MR images show a large lesion in the right parietal area and a smaller one in the left parietal region. On the right side the U fibers are involved and there is a sharp cut-off border with the cortex. There is also atrophy and enlargement of the right ventricle. The lesions in the right and left hemisphere are connected via the corpus callosum as is clearly seen on the midsagittal, contrast-enhanced T_1-weighted image in the *right bottom row*. There was no enhancement of the lesions

myelination. It is postulated that there is also an infection of the astrocytes in which the viral genome is integrated into the cellular DNA leading to cell transformation. The hypothesis that astrocytic cell transformation in PML is viral-induced is still unproven and is only indirectly supported by the known oncogenic potential of papovaviruses in hamsters, the reported simultaneous occurrence of PML and gliomas, and the demonstration of shared internal capsid antigens of a polyomavirus in the nucleus of giant astrocytes in PML.

A defect in cell-mediated immune defenses appears to be a central factor in the development of PML. The lack of cellular inflammatory reaction in white matter lesions also supports the notion of a deficit in cellular immunity. Yet this deficit alone does not provide an adequate explanation for the occurrence of PML since diseases associated with such immunological deficiency and treatment with immunosuppressive drugs are relatively frequent, while PML is rare. The problem is made more difficult by the fact that PML may even occur in the presence of apparently intact immune responses.

56.4 Therapy

At present the prognosis in PML is generally poor. Treatment with idoxuridine and vidarabine, both antiviral agents, has been shown to be non-beneficial. Cytarabine (arabinosylcytosine) administered intravenously and intrathecally has been demonstrated to be more promising in PML. The raionale for the use of this agent is that polyomaviruses are DNA viruses, and that cytarabine impairs DNA synthesis. Long-term survival of patients with cytarabine-treated PML has been reported. The improvement of the neurological condition varied from moderate to important in these patients. In some patients there was very rapid improvement, occurring within 48 h of initiation of therapy. In

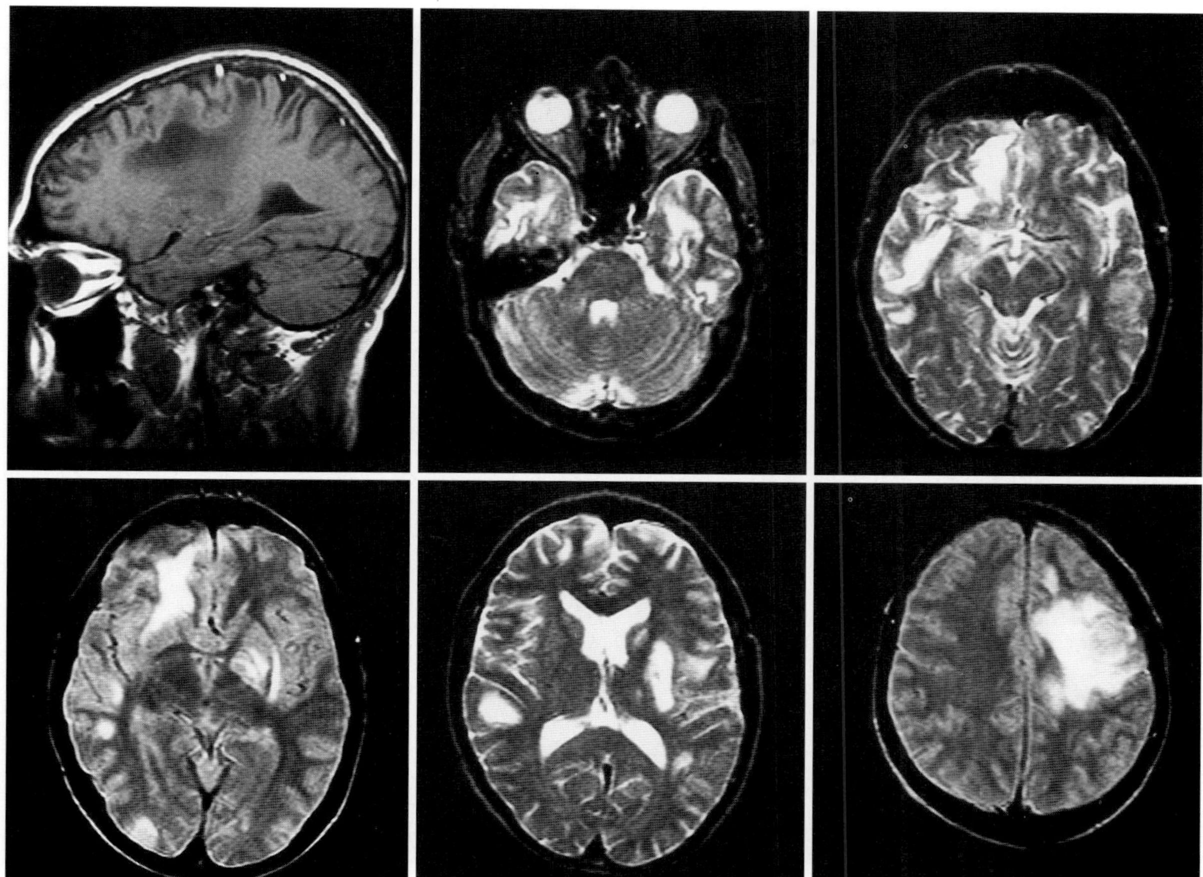

Fig. 56.2. One parasagittal T_1-weighted and a series of T_2-weighted MR images are shown in this 48-year-old man with AIDS and PML. The images show multiple lesions in the white matter. Note that gray matter structures are also involved: putamen and caudate nucleus on the *left* are affected and some lesions extend into the cortical gray matter

others there was a delay of several weeks. Sometimes cytarabine was only transiently beneficial, and sometimes it had no benefical effect at all. Neither type and duration of underlying disease nor duration and course of neurological symptoms prior to treatment appeared to yield a clue as to the different responses to therapy. Although benefit from cytarabine therapy has not yet been proven, the administration of this drug would seem appropriate in a patient with PML for whom a reasonable prognosis exists if the neurological deficit can be reversed. Successful outcome of PML has also been reported in a case treated with a combination of cytarabine and interferon-α (Steiger et al. 1993).

Therapy should not only be directed at eradication of the viral infection by specific antiviral agents but also by enhancing host immune defenses. Lowering of the immunosuppressive medication may be appropriate. Early diagnosis before actual destruction of nervous tissue has occurred may be necessary for treatment to be successful.

56.5 Magnetic Resonance Imaging

CT scan shows low density white matter lesions with characteristically scalloped lateral borders following the contours of the gray-white matter junction, whereas the medial border is smoother in outline. Enhancement of part of the lesions may be seen. Small and early lesions are not detected, and CT often shows no abnormalities in the early stages of the disease.

The JC virus causes lytic infection of oligodendroglial cells, which results in progressive demyelination of the CNS. Neurons are spared. The nature of the white matter involvement, together with local edema explain some of the characteristics of the MRI findings.

PML lesions can be found anywhere in the white matter of the cerebral hemispheres, the brainstem and the cerebellum, but most often in the cerebral subcortical area (Figs. 56.1–56.4). The lesions have an intermediate to low signal intensity on T_1-weighted images, a high or very high signal intensity on T_2-weighted images. The affected white matter appears somewhat

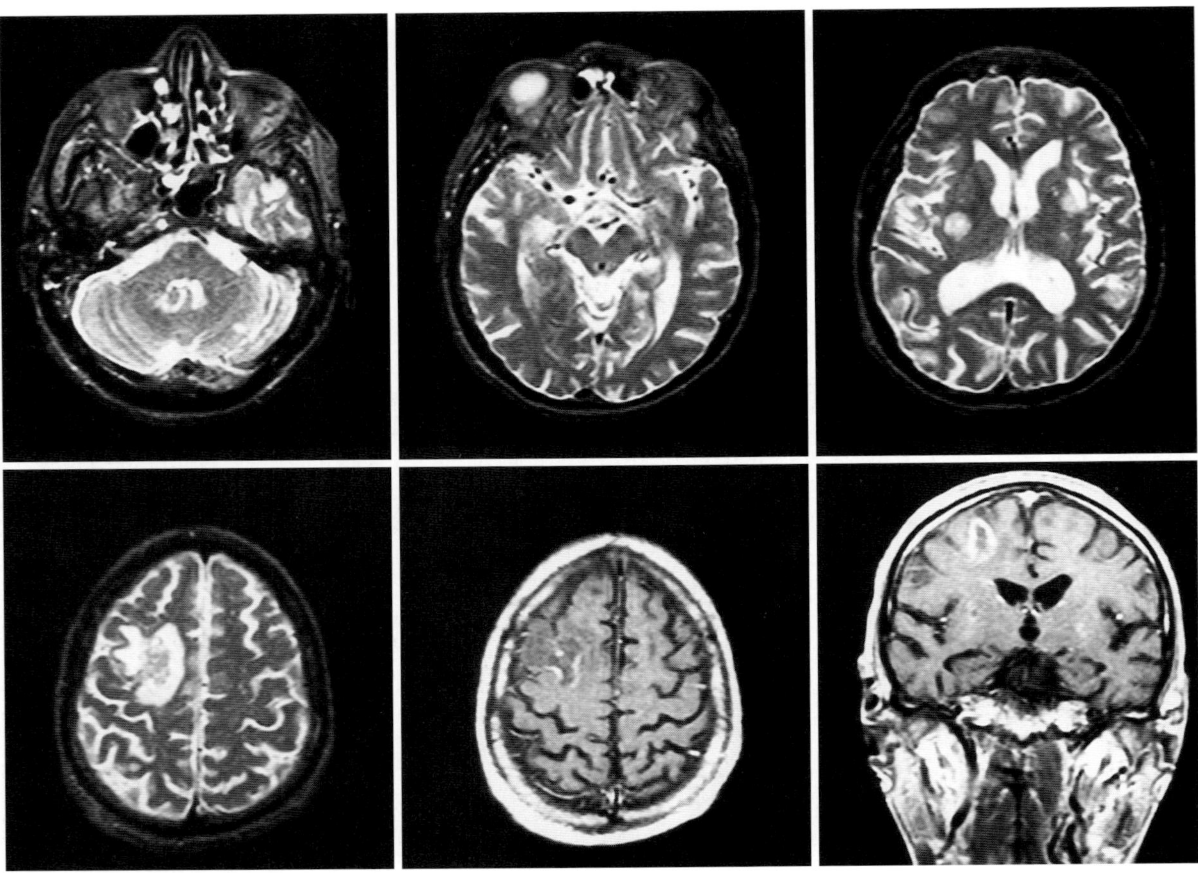

Fig. 56.3. A 63-year-old male with AIDS and PML. In this case of PML, some gray matter structures are also involved. The large frontal lesion on the *right side* shows enhancement after contrast injection, as is seen on the transverse and coronal T_1-weighted contrast enhanced images (*lower row, right*)

swollen, which becomes more evident in those areas where the U fibers are involved. The subcortical white matter lesions then have a scalloped appearance, outlining the overlying cortex and stretching it. The sharp edge between affected white matter and cortical gray matter is due to the anatomical barrier formed by the non-infected neuronal layers with its relative myelin paucity. In exceptional cases MRI shows some extension of a white matter lesion into the cortex, where probably intracortical myelin is attacked. Lesions of the external capsule have been found in 38%, posterior fossa lesions in 32% of the PML patients, less infrequently than previously thought. Isolated posterior fossa lesions have been reported incidentally. There have been reports of basal ganglia involvement. As the myelin content of thalamus and globus pallidus is relatively high, lesions would be expected to occur more often in these areas. In our cases, involvement of the corpus callosum is regularly seen (Fig. 56.1). Although the epithet "multifocal" suggests more than one lesion in all cases, this is not necessarily true. Single lesions may occur. Confluency of several lesions may cause an appearance of a widespread white matter disorder. Enhancement after the injection of gadolinium is exceptional, but it certainly may occur (Fig. 56.3). If enhancement is seen, it is usually only present in part of the lesions; it is faint and peripheral. We have observed, however, in one case more solid enhancement.

PML has to be differentiated from other multifocal white matter disorders, especially from those occurring in AIDS patients, such as cytomegalovirus infections and from HIV encephalitis itself. These latter infections, however, do not usually involve the U fibers, do have different signal intensity characteristics on T_1- and T_2-weighted images, and tend to be symmetrical. Recently, a case has been described with cerebral vasculitis lesions in systemic lupus erythematosus mimicking PML (Kaye et al. 1992), whereas in the same disease PML has been reported to occur. Multifocal white matter involvement with some swelling of the subcortical lesions and stretching of the overlying cortex may also be seen in inflammatory disorders, in particular mulitiple sclerosis and acute disseminated encephalomyelitis. Similar lesions have been reported

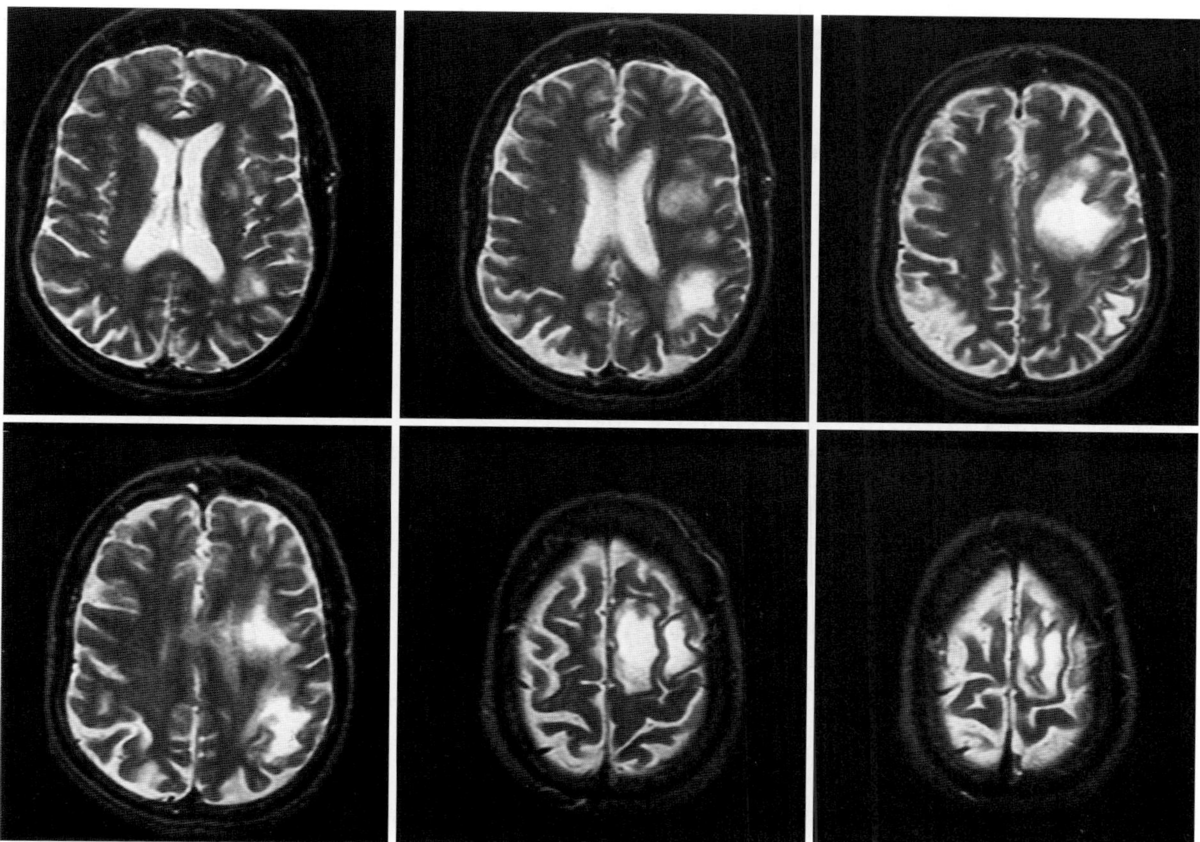

Fig. 56.4. A 57-year-old male patient with AIDS and PML. T_2-weighted series starting at the ventricular level and going upwards. Lesions are seen on the *left* and the *right side*. They vary in size, but are relatively large and confluent. They involve the U fibers and the lobar white matter

in eclampsia, based on subcortical hypoxic-ischemic lesions. In vasculitis, eclampsia and inflammatory disorders, white matter lesions are, as a rule, asymmetrical and differentiation from PML may be impossible based on MRI features alone. Clinical and laboratory information is necessary. In several inborn errors of metabolism and in several toxic encephalopathies, spongiform white matter changes occur, which result in some white matter swelling and stretching of the overlying cortex which is otherwise intact. The aspect of the white matter changes shows similarities to those observed in PML, but the white matter abnormalities are usually symmetrical and usually generalized rather than multifocal.

57 Subacute Sclerosing Panencephalitis

57.1 Clinical Features and Laboratory Investigations

Subacute sclerosing panencephalitis (SSPE) is one of the slow virus infections of the CNS. It is a rare disorder, but it is the commonest of the chronic virus infections to affect children. It is caused by measles virus. SSPE is a disease of childhood and adolescence, with an age range of 4–20 years and a peak incidence at 7–10 years. There is a racial difference in incidence of SSPE: in the United States the incidence is four times higher in Whites than in Blacks. Boys outnumber girls by 3 or 2 to 1. Children who acquire measles infection under 2 years of age are more likely to develop SSPE. The mean age of infection is 12–14 months. In exceptional cases SSPE can also occur after live measles immunization, but the rate of incidence is highly reduced after immunization. Since the introduction of measles vaccination, and since coverage in The Netherlands has reached 95%, the incidence of SSPE has gone down to one case annually. In Japan, 10–25 new cases a year are reported.

The clinical syndrome of SSPE is rather variable. The duration of the disease ranges from 3 months to more than 7 years. Although there is a marked variation in presenting signs and in the sequence of events, four clinical phases can usually be discerned. Stage 1 is characterized by an insidious deterioration of behavior and intellectual performance. The duration of this stage is usually several months, but the exact time of onset of the disease is often difficult to determine. Personality changes occur with withdrawn, timid, or aggressive behavior. These changes are followed by lethargy, drooling, slurred speech, and paucity of speech. Soon after the onset of intellectual deterioration, visual disturbances can often be detected. These are either related to progressive chorioretinitis or to lesions of the central visual pathways. In stage 2, massive, repetitive, and frequent myoclonic jerking occurs. The myoclonia develops slowly and iregularly, but gradually affects all somatic muscle groups, especially the axial muscles, in a reasonably symmetric fashion and at a regularly repetitive rate. The myoclonus may be sufficiently severe to throw the child to the floor. The jerking interferes with intentional movements, giving the impression of clumsiness. The jerking is absent during sleep. Seizures of a more conventional type may also occur, such as focal motor, generalized, and psychomotor convulsions. They may even precede the myoclonic jerking. Mental deterioration becomes progressively more obvious. At this stage, choreoathetosis, ataxia, tremor, and spasticity are common. The duration of stage 2 varies from 1 month to 1 year or more. In some patients the disease is arrested in stage 2 and remains in this stage for years. In stage 3 there is severe dementia. The spasticity increases, and the child becomes bedridden. Extrapyramidal dysfunction of the parkinsonian type is frequent. Nasogastric tube feeding is often required at this time because of progressive bulbar palsy. Hyperthermia may be found without evidence of infection. It is the rule that the myoclonia diminishes in stage 3. Stage 4 is the final stage in which the child is in a vegetative state, characterized by mutism and decorticate or decerebrate postures. There is no bladder or bowel control. Ophthalmological abnormalities occur in 50% of patients and include optic atrophy and chorioretinitis. The chorioretinitis may be most marked at the maculae, where scars are seen with characteristic pigmentation. There are signs of autonomic dysfunction, such as hyperthermia, severe perspiration, and changes in heart rate and blood pressure. The duration of stage 4 varies from 1 to 6 years. Most patients die during stage 3 or 4 from cardiorespiratory complications related to impaired central mechanisms controlling temperature, cardiac, and respiratory functions. Another common cause of death is infection.

The clinical diagnosis of SSPE is confirmed by the finding of increased levels of anti-measles virus antibody in serum and CSF. The CSF is clear, and the pressure and glucose concentration are normal. Moderate pleocytosis (5–20 mononuclear cells per ml) is often present. The protein level is usually normal or mildly elevated; a level that exceeds 0.90 g/l is uncommon. The level of IgG as percent of total protein is increased, and oligoclonal bands are seen. Measles-specific IgG antibodies represent nearly 10%–20% of total serum IgG and about 75% of the total CSF IgG. There is always an elevated CSF:serum ratio of IgG, especially of measles virus antibodies, indicating a local production of measles virus antibodies within the CNS. Another confirmatory finding is a characteristic EEG pattern of periodic complexes consisting of bilateral synchronous, symmetric, 2 to 4 Hz high amplitude sharp and slow wave bursts, which may occur every 5–7 s. These periodic complexes occur simultaneously with the involuntary myoclonic movements. In stage 1 the EEG may be normal or show only mild to moderate, nonspecific slowing. Stage 2 is characterized by the occurrence of periodic complexes; the background pattern is still relatively normal. In stage 3, the background rhythm slows, and fewer bursts of periodic complexes occur. Stage 4 has slow delta activity and rare SSPE complexes. These complexes in association with myoclonic seizures provide strong corroborative evidence of SSPE. However, periodic complexes are also seen in other diffuse cerebral disorders, such as some lysosomal storage disorders, mitochondrial encephalopathy (MERRF), cerebral anoxia, and widespread infections of the brain.

57.2 Pathology

The pathology of SSPE is restricted to the CNS. The brain may show atrophy during the terminal stages of disease but is otherwise generally normal. Microscopically, the disease appears to be multifocal in character and may involve all portions of the CNS, with the exception that the cerebellum is rarely affected. The frontal lobes are involved first, followed eventually by involvement of the parietal, temporal, and occipital lobes, the basal ganglia, brain stem, and spinal cord. The typical pathological findings include perivascular infiltration by mononuclear cells in gray and white matter and proliferation of both macroglia and microglia. Astrocyte proliferation can be particularly pronounced in white matter. Neuronal degeneration and neuronal loss may be severe. Demyelination is focal and not always conspicuous. The subcortical white matter is mostly affected, first with inflammation and then with destruction. In the later stages of the disease both cortical atrophy and demyelination are more pronounced. Intranuclear and intracytoplasmic inclusions are present in neurons, astrocytes and oligodendrocytes.

Ultrastructural examination shows the presence of paramyxovirus particles. A spectrum of viral inclusions and particles has been reported. Some inclusions fill nuclei, whereas smaller particles, nucleocapsids and virions of different configurations are found in either the nucleus or the cytoplasm of glial cells and neurons.

57.3 Pathogenetic Considerations

SSPE is caused by a measles infection of the brain. The elevated serum and CSF measles virus antibody levels are indicative of an active measles virus infection of the brain. Inclusions with paramyxovirus particles have been demonstrated in neuronal and glial cells in SSPE. The cellular inclusions have been shown to fluoresce when treated with measles virus antisera. For a long time, however, the virus could not be recovered from brain tissue by conventional methods, presumably because it is structurally incomplete and cell-associated. Successful isolation of the measles virus was finally accomplished by cocultivating brain cells of SSPE patients with cells known to support measles virus replication. After the isolation of the virus, the agent was studied extensively to determine its structural and biological characteristics. Its ultrastructural features are similar to those of measles virus. Further studies of the immune response in patients demonstrated the absence of serum antibody to the matrix (M) protein of measles virus. The M protein is associated with the inner surface of the viral membrane. It is important in the assembly of the virus particle, which occurs by a budding process from the surface membrane of the infected cell. Subsequent studies demonstrated the absence of measles virus M protein in the brain tissue of patients with SSPE. Cocultivation with permissive cells presumably makes the protein available for virus assembly. Further confirmation of the importance of M protein comes from a small animal model of experimental SSPE. In this system a defective measles virus infection of the brain develops in some of the animals that recover after intracerebral inoculation. Recovery of virus from their brain cell cultures requires similar cocultivation procedures. In these animals, viral M protein can be demonstrated to disappear from the brain coincidentally with the disappearance of infectious virus and the development of a cell-associated infection. It is interesting that an infection of this type can only be accomplished in an animal inoculated during the weaning period. As in human beings, the age at which virus is introduced into the nervous system seems to be critical to the development of SSPE. In human beings the primary infection seems to occur during a critical period in early life when passive maternal immunity has faded and before the age of approximately 2 years. Regardless of the precise explanation, the absence of M protein explains many of the virological features of SSPE. Because the M protein plays a primary role in the assembly of the virus particle at the cell membrane, lack of M protein in the cells would result in persistent, abortive infection in which no mature infectious virus is produced in the extracellular space. The internal components of the virus would accumulate in the cells, and the surface glycoproteins of the virus would be exposed on the surface of the cells to stimulate high levels of antibodies. As the measles virus infection of the brain is acquired early in life, it is remarkable that patients remain well during the prolonged interval from primary infection to the onset of SSPE symptoms. During this time it is thought that viral nucleocapsids, RNA, and probably other gene products accumulate and spread from cell to cell through the nervous system. The onset of symptoms is usually ascribed to altered cell function and cell death, resulting from excessive accumulation of viral products.

There are several theories about how a ubiquitous virus such as the measles virus establishes a persistent infection of the brain in a small minority of patients, and why the measles virus is not eradicated at first contact during the acute episode of measles or afterwards when the virus is localized in the brain. An immunological deficiency has been assumed, but never clearly demonstrated. Some still suspect there is a minor defect in cellular immunity in SSPE patients. Others believe that the measles virus enters the brain of the susceptible host during a transient, vulnerable immunological period. The immunological vulnerability may be a consequence of a combination of infancy (due to immaturity of the immune system), genetic factors (male versus female), racial factors (Whites versus Blacks), nutritional condition, and other simultaneous infections. Another theory assumes that SSPE is not caused by the common measles virus but by a mutant measles virus strain with a defect in its M protein. However, it is more probable that the failure in synthesis of this protein is due to a failure of brain cells to synthesize M protein as a general property of these cells. An observation compatible with this theory is that in acute measles encephalitis, many attempts to isolate the virus have been made over the years, but for successful isolation cocultivation with other cells is necessary. Thus, the available evidence suggests that there is a restriction of measles virus replication in the brain cells due to a lack of synthesis of M protein by these cells. Some believe that the immune response is ineffective in SSPE as the virus is harbored intracellularly in the relatively privileged CNS. The intracellular virus is never in contact with the extracellular space, as a consequence of the absence of M protein and the resulting inability of the virus to assemble and bud. The measles virus particles are probably passed from cell to cell. In the brain compact cell-to-cell contact allows the passage of virus from one cell to the other without extracellular contact. Only when cells begin to deteriorate and die, does the virus make contact with the immune system, causing a rise of anti-measles antibodies, except antibodies to M protein. These antibodies are ineffective in eradicating the intracellular virus. In addition, modulation of measles antigen on the surface of infected cells by anti-measles antibodies has been described, and this modulation might make the cell invulnerable to attack by the immune system and could alter expression of the virus within the cell. There is also evidence that lymphocytes may be involved in the pathogenesis of SSPE. Some 70%–90% of peripheral mononuclear cells from SSPE patients have been found to contain virus RNA sequences, which are also present in nerve cells and in numerous cells from the perivascular infiltrates in the brain of SSPE patients. In contrast, only a low percentage of such cells (0.1%–15%) was observed in the blood of seropositive control patients. Until now it is not clear whether there is any connection between the infection of the lymphocytes and brain cells, and what the nature of the interaction is.

In conclusion, it is probable that whether or not an individual develops SSPE, depends on the extent of seeding of the brain in the acute episode of measles, i.e., the type and number of cells that are infected at that time. Brain cells are relatively nonpermissive for viral replication as a consequence of their inability to synthesize M protein. An abortive, persistent viral infection develops. It is speculative which other factors play a role in the pathogenesis of SSPE.

57.4   Therapy

There is no effective treatment for SSPE. The disease leads to death in most cases, but there may be spontaneous temporary improvement or an arrest of further progression for a number of years. Attempts to alter the disease course with transfer factor or with an antiviral agent such as amantadine (Symmetrel), 5-bromodeoxyuridine, or inosiplex (Isoprinosine, Viruxan) have failed , which is not surprising in view of the marked cell-associated nature of the virus. A combination of intraventricular interferon and oral inosiplex seems to have a higher remission rate (Yalaz et al. 1992).

57.5   Magnetic Resonance Imaging

SPPE is a rare disease, in particular during the last few years, since the availability of adequate immunization strategies, and so neuroimaging data are scarce. CT is normal during the initial stage of the disease, shows multiple low density areas in the white matter and basal nuclei in subsequent stages, and severe atrophy in the end stage. Low density areas may show contrast enhancement.

In the earliest stage, MRI may be normal, but it shows abnormalities before CT does. Lesions in the lateral geniculate bodies have been reported as early lesions. Early changes are also multifocal and confluent white matter lesions which have a preference for hemispheral subcortical white matter (Fig. 57.1). In more extensive lesions, lobar and periventricular white matter are involved additionally. In some cases the abnormalities are asymmetrical, but in most cases they are symmetrical and rather extensive. Brain stem and cerebellar involvement has also been reported. The white matter changes may decrease or resolve, even in the presence of clinical deterioration. Large focal lesions involving white and gray matter, resembling infarctions, have also been reported. These may enhance ini-

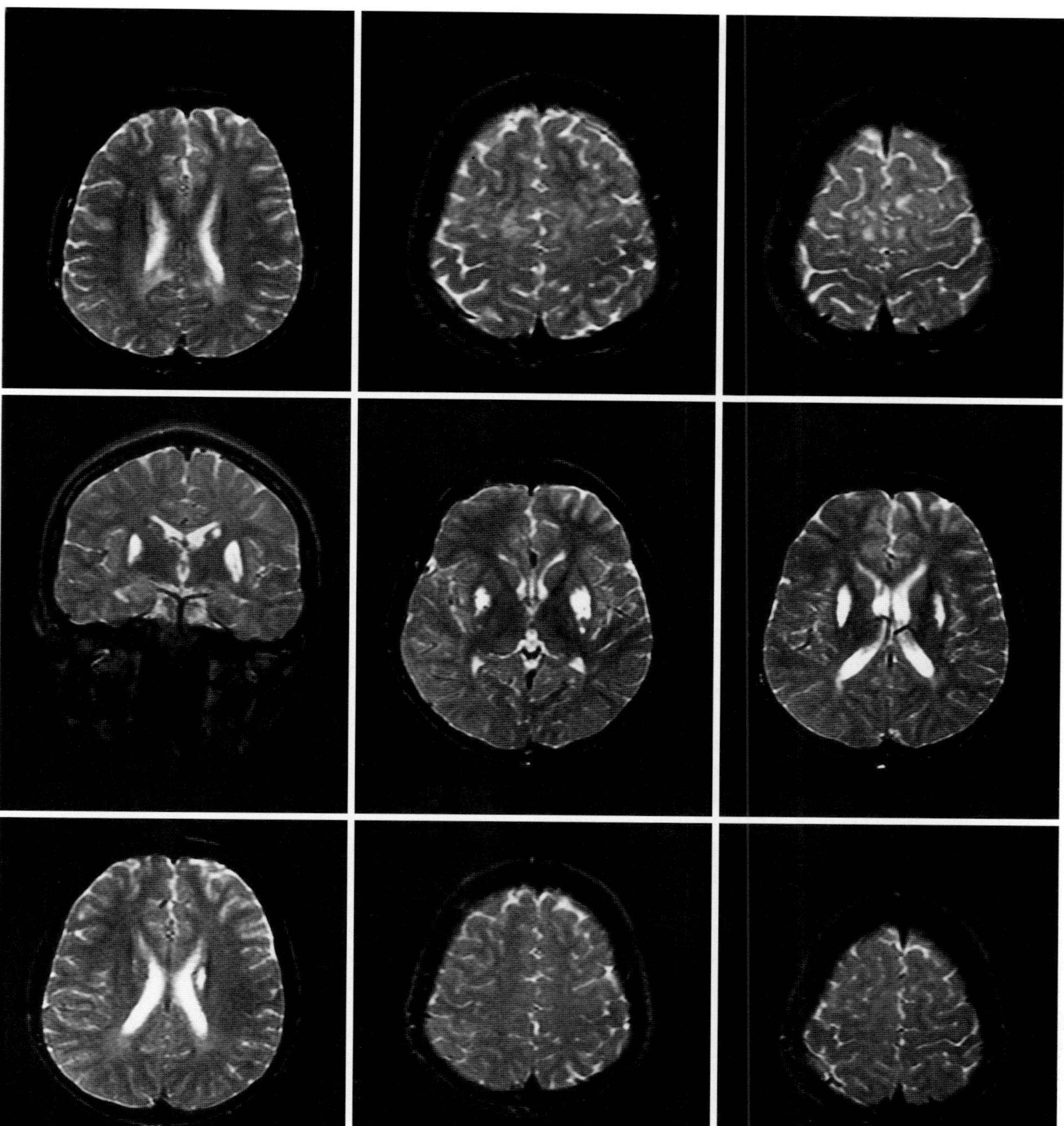

Fig. 57.1. A 9-year-old boy with SSPE. The first MRI was made when there were signs of diminution of intellectual performance and altered behavior. A few moderately hyperintense white matter lesions are seen in the centrum semiovale (images in the *upper row*). The second MRI was made 7 months later (*middle and lower rows*), when signs of neurological dysfunction were much more severe. MRI now shows lesions of the caudate nucleus and putamen on both sides. There is still a somewhat higher signal intensity of the white matter in the supraventricular slices, but this is less clear

tially and subsequently become non-enhancing. In particular in more advanced stages of the disease, bilateral striatal lesions may occur. In end stage disease, severe atrophy of cerebrum, brain stem and cerebellum is found, often with global and generalized white matter abnormality.

Differential diagnosis includes acute disseminated encephalomyelitis and Schilder's diffuse sclerosis. In some cases of SSPE, MRI shows symmetrical white matter lesions in the occipital area and splenium of the corpus callosum, simulating X-linked adrenoleukodystrophy. In cases with involvement of the basal nuclei, the differential diagnosis includes mitochondrial disorders, in particular MERRF syndrome, and other neurodegenerative disorders. EEG and laboratory findings help to establish the correct diagnosis.

58 Progressive Rubella Panencephalitis

58.1 Clinical Features and Laboratory Investigations

Progressive rubella panencephalitis (PRP) is a very rare disorder of the CNS. It is analogous to subacute sclerosing panencephalitis (SSPE) in many ways and is related to rubella virus. It may develop about a decade after congenital rubella virus infection and may also occur years after childhood rubella infection. Children infected in utero with rubella may have multiple congenital defects including cataracts, retinal pigmentation, deafness, cardiac anomalies, microcephaly and mental retardation. This condition is nonprogressive. A number of these patients, however, develop progressive neurological symptoms during the second decade. A similar picture of neurological deterioration may occur in apparently healthy teenagers. The symptomatology and course of the disease resemble those of SSPE. The major clinical features of PRP are progressive dementia and signs of cerebellar, pyramidal and extrapyramidal motor disturbances, with cerebellar ataxia and spastic paresis of the extremities, nystagmus, dysarthria and choreiform movements. Myoclonic seizures and other epileptic manifestations may occur. Decreased vision with optic atrophy has been observed. Ongoing neurological deterioration eventually leads to death. The rate of progression of the illness is slower than in SSPE.

CSF examination reveals mild mononuclear pleocytosis and increased protein levels. The level of IgG is strikingly elevated, with an elevation of the IgG index, indicative of intrathecal IgG synthesis. Electrophoretic analysis shows oligoclonal bands in the gamma-globulin fraction. These oligoclonal IgG antibodies appear to be rubella virus-specific. The same virus-specific antibodies are increased in the serum of PRP patients, but on a comparatively lower scale than in the CSF. The EEG is abnormal, with diffuse slow activity and periodic high-amplitude slow-wave complexes.

58.2 Pathology

External examination reveals a variable degree of brain atrophy, depending on the severity and duration of the illness. The pons, medulla, and cerebellum are most severely atrophic. There is thickening of the basal meninges. On sectioning, the ventricles are found to be dilated, and the white matter is diffusely shrunken and discolored. Microscopically, the cerebral cortex is relatively intact. There is widespread destruction of the white matter, with extensive demyelination, fragmentation of axons, and astrocytosis. The meninges and the perivascular spaces in gray and white matter are diffusely infiltrated by lymphocytes and plasma cells. Some vessel walls undergo fibrinoid degeneration with invasion by lymphocytes and plasma cells. Some vessel walls are fibrotic and contain mineral deposits of calcium, iron, glycogen, and acid mucopolysaccharides. Iron deposits are present not only in vessel walls but also in astrocytes, microglia, and throughout the parenchyma of the centrum semiovale. Glial nodules containing astrocytes, lymphocytes, and microglia are scattered throughout the brain parenchyma. Diffuse neuronal loss with gliosis is apparent in the basal ganglia, brain stem, and the cerebellar cortex. All layers of the cerebellar cortex show severe sclerotic atrophy in combination with diffuse white matter destruction. Purkinje cells are virtually absent. Optic nerves are also affected, and demyelination with gliosis, axonal fragmentation, and perivascular infiltrates are noted. To date, no virus particles have been revealed by electron microscopy.

58.3 Pathogenetic Considerations

Antibody titers to rubella virus are increased in serum and especially in CSF, suggesting a direct role for rubella virus in the pathogenesis of PRP. Attempts to isolate the virus from the CSF have so far been unsuccessful. In a small number of PRP patients, rubella virus could be isolated from brain cells by means of cocultivation techniques. Rubella virus has also been isolated from peripheral blood leukocytes. Persistence of the virus for 10–20 years, even in the presence of high serum and CSF antibody levels, is a noteworthy feature of the disease.

There are many analogies between PRP and SSPE (see also chapter on SSPE). However, there are also differences. Extensive cerebellar atrophy and mineral deposits in vessel walls in white and gray matter are findings that distinguish PRP from SSPE. Much less is known about PRP than about SSPE. Therefore, no definite statement can be made concerning the similarities and differences in pathogenesis between SSPE and PRP. In any case, an immune mechanism must be considered in the pathogenesis of PRP. Circulating immune complexes have been demonstrated which consist of rubella-specific IgG antibody and rubella antigen. The persistent presence of these complexes suggest continued release of virus and viral antigens into the circulation. The marked elevations of rubella-specific immunoglobulins in the CSF is indicative of their intrathecal synthesis, presumably by plasma cells seen within the lesions. Immunoglobulins have been shown in the walls of vessels in the brain with signs of vasculitis but also in vessels without apparent vasculitis. These deposits may consist of rubella-specific antibody. It is possible that they are part of the deposited rubella-antirubella immune complexes. The vasculitis produced in this way may be important in the pathogenesis of PRP.

58.4   Therapy

There is no effective treatment for PRP. The outcome of this disorder is always fatal.

58.5   Magnetic Resonance Imaging

This condition is extremely rare, and no reports on MRI findings have appeared in the literature so far. One can expect to find extensive white matter changes with a relatively preserved cerebral cortex. The cerebellum and brain stem will show severe atrophy. Lesions of the optic nerve may be visualized. This combination forms a pattern that is unusual enough to raise suspicion. The diagnosis is, however, made by the identification of high levels of rubella virus-specific oligoclonal IgG antibodies in CSF.

59 Toxic Encephalopathy

There is growing awareness that chronic intoxications by industrial, agricultural, iatrogenic, and environmental pollution may have teratogenic or oncogenic effects or may cause neurological or psychiatric syndromes.

Toxic encephalopathy (TE) is the result of the interaction between a chemical compound and the brain. Disturbance of normal brain function is caused by:
1. Depletion of oxidative energy;
2. Deficiency of substrates for cerebral processes;
3. Alteration of membrane function and stability;
4. Enzymatic dysfunction;
5. Derangement of neurotransmission;
6. Altered ion balance.

The list of examples of TEs is long and reflects the real difficulty in recognizing that slow deterioration of neurological functions may indicate poisoning by a toxin. In many cases, religious, superstitious, or racial "explanations" have been believed for a long time, before the true cause of the disorder was detected.

Well known examples of TE include:
1941 Lathyrus sativus peas, causing spastic paraparesis; the toxic agent was identified to be β-N-methylamino-L-alanine (BMAA);
1953 Guamalian type of Parkinsonism, caused by the seeds of Cycas circinalis; the toxic agent was identified as β-N-oxalylmethyl- amino-L-alanine (BOMAA);
1948 Hexachloraphene encephalopathy;
1950 Monosodium glutamate in baby food;
1953 Minamata disease, mercury encephalopathy;
1960 Housepainters dementia, organic solvents;
1983 Methylphenyltetrahydropyridine (MPTP), "synthetic heroin", causing striatal dopamine deficiency and Parkinsonism.

Other TEs have a somewhat more familiar background. In this category we find the conditions caused by alcohol abuse, such as the Marchiafava Bignami syndrome, Korsakoff syndrome, and Wernicke encephalopathy, and metabolic derangements such as the Reye syndrome.

It should also be mentioned that age can be a prominent pathoplastic factor in TE. Many fetal intoxications, such as those caused by maternal use of antiepileptic or antidepressive drugs, maternal alcohol abuse, and maternal drug abuse, lead to serious syndromes of which the fetal alcohol syndrome, and fetal hydantoin syndrome are well known examples. Fetal intoxications may result in cerebral maldevelopment, cerebral disruptions and arrest or delay of cerebral maturation, including delay of myelination. The resulting conditions are stationary and have cerebral palsy-like clinical manifestations. In adults, TE presents with one or more of the following neurological or psychiatric symptoms (Bonhoeffer types):
1. Decreased concentration and consciousness;
2. Excitability and convulsions;
3. Motor and sensory disturbances;
4. Extrapyramidal movement disorders;
5. Disturbance of specific senses;
6. Disturbance of coordination; and
7. Behavioral and psychological changes.

In many forms of TE, clinical manifestations are acute and severe, requiring immediate treatment. Imaging of the brain is often only of secondary interest, although in unsuspected cases MRI may play a leading role in diagnosis. The role of imaging is as a rule more important in cases of subacute or chronic TE with slowly progressive neurological damage. In such cases, MRI may demonstrate striking pathological changes, and can be of importance for further diagnosis and therapy monitoring. However, even in cases with histologically proven organic cerebral damage, MRI is not always positive. For example, tardive dyskinesia is a severe movement disorder due to the chronic use of neuroleptic drugs. The pathology is well known. Histology shows a decrease in the number of ganglion cells in the substantia nigra. MRI shows no abnormalities. Also in other cases, when the encephalopathy is the result of interference with neurotransmitters, for example, in the malignant neuroleptic syndrome, MRI shows no abnormalities.

Knowledge of the biomechanisms whereby toxins of endogenous or exogenous origin cause encephalopathy helps us to understand the patterns of lesions seen in imaging studies. MRI abnormalities are, as a rule, symmetrical as toxins have no left-right preference. Characteristic MRI patterns showing involvement of particular brain structures are the result of differences in regional vulnerability of brain tissue to environmental perturbations and to biochemical changes. Here, the concept of selective vulnerability comes in (see also the chapter on this subject).

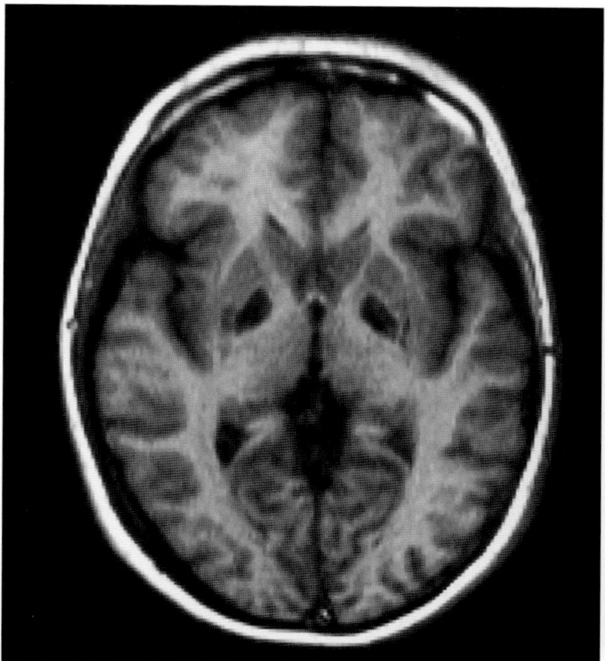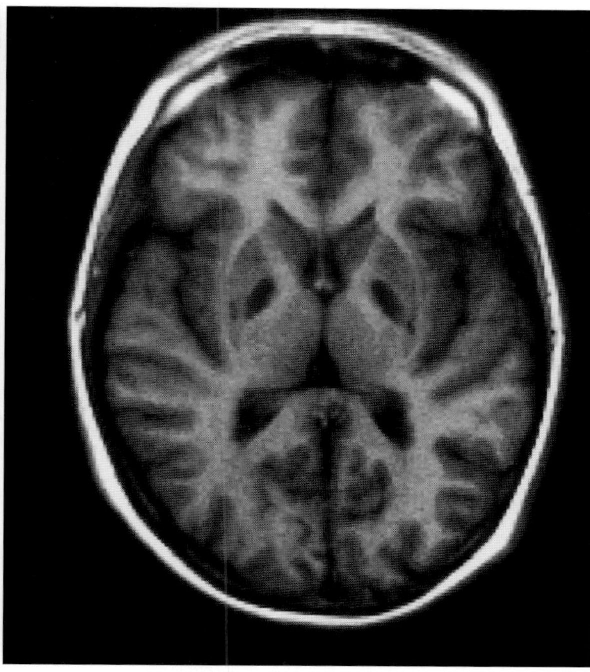

Fig. 59.1. An 18-year-old girl, admitted to a psychiatric asylum because of severe behavioral disturbances after having taken a love potion containing ecstasy. Cyst-like lesions are seen in the globus pallidus and the posterior parts of the putamina

As a general rule, specific groups of toxins tend to affect specific brain structures more than others. That is, certain regions and systems within the brain have greater affinity for and greater sensitivity to specific types of toxins. These regions of identical affinity and vulnerability were recognized by German neuropathologists who designated them the "Topistische Bezirke" or topistic areas. Topistic areas often involve more than one structure; indeed, they often encompass a whole functional chain of neurons and tracts. The principle of functionally related systems is well established in neurology. Topistic areas related to functional systems can be readily identified during normal physiological development of the brain and in systemic degenerative disorders. Thus, in 1920, Flechsig already recognized that functionally related systems myelinate at the same time. Similarly, functionally related and interdependent nuclei appear to degenerate at the same time in multiple system atrophies such as Parkinson disease and progressive supranuclear palsy.

Other mechanisms of selective vulnerability in TE are related to the similarity in particular physicochemical characteristics that make the different geographic areas equally vulnerable to a particular noxious agent. Thus, apparently diverse areas may prove to have similar oxygen requirements, chemical composition, and/or neurotransmitter dependency and density.

Gray matter structures have a higher cellular activity and a higher oxygen requirement than white matter structures and, therefore, are more vulnerable to oxygen deprivation. The damage that results from oxygen deprivation is actually mediated by toxic products, such as excitatory amino acids and free radicals inducing irreversible neuronal damage and death. The selective vulnerability of gray matter structures to energy depletion is also reflected in the preferential affliction of gray matter structures in carbon monoxide intoxication (especially the globus pallidus) and Leigh's disease (putamen, caudate nucleus, globus pallidus, periaqueductal gray matter, tectum and tegmentum of the brain stem, and dentate nuclei). Wernicke's encephalopathy, a toxic encephalopathy caused by thiamine deficiency in alcoholics, shows a similarity in pattern of involvement to Leigh's disease, presumably because thiamine deficiency also influences energy metabolism. A difference is that in Wernicke's encephalopathy the mammillary bodies are always involved and putamen and caudate nucleus are nearly always preserved. The reason for this difference is unknown.

An example of selective vulnerability resulting from specific chemical composition is found in myelin. Myelin has a high lipid content and a very slow turnover. As a result, all the myelinated tracts are particularly vulnerable to the accumulation of lipophilic substances and to lipid peroxidation. Lipophilic substances easily cross the blood-brain barrier. One instance of such intoxication has become notorious in medical literature: hexachlorophene encephalopathy, a

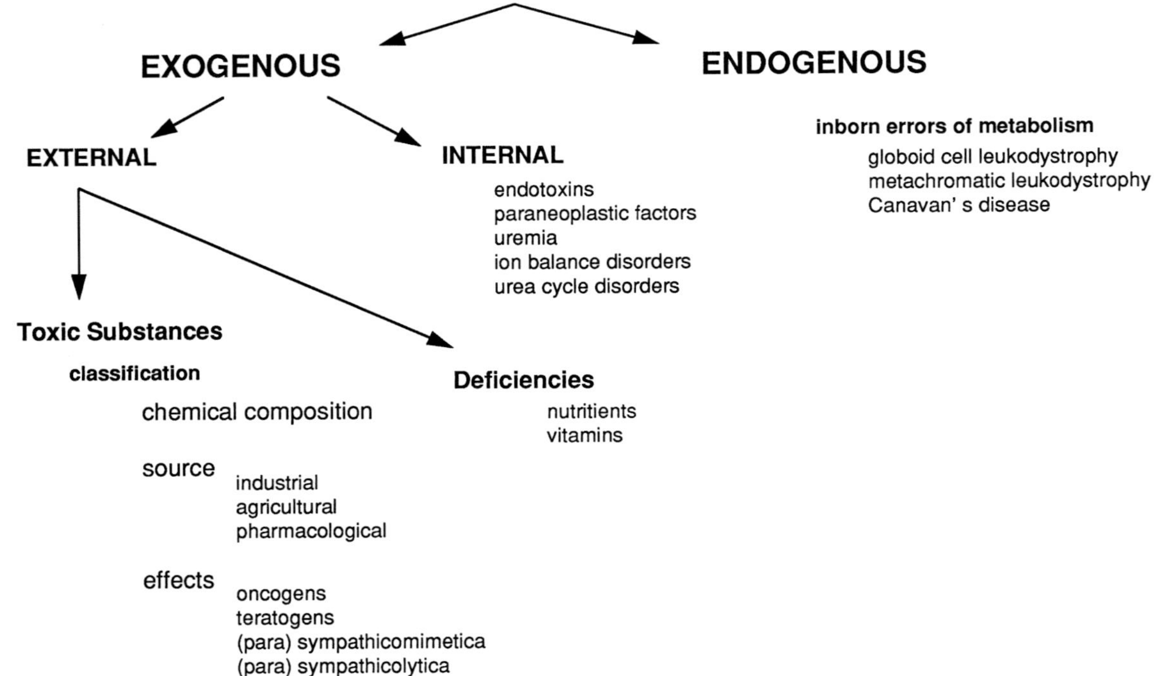

Fig. 59.2. Classification of toxic encephalopathies

vacuolating myelinopathy, was found in infants who were washed with antiseptic hexachlorophene solutions for dermal problems. The skin of preterm neonates proved to be more permeable to these agents than the more mature skin, resulting in increased absorption and toxicity. In adults, vacuolating myelinopathy has been described after the use of hexachlorophene solutions in vaginal tampons and as an antiseptic agent on burned areas. Intoxication with triethyltin has identical effects.

Topistic areas related to the distribution of a particular neurotransmitter are best visualized by positron emission tomography (PET). PET, for example, shows the distribution of [18]fluorodopa in the basal ganglia. Methylphenyltetrahydropyridine (MPTP) interferes selectively with the dopamine neurotransmitters and leads to severe Parkinsonism. Tardive dyskinesia and malignant neuroleptic syndrome are other examples of TEs in topistic areas related to specific neurotransmitters. In this kind of involvement of a neurotransmitter system, imaging modalities do not usually show abnormalities. However, in some cases MRI successfully depicts the topistic areas, as shown in a case of ecstasy intoxication (Fig. 59.1).

Selective vulnerability is also related to the level of activity during development. This concept was particularly stressed by Dobbing (1968) and has broadened the insight into the origin of congenital malformations of the CNS. The greatest impact of noxious agents is on those structures that grow and develop at the highest rate at the time of insult. Thus, migrational disorders result when toxic insults occur in the third to fifth month of gestation, the period in which neuronal migration occurs. Similarly, disorders of myelination are observed when toxic insults occur during the last trimester of pregnancy and the first year of life, because myelination of the CNS occurs at a high rate in these periods. Since normal myelination depends upon complex interactions between axons, myelin-forming oligodendrocytes and the provision of substrates by the environment, the delicate interactive process is easily disturbed by adverse factors such as nutritional deficiencies, inborn errors of metabolism and intoxications.

To facilitate the analysis of TE, we have classified them according to origin of the toxins within or outside the blood-brain barrier (endogenous vs exogenous). Exogenous TE is then further subdivided depending on whether the toxic substance originates inside or outside the body (exogenous-internal vs exogenous-external) (Fig. 59.2). This classification is imperfect because it depends, in part, on the point of view of the observer. Thus, a bacterial endotoxin can be classified either as exogenous-external, because the infection by gram-negative bacteria stems from outside the body, or as exogenous-internal because the endotoxin causing the related encephalopathy is produced by the bacteria within the body. We prefer exogenous-internal, because the toxin itself is produced within – and in interaction with – the body. The largest group of toxins are

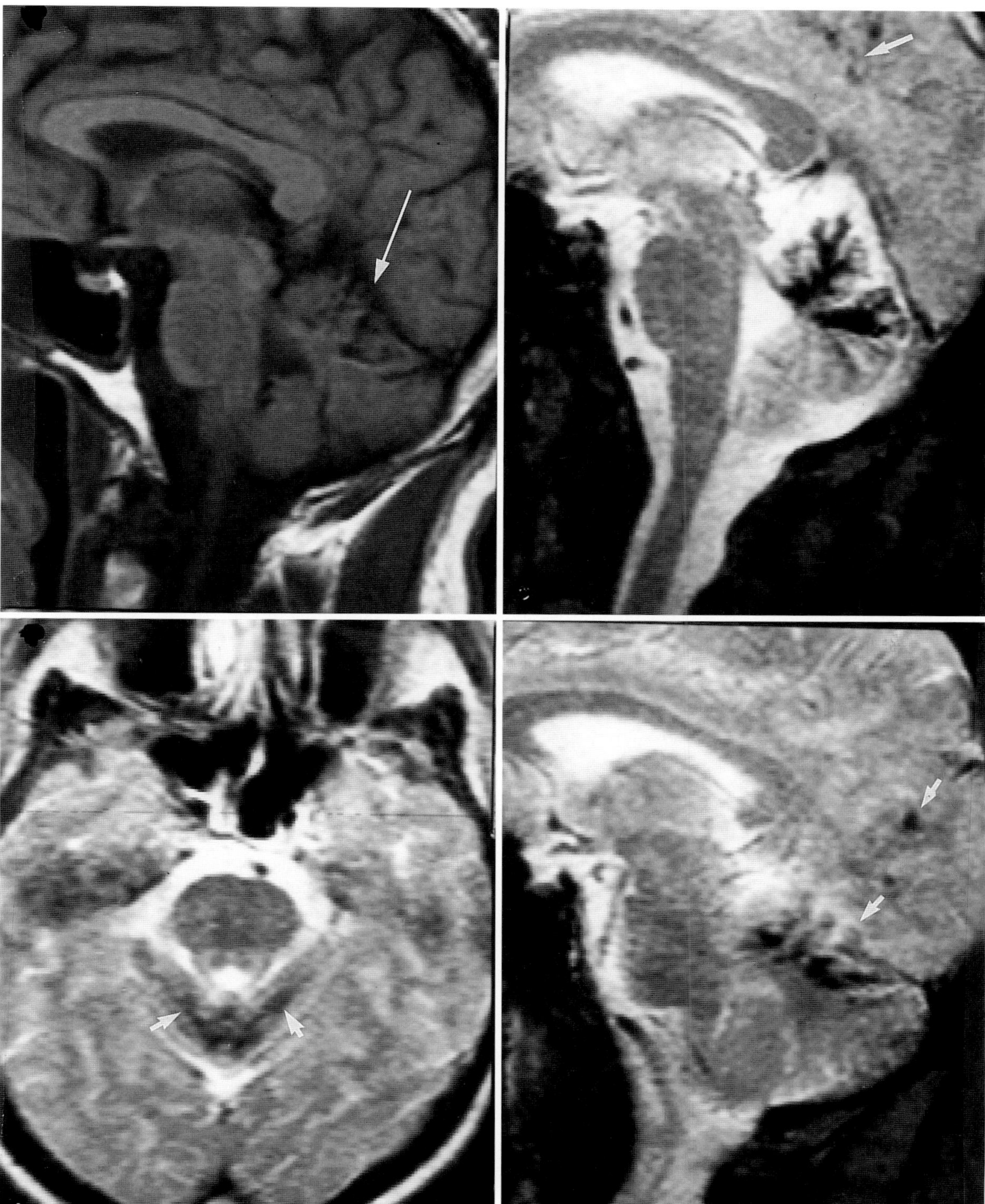

Fig. 59.3. Mercury encephalopathy in a 50-year-old male with a 2-year course of progressive cerebellar and focal cerebral signs following use of a mercury-containing compound to prevent tulip bulbs from cropping. In particular in the gradient echo techniques, more sensitive to magnetic susceptibility changes, the abnormal mineral depositions are clearly shown in cerebellar tissue and, to a less severe extent, in the occipital area

exogenous-external. Toxins within this group are usually categorized by chemical composition, source, or effect. Dietary and metabolic deficiencies may lead to abnormal bichemical processes that produce effects comparable to intoxications. They may show patterns of damage by virtue of the same selective vulnerability. These deficiency states are included among the exogenous-external TEs.

The group of *exogenous-external TEs* includes all intoxications from iatrogenic, agricultural, industrial, environmental, and social (drugs, alcohol, nicotine) sources that affect the CNS.

Belonging to this group are intoxications with the Lathyrus sativus peas, the Guamalian type of Parkinsonism, organic mercury poisoning, organic lead poisoning, and toluene exposure, as well as other well known encephalopathies associated with ethanol abuse, such as the Marchiafava-Bignami syndrome, Wernicke encephalopathy, and Korsakoff syndrome. Iatrogenic exogenous-external TEs include all TEs caused by the ingestion of prescribed drugs, such as chemotherapeutic agents, anticonvulsants, tranquilizers, and anesthetic gases, or caused by medical treatment such as progressive aluminum encephalopathy in patients undergoing dialysis. Some fetal intoxication syndromes can also be considered in this category.

Organic Mercury Poisoning. Ingestion of fish caught in the poisoned bay of Minamata led to a neurological disorder that was eventually identified as being caused by organic mercury. Mercury intoxication has also been reported following accidental ingestion of wheat that had been treated with organic mercury compounds to prevent cropping. Neuropathology shows degeneration of the granular layer of the cerebellum and patchy loss of cells in the cerebral cortex, in particular the calcarine cortex. MR images show the deposition of mercury in cerebellar structures and under the occipital cortex (Fig. 59.3).

Lead Encephalopathy. Children may have a lower tolerance to lead than adults. Acute lead intoxication is associated with convulsions, delirium, meningism and papilledema. Chronic intoxication is associated with dementia, peripheral neuropathy, anemia, and a variety of visceral features. Neuropathologically the mildest chronic form of lead intoxication is the selective, segmental demyelination of peripheral nerves. In acute cases there may be demyelination and necrosis of central and cerebellar white matter. Neuronal damage is pronounced. The neuropathological picture may resemble that of Schilder disease.

Aluminum dementia. Aluminum has been indicated as a toxic factor in dialysis dementia. The excessive aluminum was probably derived from the high aluminum concentration in the dialysate and from the phosphate binding gels which contain aluminum. It has been suggested that aluminium is of pathogenetic importance in Alzheimer's disease and a possible role has also been mentioned in amyotrophic lateral sclerosis and the Guamalian Parkinson syndrome.

Wernicke Encephalopathy. Wernicke encnephalopathy results from a deficiency of vitmain B_1 (thiamine), and, as such, is not confined to chronic alcoholics. Because vitamin B_1 is a cofactor of transketolase, thiamine deficiency causes decreased activity of this enzyme. The precise relationship of reduced enzyme activity to damage in the characteristic "topistic area" represented by Wernicke encephalopathy is conjectural. Korsakoff disease is now generally seen as a chronic stage of Wernicke encephalopathy, with consistent atrophy of the mammillary bodies and variable involvement of the dorsomedial nucleus of the thalamus.

Cytostatic Agents. Cytostatics, such as methotrexate and 5-fluorouracil can lead to severe changes in the white matter when they are used to treat extracranial tumors, or intracranial tumors (often in combination with radiotherapy).

Heroin Pyrolysite. During the 1980s, it was discovered that a group of chronic heroin addicts in Amsterdam manifested progressive neurological symptoms after sniffing heroin. On neuropathological examination, a vacuolating myelinopathy was discoverd in these cases. MR studies revealed extensive involvement of the white matter of the cerebral hemispheres and the cerebellum and clearly depicted the affected tracts from the parietal cortex to the brain stem (Fig. 59.4). The toxic substance in the heroin has not been identified. One assumes that it must be a lipophilic substance. Identical neurological findings and MRI abnormalities have been found among cocaine addicts (Fig. 59.5).

Organic Solvents. Chronic inhalation of organic solvents or other preparations containing toluene is known to cause multifocal neurological and mental disorders. Cerebral, cerebellar and brain stem atrophy, and diffuse focal white matter abnormalities are detected by MRI (Fig. 59.6–59.8). Toluene is one example of a typical lipophilic substance that persists in the myelin for a long time, leading to myelin damage.

Common to the disorders caused by *exogenous-internal toxins* is a focal or generalized process in the body outside the blood-brain barrier that produces a toxin that crosses the blood-brain barrier, enters the brain, and gives rise to encephalopathy. Paraneoplastic syndromes and parainfectious degeneration may partially belong to this category. It must be noted that tumors may contain antigens that lead to the formation of antibodies, which cannot distinguish between tumor cells and own-body cells, for example, Purkinje cells. Malignant disease anywhere in the body may have a remote effect on the peripheral nerves, the spinal cord, and on the brain, causing peripheral neuropathy, subacute necrotizing myelopathy, and encephalomyeloradiculitis. The encephalomyeloradiculitis group in-

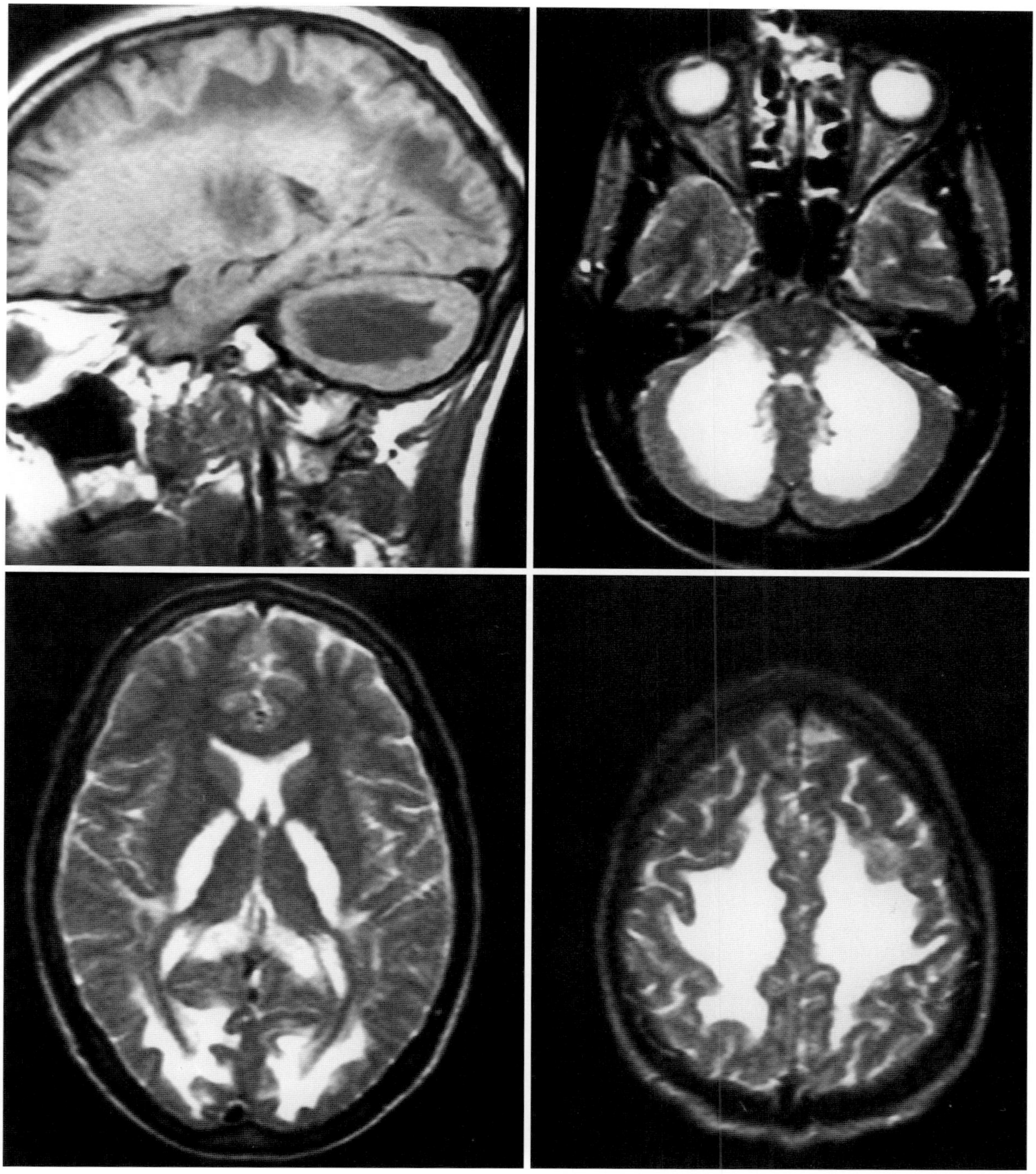

Fig. 59.4. A 26-year-old male with severe neurological disability after sniffing toxic heroin. Histologically the white matter changes are due to a vacuolating myelinopathy. There are lesions in the parietooccipital white matter, the posterior limb of the internal capsule (note the swelling), tracts in the brain stem and the cerebellar white matter. In all cases investigated in Amsterdam, the MRI pattern is identical

cludes two special forms: brain stem encephalitis, and so-called limbic encephalitis in which the changes are restricted to the limbic system. The differing manifestations presumably reflect the differing antigenic content of these brain structures. It is, however, probable that a more general toxic effect may play an additional role. The general atrophy of the brain often seen in lung cancer may be caused by toxins.

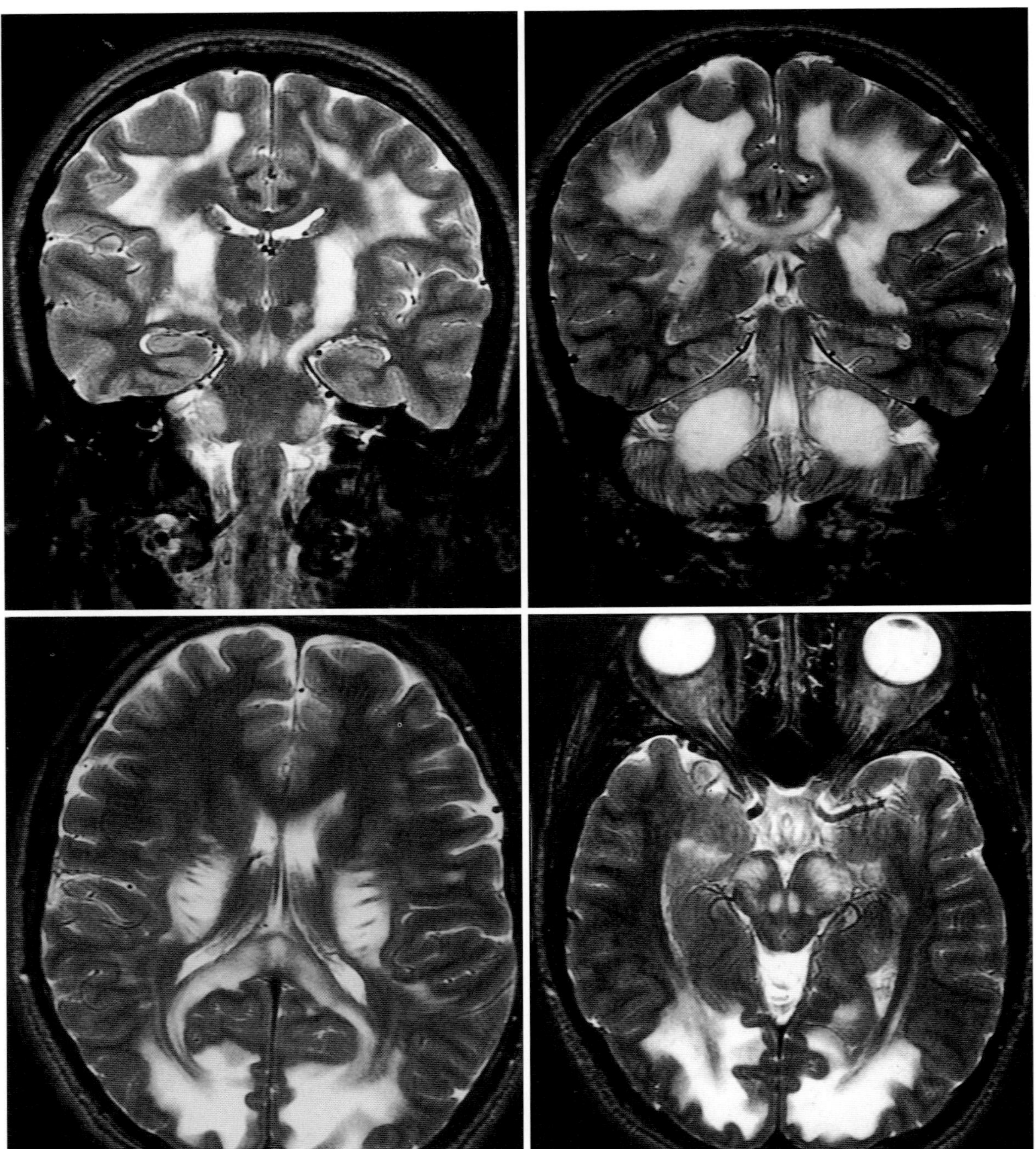

Fig. 59.5. Series of T_2-weighted MR images in transverse and coronal planes of a 22-year-old male cocaine sniffer. The abnormalities are similar to those found in patients sniffing heroin. The swelling of the white matter suggests that a vacuolating myelinopathy also exists in this case. The images demonstrate beautifully all involved structures. Courtesy of Dr. Tamraz, Paris, with permission

Parainfectious encephalopathy has been reported with Escherichia coli, Mycoplasma pneumoniae, and diphtheria infections. Here, too, the reaction may be toxic, allergic or both.

Changes in the ion balance are held responsible for central pontine and extrapontine myelinolysis. Hyponatremia is considered to be an important initial factor in these disorders, subsequently precipitated by

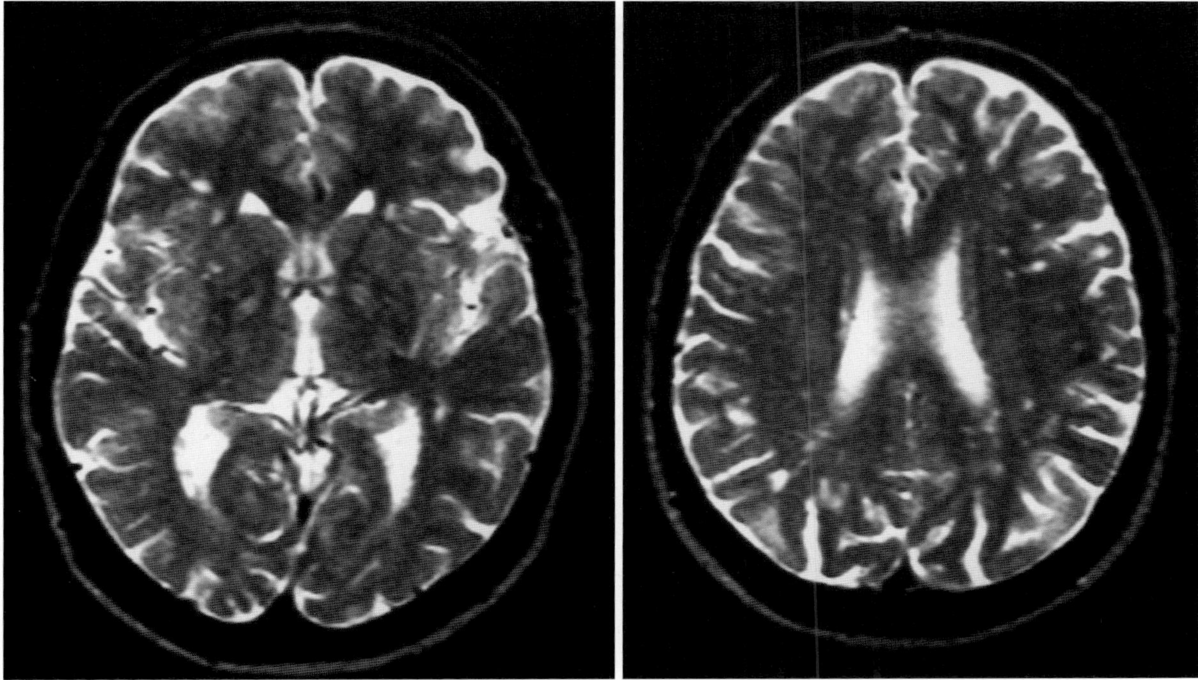

Fig. 59.6. A 58-year-old male with progressive memory loss, who worked in the paint industry for more than 40 years. The T_2-weighted MR images show widespread focal changes, disseminated throughout the white matter, and also faint changes in the basal ganglia. There is some loss of cortical tissue

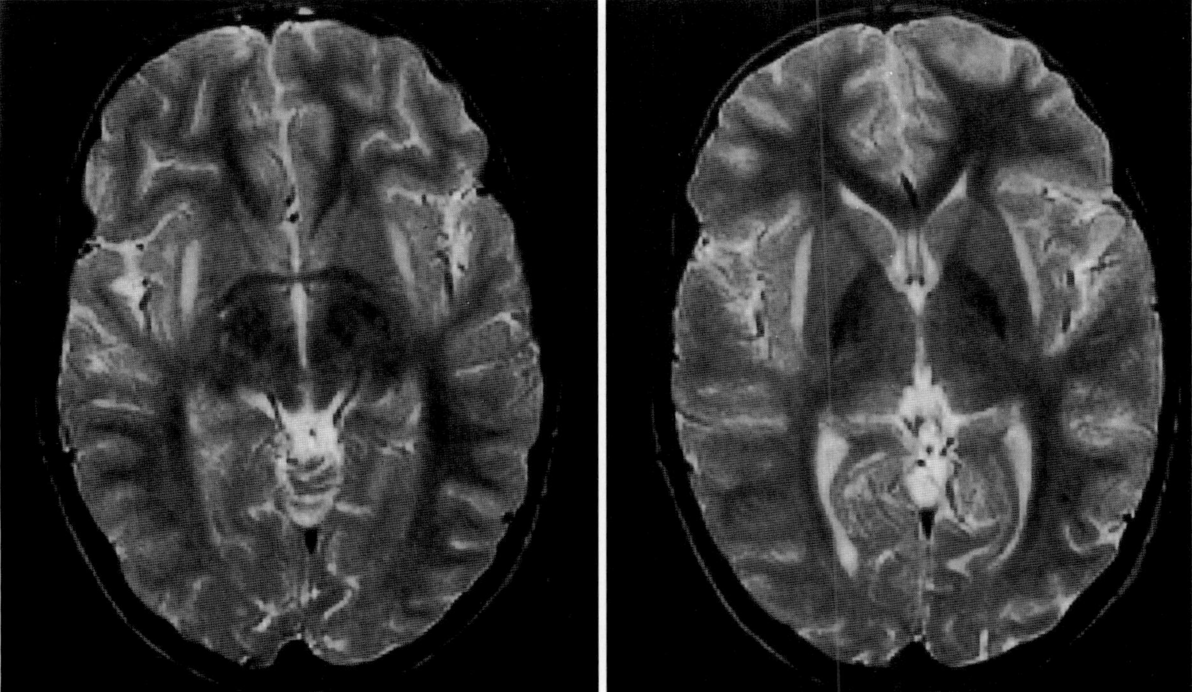

Fig. 59.7. An 18-year-old girl was admitted to the hospital with epileptic status. She had painted her new apartment during the last 3 days with closed doors and windows. The T_2-weighted images show bilateral, symmetric high signal intensity of the claustrum. This proved to be transient and disappeared in 3 weeks

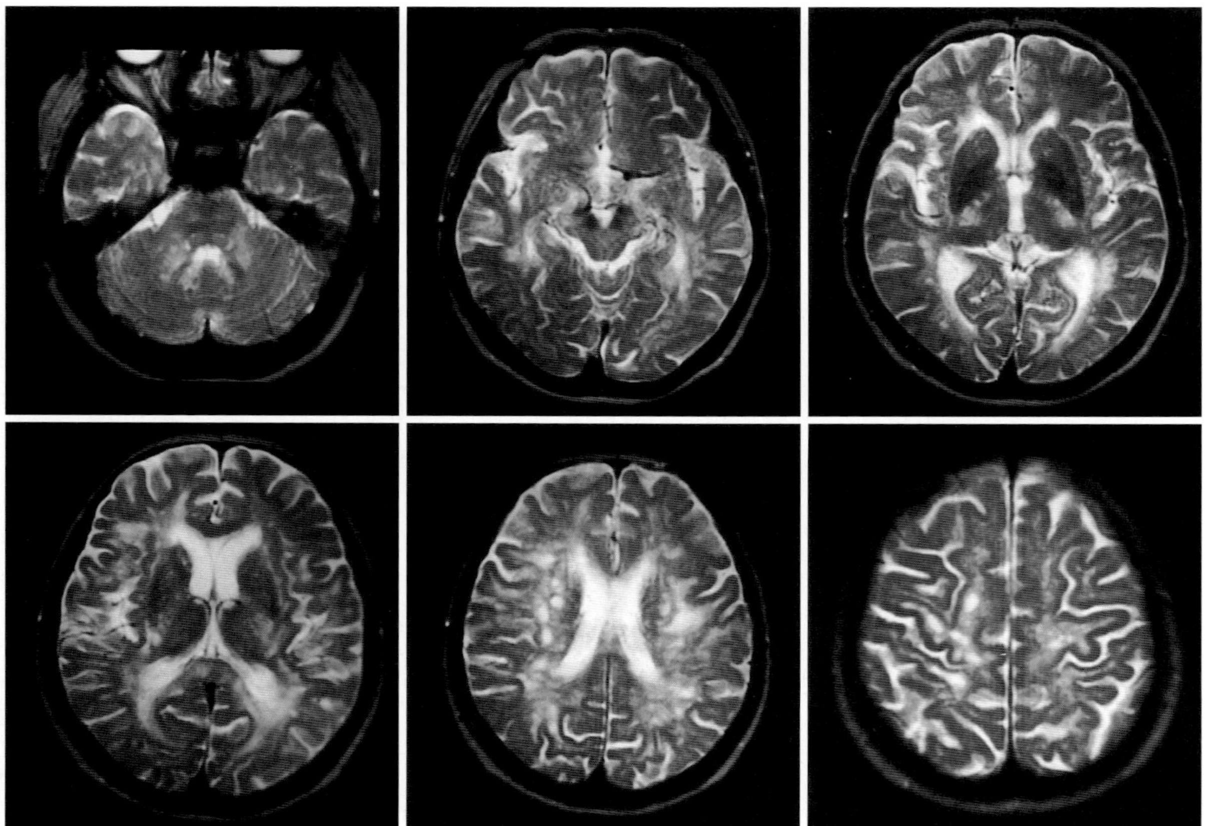

Fig. 59.8. T$_2$-weighted series of a 64-year-old female patient with progressive subcortical dementia and gait disturbances. This patient had been handling insecticides and pesticides for about 40 years. There is a widespread, focal, in some areas confluent, increased signal intensity in the white matter of the hemispheres and middle cerebellar peduncles

(too) fast restoration of the serum plasma concentration. It has often been linked to alcohol abuse, but has also been reported in postoperative cases and in psychiatric patients with excessive intake of water.

Inborn errors of metabolism may lead to accumulation of toxic substances produced outside the blood-brain barrier, crossing the blood-brain barrier and leading to toxic brain damage. Many of the disorders described in the first part of this book may be considered an exogenous-internal TE. Examples are many of the amino acidopathies and organic acidopathies, including the urea cycle disorders. In Wilson disease, the encephalopathy is related to excessive deposition of copper in the brain, especially in the globus pallidus.

Hormonal abnormalities in infants may disturb the normal process of myelination. Thyroid deficiency in the neonatal period causes disturbed development of the CNS with a decreased formation of myelin. Also hypocortisolism, hypercortisolism, cortisol treatment and a deficiency of growth hormone result in hypomyelination in infants.

Failure of internal organs may lead to exogenous-internal TEs. The most well-known examples are renal failure and hepatic failure. The so-called hepatocerebral syndromes manifest by cerebral atrophy, by changes in signal intensity in the basal ganglia, and by T$_1$-shortening of the white matter (particularly in infants and children). ^{1}H MR spectroscopy has shown an increase in glutamine and a depletion of myo-inositol. Most investigators believe that ammonia plays a key role in hepatic encephalopathy. It appears to cause neurotoxiticity by interacting with the glutamate/glutamine/GABA balance. Apart from its other roles in metabolism, glutamate is the most important excitatory neurotransmitter. Gamma-aminobutyric acid, GABA, formed by decarboxylation from glutamate, is the most important inhibitory neurotransmitter. In the presynaptic neuron glutamate is formed from glutamine by glutaminase. After neurotransmission glutamate is taken up by astrocytes where it is processed by glutamine synthetase into glutamine. Glutamine is transported to the presynaptic neuron where glutaminase catalyses the formation of glutamate available for neurotransmission. Hyperammonemia has a great impact on this cycle by stimulating glutamine synthesis via glutamine synthetase, by possible inhibition of glu-

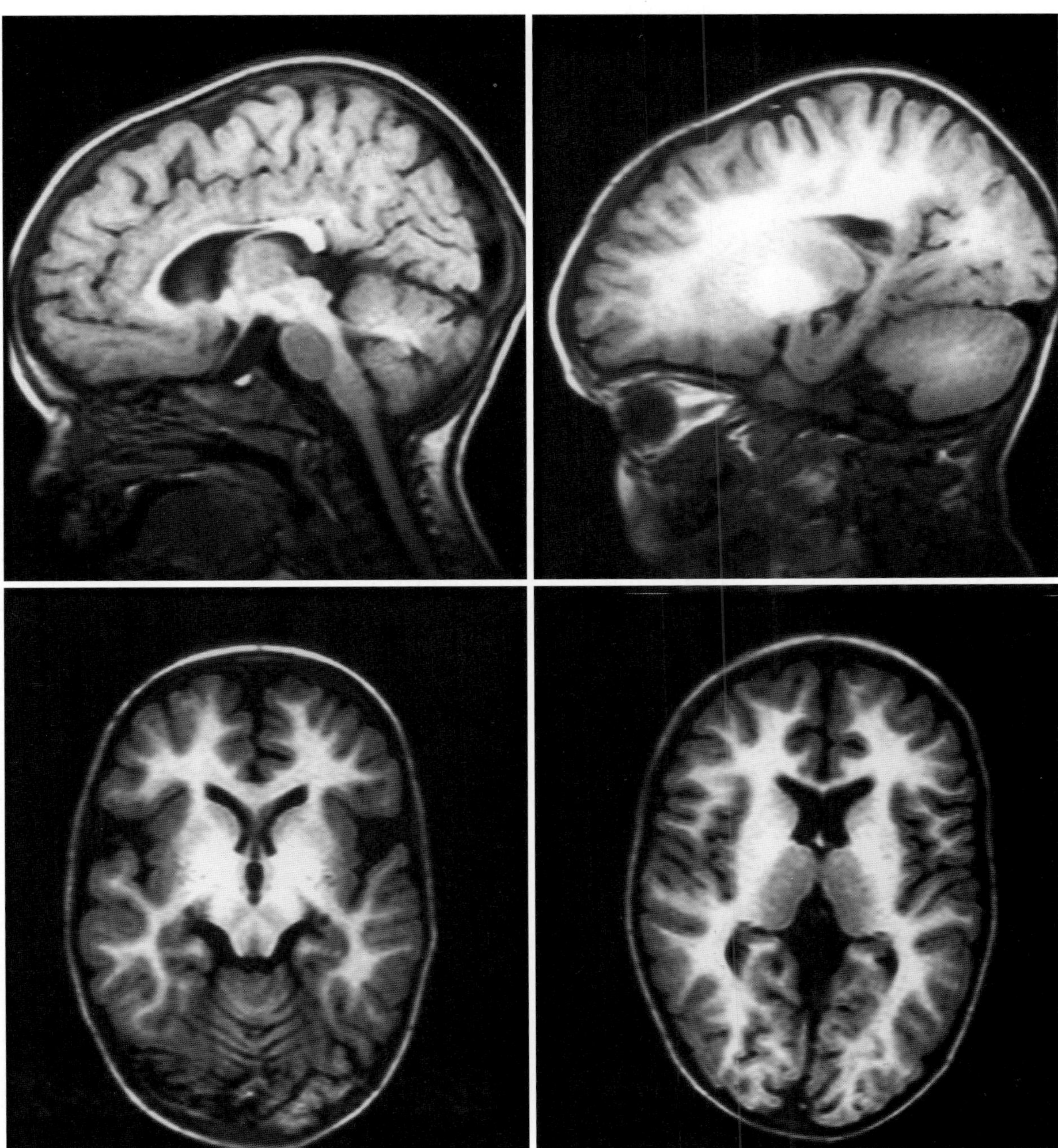

Fig. 59.9. T_1-weighted sagittal and transverse (IR) images in 3-year-old boy with hepatic failure and hepatic encephalopathy. The images show the typical T_1 shortening in the basal ganglia but also of the white matter. Due to T_1-shortening the basal ganglia can hardly be distinguished from the surrounding white matter. The pons shows T_1-shortening in the posterior part, leading to a pattern on the T_1-weighted sagittal image as seen in neonates

taminase and by inhibition of glutamate re-uptake by the astrocyte. However, the relation between the neurotransmitters changes and the T_1-shortening as seen on MR is not clear. Other explanations for the T_1- shortening of the basal ganglia have been suggested, such as accumulation of manganese or of lipid particles. A group of researchers demonstrated intracytoplasmatic lipid accumulation in glia in the caudate nucleus and putamen. In MR images, T_1-shortening in the basal ganglia can make the basal ganglia indistinguishable from white matter on T_1-weighted images (Fig. 59.9). At the same time, there is T_1-shortening in the white matter, typically sparing the pons. In older patients, this spread of T_1-shortening over the white matter is

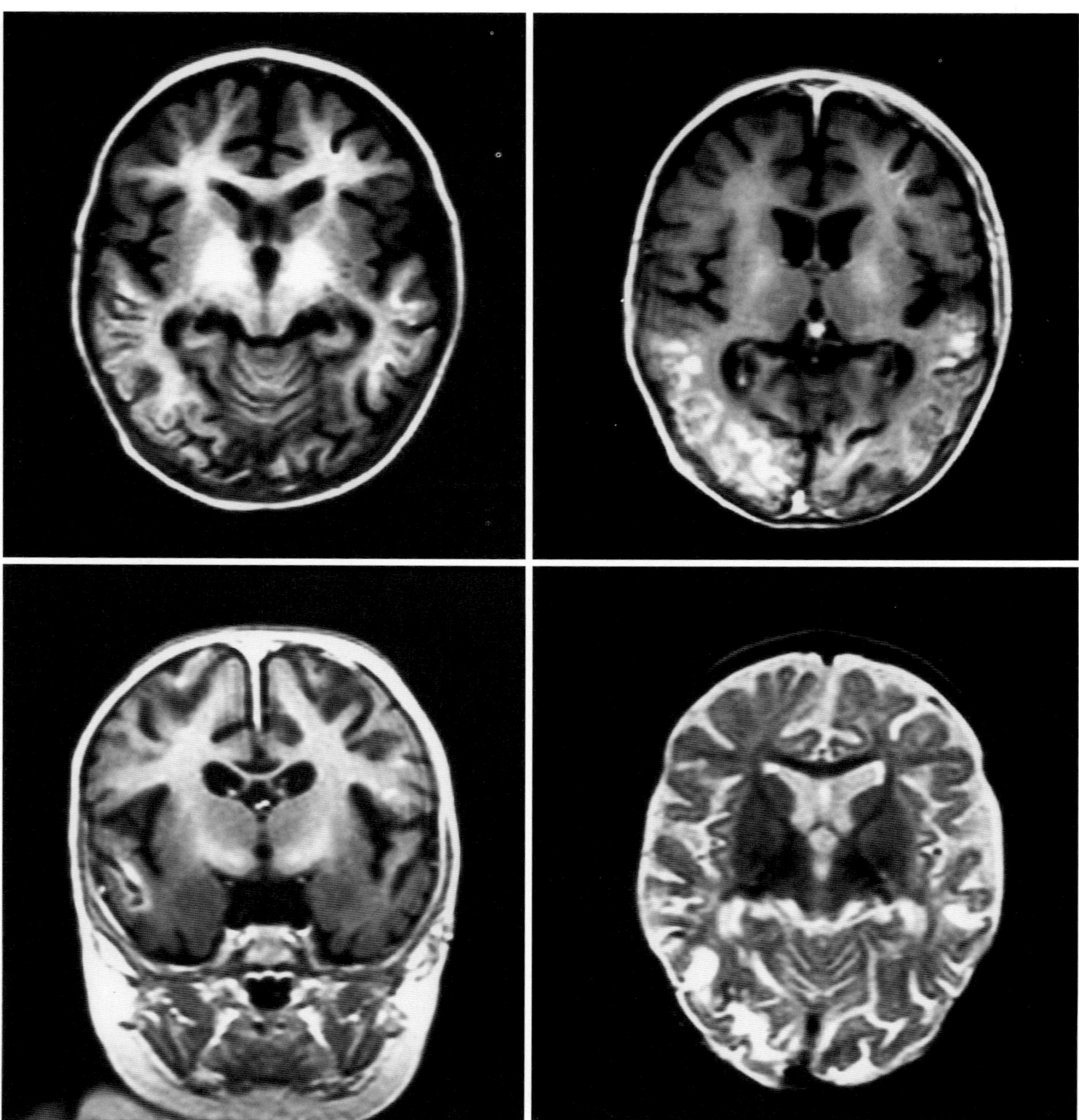

Fig. 59.10. A 7-month-old girl with a hemorrhagic shock and encephalopathy syndrome. Hemorrhagic laminar cortical lesions are seen in the occipital lobe. There is also a striking T_1 shortening in the globus pallidus on the T_1-weighted images. The T_2-weighted transverse image (*lower right*) shows generalized atrophy, presence of lesions in the occipital area, but no clear changes in T_2 relaxation time in the basal ganglia

less clear. The T_1-shortening of gray and white matter may be observed with a number of toxic-metabolic conditions, not just hepatic encephalopathy. For instance, we have seen this phenomenon in a child with a hemorrhagic shock and encephalopathy syndrome (Fig. 59.10). It has also been reported in patients who received parenteral nutrition over a long period.

The *endogenous forms of TE* are the smallest group. A number of inborn errors of metabolism should be included here, because their effects are mediated by a toxic product produced locally. In particular, this is the case in lysosomal storage disorders, such as Krabbe disease or globoid cell leukodystrophy. The primary defect is galactocerebroside-β-galactosidase deficiency. This enzyme has two functions: it normally degrades cerebroside into galactose and ceramide and it normally hydrolyzes psychosine (galactosyl sphingosine). Psychosine is a toxic metabolite that is essentially non-existent in normal brain. Presence of elevated psychosine in Krabbe's disease causes early, very rapid, almost complete death of the oligodendroglia with extensive loss of myelin sheaths maintained by these cells. In addition, inability to degrade cerebroside leads to an abnormally high concentration of this substance within the myelin membrane, eventually resulting in myelin instability and breakdown. In Krabbe disease, the disturbance of both functions of galactocerebroside-β-galactosidase contributes to the myelin loss. In metachromatic leukodystrophy it is the local storage of sulfatide that causes myelin damage and loss.

The *toxic interactions interfering with fetal development* can be considered an exogenous-external intoxication, reaching the unborn child via the mother. The fetal syndromes are unique, because the effect of the toxin depends upon the stage of development the child has reached, as well as upon the nature of the toxin, its concentration, and the duration of the exposure. Toxic or teratogenic substances have a great impact on the developing fetus. The effects are often widespread and involve multiple parts of the body or the whole body, in addition to the brain. The gamut of possible dysgeneses is extensive and ranges from lethal malformation with early spontaneous abortion to mild alteration in morphology and function. The sources of the toxins include:

1. Medical treatment. Syndromes can result from the use of established drugs prescribed to the mother, but taken during pregnancy. Most such cases are accidental. A few arise when drugs are given knowingly in desperate cases. Antiepileptic drugs are known to cause developmental damage, resulting, for example, in the fetal hydantion syndrome and the fetal valproate syndrome.

2. Alcohol and drug abuse. An important cause of fetal dysgenesis is the use of drugs or alcohol during pregnancy. The fetal alcohol syndrome has been reported extensively in the literature. These children are growth retarded, have short palpebral fissures, a low nasal bridge, epicanthus, a long convex upper lip, and mental reardation. The numerous CNS anomalies of the fetal alcohol syndrome include: derangement of neuronal and glial migration, microcephaly, hydrocephaly, porencephaly, agenesis of the corpus callosum, meningomyelocele, and Dandy Walker malformation.

3. Metabolic disorders of the mother. Fetal development may suffer if the mother has a metabolic disorder. Diabetes mellitus may be one causative factor in the caudal regression syndrome, a complex abonormality of the caudal end of the embryo with anal atresia, sacral dysgenesis or agenesis, high position of the conus medullaris, and diverse urological, neurological, and orthopedic disorders. Microcephaly can be caused by maternal phenylketonuria.

4. Teratogenic chemical substances. Compounds with teratogenic action may be encountered in the direct environment (pollution, professional contact with chemicals).

60 Central Pontine and Extrapontine Myelinolysis

60.1 Clinical Features and Laboratory Investigations

Central pontine myelinolysis (CPM) is a demyelinating disorder affecting mainly the ventral part of the pons. In some cases, CPM is accompanied by extrapontine myelinolysis (EPM, together CPM/EPM). CPM/EPM is not a primary disease but develops against a background of other, usually severe conditions, apparently as a complication of the main disease. It occurs mostly in alcoholics but has also been reported in association with diabetic ketoacidosis, psychogenic excessive water drinking, inappropriate antidiuretic hormone secretion, malnutrition, and chronic debilitating diseases. It is probable that the underlying cause of myelinolysis in all these disorders is a derangement of serum sodium concentration, particularly a rapid correction of hyponatremia.

Most of the patients are severely ill as a result of the primary disorder. It takes a period of a few days for patients to develop the clinical symptoms caused by CPM/EPM. Mental confusion is present in many but not all cases. Sometimes patients suddenly lapse into coma for no apparent reason. No particular type of mental change is specific for CPM and EPM, as there is a variety of associated clinical conditions, some of which have their own mental counterparts, such as Wernicke's encephalopathy, delirium tremens and various metabolic encephalopathies. Frequently a bulbar or pseudobulbar syndrome is present, manifesting itself in dysarthria or anarthria, dysphagia, and sometimes weakness of the neck muscles. Involvement of the facial nerve is uncommon; when present, it is of the central type and part of a hemispheric syndrome. Occasionally a limitation of conjugate movement of the eyes is found. Oculomotor or abducens nerve dysfunction is rarely observed. Pupillary disturbances may be present. The weakness of the limbs is often severe, resulting in tetraparesis or tetraplegia. The usual type of motor weakness is flaccid with hyporeflexia. Extensor plantar reflexes and abnormal bulbar reflexes are often part of the clinical picture. Due to this weakness the testing of cerebellar function is often impossible. Extrapyramidal features may occur. Sensory findings are rare.

The clinical manifestations of CPM/EPM vary, according to the extent of the lesions, from minimal to a complete locked-in syndrome or coma. The constellation of neurological findings is not specific for CPM/EPM and may also be seen in other types of brain dysfunction, particularly in pontine infarction or hemorrhage. Clinically, CPM/EPM can only be suspected, especially if the neurological condition of a patient deteriorates after correction of hyponatremia. Symptoms of the disease appear within hours or up to a week after correction of hyponatremia. Many patients with neurological manifestations of CPM/EPM die of complications or underlying disease. However, other patients survive with partial or complete recovery.

In a case of CPM the EEG is rarely abnormal, as even large lesions of the basis pontis are compatible with a normal EEG. The most frequently observed EEG abnormality is a generalized slowing, correlating with the level of consciousness. In EPM, the EEG may show focal abnormalities. BAEPs and SSEPs often show abnormalities consistent with a pontine lesion, but may also be completely normal. The abnormalities are nonspecific.

60.2 Pathology

In CPM there is usually a single symmetrical lesion, located in the central part of the basis pontis. It can be large, occupying almost the entire basis pontis, or very small. Generally the lesion is continuous and sharply defined, although an island of tissue is occasionally preserved. In exceptional cases the lesion develops unilaterally or appears to be multifocal. Rarely, the lesion spreads into the tegmentum pontis or into the middle cerebellar peduncles. It does not usually extend to the surface of the pons.

Histologically, there is a severe and sometimes complete loss of myelin in the lesion with a concomitant loss of oligodendrocytes. Demyelination affects both the long tracts (pontocerebellar transverse fibers and the long descending tracts) and the pontine nuclei. The axons are mostly well preserved, although a considerable loss of axons may occur. The most severely affected area may be cystic in nature due to almost total disappearance of myelin and axons. Axonal loss is associated with degenerative changes in nerve cells. However, on the whole, neurons of the pontine nuclei are relatively spared even in areas of severe demyelination. Reactive astrocytosis and macrophage response are usually present. Macrophages contain remnants of disintegrated myelin and lipid material. Neither vascular disease nor inflammation is seen.

In EPM, which accompanies CPM in 10% of patients, similar demyelinating lesions occur outside the pons with predilection for the white matter of the cerebellum, especially of the folia. Also affected are the mammillary bodies, the tegmentum of the midbrain, the lateral geniculate bodies, the thalamus, basal ganglia, the internal, external, and extreme capsules, the anterior commissure, the fornix, the deep layers of the cerebral cortex and subjacent white matter of the crowns, and sides of the cerebral gyri. Not all these structures are necessarily affected in any one patient; the precise localization of demyelinated lesions varies from patient to patient. In exceptional cases, histological abnormalities consistent with the diagnosis EPM occur without any pontine lesion.

60.3 Pathogenetic Considerations

CPM and EPM have been reported in quite a number of diseases: alcoholism, psychogenic water drinking, diabetic ketoacidosis, subdural abscess, brain tumor, cerebral trauma, meningitis, encephalitis, renal dialysis, malnutrition, lung infections, adrenocortical insufficiency, postoperative hyponatremia, inappropriate antidiurectic hormone secretion, extracerebral malignancy, and other chronic debilitating diseases. The etiology is not completely understood. Abnormalities in serum sodium levels have been the subject of considerable interest in this respect. There is evidence that a rapid correction of hyponatremia may cause CPM/EPM. Clinical observations strongly suggest this causal relationship as the clinical symptomatology in CPM/EPM is usually preceded by a rapid rise in serum sodium after a period of sustained hyponatremia. Usually, no neurological injury is seen when the chronic hyponatremia is corrected slowly. In all diseases inferred to be able to induce CPM/EPM, hyponatremia is a common complication, for which a rigorous treatment is often instituted after hospitalization.

There are strong indications that CPM/EPM is indeed an iatrogenic disease. The first description of this syndrome dates from the 1950s. It is inconceivable that it could have been missed by neurologists and pathologists of the nineteenth and early twentieth centuries with their strong reliance on postmortem examination. In the 1950s a more liberal use was made of intra-venous tubing, and there was interest in treating alcoholic withdrawal states by massive administration of intravenous fluid. Thiazide diuretics were introduced for clinical use at this time. These factors probably contributed to the genesis of hyponatremia. Alcohol has an antidiuretic hormone blocking effect. Alcohol withdrawal leads to a rapid return of antidiuretic hormone function, thus causing hyponatremia. With intravenous tubing aggressive treatment of hyponatremia by infusion of hypertonic solutions became possible in any of the implicated diseases. The clinical syndrome and the characteristic histological lesions of CPM/EPM can be reproduced in experimental work with dogs and rats by rapid correction of hyponatremia. In these experiments, hyponatremia in itself does not appear sufficient to induce CPM/EPM, and neither a self-correction of the serum sodium nor a rapid rise from normonatremia to hypernatremia result in CPM/EPM.

However, there are other, conflicting data. Some investigators found that the rate of increase in serum sodium in patients with CPM/EPM had been more rapid than in patients with hyponatremia but without CPM/EPM. Others found no difference in the rate of increase of serum sodium in the two groups. Sometimes patients with a slow rise in serum sodium actually develop CPM/EPM. Some authors stress that most of the patients developing CPM/EPM became hypernatremic after correction and state that it is the elevation of serum sodium to hypernatremic levels rather than the rapid correction that predisposes to CPM/EPM. Others have found that CPM/EPM can develop without overcorrection, while a mild hyponatremia still exists. In a recent discussion, attention was paid to the combined role of hyponatremia and hypoxia. The new point of view was that independent of the rate of correction of the hyponatremia, brain stem lesions develop when hypoxia is present.

The exact pathogenesis of demyelination in CPM/EPM is not clear. It is known that generalized cellular edema is the hallmark of acute hyponatremia. In cases of chronic hyponatremia, brain cells have adapted to this condition by extruding sodium, potassium, chloride, and water. The loss of more solute than water renders cellular and extracellular fluid equally hypotonic, but reduces cell swelling. Restoration of normal serum osmolality removes water from the hypotonic tissue and causes the adapted, normovolemic brain cells to shrink to volumes less than normal. As brain cells replenish lost electrolytes, the normal cellular volume is re-established. Complications may result if normoatremia is achieved too rapidly before cellular restoration of lost solute. The rapid rise in sodium level results in an osmotic endothelial injury and in opening of the blood-brain barrier. The proposed mechanisms for opening the blood-brain barrier is endothelial cell shrinkage allowing fluid into the intercapillary and pericapillary spaces. Others suggest that the barrier opening is in fact due to enhanced vesicular transport. In any case, the penetration of the blood-brain barrier is proven by the presence of biliary pigment in the myelinolytic lesion of some highly jaundiced patients. It is hypothesized that the endothelial injury leads to a release of myelinotoxic factors from the damaged cells, in turn leading to demyelination. Alternatively, and not necessarily mutually exclusively, the osmotic opening of the blood-brain barrier results in vasogenic edema. Indeed, edema has been observed in CPM lesions. It is known that edema may itself be myelinotoxic. If the presumption of this mechanism is correct, it may explain the localization of lesions, which preferentially develop at sites characterized by an extensive admixture of gray and white matter. Of all regions in the brain, the pons has the greatest degree of gray-white apposition. Areas such as the basal ganglia, thalamus, geniculate bodies, and cortex-white matter junctions also have extensive apposition of gray and white matter. Edema or related myelinotoxic factors are principally derived from the highly vascular gray matter and are thus able to affect the adjacent heavily myelinated white matter. However, the mechanism whereby edema may cause demyelination remains to be determined. An alternative hypothesis states that edema of the pons would result in strangulation of tracts and nuclear masses. In the pontine basis longitudinal and transverse fibers are interlacing. Because of this grid-like anatomy, the pons is particularly susceptible to damage when edema occurs, as the edema literally strangles the myelin sheaths and small blood vessels. If mild, this would result in a reversible physiological block of neurotransmission. If edema persisted and became more severe, irreversible demyelination would occur.

Although the summarized views seem reasonable, there are some objections. This grid pattern is not present in extrapontine localizations of myelinolysis. There are regions in the brain in which myelinated fibers are interspersed with layers of gray matter, that do not show myelinolysis. And, finally, the factor of edema, invoked in several theories of myelinolysis, is little documented.

Another variable to be considered is the role of the underlying condition. The overrepresentation of alcoholics in the myelinolysis population requires explanation. It may simply be related to the fact that alcoholics admitted to hospital are in withdrawal and at the same time vigorously treated with intravenous fluids. Another possibility is that the alcoholic state or the withdrawal of alcohol somehow makes the brain more sensitive to the rapid rise of serum sodium from hyponatremia. This is conceivable, since alcohol reportedly affects brain hydration. Thiamine deficiency may be another factor. Thiamine deficiency may cause depletion of ATP, which may affect the transport of electrolytes in the cell membranes, producing endothelial damage and making cells more vulnerable to osmotic change. The fact that CPM/EPM has been observed in the setting of a variety of medical disorders other than alcoholism suggests that seriously ill patients are in general vulnerable to the disease. Again, this fact may simply indicate that very sick patients face an increased risk of hyponatremia or a greater likelihood of undergoing vigorous correction of hyponatremia. The other possibility is that the brains of debilitated patients are less resistant to a rapid rise of serum sodium. Here too thiamine deficiency may play a role.

60.4 Therapy

No therapy is available for CPM/EPM. As soon as the neurological symptomatology has developed, only symptomatic measures can be taken. Prevention must therefore be the focus of clinical efforts. The prevention of CPM/EPM relates to the medical approach to hyponatremia, especially chronic hyponatremia. As there are different opinions about the role of hyponatremia and the rise of serum sodium level in the genesis of CPM/EPM, there are likewise many guidelines for the correction of hyponatremia. In severe hyponatremia with a serum sodium concentration below 120 mmol/l, correction is necessary. The recommended rate of correction varies between 0.5 to 2 mmol/l per hour, or 12 to 48 mmol/l per day. The fact that hyponatremia itself may lead to brain damage forms an argument against very slow correction. After reaching a concentration of 120–130 mmol/l, water restriction in combination with a diet with normal salt content is recommended. In chronic asymptomatic hyponatremia, simple water restriction and a diet with normal salt content may suffice from the beginning. Others prefer a combination of normal saline with fluid restriction. Of course, diuretics which cause salt loss are discontinued. It is advisable to avoid hypernatremia. In the light of recent discussion, one should also be aware of the influence of hypoxic-ischemic conditions and correct those as soon as possible.

In addition to the rate of sodium correction, the total osmotic load from contrast material in CT scanning must be considered. Intravenous contrast material should not be used in the immediate post-correctional period of hyponatremia.

60.5 Magnetic Resonance Imaging

CT scanning may show fairly characteristic abnormalities in CPM, consisting of a roundish or triangular hypodense area on the midline of the pons, approxi-

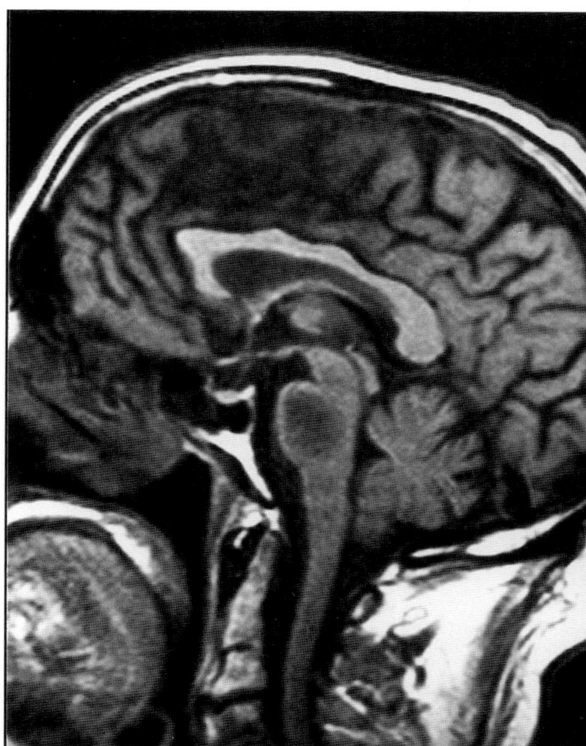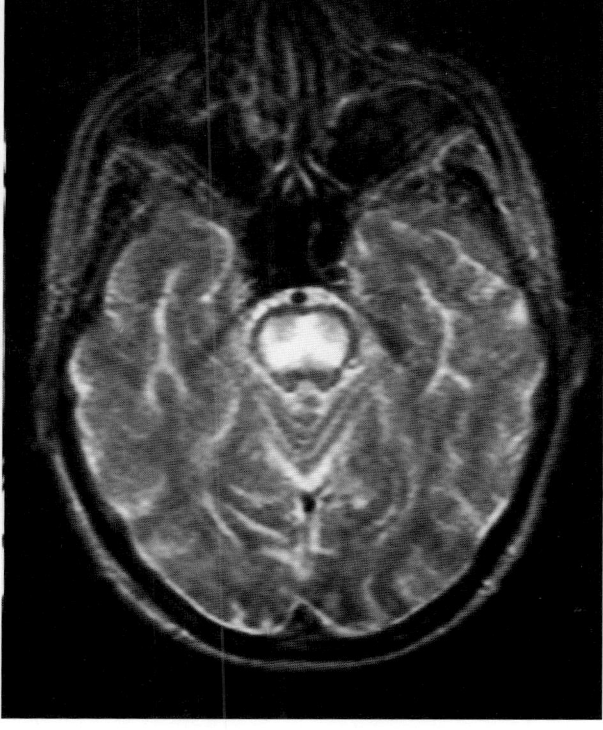

Fig. 60.1. A 56-year-old male with an episode of general malaise, vomiting and desiccation. Hyponatremia of 111.5 mmol/l was corrected in 2 days to 134 mmol/l, followed by severe neurological symptoms. Midsagittal T_1 and transverse T_2-weighted MR images demonstrate the characteristic features of CPM, typically sparing the outer rim of the pons

mately equidistant from the floor of the fourth ventricle and the ventral surface of the pons with little or no peripheral enhancement after contrast injection. The fourth ventricle shows no displacement, and the brain stem is of normal size. The CT scan can also detect abnormalities consistent with EPM. Sometimes the CT scan is found to be normal in CPM/EPM. In some patients the hypodensities of the CT scan disappear as the patient improves, but persistence of hypodensities has also been observed despite clinical cure. CT findings appear to correlate rather poorly with the clinical syndrome. Furthermore, the specificity of CT findings in CPM is not high, as differentiation between CPM and other pontine lesions, especially pontine infarction, is often difficult or impossible. It is not an infrequent occurrence that posterior fossa artefacts, characteristic on CT, prevent optimal assessment of the pontine area.

MRI is capable of showing the characteristics of CPM and EPM in more detail. MRI is normal or may show low signal intensity in the pons at onset of clinical symptoms. In classic cases of CPM, repeat MRI after a few days shows symmetric demyelination of the basis pontis, spreading centrifugally from the median raphe, characteristically leaving the outer rim of the pons un-

affected (Fig. 60.1). Hence, the ventrolateral longitudinal fibers are spared. In severe cases, necrosis and cavitation may develop. The lesions may spread into the pontine tegmentum and mesencephalon. Most reports decline a correlation between the severity of the MRI findings and the clinical condition. On the other hand, in the follow-up of patients a good correlation between clinical improvement and the fading of lesions on MRI is observed. Even with complete clinical restoration, however, abnormalities on MRI still remain visible for a long time. There has been one report showing ring enhancement of the lesions in the pons after injection of intravenous contrast. Although in MRI the quantities of injected contrast material are far less than in CT, administration of contrast should be avoided in order to avoid aggravating the patient's ionic imbalance. Enhancement of the lesions in the pons also does not contribute to the diagnosis. The findings, as described, are highly characteristic in themselves.

Sometimes lesions in the basal ganglia are seen together with the typical lesions in the pons. These cases can be considered transitional between CPM and CPM/EPM. In EPM, lesions are described of the neostriatum, thalamus, geniculate bodies, internal and external capsule and cerebellar and cerebral gyral convo-

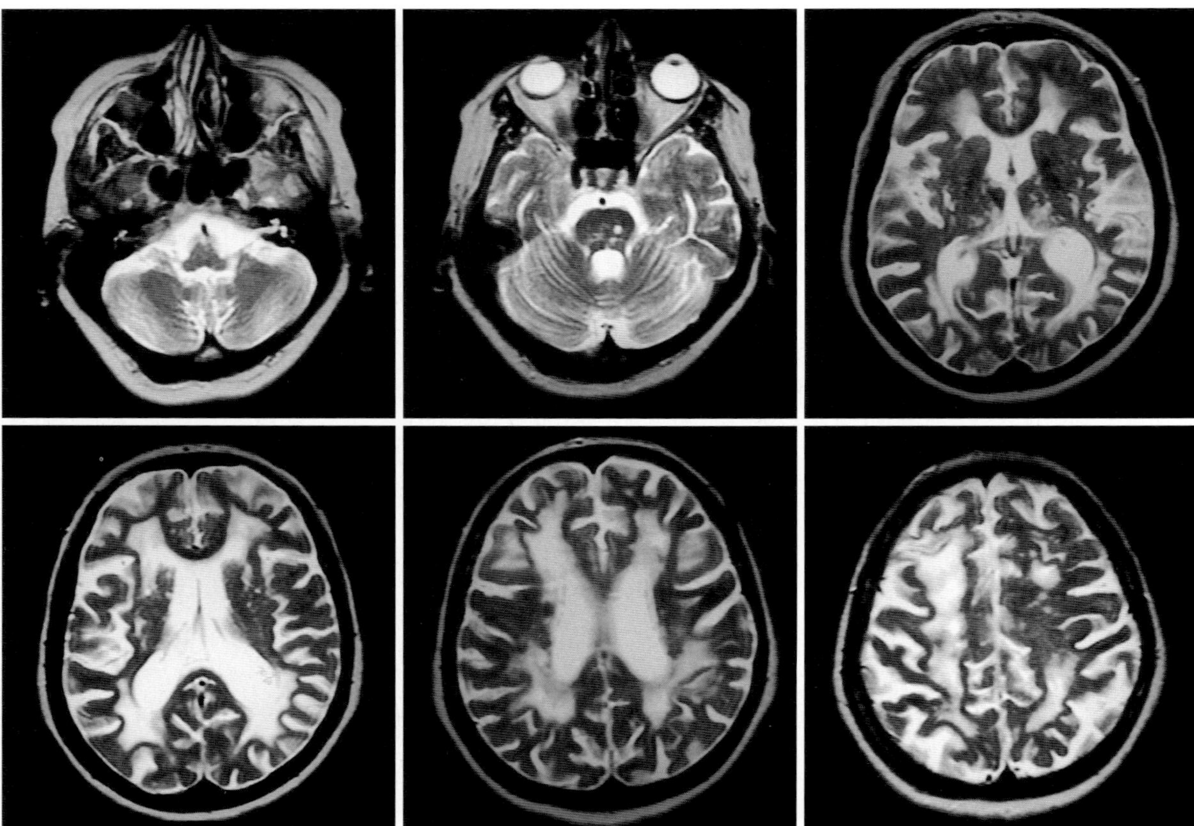

Fig. 60.2. A 61-year-old woman with terminal renal insufficiency on dialysis therapy over a period of more than 10 years with many complications. She had experienced several critical episodes with ion balance disorders. The T_2-weighted images show some focal areas of hyperintense signal in the pons, in the thalamus, basal ganglia and in the external capsule in addition to extensive confluent white matter involvement around the frontal and occipital horns and in the centrum semiovale with right-sided preponderance. Although the hypertensive crises from which this patient also suffered may have contributed to this pattern, it shows greater similarity to the pattern of EPM

lutions (Figs. 60.2, 60.3). EPM may occur in isolation or be combined with CPM. Establishing the diagnosis EPM is not difficult in the presence of the characteristic pons lesion. The differential diagnosis in EPM without a pontine lesion is more difficult and includes acute disseminated encephalomyelitis, encephalitis, and toxic-metabolic encephalopathies.

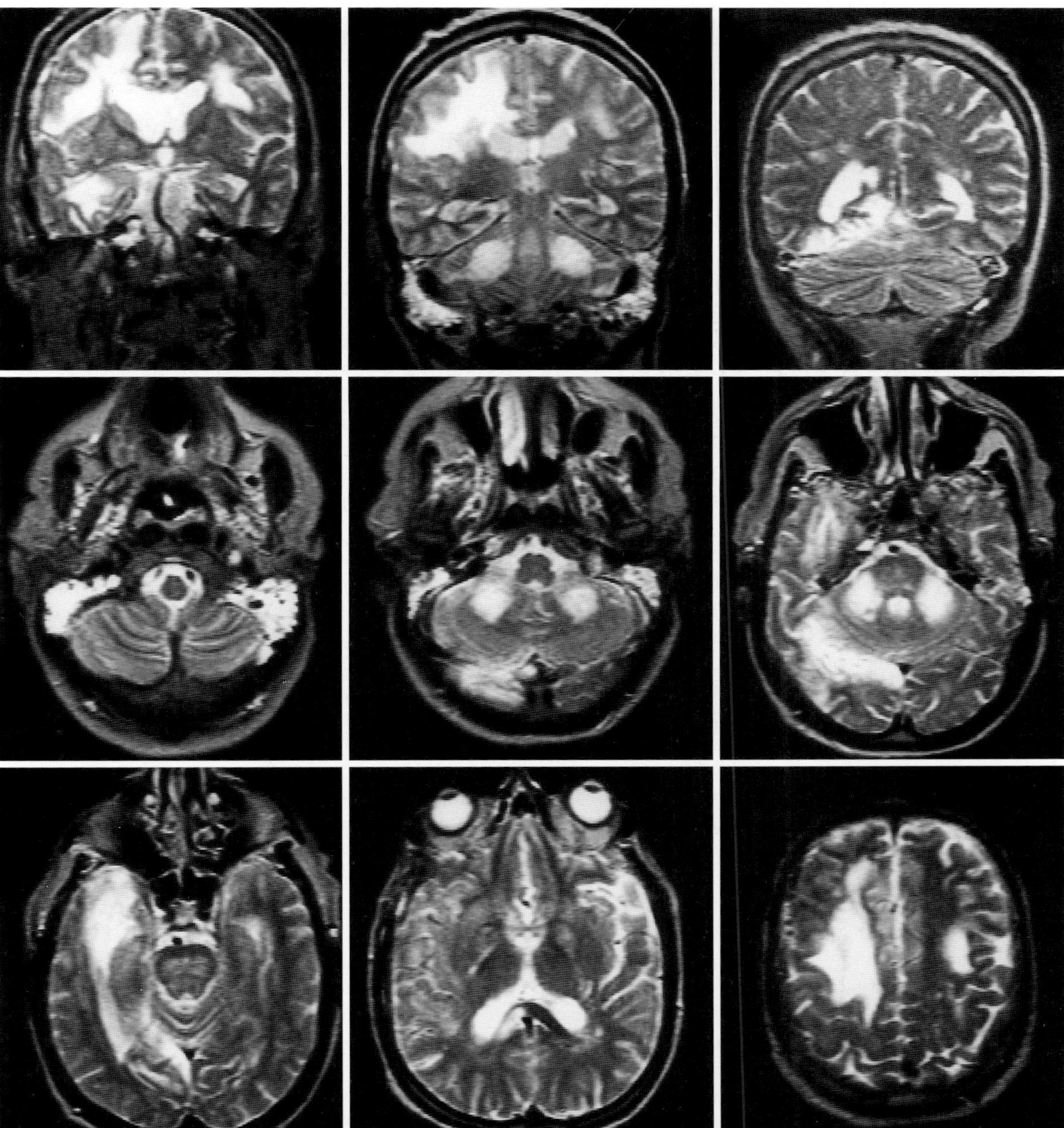

Fig 60.3. A 64-year-old man became critically ill after surgery for removal of a meningioma. Surgery and postoperative course were complicated by severe blood loss and hyponatremia, both of which were corrected. After initial good recovery deterioration of the clinical condition occurred. The T_2-weighted coronal and transverse images show the postoperative edema in the right temporal lobe. Furthermore, there is extensive myelinolysis in the cerebellar white matter, the middle cerebellar peduncles, the internal capsule and the subcortical white matter with preponderance on the right side. The pontine white matter is slightly affected. Gradual return to normal occurred in the weeks that followed

61 Marchiafava-Bignami Syndrome

61.1 Clinical Features and Laboratory Investigations

Marchiafava-Bignami syndrome (MBS) is a disorder characterized by primary degeneration of the corpus callosum in chronic alcoholics. Although a high proportion of reported cases have been Italians, drinking Italian wine, the condition has also been described in many non-Italians drinking non-Italian wine. Most affected cases were middle-aged men whose daily wine consumption had been 2 l or more for many years. The disease knows three major clinical forms: acute, subacute, and chronic. The acute form is characterized by sudden onset with severe disturbances of consciousness, sometimes heralded by convulsions. The initial phase is followed by the development of persistent coma or stupor with pyramidal signs and hypertonia. Patients are generally mute, but if they say a few words, they appear to be severely dysarthric. They die within a few days. The subacute condition is characterized by a rapidly progressive dementia, sometimes following an intial acute state with temporary coma or convulsions. The dementia has characteristics of a split-brain syndrome. The patients are usually dysarthric. Hypertonia of the limbs is quite common and marked by strong opposition to any movement, either flexion or extension. There is spastic flexion of the arms and extension of the legs with hyperreflexia and extensor plantar reflexes. A facial grimace and trismus may be present, as well as an opisthotonus. In the end-stage the patients are unable to walk or stand. Severe dementia progresses to a vegetative state and death usually occurs within a few months. In the chronic form, which is much less common, dementia progresses slowly over a number of years. Neurological examination reveals diffuse rigidity, dysarthria, and inability to stand or walk as in the subacute form. This condition progresses steadily towards death several years later.

Laboratory investigations may reveal vitamin deficiencies due to malnutrition but unrelated to MBS. There is no laboratory test for MBS.

61.2 Pathology

The principal pathological change is necrosis of the corpus callosum. The necrosis may involve the entire length of the commissure or only a part of it. The central portion is mainly affected, an upper and lower rim of unaffected callosal fibers usually being preserved. The lesion extends laterally to the edges of the corpus callosum. When necrosis is incomplete, demyelination is found, with relative preservation of axons and a moderate glial reaction. In cases of total necrosis, both myelin and axons have disappeared and are replaced by an accumulation of macrophages and perivascular cells together with a variable glial reaction. The lesion is sharply delimited. In acute cases the lesion appears in the form of a band of edematous necrosis with fresh coagulation. An upper and a lower band of normal tissue remain. In cases of long duration, the corpus callosum is thinned and atrophic with a slit or a band of demyelination in the middle. Macrophages accumulate perivascularly.

Other regions of white matter are sometimes involved, including the centrum semiovale in the frontal, parietal, and occipital region as an extension of the lesion of the corpus callosum. Sometimes the lesion includes all the white matter up to the U fibers. Furthermore, the cerebellar peduncles and the anterior commissure may be involved. The fornix is thought never to be affected. Also, these lesions are primarily characterized by demyelination with accumulation of macrophages. In complete necrosis axons are also lost. There is occasionally cortical laminar necrosis and, exceptionally, necrosis of the basal ganglia.

61.3 Pathogenetic Considerations

The pathogenesis of MBS is still unknown. A toxic factor present in cheap red wine seems to be the closest constant association, but the factor responsible has never been identified. It has been shown that vitamin deficiencies are not important in the pathogenesis as a supply of vitamins could not prevent MBS in animals. Similar lesions of the white matter, affecting the corpus callosum and anterior commissure have been described following chronic cyanide intoxication and chronic methyl alcohol intoxications. However, the pathogenetic similarities on the molecular level between MBS and these intoxications is unclear. Why the central part of the corpus callosum is preferentially affected in MBS remains obscure. The cause of the additional gray matter lesions, usually in the form of laminar necrosis of the cerebral cortex, has not been explained satisfactorily. The most attractive hypothesis would seem to be that the cortical necrosis is secondary to the callosal lesion, which leads to loss of neurons due to secondary degeneration.

61.4 Therapy

There is no effective treatment for MBS; only symptomatic treatment is possible. However, it is important not to overlook other complications of long-standing alcoholism, particularly vitamin deficiencies and disturbances of electrolytes.

61.5 Magnetic Resonance Imaging

CT scan may show abnormality of the corpus callosum with some swelling and edema in the acute form. The corpus callosum lesions in the subacute or chronic forms of the disease, which are not associated with swelling, may be more difficult to detect. Extensive hypodense areas may be found in the hemispheric white matter. Contrast enhancement has been described in the early stages of the disease. In the later stages there is atrophy of the corpus callosum, progressive and marked widening of the cerebral sulci and dilatation of the lateral ventricles.

The corpus callosum lesions are much more easily visualized by MRI (Fig. 61.1). The sagittal MR images are diagnostic: they show the typical pattern of the corpus callosum splitting into three layers, the most extensive lesion in the central part of the corpus callosum, with relative sparing of the dorsal and ventral layers. Contrast enhancement may be present, in particular in genu and splenium, in the initial stages of the disease. The middle layer may be cystic, in particular in the genu and splenium. Hemispheral white matter may be involved, with a less characteristic appearance. Apart from the corpus callosum, other interhemispheric commissural fibers may be involved. Cortical laminar necrosis and basal nuclei necrosis can be visualized by MRI. However, it is the midsagittal image showing the splitting of the corpus callosum into three layers, that leads to the correct diagnosis.

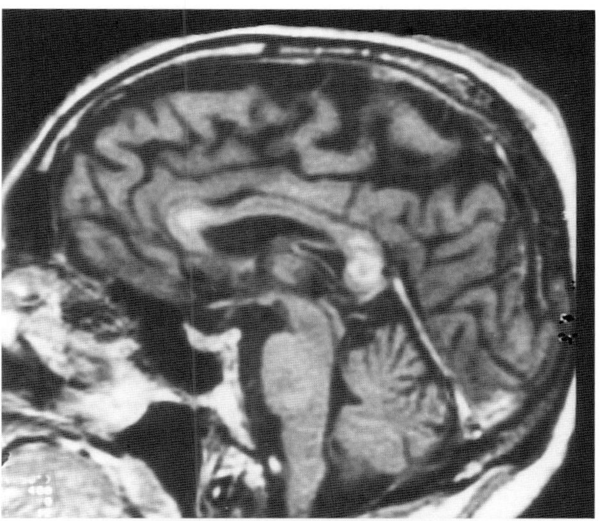
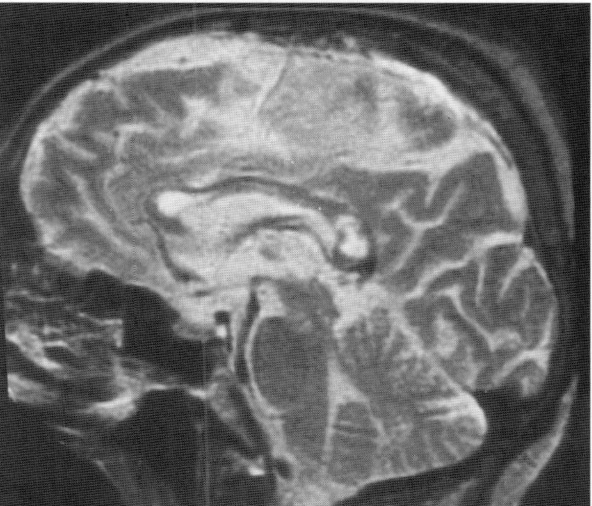
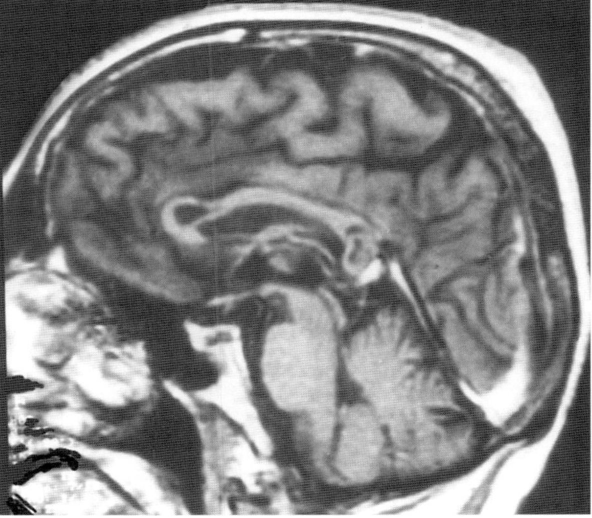

Fig. 61.1. A 53-year-old man with MBS with acute onset. MRI on the ninth day (*upper image*) shows contrast enhancing lesions in the genu and the splenium of the corpus callosum. At 3 weeks the images (*middle and lower images*) show affection of the middle layer of the corpus callosum, in particular in splenium and genu, but no contrast enhancement. Courtesy of Caparros-Lefebvre et al. 1994, with permission

62 Posthypoxic-Ischemic Damage

62.1 Pathogenetic Factors

In hypoxic and ischemic conditions the supply of oxygen and nutrients to brain tissue is compromised. If this condition lasts for some time, changes occur in cells and tissues, eventually leading to cell death.

The first change to occur at molecular level is the replacement of the highly efficient aerobic glycolysis, which delivers 38 molecules of adenosine triphosphate (ATP) for one molecule of glucose, by inefficient anaerobic glycolysis with only 2 molecules of ATP for one molecule of glucose. Under aerobic conditions the major product of glycolysis is pyruvate, which is metabolized to acetyl-CoA (activated acetate) which enters the citric acid cycle. Under anaerobic conditions, pyruvate is not converted into acetyl-CoA, but into lactate, a potentially harmful compound.

Energy depletion leads to membrane depolarisation, and disturbed transport of ions across membranes of organelles and cells. Concentration and voltage gradients are no longer maintained; water is osmotically drawn into the organelles and cells, causing them to swell. These changes may be reversible, but if the hypoxic condition lasts too long, irreparable damage with cell death will occur. Morphologically this point of no return is indicated by the appearance of cloudy precipitations within the mitochondria. Apparent changes in the inner membrane of the mitochondrion, where oxidative phosphorylation takes place, occur much later.

62.2 Reperfusion Damage

Repair of the condition that has caused the hypoxic-ischemic changes, with restoration of blood circulation and oxygen supply, can lead to the introduction of new damage in ischemic cells. This means that cells that are reversibly damaged are again threatened, now by the harmful effects of reperfusion. Two factors are assumed to play a critical role as causative agent in this additional damage: the calcium factor and the oxygen paradox.

The concentration of Ca^{2+} in blood is much higher than in the cell. A Ca^{2+} gradient is maintained across the cell membrane with ATP as energy donor. Lowering of the ATP concentration causes influx of Ca^{2+} and Na^+ into the cell. First of all, Ca^{2+} is stored in organelles, such as the endoplasmic reticulum and mitochondria, and it is not until these are flooded that the cytosol concentration of Ca^{2+} will increase. Ca^{2+} is a co-factor for certain enzymes, including proteases and phospholipases, which will attack functional components of the cell, such as lipids and proteins. High Ca^{2+} levels in the cytosol are at the core of many detrimental biochemical cascades.

The oxygen paradox is based on the observation that oxygen supplied after a hypoxic episode causes additional damage. This is explained by the action of oxygen radicals. Free radicals are compounds with a lone electron in an outer orbital, which are, therefore, highly reactive. They are normally present in the mitochondrial electron transport chain of all cells and are kept under control by physical and chemical coupling. The defense mechanisms against the toxic effect of oxygen radicals include a low oxygen pressure at the cellular level, and enzymatic decomposition of active oxygens by enzymes and scavengers, such as superoxide dismutase and catalase, as well as anti-oxidants, such as α-tocopherol (vitamin E) and ascorbic acid (vitamin C). The latter compounds are fat-soluble and water-soluble, respectively. Superoxide dismutase snatches away the superoxide ion; catalase counteracts the effects of hydrogen peroxide. However, under conditions of hypoxia-ischemia, and in particular after restoration of oxygen supply, these defense mechanisms may be overwhelmed. One of the cascades then becoming active is the xanthine oxidase reaction. Under anaerobic conditions ATP is broken down in larger than usual quantities via ADP, to AMP, to inosine and hypoxanthine and finally to uric acid under the enzymatic influence of xanthine dehydrogenase. The raised Ca^{2+} concentration in the cytosol activates proteases which convert xanthine dehydrogenase into xanthine oxidase, thereby producing a superoxide anion (O$\cdot$). Superoxide anions, once formed from this xanthine oxidase system, react with iron salts to form perhydroxyl radicals (OH$\cdot$). This chemical process is described as the superoxide driven, iron promoted Haber-Weiss reaction. This reaction occurs when free Fe^{2+} is present: under hemorrhagic conditions or in structures whose natural iron content is high. Targets for the perhydroxyl radicals are polyunsaturated fatty acids, compounds that are highly vulnerable to peroxidation. Polyunsaturated fatty acids reside in the midzone of biomembranes, spatially separated from the site of generation of active oxygen. Under hypoxic ischemic conditions, with activation of Ca^{2+}-dependent enzymes in the cells, in particular proteases and phospholipases, this is no longer the case. The polyunsaturated fatty acids in the cell membrane come under attack and become new sources of oxygen radicals. The superoxide anion withdraws a proton from a polyunsaturated fatty acid, creating a lipid with an unpaired electron. This newly created lipid radical (L·) reacts with O_2 (reperfusion) and forms a lipid peroxyl radical (LOO·). This compound will withdraw a proton from a nearby polyunsaturated fatty acid, creating a new radical and initiating a chain reaction. Iron plays a very important catalytic role in lipid peroxidation. In a normal adult about 4 g iron is present in hemoglobin. Myoglobin contains 10% of total body iron and a small part is present in enzymes and in the transport protein transferrin. The remaining iron is found in storage proteins such as ferritin. Free iron is not usually present in peripheral blood. Iron from ferritin is liberated at pH values lower than 6, which may occur under conditions of severe hypoxia. Superoxide anions are also capable of dissociating the iron-ferritin complex. Lipid peroxyl radicals can even dissociate iron from hemoglobin molecules. Hemorrhagic conditions, such as hemorrhagic infarctions, infections, contusions, and subarachnoid hemorrhages create the optimal environment for these deleterious reactions.

In the formation of free radicals the polyunsaturated fatty acid arachidonic acid, abundant in cell membranes, has a special place. Arachidonic acid is metabolized by at least three enzymes: cycloxygenase, lipoxygenase and cytochrome-D450 oxygenase. All three pathways are capable of producing superoxide radicals. The cycloxygenase pathway leads to the formation of prostaglandins and thromboxanes, which influence, amongst others, the microcirculation. The lipoxygenase pathway leads to the formation of leukotrienes, which may induce edema, necrosis and further inhibit microcirculation. Cytochrome-D450 oxygenase leads directly to the formation of oxygen radicals. There is interaction at each level of the components of this cascade, leading to either stimulation or inhibition of effects of the other components.

Free radicals are formed by many other mechanisms. They can be formed by membrane-bound enzymes on the surface of neutrophils and phagocytes, which are activated by endotoxins from bacteria, or by cytokines, inducing the so-called oxygen burst of phagocyte membrane compounds in the acute phase of infections.

Nitric oxide (NO·) is a reactive free radical which can inhibit mitochondrial respiration. It is one of the major defense molecules against microbes and malignant cells. It has recently been reported to act as a highly unorthodox messenger molecule within the CNS and there is evidence that it may contribute to excitotoxicity. It is a simple molecule which is synthesized from L-arginine by the enzyme nitric oxide synthetase. Nitric oxide synthetase is present in endothelial cells. There are several isoforms and the neuronal isoform is activated by high cytosol Ca^{2+}. Once formed nitric oxide diffuses to neighboring cells and reacts with guanylate cyclase, inducing the formation of cyclic guanosine monophosphate from guanosine triphosphate. Cyclic guanosine monophosphate influences the relaxation of smooth muscles, including blood vessels. Nitric oxide preferentially combines with superoxide anions when present, leading to the formation of highly reactive peroxynitrite, which causes cell damage. The resulting drop in cyclic guanosine monophosphate leads to vasoconstriction. On the other hand, nitric oxide can be changed to a chemical state that has the opposite effect, i.e., a protective effect. In the presence of electron donors such as ascorbate or cysteine, nitric oxide becomes nitrosonium ion (NO^+), which binds to a regulatory site on the most prominent receptor of excitatory amino acids, resulting in decreased activity of this receptor.

The deleterious action of free radicals, as mentioned before, is dependent on the presence of oxygen. Therefore, most of the damage occurs during reperfusion after ischemia. The capacity of tissue to neutralize free radicals is called the anti-oxidance capacity. During ischemia and reperfusion, this capacity decreases rapidly. The decrease is greater in experiments in which some blood is still perfusing the ischemic area, than when the oxygen supply is totally arrested. This is understandable because of the necessary presence of oxygen for free radical damage to occur.

The recognition of the harmful effects of free radicals has induced a worldwide search for counteracting compounds. Several pharmaceutics are under consideration as cerebro-protective agents. Free radical scavengers are used to diminish negative effects of cranial trauma or cerebral hypoxia. Substances such as vitamin E, N-acetylcysteine, and dimethylsulfoxide are used for this purpose. Vitamin E works by offering a competitive binding site to superoxide anions. Allopurinol counteracts the effects of xanthine-oxidase, and is effective in diminishing the influence of one of the cascades. The newly developed 21-amino steroids (lazaroids) have been proven to be potent inhibitors of lipid peroxidation. Calcium entry blockers are considered to prevent high Ca^{2+} concentrations in the cytosol and inhibit the formation of Ca^{2+}-dependent enzymes. Not all newly conceived drugs have met the theoretical expectations. Often, of course, in clinical situations the therapy starts when most of the damage has already been done. Also the processes behind posthypoxic-ischemic encephalopathy are complicated.

Free radicals are not the only factors that have to be taken into account.

62.3 Excitatory Amino Acids

Overstimulation of neurons by excitatory amino acids (EAAs), in particular glutamate and aspartate, can lead to cell dysfunction and, eventually, neuronal death. EEAs serve as excitatory neurotransmitters, as opposed to inhibitory neurotransmittters, of which γ-amino butyric acid (GABA) is the most prominent. These amino acids play a role in the normal messenger system of the CNS. Under normal circumstances the potentially harmful accumulation of EAAs is prevented from happening. After conversion from glutamine, glutamate is released in the synapse, making contact with glutamate responding receptors. On the distal side of the synapse, glutamate is broken down to glutamine, which re-enters the presynaptic side, or is taken by a glutamate transporter into a nearby astrocyte for further transformation. The ensuing neuronal depolarization is very short-lived. This glutamate re-uptake chain is energy dependent. In energy deprived conditions glutamate accumulates in the extracellular space and causes neuronal overstimulation. There are several mechanisms leading to pathological glutamate accumulation. For example, the role of the glutamate transporter in the astrocyte may be compromised, because of the collapse of the gradients for Na^+ and K^+ across the cell membrane. Its function may even be reversed and the transporter may become a source of extracellular glutamate. Or, in case of cell injury, glutamate may leak out of damaged cells. Every cell contains enough glutamate to cause damage to many neighboring cells.

Further analysis of the excitatory synapses reveals that at least three types of glutamate receptor can be distinguished. The EAA receptors are classified according to their typical agonists: N-methyl-D-aspartate (NMDA), quisqualate (QA) and kainate (KA). Recently a new class of receptor has been described: 2-amino-4-phosphonobutyrate (AP_4). Each class of receptors has distinct pharmacological properties and anatomical distribution. The NMDA receptor is the best understood. It contains an NMDA recognition site, and a cationic ionophore, allowing Na^+ and Ca^{2+} to enter the cytosol. Other sites are an Mg^{2+} binding site and a Zn^{2+} binding site, probably for non-competitive inhibition of the ionophore. A glycine site has also been recognized for positive allosteric modulation at the receptor site. Agonists and antagonists of each of these sites are known. For example, agonists for the NMDA site are l-glutamate and l-aspartate; an antagonist is

carboxypiperazine propyl 1-phosphonate. At the ionophore site antagonists are phencyclidine, inimemaleate (MK 801), ketamine and dextromethorphan. At the glycine site, glycine and D-serine are agonists; kynurenate is an antagonist.

Agonists and antagonists for the quisqualate and kainate receptors have also been identified. They are directly involved in the regulation of Ca^{2+} and Na^+ concentration in the cell. These non-NMDA receptors open channels to allow Na^+ en Cl^- into the cell under anoxic conditions, passively causing the entrance of H_2O and cell edema.

The action of these EAA receptors is basic in the concept of excitotoxicity. Lately, effects of overstimulation by EAAs have been considered to play a role in many different neurological disorders, for example, in epilepsy, hypoglycemia, trauma, AIDS dementia complex, Huntington's chorea, amyotrophic lateral sclerosis, toxic encephalopathies and perhaps Alzheimer's disease, making the described mechanism a "final common pathway" of neuronal injury.

Although the ideas on the action of EAAs change frequently, evidence is emerging to support the concept that in vivo high levels of endogenous EAAs, such as glutamate and aspartate, also play a critical role in brain damage caused by hypoxic-ischemic insults. As has already been stressed, glutamate reclaim after the synaptic release is highly energy-dependent. In low energy states glutamate accumulates in the extracellular spaces, leading to neuronal overstimulation with excessive anionic and cationic fluxes and, in the acute phase, to intracellular edema and osmotic lysis, which may be the cause of instant cell death. Resulting high concentrations of Ca^{2+} in the cytosol contribute to delayed cell death. In vitro tests have shown that these two processes, the osmotic instant lysis and the delayed Ca^{2+}-dependent neuronal death, can be separated by manipulating the conditions. Also the possible prevention of each type of damage by different biochemical environments shows this difference. This knowledge is potentially of use in therapeutic interventions.

Antagonists of EAAs have been tested in cell cultures, animal experiments and clinical trials of their "cerebroprotective" properties. In the clinical tests especially, the results have so far been disappointing. This may be because the whole process is extremely complicated and an antagonist interferes somewhere in this complex process with unexpected reactions and effects, or because of insufficient passage through the blood-brain barrier, or because the administration of drugs in humans usually occurs when the damage has already been done.

62.4 Patterns of Morphological Changes of White Matter in Hypoxic-Ischemic Encephalopathy

Hypoxemia, a reduced oxygen content of the arterial blood, occurs clinically in many conditions, including asphyxia, severe pulmonary failure, respiratory insufficiency, arrest, and incorrect anesthesia. Ischemia or oligemia means a reduction in blood flow. This condition exists in occlusion of arteries, in exsanguination and in cardiac arrest. Hypoxia, ischemia and hypoglycemia have the same effect on the brain. Neurons are usually most susceptible, but there is also a hierarchy of vulnerability within the group of neurons, as is discussed in the chapter on selective vulnerability. Under certain conditions, however, for example an early stage of development, white matter may be more vulnerable than gray matter. This is in particular the case in preterm infants.

Several patterns of morphological posthypoxic-ischemic damage can be distinguished:

I. Focal lesions, the distribution also depending on vascular patterns:

1. Arterial territorial pattern. If the perfusion through one major artery fails, the territory nurtured by this artery is compromised. The initial cytotoxic edema affects all structures, gray and white.

2. The arterial border zone pattern, due to diminished perfusion, mostly leads to changes in the parietal region, or along the frontal parasagittal border between middle and anterior cerebral arteries. Other border zones may, however, also be involved.

3. Focal symmetrical abnormalities occur preferentially in the basal ganglia in patients with hypertension and concurrent vascular changes. "Etat lacunaire" is the ancient notation of a condition in which multiple small, old, cystic infarcts are seeded through the basal ganglia, leading to a highly characteristic appearance. This condition is difficult to separate from the "état criblé" (cribiform atrophy), caused by the widening of the Virchow-Robin spaces around tortuous vessels.

4. Periventricular leukomalacia occurs in older patients in subcortical arteriosclerotic encephalopathy, also referred to as Binswanger's disease. Periventricular leukomalacia also occurs in prematurely born infants.

II. Lesions due to generalized hypoxia-ischemia:

5. Cortical and subcortical gray matter damage. Typical involvement of the "topistic" areas as described by Vogt en Vogt is the result of generalized hypoxia-ischemia. Morphologically changes occur in the most vulnerable areas, resulting in cortical laminar necrosis, Sommer's sector necrosis (hippocampus necrosis), striatum necrosis, and Purkinje cell necrosis (Figs. 62.1, 62.2). At least two factors are involved in this selective involvement of particular brain structures. First, the distribution of excitatory amino acid receptors is important. The differences in concentration of EAA receptors can lead to focal damage in areas with higher receptor density. These areas are to a large extent the areas involved as mentioned above. Secondly, a role is also played by reperfusion damage and free radical action. As has been explained, the Haber-Weiss reaction occurs especially in areas with a high iron concentration including the thalamus, globus pallidus, substantia nigra, and several cortical layers.

6. Specific involvement of zones of active myelination. Following asphyxia in term-born neonates lesions are frequently seen in the dorsal part of the putamen, the ventrolateral nucleus of the thalamus, and in the hippocampus. They are often combined with damage in the white and gray matter bordering the sulcus centralis, leading to local atrophy and sclerotic ulegyria. The explanation for the vulnerability of these affected areas at this period of time is the active myelination, taking place at term in these areas, with high chemical turnover and high regional blood flow.

7. Diffuse white matter injury. In delayed posthypoxic-ischemic demyelination there is usually diffuse involvement of all the white matter. This is seen in rare cases after cardiac arrest, errors in anesthesia and in toxic encephalopathies, in particular after carbon monoxide and cyanide poisoning. The same pattern is seen in diffuse white matter injury after irradiation and chemotherapy, in which diffuse vascular changes play an intermediary role.

III. Miscellaneous lesions affecting both gray and white matter:

8. A number of congenital conditions such as encephaloclastic schizencephaly, hydranencephaly and porencephaly are probably the result of hypoxic-ischemic conditions during pregnancy.

Those conditions which primarily lead to white matter changes will be discussed in separate chapters.

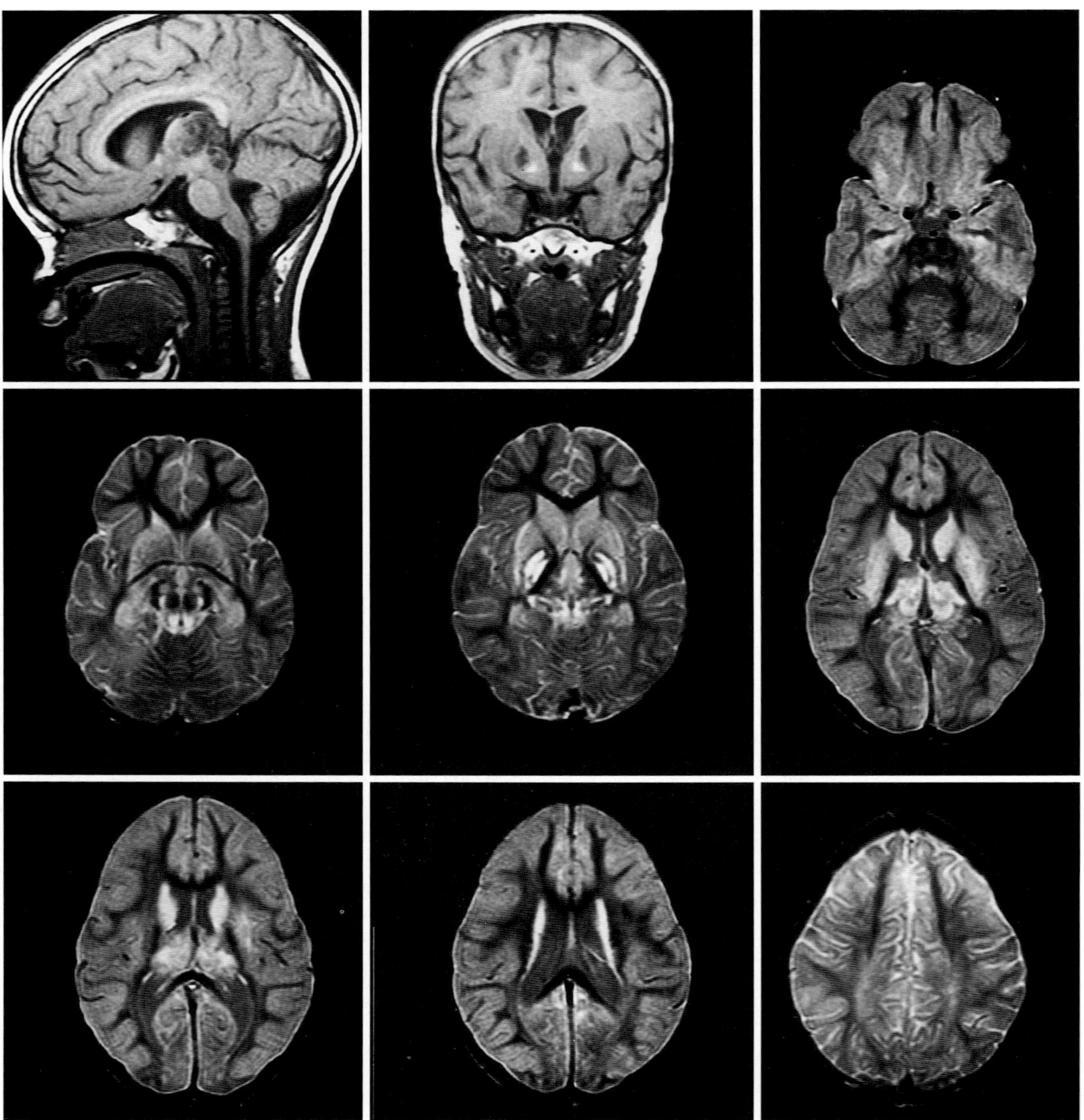

Fig. 62.1. Sagittal and coronal T_1-weighted and transverse T_2-weighted images in a 3-year-old child who nearly drowned. There are partly hemorrhagic, partly necrotic lesions in the globus pallidus, but also severe involvement of the putamen, caudate nucleus, thalamus and periaqueductal gray matter. The white matter is least affected. In the highest slice, cortical laminar necrosis is visible in the frontal area

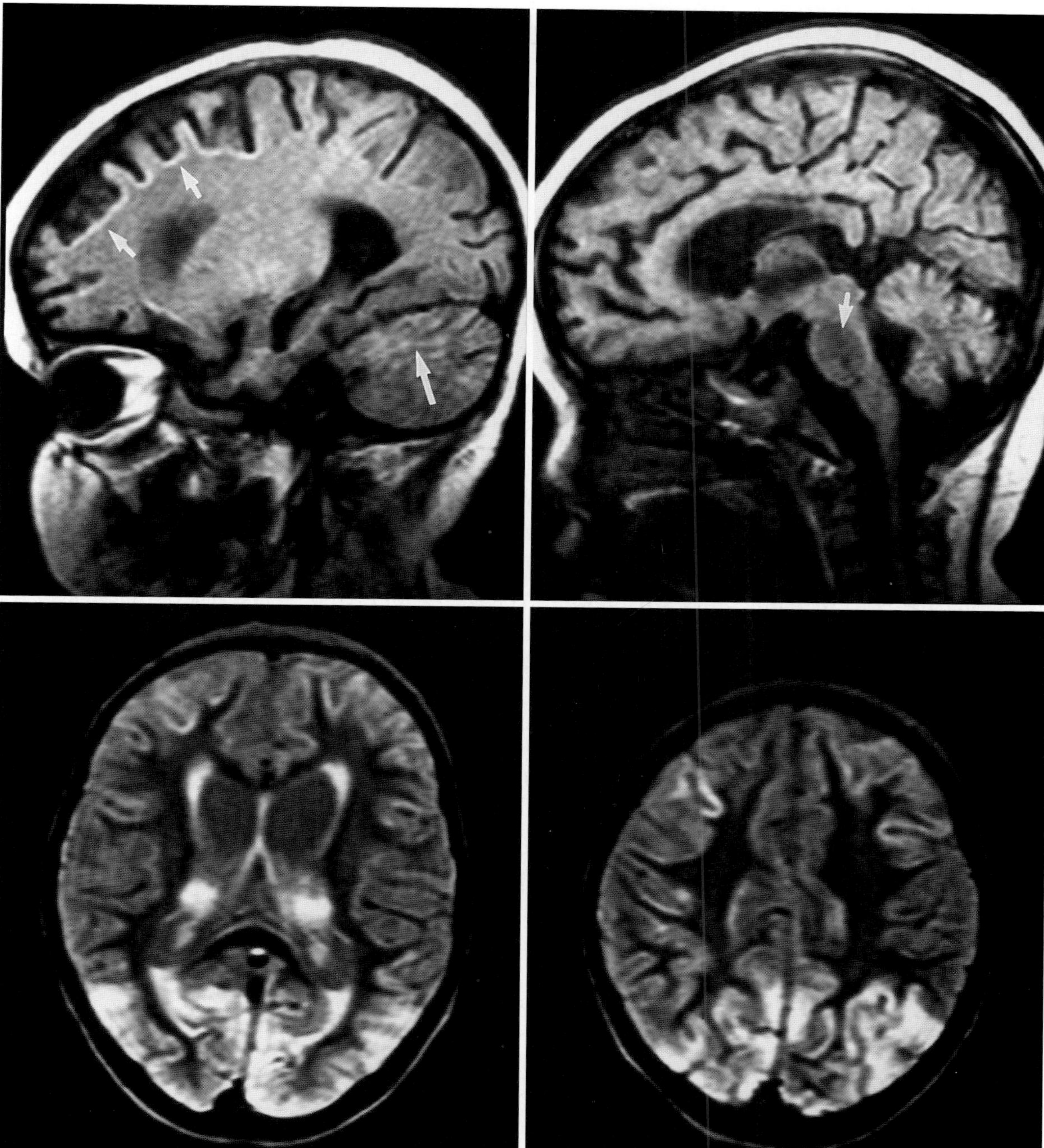

Fig. 62.2. This 7-year-old girl suffered from a long-standing epileptic status leading to cortical energy depletion, a condition comparable in effect to hypoxia-ischemia. The cortical laminar necrosis is evident. In the sagittal images there is a high signal linear lesion intracortically, probably caused by hemorrhage. Also in the cerebellum the cortex is affected (*arrow*). The proton density images on the lower row show the central lesions and the lesions in the cortex with high signal intensity

63 Posthypoxic-Ischemic Leukoencephalopathy of Neonates

63.1 Clinical Features and Laboratory Investigations

Periventricular leukomalacia (PVL) is a posthypoxic-ischemic leukoencephalopathy resulting from a pre- or perinatal hypoxic-ischemic insult. Little (1861) was the first to describe the clinical picture of the condition. It occurs in particular in preterm neonates with a gestational age of 32–36 weeks. Before that period, at a gestational age of 28–32 weeks, germinal layer, intraventricular and intraparenchymal hemorrhages prevail. PVL is rarely seen in term neonates; if present it is in combination with cardiac disorders, intrauterine growth retardation, or any other sign of an intrauterine incident. There is a distinct relationship between PVL and the clinical concept of "infantile encephalopathy" or "cerebral palsy". The typical location of PVL in the periventricular region, interfering with the corticospinal tracts of the legs more than of the arms, is responsible for the resulting spastic diplegia, tetraplegia (legs more severely affected than arms) or hemiplegia (leg more severely affected than arm). Because the disorder is limited to the white matter, seizures are not a prevalent feature of PVL. Mental development is relatively better preserved. Extension of the leukomalacia into the optic radiation may lead to cerebral blindness or, more often, delayed visual maturation. The CNS manifestations of the disorder take 1 or 2 years to show full clinical development.

In older preterms the white matter damage tends to have a more peripheral, subcortical location. This condition is known as subcortical leukomalacia (SCL). In fact, PVL and SCL form a continuum, and SCL as a rule includes periventricular white matter damage. Clinically, so-called SCL leads to a more severe handicap than PVL. The children have a spastic tetraplegia, are mentally more severely retarded and often have epilepsy. Delayed visual maturation and cerebral visual failure are usually present.

A very special clinical picture is seen in perinatal asphyxia in term or postterm babies. In the course of the first year of life an extrapyramidal movement disorder becomes apparent with choreoathetosis, dystonia and orobuccolingual dyskinesia in combination with variable spasticity and variable mental retardation, although mental capacities may be relatively better pre-served. The motor handicap is often very severe, the combination of extrapyramidal and pyramidal abnormalities leading to serious impairment of intentional movements. This clinical picture is associated with lesions of the basal nuclei and the central, perirolandic cortical and subcortical area.

To predict the outcome of the pre- and perinatal injury one has to rely in the early phase on clinical symptomatology and paraclinical test results available at the time. A classification of the severity of the posthypoxic-ischemic encephalopathy was proposed by Sarnat and Sarnat (1976) for neonates with a gestational age of over 36 weeks. This classification, based on clinical and EEG findings, has been shown to have prognostic significance. Stage I usually occurs during the first 24 h of life and is characterized by jitteriness, a state of irritability, hyperalertness, sympathetic nervous system preponderance, uninhibited reflexes and a normal EEG. Stage II consists clinically of hypotonia, lethargy or obtundation for at least 12 h after birth, strong distal flexion, parasympathetic predominance and multifocal seizures. EEG displays periodicity, sometimes preceded by continuous delta wave activity. The period between 48 and 72 h is critical, during which the encephalopathy either worsens or improves. Stage III is characterized by suppression of brain stem and autonomic functions, stupor or coma and generalized flaccidity. Mechanical ventilation is necessary. The EEG is isopotential or shows a burst-suppression pattern. Persistence of stage II for less than 5 days and no entry in stage III are associated with favorable outcome. Entry in stage III, failure of the EEG to return to normal or persistence of stage II for longer than 7 days predicts a poor neurological outcome.

CSF and blood tests are not informative in predicting outcome. Abnormal VEP and SSEP results carry some negative prognostic value.

Ultrasound (US), bedside, versatile, is the imaging modality of first choice in the neonatal intensive care unit. It can help to identify areas of hyperechogenicity located around the trigonum or the frontal horns with onset 3–7 days after the hypoxic-ischemic incident. This hyperechogenicity is either transient or progresses into cysts. It takes about 7–14 days before cysts develop in the hyperechogenic areas. This time delay is also reported in histological studies. US can be helpful in demonstrating SCL, depending on the type of equipment. US is also helpful in demonstrating germinal layer hemorrhage, intraventricular hemorrhage, ventricular dilatation, intraparenchymal hemorrhage, focal infarctions, porencephalic cysts and lesions in the basal nuclei. An important acquisition is the possibility to measure flow velocity and pulsatility index in major cerebral vessels with echo-Doppler.

Near infrared spectroscopy is a method with potential to measure the oxy-deoxyhemoglobin ratio in the brain and to estimate cerebral blood flow. The method has not yet reached the level of routine clinical examination and it is, at this moment, too early to assess its true clinical value.

PET studies have been used to determine the metabolic rate and the cerebral blood flow of the various brain regions. This is rather a research than a clinical tool for posthypoxic-ischemic encephalopathy in neonates.

Clinical signs, EEG, US, and evoked potentials are of importance as predictors of the outcome of perinatal asphyxia in the acute stage, especially in those newborns who require intensive treatment to survive. So far, MRI has usually proven to be of value later in the course of disease. The extent of lesions on MRI, in particular the presence of subcortical damage, glial retraction and ulegyria, the presence of secondary phenomena, such as atrophy and hydrocephalus, and the disturbance of myelination are helpful in predicting the degree of disability in the future.

63.2 Pathology

PVL was described histologically for the first time in 1867 by Virchow and in 1868 by Parrot. They described "pale" infarcts in the periventricular white matter as yellowish or chalky plaques, 1–6 mm in diameter, 1–15 mm from the ependymal surface of the lateral ventricles. Softening of the plaques forms cavities filled with a milky fluid. The most common localizations are the area anterior to the frontal horn, the superolateral angles of the lateral ventricles, the peritrigonal area and the area around the occipital horns.

Microscopically the lesions initially show coagulation necrosis, with nuclear pyknosis and sponginess of the tissue. Astrocytic proliferation at the borders sets in after a few days and varicose axon swellings develop. Microglia proliferate and lipid-laden macrophages accumulate. The organizing lesions are delineated by active gliosis. Cavitation forms within a few weeks. The cavities are lined by fibrillary glial scar tissue. Swollen axons mineralize quickly and persist for many months. Most of the infarcts are ischemic and lack hemorrhage. Vasculo-occlusive changes are usually absent. Occasionally hemorrhages are found with a distribution similar to that of the leukomalacia. They are due to secondary hemorrhages into periventricular infarcts. Under certain circumstances these hemorrhages may become massive.

The severity of the gliotic reaction and its extent depend on age. Before 24–28 weeks gestational age, the immature brain cannot respond to insults with astrogliosis. In premature neonates of 28–32 weeks gestational age, gliosis is usually limited to the periventricular area. In older premature neonates gliosis extends more often into the subcortical area (SCL). This subcortical extension of the gliotic lesion is probably related to both gestational age and the severity of the hypoxic-ischemic insult. If subcortical cysts develop and the child dies during this stage, multicystic subcortical degeneration is found at autopsy. If the child survives, the cysts usually disappear and gliotic scarring occurs with retraction of white matter deforming ventricular system and cortex. The distribution of these lesions follows a pattern parallel to the periventricular area, closer to the cortical lining, extending from the frontal to the occipital region. The scars of PVL and SCL remain visible throughout life. The residual lesions of PVL are characterized by irregular borders of the ventricles, where periventricular cysts have made contact with the lumen of the ventricles, with glial retraction often at the level of the trigonum, focal loss of white matter, and deep sulci abutting the walls of the ventricles. In case of SCL, glial retraction disfigures the centrum semiovale and causes crowding of gyri, eventually leading to parietal and occipital ulegyria (=sclerotic polymicrogyria).

In term neonates the pattern of damage is different. The posthypoxic-ischemic lesions occur preferentially in a triangular area in the parasagittal, cortical and subcortical region bordering the sulcus centralis. The resulting gliotic scar has a typical triangular shape with retraction of the parietal cortex, leading to local ulegyria. This is often combined with lesions in the dorsal part of the putamen and the ventrolateral part of the thalamus. In some cases, the hippocampus is also involved. The nuclei of the brain stem may also be involved in this condition and pontosubicular necrosis, a histological entity, could fit as well in this gamut of posthypoxic-ischemic damage of the term neonate.

63.3 Pathogenetic Considerations

PVL and germinal layer related hemorrhage are considered to be due to hypoxic-ischemic insults of the preterm neonate, acquired in the pre-, peri- or postnatal period. Age seems to be the pathoplastic factor. The incidence of germinal layer related hemorrhage is highest before the 32nd week gestational age; the highest incidence of PVL lies between the 32nd and

36th week gestational age. Both conditions are rare in term neonates. The high incidence of germinal layer hemorrhage before the age of 32 weeks gestation can be explained by the presence of the germinal layer up until that time. After the 32nd week of gestation the germinal layer rapidly disappears. This germinal layer or matrix layer is considered to be the nurturing bed for the neuronal and glial cells of the developing brain. It is extremely well vascularized, whereas the vascular channels have thin endothelial walls without supportive tissue. The germinal layer therefore bleeds easily. A hemodynamic contribution stems from the pressure-passive cerebral blood flow in stressed premature children, causing a direct dependency of the cerebral blood flow on the systemic blood pressure and blood flow. The existence of a still open ductus Botalli and a drug-induced (indomethacin) closure can have a profound influence on the cerebral circulation, lacking a regulatory mechanism to buffer these changes. All these factors explain the relative high frequency of development of germinal layer hemorrhage in early preterm babies. The hemorrhages potentially break through into the ventricles, which may or may not expand. Under certain conditions there is also a breakthrough of hemorrhage into the parenchyma. The intraparenchymal hemorrhages have a poor prognosis. There is growing evidence that the intraparenchymal extension of the hemorrhage occurs in tissue that has already suffered from hypoxia. In other words, the hemorrhage occurs in infarcted tissue. Combinations of PVL and germinal layer hemorrhage are frequently observed.

The selective vulnerability of white matter versus gray matter in PVL and SCL is more difficult to understand, because there is a less clearly defined anatomical basis for this selectivity than in germinal layer hemorrhage. Suggestions have been made about the possible role of arterial borderzones around the ventricles, defined by branches of perforating arteries turning backwards at the ventricular wall and arteries from the choroid plexus penetrating the ventricular wall. Whether such a borderzone exists is, according to recent research data, doubtful. Newer data make it highly probable that in the early research on this subject veins have been wrongly identified as arteries. Another explanation originates from animal experimentation. In newborn dogs hypotension was induced either by exsanguination or administration of Escherichia coli endotoxins. The regional cerebral blood flow to gray matter was preserved under severe hypotension whereas the regional flow to periventricular white matter decreased significantly. What causes this difference in regional blood flow and how this pattern changes during maturation remains to be elucidated. Hypocarbia leading to vasoconstriction has been shown to be a contributing factor to the selective involvement of white matter in premature neonates. This finding may be of clinical importance, since premature children with respiratory distress supported by artificial ventilation are at risk of developing hypocarbia.

The pathophysiology of encephalopathy in prematurely born neonates differs in many respects from that of term born neonates. As has been mentioned, also from a clinical point of view, the pathology of asphyxiated preterm babies differs from the pathology of asphyxiated term or postterm babies. In the postnatal period the preterm neonate with a low birth weight is going through an extremely stressful period, in which the baby depends on a special environment, monitoring and life support systems. These include artificial ventilation, administration of surfactant, gastric tube feeding, and drug-induced closure of the ductus Botalli, to mention a few. Often there were already prenatal problems, which, after preterm birth, continue into postnatal problems. It is often not possible to pinpoint one exact hypoxic-ischemic incident as the cause of brain damage. In term born neonates, most cases of hypoxia-ischemia are due to a single, severe, perinatal incident. The cerebral damage as a result of such an incident at this time is completely different from the cerebral damage in premature neonates. Selective vulnerability of the brain in term babies is apparently dictated by the biochemically most active parts of the brain which demand the most glucose and oxygen: the zones of active myelination. The resulting damage has the form of the so-called central cortico-subcortical pattern, with leukomalacia in the myelination zone, extending band-shaped from the basal ganglia into the pre- and postcentral gyri. Often there are additional lesions in the dorsal part of the putamen, the ventrolateral part of the thalamus and the hippocampus, also actively myelinating at that time. It may be that, as far as lesions in the basal ganglia and hippocampus are concerned, excitotoxicity and the high local density of glutamate receptors also play a role. The pattern as described is well-established and may, in reverse, be used to date the time of the original incident.

The concept of secondary energy failure has been given special attention in the literature. It has been noted that neonates, after an initial period of suboptimal responses, improve to a much better functional level within the first day, only to present with a catastrophic reaction about 24 h after the first episode. The explanation for the first episode may be found in the acute reaction of neurons to energy depletion and cell membrane paralysis with edema and swelling and impaired function. When the cell survives, a second, calcium-dependent mechanism is triggered, leading via activation of enzymes, formation of free radicals, lipid peroxidation and accumulation of excitatory amino acids to delayed cell death. The sequence of events, however, does not differ essentially from the general cascades triggered whenever energy failure occurs.

63.4 Therapy

Because of the serious consequences of posthypoxic-ischemic damage, many attempts have been directed at preventing PVL or other posthypoxic-ischemic damage from happening. Intensive controls during pregnancy, early diagnosis in utero of congenital abnormalities, electronic fetal monitoring during deliveries, and even technically advanced neonatal intensive care units have not, however, led to a reduction in the incidence of cerebral palsy, 1 or 2 per 10 000 newborns. This is at least partly due to a population shift. Neonates of very low birth weight can now be kept alive and carry high risk factors for the development of posthypoxic-ischemic damage. Preventive measures which were applied in the past to reduce brain metabolism and thus to increase the resistance against hypoxia, such as the use of phenobarbital or low body temperature, have failed to improve the outcome. Better understanding of the pathophysiological mechanisms underlying posthypoxic-ischemic encephalopathy has triggered new efforts to develop cerebroprotective drugs. Various pharmacological entries are now made in this field. It has become clear that disrupted calcium homeostasis within ischemic cells is an essential factor in delayed cell death. Energy depletion leads to high calcium concentration within the cytosol, triggering many other cascades that can damage the cell. Calcium entry blockers would seem to be a logical answer to this problem. Results of trials, however, have not been satisfactory. One of the cascades triggered by high cytosol calcium is the xanthine dehydroxygenase transformation into xanthine oxidase, enzymes of the adenosine-nucleotide biochemical pathway. The xanthine oxidase formation leads to free radical formation and cell damage by lipid peroxidation after reperfusion. Blocking of this cascade was supposed to improve the outcome. Also free radical scavengers have been tested for their ability to prevent reperfusion damage. Substantial results have not as yet been reported. Energy depletion of cell membranes leads to the accumulation of excitatory amino acids, glutamate in particular. Glutamate exerts its stimulating action via at least three different receptors, which have unequal topographical distribution. Of the glutamate receptors, the pharmacological properties of the NMDA receptor are best understood. An attempt has been made to counteract excitotoxicity by the administration of antagonists for specific sites of the NMDA receptor. Although in vitro neuroprotective effects have been obtained, the first clinical trials in preterm neonates have been disappointing. This is probably because glutamate is the working horse of neurotransmission in the brain, extremely important for many reactions. Nonselective inhibition may lead to tampering with the other functions of this neurotransmitter. For instance, maturing neuroreceptors in devel-oping neurosynapses also play a role in the maturation of brain parts and brain functions; they are intermediates in the fetal period in cell plasticity and processes of memory and learning.

This is not the context for analyzing in depth the many pharmacological approaches which are still open. One can, however, expect many new propositions in this field.

Once a static encephalopathy has developed the child should be given physiotherapeutic help, where necessary special education, and neurological treatment for secondary sequelae, such as epilepsy.

63.5 Magnetic Resonance Imaging

CT can be helpful in estimating the extent of hemorrhages and in giving an impression about gyration. CT may also demonstrate the presence of hyperdensities, in particular in the basal ganglia, related to mineralization. Calcium depositions are more difficult to appreciate on MRI.

Generally speaking, however, the superior tissue contrast of MRI makes this modality the logical next step. MRI can identify PVL and SCL at an early stage and can depict the remaining damage in the chronic stage. A very good MRI-pathology correlation has been found in neonates in the first 2 weeks after birth. In the early stage of PVL, MRI can show periventricular damage. In many cases this is facilitated by tiny, punctuate hemorrhages in the lesions ($> 30\%$) with characteristic signal intensities of acute-subacute hemorrhage (Fig. 63.1).

Schouman-Claeys et al. (1993) described four types of different bilateral and usually symmetrical signal abnormality changes in the periventricular areas in neonates with histologically confirmed PVL. Imaging was performed on 0.5 T scanners and T_1-weighted SE or T_1-weighted gradient-echo sequences were used. All images were made in the coronal plane. First of all, lesions were seen at the upper lateral edge of the lateral ventricles, isointense to CSF; they were roundish, sharply demarcated, and corresponded to cysts on autopsy. Secondly, lesions were seen with a somewhat higher signal intensity than CSF. They were homogeneous, sharply demarcated and had the same topographical distribution but extending anteriorly beyond the periventricular area. They corresponded histologically to translucent "watery" patches, with loose cellular aspect and reactive astrocytes, macrophages and edema. Thirdly, lesions were seen with a high signal intensity even compared to cortical gray matter; they were usually fairly large, crescent-shaped, and situated in the same place or at the periphery of the first type of lesion. These lesions corresponded in all cases to severely hemorrhagic cavities. Fourthly, lesions were

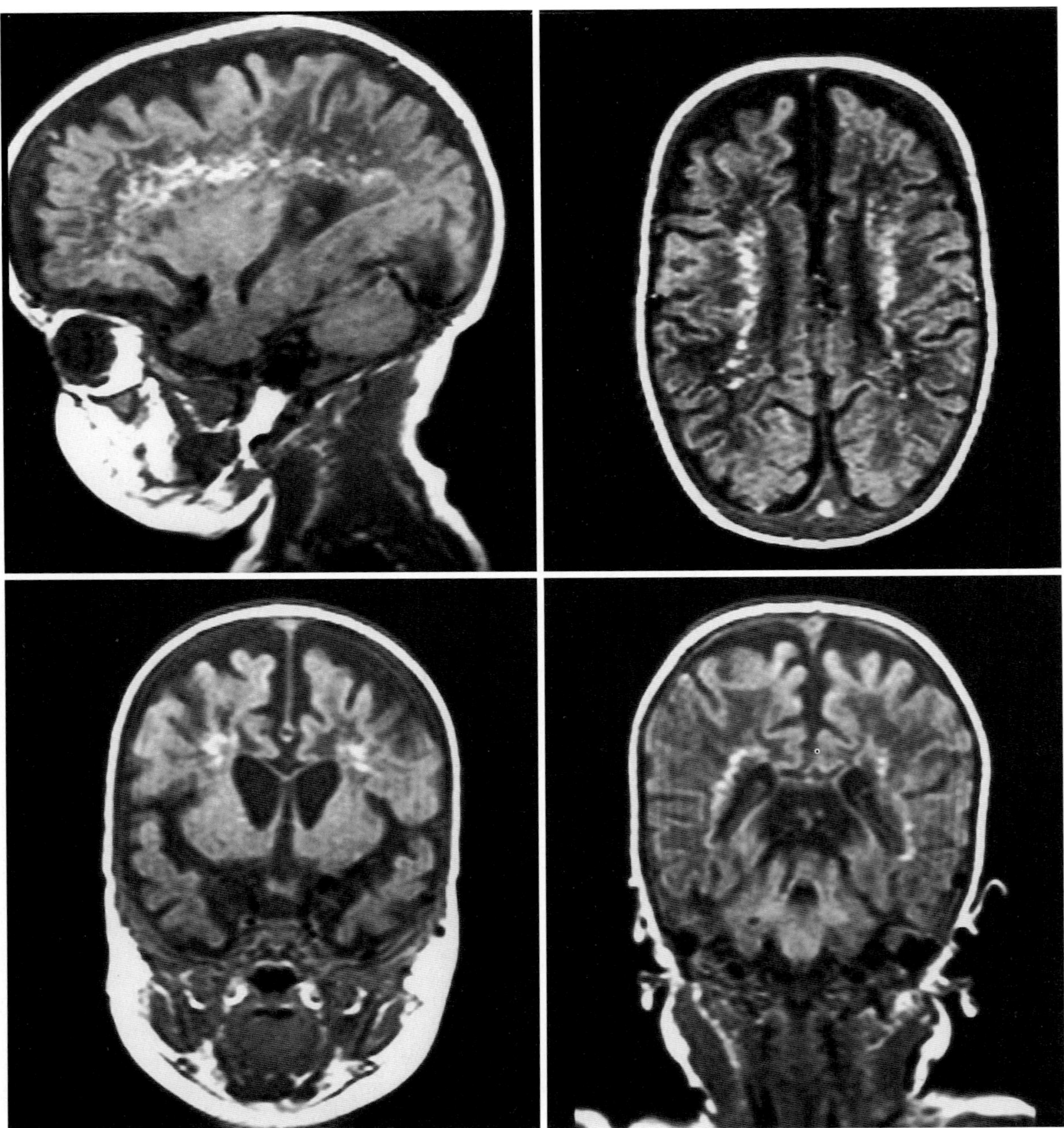

Fig. 63.1. Premature baby-boy (34 weeks postconceptional age), now 6 weeks of age. Multiplanar representation of T_1-weighted images showing brain hemorrhagic PVL over the entire ventricular range

seen with moderately high signal intensity, isointense with cortical gray matter; they appeared as streaks or punctate areas, farther from the ependymal lining than the first three types of lesions. They corresponded to hypercellular regions with or without macrophages. Certain histologically proven lesions extending towards the peripheral white matter, into the optic radiation, and into the internal capsule were isointense with the surrounding unmyelinated white matter on the T_1-weighted images. This stresses the necessity for also obtaining high-quality T_2-weighted images.

In MR imaging of premature children other abnormalities may be found apart from the periventricular lesions described above. Associated abnormalities are often noted: germinal layer related hemorrhage; hemorrhages in the basal ganglia; retarded myelination, mostly observed as too high signal intensity in the posterior limb of the internal capsule on T_2-weighted

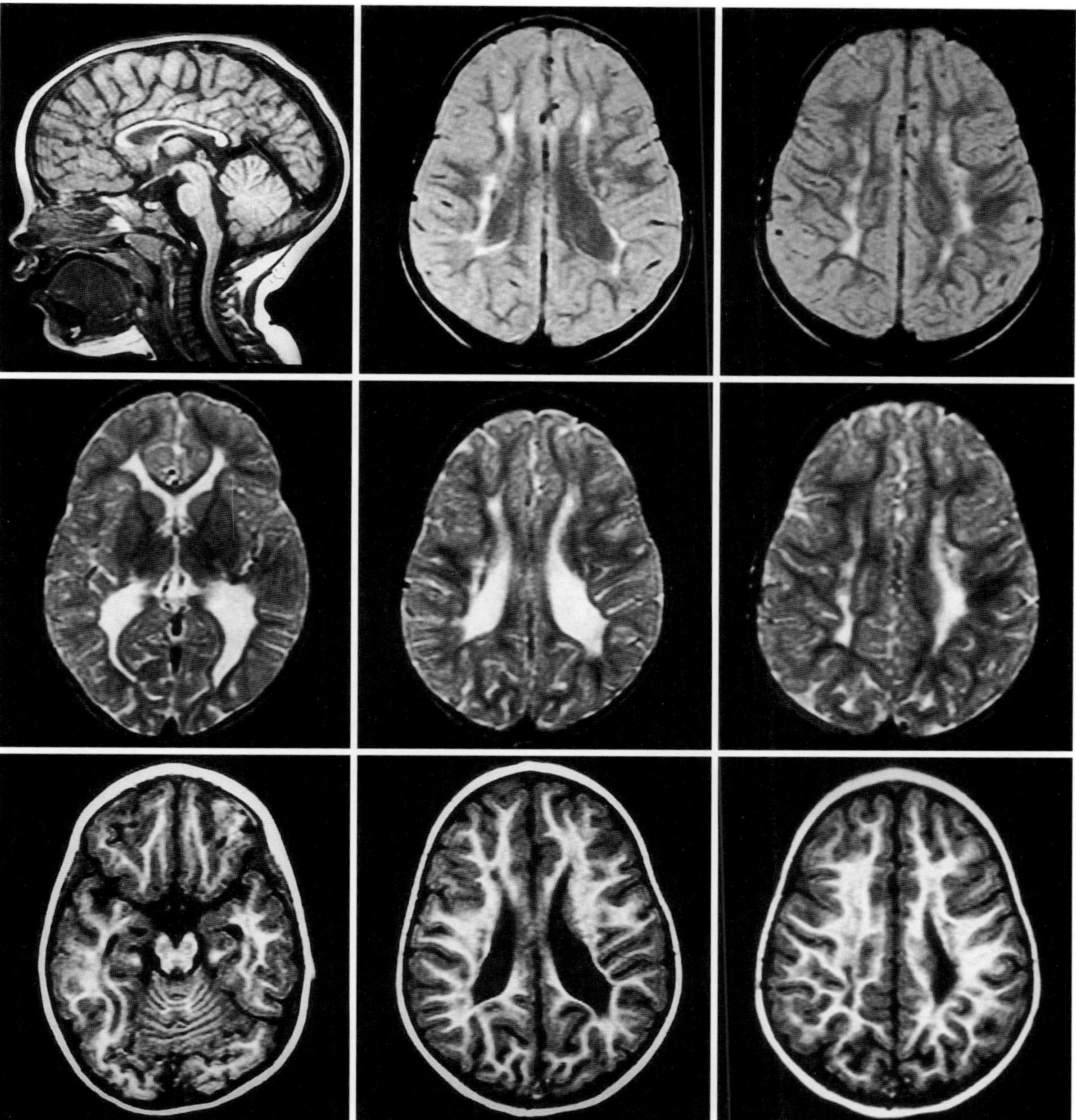

Fig. 63.2. PVL in a girl, 2 years of age with spastic diplegia. The characteristic triad of PVL is present: somewhat enlarged ventricles with irregular borders, especially around the trigonum, loss of white matter, and deep sulci nearly abutting the ventricular walls

images; and posthypoxic-ischemic edema, which may be limited to areas with unmyelinated white matter.

All authors stress the necessity of follow-up examinations in cases with, and sometimes without, pertinent MRI findings. As is known from neurosonography, periventricular cysts may completely disappear or they may grow and make contact with the lateral ventricles, leading to the characteristic appearance of PVL in chronic static cases. Loss of white matter and re-placement by gliosis further assist in shaping the typical image. Due to gliotic retraction and white matter disappearance the cortical sulci become very deep, in particular in the insular/peri-insular region, where sulci abut the ventricular wall. The ventricular wall is irregular and often shows retraction at the level of the trigonum. These features form the triad of MRI characteristics in chronic cases of PVL: (1) dilated ventricles with irregular lateral borders; (2) a periventricular rim

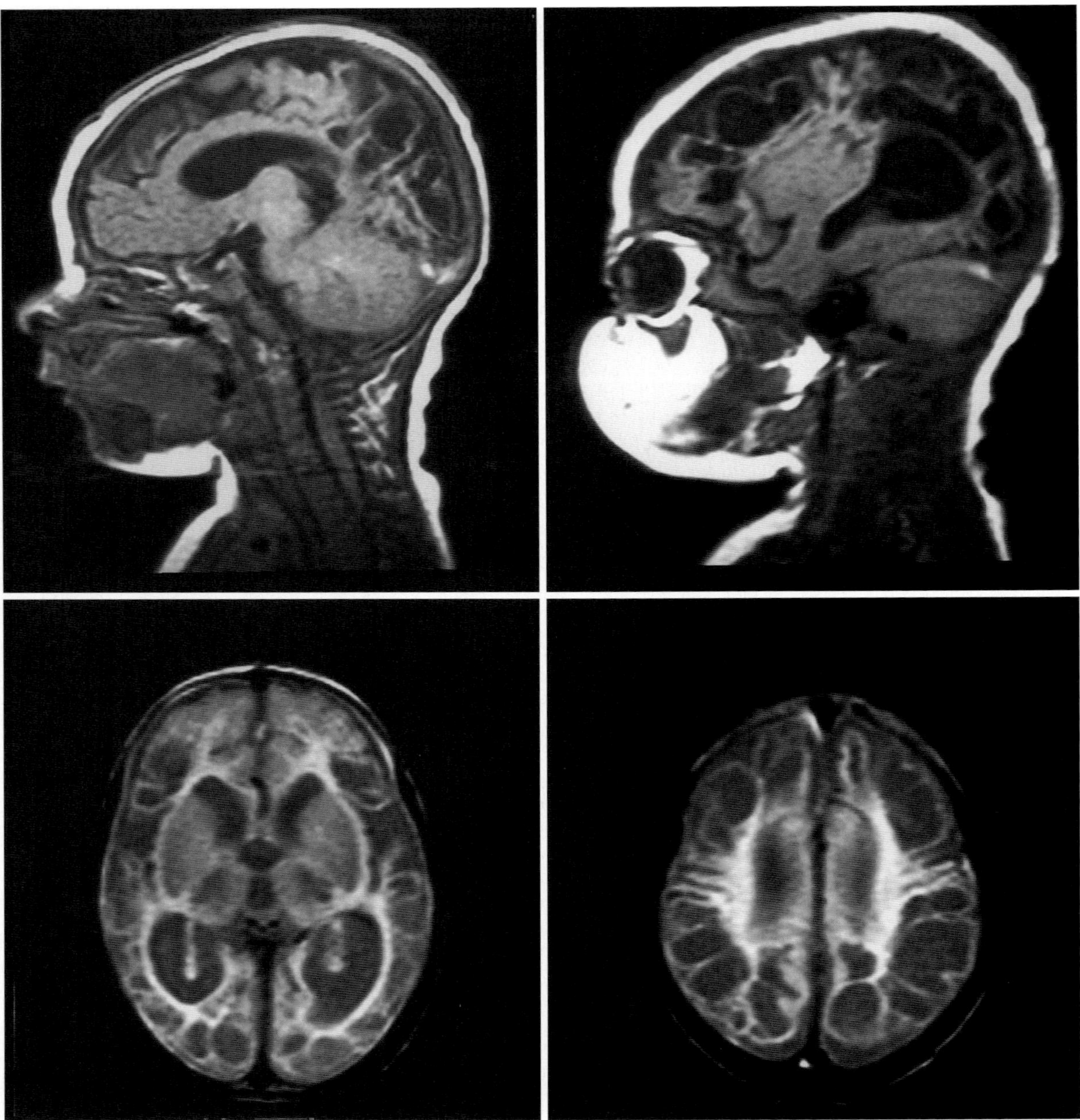

Fig. 63.3. T_1-weighted images in sagittal and transverse planes in a neonate, born at 36 weeks postconceptional age, now 6 weeks, showing multicystic subcortical degeneration. The myelinated areas seem to be spared

of high signal intensity on T_2-weighted and proton density images, representing replacement of white matter by gliosis; (3) deep sulci in the parietal region, nearly abutting the ventricular wall (Fig. 63.2).

The amount of periventricular gliosis depends upon the gestational age at the time of the insult. Prior to week 24 of gestational age, reactive astrogliosis has not yet developed in the brain. Before this stage, ischemic-necrotic tissue will undergo liquefaction and disappear. With increasing gestational age, astrogliosis be-

comes more and more prominent in tissue repair and replacement. The extent of the periventricular gliotic rim, therefore, corresponds roughly with gestational age. In older preterm children, the leukomalacia extends more often towards the subcortical region. Subcortical cysts may develop and subsequent scarring may lead to cortical disfiguration (Figs. 63.3, 63.4). The lesions are most conspicuous in the centrum semiovale extending in a fronto-occipital direction. The lesions of SCL are always accompanied by PVL.

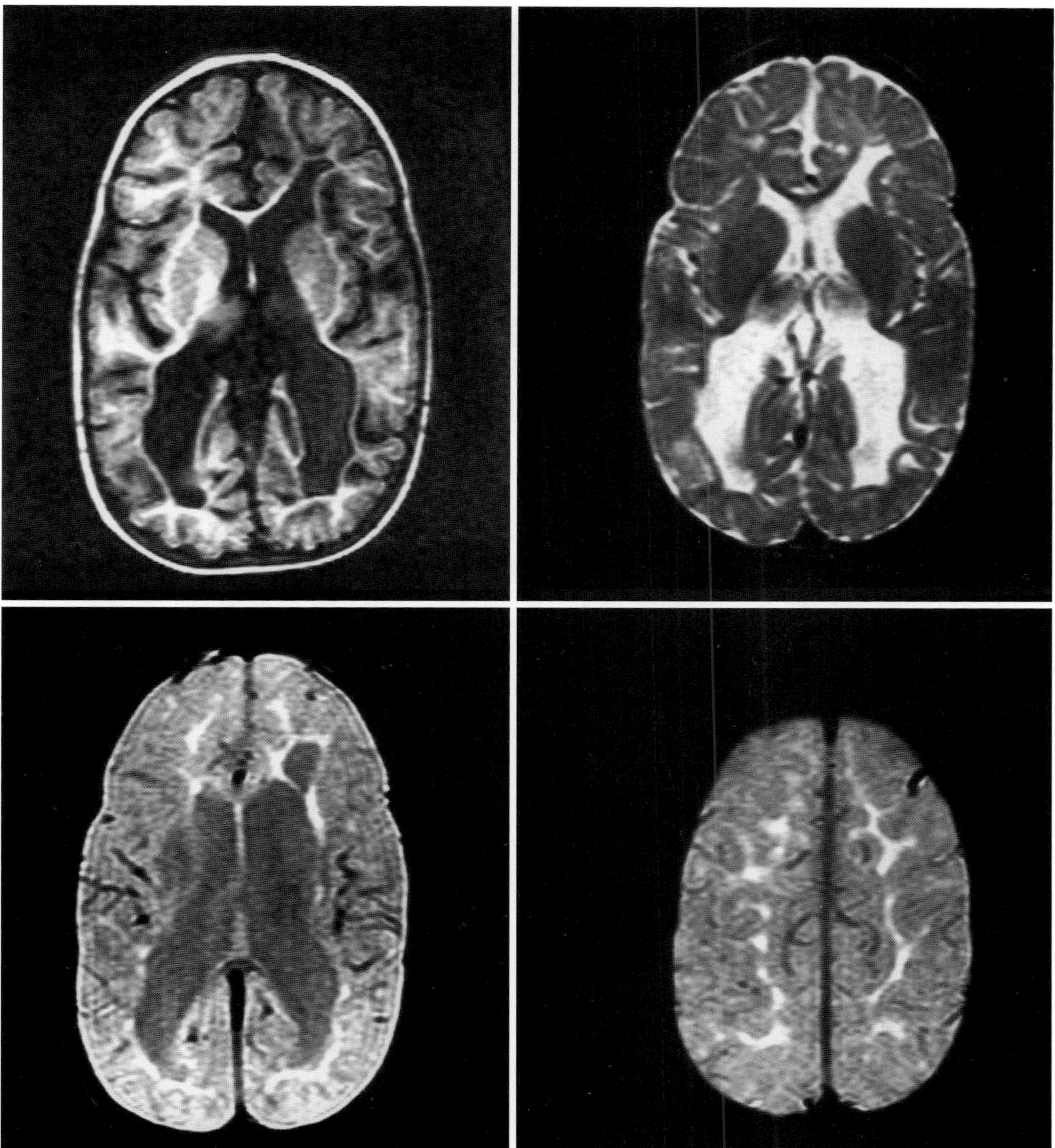

Fig. 63.4. A 2-year-old ex-premature girl with severe tetraplegia and mental retardation. The extension of the leukomalacia into the subcortical area is prominent and there is cyst formation, surrounded by gliosis in the left frontal lobe

With increasing maturity the pattern of lesions changes. Asphyxia in term neonates leads to leukomalacia affecting especially the cortico-subcortical central region, affecting the tracts that are normally shown to be partially myelinated at that time. The permanent damage consists of local gliosis and white matter loss, crowding of parietal gyri, leading to parietal ulegyria. On MRI the lesions have a typical triangular aspect, symmetrical, with a left-right orientation (Fig. 63.5, less severe in Fig. 63.6). This pattern may be combined with highly characteristic abnormalities in the dorsal part of the putamen and the ventrolateral parts of the thalamus, nearly always perfectly symmetrical. In some cases, the hippocampus is involved bilaterally. Often mild periventricular white matter changes are also seen.

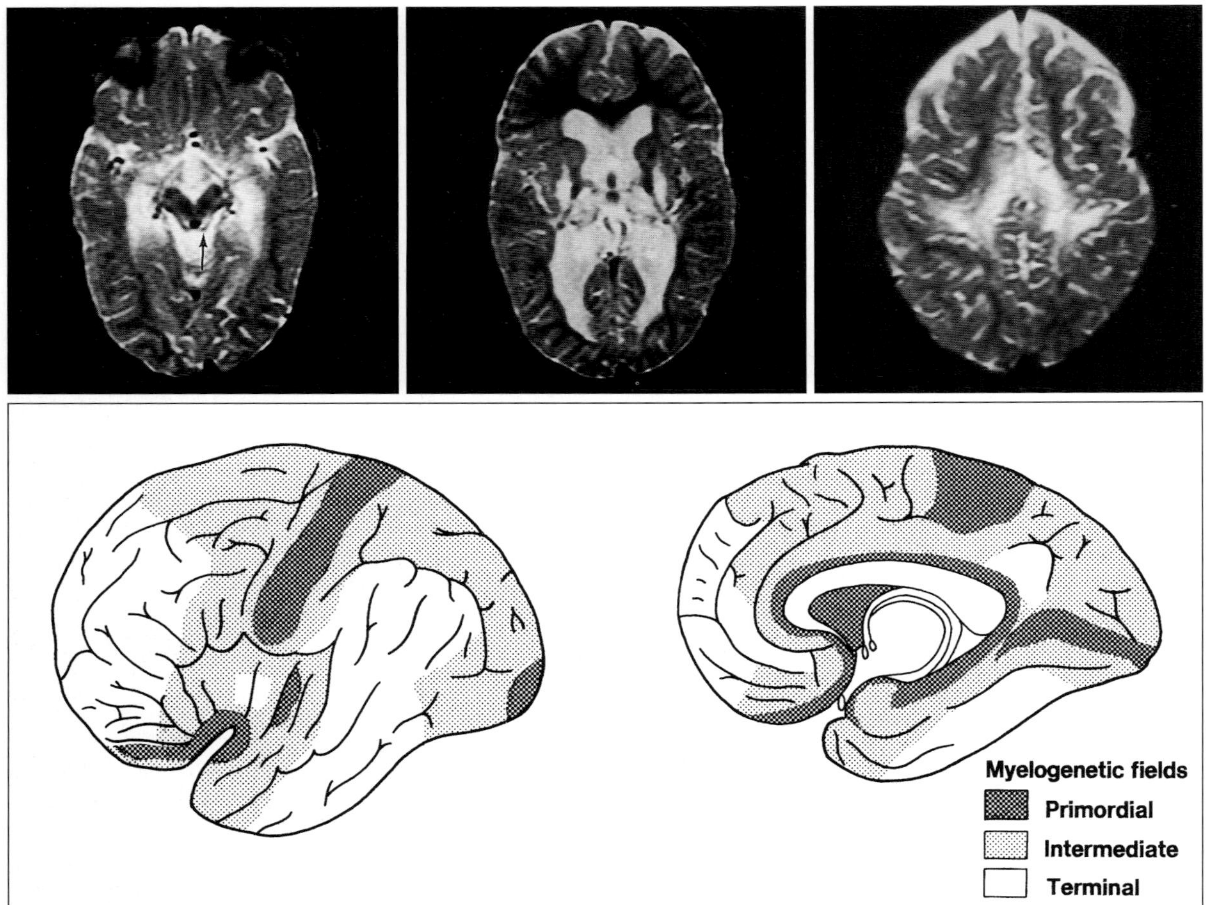

Fig. 63.5. The features of MR in term-born neonates with asphyxia are different from the pattern in prematures. In this 2-year-old term-born girl with a history of severe birth asphyxia, there is necrosis in the central cortico-subcortical re- gion, corresponding to a primordial myelogenetic field (see diagram after Paul Flechsig). There is also necrosis of the basal ganglia and hippocampus. Note the lesions in the dorsal part of the mesencephalon (*arrow*)

MRI is the modality of choice for surveying residual lesions at a later age. The typical aspects of PVL make the diagnosis easy. Proton density images allow the assessment of gliosis in the process, the identification of gliotic cysts and the pattern of subcortical retrac- tion. Unusual features can sometimes be observed such as loss of white matter, gliotic scarring and deformity of the ventricles in one region of the brain, for example the occipital or the frontal lobe (Fig. 63.7), with, of course, a different clinical presentation. The typical features of PVL, as described, will lead to the correct diagnosis.

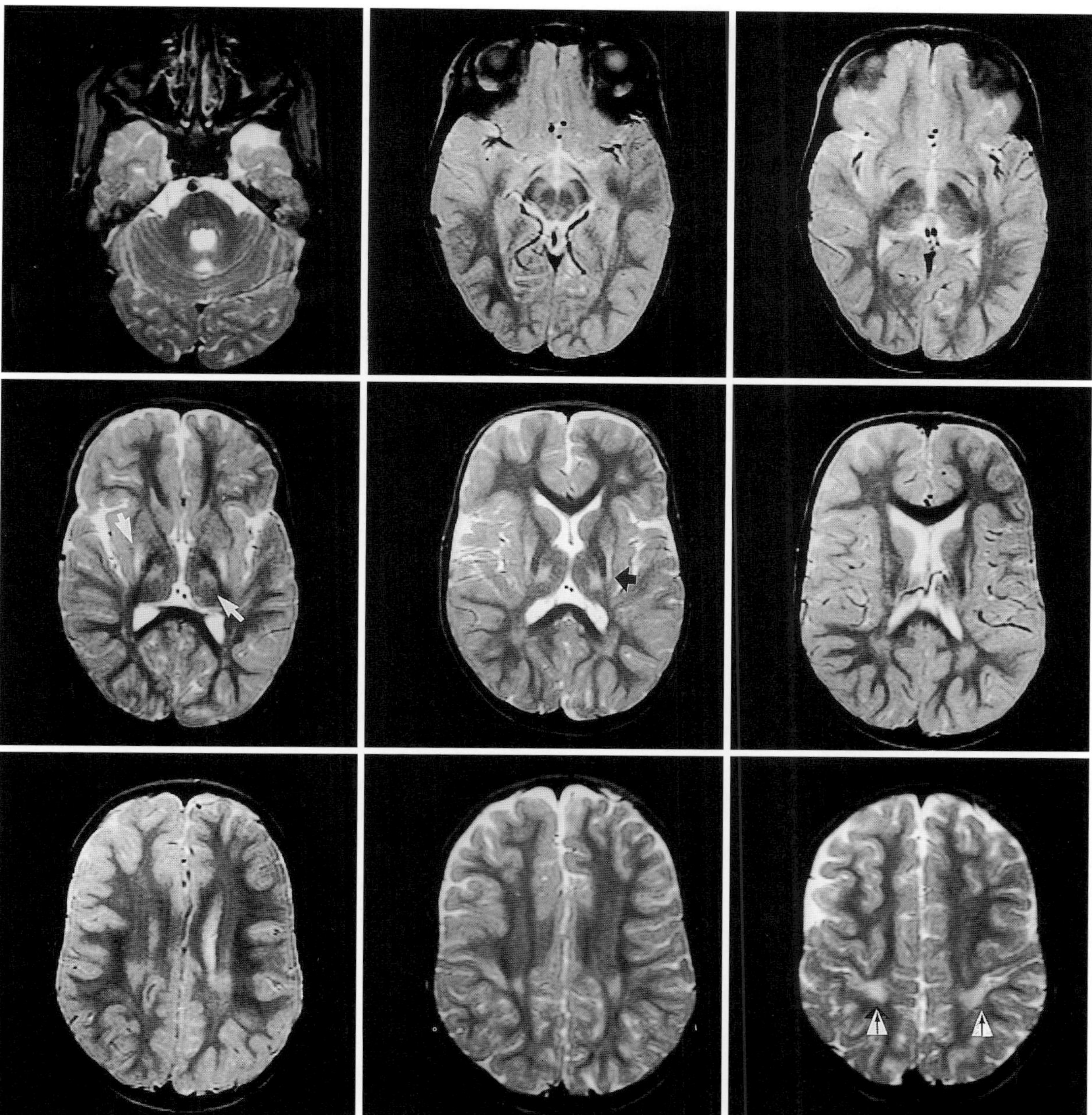

Fig. 63.6. A 3-year-old girl with spastic tetraplegia and severe dystonia. She was born at term with severe asphyxia. Typical lesions are seen in the lateral part of the thalamus and the dorsal part of the putamen (*arrows, middle row*). The white matter lesions of the central cortico-subcortical pattern are seen in the fronto-parietal region (*arrows, lower row*)

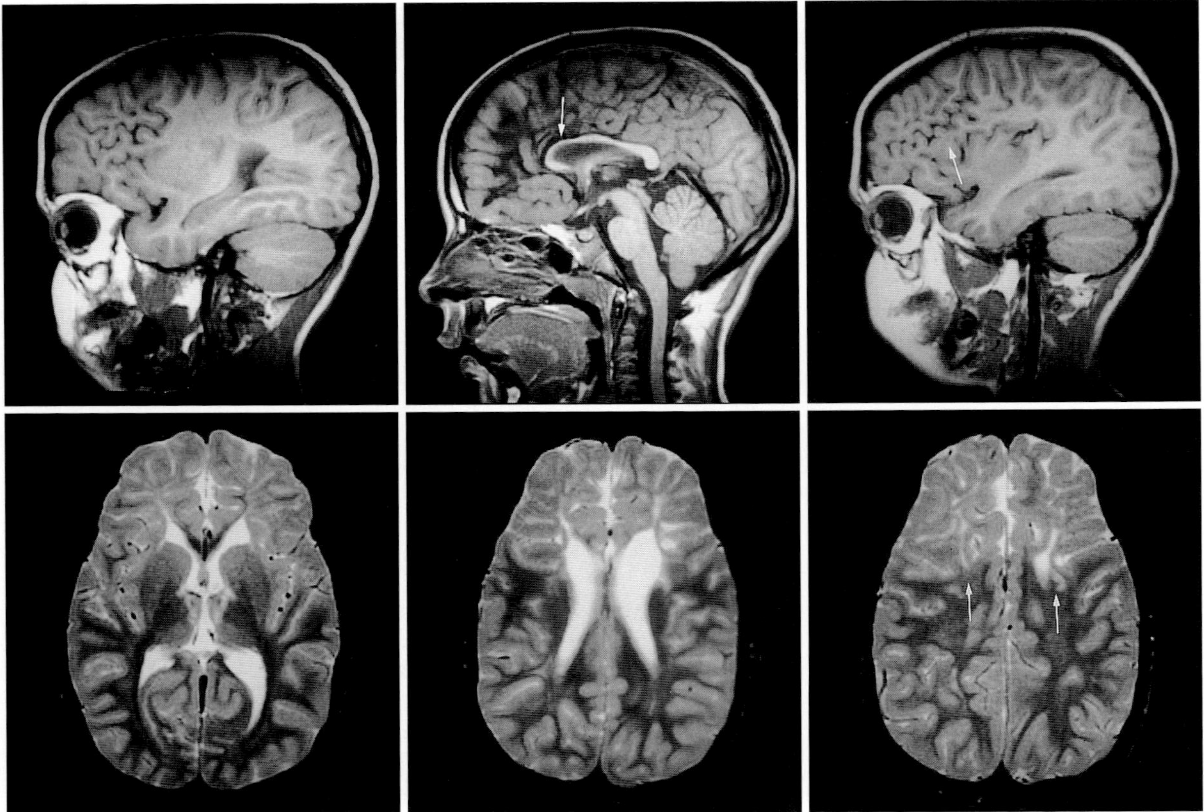

Fig. 63.7. In this 6-year-old girl only the frontal horns are widened and irregular. There is severe loss of white matter in the frontal lobe, which has diminished in size. This pattern is highly unusual, but fits the PVL criteria

64.1 Clinical Features and Laboratory Investigations

The usual pathological sequela of hypoxia in the CNS consists of damage to the neurons of the cortex and the subcortical gray matter structures. Selective injury to the cerebral white matter as a consequence of hypoxia-ischemia after the neonatal period is far less common. Posthypoxic leukoencephalopathy may occur immediately subsequent to the hypoxic-ischemic event, but there is usually an early phase of improvement from the initial stage of lowered consciousness. In these cases improvement is followed several days or weeks later by recurrence of impaired consciousness and other neurological signs. This condition is called delayed posthypoxic leukoencephalopathy (DPHL). The neurological abnormalities in DPHL vary from patient to patient and include spastic paresis of the extremities, a parkinsonian syndrome, choreiform movements, visual failure, myoclonus, seizures, psychosis, and mental deterioration. The condition results in a chronic state of global dementia, a vegetative state, or death, but recovery may also occur.

Laboratory tests in the acute phase include, first of all, determination of blood gases to assess oxygenation and acid-base status, since acidosis frequently accompanies the hypoxia. In a case of suspected carbon monoxide poisoning, the level of carboxyhemoglobin is determined. In cases of carbon monoxide poisoning, the ECG often shows signs of ischemia with inverted T waves and ST wave depression. If other intoxications are suspected, specific laboratory estimations of the level of toxic agents are necessary. The diagnosis of DPHL is established at a later stage with the help of clinical history, physical findings, and imaging techniques. The EEG contains diffuse bilateral slow wave activity with low voltage.

64.2 Pathology

The neuropathological findings are highly variable, depending on the severity of the insult and the time between the event and the pathological examination of the brain. Here only the neuropathological findings of DPHL in the more chronic stage of the disease are described.

The external appearance of the brain is normal. On sectioning, confluent white matter lesions are found bilaterally, with a fairly symmetrical distribution. Microscopically, the central white matter of both hemispheres contains areas of diffuse demyelination with loss of oligodendroglial cells and proliferation of astrocytes. The axons are relatively spared, but areas of extensive necrosis may occur with loss of both myelin and axons. Such necrosis is seen predominantly in arterial end and border zones of the deep white matter, while in the less distant arterial end fields of the white matter only demyelination is observed. The arcuate fibers and white matter underneath the ependyma are preserved. Patches of myelin persist around numerous vessels.

The cortex is also spared, but concomitant areas of necrosis may be present in the cerebral cortex, especially in an arterial border zone distribution. Necrotic areas are regularly present in the basal ganglia. The brain stem and cerebellum are usually, but not always, unaffected.

64.3 Pathogenetic Considerations

The susceptibility of tissues to anoxic-ischemic damage depends on the extent of vascular supply, the presence and quality of collateral circulation, the metabolic activity, and, with this, the energy demands of the particular tissues. In the brain anoxic-ischemic processes most commonly affect the cerebral cortex, while the white matter is completely or relatively spared. This observation can be explained by the fact that the white matter is metabolically less active than the cortex. Other explanations are found in the distribution of excitatory amino acid synapses and local physicochemical factors at cellular level. However, a diffuse injury of the white matter is seen in DPHL. DPHL occurs under circumstances of prolonged hypoxia, hypotension, and metabolic imbalance. The underlying causes comprise respiratory failure, cardiac arrest, and systematic hypotension. Precipitating events are carbon monoxide poisoning, cyanide poisoning, carbon disulfide poisoning, heroin overdose, morphine intoxication, anesthetic accidents, postoperative states of shock, and many other events.

The white matter lesions of DPHL are located in arterial end and border zones. For their arterial blood supply, the cerebral cortex and arcuate fibers depend on cortical branches of the major cerebral arteries and their leptomeningeal anastomoses. The white matter immediately beneath the ependyma depends on branches of the choroid arteries, perforating and medullary branches of the major cerebral arteries and their leptomeningeal anastomoses. These arteries form a border zone in the deep white matter. The basal ganglia receive their supply from end-arteries. The deep white matter lesions of DPHL are frequently accompanied by lesions in the basal ganglia, as well as in border zones of the cerebral cortex. However, there is no clear correlation between gray and white matter damage, and white matter damage does not appear to depend directly on the degree of anoxia. Although some consider the white matter lesions to be merely a border zone effect, it is probable that something other than hypoxia alone is required for lesions of this kind to be produced. There are several reasons for this assumption. Cerebral DPHL occurs only rarely, in contrast to the much more frequent anoxic-ischemic gray matter damage. In addition, gray matter structures are relatively spared in DPHL, which suggests that the hypoxic-ischemic process in itself is not profound as these structures are rather sensitive to lack of oxygen. One has the impression that white matter damage is particularly likely to occur under conditions of prolonged depression of both oxygenation and circulation. Acidosis may be another adverse factor in this context. Drug overdose, for instance morphine intoxication, leading both to a depression of respiration and to hypotension, is particularly apt to lead to DPHL, much more often than, for instance, a cardiac arrest without antecedent impairment of respiration.

Carbon monoxide intoxication relatively frequently leads to DPHL. It causes tissue hypoxia by reversibly binding to hemoglobin in red blood cells, thereby reducing the oxygen-carrying capacity of the blood. The presence of carboxyhemoglobin shifts the oxyhemoglobin dissociation curve to the left, and tissue oxygen tension must therefore fall to much lower levels before the remaining oxyhemoglobin can give up its oxygen, a factor aggravating the tissue hypoxia. Moreover, carbon monoxide inhibits cellular respiration by binding to cytochrome oxidase. In addition to hypoxia, carbon monoxide often causes a general hypotension by the formation of carboxymyoglobin in the myocardium, which in turn leads to myocardial dysfunction. This combination of hypoxia and general circulatory collapse probably explains why DPHL is so often seen in carbon monoxide poisoning.

Cyanide may also lead to DPHL. Cyanides have specific inhibitory effects on the cytochrome oxidase respiratory enzyme system of cells due to a strong affinity of cyanides for the iron core of the cytochromes. In this way cyanides lead to tissue hypoxia despite the presence of sufficient amounts of oxygen.

64.4 Therapy

Prevention of cerebral hypoxia and ischemia and the prompt restitution of normal oxygenation, blood pressure, and acid-base balance after any hypoxic-ischemic insult are the only possible measures in the prevention and treatment of DPHL.

The treatment of choice for patients with carbon monoxide poisoning is exposure to hyperbaric oxygen in order to wash out the carbon monoxide as soon as possible.

Cyanide poisoning can be treated with hydroxycobalamin and sodium thiosulfate in the acute stage. Adequate treatment of the acute poisoning may prevent the occurrence of DPHL.

Once DPHL has developed, the only option is to provide supportive care.

64.5 Magnetic Resonance Imaging

In DPHL, the involvement of the white matter is generally symmetrical and confluent and located in arterial border and end zones, due to the underlying systemic cause. In carbon monoxide poisoning, extensive, confluent deep white matter involvement with late occurrences has been reported (Fig. 64.1), but more focal and asymmetrical white matter involvement has also been reported. We have observed DPHL after cardiac surgery in a 6-year-old boy (Fig. 64.2).

White matter lesions may be accompanied by lesions in gray matter structures in arterial end and border zones of the cortex and in the basal ganglia. In carbon monoxide intoxication, the globus pallidus is preferentially affected. The pattern of the lesions may suggest the diagnosis, or, more often, sustain the clinical suspicion.

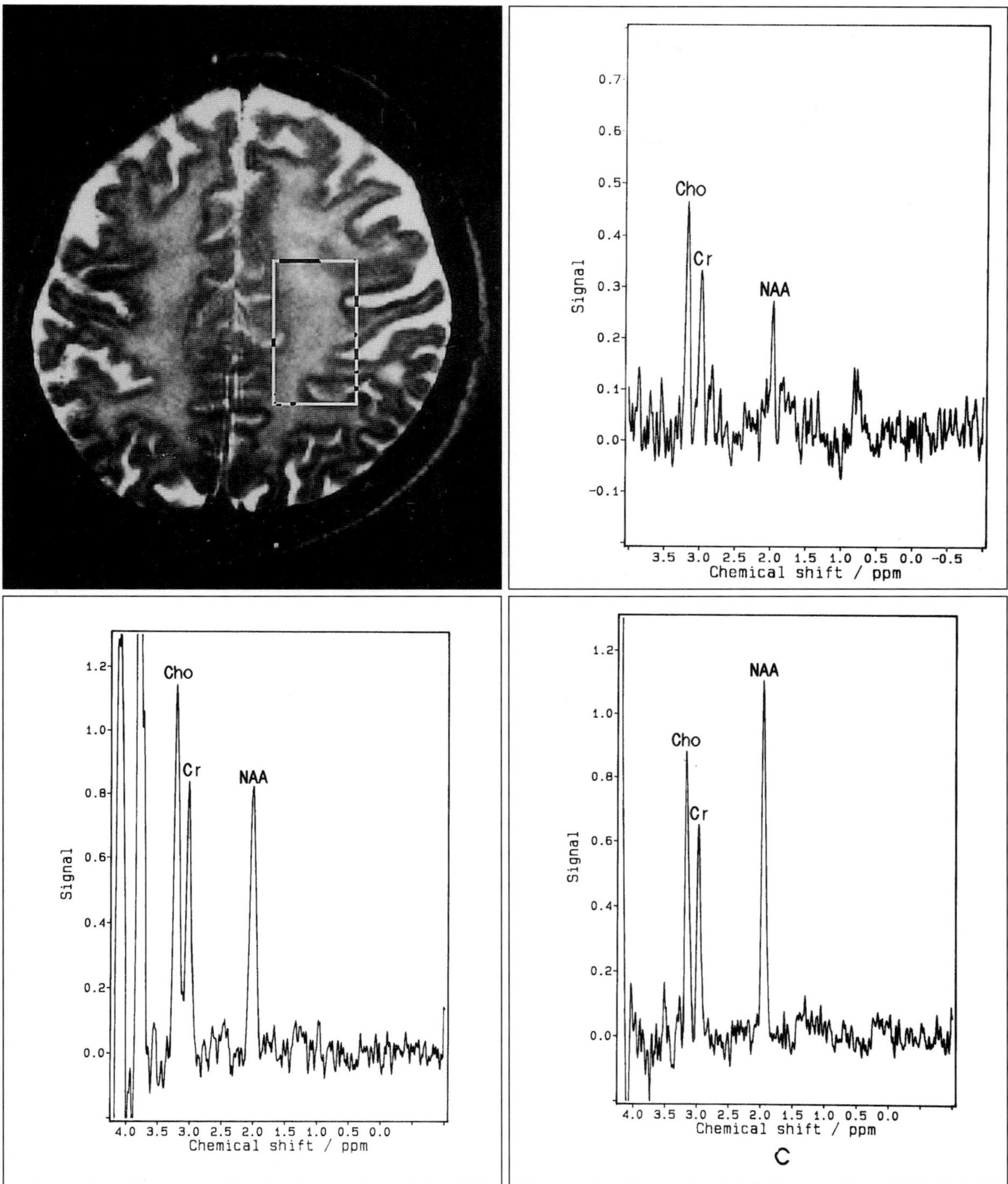

Fig. 64.1. A 55-year-old woman with DPHL after carbon monoxide poisoning. A T$_2$-weighted axial image on the 45th day after poisoning shows marked bilateral high signal intensity in the hemispheral white matter (*upper left*). There are signs of atrophy. The globus pallidus is also involved bilaterally. The ^{1}H spectra were taken on the 29th (*upper right*), the 42nd (*lower left*) and 151th (*lower right*) days after poisoning. At the first two examinations, the N-acetylaspartate peak was relatively low with high choline/creatine ratios. At the last examination, the N-acetylaspartate/creatine ratio had returned to normal, whereas MRI was more or less unchanged. For details on spectroscopy, see Chap. 71. Courtesy of Kamada et al. 1994, with permission

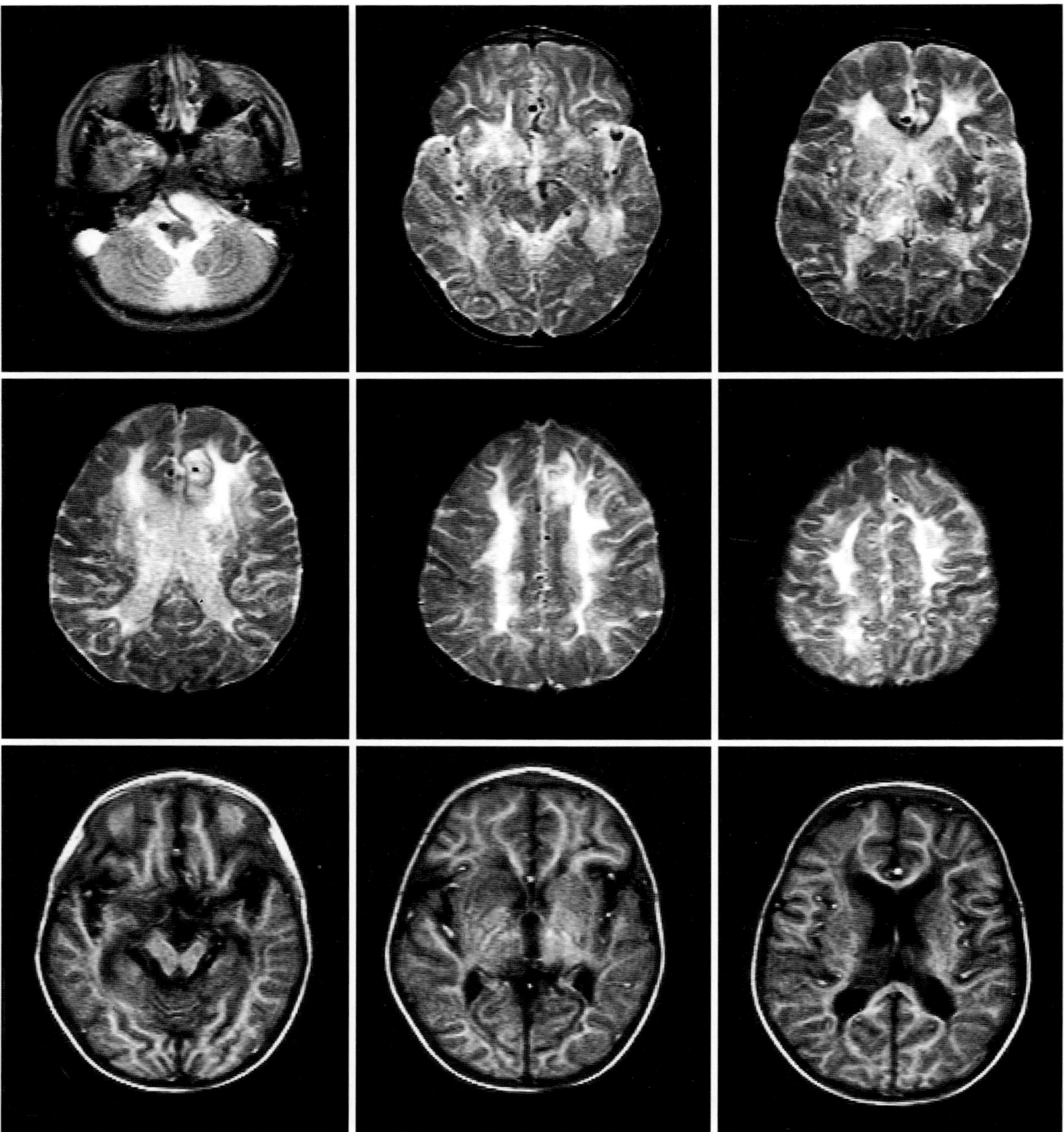

Fig. 64.2. Boy, 6 years of age, underwent surgery for a congenital cardiac defect. Postoperatively he did well. Four weeks later he started to behave strangely. He suffered two cardiac arrests, necessitating resuscitation, after which he remained subcomatose. Neurological recovery was slow and only partial. He could follow objects with his eyes. He could not speak. He showed signs of a spastic tetraplegia. MRI shows extensive changes in the white matter, largely sparing the arcuate fibers. There are also lesions in the internal capsule, basal ganglia and mesencephalon. The cerebellum is not affected

65 Subcortical Arteriosclerotic Encephalopathy

65.1 Clinical Features and Laboratory Investigations

In 1894, Binswanger was the first to describe encephalitis subcorticalis chronica progressiva, later renamed by Olszewski (1962) as subcortical arteriosclerotic encephalopathy (SAE). SAE is frequently called Binswanger's disease, or Binswanger's microangiopathic leukoencephalopathy. The age at onset is usually between 50 and 70 years, but sometimes earlier or later in life. SAE is a relatively rare affliction of elderly patients, most of whom have risk factors for arteriosclerosis. It is clearly associated with a history of hypertension, although there are also reports of patients whose necropsy examinations reveal SAE but who did not have hypertension during life.

The patients usually present with a slowly developing dementia with or without motor deficits, but sometimes the motor deficits precede the dementia. The dementia begins with insidious memory loss and progresses to global intellectual impairment. Psychological disturbances are frequent, ranging from loss of interest, lack of drive, and mild depression to severe alterations in mood and personality. Clinical features include acute strokes with focal neurological deficits followed by a variable degree of improvement. More often, neurological deficits develop subacutely over periods of weeks or months. There are long plateau periods without further deterioration. Neurological signs include dysarthria, clumsiness of the arms, and disturbances of gait due to pyramidal or extrapyramidal motor deficit, ataxia, or apraxia. Also aphasia, hemianopia, sensory disturbances, and urinary incontinence are common. Seizures occur occasionally. The clinical features of SAE are common to other disorders, such as multi-infarct dementia, or even Alzheimer's dementia. Clinical differentiation is often difficult or impossible.

Recently, an autosomal dominant cerebral arteriopathy with subcortical leukoencephalopathy and infarcts has been described by Tournier-Lasserve et al. (1991). The disease is characterized by recurrent subcortical ischemic strokes in the absence of hypertension. It starts in early mid-adulthood and leads in some patients to dementia. The disease is called CADASIL (cerebral autosomal dominant arteriopathy with subcortical infarcts and leukoencephalopathy).

Laboratory investigations in SAE yield normal hematological and biochemical findings. CSF is normal except for an elevated protein level in some cases. CSF pressure is normal. Carotid angiography is usually negative but may show arteriosclerosis of the extra- and intracranial vessels. The EEG shows moderate or marked slow-wave activity bilaterally. Focal abnormalities may be found and, rarely, periodic complexes. Psychometric testing confirms the subcortical type of dementia but does not yield specific information.

65.2 Pathology

External examination of the brain shows either no abnormalities or some degree of atrophy. On sectioning, an enlarged ventricular system is found. The cerebral cortex appears normal. The white matter in the vicinity of the lateral ventricles contains grayish, ill-defined lesions in both hemispheres. Cystic lesions may be present in the basal ganglia, thalami, brain stem, cerebellum, and cerebral white matter.

Histological examination shows that the small cystic lesions contain a few macrophages and some hemosiderin deposits and are surrounded by a moderate gliosis. In addition, there is bilateral involvement of the white matter, extending from the frontal to the occipital lobe with variable severity from region to region. Pallor of the myelin predominates in the periventricular region and decreases in intensity as the convolutions are approached. The U fibers are spared. The more uniform pallor is peppered with dots, spots, and streaks of accentuated pallor. Diffusely scattered through the affected white matter are foci showing every degree of destruction, from typical lacunar infarcts, 3–6 mm in diameter at one end of the spectrum, down to merely a spongy looseness of the tissue with loss of myelin sheaths and astrocytic proliferation without necrosis. Between these two extremes every gradation of severity and size of lesions may be found. Myelin may be destroyed along with the contained axons, or myelin sheaths may be swollen and pale and the axons preserved. The most severely affected periventricular regions may show zones of frank necrosis, 3–4 mm in extent. Etat criblé, i.e. a widening of the Virchow-Robin spaces, is an almost constant feature. The intracranial cerebral arteries show signs of arteriosclerosis with superimposed hypertensive changes consisting of media hypertrophy with fibrosis and hyalinosis. These changes affect predominantly the perforating small arteries and arterioles of the deep white matter, basal ganglia, and thalami. They lead to narrowing and occlusion of the lumina especially at the sites of origin of capillaries.

65.3   Pathogenetic Considerations

The cause of SAE is arteriosclerosis and hypertensive vessel wall changes leading to narrowing and occlusion of the deep perforating arteries and their branches. These vessels appear to be affected preferentially. An important factor is that these arteries and arterioles are end vessels, without collateral circulation. These vessels form an arterial end and border zone in the periventricular region, and it is in this area that the microscopic features of microinfarction, focal or diffuse demyelination with associated gliosis are found. The cortex and subcortical U fibers are relatively well preserved, as they are within the territory of supply of the cortical vessels and their leptomeningeal anastomoses. Thus, the pathogenesis of white matter degeneration is probably related to chronic hypoperfusion and ischemia.

The preferential involvement of deep white and gray matter with sparing of the cerebral cortex leads to the clinical picture of subcortical dementia. However, not infrequently one also finds signs of cortical dysfunction due to the presence of cortical infarcts. The occurrence of cortical infarcts in a large number of patients with SAE suggests a relationship between these lesions and SAE. Arteriosclerosis probably underlies both types of lesion. There is good reason to consider SAE and multi-infarct dementia to be two variants of the same vascular disease.

The finding of a genetic disease with clinical and pathological characteristics similar to SAE and without a history of hypertension sheds a new light on the genesis of SAE. Genetic linkage analysis was performed in two unrelated families with CADASIL patients. The locus of the disease was assigned to chromosome 19q12. Insight into the gene product of this gene could provide new insights into understanding the disease mechanisms of SAE and other vascular disorders.

The term leuko-araiosis was coined by Hachinski et al. (1987) to indicate the periventricular white matter changes in elderly people. "Araios" means "rarefied, with its units far apart". The distinction between leuko-araiosis and SAE was made to separate inciden-

tal findings of periventricular white matter changes, found in abundance in asymptomatic elderly people on CT (and later even more on MRI), from the true cases of SAE with clinical symptoms which is considered to be rare. The relatively neutral term "leuko-araiosis" allows further investigations into risk factors, clinical and pathological correlations of the neuroimaging finding. As a result of this method of definition, there is not a clinical entity which is directly associated with the concept leuko-araiosis.

In SAE there is often compensatory ventricular dilatation due to loss of white matter substance. However, the ventricular dilatation may also be caused by normal pressure hydrocephalus, which has been repeatedly reported in association with SAE. In these cases the neurological symptoms improve after ventricular shunting.

65.4   Therapy

Treatment of already acquired structural damage is, of course, impossible. Adequate treatment of hypertension is helpful in preventing SAE. When SAE becomes clinically manifest, antihypertensive treatment is no longer helpful. It has even been suggested that tolerance of lowering the blood pressure is reduced in SAE. The arteriosclerotic vessel wall changes impair vascular autoregulation so that normalization of blood pressure leads to poor perfusion of deep white matter, thus worsening the white matter damage. In the case of coexisting normal pressure hydrocephalus, patients benefit from ventricular shunting.

65.5   Magnetic Resonance Imaging

In patients with dementia and a history of hypertension the diagnosis SAE depends on two parameters: the clinical establishment of a subcortical type of dementia and the establishment of diffuse damage to the deep white matter by an imaging modality, CT or MRI. In uncomplicated cases of SAE, CT and MRI identify a relatively well preserved cortex, somewhat enlarged ventricles (note that a normal pressure hydrocephalus sometimes coexists) and an area of reduced density around the ventricles on CT or, on MRI, a periventricular rim with high signal intensity on T_2-weighted images (Figs. 65.1 and 65.2). In some cases cavities are seen within this rim, residues of infarcted areas, in agreement with the neuropathological findings. In most cases the U fibers are spared. In cases of longer standing the white matter disorder may also involve the subcortical area. Apart from the periventricular rim there are often isolated lesions scattered through the basal ganglia, the pons, and midbrain, representing

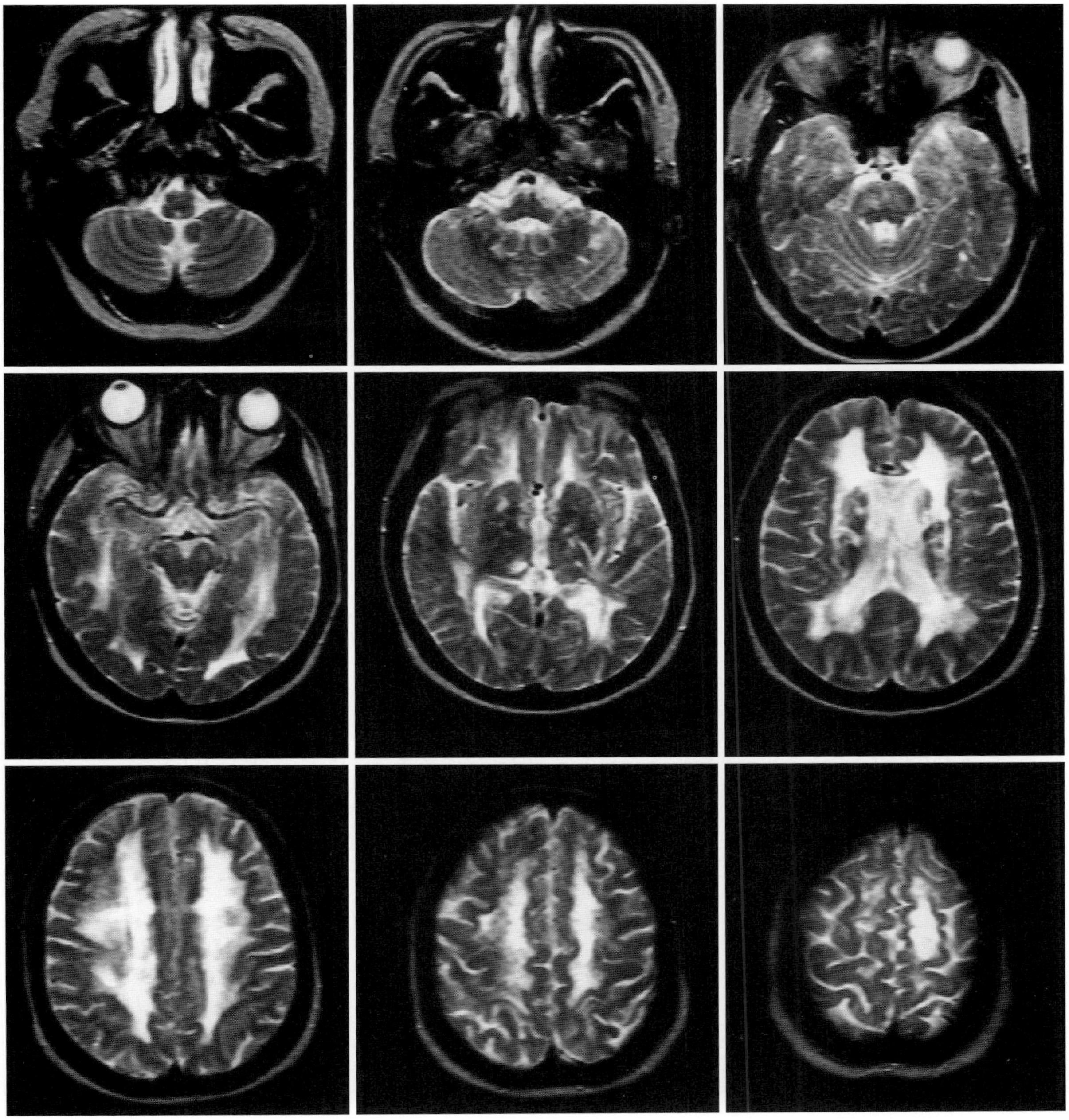

Fig. 65.1. A 58-year-old man with progressive subcortical dementia and transient ischemic attacks. The T$_2$-weighted series shows small lesions in the left cerebellar hemisphere, diffuse hyperintensities in the pons small punctate lesions in the basal ganglia and periventricular leukencephalopathy, extending into the centrum semiovale. Lesions are also present in the corpus callosum

lacunar infarctions. The corpus callosum is usually less affected than in multiple sclerosis, but this is a rule with exceptions. The anterior commissure is usually spared. In cases with a history of chronic hypertension, treated or untreated, and clinically a subcortical dementia one can assume that the periventricular rim confirms the clinical suspicion of SAE.

The MR presentation can be unusual and one may see a combination of état criblé, état lacunaire and more confluent periventricular white matter changes (Fig. 65.3). The patients present with neurological deficits related to transient ischemic attacks or cerebral infarcts, although initially the neuropsychological deficits are inconspicuous. The MR images are striking.

The sensitivity of MRI for white matter changes is impressive. This high sensitivity has led to the discovery of an abundance of deep white matter changes,

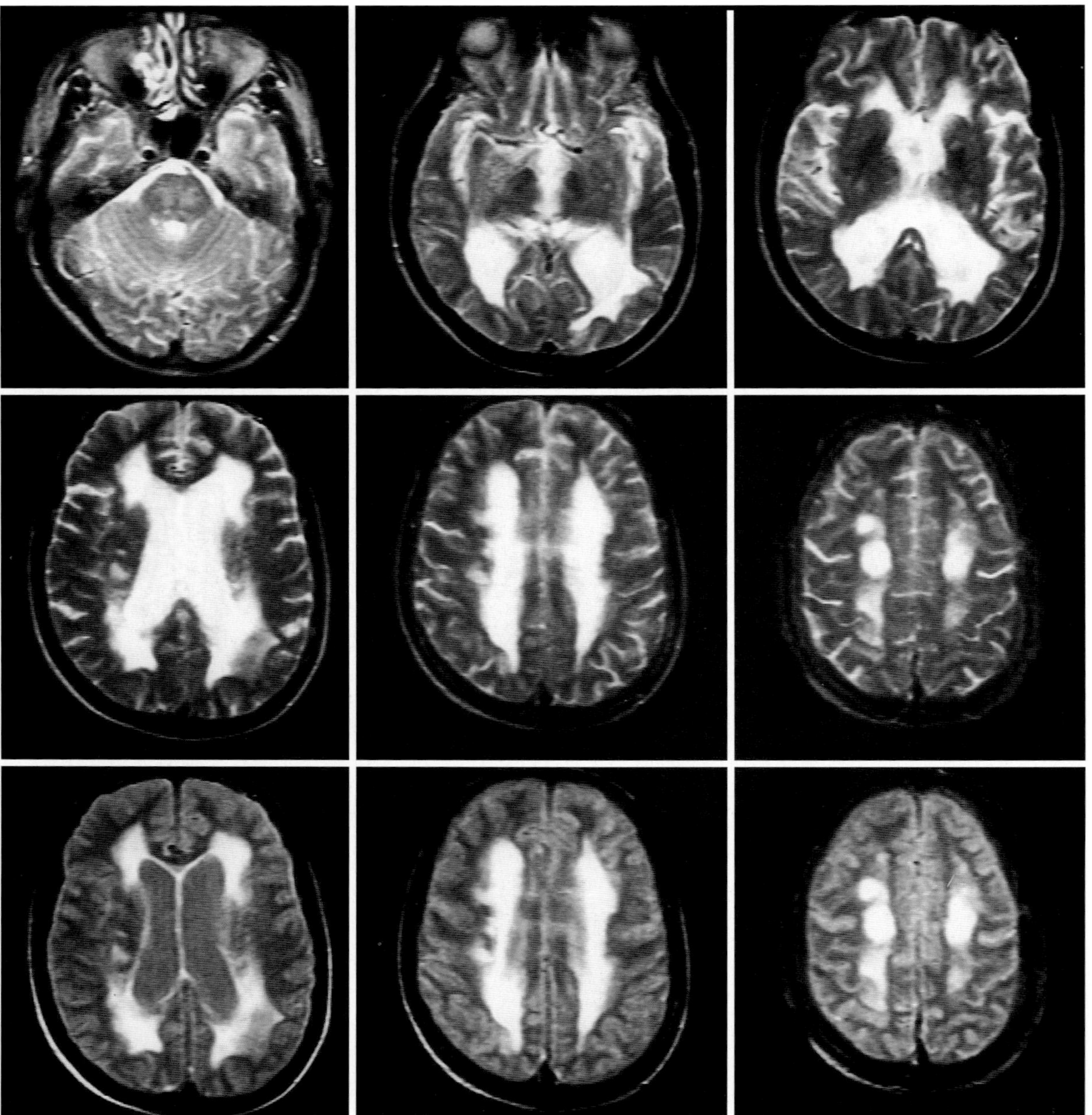

Fig. 65.2. A 64-year-old man with subcortical dementia. Features of these MR images are very similar to the previous case, with somewhat less severe involvement of the basal ganglia. This case also shows there are multiple lesions in the corpus callosum

particularly in elderly people, and to a steep increase in the diagnosis of "SAE". Until the introduction of MRI only 50 cases of SAE with histological confirmation had been reported in the literature. In view of this development, Hachinski et al. (1987) decided to introduce the term leuko-araiosis, describing the abnormalities as found on CT and MR with a neutral term and creating the opportunity to study the connection between the radiological findings, histology and clinical presentation. Deep white matter changes proved to be

common in the elderly, and both age and previous vascular incidents were shown to stand out significantly as risk factors in nearly all studies. In some reports the focal and confluent areas of periventricular hyperintensity occur in 30% of patients over 60 years of age. Several authors have reported comparisons between MRI and neuropathological findings. In nearly all these studies the lesions on MRI were found to represent myelin pallor, demyelination, gliosis, widened perivascular spaces, lacunar infarctions, and, with cortical in-

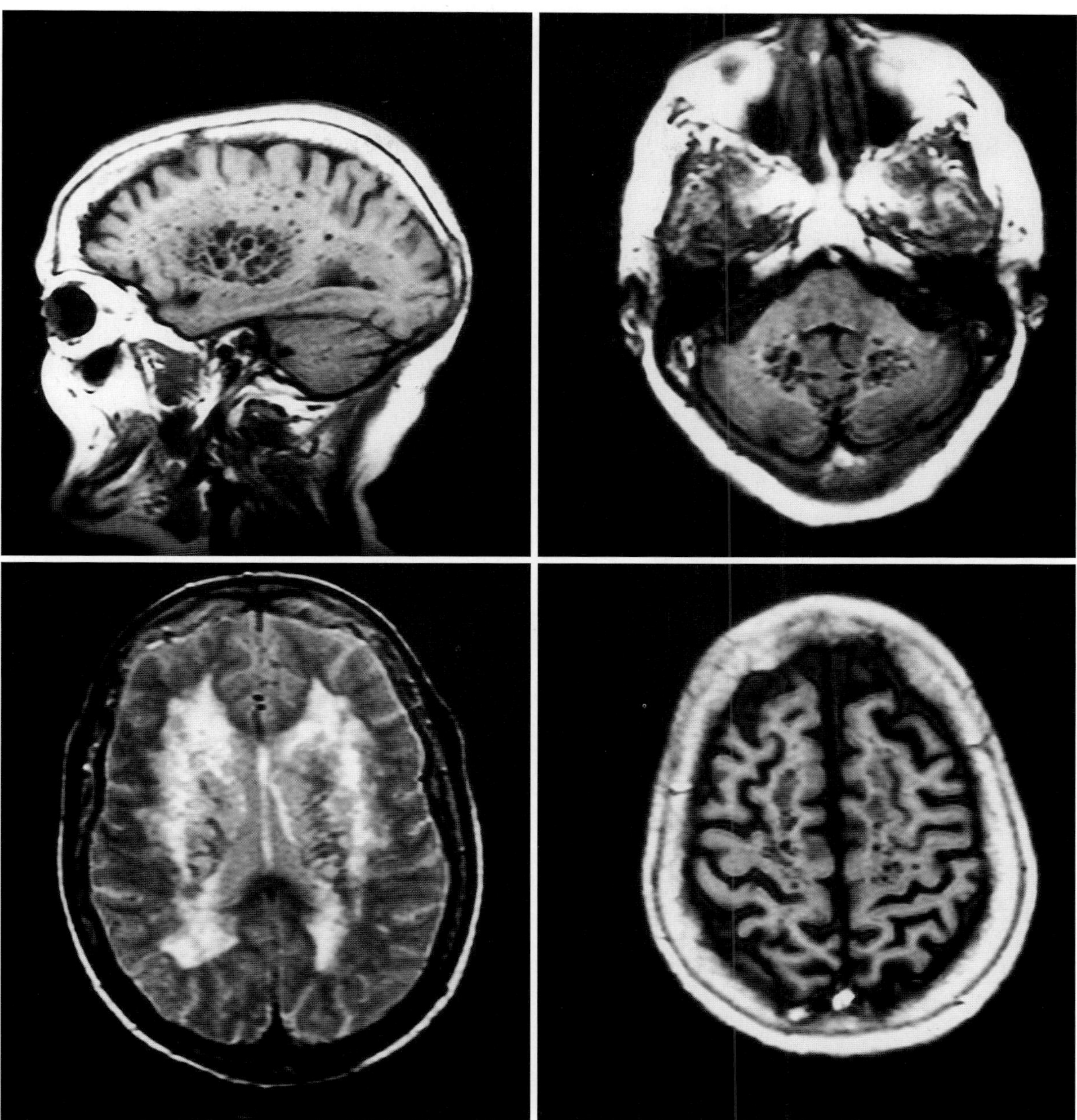

Fig. 65.3. 67-year-old female with subcortical dementia. Although there is evidently a periventricular leukoencephalopathy, there is also a striking enlargement of the Virchow-Robin spaces in the basal ganglia, centrum semiovale, and, which is less common, in the dentate nucleus and corpus medullare of the cerebellum

farctions present, Wallerian degeneration. A recent study compared antemortem and postmortem MRI investigations with neuropathological findings. The presence of lesions with high signal intensity on proton density MR images showed a strong correlation with demyelination and gliosis in the same area in histopathology. Dilation of perivascular spaces was strongly but not perfectly correlated with demyelination and arteriosclerosis. In true SAE, the common factors are probably still arteriolar disease, microangiopathy, with hypoperfusion in perforating, non-collateralizing vessels. We would agree with Drayer (1988a,b) that we are looking at a continuum of MRI abnormalities, with SAE as the most severe clinical expression and, at the other extreme, the so-called UBOs (unidentified bright objects) as the clinically silent first indication of arteriolar change. There is growing evidence that, generally speaking, the extensiveness of the white matter lesions corresponds with the severity of the clinical disease.

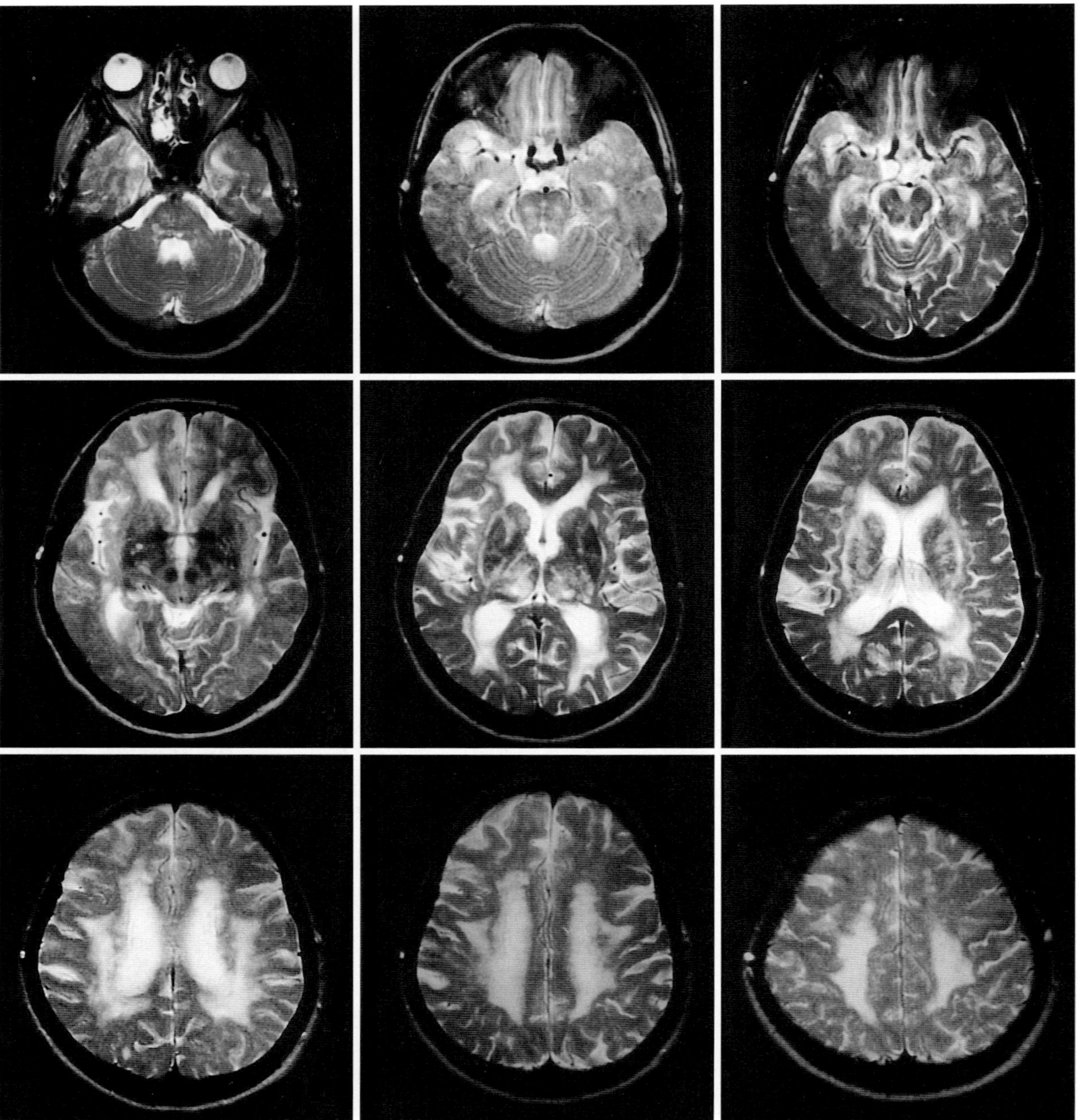

Fig. 65.4. Patient from the CADASIL group. Although in many respects similar to the SAE cases, some features remain that may distinguish the two conditions: the temporal white matter is always involved; the basal ganglia show an état criblé; the external capsule is always more involved than the internal capsule in CADASIL patients. Courtesy of Ph. Scheltens, Amsterdam, The Netherlands

The finding of a zone of periventricular high signal intensity on MRI in asymptomatic patients leads to a differential diagnosis including asymptomatic normal pressure hydrocephalus with periventricular CSF effusion; age-related changes in the deep white matter probably on a vascular basis; chronic white matter disease as in multiple sclerosis, and postinfectious and posttraumatic conditions. At the symptomatic stage the differential diagnosis would include: symptomatic normal pressure hydrocephalus; infections, such as Lyme's disease; generalized or isolated cerebral vasculitis; toxic encephalopathies; and inborn errors of metabolism of very late onset, such as metachromatic leukodystrophy. The combination of periventricular white matter changes and spots in the basal nuclei is, however, rather special and argues in favor of SAE.

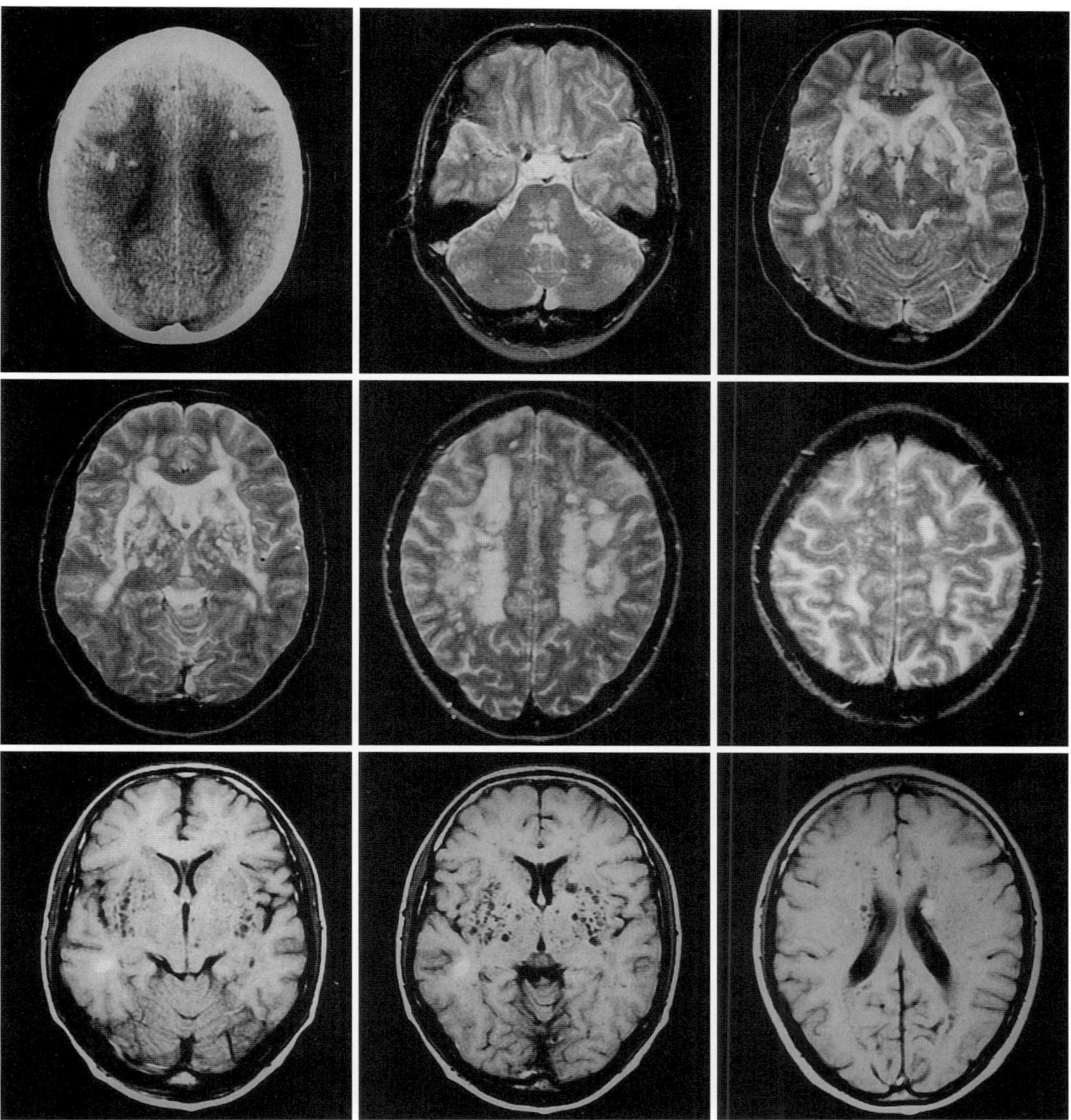

Fig. 65.5. Other typical aspects of the CADASIL cases. In this 45-year-old female the CT and T_1-weighted images (*lower row*) show hemorrhages and dilated Virchow-Robin spaces more or less throughout the brain. The T_2-weighted images (*upper rows*) show the état criblé of the basal nuclei bilaterally and white matter lesions, less symmetrical than usual. Pontine and cerebellar lesions are present as well. Courtesy of Ph. Scheltens, Amsterdam, The Netherlands

Standard MRI series are fully capable of displaying the cerebral abnormalities. Fast imaging sequences can often be used to advantage. In cases in which segmentation is demanded for postprocessing purposes, special techniques, such as the FLAIR technique, can be applied with differentiation between pathological and normal tissue.

Although the MR images of patients with CADASIL have many features in common with those of SAE pa-
tients, there are some special characteristics, at least in the patients examined by us. First of all, the external capsule is involved in an early stage in all cases; secondly, the white matter of the temporal lobe is preferentially involved; thirdly, there is an extensive état criblé, involving the basal ganglia, the centrum semiovale and the temporal lobes; and fourthly, small hemorrhages dispersed throughout the brain, are seen more commonly (Figs. 65.4 and 65.5).

66 Vasculitis

66.1 Disease Categories

Apart from arteriosclerotic vessel disease and its consequences, other, usually rare, disorders of the cerebral blood vessels exist which can lead to focal changes in white matter, sometimes in white and gray matter, with a variety of clinical presentations. These disorders may be of infectious origin, as in syphilitic infections, but more commonly they are the expression of a generalized autoimmune disease, such as rheumatoid arthritis, Sjögren disease, systemic lupus erythematosus, periarthritis nodosa and temporal arteritis. Treatment and secondary prevention in these disorders may be quite important, making correct diagnosis essential.

The vasculitic disorders of the CNS can be subdivided into (1) primary CNS vasculitides, (2) systemic necrotizing vasculitides with CNS involvement, (3) rheumatological syndromes associated with CNS disease due to vasculitis, (4) infectious vasculitides.

The most important representative of *primary CNS vasculitis* is the granulomatous angiitis of the nervous system. Delayed hemiplegia following herpes zoster ophthalmicus has often been considered to be the equivalent of granulomatous angiitis. Sufficient clinical differences, however, exist to justify the assumption of two distinct entities.

The presenting clinical signs of granulomatous angiitis are nonspecific, often suggesting global dysfunction of the CNS. Acute or subacute onset confusion, headache, change of personality, paresis, cranial neuropathy or loss of consciousness may suggest a variety of presumed diagnoses at first evaluation. The most frequent presenting symptoms of granulomatous angiitis are headache (68%), paresis (56%) and confusion (55%). In almost 25% of the patients fever and elevated blood pressure are noted. Dermatological abnormalities are rare. Funduscopy reveals vascular changes in 25% of patients. The erythrocyte sedimentation rate is usually accelerated. CSF pressure is usually elevated and CSF is nearly always abnormal with increased total protein, lymphocytic pleiocytosis and in 30% decreased glucose levels. The EEG is abnormal in most patients. CT and angiography are helpful in revealing the CNS lesions and changes of caliber in the cerebral vessels (Fig. 66.1). Postmortem examination of brain tissue and examination of brain biopsy material show an inflammatory process of small arteries and arterioles, preferentially involving deep white matter and leptomeningeal vessels. Intima proliferation and fibrosis are frequent, with multinuclear giant cells of the Langhans type and foreign body type. In comparison with the other vessel layers, the media is relatively spared. Granulomata with macrophages, and lymphocytes are present. Without treatment the disease is usually fatal. However, granulomatous angiitis responds to high dose steroids and cytotoxic agents, such as cyclophosphamide and azothioprine. The cause of the disease is unknown.

Delayed contralateral hemiplegia following herpes zoster ophthalmicus tends to occur at middle age (mean age 55 years, range 7–96). The hemiplegia occurs 1 week to 2 years after the onset of the herpes zoster ophthalmicus. Symptoms tend to be milder in this disorder than in granulomatous angiitis of the nervous system. Microscopic tissue examination reveals the same histological abnormalities in both disorders. Most patients with this disorder survive, even without steroids.

Other primary CNS vasculitides are Cogan's syndrome and Eales disease. Cogan's syndrome consists of episodes of acute interstitial keratitis or scleritis-episcleritis with vestibulo-auditory dysfunction, usually in young adults. Eales disease, also an affliction of young adults, is an isolated peripheral retinal vasculitis, often leading to visual loss. The symptoms of both disorders occur also frequently in other vasculitides, including polyarteritis nodosa, Wegener's granulomatosis, rheumatoid disease, Behçet's syndrome and systemic lupus erythematosus.

The group of *systemic necrotizing vasculitides with involvement of CNS* includes the polyarteritis nodosa group, giant cell arteritis, Takayasu arteritis, Wegener granulomatosis, lymphomatoid granulomatosis, Henoch-Schönlein purpura and cryoglobulinemia.

CNS manifestations of periarteritis nodosa mostly develop in patients that have had systemic disease for several years. Clinically two main groups are usually distinguished: one with general signs of CNS involvement, including changes of consciousness and epileptic seizures; the other with focal or multifocal symptoms, including ataxia, aphasia, hemiparesis, sensory disorders, ophthalmoplegia, and visual disorders. CSF is of-

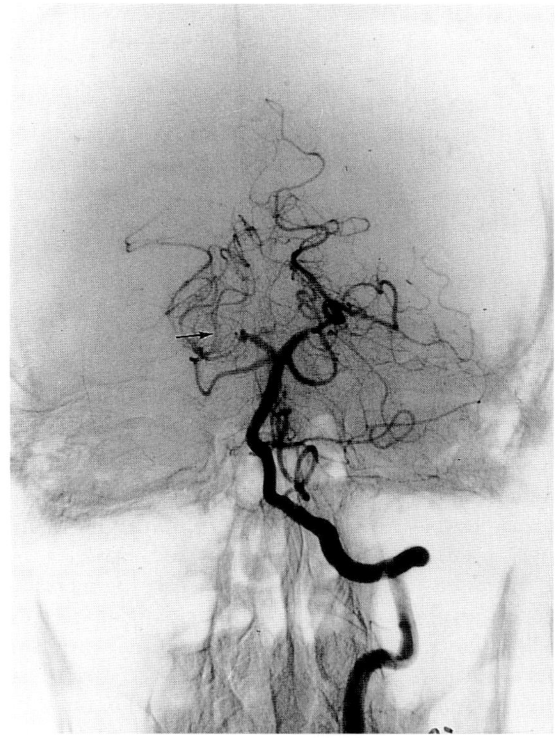

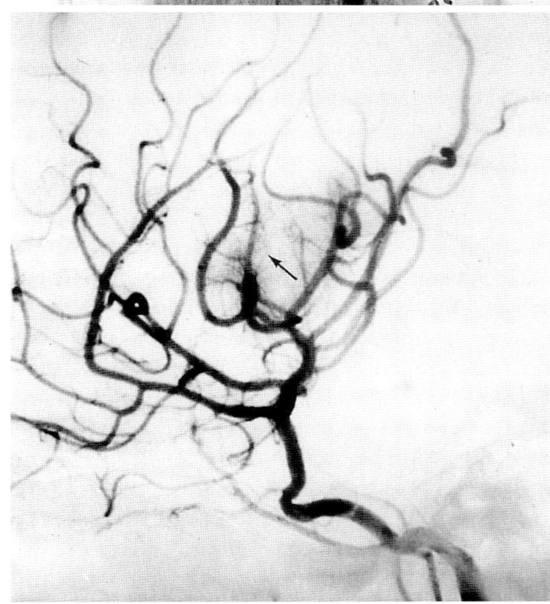

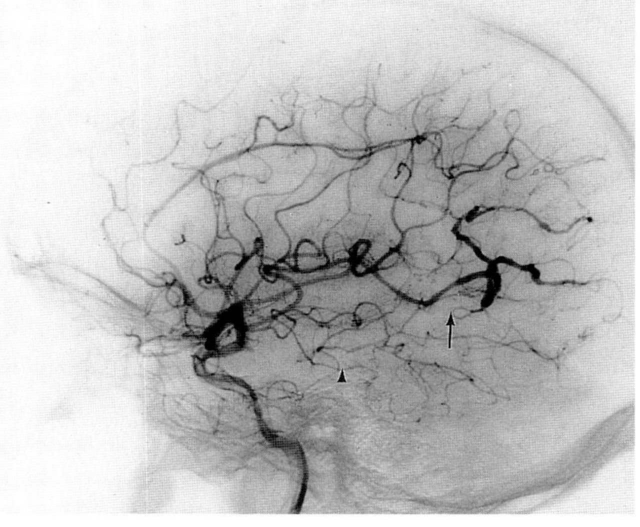

Fig. 66.1. Three different angiographic patterns of intracerebral arteritis: obstruction of larger secondary branches (*upper left*) with occlusion of the posterior cerebral artery; caliber changes with narrowing and widening of the vessels (*upper right*); perivascular blushes (hyperemia) and ensuing thrombosis in acute inflammatory reactions (*lower left*). In none of these cases was there systemic vasculitic involvement

tion of small aneurysms. The parenchymatous lesions are small infarctions, multiple and disseminated, sometimes hemorrhagic. Part of the periarteritis nodosa group are the abuse-associated vasculitis, best described in intravenous metamphetamine users, and hepatitis B virus-associated vasculitis. Also in these cases the disorder is systemic.

Giant cell arteritis or temporal arteritis usually occurs in patients, male and female, older than 55 years. It often involves the superficial temporal arteries, which become swollen, tortuous, tender and nodular. Pulsations are usually diminished. Eventually the vessels become hardened and shrink. Clinical problems most often consist of acute visual failure of one eye. Signs of CNS dysfunction are relatively rare. However, all larger and medium-sized vessels of the head and neck may be involved. Of particular interest are the carotid, vertebral and ophthalmic arteries, including the ciliary arteries and the central artery of the retina. The cervical portions of the carotid and vertebral arteries are usually involved, the intracranial arteries to a lesser extent and the spinal arteries least of all. Histologically a segmental, multifocal panarteritis is found. The intima of the vessels is thickened by a subendothelial fibrosis, narrowing or occluding the lumen. The internal elastic lamina is severely, but irregularly fragmented. The media is infiltrated by small and large

ten normal. The sedimentation rate of erythrocytes is accelerated. Histologically the small arteries and arterioles are most affected, especially of the leptomeninges, the deep white and gray matter, and the choroid plexus. The affected vessels show a fibrinoid or hyaline necrosis of the media and destruction of the internal elastic lamina. There is an inflammatory granuloma of the whole thickness of the vessel wall, eventually obstructing the vessel lumen with secondary intima lesions. Segmentary vessel wall necrosis may lead to the forma-

mononuclear cells, some of the "epithelioid" type. Giant cells of either Langhans or foreign body type are almost invariably present, either in the media close to the damaged internal elastic lamina or in the adjacent intima. With healing there is scarring and occasionally aneurysm formation. In some cases the vessels are occluded by organizing thrombus. Diagnosis is usually by biopsy of the temporal vessels. A negative biopsy does not exclude the diagnosis.

Takayasu arteritis affects the aortic arch and its branches, in particular in young women of Asiatic origin. The smaller intracranial vessels are not usually involved. The neurological symptoms are necessarily variable and depend on the extent of abnormalities of the aortic arch and brachiocephalic artery abnormalities, in particular on the involvement of the carotid and vertebral arteries. Visual problems are relatively frequent, mostly as one-sided amaurosis fugax. Many other neurological symptoms are possible, including hemiparesis, aphasia, cranial nerve palsies, coordination disorders and vertigo. Histologically the lesions in the media and adventitia of the vessels are predominant. In the adventitia sclerosis is formed with collagenous proliferations and perivascular lymphocyte infiltration; the media shows an inflammatory granulomatous reaction, narrowing the lumen. The cerebral lesions are secondary to either diminished perfusion or emboli. Angiography is necessary to assess the changes of the aortic arch and brachiocephalic vessels. MR angiography could serve as a first orientation, but lacks the detailed functional information digital subtraction angiography provides.

Wegeners's granulomatosis may lead to cerebral lesions, either by extending intracranially from nasal and sinus lesions, or as necrotizing cerebral vasculitis, nearly always in the presence of active sinusitis, otitis, or lung disease. The clinical features are protean, but ocular manifestations are common. Histologically Wegener's disease is characterized as a necrotizing panarteritis of the middle great vessels. Multiple foci of arteritis develop in the nasal sinuses, the respiratory tract and the kidneys. There is much similarity between Wegener's granulomatosis and involvement of the CNS by other granulomatous and arteritic diseases, including periarteritis nodosa.

Neurological symptoms are seen in about 30% of patients with lymphomatoid granulomatosis. CNS disease imparts a poor prognosis, because it may progress even where lung and other manifestations respond to therapy. Neurological symptoms depend on the affected areas in the CNS. CNS pathology at autopsy reveals the classic triad of angiitis, lymphoreticular infiltration of abnormal neoplastic appearing cells, and necrosis of meninges, parenchyma and vessels.

Patients with Henoch-Schönlein purpura have been described with neurological symptoms. Extensive lesions in the brain stem and in the lobar gray and white matter have been found, with concurrent neurological symptoms.

The *rheumatological syndromes associated with CNS disease* due to vasculitis include a broad spectrum of autoimmune diseases. At one end of this spectrum one finds organ-specific diseases with organ-specific antibodies, for example Hashimoto's disease of the thyroid. In the middle of the spectrum the lesions tend to be localized in one organ but the antibodies are not organ-specific. A typical example is primary biliary cirrhosis, where the small bile ductules are the main target of inflammatory cell infiltration but the serum antibodies, mainly anti-mitochondrial, are not organ specific. At the other end of the spectrum the disorder is non-organ-specific. Lesions and antibodies are not confined to a single organ. In systemic lupus erythematosus, lesions are seen in the skin, renal glomeruli, joints, serous membranes and blood vessels. In Sjögren's disease, the salivary glands and the lacrimal gland are involved. Rheumatoid arthritis primarily affects the joints. In the non-organ-specific disorders a cerebral vasculitis may develop. Among the disorders in this group there is much overlap in auto-antibodies and clinical disease. There is however, no overlap between the organ-specific and the non-organ-specific disorders. The clinical signs of vasculitis are nonspecific. They depend on the location and extent of the lesions.

In rheumatoid disease, vasculitis occurs relatively rarely. In all cases joint disease is apparent. Patients may have demonstrable rheumatoid arthritis for between 1 and 30 years prior to the onset of their neurological problems. CNS disease manifests itself nonspecifically by a multitude of possible neurological signs and symptoms, including seizures, dementia, hemiparesis, cranial nerve palsies, blindness, cerebellar ataxia, and dysphasia. Serum rheumatoid factors are present and the erythrocyte sedimentation rate is elevated. In a number of cases amyloid deposits are formed together with signs of vasculitis.

In patients with systemic lupus erythematosus with cerebral involvement, neuropsychiatric symptoms are common. Neurological disease is the second or third leading cause of death after renal disease. Neurological manifestations mostly follow systemic manifestations by more than a year. Neurological symptomatology is related to site of CNS involvement. Also, there may be spinal cord involvement with transverse myelitis. The disease occurs preferentially in adolescent and young women. True vasculitis of the CNS is rare; vasculopathic changes are common. Immune complexes and diminished levels or altered metabolism of the fourth component of the complement cascade have been found in the CSF of patients with CNS disease. Antibodies to neuronal antigens, often cross-reacting with lymphocytic antigens, are preferentially seen in the serum and CSF of patients with neurological manifestations. Microscopic changes are most marked in small vessels and consist of acute fibrinoid necrosis and marked thickening of the vessel wall with minimal inflammatory cell infiltration. Some vessels are occluded by thrombi with corresponding micro-infarcts.

In Sjögren syndrome, trigeminal neuropathy, recurrent aseptic meningoencephalitis, necrotizing spinal arteritis and unifocal and multifocal cerebral disease have been reported. The involvement of the salivary and lacrimal gland is usually manifest before CNS symptoms, but may also appear later. This disease has much in common with rheumatoid arthritis and systemic lupus erythematosus.

Behçet's disease is a systematic vasculitis involving many organs. Originally it was described as a clinical case of oral and genital aphthosis and relapsing uveitis. It is now known to cause arthritis, venous thrombosis, cutaneous lesions, rectocolitis and lesions of the CNS. The disease is frequently encountered in a geographic distribution extending from Japan to the eastern Mediterranean countries, passing through China and Iran, the area that was supposedly the ancient silk route. CNS involvement is estimated to occur in 4%–49% of the cases. Involvement of the CNS leads to quadriparesis, pseudobulbar palsy, cranial nerve palsies, cerebral ataxia, aseptic or chronic recurrent meningitis and various vascular syndromes, including cerebral venous thrombosis, mostly of one or more of the large sinuses. Brain stem lesions are rather common.

A number of *infectious disorders* give rise to vasculitis and related cerebral lesions. Lyme disease, caused by Borrelia burgdorferi, leads to neurological disease in about 20% of the cases. Findings vary from fluctuating meningoencephalitis to demyelinating radiculoneuropathy and encephalopathy. The diagnosis is important because of the good response of the disease to antibiotic therapy. Histologically Lyme's disease is not a real vasculitis but rather a perivascular inflammation.

In tuberculosis the most common finding is arteritis at the base of the brain, the predominant location of the purulent arachnoiditis. Mycotic aneurysms may develop. Tuberculosis also has affinity for the supraclinoid portion of the internal carotid artery and the horizontal portion of the middle cerebral artery. Eventually infarctions may result from vascular occlusion, or subarachnoid or intraparenchymal hemorrhage from the burst of a mycotic aneurysm.

In syphilitic angiitis, both arteries and veins are affected with a predilection for branches of the middle cerebral artery. Vessel abnormalities develop in the third stage of lues as tertiary meningovascular disease. Luetic arterial lesions are generally diffuse and affect all leptomeningeal vessels, obstructing the leptomeningeal anastomoses.

66.2 Magnetic Resonance Imaging

Vasculitis can lead to a variety of MRI patterns. The lesions can be distinct, asymmetrically distributed throughout the brain parenchyma, sometimes mimicking multiple sclerosis, or lesions can become more confluent. Infarctions may occur in vascular territories or present as small or lacunar infarctions (Fig. 66.2). Involvement of the basal ganglia, thalamus, mesencephalon, pons, medulla oblongata and leptomeninges is often seen (Figs. 66.3, 66.4). Lesions may become hemorrhagic. In later phases of the disease, atrophy may become apparent. It is obvious that the pattern is not specific. Disorders which may share this pattern are: multiple sclerosis, acute disseminated encephalomyelitis, extrapontine myelinolysis, progressive multifocal leukoencephalitis, neurosarcoidosis, radiation vasculopathy, migraine, subcortical arteriosclerotic encephalopathy (Binswanger disease), eclampsia, neoplasms and emboli. Clinical and laboratory data are helpful in further differentiation of these disorders. There is still a place for angiography (Fig. 66.1).

Some of the vasculitic disorders may present with a more characteristic MRI-pattern. Vasculitis in systemic lupus erythematosus can lead to extensive calcifications, which may be prominent in the basal ganglia, the geniculate bodies, and the dentate nucleus. On T_1-weighted images this may lead to a high signal intensity in the involved areas, sometimes blotting out the basal ganglia. This phenomenon may also be seen in such disorders as hypoparathyroidism, pseudohypoparathyroidism, liver failure, and parenteral nutrition. The signal intensity on T_2-weighted images is decreased. These calcifications are largely symmetrical but there seem to be exceptions to this rule. In Behçet's disease, cerebral venous thrombosis is a frequent occurrence leading to venous infarctions, sometimes hemorrhagic. Other patterns are also seen: periventricular leukomalacia with corpus callosum involvement, patterns similar to multiple sclerosis, and pontine infarctions or demyelination.

In unusual MR patterns (Fig. 66.5) vasculitis should be always be considered as a possible cause, especially with clinical suspicion. The combination of MRI findings with the clinical and laboratory data may lead to the correct diagnosis (Fig. 66.6).

It should be noted that in most of the vasculitic disorders, but in particular in systemic lupus erythematosus, Beçet's disease and Cogan's syndrome, mild to extensive white matter disease can be found in absence of clinical neurological abnormalities. The reverse is also true: in systemic lupus erythematosus, despite evident neurological manifestation, the findings at autopsy may be disappointing.

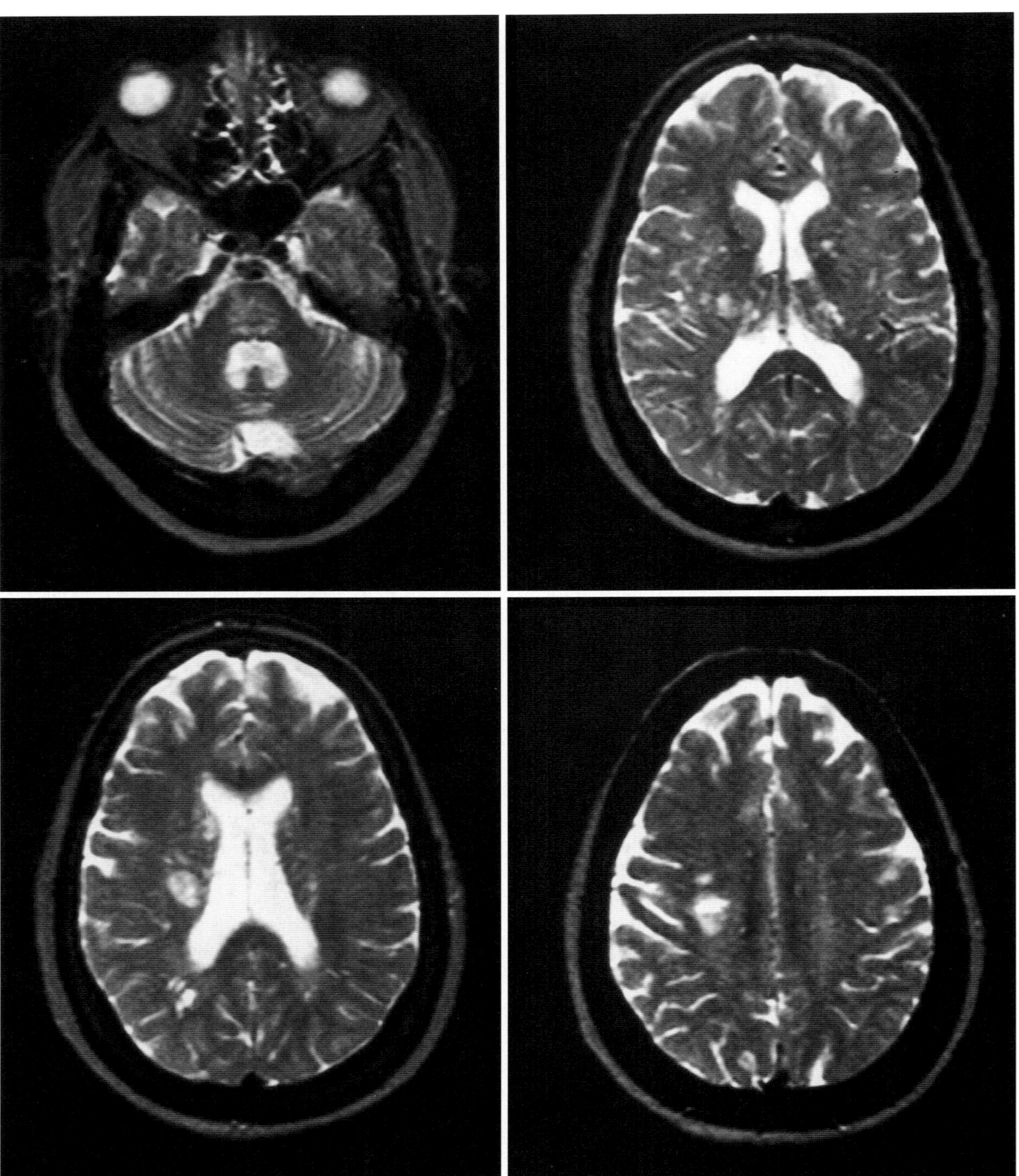

Fig. 66.2. Pattern of MRI abnormalities in a 52-year-old female with granulomatous angiitis of the CNS. The T_2-weighted images show multiple lesions, particularly on the right side, in both the white matter and the basal ganglia. There is also some loss of cortical tissue

Fig. 66.3. In this case of angiitis of the CNS in a 48-year-old male, the T_1-weighted images with contrast (*upper row*) show the elongated large vessels, especially the dolichobasilar artery (*arrow*). The *lower row* shows the lesions in the globus pallidus and multiple lesions around the ventricles and in the centrum semiovale. Remnants of a hemorrhage are seen in the right parieto-occipital area

Fig. 66.4. A 62-year-old woman without risk factors for arteriosclerosis developed severe neurological signs with episodic (sub)acute worsening. Lesions are dispersed through the brain, affecting the white matter of the temporal lobes and the centrum semiovale. The pons is also involved. The pattern of the lesions is compatible with vasculitis. It is, of course, necessary to differentiate this condition from arteriosclerotic disease, because the treatment is different

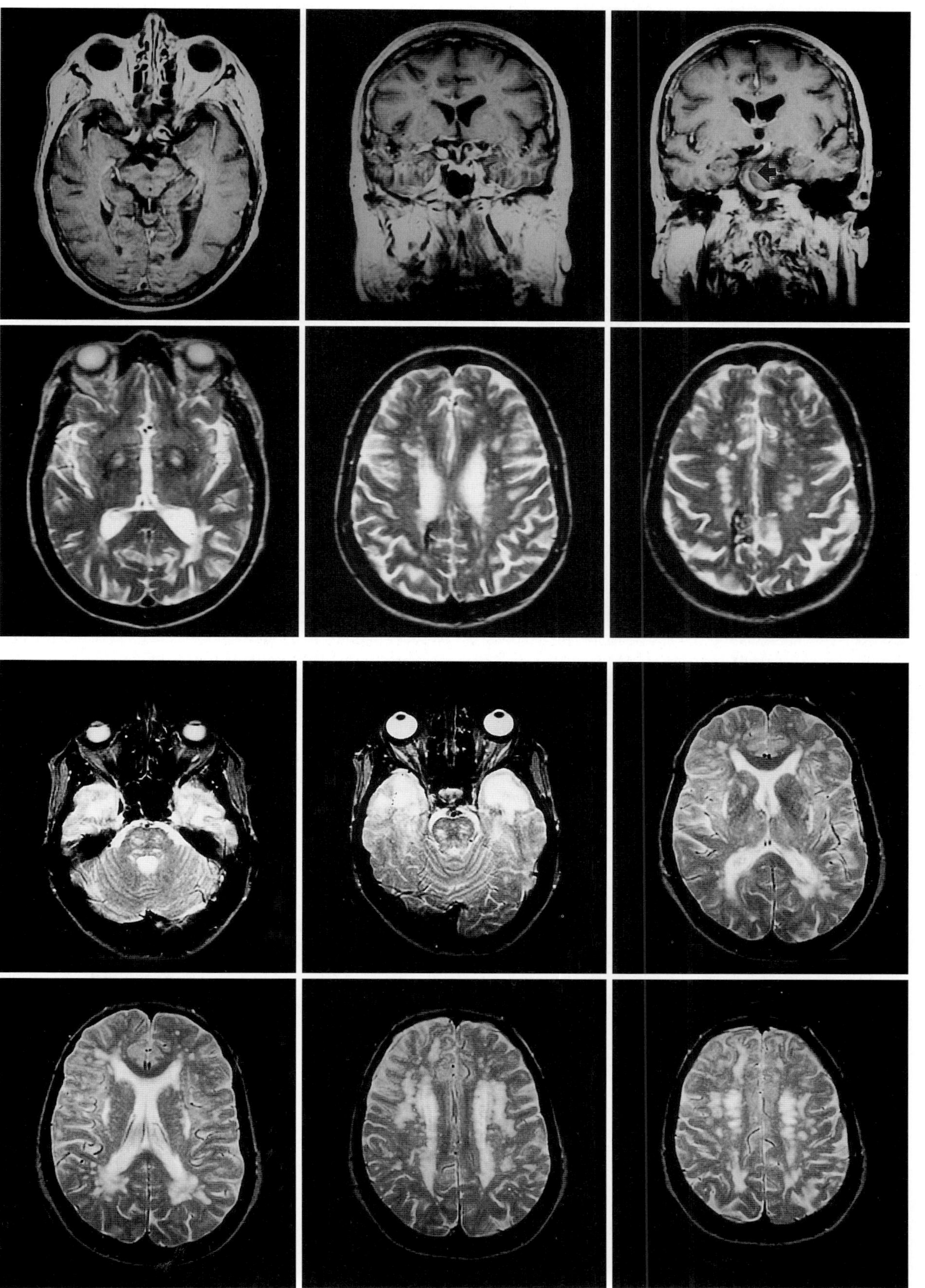

Fig. 66.3

Fig. 66.4

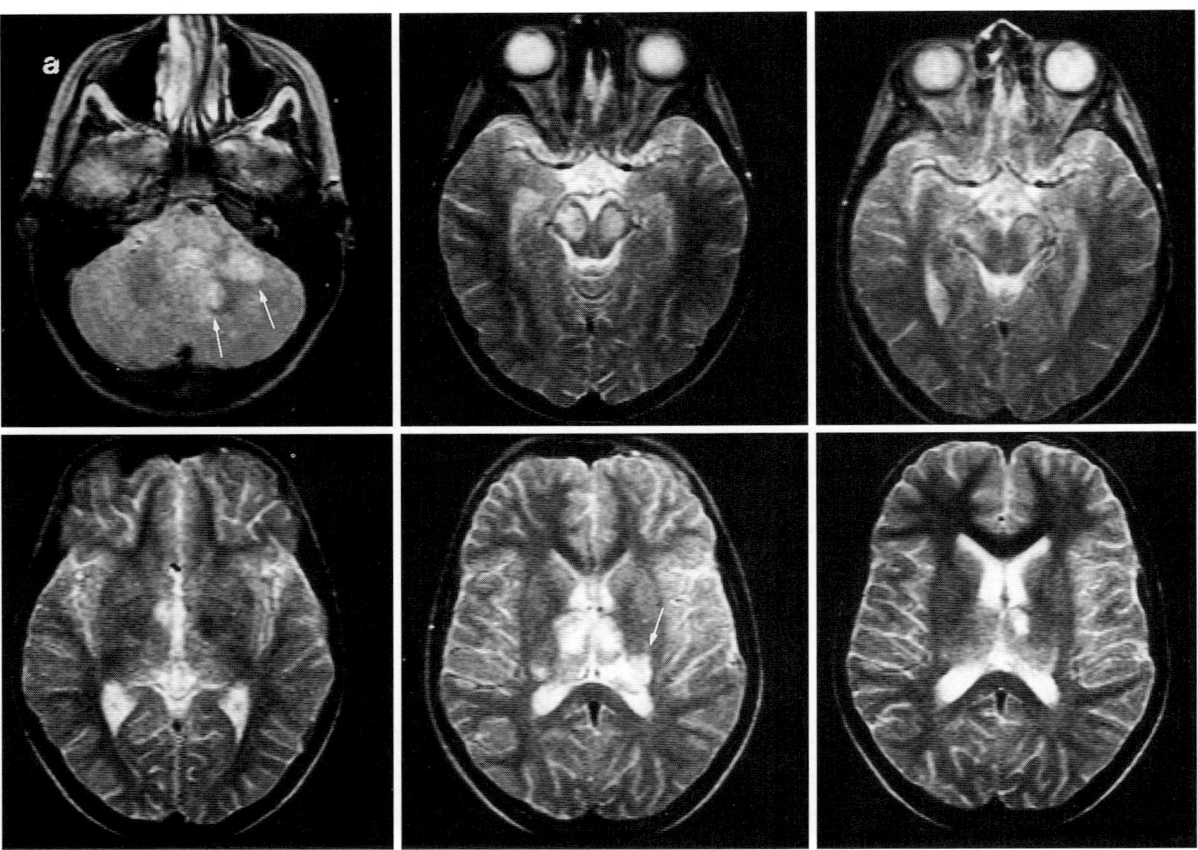

Fig. 66.5. Unusual form of vasculitis, involving mainly the perforating basal arteries in a boy, 14 years of age. Lesions are seen in the cerebellum, the mesencephalon, the thalamus, and the lateral geniculate bodies. Angiography showed irregular vessels in the vertebro-basilar territory. Improvement occurred after treatment with corticosteroids

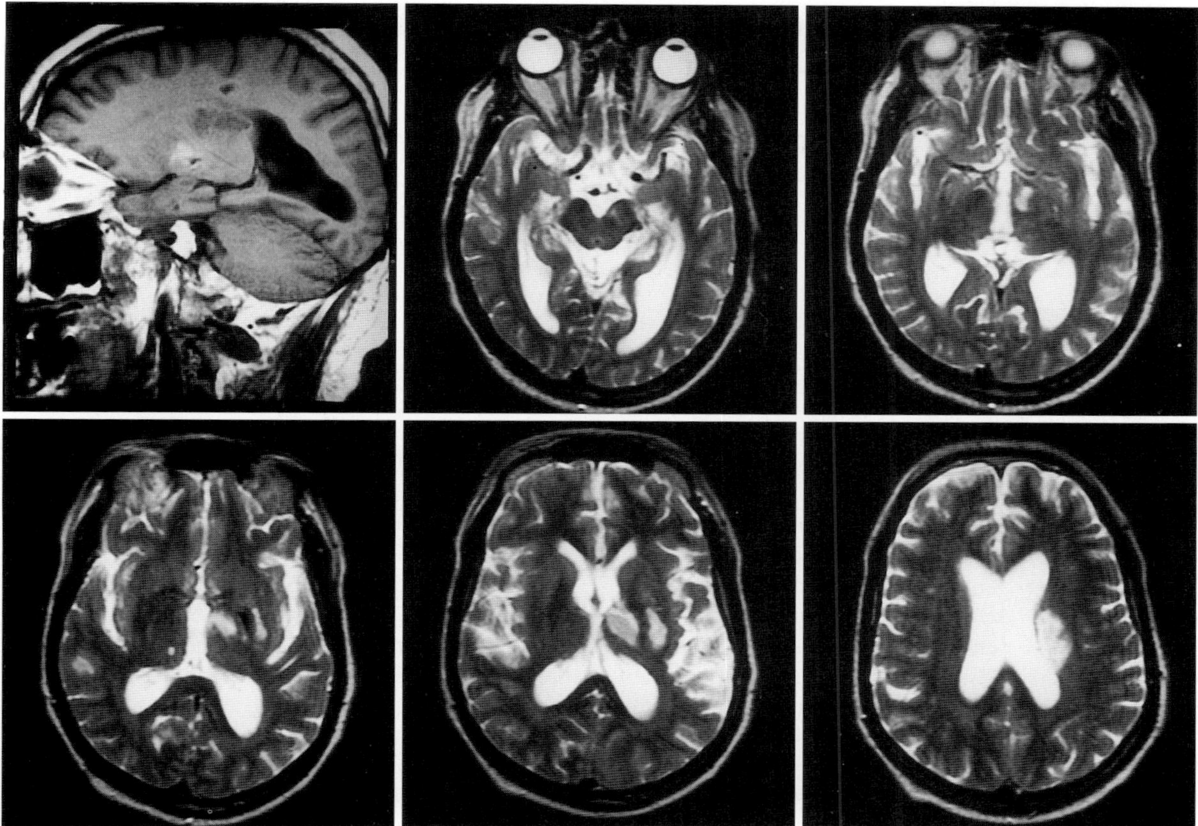

Fig. 66.6. A 62-year-old male who developed a hemiparesis several weeks after he had suffered a herpes zoster ophthalmicus infection. Without this clinical fact the correct diagnosis of granulomatous angiitis would not have been possible. The images show partly hemorrhagic (see T_1-weighted parasagittal image, *left, upper row*) infarctions in the left basal ganglia, and a small lesion on the right side

67 Leukoencephalopathy After Chemotherapy and/or Radiotherapy

67.1 Clinical Features and Laboratory Investigations

In the treatment of malignancies three modalities play a major role: surgery, radiotherapy, and chemotherapy. Other treatment modalities, such as hyperthermia and laser coagulation, are also important, but to a lesser extent. Radiotherapy and chemotherapy are not only applied in the approach to primary brain tumors and brain metastases, but intrathecal and intravenous administration of chemotherapeutic drugs, together with cranial or total neuraxis irradiation are also widely used in the prophylaxis of cerebral metastases in extracerebral malignancies. Furthermore, systemic chemotherapy, used for malignancies elsewhere in the body will also reach the brain. For many years the brain was considered to be relatively resistant to therapeutic doses of chemotherapy and irradiation, because neurons do not multiply and the turnover of glial tissue is relatively low. This concept had to be modified because it was established that adverse effects are not exceptional.

The effects of chemotherapy and irradiation on the brain are rather stereotyped and demonstrate the whole gamut from mild and transient white matter changes, to more permanent diffuse or focal white matter injury with demyelination and gliosis, to the most severe forms of coagulation necrosis with cavitation. In the classical description, types of damage are distinguished according to their time of occurrence: acute reactions, occurring during the course of treatment, potentially changing the treatment schedule; early delayed reactions, usually transient and appearing from a few weeks to a few months after treatment; and late delayed reactions, with onset from several months to several years later.

Acute reactions are usually mild and of little consequence, but also severe reactions may occur. The acute reactions are generally manifested by mild signs of increased intracranial pressure. The patient may become confused, disorientated, or incoherent. In more severe cases the patient suffers from headaches, nausea, vomiting, and sometimes elevations of temperature. Seizures occasionally occur, and the patient may lapse into coma. The acute reaction may even be fatal due to cerebral herniation. Discontinuation of the treatment regimen and corticosteroid administration may be necessary and life saving. Patients usually recover but do not always return to their baseline status.

Early delayed reactions are usually transient and disappear without treatment. Various clinical symptoms have been described: somnolence, nausea, vomiting, dysarthria, dysphagia, cerebellar ataxia, and nystagmus.

Late delayed reactions are generally irreversible. The process begins insidiously with personality changes that gradually progress over several months. Initially there is excessive drowsiness and loss of initiative and interest. In the course of time there is a decrease in intellectual function, with confusion, disorientation, memory loss, loss of abstract thinking, and eventually a global dementia. Signs of spasticity and cerebellar ataxia develop, and death from brain necrosis may ensue.

This classical classification is still used to describe time-linked reactions after chemotherapy and/or radiotherapy. However, specific kinds of treatment, such as focal irradiation as in gamma-knife surgery or stereotactic radiosurgery with linear accelerators, and treatment of special populations, such as children with acute lymphatic leukemia who are treated prophylactically with cranial irradiation and intrathecal and/or intravenous methotrexate, have prompted descriptions of post-irradiation/post-chemotherapy damage, usually not grouped under the heading of one of the classical types described above. Terms such as "focal radiation injury" and "diffuse white matter injury" have been proposed, but in fact the clinical signs and symptoms and the histological findings often fit the spectrum of abnormalities as described in the classical concept. Mineralizing angiopathy is a reaction seen far more often seen in children than in adults, but it is in fact part of the late delayed damage. Focal irradiation, for example in the irradiation of sellar or parasellar tumors, may damage the greater cerebral vessels, in some cases leading to obstruction and stroke-like episodes. Focal radiation injury may develop in areas which have received a surdosage during irradiation. The damage presents as a mass lesion, with focal neurological abnormalities and evidence of raised intracranial pressure. The clinical course is unpredictable. Often the changes are progressive and extension of necrosis may lead to death.

Clinically it is important to realize that neurological and neuropsychological consequences of irradiation of the brain, in particular in combination with chemotherapy, may be much more severe in infants and children than in adults. In as much as the consequences for the immature brain may differ from those for the mature brain, the age of the patients with acute lymphatic leukemia (usually 1–12 years) justifies a separate consideration. In a postmortem comparison of children with childhood leukemia who showed leukoencephalopathy with those who did not show leukoencephalopathy, it became clear that the development of white matter damage did not correlate with age, despite the different stages of myelination and neuronal differentiation in the age group of children. Nor was there a relationship with intercurrent infections, nutrition or the presence of CNS leukemia. There was a clear relationship with the radiation dose the child had received (lower than versus more than 20 Gray) in combination with intrathecal methotrexate. The total amount of intrathecally administered methotrexate seemed less important. The dose of methotrexate was important when given intravenously: the incidence of leukoencephalopathy increased with the total dose of intravenous methotrexate. Patients who received cranial irradiation of less than 20 Gray did not develop leukoencephalopathy, irrespective of the methotrexate dose given.

67.2 Pathology

Neuropathological findings in acute reactions are primarily characterized by cerebral edema with flattening of gyri, obliteration of sulci, and signs of tentorial herniation. The lateral ventricles are compressed. Vascular changes are present and consist of fibrinoid necrosis and thickening of the endothelium with extravasation of fibrinous material and perivascular lymphocytic infiltration.

Because of the usually transient and nonlethal nature of the early delayed reaction, the amount of information available on the histopathological features is limited. Foci of demyelination with central necrosis and petechial hemorrhages have been described. Lymphocytes and plasma cells are found in the perivascular spaces, and there is a pronounced microglial and astrocytic proliferation in the affected areas. Vascular abnormalities are not prominent in these lesions, but sometimes the changes are more marked and consist of fibrinoid necrosis, fibroproliferative vessel thickening, enlargement of endothelial cells, and capillary proliferation. The cytoarchitecture of the gray matter is usually intact.

The neuropathological findings of late delayed leukoencephalopathy are rather specific. The changes consist of demyelination, astrogliosis, multifocal coagulative necrosis, and cavitation. The periventricular white matter and the centrum semiovale are involved bilaterally, whereas the cerebral cortex, subcortical arcuate fibers, and deep-seated gray matter structures are usually spared. Within and around the necrotizing lesions conspicuous swelling of axons occurs. An inflammatory response is usually absent. There are marked vascular lesions, characterized by hyalinization, fibrosis, and necrosis of vessel walls and vascular thrombosis. Areas of endothelial proliferation and varying degrees of adventitial fibroblast proliferation occur. Obliteration of the lumen may result. At times, deposition of iron salts and calcium occurs in vessel walls. Protein-rich fluid is deposited in the perivascular spaces and adjacent parenchyma. In general, the areas with the most severe vascular injury are the most necrotic and cavitated. The most prominent vasculopathic changes involve small arteries and arterioles. In particular in children a mineralizing microangiopathy may develop, leading to vessel changes with deposition of minerals, such as calcium salts, in the vessel wall. This calcification may be very extensive and be present in the basal ganglia and the subcortical regions, less commonly in the pons.

Radiation injury and chemotherapy-induced damage closely resemble each other. There seem to be some slight differences between the two conditions as far as vascular changes are concerned. The gray matter is affected more often in chemotherapy lesions than in radiation changes. In postradiation leukoencephalopathy lesions in the cerebral hemispheres are either symmetrical or asymmetrical, depending on the field of irradiation.

Focal radiation injury occurs in and around the tumor in the zones of highest radiation dose. The lesion consists of tissue necrosis associated with vasogenic edema and may occur in the acute stage as well as after a delay of many months.

If damage occurs to the large vessels, this usually develops slowly. The vessel walls are thickened, which eventually leads to complete occlusion and Moya-Moya formation, as an expression of collateral circulation.

67.3 Pathogenetic Considerations

Cranial irradiation and systemic, intracarotid, intravenous, or intrathecal chemotherapy alone, as well as a combination of cranial irradiation and chemotherapy, may result in leukoencephalopathic changes. It has been impossible to delineate the relative contribution of radiation and chemotherapy to the development of cerebral lesions. Treatment factors important in the causation of leukoencephalopathy include the dose and fraction size of the cranial irradiation, the dose and neurotoxicity of the chemotherapeutic agents, and the interaction between irradiation and chemotherapy. Some chemotherapeutic agents, including methotrexate and cisplatin, are radiation sensitizers. On the other hand, radiation may induce acute changes in the permeability of the blood-brain barrier increasing the cerebral delivery of potentially toxic agents. Other factors in the patients, such as nutritional status, type of primary malignancy, peritumoral edema, and the presence of a paraneoplastic syndrome, may well contribute to the development of cerebral lesions.

The acute encephalopathic syndrome in anticancer therapy is thought to be due to vasogenic edema resulting from damage to the capillary endothelium. A direct and immediate effect of the treatment on neurons cannot be excluded.

Early delayed effects are presumed to be due to demyelination and may be reversible. There is some suggestion that they may represent an autoimmune reaction following sensitization for some myelin antigen which has become exposed by therapy-induced tissue necrosis. Damaged glial cells and myelin release antigens into the extracellular spaces which may elicit a hypersensitivity response. This hypothesis has never been proven, but the perivascular inflammatory reaction may form an argument. Another mechanism which may account for the observed demyelination in the absence of marked vascular alterations in early delayed leukoencephalopathy is primary damage to glial cells, particularly oligodendroglial cells. Sometimes striking glial proliferation is observed associated with bizarre cells and giant multinucleated astrocytes, and this observation lends support to the hypothesis of a primary effect of radiation on glial cells.

In late delayed leukoencephalopathy, damage to oligodendroglial cells and their subsequent inability to maintain the integrity of myelin sheaths has been proposed, but primary vascular damage and tissue damage secondary to ischemia form a more likely explanation. It is probable that white matter lesions begin as endothelial damage followed by endothelial proliferation and more extensive changes in the vessel walls. Small arteries and arterioles are preferentially affected. The endothelium is one of the most radiosensitive tissues of the brain. Similar endothelial reaction is seen in chemotherapy. White matter changes are probably secondary to a resultant chronic ischemia. The most severe changes occur in deep locations where the blood supply is most tenuous. The slow evolution of the syndrome and the close relationship between the degree of vascular damage and the profundity of demyelination or necrosis also form arguments in favor of the vascular hypothesis. It is assumed that the impairment of blood supply is followed first by more or less diffuse demyelination, subsequently by axonal loss, necrosis, and liquefaction, and finally by cyst formation.

In the case of leukoencephalopathy following combined therapy with cranial irradiation and methotrexate, several other factors probably play a role. First of all, irradiation and methotrexate synergistically inhibit synthesis of macromolecules and DNA repair. Secondly, irradiation alters the distribution of methotrexate in the CNS in such a way that certain areas of the brain accumulate increased amounts of the antifolate. Thirdly, methotrexate acts as a radiosensitizer and increases the sensitivity of CNS cells to irradiation. Fourthly, irradiation increases the permeability of the blood-brain barrier, allowing methotrexate to enter the brain.

67.4 Therapy

In acute reactions corticosteroids are useful in alleviating cerebral edema and may in this way ameliorate the clinical symptoms, and may even be life saving in cases of threatening tentorial herniation. However, apart from this transitory beneficial effect there is no evidence of long-term benefit.

The importance of recognizing the early delayed syndrome resides in the fact that it is generally transient, and that it does not indicate treatment failure or the need for a change in therapy.

In the late delayed syndrome corticosteroids may only have some beneficial effect if edema is part of the problem. A favorable influence of intravenous heparin administration has also been reported. However, therapeutic possibilities are poor in the late delayed leukoencephalopathy, as one might expect on the basis of histopathological data.

In focal radiation necrosis, neurosurgical resection of the necrotic area is often efficacious and may be life saving. Administration of corticosteroids is an effective adjunct to surgical therapy and may in some instances be sufficient and effective as primary therapy.

67.5 Magnetic Resonance Imaging

In all types of white matter lesions after irradiation and chemotherapy, acute, early delayed, and late delayed, CT may demonstrate hypodensities in the white matter. The threshold for detection of these lesions is much higher on CT than on MRI. Because comparable abnormalities on CT are, with the exception of (micro)calcifications, seen more easily and better on MRI, this latter modality is now generally the first choice for follow-up in patients. All stages of radiation injury have in common an increase in free tissue water in the involved areas. This may result from endothelial dam-

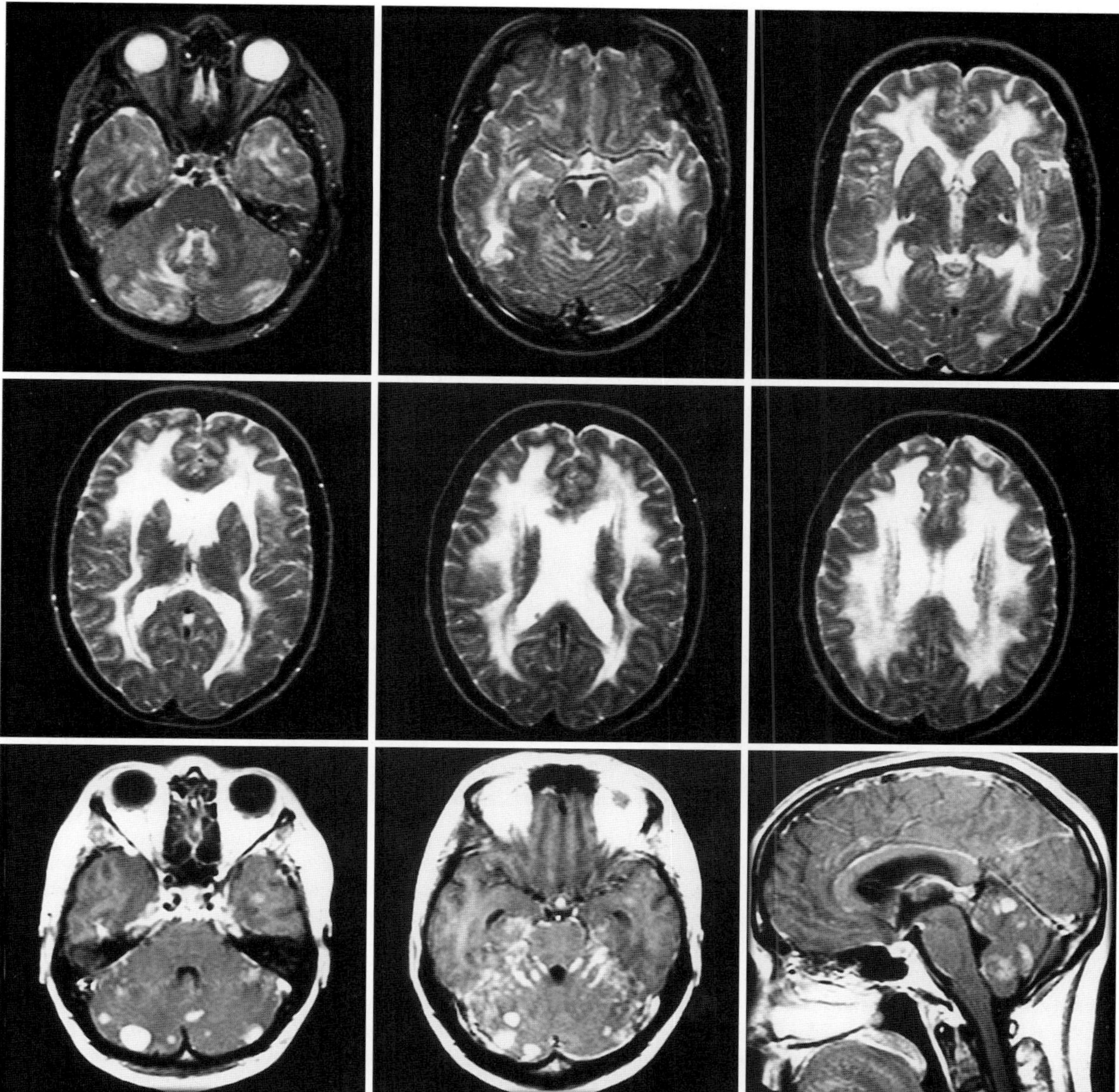

Fig. 67.1. A 29-year-old female treated for disseminated breast carcinoma. Metastases in the brain were treated with radiotherapy and patient received systemic cytostatic therapy. The T_2-weighted transverse MR series (*upper and middle rows*) 6 months after radiotherapy show some irregular bright spots in the posterior fossa and diffuse white matter injury in the supratentorial area, with a symmetrical distribution, sparing the U fibers and involving the posterior limb of the internal capsule. The *lower row* of contrast-enhanced T_1-weighted images show recurrence of metastases and leptomeningeal carcinomatosis

age, causing increased capillary permeability and vasogenic edema, or from demyelination, leading to replacement of hydrophobic myelin by scar tissue with a higher water content. The increase in water content may reflect many conditions from minimal change to coagulation necrosis. Separation of edema from demyelination, gliosis or coagulation necrosis by means of MRI is difficult. The correlation of the MRI findings with the clinical condition of the patient is generally speaking limited.

In acute reactions occurring during course of treatment the MRI findings are nonspecific. The images may be completely normal, or subtly abnormal with poorly defined multifocal hyperintense areas on T_2-weighted images, mostly in both hemispheres. The abnormalities usually disappear spontaneously, given an uneventful clinical course.

In early delayed reactions occurring a few weeks to a few months after treatment, the white matter changes are usually also transient. Changes on MRI may be

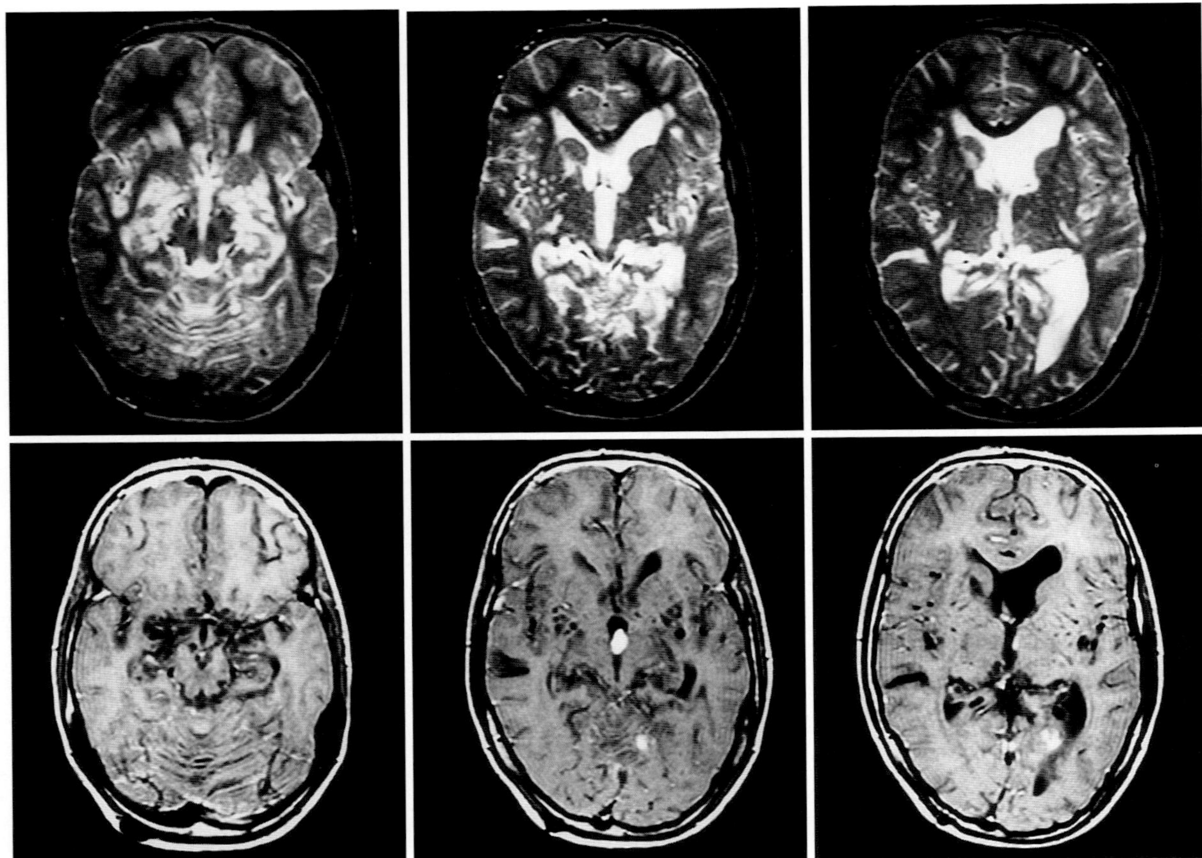

Fig. 67.2. A 4-year-old boy treated prophylactically with cerebral irradiation and intrathecal methotrexate because of acute lymphatic leukemia. The T_2-weighted images at the level of the mesencephalon and third ventricle (*upper row*) show that this treatment does not always lead to diffuse white matter injury. In this case a diffuse cystic necrosis has developed in the basal ganglia. After contrast injection, recurrent tumor is seen in the third ventricle (*lower row*)

seen by higher signal intensities on T_2-weighted images in the basal ganglia, the cerebral peduncles and the deep white matter. These abnormalities resolve completely without treatment.

Transient diffuse white matter injury is seen in children with acute lymphatic leukemia who have been given preventive cranial irradiation and chemotherapy. On MRI, these children show transient periventricular white matter abnormalities of different severity occurring within 2–10 weeks of treatment. In some patients there are limited areas of changed signal intensity around the frontal and occipital horns of the ventricles; in others the periventricular leukoencephalopathy is extensive. There is no correlation with clinical manifestations and the finding has no clear prognostic significance. This reaction does not basically differ from an early delayed reaction in the classical concept.

Late delayed reactions occurring several months to several years after treatment are also known under the name diffuse radiation injury. This type of injury is characterized by a periventricular leukoencephalopathy, with high signal intensity on proton density and T_2-weighted images (Fig. 67.1; cf. Fig. 67.2). There is no enhancement after gadolineum injection. These white matter changes are permanent. The pattern of the lesions is sometimes difficult to distinguish from the periventricular leukoencephalopathy in older people and in patients with risk factors for vascular disease. The severity of the abnormalities increases with age, volume of the brain irradiated, radiation dose, and interval between irradiation and imaging. Despite the sometimes dramatic appearance of the deep white matter changes, the patients may be asymptomatic. In cases with neurological symptoms the MRI abnormalities are usually severe. The most severe form of the late delayed reaction is a necrotizing leukoencephalopathy, in which areas of focal necrosis are seen. The borders of these lesions may enhance with gadolinium.

Mineralizing microangiopathy with dystrophic calcification is the most commonly seen neuroradiological abnormality in children treated for cancer. This, evidently, is best seen on CT. Calcifications occur in the basal ganglia, in particular in the putamen. Also (sub)-cortical calcifications may be seen.

Damage to large arteries is rare in comparison to small vessel injury. The changes in the large vessel resemble arteriosclerotic vessel disease, may be slowly progressive and lead to gradual occlusion. In patients irradiated for craniopharyngiomas or optic nerve gliomas this may lead to Moya-Moya formation. MR angiography may be helpful in establishing the diagnosis.

Focal radiation injury without a more generalized leukoencephalopathy presents as a mass lesion. On MRI the mass lesion is easily identified. It is preferentially located in the white matter, with high signal intensity on proton density and T_2-weighted images. After injection of gadolineum there may be enhancement, sometimes solid, more often ring-like or irregular, around a necrotic center. Occasionally the lesions become hemorrhagic, and this can also be easily identified on MRI. MRI, however, cannot with certainty differentiate between tumor recurrence and focal radiation injury. This can be successfully done by positron emission tomography because glucose consumption in focal radiation injury is supposed to be decreased and in tumor recurrence increased. MR spectroscopy may also have potential in this differentiation. Recently it has been shown that MR perfusion studies with good time resolution are capable of the same differentiation.

Lesions after stereotactic (localized) radiosurgery are also focal, and basically no different from the lesions described above. Also in these cases, the whole gamut of reactions from mild and transient to severe and cavitating is possible. In the early phase one may encounter rather extensive white matter changes near the target of irradiation, most probably caused by edema. Many of the changes seen in the early period after the treatment are transient. Occasionally, however, a white matter lesion outside the target area remains permanent. Here again, the correlation with the clinical condition is not straightforward.

An abnormal increase in water content in the extracellular compartment of the brain is usually referred to as cerebral edema. There are, however, many other compartments in the brain, enlargement of which may lead to local or generalized swelling of the brain and to changes in tissue parameters on MR images. It is, therefore, important to identify the different fluid compartments of the brain and to relate them, if possible, to clinical disease conditions (Table 68.1).

The vascular compartment consists of arteries, veins and capillaries. This compartment may undergo swelling as a result of arterial and capillary dilatation or venous obstruction.

The intracellular compartment consists of the various cells and their extensions present in the CNS. These cells and their extensions may swell either individually or together, depending on the cause of the changes. The following cellular elements are present: astrocytes, probably acting as a go between in the nutritional chain between the vascular compartment and the neurons; oligodendrocytes and their extensions, the myelin membranes; microglia, which form an important part of the immune system; and neurons and their extensions, dendrites and axons.

The extracellular compartment, formed by interstitial spaces between the elements of the CNS, practically virtual in adults, grossly visible in preterm infants.

Table 68.1. Compartments in the CNS

1. Vascular		
Arteries	→	Increasing volume
Veins	→	Venous obstruction
Capillaries	→	Blood-brain barrier leakage
2. Intracellular compartment		
Astrocytes	→	Astrocytic swelling
Neurons	→	Storage disorders, cytotoxic
Axons, dendrites		edema, vacuolation
Oligodendrocytes		
Cell body	→	Cytotoxic edema, vacuolation
Myelin	→	Vacuolating myelinopathy
3. Extracellular compartment		
CSF	→	Hydrocephalus
Extracellular space	→	Extracellular vasogenic or
		Osmotic edema
Virchow-Robin space	→	Widened VR spaces

This compartment is generally referred to as the extracellular space. The extracellular compartment also includes the Virchow-Robin spaces, the perivascular extension of the pia mater perforating the brain tissue as a tapering manchet, at the end in continuity with the interstitial compartment of the brain. The parenchymal extracellular spaces are in open contact with the CSF spaces, which can be subdivided into the ventricular spaces and the extracerebral CSF spaces.

On MRI the various kinds of edema will display a low signal intensity on T_1-weighted images, a high signal intensity on T_2-weighted images, compared to brain tissue. It is important to realize that there is a difference between the signal intensities characteristic of edema in general and signal intensities of CSF on MR images. CSF, behaving as nearly pure water (H_2O), has a very long T_1 and very long T_2. Edema, because of the formation of hydration layers around proteins, has a shorter T_1 and T_2. With a TR of 2000–3000 ms, H_2O will not be fully relaxed (still partially saturated) and will therefore have a lower magnetization in the Z-direction (M_z) than edema at the moment of excitation. H_2O will, therefore, have a lower signal intensity than edema at short echo times, the cross-over lying between 100 and 150 ms (on 1.5 T MR equipment). Signal intensity alone cannot differentiate between the different kinds of cerebral edema. Other morphological criteria are helpful in making further differentiation.

From the description of the fluid compartments of the CNS the various types of edema can be inferred. *Vasogenic Edema.* Accumulation of fluid occurs in the interstitial spaces, spreading according to the rule of least resistance (Fig. 68.1). Vasogenic edema surrounds a lesion, such as a tumor, metastasis, abscess, hemorrhage or contusion, and extends into the white matter tracts, because the extra interstitial fluid has to find its way (pressure gradient) and follows the pathways offering the least resistance. On MRI, vasogenic edema shows characteristic digitation in the subcortical area, where the gray matter structures offer greater resistance (Fig. 68.2).

There has been much discussion about the cause of vasogenic edema. The most likely explanations are (1) extra fluid produced by the lesion, (2) leakage of the blood-brain barrier, and (3) toxic factors, not yet identified, produced by the initial lesion. It is remarkable

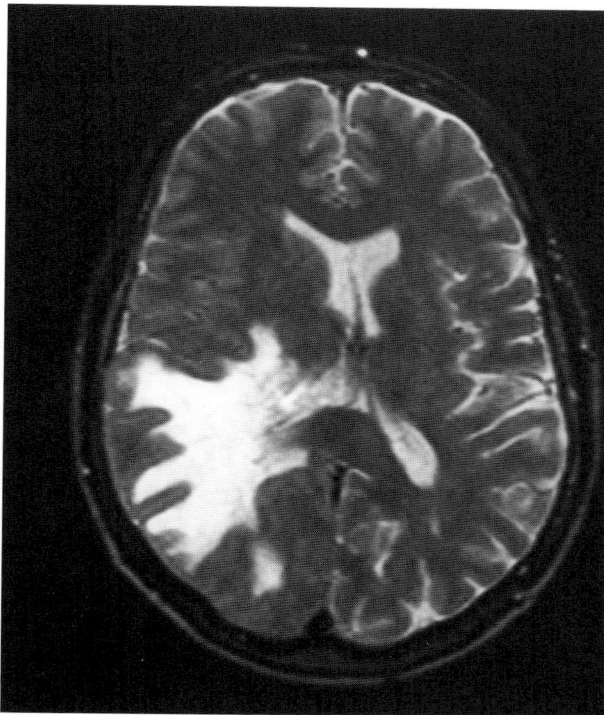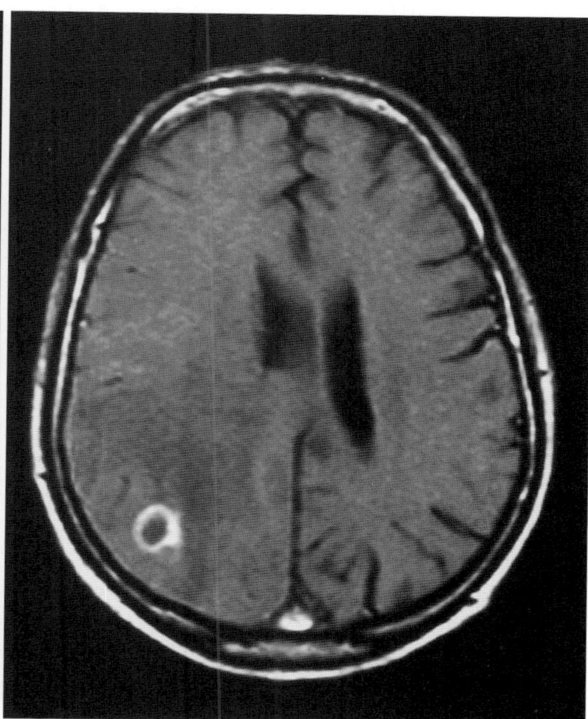

Fig. 68.1. On the T_2-weighted image on the *left*, vasogenic edema is seen in the right temporo-occipital region with typical digital extensions towards the cortex and into the central white matter. The gray matter is spared. After gadolinium injection, the underlying metastasis becomes visible

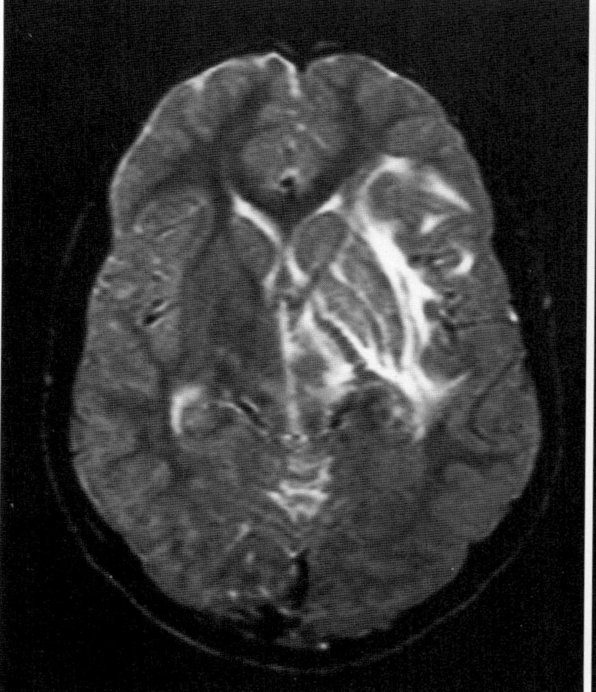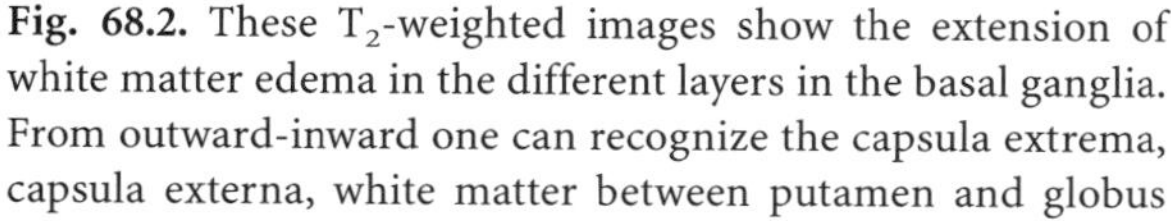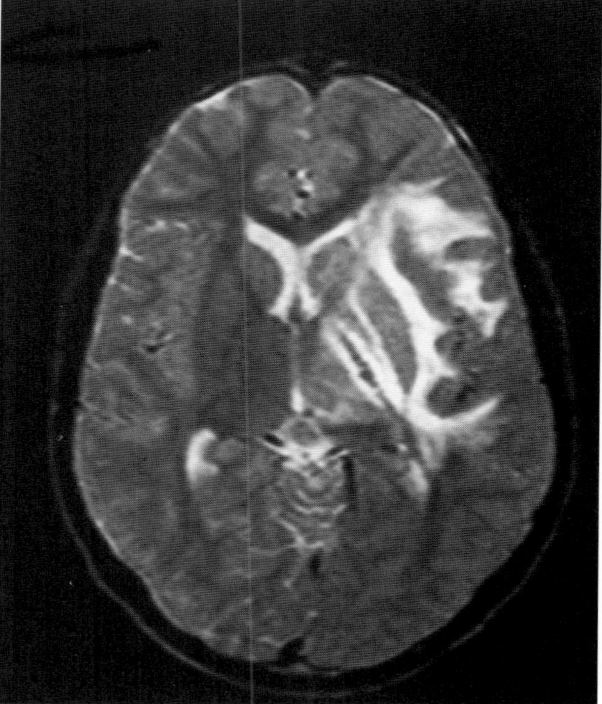

Fig. 68.2. These T_2-weighted images show the extension of white matter edema in the different layers in the basal ganglia. From outward-inward one can recognize the capsula extrema, capsula externa, white matter between putamen and globus pallidus, the internal white matter band in the globus pallidus and the capsula interna. Vasogenic edema follows the paths of lowest resistance and spares gray matter structures

that meningiomas, which are extracerebral tumors, induce in many cases extensive vasogenic edema. In this case the presently favored explanation lies in the extra fluid production by the tumor cells, which leads to a much higher pressure gradient at the tumor-brain interface than normally present in the interstitial fluid of the brain. Sometimes leakage through the blood-brain barrier is suggested as being causative in vasogenic edema. This, then, should occur in the primary lesion, because the area of vasogenic edema does not show contrast enhancement after administration of gadolinium, which makes local leakage of the blood-brain barrier improbable. Although it may occasionally be difficult to find the underlying lesion, the identification of vasogenic edema should induce a search for one.

Osmotic Edema. Despite the same appearance on MRI it is reasonable to distinguish another entity from vasogenic edema, which is caused by differences in osmolarity on both sides of the intact blood-brain barrier. Both hypo- and hyperosmolarity may be an inducing factor. This kind of edema is seen under conditions such as water-intoxication due to polydypsia, or other states of dilution, as caused by inappropriate secretion of antidiuretic hormone. Hyponatremia is the most common electrolyte abnormality in a general hospital population. In patients dying from hyponatremic encephalopathy the brain weight is increased. Although the explanation of the brain swelling in hyponatremia seems simple, it is in fact complicated and many processes play a role in undoing the effects of hyponatremia on the brain. Hyponatremic encephalopathy leads to movement of water into brain cells, a process which can begin as little as 20 min after the serum sodium drops below 130 mmol/l. Endogenous release of vasopressin into the CSF and into the cerebral circulation appears to facilitate direct movement of water into brain cells independent of the effects of hyponatremia. As edema progresses, compensatory mechanisms become active, for example resulting in extrusion of sodium from neural tissues, and the extrusion of osmotically active cations in an attempt to lower the osmolality. Many hormones play an additional role in the defense of the CNS against the influx of water. The swelling of the brain eventually leads to decrease of cerebral perfusion and hypoxia adds to the deleterious effect of hyponatremia. Further progression of edema leads to either death or severe brain damage.

It is even more difficult to understand that hypernatremia can also cause brain swelling, where one would expect the opposite. According to the laws of osmolality, one would expect shrinkage of brain cells under hypernatremic conditions. Even though this is possibly the case initially, this phase is rapidly – in the course of a few hours – followed by swelling of parts of the brain, probably largely due to cytotoxic edema. An additional contributing factor could be that after the initial hypo-

osmolality of the brain, restoration of the osmotic condition of the blood is achieved faster than restoration of the osmotic condition of the brain. After a while, therefore, the brain is again relatively hyperosmotic. In children the mortality of acute hypernatremia (plasma sodium above 160 mmol/l) exceeds 40%. It is usually the result of acute solute loading. In a baby, only a few weeks old, with sodium intoxication, we have observed that the brain was swollen in the unmyelinated areas, which probably offered the least resistance (Figs. 68.3, 68.4). Follow-up showed development of severe atrophy in the same area, a finding described in histology of acute hypernatremia.

The problems of hypo/hyperosmolality, and hypo/hypernatremia are closely related to entities such as central pontine myelinolysis and extrapontine myelinolysis. It is unclear which conditions cause the selective vulnerability in central pontine myelinolysis, and what pathogenetic mechanisms underly the process, although fast suppletion with sodium in hyponatremic states is often mentioned as the most important factor. Although an initial edema possibly exists in these conditions, the eventual histological lesion is demyelinating.

Cytotoxic Edema. In this condition fluid accumulates in the cells present in both gray and white matter (Fig. 68.5). The MRI characteristics of slightly swollen brain tissue with intermediate signal intensity on T_1-weighted images, high signal intensity on T_2-weighted images, with sharp margins and moderate mass effect usually make the diagnosis possible. This is important because cytotoxic edema occurs mainly in three disease categories (the three "i's"): infarction, infection, and intoxication. In infarctions the involvement of a vascular territory may be helpful in making the correct diagnosis (Fig. 68.5). In infections the cytotoxic edema occurs in the cerebritis phase, the early phase of inflammation (Fig. 68.6). Identification is important, because with the appropriate therapy the abnormalities may be transient and not progress to abscess formation. In intoxications cytotoxic edema is only one of the kinds of edema that may occur. The involvement of particular topistic areas and a symmetrical distribution of the involved areas may be helpful in diagnosis. In some inborn errors of metabolism, for example, methylmalonic aciduria and glutaric aciduria type 1, cytotoxic edema may occur, probably due to toxic effects of abnormal products of metabolism.

Selective Astrocytic Swelling. In some conditions the accumulation of water occurs selectively in astrocytes. Although astrocytic swelling is described in many neuropathological conditions, it is known to occur particularly in Alexander's disease, where the underlying disease is probably a dysfunction of the astrocytes themselves. The second condition where astrocytic swelling is a prominent pathological issue, is posthypoxic-is-

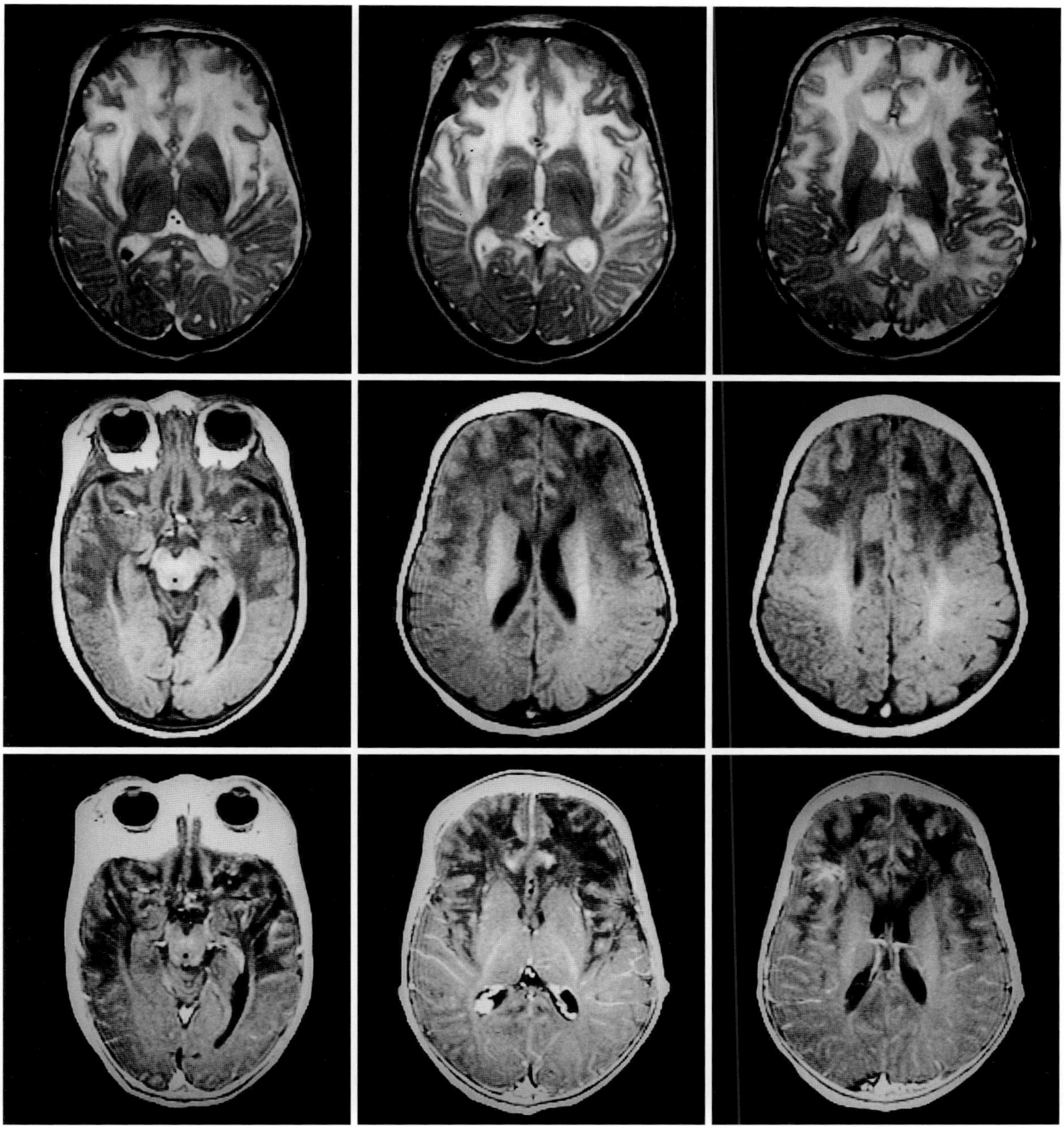

Fig. 68.3. The *upper row* of T_2-weighted images shows the findings at admission of this 2-month-old baby-girl with salt intoxication. There is severe swelling of the frontal and temporal white matter. The *middle and lower rows* show T_1-weighted images without (*middle*) and with (*lower*) injection of contrast. There are local deficits in the blood-brain barrier considering the presence of contrast enhancement. Probably the selectivity of the structural involvement is related to the fact that the affected areas are still unmyelinated. This type of edema can be regarded as osmotic edema

chemic encephalopathy in infants. In these cases the swelling is the consequence of energy depletion of the cells. The depolarisation of cell membranes, caused by energy depletion leads to a number of deleterious cascades. Ion channels will open and Ca^{2+} and Na^+ will enter the cell, K^+ will be forced outside the cell. The interstitial concentration of K^+ increases. When this reaches a critical level, Na^+, Cl^- and H_2O will enter the astrocytes. Astrocytes, or more likely all glial tissue elements, are probably singled out because their membrane properties make them more liable to swell. Astrocytic swelling causes a volume increase of the in-

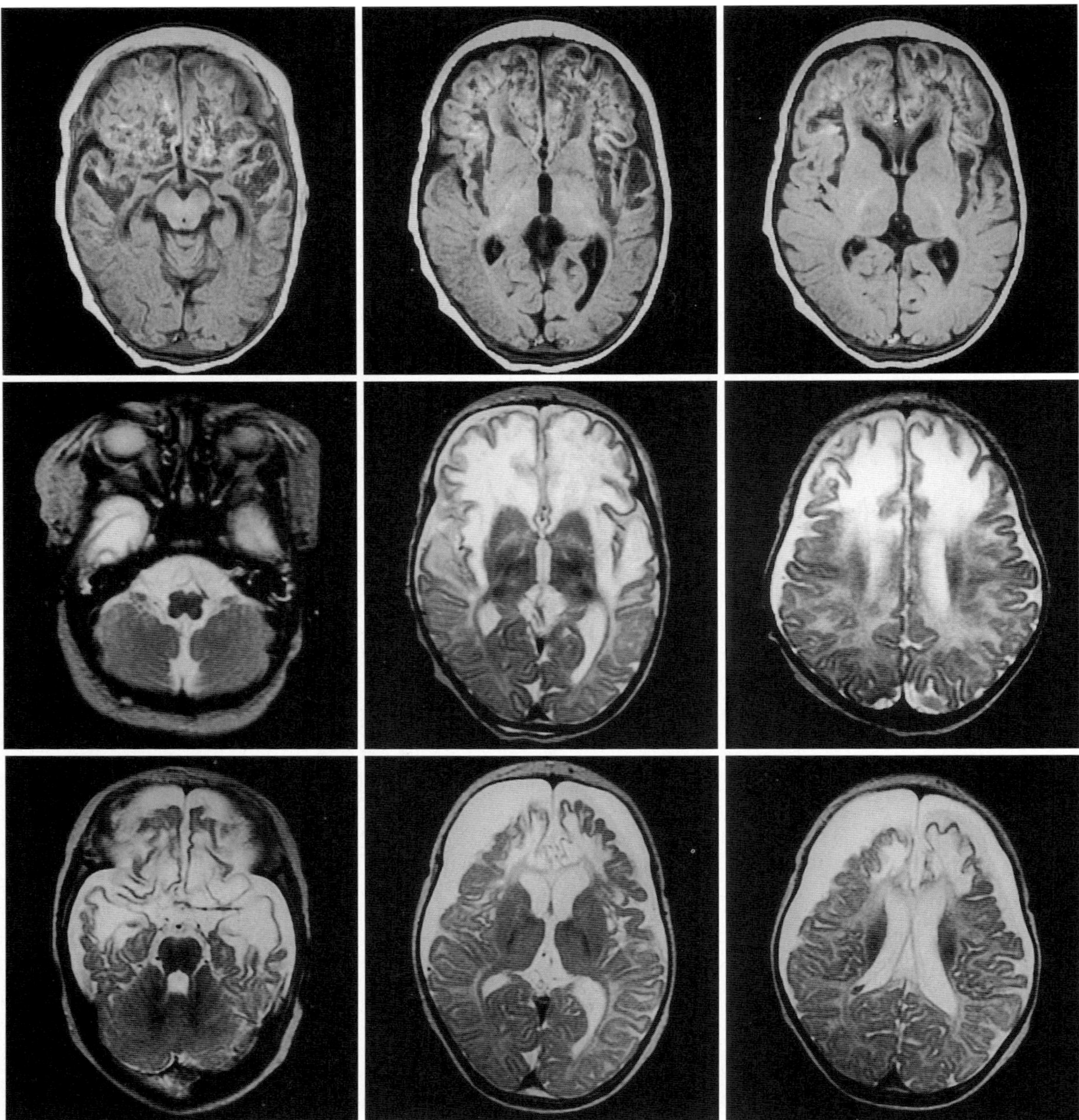

Fig. 68.4. (continued from Fig. 68.3) Two weeks later, the T$_1$-weighted images show a hemorrhagic component (*upper row*) and initial stages of atrophy of the involved structures. The T$_2$-weighted images (*middle row*) also show an increase in the pericerebral space and still a high signal from the involved areas. Finally, 2 months later, severe frontotemporal atrophy results (*lower row*)

volved brain areas. Swelling of astrocytes is also typically seen following exposure to methionine sulfoximine, cuprizone, and in conditions of metabolic derangement such as liver failure, Reye syndrome and several inborn errors of metabolism. In histology, this condition is referred to as metabolic astrocytosis. Astrocytic swelling has also been reported in infections with transmissible viruses, such as Creutzfeld-Jakob disease.

Selective Neuronal Swelling. In some disorders uptake or accumulation of abnormal substances takes place in neurons, in particular in some of the inborn errors of metabolism, lysosomal storage disorders. These disorders include glycogen storage disorders (Pompe's disease), mucopolysaccharidoses, GM$_2$ gangliosidoses, glycosyl ceramidosis (Gaucher's disease) and sphingomyelin storage disorder (Niemann-Pick disease).

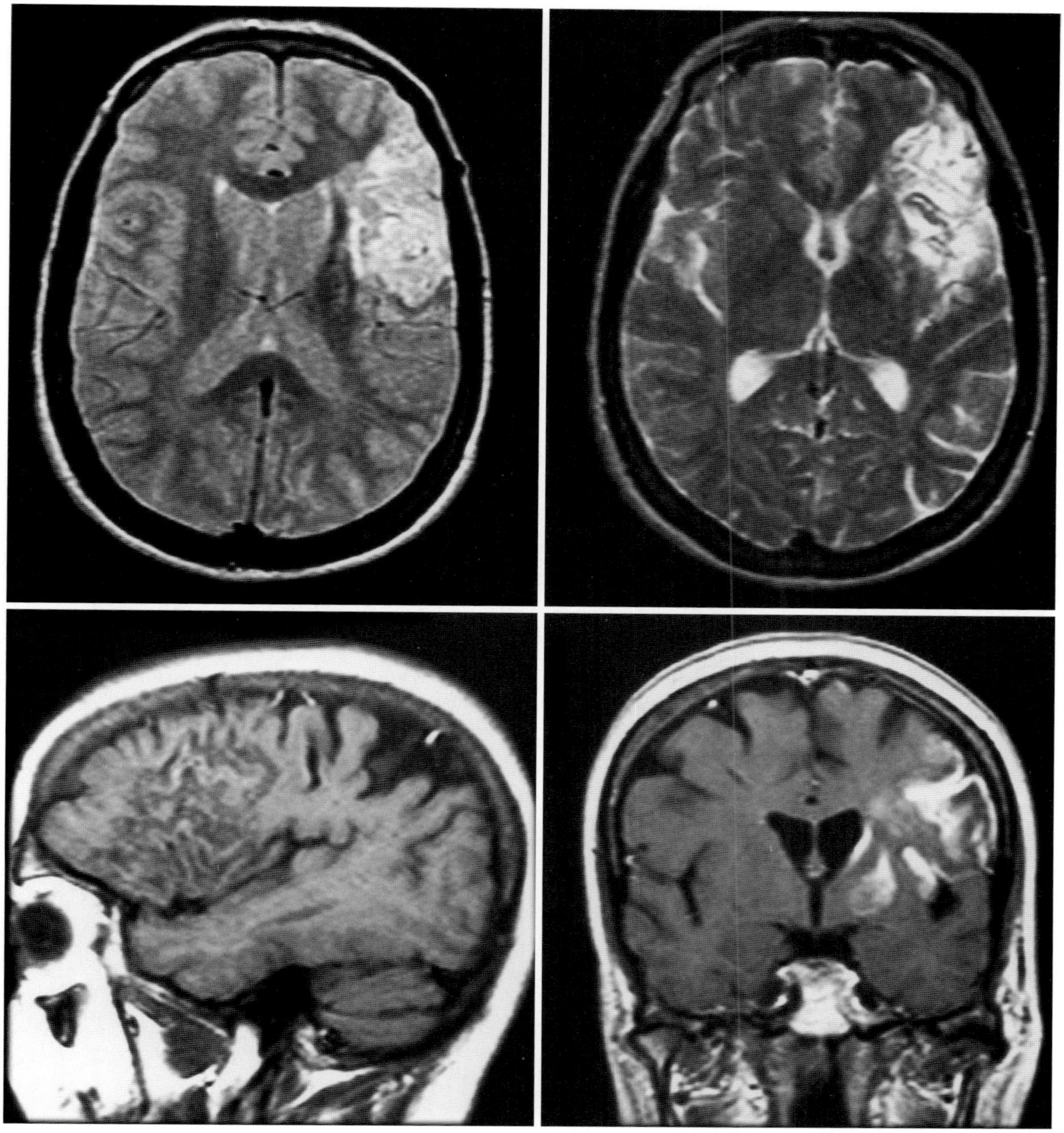

Fig. 68.5. Cytotoxic edema in the early phase of a left opercular middle cerebral artery infarction. The *upper row* shows a proton density and a T$_2$-weighted image at the level of the frontal operculum. The lesion involves gray and white matter, and has hardly any mass effect. The parasagittal image (*left, lower row*) shows the hemorrhagic gyral pattern of the lesion. The coronal image (*lower row, right*) after contrast injection shows gyral enhancement and enhancement of the striatum

Vacuolating Myelinopathy. So far we have described fluid accumulation in pre-existent spaces or cell bodies. Compartments within the brain tissue can, however, be formed in previously non-existing spaces. Vacuolating myelinopathy refers to such a condition. Before the age of electron microscopy, this condition was known as white matter spongiosis. Electron microscopy has demonstrated that the condition is produced by splitting of the myelin membrane at the intraperiod line. In this newly created space, fluid accumulates, vacuoles appear and eventually coalesce into larger cavities. In light microscopy studies, this gives the affected brain a spongy appearance. Vacuolating myelinopathy has been described in a number of conditions, in particular

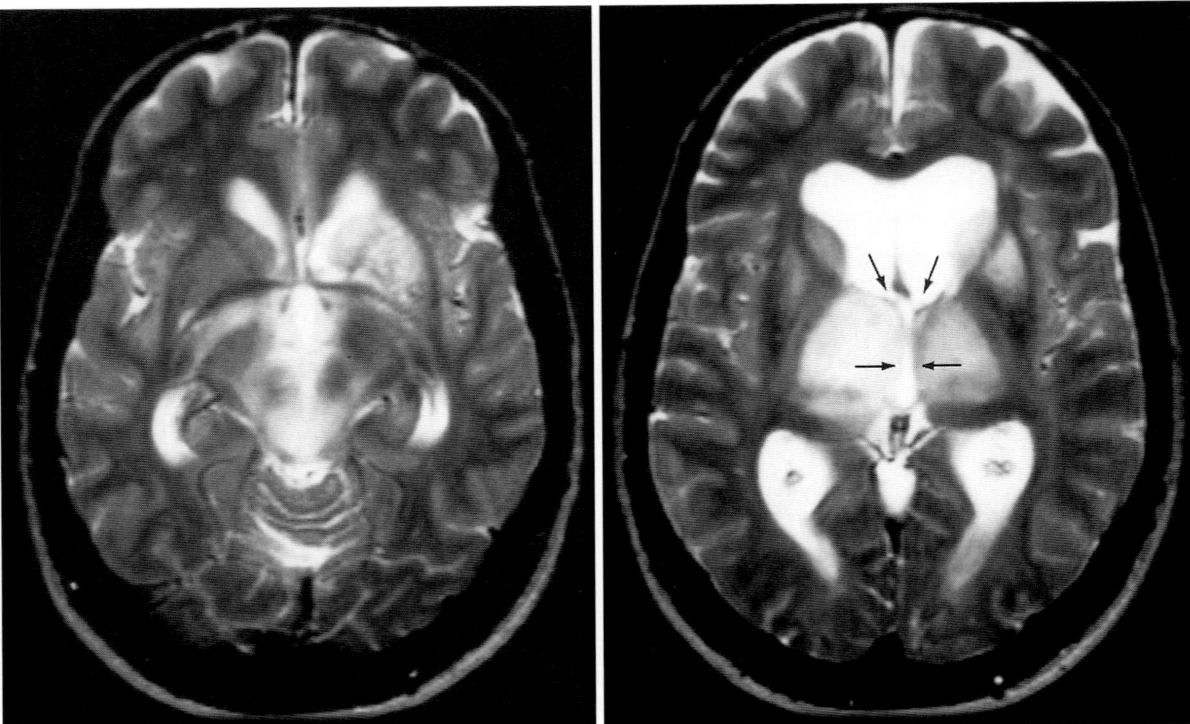

Fig. 68.6. Cytotoxic edema in an acute encephalitis of unknown origin. Acute swelling of the thalamus, periaqueductal gray matter and on both sides the caudate nucleus and puta- men. Though the swelling is moderate and the third ventricle and foramina of Monro are still open (*arrows*), the periaque- ductal swelling is sufficient to cause a hydrocephalus

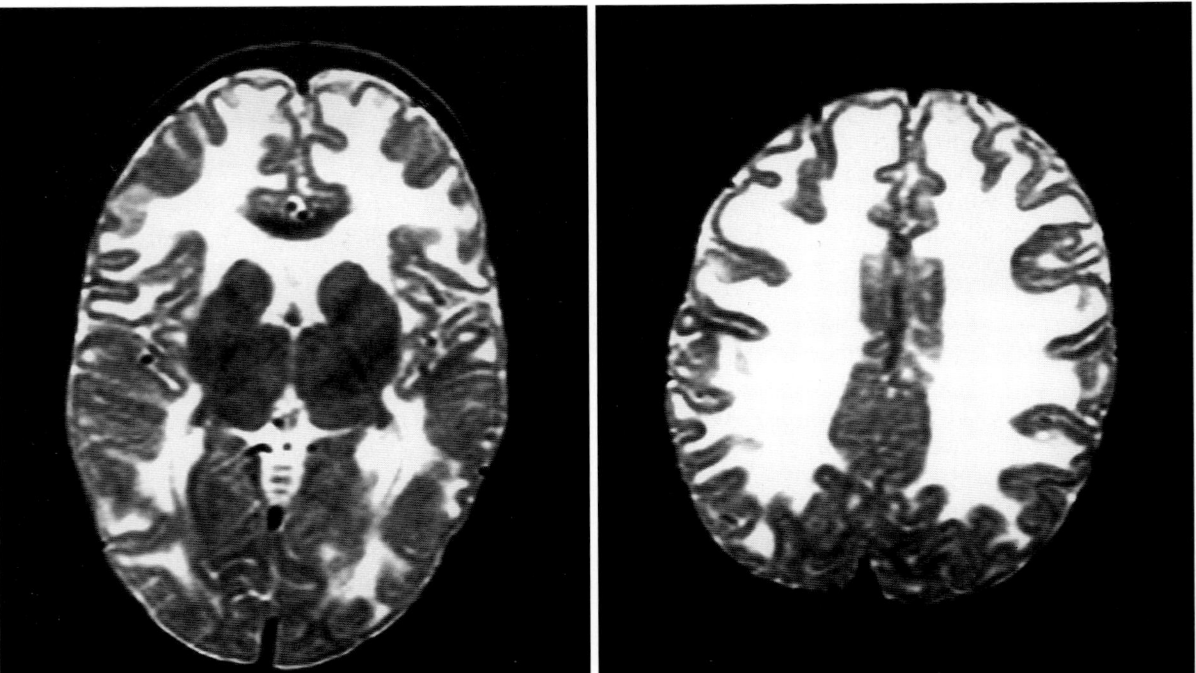

Fig. 68.7. Vacuolating myelinopathy, caused by splitting of the myelin membrane causes a mild swelling of the white matter, as illustrated in these T_2-weighted images

in inborn errors of metabolism and intoxications. The classical example of this disease is Canavan disease. It has, however, been found, though often less extensive, in other inborn errors of metabolism such as maple syrup urine disease, pyruvate carboxylase deficiency, Kearns-Sayre syndrome, and Leigh syndrome. Hexachlorophene encephalopathy is a well-known example of toxic encephalopathies with myelin splitting. Other toxins, such as triethyltin and poisonous heroin, can also lead to vacuolating myelinopathy. The MR appearance of vacuolating myelinopathy is rather characteristic (Fig. 68.7). The white matter is swollen, the arcuate fibers are involved, often the lesions even start in the arcuate fibers, and the cortex is stretched over the swollen white matter. If vacuolating myelinopathy occurs in neonates, the distribution of the lesions is very special. As the presence of formed myelin sheaths is a prerequisite for the development of vacuolating myelinopathy, the white matter sponginess and swelling is limited to the myelinated areas.

Accumulation in Virchow-Robin Spaces. The blood vessels penetrating the brain are covered by a pial sheath and a small amount of CSF, the Virchow-Robin spaces. In normal aging and under certain pathological circumstances these spaces can enlarge and become visible on MR images (Fig. 68.8). Elongation of the arteries in arteriosclerotic patients may expand the Virchow-Robin spaces. More CSF will fill the expanded Virchow-Robin spaces. This will be visible on MR scans as bright spots on T_2-weighted images, and low signal intensity spots on T_1-weighted images. Or, more generally stated, the signal intensity of these expanded Virchow-Robin spaces follows the signal intensity of CSF on all sequences. Therefore it is possible to differentiate the widened Virchow-Robin spaces from lacunar infarction, which have either a high signal intensity on mildly T_2-weighted or proton density images (where CSF is intermediate) or a very low signal intensity on T_2-weighted images if necrotic material is present with prevalent T_2 shortening. Small, isolated multiple sclerosis lesions differ from widened Virchow-Robin spaces, because the multiple sclerosis lesions have a high signal intensity on mildly T_2-weighted images as compared to CSF. In some conditions the contents of the expanded Virchow-Robin spaces are not CSF but other substances. The Virchow-Robin spaces are not just a passive CSF sheath around the blood vessels, but play an intermediary role in the transportation of water soluble products, both normal and abnormal. In a number of the polymucosaccharidoses the water soluble mucopolysaccharides accumulate in macrophages within the Virchow-Robin spaces.

CSF Spaces/Edema in Hydrocephalus. The edema of hydrocephalus, more than any other type of cerebral edema, resembles lymphedema in general body tissues. Both result from the obstruction of the normal drainage, which leads to distension of the channels proximal to the block, with retrograde flooding of the extracellular compartment. In acute hydrocephalus the earliest finding involving the brain parenchyma is periventricular edema (Fig. 68.9). The invaded tissues are spongy in appearance and glial cells and axons are widely separated, indicating extracellular edema. Astrocytes are particularly susceptible to the fluid and ion changes in the interstitial spaces and undergo selective swelling, followed by gradual development of permanent damage, atrophy and cell loss. In chronic hydrocephalus, axons are destroyed, myelin sheaths are gradually broken down, and phagocytosis of lipid by microglia occurs. The two mechanisms involved in this process are well documented: stasis of interstitial fluid, because the normal bulk flow channels are blocked and, secondly, reflux of CSF into periventricular tissues.

Normal pressure hydrocephalus or chronic communicating hydrocephalus is a special form of hydrocephalus and an important entity in so far as it represents a treatable form of dementia. It has attracted attention from clinicians and radiologists ever since its description in 1964 by Salomon Hakim. He described the clinical triad of gait apraxia, incontinence and dementia in adults with hydrocephalus and "normal" CSF pressure. The application of a ventriculo-peritoneal or atrial shunt can lead to dramatic improvement. A correct diagnosis, therefore, is clearly important, especially for predicting of which patients have the best chance of improving after drainage and which ones will not profit from this treatment. To predict the outcome of shunting has proved to be extremely difficult, even in cases with radiological evidence of a communicating hydrocephalus with excessive pulsations (flow void) on MRI studies in the aqueduct, and a rim of high signal intensity around the ventricles on T_2-weighted images. In patients with this combination, it is not only the differentiation from Binswanger's disease which is difficult, but also the question arises whether periventricular gliosis, demyelination or infarction is a contra-indication for shunting. The theoretical difference between the periventricular white matter changes in normal pressure hydrocephalus and Binswanger disease is obvious: in normal pressure hydrocephalus the changes are due to the backflow of CSF into the extracellular brain spaces or to concurrently present microvascular periventricular changes in the elderly; in Binswanger's disease they represent infarctions. In the former condition, one might expect improvement after shunting, in the latter obviously not. The differentiation between the conditions is not always easy to make on MRI, and even more difficult because both conditions may coexist. Some have recently tried to explain the hydrocephalus as a consequence of deep white matter changes, rather than as its cause. There is a decrease

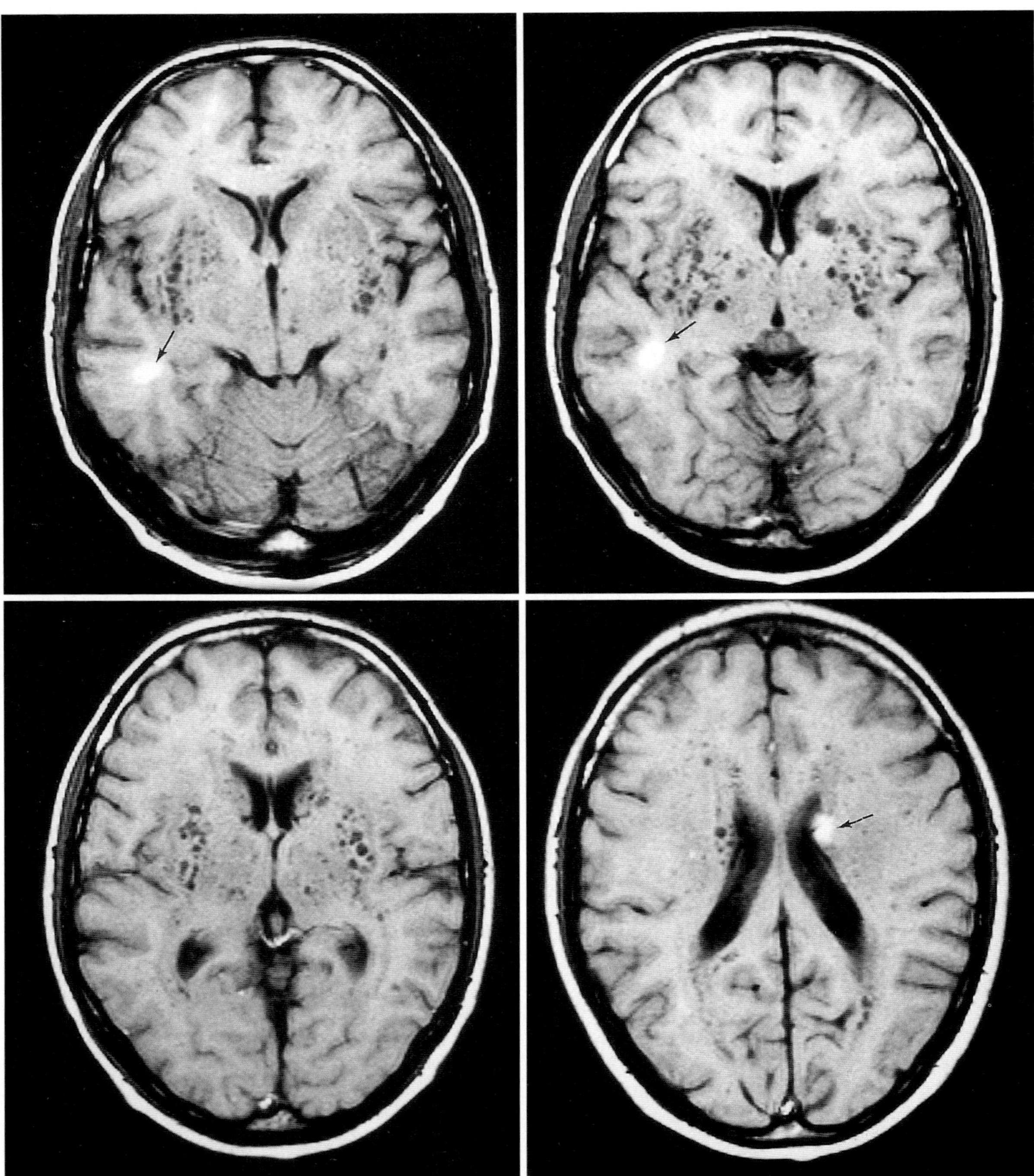

Fig. 68.8. Patient with CADASIL (see chapter on subcortical arteriosclerotic encephalopathy, Chap. 65), a hereditary angiopathy, with white matter involvement, focal hemorrhages (*arrows*), and, as demonstrated on these T_1-weighted images, widening of the Virchow Robin spaces

in compliance of the brain because of the white matter changes, and the inner table of the skull forms an obstruction for the brain to expand in that direction during the systolic expansion. The combination of both factors would result in a large centripetally directed pulse wave, leading to the enhanced aqueductal pulsatile flow, as seen on MR flow studies. The greater aqueductal to and fro CSF shift would predict presence of communicating hydrocephalus and therefore a more important beneficial effect of shunting. One has to be

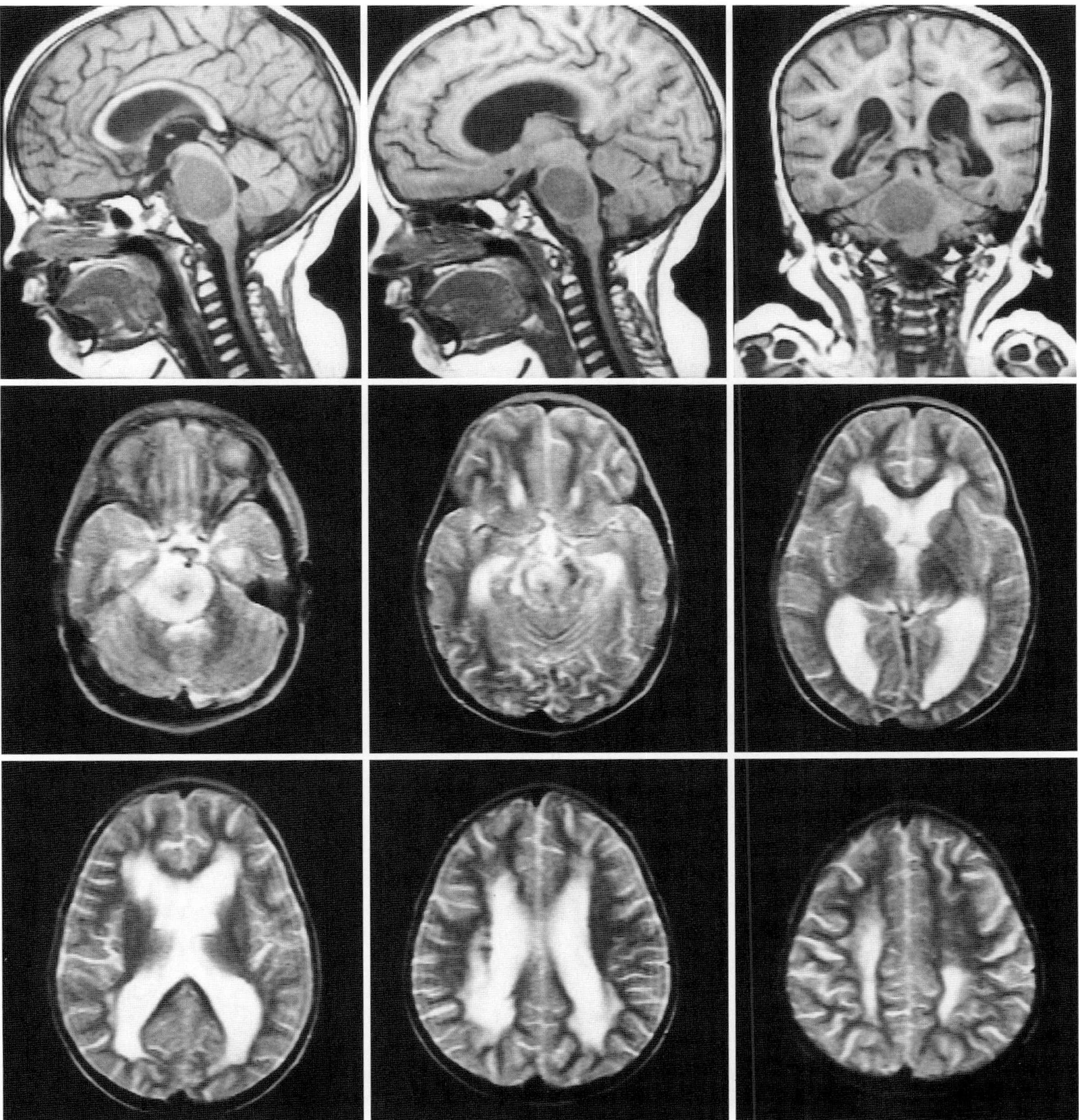

Fig. 68.9. In this 4-year-old boy with a large pons glioma an obstructive hydrocephalus has developed. On the T_2-weighted images (*middle and lower rows*) a high signal intensity rim is seen around the ventricles, representing transependymal exudation of CSF in the extracellular spaces

cautious, however. Others have reported no predictive value from the same sign, as so many tests have failed to make a good selection of patients for treatment. Some have claimed that improvement of periventricular circulation and metabolism after CSF taps in cases with radiological evidence of a communicating hydrocephalus, with or without deep white matter abnormalities, carries the best prognosis. In our experience the best results after shunting are obtained in patients with a relative (or absolute) aqueduct stenosis. The discussion is still open.

69 Wallerian Degeneration and Myelin Loss Secondary to Neuronal and Axonal Degeneration

69.1 Introduction

There are basically two causes of Wallerian degeneration in our definition: neuronal cell death and axonal lesion. It should be noted, that our definition is wider than usual and not only includes acute axonal lesions, but neuronal and axonal lesions of any kind. Degeneration of the entire arborization of a neuron with its axon and axonal branches inevitably follows necrosis of the neuronal cell body. Examples are degenerative diseases affecting neuronal cell bodies and axons, such as Friedreich's disease, olivopontocerebellar atrophy, and neuronal ceroid lipofuscinosis. A lesion of the axon that leads to an interruption of its continuity gives rise to degeneration of the distal part, whereas the proximal portion survives. The myelin in the distal portion undergoes dissolution as a consequence of the axonal degeneration, as the integrity of the myelin sheaths depends on continued contact with a viable axon. The changes in the distal part of the interrupted nerve are called Wallerian degeneration in a narrower sense, following Waller's original description of the changes that he observed after cutting the glossopharyngeal and hypoglossal nerves in the frog in 1850.

Any lesion of the axons that leads to an interruption, and any lesion of the nerve cell bodies that leads to cell death is followed by Wallerian degeneration. In the CNS common causes are infarctions, hemorrhages, tumors, and head injury with shearing of nerve fibers. In all white matter disorders, Wallerian degeneration eventually plays a role, as myelin loss is followed by secondary axonal degeneration, which in turn is followed by Wallerian degeneration of the distal parts of the axons and their myelin sheaths. Wallerian degeneration as such cannot be considered to be a condition which primarily affects myelin. Nevertheless, Wallerian degeneration with demyelination secondary to neuronal and axonal degeneration are discussed here as a component of all disorders and because their MRI appearance may be mistaken for primary white matter affections. This is especially the case when the cortex and the neuronal cell bodies are unaffected. An example is the traumatic shearing of nerve fibers, which may lead to bilateral extensive white matter degeneration whereas the cortex is remarkably normal.

69.2 Pathology

A characteristic of Wallerian degeneration is the fact that the sequence and timing of its changes are highly stereotyped. Degeneration is much faster in the PNS than in the CNS. Most studies of Wallerian degeneration in the CNS have been carried out in the optic nerve, degenerating as a result of enucleation of the eye. Tract degeneration in the dorsal column of animals has also been studied after myelotomy.

Abnormalities in axons severed from their neuronal perikarya precede changes in the myelin sheath. There is no spatiotemporal gradient of degradation. Abnormalities appear over the whole length of the axons simultaneously. About 8–15 days after the event the axons have disintegrated, whereas the myelin still appears normal. Most axonal debris disappears from degenerating tracts within about 1 month. Increased cellularity in the degenerating tracts is due to the greater number of astrocytes. In the process of Wallerian degeneration, degradation of myelin sheaths becomes apparent after 30 to 90 days. Myelin sheaths collapse and the lamellae become loose. The myelin sheaths then lose their regular smooth outline and split into ovoids, which break down into smaller globules. The breakdown of myelin into simpler lipids does not start until after about 100 days and takes place in the cytoplasm of phagocytic cells.

Electron microscopy reveals the degenerating axons and axonal debris to be surrounded by myelin sheaths, occasionally irregularly folded. The myelin sheaths initially show a regular structure with major and minor dense lines and a periodicity of 105 Å. Splitting of myelin lamellae is noted. The structure of myelin lamellae continues to change with time, developing into uniformly layered structures with a periodicity of 40–50 Å. At this stage, the myelin degradation products become smaller and are phagocytosed. Unstructured lipid droplets as well as complex lamellar inclusions are typically found in phagocytic cells during the later stages of degeneration. Inclusions of unstructured lipid crystals are sometimes seen. In the final stages, numerous different inclusions are seen.

In the damaged peripheral nerve, Schwann cells appear to be involved in myelin destruction in Wallerian degeneration. The role of oligodendrocytes in Walleri-

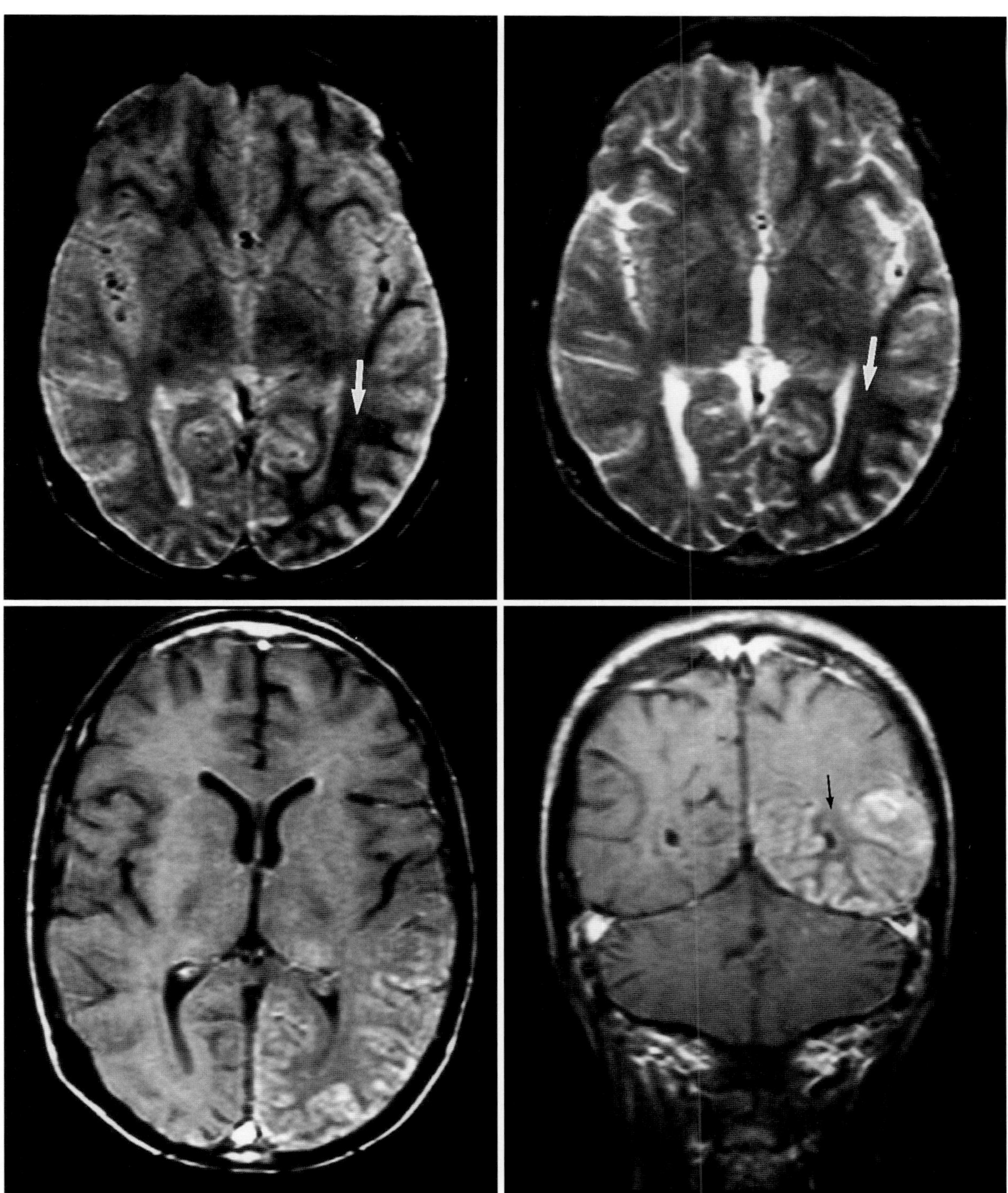

Fig. 69.1. A patient with a subacute meningo-encephalitis, involving the leptomeninges over the left hemisphere and the cortex in the occipital region. On the T_2-weighted images (*upper row*) the white matter underneath has a lower signal intensity than the white matter elsewhere. This represents the second stage of Wallerian degeneration. The *lower row* shows T_1-weighted images after Gadolinium injection with cortical enhancement occipitally

an degeneration in the CNS is less clear. It is probable but not certain that the oligodendrocyte does not participate, or participates only to a minor extent. Macrophages, astrocytes, and multipotent glial cells have been observed to contain myelin debris.

Histological evidence indicates that Wallerian degeneration takes place at different rates depending on a number of variables. The time course of myelin degradation, as well as the cellular reaction, depends on the localization of the trauma, type of noxious agent, and distance from the site of injury, the reaction in the peritraumatic area being more enhanced and pronounced than in sites distal from the site of injury. However, the most important factor in determining the course of the Wallerian degeneration is whether the axonal or neuronal lesion is acute and monophasic or chronically progressive.

69.3 Chemical Pathology

Biochemical analysis of CNS myelin undergoing Wallerian degeneration shows a gradual decrease in all myelin constituents but otherwise a remarkable normality in composition of the remaining myelin. Only an increase in cholesterol esters and a slight decrease of ethanolamine phosphoglycerides have been demonstrated. Also, no major abnormalities are found in the protein constituents. Basic protein is lost from the myelin sheath relatively early in the process of myelin degradation due to an increase in proteinase activity. This occurs before phagocytosis of myelin by macrophages and astrocytes and results in transformation of myelin sheaths in uniformly layered lipid structures.

Cholesterol esters are the major constituents of the lipid droplets and the crystal inclusions of phagocytic cells.

The change in biochemical composition of whole white matter depends on the extent of myelin loss. Cholesterol esters are relatively elevated.

69.4 Pathogenetic Considerations

The isolation of myelin with almost normal protein and lipid composition despite Wallerian degeneration as late as 90 days after the injury is consistent with the morphological evidence that in Wallerian degeneration in the CNS the breakdown of myelin occurs mainly within the cytoplasm of phagocytic cells. It would seem that the myelin sheath is degraded as a unit, cholesterol esters being the only residual constituents. There seems to be nonselective digestion of myelin constituents, as the composition of the remaining myelin is normal.

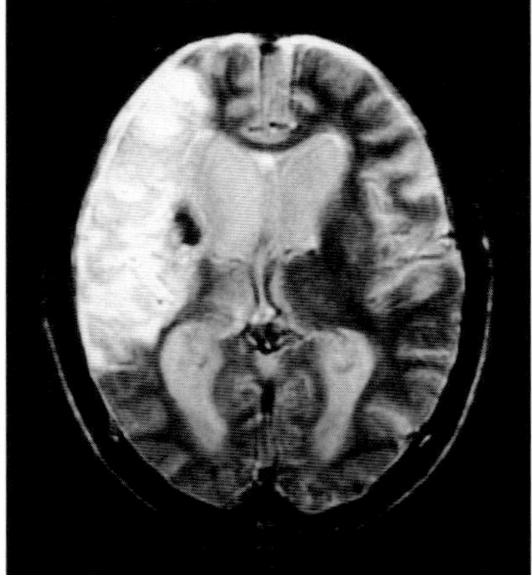
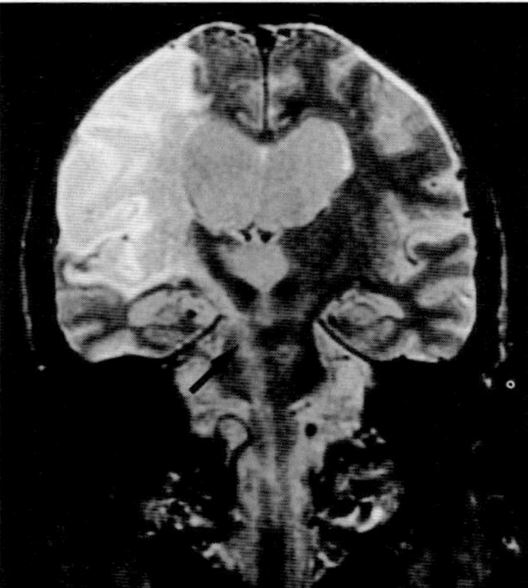
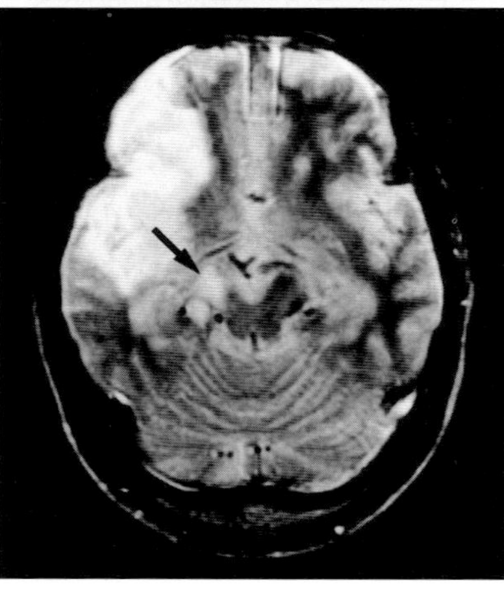

Fig. 69.2. The third phase of Wallerian degeneration is beautifully displayed in these T_2-weighted images, showing the initial lesion and the corticospinal tracts all the way down into the brain stem. Courtesy of Waragai et al. 1994, with permission

A hypothetical model of four stages of myelin degradation in Wallerian degeneration has been proposed (Lassman et al. 1978):

1. The stage of mechanical deterioration of myelin sheaths showing a normal myelin periodicity under the electron microscope.

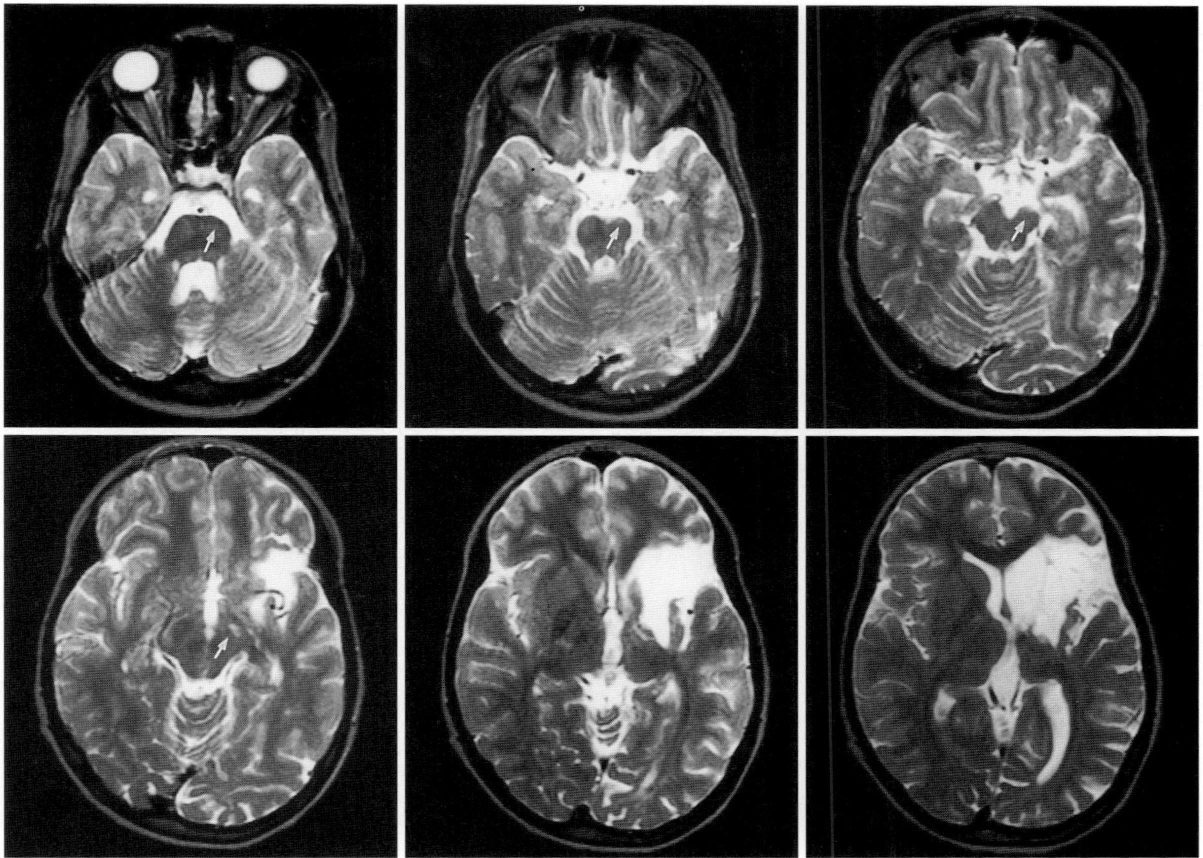

Fig. 69.3. T$_2$-weighted transverse series showing a left opercular infarction. In the fourth stage of Wallerian degeneration, atrophy results, as is shown in the brain stem (*arrows*)

2. The stage of degradation of digestible proteins restulting in the transformation of myelin sheaths into uniformly layered structures.

3. The stage of lipid degradation accompanied by the occurrence of unstructured lipid droplets and crystals in phagocytic cells.

4. The stage of deposition of poorly digestible lipids or lipoproteins, resulting in numerous different electron-microscopic inclusion types in phagocytic cells. Resolution of tissue debris and atrophy.

69.5 Magnetic Resonance Imaging

In the CNS Wallerian degeneration of long tracts can usually be very well depicted, as shown in patients with hemorrhages and infarctions. As a multiplanar modality, the MR plane can be chosen to depict the signal changes over their full length. Depending on the location of the primary lesion or lesions, Wallerian tract degeneration can be unilateral or bilateral, and, if bilateral, symmetrical or asymmetrical. Normally the long tracts of packed white matter have a somewhat lower signal intensity on proton density and T$_2$-weighted images than the remainder of the white matter. In Wallerian degeneration the signal in the tract is lower or higher than usual compared to the normal white matter tracts depending on the stage of degeneration. In fact MRI can help to distinguish the four stages of Wallerian degeneration, each resulting from a rather well-defined phase in the process of degeneration:

1. Physical degeneration of the axon occurs first with only mild biochemical changes. This happens in the first 4 weeks after the incident. This stage is not visible on MRI.

2. The first stage is followed by myelin protein breakdown without myelin lipid breakdown. The resulting material with high lipid content is considered to be hydrophobic, causing a low signal intensity on proton density and T$_2$-weighted images. This occurs between 4 and 14 weeks (Fig. 69.1).

3. Subsequently myelin lipid breakdown starts to take place, with gliosis and increased water content, leading to a higher signal intensity of the involved tracts on proton density and T$_2$-weighted images (Fig. 69.2).

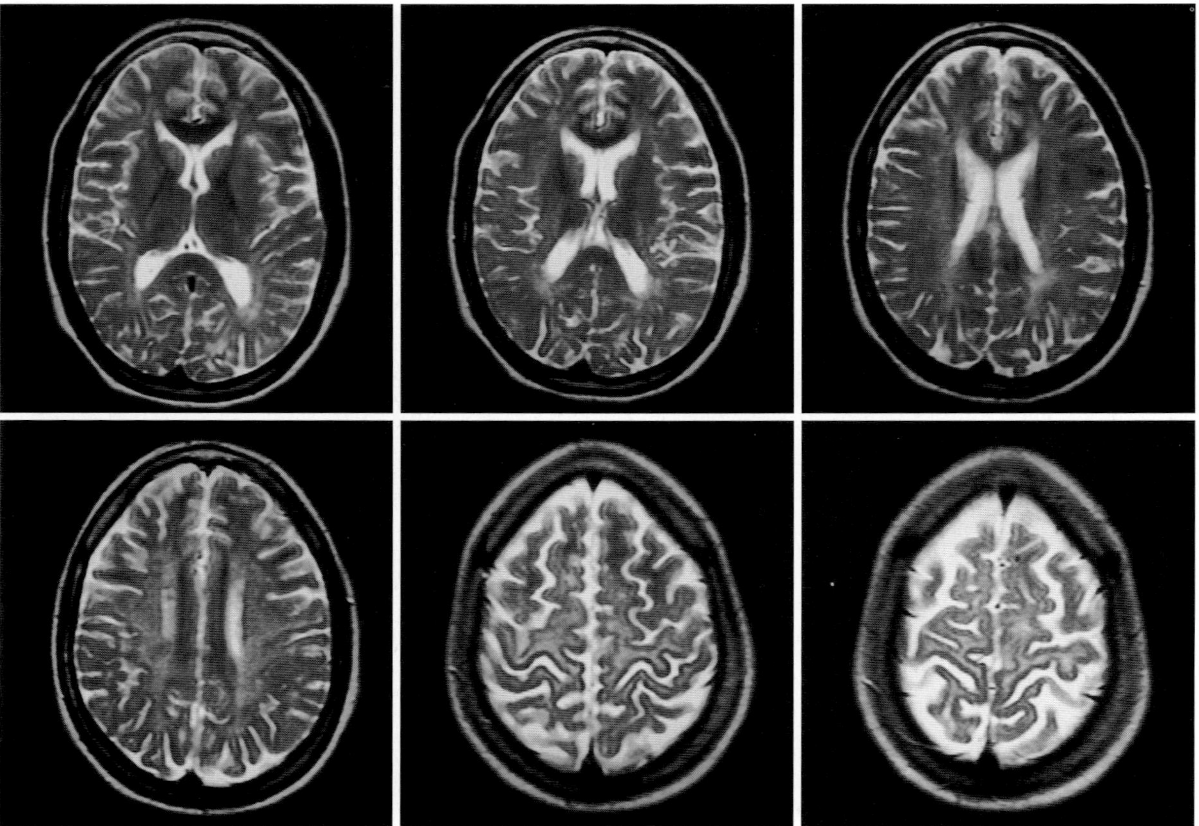

Fig. 69.4. A 19-year-old female with a slowly progressive neurodegenerative disorder and diffuse loss of neurons. There is a diffuse slight hyperintensity of the subcortical white matter as an expression of Wallerian degeneration. This type of change in signal intensity of the white matter is often seen in slowly progressive neurodegenerative disorders involving the cortex

4. Finally, after a number of months to years, the abnormal tissue constituents are removed and atrophy results (Fig. 69.3).

It will be obvious that there is a cross-over of contrast between the degenerating tract and the surrounding tissue between stages 2 and 3, "fogging" the MR depiction of Wallerian degeneration.

The four stages of Wallerian degeneration have been well described, and although there is considerable overlap in time, each phase has been recognized by several authors. To improve the detection of Wallerian degeneration on MR special techniques, such as diffusion weighted imaging and Magnetization Transfer ratio calculations may be used. With these techniques changes can be detected even earlier.

Most attention has been paid to local Wallerian degeneration following focal lesions. Two types of diffuse Wallerian degeneration can be distinguished. In the first place diffuse, low-grade Wallerian degeneration occurs in neurodegenerative disorders with loss of cortical neurons. In these disorders MRI shows atrophy and often, in addition, a slight moderate increase of signal intensity in the hemispheral white matter (Fig. 69.4). In the second place acute diffuse Wallerian degeneration occurs in cases of diffuse axonal injury, for instance after cerebral trauma. The most striking example is found in white matter shearing injuries with disruption of corticomedullary connections. The Wallerian degeneration leads to diffuse white matter degeneration in the course of weeks (Fig. 69.5).

Wallerian degeneration has also been reported in the spinal cord, in particular in the posterior columns. It is possible to see a gap between the original myelopathic lesions, degenerative, or traumatic, and the Wallerian degeneration several segments higher in the afferent tracts. Given time, the parts in between eventually also show signal intensity changes.

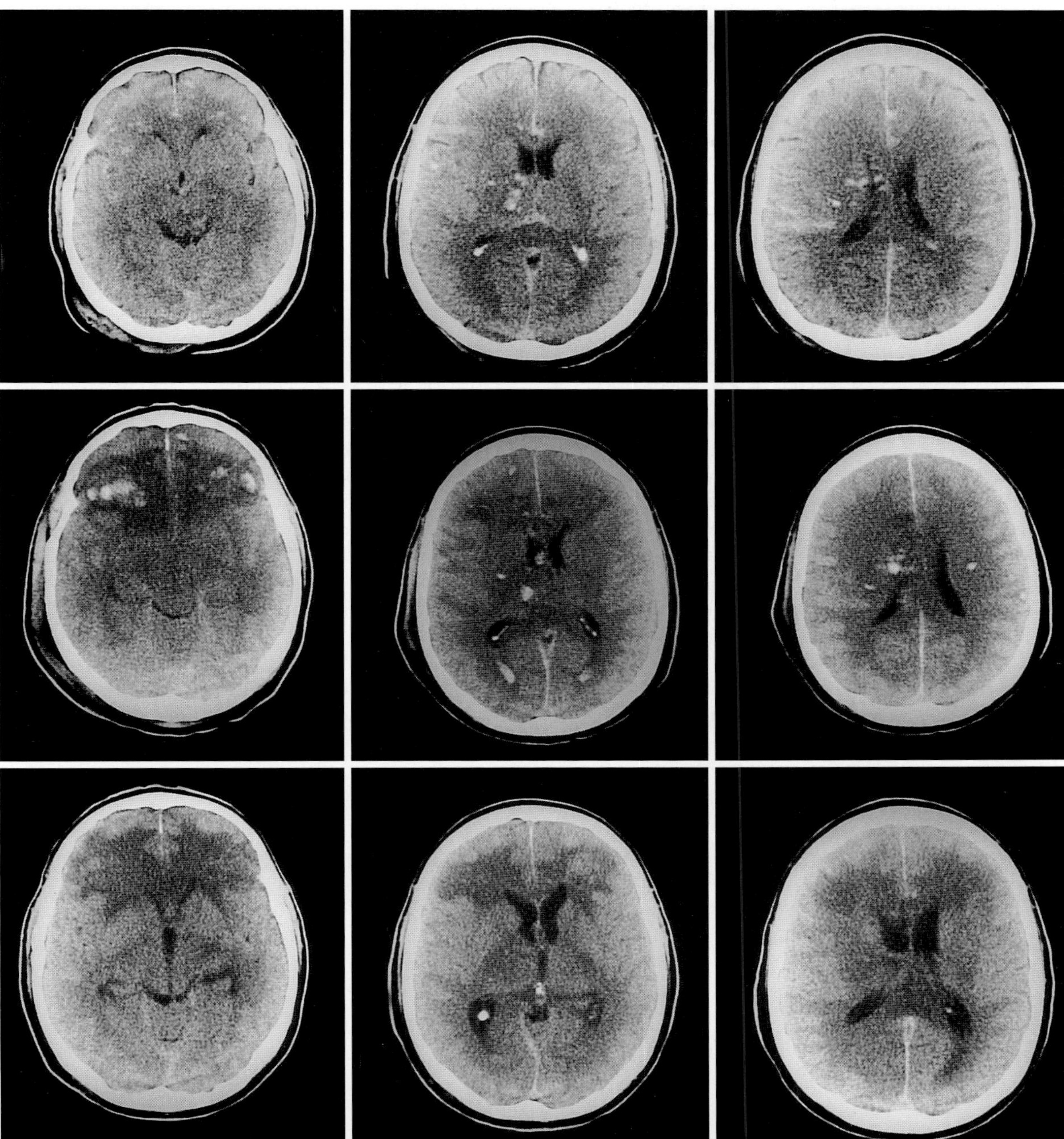

Fig. 69.5. A 36-year-old man with severe head trauma. The *upper row* of images, made on admission, shows evidence of white matter shearing in the subcortical region frontally, in the corpus callosum and basal ganglia with presence of small hemorrhages. The *middle row* of images, taken 1 week later, shows the hemorrhages to be more pronounced and the development of leukencephalopathy in the frontal region. The *lower row* shows images 6 weeks after the accident. The hemorrhages have now disappeared. In the frontal area the cortex is still intact, Wallerian degeneration has progressed in an antegrade axonal direction

70.1 Introduction

MR imaging is highly sensitive in the detection of white matter lesions. A close association has been demonstrated between the occurrence of white matter abnormalities observed with MRI and those found at autopsy. It has been generally assumed that the specificity of MRI is much lower than its sensitivity. However, the specificity of MRI depends not only on the potential and limitations of the method, but also on the capabilities of the person interpreting the MR images (Fig. 70.1). Hence, optimization of the specificity of MRI for white matter disorders is achieved by optimizing the quality of both MR images and MRI interpretation.

Aids to the perceptual and decision processes can be constructed to support the interpretative process. Such an aid is a systematic and detailed image analysis. A checklist or scorelist which prompts the image reader to assess and record a scale value for each feature is helpful in this respect. A second aid is a computer program that integrates these scale values, compares the pattern obtained with the known patterns in a data base and then reaches a differential diagnosis. The reader of the images can use the computer estimates of the likelihood of various disease conditions as a guide.

It is important is to realize that MRI pattern recognition has its limitations. In the first place, MRI patterns have characteristic features only during a certain period of development of progressive disorders. This is well illustrated in Fig. 70.2. In the early phase of the disease the MRI pattern is diagnostic; in the end-phase all characteristics have been lost. A second problem is seen in Fig. 70.3 where the pattern, for reasons unknown, is the inverse of the pattern commonly observed in this disease. The computer program should allow for these exceptions to the rule when they are known to occur. The third illustration (Fig. 70.4)

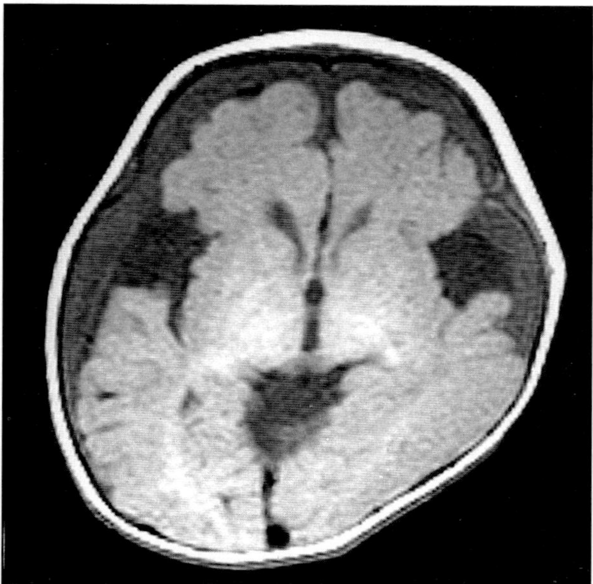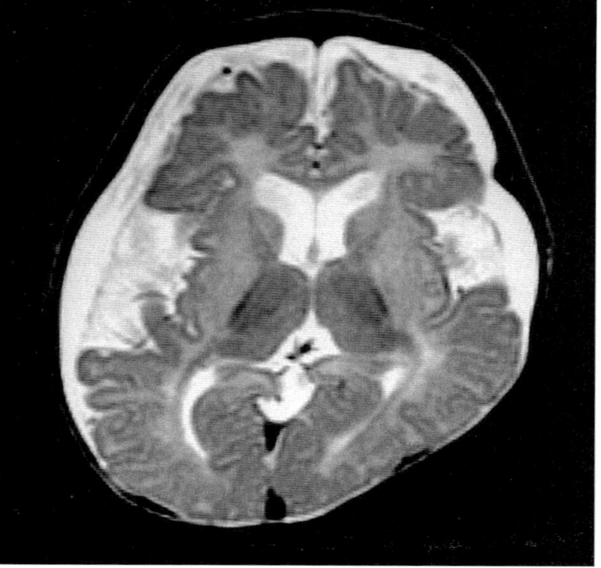

Fig. 70.1. T_1 and T_2-weighted image of a 10-month-old male with glutaric aciduria type I. The images show diffuse bilateral subdural hygromas and frontotemporal hypoplasia. Myelination is severely retarded. Note that the arachnoid and subdural spaces can be clearly separated. The presence of bilateral subdural hygromas could be wrongly interpreted as evidence of child battering. Knowledge of the specific features of glutaric aciduria type I with presence of frontotemporal opercular hypoplasia precludes this mistake. Courtesy of Osaka 1993, with permission

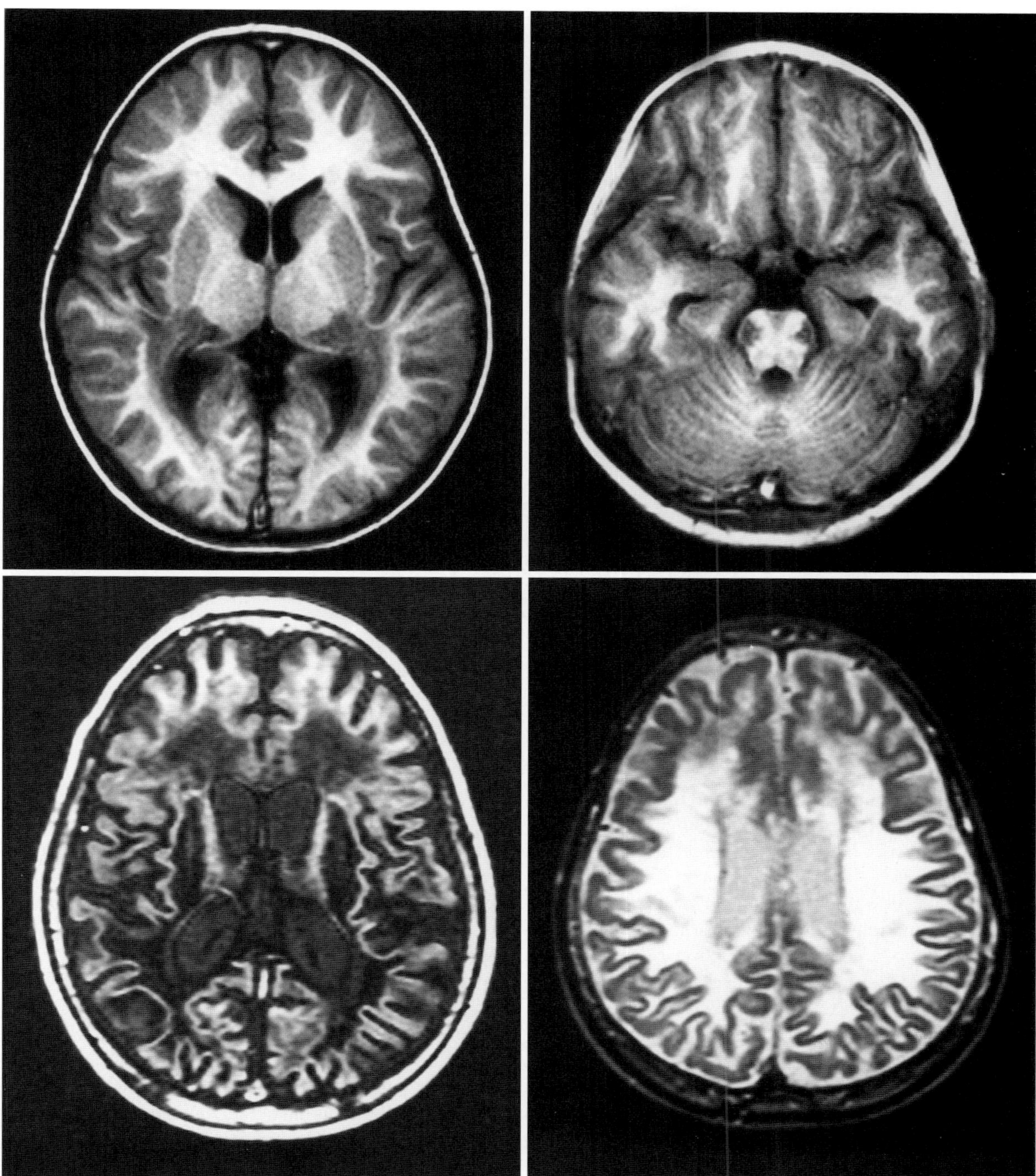

Fig. 70.2. The *upper row* of T_1-weighted (IR) images in this 3-year-old boy show the pattern that is typical for the childhood cerebral form of X-linked adrenoleukodystrophy: peritrigonal and occipital leukoencephalopathy, sparing the U fibers, involving the geniculate bodies and the splenium of the corpus callosum with typical involvement of corticospinal tracts in pons and mesencephalon. The *lower row* of one T_1 and one T_2-weighted image are of the same child, 3 years later. No pattern is recognizable as all white matter structures are involved and all characteristic features of the disease are lost

shows the difficulty of discriminating disorders on the basis of the pattern recognition programme alone, when only some and not all main MRI features of a disease are present.

70.2 Noncomputerized Pattern Recognition

Pattern recognition in the daily practice of medical imaging involves three levels of action which must be

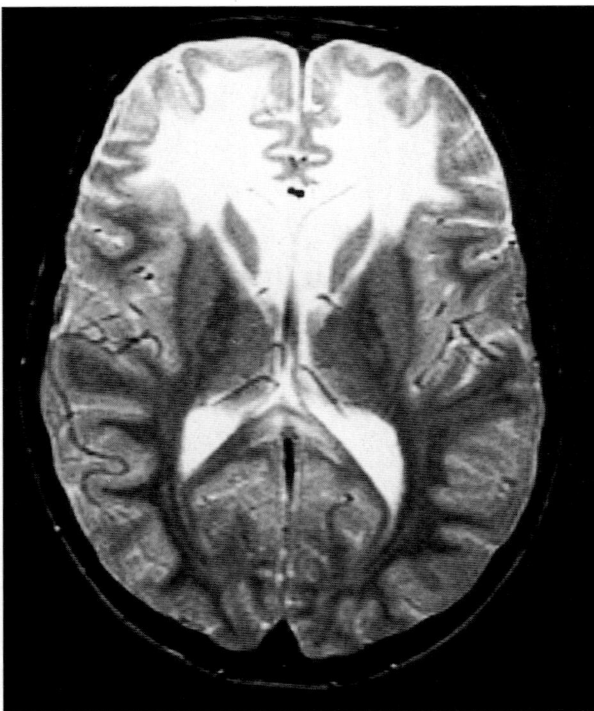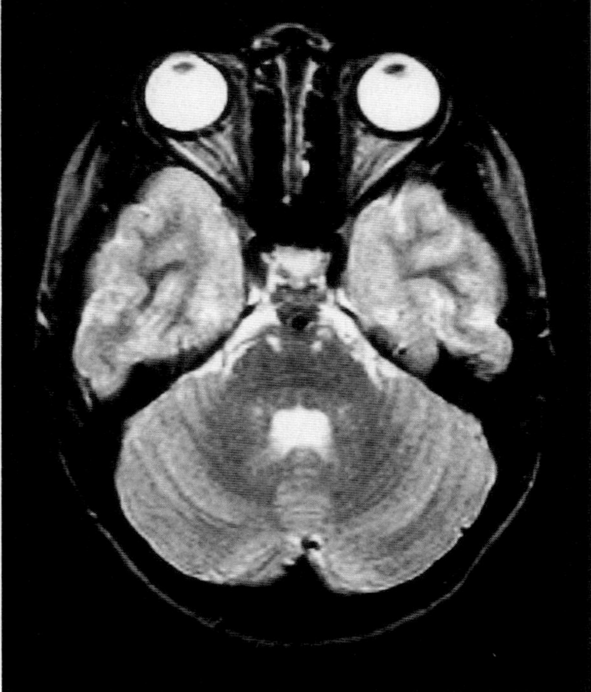

Fig. 70.3. T$_2$-weighted images in a 6-year-old boy show bilateral, symmetrical involvement of the frontal white matter and the fronto-spinal tracts in the anterior limb of the internal capsule, which can be followed in the brain stem. The spread of the disease is evidently in a ventro-dorsal direction. Diagnosis: X-linked adrenoleukodystrophy (with reversed pattern). Courtesy of P. Hoogland and W.F.M. Arts, the Hague, the Netherlands, with permission

integrated to permit optimal interpretation of the image. These levels can be described as image formation, image analysis, and image interpretation (see Table 70.1).

The first level is the technological level and has to do with the formation of the image. Although the reader of the image can consider large parts of the components of an MR system as a "black box", he/she certainly needs to have a general knowledge of the imaging process, the parameters involved (repetition time, echo time, inversion time, number of excitations, slice thickness, flip angle), the influence of parameter settings on the image, the possible artefacts, and the ways of improving quality when special answers are required.

The second level is the level of image analysis, in which the structural elements of the image are analyzed, weighted as to their normality or abnormality, and described as such. This is an important step in the process of teaching and learning, because the analysis of structural elements depends very much on experience, knowledge of anatomy, knowledge of normal brain maturation and knowledge of pathology.

The first and second levels lay the foundation for the third level, the interpretation of the image. In this process the image as such is transcended. Interpreting of the image requires a combination of acquaintance with the image formation, analysis of the structural elements, experience, knowledge of disease entities, histopathology, pathophysiology, biochemistry, toxicology and potentially knowledge from still other sources in an assessment that aims at answering the clinical question.

The first level, image formation, will not be discussed in this chapter.

The second level is the analytical level, which includes a systematic analysis and classification of structural elements of the image (see Tables 70.2–70.4). The identification of the structural elements of an image which are to be evaluated, depends on many factors. For example, if one was not aware from previous experience and histopathological studies that the arcuate fibers are spared in many demyelinating disorders, but that, for example, Canavan's disease starts in the arcuate fibers, it would be senseless to make the involvement of the arcuate fibers a point of discrimination in the decision-making process. Structural elements that have been identified by us as having discriminating value are: the general distribution of lesions in the brain, the involvement or sparing of specific structures, symmetry of lesions, appearance of lesions, additional components of the lesion including the possible en-

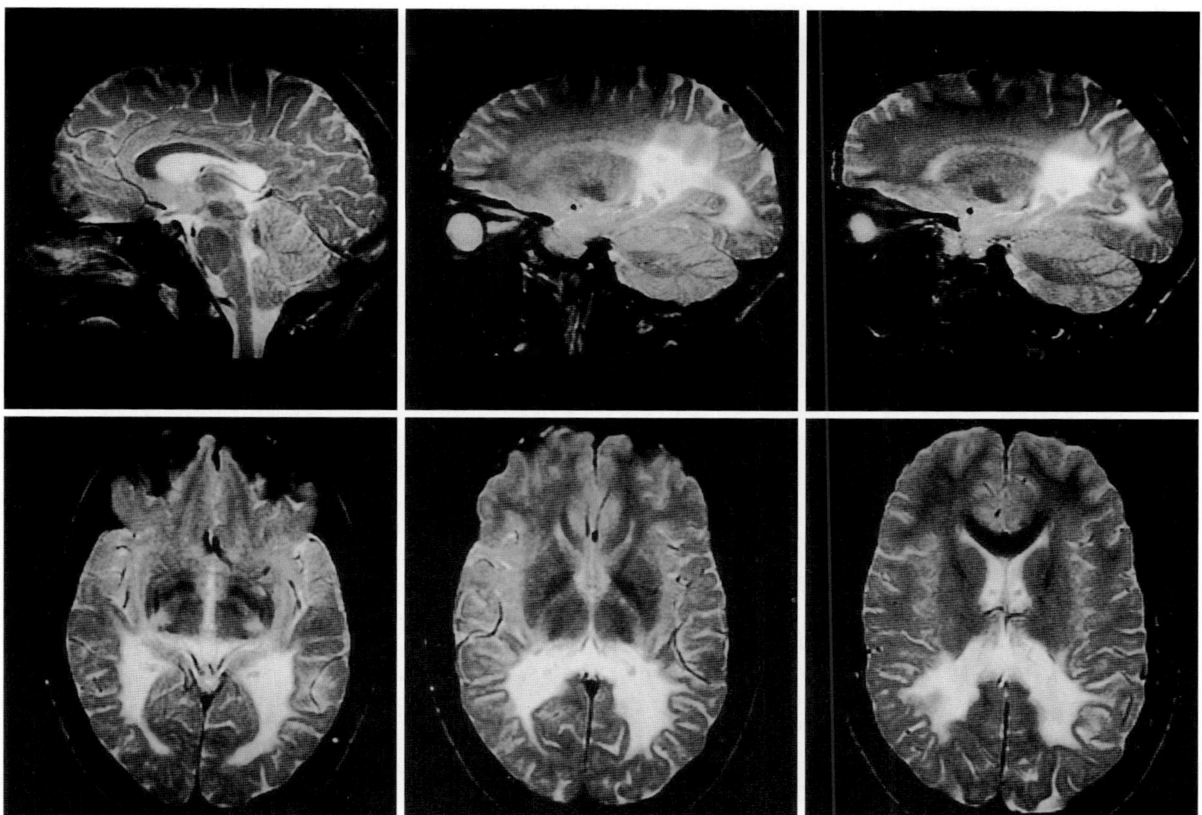

Fig. 70.4. A 23-year-old man who had experienced progressive disturbances of gait for the last 2 years and moderate psychomotor retardation from birth onwards. The T_2-weighted sagittal and transverse images show bilateral peritrigonal and occipital involvement of the white matter, with affliction of the splenum of the corpus callosum, and of the posterior limb of the internal capsule. There is no enhancement after gadolinium injection, forming an argument against X-linked adrenoleukodystrophy and Schilder's disease. There was no laboratory evidence for a peroxisomal disorder. Although the changes in the peritrigonal area and occipital lobe could be the remnants of a periventricular leukomalacia, the involvement of the internal capsule and the involvement of the splenium of the corpus callosum make that diagnosis highly improbable. Despite the highly characteristic image and perfect symmetry this remains an unsolved case which needs to be followed up

Table 70.1. Pattern recognition

1. Image formation	2. Image analysis	3. Image interpretation

Influence parameter settings on image:
  TR, TE, TI, SLT, NEX, FA
  Gradient compensation
  Triggering
	Perceptual process + structural elements
	of the image:
	  Define
	  Classify
		Pattern recognition:
		  Diagnostic
		  Highly suggestive
		  Suggestive
		  Possible
		  Atypical
		  Impossible

TR, repetition time; TE, echo time; TI, inversion time; SLT, slice thickness; NEX, number of excitations; FA, flip angle

hancement with Gd-DTPA and the presence of calcifications.

At the third level, a global survey of the distribution of the lesion may already give an indication of the kind of disorder we are dealing with. Sparing of the U fibers is seen in most inherited myelin disorders and in subacute HIV encephalitis. Some organic and amino acidopathies, contrariwise, are preferentially located in the U fibers. In many cases, symmetry is a striking feature of inherited myelin disorders and toxic en-

Table 70.2. List of structural elements to be analyzed

Cerebral cortex	Occipital/frontal/parietal/temporal
Arcuate fibers	Occipital/frontal/parietal/temporal
Lobar white matter	Occipital/frontal/parietal/temporal
Periventricular white matter	Occipital/frontal/parietal/temporal
Internal capsule	Anterior limb/posterior limb
External capsule+extreme capsule	
Caudate nucleus	
Putamen	
Globus pallidus	
Thalamus	
Corpus callosum	Rostrum/genu/corpus/splenium
Cerebellar cortex	
Cerebellar white matter	
Cerebellar pedunculi	
Nucleus dentatus	
Mesencephalon	Central part/peripheral rim/corticospinal tracts/tectum and tegmentum
Pons	Central part/peripheral rim/corticospinal tracts/tegmentum

Scoring: no affection/slight to mild affection/severe affection

Table 70.3. List of characteristics of the lesions to be analyzed

Symmetry	Perfectly symmetrical/slightly asymmetrical/asymmetrical
Extension	Small isolated lesions/large isolated lesions/irregularly confluent lesions/highly confluent lesions/combination of these
Signal intensity	Slightly to mildly abnormal/severely abnormal/mixed
Homogeneity	Homogeneous/inhomogeneous/two zones
Demarcation	Sharp/vague/mixed

Table 70.4. List of extra elements to be analyzed

Calcium deposition	Absent/present
Enhancement with gadolinium – DTPA	Absent/present
Ventricular enlargement	No/slight to mild/severe
Enlargement of pericerebral subarachnoid spaces	No/slight to mild/severe
Cerebellar atrophy	No/slight to mild/severe
Myelination	Normal/delayed/no or hardly any myelin present

cephalopathies, and much less so of acquired demyelinating disorders. Appearance of the lesions is important: are they isolated, or confluent, or both? In X-linked adrenoleukodystrophy, in metachromatic leukodystrophy, in Alexander's disease, Canavan's disease, and in diffuse white matter injury after irradiation and chemotherapy the lesions are confluent; as a rule no isolated lesions are seen. In multiple sclerosis a mixture of isolated and confluent lesions is the rule. The same is true for Binswanger's disease. Extra components are such features as calcifications, which occur in patients with Cockayne's disease, a minority of patients with X-linked adrenoleukodystrophy, in malignant phenylketonuria, in some patients with a mitochondrial leukoencephalopathy and in some children after cranial irradiation and chemotherapy. In some white matter disorders enhancement with Gd-DTPA is seen in part of the lesion, mostly in the active border. This observation can be very helpful. In X-linked adrenoleukodystrophy this enhanced border separates the area of complete demyelination from the area in which part of the brain structure is still recognizable. Enhancement is also a prominent feature of Schilder's disease, Balò's disease and Alexander's disease.

Perhaps other criteria could also be used in the recognition of patterns of white matter disorders on the images, such as measurements of the absolute signal intensities, or T_1 and T_2 measurements. For instance, in subacute HIV encephalitis, the signal intensity of the white matter lesion, at least in the beginning of the disease, is not as high on T_2-weighted images as it is in most other white matter disorders. Neuropathological examinations confirm that demyelination in subacute HIV encephalitis is only partial and mild. On the MR images the involved white matter has a coarse, granular texture which also corresponds very well with histological findings of numerous small foci of more complete demyelination. In the differentiation between small or lacunar infarctions, widened Virchow-Robin spaces, gliosis, and demyelination, estimations of T_1 and T_2 may be of some value.

Authors have frequently praised the sublime sensitivity of MRI but indicated the lack of specificity. Although this is at least partially due to overrating the role of MRI as a paraclinical test, this opinion testifies also to an "all or nothing" concept with respect to specificity. In our definition, specificity exists in degrees. The pattern emerging from the image can be expressed as being pathognomonic, characteristic, typical, or atypical. Although these terms have been used by some authors, we have graded the patterns in a somewhat different scale, closely related to what is used in clinical scales for the probable presence of a disease: diagnostic, highly suggestive, suggestive, possible, atypical, and impossible. It is only in the first category that, if the typical MRI pattern is present, it is

Table 70.5. Specificity of MRI patterns

Diagnostic
X-linked adrenoleukodystrophy, cerebral early childhood form
Zellweger cerebrohepatorenal syndrome
Cerebrotendinous xanthomatosis
(if fat deposits are present)
Periventricular leukomalacia
Canavan's disease
L-2-hydroxyglutaric aciduria
Alexander's disease
Some toxic encephalopathies
Kearns-Sayre syndrome

Highly suggestive
Metachromatic leukodystrophy
Globoid cell leukodystrophy
Mucopolysaccharidoses
Leigh's disease
MELAS
Pelizaeus-Merzbacher disease
Cockayne's disease
Phenylketonuria
Glutaric aciduria type 1
Schilder's disease
Wilkson disease
Central pontine myelinolysis

Suggestive
Lowe syndrome
Multiple sclerosis
Schilder's disease, less advanced cases
Subacute HIV encephalitis
Binswanger's disease
Border zone infarctions
Wallerian degeneration
Toxic encephalopathies

Possible
Multiple sclerosis, less advanced cases
Acute disseminated encephalomyelitis
Progressive multifocal leukoencephalitis
Extrapontine myelinolysis

Atypical
Unusual appearance with established diagnosis, for example, X-linked adrenoleukodystrophy asymmetric or starting frontally, Alexander's disease starting in the cerebellum

Impossible
The exclusion by MRI of a clinical diagnosis or suspicion is not a frequent occurrence. It can happen in cases in which a space-occupying lesion is considered, and the images show a demyelinating disorder

pathognomonic for one specific disorder. In the other categories, clinical or laboratory evidence is necessary to complete the diagnosis. The lists given should be considered as examples; they are by no means complete (Table 70.5).

Quite a few myelin disorders can be listed under the categories "diagnostic" or "highly suggestive", imply-

ing that MRI makes a firm contribution to the diagnostic process in these disorders. Very often, by adding clinical information or laboratory data, a higher diagnostic category can be achieved.

70.3 Computer-Assisted Pattern Recognition

Until now expert systems have played a minor role in medicine. With the increasing complexity of diagnostic processes and with the increase in number of recognized, rare disorders, the need to implement expert systems is felt. To develop these, it is essential to collect data systematically and quantitatively and to set up large data banks. We decided to create a data base that could be used for a computer-assisted pattern recognition program in white matter disorders with the exception of arteriosclerosis -related ischemic white matter disease. Over a certain period of time, the MR images of all patients under the age of 50 years or, when risk factors for vascular disease were present, under the age of 40 years, with lesions exclusively or predominantly in the white matter, were scored with the help of a detailed scoring list (see Tables 70.2–70.4). The total study population was 1483. The patients were grouped in diagnostic categories, according to the classification we proposed, that stresses etiological and histological similarities between disorders of the same category.

The data obtained were analyzed. Per disease category or subcategory the frequency of occurrence of image abnormalities and features were counted and presented as histograms (examples in Figs. 70.5–70.8). The outlines of the histograms, the "skylines", can be considered as characteristic for the disease or disease category.

In addition, a computer program was developed to estimate post-MRI probabilities of white matter disorders in new patients. The computer program was based on Bayes' theorem. Prevalences of the different disease categories and subcategories and frequencies of image abnormalities per disease were estimated from the data of this study. In this way a differential diagnosis for new MRI patterns of white matter abnormalities could be obtained. For each possible diagnosis the positive predictive value and a two-sided 95% confidence interval could be computed.

Of course, there are several limitations to the practical use of a computer-assisted diagnostic system. The large amounts of data involved make clustering necessary; for example, a two-points scale (yes – no) had to be used instead of a three-points scale indicating the severity of involvement of the structures. Also, disease groups had to be clustered to some extent. This would seem to be sensible, because it is practically impossible to differentiate on MR criteria alone all individual conditions. Another limitation of such a computer pro-

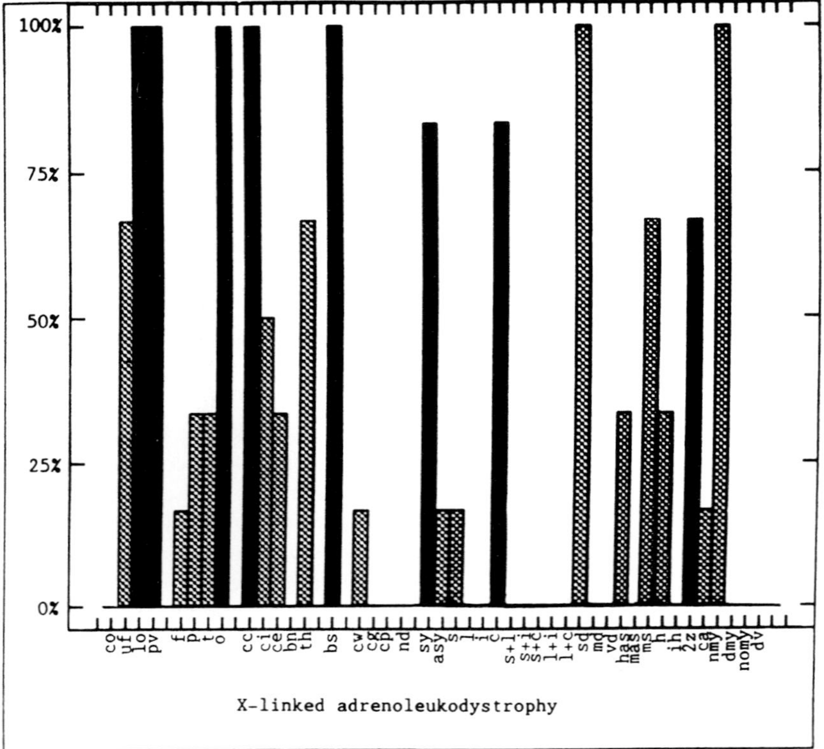

Fig. 70.5. Histogram showing the frequency of involvement of the structural elements for X-linked adrenodystrophy. (*co,* cortex; *uf,* arcuate fibers; *lo,* lobar white matter; *pv,* periventricular white matter; *f,* frontal; *p,* parietal; *t,* temporal; *o,* occipital; *cc,* corpus callosum; *ci,* internal capsule; *ce,* external and extreme capsules; *bn,* basal nuclei (globus pallidus, putamen, nucleus caudatus); *th,* thalamus; *bs,* brain stem; *cw,* cerebellar white matter; *cg,* cerebellar gray matter; *cp,* cerebellar pedunculi; *nd,* nucleus dentatus; *sy,* symmetrical distribution; *asy,* asymmetrical distribution; *s,* small isolated lesions; *l,* large isolated lesions; *i,* irregularly confluent lesions; *c,* highly confluent lesions; *sd,* sharp demarcation; *md,* mixed demarcation; *vd,* vague demarcation; *has,* highly abnormal signal intensity; *mas,* mildly abnormal signal intensity; *ms,* mixed signal intensity; *h,* homogeneous signal intensity; *ih,* inhomogeneous signal intensity; *2z,* two zones discernible in the lesion; *ca,* calcification; *nmy,* normal myelination; *dmy,* delayed myelination; *nomy,* no or hardly any myelin present; *dv,* deformation of the ventricular system)

gram is that its quality is highly dependent on the quantity and quality of the data it contains. To improve the quality of the program in this respect a multi-center data base with well-defined criteria for inclusion of cases would be extremely helpful in narrowing the confidence intervals in rare disorders.

Of course, such a computer system cannot compete with the flexibility and speed which the human brain possesses in pattern recognition. Computer systems are, therefore, not to be regarded as competitive, but as complementary: support to the experienced and learning tool for the inexperienced.

70.4 Practical Application of Pattern Recognition

Usually MR images are interpreted without the help of a computer program. However, in daily practice, our approach should also be systematical and we should progress logically through the diagnostic process. We will analyze the logical steps involved in systematically reading the MR image, well aware that several steps may occur synchronously and that the sequence is variable.

The first step identifies the nature of the cerebral abnormalities. In the analysis of MR images of the brain, the first consideration should concern the structures involved: gray matter, white matter or both. Subsequently, the examiner should try to identify the nature of the disorder with which he/she is confronted. If gray matter is involved, are there signs of a congenital anomaly with ectopic gray matter? Is there gray matter atrophy or are there parenchymatous lesions? If there is a white matter disorder, what is its nature? Is it demyelination, disturbed myelination, delayed myelination, or amyelination? Is there white matter swelling? Are there white matter cysts? Is there a loss of white matter volume or gliotic retraction?

Fig. 70.6. Histogram showing the frequency of involvement of the structural elements for Pelizaeus Merzbacher disease (for key to abbreviations, see Fig. 70.5)

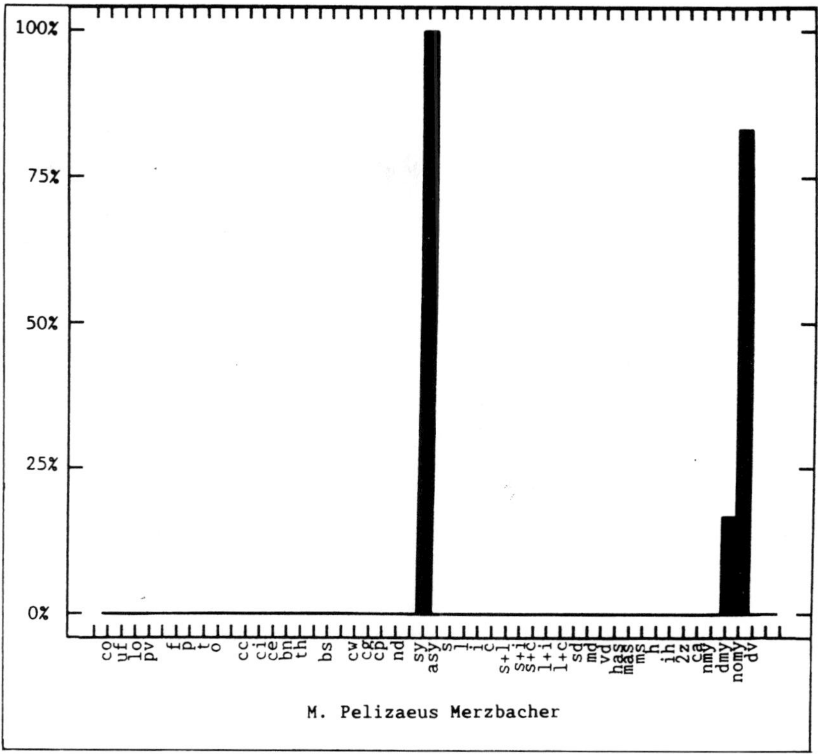

Fig. 70.7. Histogram showing the frequency of involvement of the structural elements for multiple sclerosis (for key to abbreviations, see Fig. 70.5)

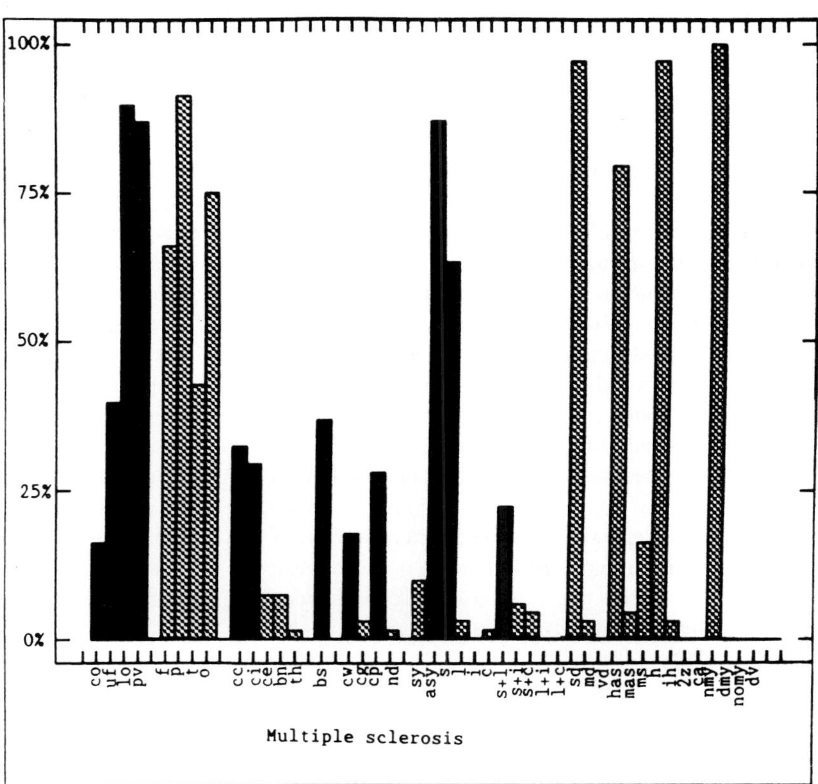

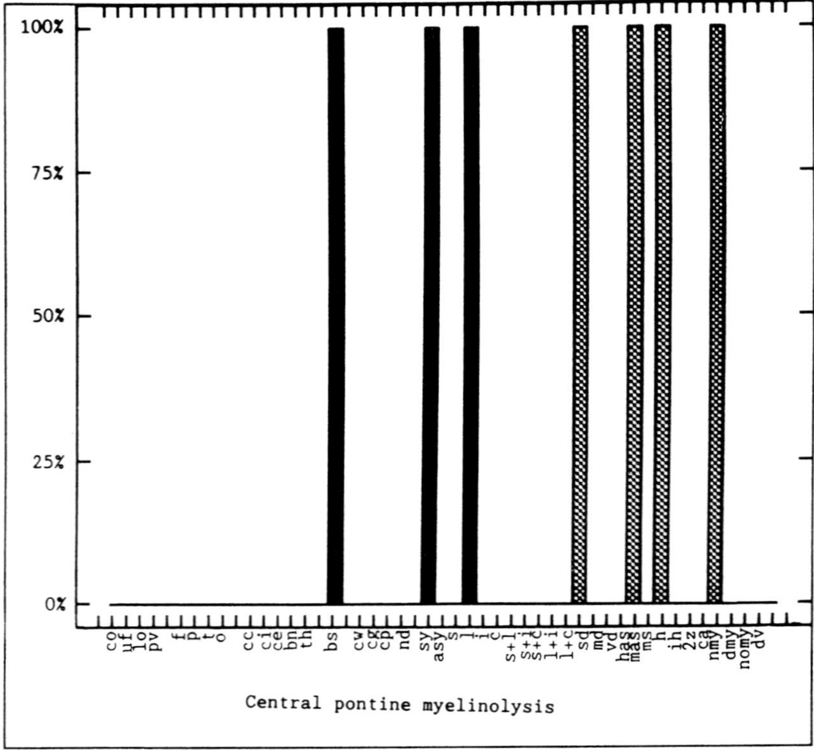

Fig. 70.8. Histogram showing the frequency of involvement of the structural elements for central pontine myelinolysis (for key to abbreviations, see Fig. 70.5)

The second step considers the symmetry or asymmetry of the cerebral abnormalities. Symmetrical white matter affection occurs in most of the inherited myelin disorders, toxic encephalopathies, and some of the other acquired white matter disorders. Many of the acquired disorders are asymmetrical, with some exceptions. A tendency towards symmetry is present in periventricular leukomalacia, subcortical arteriosclerotic encephalopathy and subacute HIV and CMV encephalitis.

The third step defines the aspect of the lesions. Are they confluent, isolated or both, diffuse or multiple? In the inherited myelin disorders lesions are often confluent and diffuse. Multiple sclerosis, of course, is the prototype of a disease with lesions which are usually asymmetrical, partly confluent, mostly isolated and confined to rather specific areas of the brain. Conditions that mimic multiple sclerosis will present similar findings and one has to look for other lesion characteristics.

The fourth step establishes the exact location of the lesions. Confluent, symmetrical lesions in the periventricular area narrow the number of diagnostic possibilities considerably. Sparing the arcuate fibers is characteristic for the sphingolipidoses, whereas the reverse is true for some of the organic and amino acidopathies, starting in the U fibers. Lesions confined to the cerebellar white matter are rare. Cerebrotendinous xanthomatosis, adrenomyeloneuropathy and Refsum disease are examples. Multiple sclerosis has preference for the upper edges of the lateral ventricles and the centrum semiovale. X-linked adrenoleukodystrophy usually presents in the occipital lobes; Schilder's disease in the fronto-parietal transition zone. Herpes simplex virus infections favor the frontal and temporal lobes.

The fifth step defines the pattern of spread of the disease. Adding the pattern of spread to the analysis further helps to distinguish certain entities. X-linked adrenoleukodystrophy usually spreads in a dorso-ventral direction; the direction of spread of Alexander's disease is ventro-dorsal, of Canavan's disease centrepetal, and of metachromatic leukodystrophy centrofugal. Of course, we are looking at major trends; there are exceptions to nearly all these usual patterns of spread.

The sixth step weighs the contribution of gray matter involvement relative to white matter involvement. Is the gray matter involvement a major or a minor part of the disease? Are cortical or central gray matter structures involved? Gray matter is often involved in mitochondrial disorders, in Binswanger's disease, in vasculitis, in glutaric aciduria type I and many other organic acidurias, in toxic encephalopathies such as carbon monoxide intoxication, cyanide intoxication, amphetamine-intoxication, and in posthypoxic-ischemic conditions. Involvement of the basal ganglia is rare in multiple sclerosis.

The seventh step evaluates whether the lesions en-

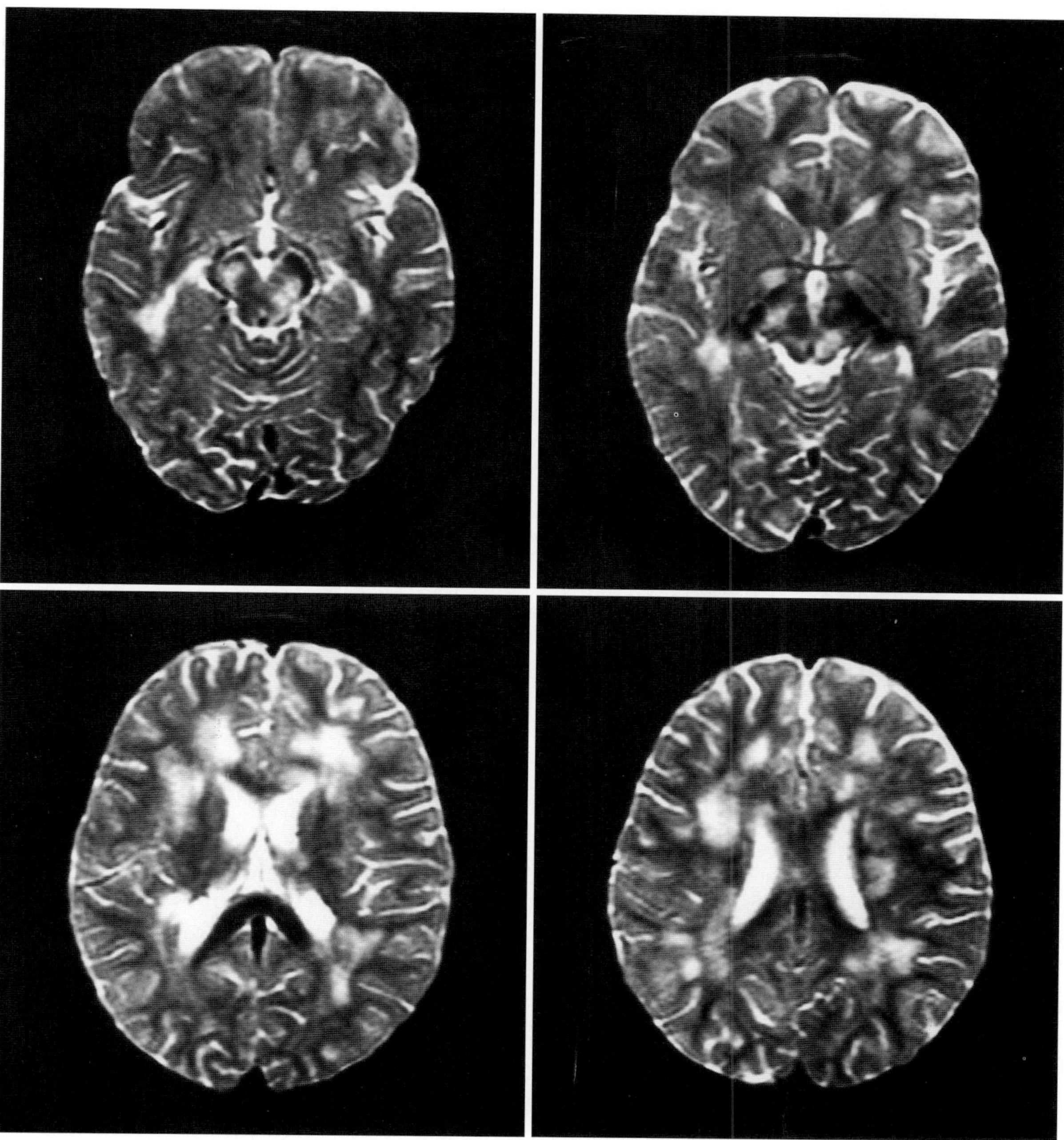

Fig. 70.9. Four T_2-weighted transverse images of a 5-year-old boy. (For details, see text)

hance after contrast injection. Sometimes enhancement of the active border of a lesion leads to a characteristic pattern, as in X-linked adrenoleukodystrophy, Schilder's diffuse sclerosis, and Alexander's disease. Active lesions in multiple sclerosis also enhance; in acute disseminated encephalomyelitis not all lesions enhance; in progressive multifocal leukoencephalitis enhancement occurs occasionally.

The following examples can be used as illustrations of the described approach.

Example I

Figure 70.9 shows four T_2-weighted transverse images of a 5-year-old boy starting at the level of the mesencephalon and moving upwards to the ventricular level. The first impression is that we are dealing with a disorder involving both white and gray matter, with preponderance of white matter involvement. Lesions are seen in the brain stem, the basal ganglia and around the ventricles. The lesions vary in size, are moderately

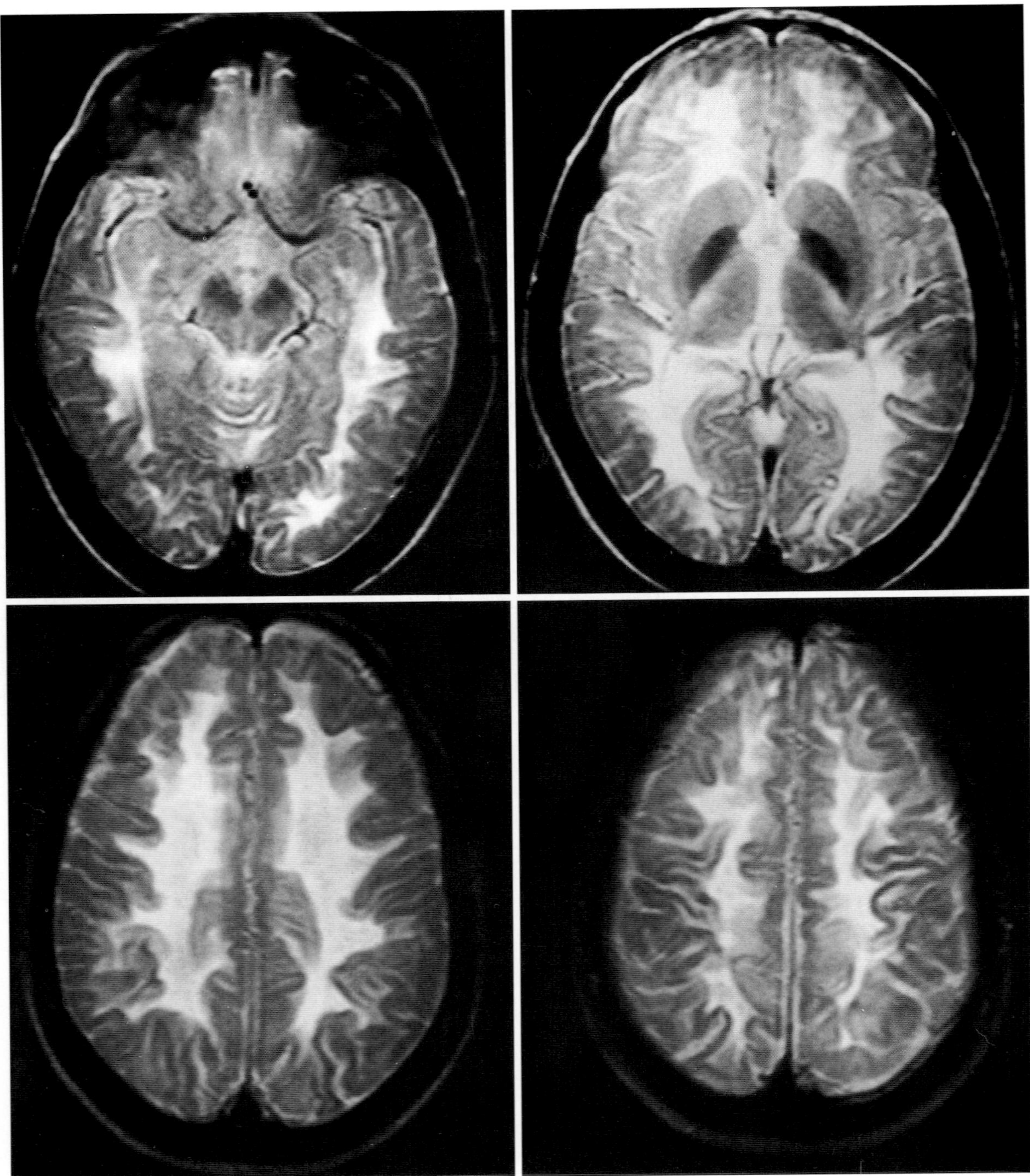

Fig. 70.10. Four T_2-weighted transverse images of a 16-year-old girl. (For details, see text)

sharply demarcated from the surrounding tissue and are asymmetric in distribution. The lesions in the white matter break into the normal pattern of myelination and therefore probably represent demyelination. This first impression rules out most of the hereditary metabolic disorders. Also the images do not suggest posthypoxic-ischemic encephalopathy. The asymmetry suggests the group of inflammatory-infectious disorders. This is a very heterogeneous group and only occassionally can one make a more precise diagnosis, when, for instance, the infection has a typical distribution as in subacute HIV encephalitis, in herpes simplex encephalitis, and in Cryptococcus neoformans infections. Also, the question whether we are dealing with a

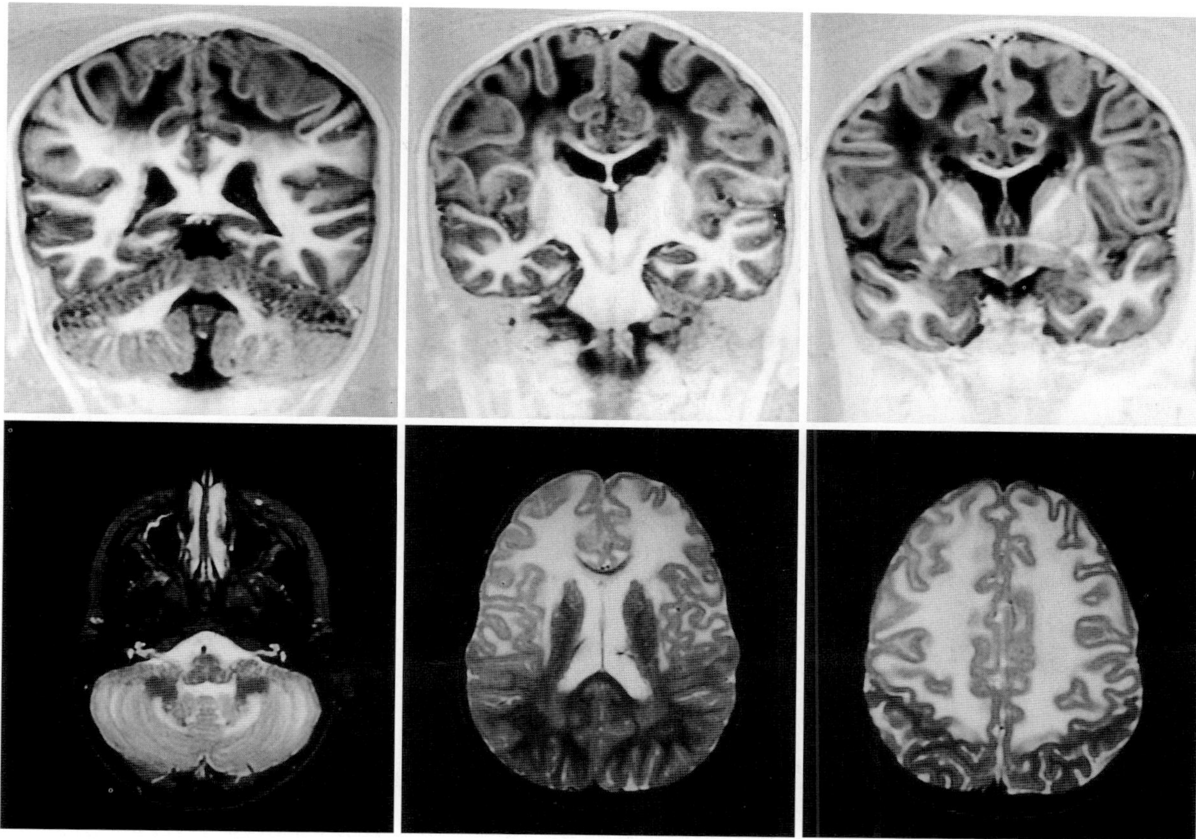

Fig. 70.11. Three T_1-weighted coronal images (*upper row*) and three T_2-weighted transverse images (*lower row*) from a 6-year-old boy. (For details see text)

noninfectious inflammatory disorder or with an infectious inflammatory disorder, cannot be answered from the images alone. Anti-Mycoplasma pneumoniae antibody titers rose to high values in this case. Mycoplasma pneumoniae infections are by no means rare and the cerebral involvement is probably an allergic-immunologic reaction, resulting in an acute disseminated encephalitis.

Example II

Figure 70.10 shows four T_2-weighted transverse images of a girl, 16 years of age, quite different from the previous example. The first impression is that of symmetrical involvement of the hemispheral white matter, relatively but not completely sparing the U fibers. This pattern suggests a demyelinating disorder. Further analysis establishes the confluency of the lesion, the spread from central areas to the periphery, the noninvolvement of the basal ganglia and mesencephalon. Although some infections (CMV, AIDS) have a pattern of symmetrical white matter involvement, the image is not really similar to this. The abnormality in signal

intensity is too severe. Evidently we have to classify this disorder under the toxic or inherited white matter disorders. Toxic disorders affecting the hemispheral white matter are known, but are rarely so extensive. Of the inherited disorders, the pattern shown in the images is seen in lysosomal disorders, especially in the sphingolipidoses.

Example III

Figure 70.11 shows three T_1-weighted coronal (IR) images are shown (upper row), together with three T_2-weighted transverse images (lower row), taken from a 6-year-old boy with macrocephaly and nonprogressive learning and behavioral problems. The images show a symmetrical involvement of the frontal white matter, with some swelling, involvement of the arcuate fibers, sparing of the corpus callosum, together with involvement of the corpus medullare of the cerebellum. There is a ventro-dorsal gradient. Categorical diagnosis would place this pattern in the toxic or hereditary group of disorders. Since toxins with this kind of selectivity are not presently known, an inherited disorder

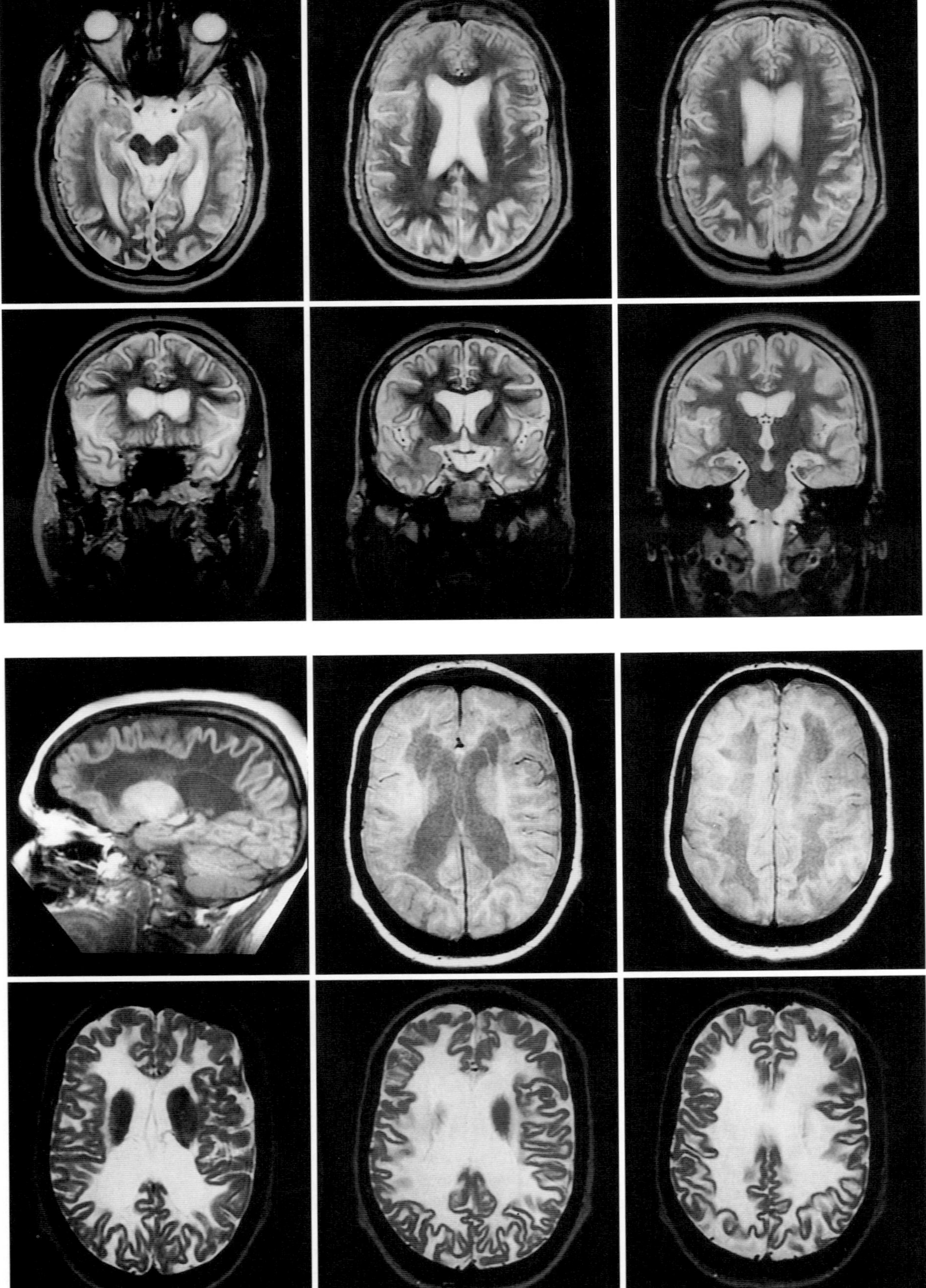

70.12

70.13

would appear to be top of the list in the differential diagnosis. Because of the spread of the disease and the suggestion of swelling, juvenile Alexander's disease must be considered, although the pattern is uncommon for that disease. Cerebellar involvement in Alexander's disease has been reported in the literature, but usually in more advanced cases. Congenital muscular dystrophy may present with similar findings, usually with less pronounced sparing of the occipital white matter. Muscular dystrophy, however, could not be found in this patient. Metabolic screening so far has not shown any positive finding.

Example IV

Figure 70.12 shows a 46-year-old woman with rapidly progressive dementia in the last year. CT scan was reported to be normal. On the T_2-weighted transverse and coronal images, thinning of the cortex is seen, with high signal intensity of the subcortical white matter. The ventricles are somewhat enlarged, in particular in the frontal and temporal region. The topographic distribution, and the combined cortical-subcortical pattern lead to the diagnosis Pick's disease, in agreement with the clinical presentation. In this disease there is a combination of cortical and subcortical gliosis in the frontal and temporal lobes, as known from histopathology.

Example V

Figure 70.13 shows MR images of a 18-year-old girl with a leukoencephalopathy with maximum in the fronto-parietal region. She is considerably disabled by spasticity and ataxia. Despite the severe "undercutting" of the cerebral cortex by the leukoencephalopathy, the mental functions are relatively well preserved. Her younger brother has an identical leukoencephalopathy. Metabolic screening was negative for all known hereditary disorders. Proton spectroscopy (Fig. 70.14) was performed using the PRESS sequence (TR 2500 ms, TE 13 ms) (a) and STEAM sequence (TR 2500 ms, TE 20 ms) (b and c). Spectra obtained from a large voxel (a,b), containing both gray and white matter, show a relatively normal pattern of N-acetylaspartate, choline and creatine. Lactate is present (inversed doublet at 1.33 ppm in a). Glutamine/glutamate (2.1–2.5 and 3.8 ppm in b), scyllo-inositol (3.35 ppm in b) and myo-inositol (3.56 ppm in b) are elevated. In the

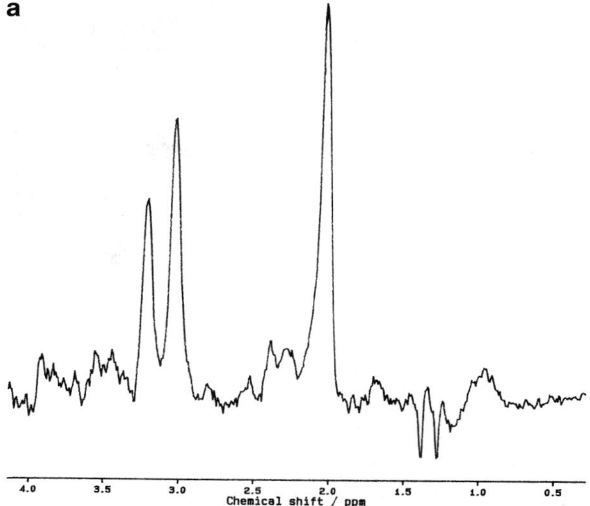

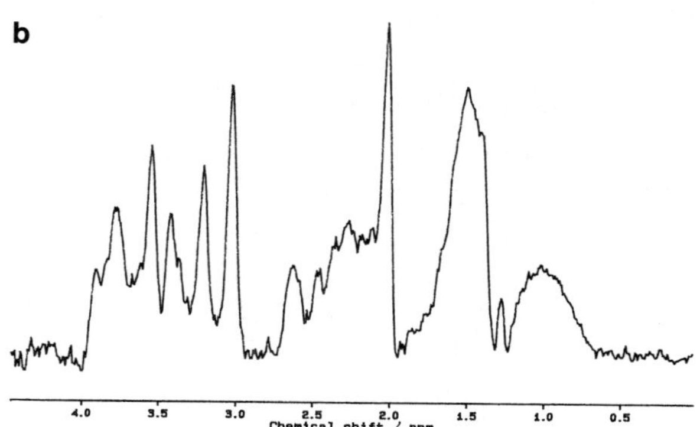

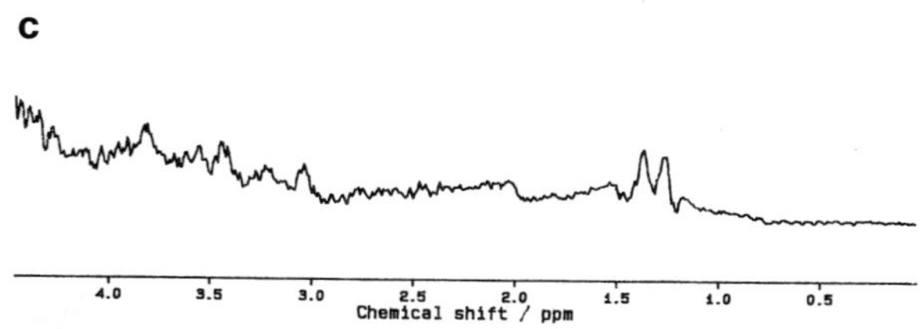

Fig. 70.14 a–c. Data from proton spectroscopy. (For details, see text)

STEAM spectrum from a small voxel, containing white matter only (c), most metabolite concentrations have decreased to a level which can no longer be detected by MRS. Only some signals from lactate (doublet at 1.33 ppm) and glucose (signals at 3.43 and 3.80 ppm) remain, probably present in the CSF. For comparable normal spectrum, see Chap. 71. Although this could be

Fig. 70.12. T_2-weighted transverse and coronal images from a 46-year-old woman. (For details, see text)

Fig. 70.13. MR images of an 18-year-old girl. (For details, see text)

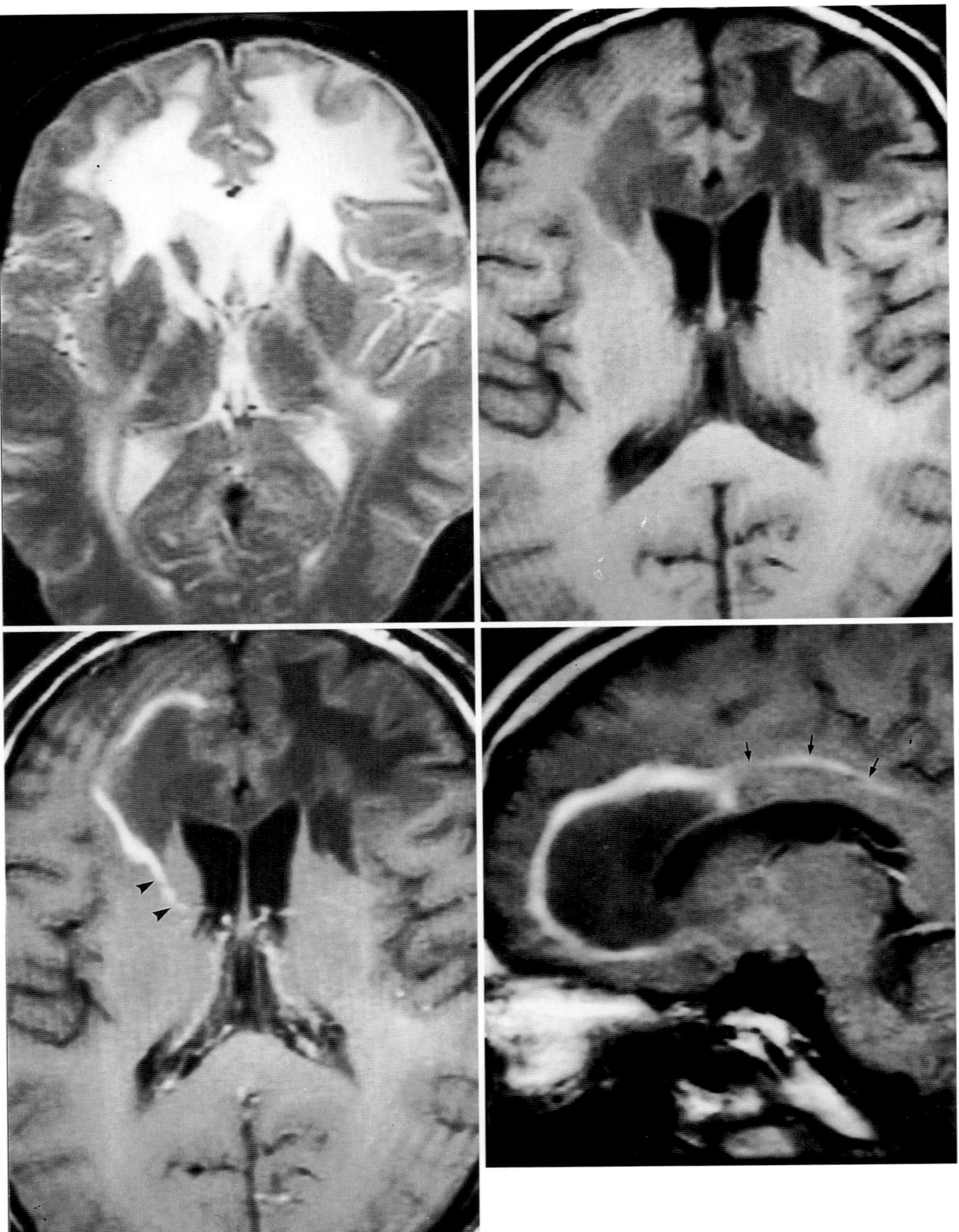

Fig. 70.15. Four MR images in a 6-year-old boy. (For details, see text)

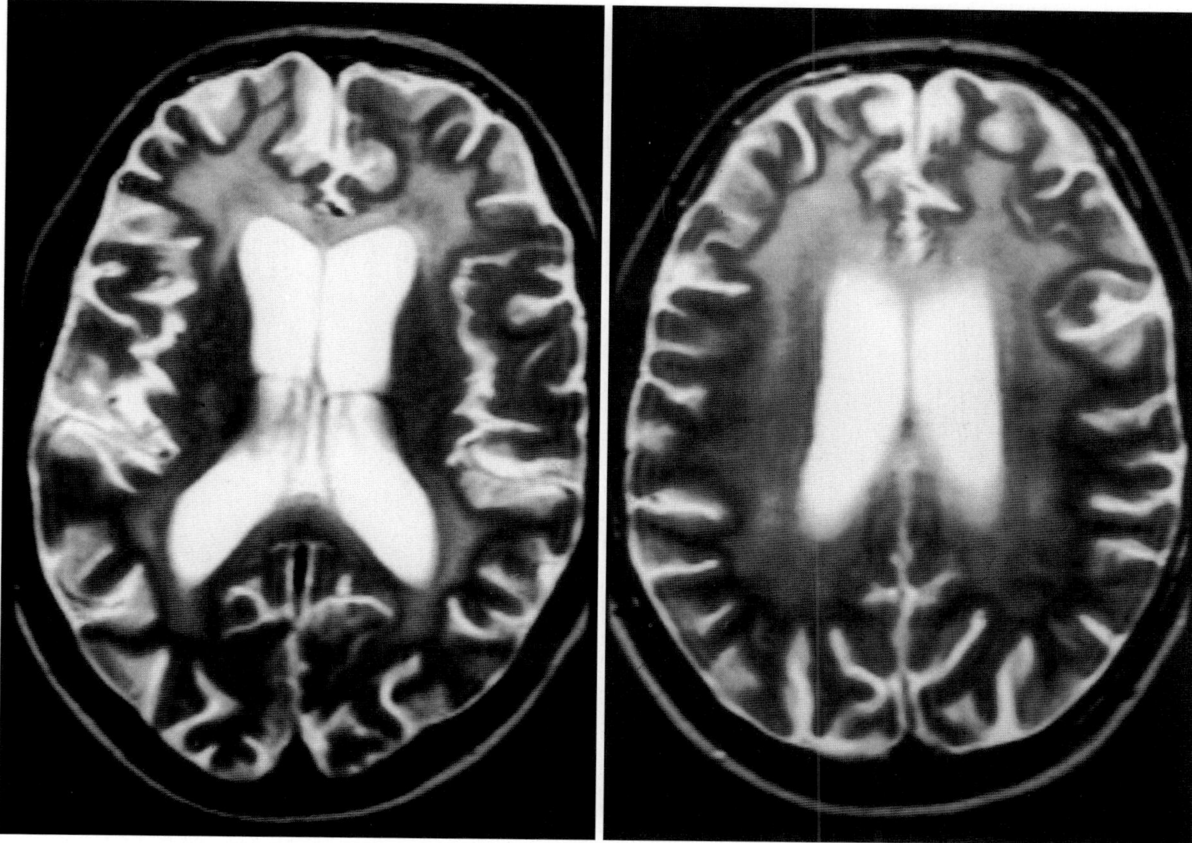

Fig. 70.16. T_2-weighted transverse images from a 36-year-old man. (For details, see text)

regarded as one of the (many) cases of unidentified leukodystrophy, similar cases have been described in the literature by Hahnefeld et al. (1993). Clustering these cases may eventually lead to the collection of sufficient data to classify this as a new entity, so that further work can be done on a larger group. See also Chapter 49.

Example VI

In the upper row of Fig. 70.15, a T_2- and T_1-weighted image show bilateral symmetric signal changes in the white matter, reaching into the arcuate fibers. There is also involvement of the anterior limb of the internal capsule, to a lesser extent of the posterior limb of the internal capsule and of the optic radiation. After contrast enhancement a very typical pattern of enhancement is seen around the lesion in the right frontal lobe, extending towards the anterior limb of the internal capsule (arrowheads) and along the cingular-callosal junction. The lesions are confluent, and have a ventrodorsal gradient. With this pattern only two diseases remain in this 6-year-old boy: Schilder's disease or X-

linked adrenoleukodystrophy. In X-linked adrenoleukodystrophy one could expect a dorso-ventral gradient; there are, however, many exceptions. Histologically Schilder's disease and X-linked adrenoleukodystrophy cannot be distinguished. In this case the laboratory data confirmed the diagnosis X-linked adrenoleukodystrophy. Courtesy Sartor and Meyding 1993, with permission.

Example VII

Figure 70.16 shows T_2-weighted transverse images of a 36-year-old male. The images show enlarged ventricles and also tissue loss at the brain surface. The frontal white matter has a high signal intensity, spreading in a dorsal direction. The white matter affection is symmetric, confluent, just leaving the U fibers intact, involves the corpus callosum and has a less high signal intensity than CSF. This white matter pattern can be seen in cytomegalovirus infections, in HIV-encephalitis and in some inherited leukodystrophies. The combination of atrophy, the mildly abnormal signal intensity and this

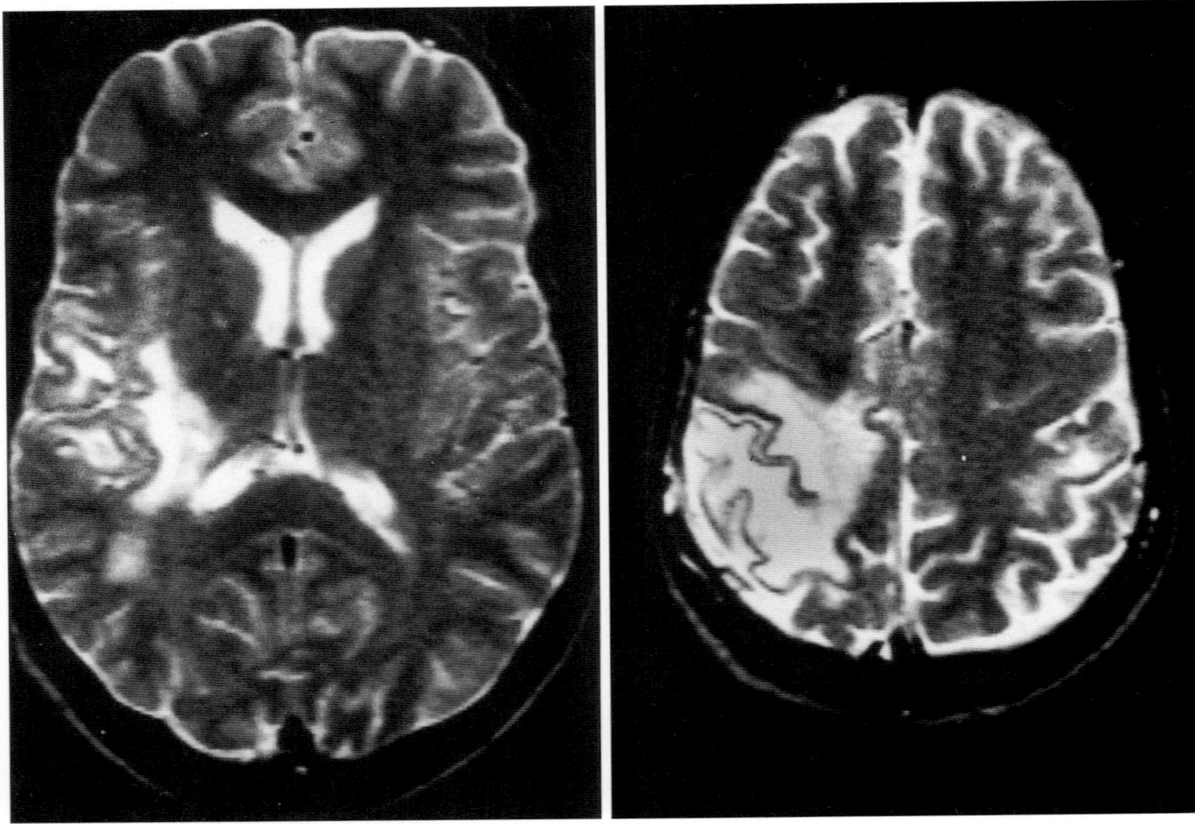

Fig. 70.17. T$_2$-weighted transverse images from an HIV-seropositive 42-year-old man

distribution of white matter involvement makes it highly suggestive of AIDS-encephalitis.

Example VIII

T$_2$-weighted transverse images of an HIV-seropositive 42-year-old man are shown in Fig. 70.17. The images show a large white matter lesion in the right posterior-temporal and parietal region and a smaller one in the left rolandic area. The U fibers are involved and there is a sharp demarcation between cortex and white matter. These features are highly suggestive of progressive multifocal leukoencephalitis. Other infections or acute disseminated encephalomyelitis are less probable: the involvement of gray matter is often more pronounced in acute disseminated encephalomyelitis and in most infections. Lesions in other infections are not usually limited to a small number of large foci.

71 Magnetic Resonance Spectroscopy, Basic Principles, and Application in Myelin Disorders

71.1 Basic Principles

In 1924, Pauli was the first to suggest that electrons spin at high speed. Because the spinning electrons have mass, they have a certain angular moment and, thus, as spinning electric charges, a magnetic moment. Later, it was observed that certain nuclei also have magnetic moments. What these nuclei have in common is the fact that they are isotopes with an odd atomic mass and/or odd atomic number, whereas nuclei with both an even atomic number and atomic mass do not have a magnetic moment. Subsequently it was noted that when these nuclei are placed in a powerful magnetic field, they show a precessional motion about the axis of the field. In 1946, Bloch et al. and Purcell et al. simultaneously discovered the possibility of resonant energy absorption and emission of precessing nuclei, the basis of magnetic resonance imaging (MRI) and of spectroscopy (MRS). For this work they were awarded the Nobel Prize in 1952. MRS has developed into a very important tool in molecular chemistry and physics to reveal molecular structure, chemical reaction rates, and diffusion processes. The first spectroscopy experiments on living systems were performed on small-bore systems with tiny objects, such as red blood cells and excised tissue. Wider bores have since been developed, allowing the study of muscle disorders and experimental work with small animals. Subsequently, in vivo MRS of human brain and other organs has also become possible.

Atomic nuclei are composed of protons and neutrons. These nuclear particles exhibit spin. A proton is positively charged, and this spinning charge generates a small magnetic field. Although a neutron is electrically neutral, its component electrical charges are not uniformly distributed within its volume, and thus the neutron also generates a magnetic field when spinning, but smaller than that produced by a spinning proton. The magnetic moments of these particles are directed randomly, and they cancel each other out in nuclei with an even number of protons and neurons. When the nucleus has an odd number of neutrons and/or protons, the nucleus has a net spin, and this spinning charge has a magnetic moment. These nuclei exhibit the magnetic resonance phenomenon. Nuclei of interest for in vivo spectroscopy are ^{1}H, ^{31}P, ^{23}Na, and also ^{13}C, ^{17}O, and ^{19}F as markers of biochemically interesting compounds. If there is no external magnetic field, the nuclear magnetic moments have a random direction and there is no net magnetic vector. The intrinsic magnetic phenomena can be detected by applying an external magnetic field. The nuclear magnetic moments tend to align themselves parallel or antiparallel to the external magnetic field. On the other hand, however, nuclei tend to be in constant random motion due to thermal effects. The percentage of nuclei that align with the external magnetic field depends on the strength of the magnetic field relative to the random thermal effects. Slightly more nuclei align with the external magnetic field than against it, because the first position is more stable than the second. Stability is related to the amount of energy that a nucleus possesses. Stability is greater at low energy levels. In fact, there is a continuous transition of nuclei between high- and low-energy positions, but there is a slight net surplus in the low energy position ($1:10^5$ at 1.5 T).

A spinning nucleus precesses about the axis of the magnetic field. This motion is called Larmor precession, and its frequency the Larmor frequency. The Larmor frequency (ω) depends on the magnetic field strength H_o and characteristics of the particular nucleus, as expressed in the gyromagnetic ratio γ. This dependency is represented in the Larmor equation $\omega = \gamma\, H_o$. Resonance is a property of physical systems to oscillate at a preferred frequency which is characteristic of the system. The characteristic frequency is referred to as resonance frequency. The most efficient energy transfer to atomic particles precessing in magnetic fields occurs in their resonance frequency, the Larmor frequency. For magnetic field strengths used in MRS these resonance frequencies are within the radio frequency (RF) band of the electromagnetic spectrum. A short burst of radio frequent energy is known as an RF pulse. When an RF pulse is administered, this energy is absorbed, and more nuclei move into the high-energy position. When the RF pulse is terminated, the nuclei return to equilibrium and energy is released at the same frequency. The RF signal emitted can be detected.

The basis of MRS is the chemical shift phenomenon. The atomic nucleus is surrounded by an electron cloud and other atomic nuclei. If an external magnetic field is applied, precession is also induced in this electron cloud resulting in a small magnetic field. This small magnetic field has an influence on the atomic nucleus and modifies the effect of the external magnetic field at the site of the nucleus. Because of this slight change in the local magnetic field, the nucleus resonates at a slightly different frequency. This shift in frequency is called chemical shift. The chemical shift is determined by the electrochemical environment of the resonating nucleus, and therefore the precise shift is characteristic of a particular atomic nucleus in a particular compound. The band width of the RF pulse, of course, must contain all the frequencies that are necessary to excite the particular atomic nucleus in compounds of interest. The radio frequent signal, which is obtained in an MRS experiment, contains many slightly different frequencies. Fourier transformation of the signal transforms a time versus amplitude display into a frequency versus amplitude display. The resulting spectrum depicts all the nuclear resonance frequencies as a function of their amplitude. Each peak in the spectrum represents the atomic nucleus in a particular compound. The area under each peak is proportional to the number of nuclei producing that peak. MR spectra can be calibrated to yield absolute concentrations of the metabolites represented. The chemical shift depends on the magnetic field strength. However, in MRS the resonance frequencies are not expressed in absolute units (Hertz) but in relative units (parts per million, ppm) related to the resonance frequency of a given reference compound. The relative units, ppm, are independent of magnetic field strength. In this way the results obtained in experiments which are performed at different magnetic field strengths become directly comparable.

MRS methods are relatively insensitive. Weak MR signals are measured from relatively low-concentration compounds. It is therefore essential to use MR instruments with optimal technical equipment to ascertain an optimal primary sensitivity. The magnetic field should be extremely homogeneous over the volume analyzed. Any significant inhomogeneity in the magnetic field spreads out and blurs chemical shift spectral lines due to the spread of Larmor frequencies across the volume. The resulting spectral line broadening is undesirable because it reduces the signal to noise ratio and hampers the ability to distinguish two closely neighboring resonance lines. The frequencies and frequency separations increase linearly with field strength. High magnetic field strengths are therefore necessary to optimize spectral resolution. High spectral resolution is particulary important for proton spectroscopy, where most interest is focussed on metabolites with a narrow chemical shift range, and where the peaks of the metabolites often overlap. For MRS in human beings, a magnetic field strength of 1.5–2 T is used. In experimental work with animals, magnetic field strengths of 4–8 T or even higher are preferred. A further improvement of the spectral signal to noise ratio is obtained by signal averaging. For purposes of cleaning the final spectrum or obviating unwanted resonances, the spectroscopist has access to many suppression and editing techniques.

MRS requires concentrations at least in the millimolar range. Many important but too diluted compounds have until now remained undetectable by in vivo MRS. In addition, only molecules sufficiently small and mobile to tumble freely render MR signals useful for in vivo work. No useful signals can be obtained from large molecules such as proteins, even soluble ones, nor from most membrane compounds or small molecules bound to larger ones. The broadening of sprectral lines makes differentiation of these molecules impossible.

For in vivo MRS it is important that a volume of interest can be selected from which the spectrum is derived. A simple and commonly used technique is the placement of a surface coil over the volume of interest. The spatial definition of such coils is rather poor since the intensity of signal reception decreases with distance. Several techniques have been devised to improve the spatial response of surface coils and to make positioning of the volume of interest more accurate. A major disadvantage remains, i.e., that surface coils are only suitable for volumes of interest near the surface. Image-localized spectroscopy by gradient control allows direct and precise definition of a volume of interest on a proton image. Major advantages are the possibility to select volumes located in the deeper parts of the brain and the possibility to define a volume of interest guided by the abnormalities seen on the image, avoiding contamination of the spectrum by signals from undesired regions.

The nuclei that one would like to observe can be selected by using the appropriate RF pulse. MRI most commonly makes use of the magnetic properties of protons and is in fact ^{1}H MRI. The protons that contribute to the signal intensity on the images are mainly present in water. MRS, however, focusses not only on protons (^{1}H MRS), but also on phosphorus (^{31}P MRS)

Table 71.1. Resonance frequencies and relative MR sensitivities at 1.5 T

Nucleus	Larmor frequency in MHz	Relative MR sensitivity
^{1}H	63.86	1
^{31}P	25.85	0.066
^{19}F	60.08	0.83
^{23}Na	16.89	0.093
^{13}C	16.06	0.016

and, less frequently, on other nuclei such as ^{19}F, ^{23}Na, and ^{13}C. In human tissues, these nuclei are present in much lower concentrations in human tissues than protons, and the overall sensitivity of the nuclei is much lower than that of water protons. Table 71.1 lists the resonant frequencies and relative MR sensitivities of various nuclei at a magnetic field strength of 1.5 T.

71.2 Metabolites

In a spectrum from the human brain, ^{31}P MRS reveals seven major peaks (Fig. 71.1): phosphomonoesters (PME), inorganic phosphate (Pi), phosphodiesters (PDE), phosphocreatine (PCr), and the γ, α, and β phosphate groups of adenosine triphosphate (ATP), resonating at 6.5, 4.9, 2.6, 0, –2.6, –8.0 and –16.5 ppm, respectively. ADP contributes to the γ and α-ATP peaks. NAD and NADH contribute to the α-ATP peak.

The main component of the PME peak is phosphoethanolamine. Other components are phosphocholine, glycerol-3-phosphate and sugar phosphates. Minor components are phosphoserine and phosphoinositol. Phosphoethanolamine is a precursor in the anabolism of phosphatidylethanolamine and a product in the catabolism of sphingomyelin. Phosphocholine is a precursor of phosphatidylcholine and sphingomyelin and a product in the catabolism of sphingomyelin. Glycerol-3-phosphate is a precursor of phosphatidylethanolamine, phosphatidylcholine and plasmalogens and a product in the catabolism of the same compounds. The PME peak is elevated in all rapidly growing tissues with rapid membrane synthesis, such as tumors and the growing brain. It is probable that the elevation is caused by the enhanced presence of compounds meant for the production of membrane phospholipids. Generally, the PME peak is considered to reflect phospholipid anabolic activity. This notion has been confirmed by the finding that the level of PME is linearly correlated with the rate of phospholipid synthesis.

The ^{31}P spectrum of the brain contains a large, broad peak centered in the PDE region, underlying the remainder of the spectrum (Fig. 71.2). This large, broad peak originates from large, relatively immobile membrane phospholipids. This broad component is commonly removed from the spectrum by filtering techniques as a standard processing procedure. The remaining PDE peak contains mainly contributions from more mobile phospholipids and relatively minor contributions from phospholipid breakdown products, including glycerophosphocholine and glycerophosphoethanolamine, freely soluble molecules. These latter compounds are catabolic products of phosphatidylcholine, phosphatidylethanolamine and plasmalogens.

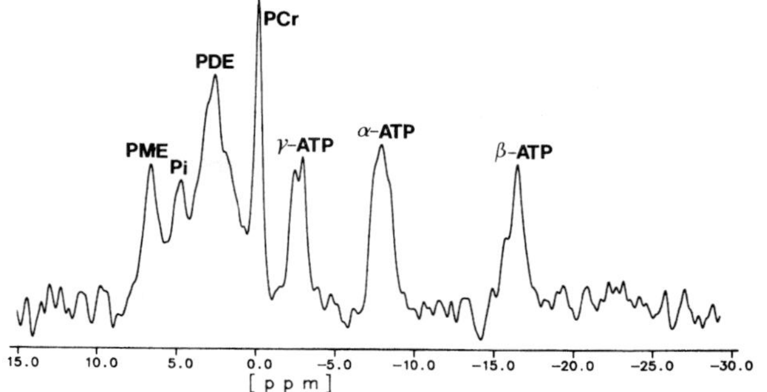

Fig. 71.1. ^{31}P spectrum of the human brain

The ^{31}P spectrum contains multiple peaks representing high-energy phosphorus compounds (ATP and PCr) and Pi. Intracellular PCr acts via the creatine kinase reaction as a buffer to maintain a constant ATP level in the face of variable energy demands. In conditions of decreasing ATP, PCr reacts with ADP to produce ATP and creatine with creatine kinase as catalyzing enzyme. The reaction is reversible and PCr can be resynthesized from creatine and ATP. This so-called creatine phosphate shuttle facilitates energy distribution and responds to energy demands. The PCr/Pi ratio is often used as a measure of the energy status of the brain. The ATP level only drops when PCr is exhausted. In view of the metabolic stability of ATP, it has often been used as an internal reference for quantitation. In particular the β-ATP peak, which does not contain any contributions of other compounds known to be present in brain tissue in significant amounts, is used as a reference.

The chemical shift of Pi relative to PCr is a function of pH. The pH determines the relative amounts of $H_2PO_4^-$, and HPO_4^{2-} in the equilibrium $H_2PO_4^- \Leftrightarrow HPO_4^{2-} + H^+$, and the precise resonance frequency of Pi as a whole. Using the equation of Petroff et al. (1985), the pH can be deduced from the chemical shift of Pi relative to PCr. This pH holds for the compartment in which these phosphates are present, which in the brain is the intracellular compartment.

Peak assignment in ^{1}H spectroscopy is more problematic because of overlapping. Straightforward assignment is possible for the singlet methyl resonances of N-acetylaspartate (NAA) at 2.02 ppm, total creatine (Cr), including free creatine and phosphocreatine, at 3.02 ppm, and choline-containing compounds (Cho) at 3.22 ppm. Since these metabolite resonances exhibit relatively long T_2 relaxation times, they may be specified in spectra at long echo times (135 or 270 ms) (Fig. 71.3). When shorter echo times (15–30 ms) are used, a considerably increased number of resonances with short T_2 relaxation times can be visualized (Fig. 71.4). Most obvious are the appearance of the

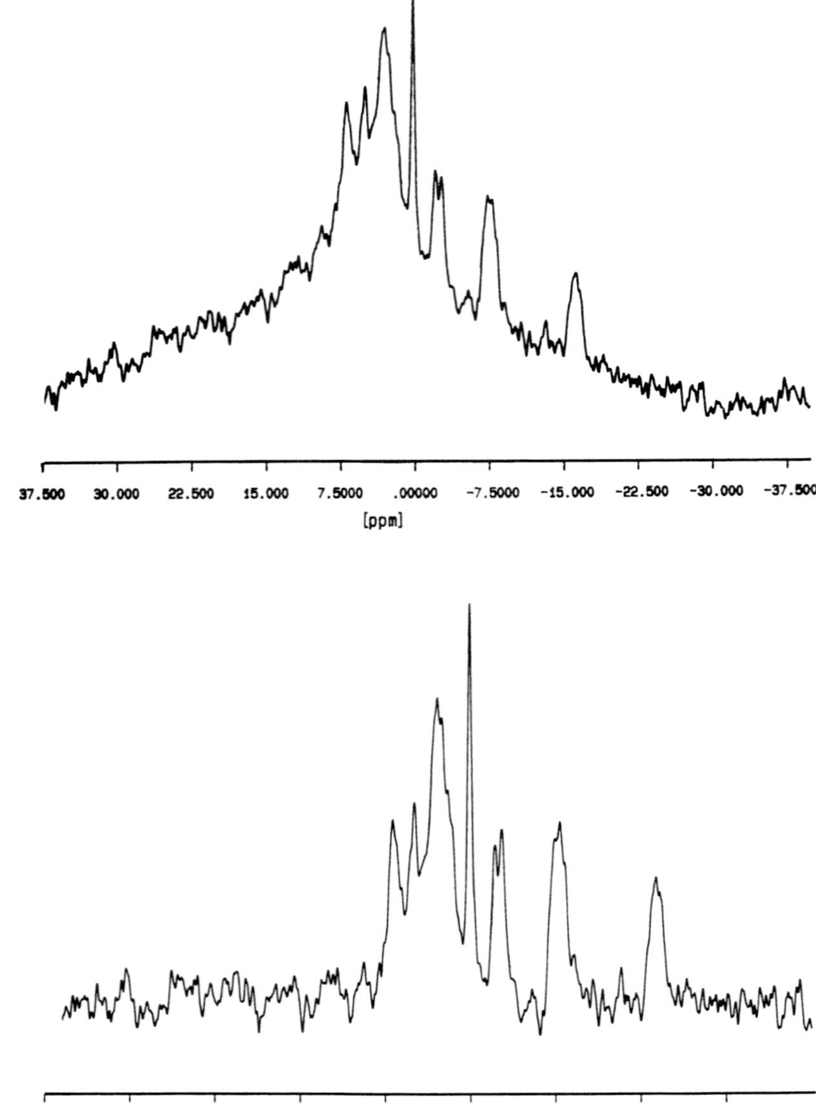

Fig. 71.2. An unfiltered ^{31}P spectrum of the brain at the *top*. The same spectrum after filtering *below*

methylene singlet resonance of Cr at 3.94 ppm and a strong signal from multiple collapsed resonances of myo-inositol (mI) at 3.56 ppm. A complex pattern of coupled resonances between 2.1 and 2.5 ppm together with a further group of resonances around 3.8 ppm are assigned to glutamine and glutamate. Resonances of γ-amino butyric acid (GABA) are overlapped by the larger resonances of Cr, glutamate and NAA (GABA resonances at 1.90, 2.30 and 3.03 ppm). Special techniques are necessary to quantify glutamine, glutamate and GABA separately. Additional resonances are seen originating from the aspartyl group of NAA (2.48, 2.60 and 2.66 ppm), glucose (3.43 and 3.80 ppm) and scyl-

lo-inositol (3.35 ppm). The glycine peak (3.55 ppm) overlaps with the mI peak; the taurine peak (3.35 ppm) overlaps with scyllo-inositol. Lactate is not usually visible under normal conditions, but can be visualized as a doublet centered at 1.33 ppm if elevated. In case of elevated tissue levels of free lipids, for instance as a result of myelin breakdown or spectral contamination by fat from the skull, broad resonances are seen at 0.9 and 1.3 ppm originating from the methyl and methylene groups of the lipids.

NAA is a compound found in high concentration in the CNS, whereas only traces are found in other tissues. In the mature brain NAA is confined to neurons. In cell

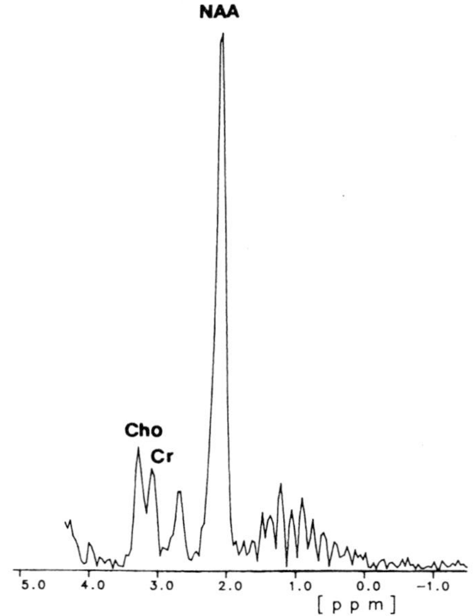

Fig. 71.3. ^{1}H spectrum acquired with a long echo time of 270 ms

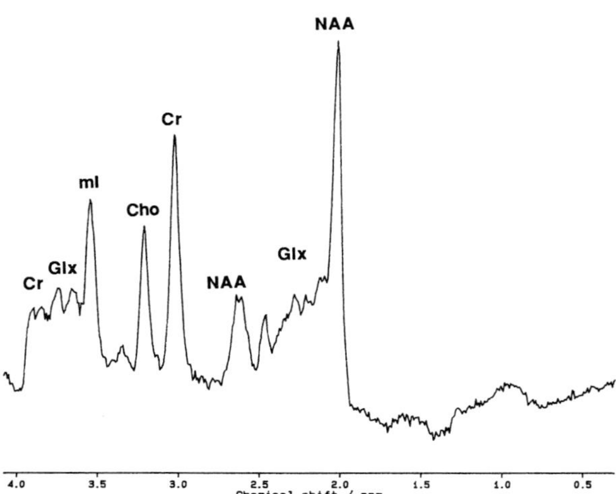

Fig. 71.4. Short echo time (20 ms) ^{1}H spectrum. *Glx* stands for glutamine and glutamate

cultures NAA has also been demonstrated in oligodendroglial precursor cells. Little is known about its role in normal function or disease states. Possible functions include a role as precursor of the putative neurotransmitter N-acetylaspartylglutamate, as storage form of the neurotransmitter aspartate, as acetyl donor in lipid synthesis (important in myelin synthesis), as stabilizer of the concentration of acetyl-CoA, or as having a role in osmotic regulation or protein synthesis. N-acetylaspartyl glutamate co-resonates with the acetyl group of NAA at 2.02 ppm and is responsible for about 10%–20% of the NAA peak. NAA is usually considered as a

neuronal marker. In disease conditions NAA is often low, related to neuronal dysfunction or loss. As some recovery of NAA level has been described in improving cerebral disorders, it is not correct to interpret a decrease in NAA as a straightforward indication of irreversible neuronal loss. In one disorder, Canavan disease, a relative elevation of NAA is present due to a disturbance of its breakdown. The relationship between accumulation of NAA and vacuolating myelinopathy, as occurs in Canavan disease, has not been elucidated.

The Cr peak represents the total amount of creatine and phosphocreatine present in the creatine kinase shuttle. The total creatine pool remains rather constant under a variety of conditions. For this reason Cr has often been used as internal reference for quantitation. However, since Cr is not constant under all conditions, other means of referencing are preferable.

The Cho peak contains contributions from various compounds. The largest contribution to the peak comes from choline-containing phospholipids, including sphingomyelin and phosphatidylcholine. Water soluble choline-containing compounds in the brain, including choline, glycerophosphocholine, phosphocholine, and acetylcholine, are responsible for a smaller part of the peak. Elevated Cho is seen in conditions of enhanced membrane turnover, such as brain growth, myelination, demyelination, inflammation and tumor growth.

Lactate occupies a special position in energy metabolism. Being the end-product of glycolysis, it must rise in concentration whenever the glycolytic rate in a volume of tissue exceeds the tissue's capacity to catabolize lactate or export it to the blood stream. Lactate levels are increased under conditions of anaerobic glycolysis, for example in failure of energy supply or a respiratory chain defect.

Glutamate is the most important excitatory neurotransmitter, whereas GABA, formed by decarboxylation from glutamate, is the most important inhibitory neurotransmitter. In the presynaptic neuron glutamine is converted to glutamate and ammonia by glutaminase. Glutamate can either be converted to GABA by glutamic acid decarboxylase or be released in the synaptic cleft. After release by the presynaptic neuron, glutamate is taken up by the astrocyte in which it is processed by glutamine synthetase into glutamine, which is transported back to the presynaptic neuron. This cycle operates between the presynaptic neuron, the neuronal cleft, and the astrocyte. Hyperammonemia has a great impact on this cycle by stimulating glutamine synthesis via glutamine synthetase, by possible inhibition of glutaminase, and by inhibition of glutamate re-uptake by the astrocyte. In hyperammonemia glutamate decreases, glutamine increases. Glutamate may be elevated in conditions of active tis-

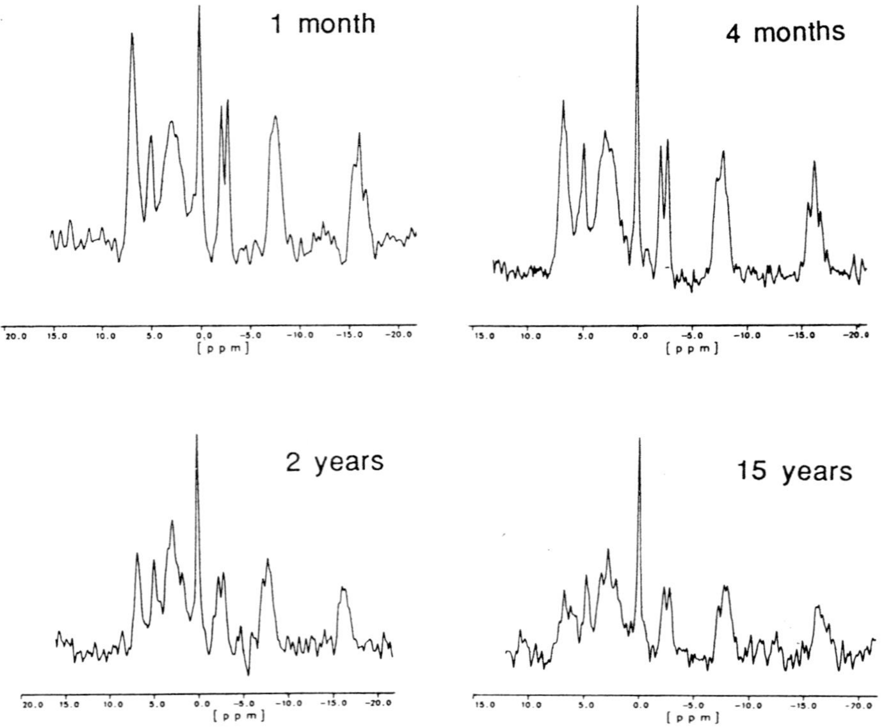

Fig. 71.5. Four ^{31}P spectra of the brain obtained at different ages after birth at term. Note the decrease in PME and increase in PDE and PCr relative to β-ATP with increasing age

sue damage, such as hypoxia-ischemia, as one of the so-called excitatory amino acids. Apart from its role as neurotransmitter and precursor of GABA, glutamate is important as a Krebs cycle component via α-ketoglutarate. Considering its predominantly glial localization, glutamine may be considered a glial marker.

The mI peak is also a composite peak, containing contributions from myo-inositol as main component, and, additionally, inositol monophosphate, phosphatidyl inositol (a membrane phospholipid), and inositol diphosphate as minor components. Inositol diphosphate is, however, a very important component, functioning as a second or third messenger for various hormone actions. Inositol diphosphate is active in releasing calcium from the endoplasmic reticulum and mitochondria. Many enzymes are dependent upon the inositol induced calcium release. The function of myo-inositol itself is still largely unknown, but it may be the storage form of the inositol-dependent messenger system. Another function of myo-inositol may be that of osmoregulator. In diabetes mellitus, inositol phosphate has been considered as a mediator of some of the secondary complications, in particular polyneuropathy. In galactosemia some of the late complications have been attributed to depletion of myo-inositol. Also in hepatic encephalopathy a depletion of myo-inositol is seen. The glial specificity of mI is under discussion; some

consider mI to be glial marker. Scyllo-inositol is a stereoisomer of mI.

Taurine is a key component of the cytosol buffer and serves to optimize cytosol buffering capacity at physiological pH. It is involved in neurotransmission, osmoregulation and brain growth. It controls magnesium homeostasis and calcium homeostasis.

71.3 Normal Values: Age-dependency and Regional Variability

The major biochemical changes related to processes of brain maturation are reflected in spectroscopic changes (Figs. 71.5–71.7).

The most striking finding in ^{31}P MRS of neonatal brain is a very high PME peak, in particular in fetuses and preterm babies in whom the PME peak is higher than all other peaks in the spectrum. Relative to β-ATP, PME decreases with ongoing brain maturation, to reach final values at about 2 years of age. Also when absolute metabolite concentrations are obtained, PME is shown to decrease with increasing age. The elevation of the PME peak in early development is largely attributable to elevation of phosphoethanolamine. The elevation of the PME peak can be attributed to active membrane phospholipid synthesis, mostly active

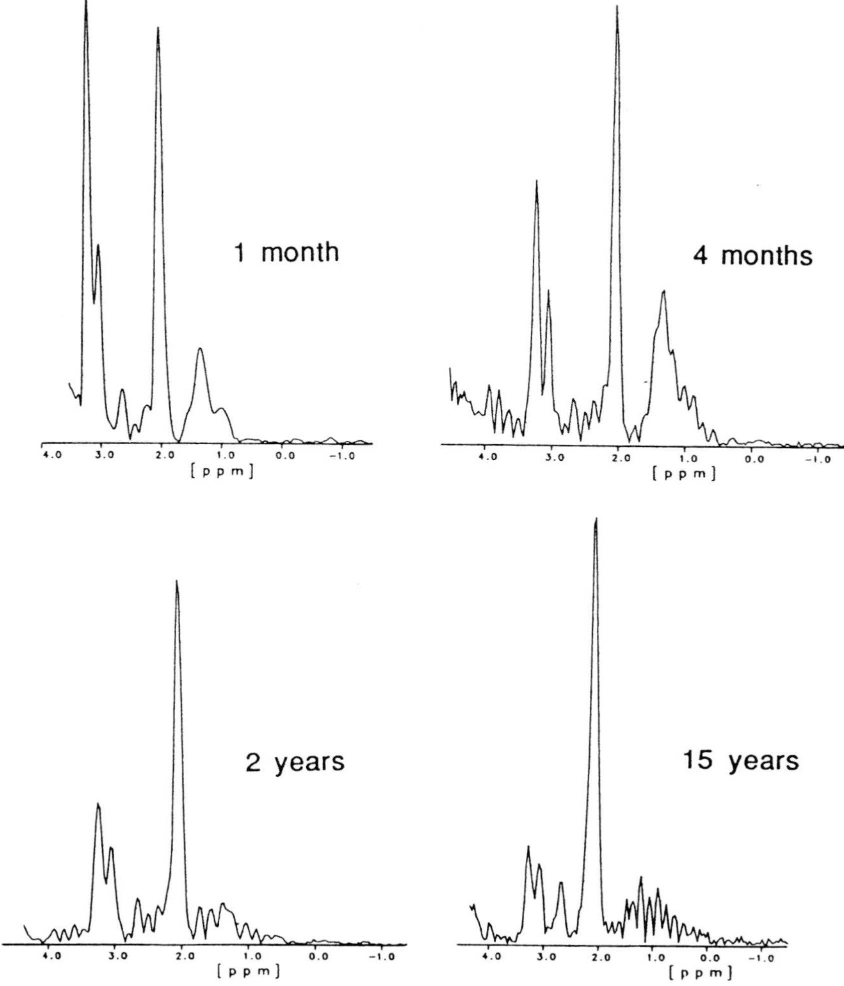

Fig. 71.6. Four ^{1}H spectra of the brain acquired using a long echo time of 270 ms and obtained at different ages after birth at term. Note the increase in NAA and decrease in Cho relative to Cr with increasing age

myelination. Myelination is almost completed at the age of 2 years.

PDE is very low in fetal brain. PDE increases with ongoing brain maturation, but is still relatively low in term neonates. The ratio PDE/β-ATP and absolute concentrations of PDE increase with age. Final values are reached at the age of about 2 years. PDE originates to a large extent from phospholipids and to a smaller extent from low molecular weight soluble metabolites in phospholipid breakdown. The increase in PDE with increasing brain maturation is most probably primarily related to the increasing membrane density of the brain, to a large extent caused by progressing myelination. With increasing membrane content, membrane turnover also increases and accordingly the concentration of intermediary products of phospholipid breakdown, contributing to the height of the PDE peak.

The ratio PME/PDE can be used as a maturation index for brain development.

There are major changes in energy metabolism related to brain maturation. On the basis of findings in animal experimental research it is usually assumed that the cerebral concentration of ATP, reflected in β-ATP, does not change with age and is constant irrespective of maturational stage. However, recently some evidence was provided by Buchli et al. (1994) that the ATP concentration in human brain increases with age. Relative to β-ATP, PCr increases rapidly after birth and final values are reached after a few months. Pi/β-ATP does not undergo significant changes. Buchli et al. (1994), using absolute quantitative data, found some postnatal increase in Pi, a more marked increase in PCr and some increase in ATP. Evidence has been found for a maturational increase in the creatine kinase reaction

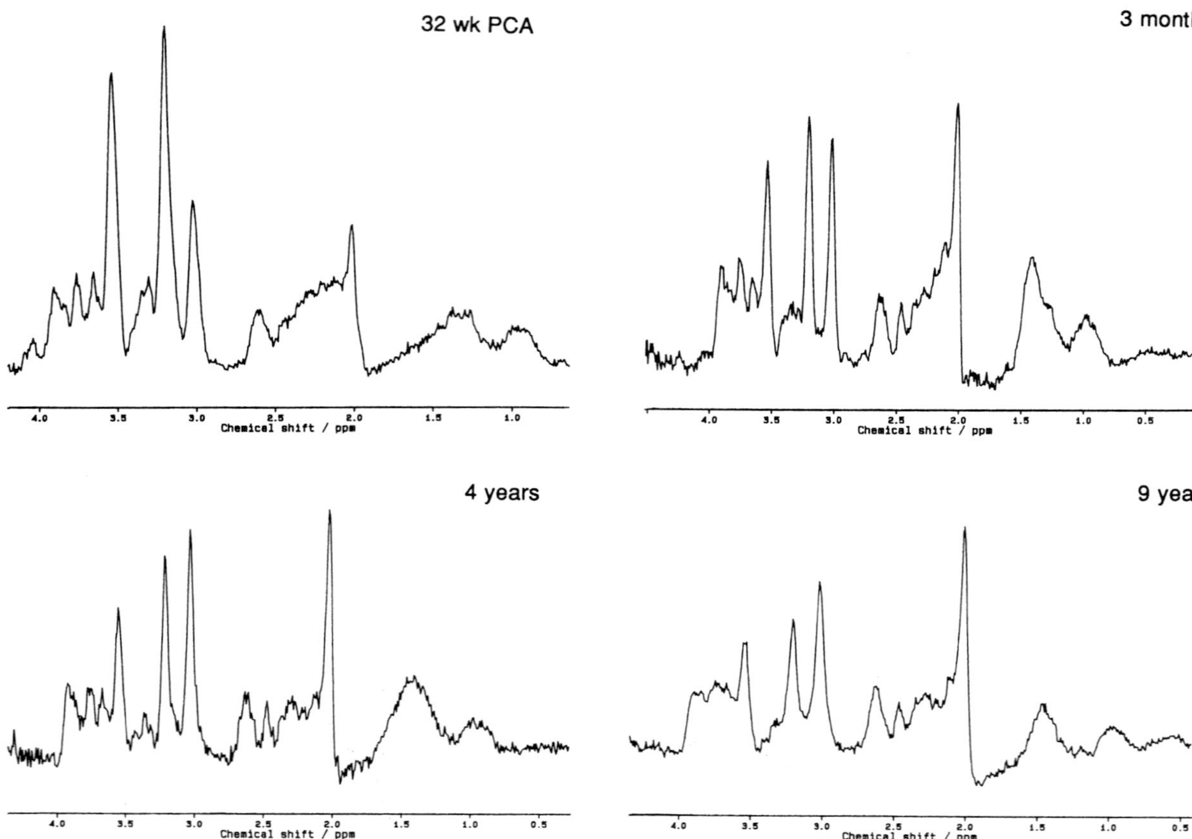

Fig. 71.7. Four ^{1}H spectra of the brain acquired using a short echo time of 20 ms, and obtained at different ages (*PCA*=postconceptional age; other ages are related to term birth). Note the increase in NAA and decrease in Cho and mI relative to Cr with increasing age

rates with age. PCr/Pi is considered a measure of the phosphorylation potential and energy status of the examined tissue; the increase may, therefore, imply an increase in energy reserve in infant brain tissue. This increase would be compatible with the increase in rate of energy metabolism observed in postnatal cerebral maturation.

Human cerebral pH shows some decrease with ongoing cerebral maturation.

Also, ^{1}H spectra undergo major developmental changes. In neonates, in particular in preterms, the spectrum is dominated by Cho and mI peaks, whereas in the adult the NAA peak is largest.

NAA is low at birth. NAA/Cr and absolute NAA values have been shown to increase after birth. The steepest increase occurs during the first year of life and final values are reached at 3–5 years. The increase in NAA can be attributed to processes of neuronal maturation, including increase in number of axons, dendrites and synaptic connections.

Cho is high in neonates and decreases thereafter. Decrease in Cho/Cr and in absolute Cho values with increasing cerebral maturation has been reported re-

peatedly. Final values are reached after 3–5 years. The high Cho peak in early development can be attributed to a high rate of membrane synthesis and turnover, in particular related to the process of myelination.

The mI peak is high at birth and decreases rapidly. Final values are reached within the first year of life. The significance of the high mI peak in early development is not known.

The peak originating from scyllo-inositol, formerly mainly attributed to taurine, decreases after birth.

The peaks originating from glutamine and glutamate do not change significantly.

In studies of brain extracts of rats, an increase in Cr has been found with increasing cerebral maturation (Bates et al. 1989a). In an in vivo study of human neonates using absolute quantitative data, Kreis et al. (1993) found a rapid increase in the cerebral Cr concentration before and around term. Final values are reached after a few months. The difference from adult values was small but significant. Hence, it is clear that Cr is an internal reference of limited value in early development.

Metabolite concentrations show regional variability,

depending on the structures included. Due to the cortical foldings it is not possible to obtain spectroscopic data from a voxel containing cortex only and it is difficult to choose a voxel containing white matter only. The impact of the problem is more severe on ^{31}P MRS than ^{1}H MRS; because of the low inherent sensitivity, larger voxels are required for ^{31}P MRS. In ^{1}H MRS it is possible to obtain spectra from voxels containing mostly cortex or white matter or central nuclei. It has been shown that NAA, Cr, mI, glutamate and glutamine are higher in gray matter spectra than in white matter spectra, whereas Cho is higher in white matter spectra.

These regional and age-dependent spectra changes make it necessary to obtain region-specific normal values for different ages. In the absence of normal values, including a measure of normal variability, ^{31}P and ^{1}H spectra of the brain cannot be appraised.

71.4 MRS in White Matter Disorders

Until now a limited number of disorders has been investigated by MRS. Two types of spectroscopic abnormalities are seen in white matter disorders:

1. Nonspecific spectroscopic abnormalities related to cerebral damage, inclu- ding demyelination and neuronal loss, as observed in inherited leukodys- trophies, AIDS encephalopathy and leukoencephalopathy after cranial irradia- tion.
2. Specific spectroscopic changes directly related to the specific disorder under investigation, such as loss of high energy metabolites in conditions of energy depletion, changes in glutamine/glutamate in hyperammonemia and elevation of glycine in hyperglycinemia.

Nonspecific cerebral damage may consist of disturbance of brain maturation, demyelination, or neuronal degeneration. In demyelinating disorders, it is primarily the myelin sheath that is lost; secondarily, axonal damage and loss occurs. Histologically, demyelinating disorders are characterized by rarefaction of the white matter with respect to its normal constituents. Gliotic scar tissue fills in the free spaces that arise as a consequence of myelin and axonal loss. Consequently, demyelinating disorders do not lead to significant cerebral atrophy, unless demyelination is severe and longstanding. In primary neuronal degenerative disorders, neurons undergo degenerative changes, die, and disappear, together with their axons and myelin sheaths. White matter rarefaction is not the rule and gliosis is usually absent or inconspicuous. Tissue loss is primarily evident as atrophy.

In demyelinating disorders, the rarefaction of white matter implies that the total amount of membrane phospholipids per volume of brain tissue decreases, resulting in a decrease in PDE in the ^{31}P spectrum (Fig. 71.8). The decrease in the ratio of PDE/β-ATP

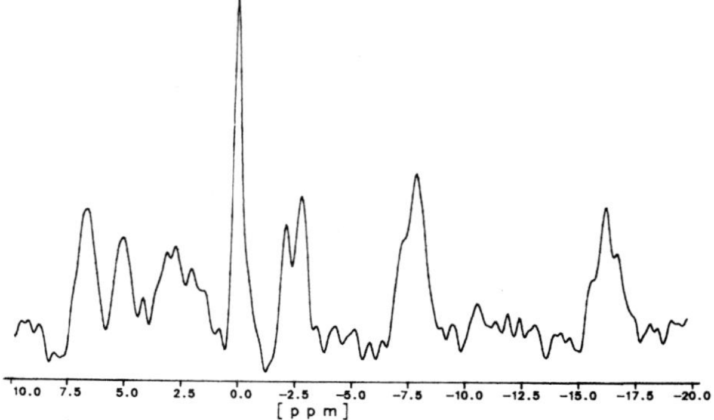

Fig. 71.8. ^{31}P spectrum of a patient with severe demyelination. Note the very low PDE. Compare this spectrum to that of Fig. 71.1, which was obtained from a normal child of the same age

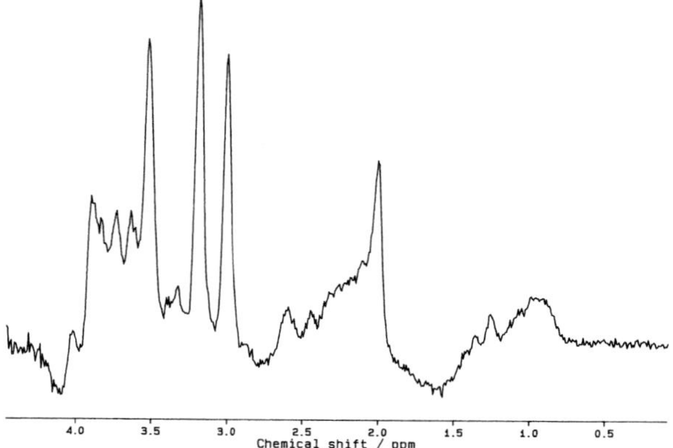

Fig. 71.9. ^{1}H spectrum (echo time 20 ms) of a 4-month-old patient with Krabbe's disease and severe demyelination. Note the decrease in NAA, and increases in Cho and mI compared to the spectrum of the 3-month-old control shown in Fig. 71.7

has been shown to be proportional to the extent of the demyelination. The PME peak, which is proportional to the rate of membrane phospholipid synthesis, remains normal until demyelination is very severe. In these conditions a variable decrease in PME/β-ATP has been observed. The neuronal damage and loss accompanying demyelination are reflected in a decrease in NAA in the ^{1}H spectrum (Fig. 71.9). In active demyelination an elevation of Cho has been reported repeatedly, in addition to elevation of fatty acids, presumably related to enhanced membrane lipid turnover and enhanced presence of myelin breakdown products, respectively. In severe chronic demyelination some decrease in Cho may be observed. In active demyelination, a variable increase in lactate, in glutamate/glutamine and in mI have been observed. The elevations of lactate and glutamate/glutamine may be related to processes of active tissue degeneration and inflammation. The cause of the elevation of mI is not clear but may be found in gliosis.

In neuronal degenerative disorders, no white matter rarefaction occurs. As expected, PDE/β-ATP has been found to remain within the normal range, even in cases of far advanced disease. The neuronal damage is reflected in a decrease in NAA. The decrease is proportional to the cerebral atrophy as visualized on MRI, with the restriction that NAA decrease occurs before evident atrophy on MRI. So, in this respect, MRS is more sensitive than MRI.

MRS, undergoing age-dependent changes, can be used to provide quantitative measures for processes of cerebral maturation. Disturbances of maturation as part of the disease process can be assessed and monitored by MRS.

Specific changes, related to the specific disorder, can be found in particular in some of the inborn and acquired errors of metabolism.

As MRS allows an in vivo assessment of cerebral energy metabolism, it can be applied to evaluate cerebral consequences of cellular energy failure in mitochondrial defects. Inborn errors involving mitochondrial oxidative phosphorylation and electron transport may lead to failure to synthesize sufficient ATP, accumulation of ADP and failure of PCr synthesis from Cr. In addition, mitochondrial dysfunction may lead to accumulation of unoxidized reducing equivalents in the form of NADH, NADPH, lactate and glutamate. The pattern of metabolic disturbances in case of mitochondrial disorders is, in most respects, indistinguishable from that of hypoxia. In ^{1}H MRS in a variety of mitochondrial encephalopathies, including Leigh syndrome, Kearns-Sayre syndrome, MELAS, MERRF and Leber's hereditary optic atrophy, variable elevations of cerebral lactate have been found (Fig. 71.10). Lactate is not elevated in all patients. Cross et al. (1993) found a good correlation between CSF levels of lactate: when the CSF lactate was below 2.5 mmol/l, no lactate was seen in ^{1}H spectra of the brain, whereas in all cases with a CSF lactate above 4.0 mmol/l, elevated lactate was found in MRS. However, patients have been described repeatedly with absence of lactate in ^{1}H spectra of the brain, while CSF lactate was high, as well as patients with elevated lactate in ^{1}H spectra of the brain while CSF lactate was normal. There is a regional variability in elevations of cerebral lactate, lactate being most pronounced in regions where MRI shows structural abnormalities. Repeatedly, but not invariably, a decrease in PCr and an increase in Pi have been described in ^{31}P MRS. Similarly, an elevation of ADP and a decreased phosphorylation potential could be calculated in these cases. The pH was normal. These spectroscopic features are a measure of the derangement of cerebral energy metabolism and can be used to moni-

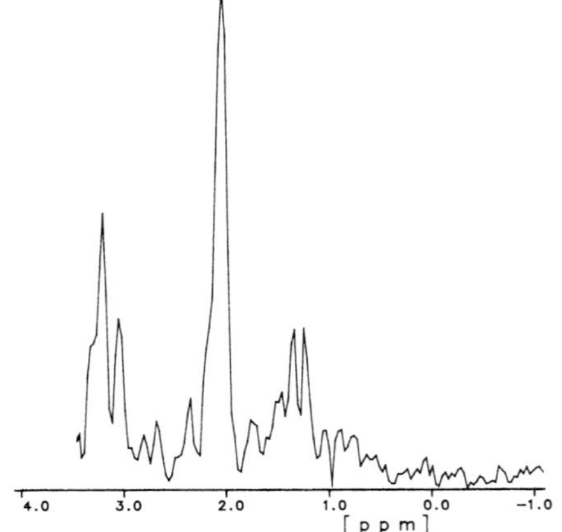

Fig. 71.10. ^{1}H spectrum of the brain (echo time 270 ms) of an adolescent with Kearns-Sayre syndrome. Note the relative decrease in NAA and increase in Cho. A lactate doublet is present at 1.33 ppm with a 7 Hz spin-spin splitting

tor the course of disease in mitochondrial disorders, in particular to evaluate effects of treatment. In addition, nonspecific spectroscopic changes can be present in mitochondrial disorders, in particular a decrease in NAA in lesions, related to neuronal dysfunction and loss.

Similar spectroscopic changes related to cellular energy failure are present in hypoxic-ischemic encephalopathy of neonates. In the acute phase of cerebral hypoxia-ischemia, acute reciprocal changes occur in the concentrations of PCr and Pi, so that the PCr/Pi ratio falls. Only when PCr/Pi reaches a low value, does the concentration of ATP also decline. Intracellular pH is reduced. These changes are rapidly reversed when cerebral perfusion and oxygenation are restored. Over the subsequent few days, spectral abnormalities develop again in spite of absence of any ongoing hypoxia-ischemia. Again there are roughly reciprocal changes in PCr and Pi and, in severely affected infants, a fall in ATP. However, intracellular pH tends to rise rather than to fall. Later Pi increases, well out of proportion to the fall in PCr, and in severely damaged brains, PCr and ATP are absent, leaving only a large residual Pi peak in the spectrum. In less severely affected infants who recover, the ^{31}P metabolite ratios return to normal over the course of about 2 weeks, but sometimes the total phosporus signal is reduced, indicating permanent loss of cells. The explanation of the presence of two stages is that the initial acute hypoxic-ischemic episode initiates a series of reactions which later cause progressive disruption of oxidative phosphorylation in brain tissue. This disruption is termed secondary energy failure. This course of events explains why ^{31}P MRS findings are often normal on the first day of life, to become abnormal over the subsequent few days. The

^{31}P MRS findings appear to have prognostic value. Of the children whose PCr/Pi falls below the 95% confidence limits for normal infants, two-thirds die and almost all survivors have a serious neurological handicap. Nearly all infants with a decrease in ATP die. With respect to ^{1}H spectroscopic findings, it has been shown that NAA begins to decrease several hours after the hypoxic-ischemic episode. In contrast to the normalization of the ^{31}P spectra, ^{1}H spectra remain abnormal with low NAA. Also ^{1}H spectroscopic findings have prognostic value. The lowest NAA/Cr levels are found in the children with the poorest outcome. The presence of elevated lactate also carries a poor prognosis with respect to survival and neurological handicap. Glutamate may be relatively elevated for a while after the acute hypoxic-ischemic incident, suggesting excitotoxic effects.

In chronic conditions of hypoxia-ischemia, such as subacute arteriosclerotic encephalopathy, only aspecific spectroscopic abnormalities are found and no spectroscopic evidence of ongoing ischemia.

In cases of hyperammonemia of whatever origin, including urea cycle defects, propionic acidemia, Reye syndrome and other causes of hepatic failure, ^{1}H spectra show changes directly related to the high levels of ammonium. Hyperammonemia has a great impact on the equilibrium between glutamate, glutamine and GABA by stimulating glutamine synthesis, resulting in an accumulation of glutamine and a depletion of glutamate. Elevated levels of glutamine can be visualized easily by ^{1}H MRS (Fig. 71.11). Other spectroscopic changes have been found in hyperammonemia, of which the cause is less clear. Depletion of mI has been found (Fig. 71.12) and the relationship between mI depletion and hyperammonemia is quite unclear. As mI could be an osmolyte, depletion of mI could be an osmotic response to glutamine accumulation. An alternative role for mI could be as precursor of glucuronic acid, which helps to detoxify xenobiotics by conjugation. Depletion of mI could be the result of excessive detoxification. A decrease in Cho has been found, the cause of which is unknown. The decrease in total Cr observed in some cases of hepatic dysfunction has been ascribed to failure of the severely damaged liver to synthesize adequate amounts of the substance. In cases of neuronal damage, NAA is decreased. The spectroscopic changes directly related to hyperammonemia are reversible after normalization of ammonia levels, implying that ^{1}H MRS is a very useful tool for monitoring cerebral abnormalities in hyperammonemias.

The relative increase in NAA in Canavan's disease is well known. It is specifically the metabolism of NAA that is disturbed in this disorder. However, when absolute quantitation is used, Cho and Cr appear to be low and NAA within the normal range or only mildly elevated. In direct biochemical measurements, the level of

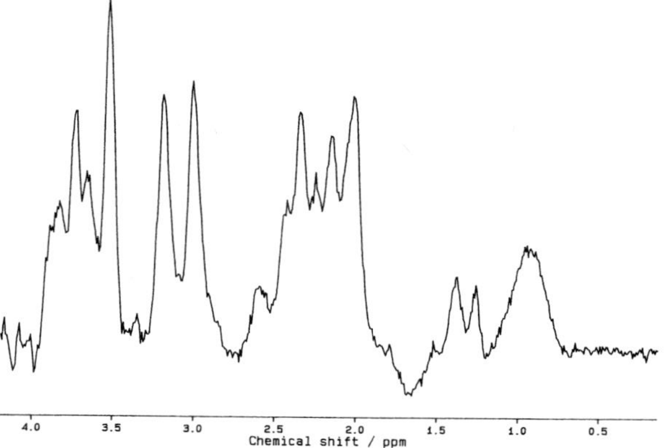

Fig. 71.11. [1]H spectrum (echo time 20 ms) of a neonate in a poor condition, suffering from argininosuccinate lyase deficiency (urea cycle defect). Note the highly elevated glutamine and the presence of lactate

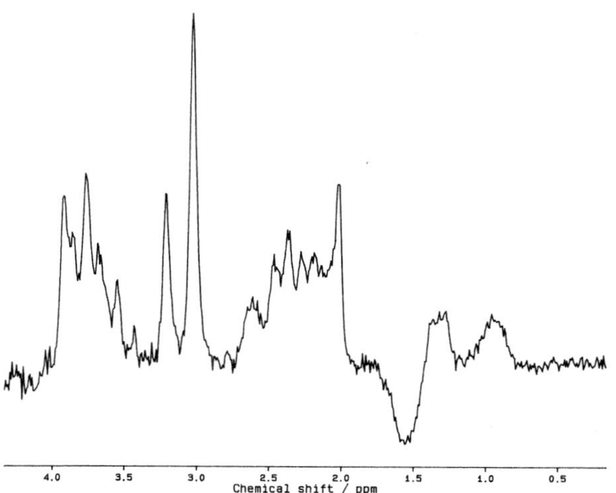

Fig. 71.12. [1]H spectrum (echo time 20 ms) of a 4-year-old boy with hyperargininemia (urea cycle defect), just recovering from an episode of metabolic derangement induced by protein-rich gavage feeding. Note the elevation of glutamine, the decrease in NAA and the depletion of mI

cerebral NAA in micromoles per milligram protein is markedly increased. The apparent discrepancy between biochemical and MRS findings can be explained, at least in part, by the reduction in myelin content and cellularity observed in Canavan's disease, where the white matter is converted into a loose, vacuolated meshwork with glia and bare axons left as tissue elements. These histological characteristics imply that a larger part of the selected volume of interest consists of water. The low Cho with low Cho/Cr ratio in Canavan's disease is probably related to the very low membrane content of the white matter. In itself the elevation of

NAA/Cr is specific for Canavan's disease, as in all other conditions NAA is normal or decreased, but never increased. In some of the Canavan patients, lactate is elevated.

In maple syrup urine disease, ^{1}H MRS during acute metabolic decompensation shows elevated lactate and resonances at 1 ppm corresponding to cerebral accumulation of branched-chain amino acids and keto acids. NAA is decreased. With treatment and clinical recovery the ^{1}H spectra normalize.

In nonketotic hyperglycinemia, ^{1}H spectra show an elevated glycine signal at 3.55 ppm. There is evidence that the time course of glycine content in brain tissue, as shown by MRS, is more closely correlated with the clinical course than plasma and CSF glycine values are.

Specific MRS findings may not only be used in the diagnosis and monitoring of particular disorders, but may also contribute to the elucidation of disorders of as yet unknown origin. A striking example is found in creatine deficiency, described by Stöckler et al. (1994). In a patient with a developmental arrest from the age of 5 months onwards and a severe extrapyramidal movement disorder, ^{1}H MRS unexpectedly revealed a complete deficiency of Cr and an unknown resonance at 3.78 ppm, subsequently identified as guanidinoacetate. The metabolic block could be pointed out as a deficiency of guanidinoacetate methyltransferase. Creatine substitution led to striking improvement of the symptoms of the patient.

Also aspecific spectroscopic findings can be very useful in monitoring disease. MRS is most often used for this purpose in multiple sclerosis (MS) for several reasons. The course of disease is fluctuating. Changes at structural cerebral level do not always correlate with clinical changes. Treatment schedules may influence the course of disease. In particular therapeutic trials require objective measures of changes in disease. Short echo time spectra obtained from acute MS lesions, as identified by gadolinium enhancement on MRI, show a reduction of NAA, an increase in Cho and mI, and large resonances at 0.9 and 1.3 ppm originating from methyl and methylene groups of lipid (Davie et al. 1994). In part of the acute lesions elevated lactate is found. In a longitudinal study it was shown that the earliest spectroscopic changes, 3 days after onset of symptoms, consist of increased Cho and lactate and

that the decrease in NAA occurs several days later (Arnold et al. 1992). Lactate disappears in a matter of weeks. Enhanced Cho returns to normal in some of the lesions within a couple of months. In some lesions, a partial recovery of NAA is seen over a period of months after acute onset of the lesion. The lipid resonances remain elevated for several months. The rise in mI is probably permanent; at least, no return to normal levels has been found during a follow-up of 9 months (Davie et al. 1994). Spectroscopic findings reflect the changes at histological level. The hypothesis is that metabolic ratios are unchanged in hyperacute, edematous plaques. Correlation with pathological findings in biopsy specimens confirms an association between acute inflammation, hypercellularity due to a mixed macrophage – astrocyte response and demyelination with increased levels of Cho and lactate. In acute lesions myelin sheaths show signs of disintegration and breakdown accompanied by liberation of neutral fat, reflected in elevated lipid signals in MRS. Initially axons are preserved, but become secondarily damaged, with decreasing NAA. Chronic and inactive lesions are hypocellular, demyelinated and gliosed. Inflammation is no longer present. Several studies suggest that normal appearing white matter in MRI of MS patients is not completely normal in MRS. A decrease in NAA in ^{1}H MRS and a decrease in total ^{31}P peak integrals in ^{31}P MRS has been described, as well as a reduction in the broad component of the ^{31}P spectrum, consistent with some demyelination and neuronal damage, too subtle to be detected by MRI.

Reviewing the information provided by MRS about brain metabolism in normal cerebral maturation, in disturbed maturation and in disease conditions, MRS has proven itself to be a tool of limited but significant use in clinical medicine and of great potential for research purposes. For clinical applications, the greatest power of MRS is found in monitoring disease processes, in particular in view of evaluating therapeutic interventions and establishing prognosis. In particular in the early stages of disease processes, MRS often appears to be more sensitive than MRI. For research applications, the greatest potential of MRS may be found in contributing to the elucidation of pathophysiological processes in cerebral disorders.

Acknowledgements

The preparation of a book is a project which relies on the support and collaboration of many people. First of all we would like to thank the specialists who referred their patients to us. Our special thanks go to Leo Smit (Free University Hospital, Amsterdam) and Peter Barth (Academic Medical Center) who discussed many patients with us. We are also extremely grateful for the kind and positive responses of colleagues whose permission we requested to use illustrations of their rare cases. There is no doubt that these widen the scope of this book. It is a continuing positive experience to work with an MRI crew, who ensure constant high quality: Ronald Prinsze, Karin Molleman-van der Vegt, Willy Rood-Admiraal, Adrie Verburg-Mast, José Sluitman, Ton Schweigmann, radiographers. In producing a book, a large load always rests on the shoulders of secretaries. Confronted with many revisions and major and minor changes, we were fortunate in being able to count on the support of Lenie de Vries. Data from the MR archive and teaching files were always available in the shortest possible time thanks to the administrative talent of Els van der Straten and Annemarie Hagedorn. Els van Deventer, Cisca Frederiks and Linda Glas did a superb job in obtaining the literature reprints we needed. The audiovisual center of the Free University Hospital, in particular Patrick Dekker and Ton Dijkstra, helped us to obtain high image quality. The language supervision was in the skilled hands of Brenda Vollers-King, who performed in her usual perfect way.

References

1 Myelin and White Matter

Asotra K, Macklin WB (1993) Protein kinase C activity modulates myelin gene expression in enriched oligodendrocytes. J Neurosci Res 34:571–588

Benjamins JA, McKhann GM (1981) Development, regeneration, and aging of the brain. In: Siegel GJ, Albers RW, Agranoff BW, Katzman R (eds) Basic neurochemistry, 3rd edn.: Little Brown, Boston, pp 445–469

Benjamins JA, Iwata R, Hazlett J (1978) Kinetics of entry of proteins into the myelin membrane. J Neurochem 31:1077–1085

Benveniste EN, Merrill JE (1986) Stimulation of oligodendroglial proliferation and maturation by interleukin-2. Nature 321:610–613

Berlet HH, Volk B (1980) Studies of human myelin proteins during old age. Mech Ageing Dev 14:211–222

Berndt JA, Kim JG, Hudson LD (1992) Identification of cis-regulatory elements in the myelin proteolipid protein (PLP) gene. J Biol Chem 267:14730–14737

Beuche W, Friede RL (1985) A new approach toward analyzing peripheral nerve fiber populations. II. Foreshortening of regenerated internodes corresponds to reduced sheath thickness. J Neuropathol Exp Neurol 44:73–84

Boiron F, Spivack WD, Deshmukh DS, Gould RM (1993) Basis for phospholipid incorporation into peripheral nerve myelin. J Neurochem 60:320–329

Bologa L (1985) Oligodendrocytes, key cells in myelination and target in demyelinating diseases. J Neurosci Res 14:1–20

Brody BA, Kinney HC, Kloman AS, Gilles FH (1987) Sequence of central nervous system myelination in human infancy. I. An autopsy study of myelination. J Neuropathol Exp Neurol 46:283–301

Brown MC, Moreno MB, Bongarzone ER, Cohen PD, Soto EF, Pasquini JM (1993) Vesicular transport of myelin proteolipid and cerebroside sulfates to the myelin membrane. J Neurosci Res 35:402–408

Burger D, Steck AJ, Bernard CCA, Kerlero de Rosbo N (1993) Human myelin/oligodendrocyte glycoprotein: a new member of the L2/HNK-1 family. J Neurochem 61:1822–1827

Campagnoni AT (1988) Molecular biology of myelin proteins from the central nervous system. J Neurochem 51:1–14

Campagnoni AT, Verdi JM, Verity AN, Amur-Umarjee S (1990) Posttranscriptional events in the expression of myelin protein genes. Ann NY Acad Sci 605:270–279

Carson MJ, Behringer RR, Brinster RL, McMorris FA (1993) Insulin-like growth factor I increases brain growth and central nervous system myelination in transgenic mice. Neuron 10:729–740

Cervós-Navarro J (1993) Nonvascular intracerebral fluid spaces. In: Lasjaunias P, Leonardi M (eds) ESNR refresher course. Edizioni del Centauro, Udine, pp 25–34

Dambska M, Laure-Kaminowska M (1990) Myelination as a parameter of normal and retarded brain maturation. Brain Dev 12:214–220

Davison AN, Dobbing J (1966) Myelination as a vulnerable period in brain development. Br Med Bull 20:40–44

De Vries GH, Norton WT (1974) The fatty acid composition of sphingolipids from bovine CNS axons and myelin. J Neurochem 22:251–257

De Vries LS, Connell JA, Dubowitz LMS, Oozeer RC, Dubowitz V, Pennock JM (1987) Neurological electrophysiological and MRI abnormalities in infants with extensive cystic leukomalacia. Neuropediatrics 18:61–66

Debuch H (1970) Biochemistry of normal lipid metabolism in the brain. In: Vinken PJ, Bruyn GW (eds) Handbook of clinical neurology, vol 10. North Holland, Amsterdam, pp 233–264

Deshmukh DS, Vorbrodt AW, Lee PK, Bear WD, Kuizon S (1988) Studies on the submicrosomal fractions of bovine oligodendroglia: lipid composition and glycolipid biosynthesis. Neurochem Res 13:571–582

Dietrich RB, Bradley WG, Zaragoza IV, Otto RJ, Taira RK, Wilson GH, Kangerloo H (1988) MR evaluation of early myelination patterns in normal and developmentally delayed infants. AJNR 9:69–76

Dobbing J (1968) Vulnerable periods in developing brain. In: Davison AN, Dobbing J (eds) Applied neurochemistry. Blackwell, Oxford, pp 287–316

Dobbing J, Sands J (1973) Quantitative growth and development of human brain. Arch Dis Child 48:757–767

Duhamel-Clerin E, Villarroya H, Mehtali M, Lapie P, Besnard F, Gumpel M, Lachapelle F (1994) Cellular expression of an HMGCR promoter-cat fusion gene in transgenic mouse brain: evidence for a developmental regulation in oligodendrocytes. Glia 11:35–46

Farrer RG, Benjamins JA (1992) Entry of newly synthesized gangliosides into myelin. J Neurochem 58:1477–1484

Fishman MA, Agrawal HC, Alexander A, Golterman J, Martenson RE, Mitchell RF (1975) Biochemical maturation of human central nervous system myelin. J Neurochem 24:689–694

Flechsig P (1901) Developmental (myelogenetic) localisation of the cerebral cortex in the human subject. Lancet II:1027–1029

Flechsig P (1920) Anatomie des menschlichen Gehirns und Rückenmarks. Thieme, Leipzig, pp 7–119

Fors L, Hood L, Saavedra RA (1993) Sequence similarities of myelin basic protein promoters from mouse and shark: implications for the control of gene expression in myelinating cells. J Neurochem 60:513–521

Futerman AH, Stieger B, Hubbard AL, Pagano RE (1990) Sphingomyelin synthesis in rat liver occurs predominantly at the cis and medial cisternae of the Golgi apparatus. J Biol Chem 265:8650–8657

Gilles FH (1976) Myelination in the neonatal brain. Hum Pathol 7:244–248

Gilles FH, Shankle W, Dooling EC (1983) Myelinated tracts:growth patterns. In: Gilles FH, Leviton A, Dooling EC (eds) The developing human brain. Wright, Boston, pp 117–192

Goodrum JF, Earnhardt T, Goines N, Bouldin TW (1994) Fate of myelin lipids during degeneration and regeneration of peripheral nerve:an autoradiographic study. J Neurosci 14:357–367

Gould RM, Spivack W, Cataneo R, Holshek J, Konat G (1987) Lipids and myelination. In: Crescenzi S (ed) A multidisciplinary approach to myelin diseases. Plenum, New York, pp 87–102

Guit GL, van de Bor M, den Ouden L, Wondergem JHM (1990) Prediction of neurodevelopmental outcome in the preterm infant: MR-staged myelination compared with cranial US. Radiology 175:107–109

Gupta SK, Pringle J, Poduslo JF, Mezei C (1993) Induction of myelin genes during peripheral nerve remyelination requires a continuous signal from the ingrowing axon. J Neurosci Res 34:14–23

Hasegawa M, Houdou S, Mito T, Takashima S, Asanuma K, Ohno T (1992) Development of myelination in the human fetal and infant cerebrum:a myelin basic protein immunohistochemical study. Brain Dev 14:1–6

Haataja L, Parkkola R, Sonninen P, Vanhanen SL, Schleutker J, Aarinaa T, Turpeinen U, Renlund M, Aula P (1994) Phenotypic variation and magnetic resonance imaging (MRI) in Salla disease, a free sialic acid storage disorder. Neuropediatrics 25:238–244

Jacoby CG, Yuh WTC, Afifi AK, Bell WE, Schelper RL, Sato Y (1987) Accelerated myelination in early Sturge-Weber syndrome demonstrated by MR imaging. J Comput Assist Tomogr 11:226–231

Jeckel D, Karrenbauer A, Birk R, Schmidt RR, Wieland F (1990) Sphingomyelin is synthesized in the cis Golgi. FEBS Lett 261:155–157

Kamholz J, Toffenetti, Lazzarini RA (1988) Organization and expression of the human myelin basic protein gene. J Neurosci Res 21:62–70

Keene LMF, Hewer EE (1931) Some observations on myelination in the human central nervous system. J Anat 66:1–13

Kinney HC, Brody BA, Kloman AS, Gilles FH (1988) Sequence of central nervous system myelination in human infancy. II. Patterns of myelination in autopsied infants. J Neuropathol Exp Neurol 47:217–234

Kinney HC, Karthigasan J, Borenshteyn NI, Flax JD, Kirschner DA (1994) Myelination in the developing human brain:biochemical correlates. Neurochem Res 19:983–996

Kocsis JD, Waxman SG (1985) Demyelination:causes and mechanisms of clinical abnormality and functional recovery. In: Koetsier JC (ed) Handbook of clinical neurology, vol 3. Elsevier, Amsterdam, pp 29–47

Konola JT, Yamamura T, Tyler B, Lees MB (1992) Orientation of the myelin proteolipid protein C-terminus in oligodendroglial membranes. Glia 5:112–121OR (1933) Development of behavior patterns and myelinization of the nervous system in human fetus and infant. Contrib Embryol XXIV:1–57

Lemke G (1988) Unwrapping the genes of myelin. Neuron 1:535–543

Lemke G (1993) The molecular genetics of myelination:an update. Glia 7:263–271

Ludin HP (1984) Function of myelin in the normal nerve fibre. Neuropediatrics 15 [Suppl]:21–23

Ludwin SK (1988) Remyelination in the central nervous system and the peripheral nervous system. In: Waxman SG (ed) Advances in neurology: functional recovery in neurological disease, vol 47. Raven, New York, pp 215–254

Lütschg J (1984) Pathophysiological aspects of central and peripheral myelin lesions. Neuropediatrics 15 [Suppl]:24–27

Martin DW (1985) Membranes. In: Martin DW, Mayes PA, Rochwel VW, Granner DK (eds) Harper's review of biochemistry, 20th edn. Lange Medical, Los Altos, pp 448–463

Martin E, Boesch C, Zuerrer M, Kikinis R, Molinari L, Kaelin P, Boltshauser E, Duc G (1990) MR imaging of brain maturation in normal and developmentally handicapped children. J Comput Assist Tomogr 14:685–692

Matthieu JM (1993) An introduction to the molecular basis of inherited myelin diseases. J Inherit Metab Dis 16:724–732

Matthieu JM, Comte V, Tosic M, Honegger P (1992) Myelin gene expression during demyelination and remyelination in aggregating brain cell cultures. J Neuroimmunol 40:231–234

McLaurin J, Ackerley CA, Moscarello MA (1993) Localization of basic proteins in human myelin. J Neurosci Res 35:618–628

Menkes JH (1990) The leukodystrophies. N Engl J Med 322:54–55

Mickel HS, Gilles FH (1970) Changes in glial cells during human telencephalic myelinogenesis. Brain 93:337–346

Mikol DD, Rongnoparut P, Allwardt BA, Marton LS, Stefansson K (1993) The oligodendrocyte-myelin glycoprotein of mouse:primary structure and gene structure. Genomics 17:604–610

Mitchell LS, Gillespie SC, McAllister F, Fanarraga ML, Kirkham D, Kelly B, Brophy PJ, Grittiths IR, Montague P, Kennedy PGE (1992) Developmental expression of major myelin protein genes in the CNS of X-linked hypomyelinating mutant rumpshaker. J Neurosci Res 33:205–217

Morell P (ed) (1984) Myelin, 2nd edn. Plenum, New York

Morell P, Wiesmann U (1984) A correlative synopsis of the leukodystrophies. Neuropediatrics 15 [Suppl]:62–65

Morell P, Quarles RH, Norton WT (1989) Formation, structure, and biochemistry of myelin. In: Siegel GJ, Agranoff BW, Albers RW (eds) Basic neurochemistry: molecular, cellular and medical aspects, 4th edn. Raven, New York, pp 109–136

Norton WT (1984) Recent advances in myelin biochemistry. Ann NY Acad Sci 436:5–10

Norton WT, Autilio LA (1966) The lipid composition of purified bovine brain myelin. J Neurochem 13:213–222

Norton WT, Cammer W (1984) Isolation and characterization of myelin. In: Morell P (ed) Myelin. Plenum, New York, pp 147–195

Notterpek LM, Rome LH (1994) Functional evidence for the role of axolemma in CNS myelination. Neuron 13:473–485

Pagano RE (1990) The Golgi apparatus:insights from lipid biochemistry. Biochem Soc Trans 18:361–366

Patsalos PN, Wiggins RC (1982) Brain maturation following administration of phenobarbital, phenytoin, and sodium valproate to developing rats or to their dams:effects on synthesis of brain myelin and other subcellular membrane proteins. J Neurochem 39:915–923

Percy AK, McKhann GM (1970) The biochemistry of myelin and the leukodystrophies. In: Vinken PJ, Bruyn GW (eds) Handbook of clinical neurology, vol 10. North Holland, Amsterdam, pp 134–149

Poduslo SE, Jang Y (1984) Myelin development in infant brain. Neurochem Res 9:1615–1626

Pope A (1977) Neuroglia:quantitative aspects. In: Schoffeniels E, Franck G, Hertz L, Tower DB (eds) Dynamic properties of glia cells. Pergamon, New York, pp 13–20

Poser CM (1957) Discussion des rapports sur les maladies démyélinisantes. Proceedings of the 3rd international congress of neuropathology. Editions Acta Medica Belgica, Brussels, pp 106–111

Poser CM (1961) Leukodystrophy and the concept of dysmyelination. Arch Neurol 4:323–332

Poser CM (1978) Dysmyelination revisited. Arch Neurol 35:401–407

Probstmeier R, Fahrig T, Spiess E, Schachner M (1992) Interactions of the neural cell adhesion molecule and the myelin-associated glycoprotein with collagen type I: involvement in fibrillogenesis. J Cell Biol 116:1063–1070

Richardson EP (1982) Myelination in the human central nervous system. In: Haymaker W, Adams RD (eds) Histology and histopathology of the nervous system. Thomas, Springfield, pp 146–173

Rodriguez M (1992) Central nervous system demyelination and remyelination in multiple sclerosis and viral models of disease. J Neuroimmunol 40:255–264

Rodriguez M, Prayoonwiwat N, Howe C, Sanborn K (1994) Proteolipid protein gene expression in demyelination and remyelination of the central nervous system: a model for multiple sclerosis. J Neuropathol Exp Neurol 53:136–143

Rorke LB, Riggs HE, Showers MJC, Cabrera CV, Cohn M (1969) Myelination of the brain in the newborn. Lippincott, Philadelphia, pp 1–105

Royland J, Konat GW, Kanoh M, Wiggins RC (1992) Down regulation of myelin-specific mRNAs in the mechanism of hypomyelination in the undernourished developing brain. Dev Brain Res 65:223–226

Royland JE, Konat G, Wiggins RC (1993a) Abnormal upregulation of myelin genes underlies the critical period of myelination in undernourished developing rat brain. Brain Res 607:113–116

Royland JE, Konat GW, Wiggins RC (1993b) Myelin gene activation: a glucose sensitive critical period in development. J Neurosci Res 36:399–404

Saito M, Yu RK (1992) Role of myelin-associated neuraminidase in the ganglioside metabolism of rat brain myelin. J Neurochem 58:83–87

Seitelberger F (1984) Structural manifestations of leukodystrophies. Neuropediatrics 15 [Suppl]:53–61

Shine HD, Readhead C, Popko B, Hood L, Sidman RL (1992) Morphometric analysis of normal, mutant, and transgenic

CNS: correlation of myelin basic protein expression to myelinogenesis. J Neurochem 58:342–349

Sinoway MP, Kitagawa K, Timsit S, Hashim GA, Colman DR (1994) Proteolipid protein interactions in transfectants: implications for myelin assembly. J Neurosci Res 37:551–562

Skoff RP (1980) Neuroglia: a reevaluation of their origin and development. Pathol Res Pract 168:279–300

Smith R (1992) The basic protein of CNS myelin:its structure and ligand binding. J Neurochem 59:1589–1608

Stryer L (1981) Introduction to biological membranes. In: Stryer L (ed) Biochemistry, 2nd edn. Freeman, New York, pp 205–230

Svennerholm L (1963) Some aspects of the biochemical changes in leukodystrophy. In: Folch PJ, Bauer H (eds) Brain lipids and lipoproteins and the leukodystrophies. Elsevier, Amsterdam, pp 104–119

Thompson EB (1970) The biochemistry of the lipids and proteins of white matter. In: Vinken PJ, Bruyn GW (eds) Handbook of clinical neurology, vol 9. North Holland, Amsterdam, pp 1–22

Van de Bor M, Guit GL, Schreuder AM, Wondergem J, Vielvoye GJ (1989) Early detection of delayed myelination in preterm infants. Pediatrics 84:407–411

Van der Knaap MS, Valk J, Bakker CJ, Schooneveld M, Faber JAJ, Willemse J, Gooskens PHJM (1991) Myelination as expression of the functional maturity of the brain. Dev Med Child Neurol 33:849–857

Vogel US, Thompson RJ (1988) Molecular structure, localization, and possible functions of the myelin-associated enzyme 2′,3′-cyclic nucleotide 3′-phosphodiesterase. J Neurochem 50:1667–1677

Vogt O (1910) Quelques considérations genérales sur la myélo-architecture du lobe frontal. Rev Neurol 20:405–420

Waxman SG, Sims TJ (1984) Specificity in central myelination: evidence for local regulation of myelin thickness. Brain Res 292:179–185

Waxman SG, Ritchie JM (1993) Molecular dissection of the myelinated axon. Ann Neurol 33:121–136

Weimbs T, Stoffel W (1992) Proteolipid protein (PLP) of CNS myelin:positions of free, disulfide-bonded and fatty acid thioester-linked cysteine residues and implications for the membrane topology of PLP. Biochem 31:12289–12296

Wiggings RC (1986) Myelination:a critical stage in development. Neurotoxicology 7:103–120

Williams KA, Deber CM (1993) The structure and function of central nervous system myelin. Crit Rev Clin Lab Sci 30:29–64

Wisniewski KE, Schmidt-Sidor B (1989) Postnatal delay of myelin formation in brains from Down syndrome infants and children. Clin Neuropathol 8:55–62

Wood PM, Bunge RP (1991) The origin of remyelinating cells in the adult central nervous system: the role of the mature oligodendrocyte. Glia 4:225–232

Yakovlev PI, Lecours AR (1967) The myelogenetic cycles of regional maturation of the brain. In: Minkowski A (ed) Regional development of the brain in early life. Blackwell, Oxford, pp 3–70

Zurbriggen A, Vandevelde M, Steck A, Angst B (1984) Myelin-associated glycoprotein is produced before myelin basic protein in cultured oligodendrocytes. J Neuroimmunol 6:41–49

2 Classification of Myelin Disorders

Adams RD, Kubik CS (1952) The morbid anatomy of the demyelinative diseases. Am J Med 12:510–546

Adams RD, Richardson EP (1961) The demyelinative diseases of the human nervous system. In: Folch PJ (eds) Chemical pathology of the nervous system. Pergamon, Oxford, pp 162–194

Allan VI (1984) Demyelinating diseases. In: Adams HJ, Corsellis JAN, Duchen LW (eds) Greenfield's neuropathology. Arnold, London, pp 338–384

Alzheimer A (1910) Beiträge zur Kenntnis der pathologischen Neuroglia und ihrer Beziehungen zu den Abbauvorgängen im Nervengewebe. Nissl Alzheimer Arbeiten 3:401–562

Austin J, McAfee D, Armstrong D, O'Rourke M, Shearer L, Bachhawat B (1964) Low sulfatase activities in metachromatic leukodystrophy. Trans Am Neurol Assoc J 89:147–150

Bérard-Badier M, Paillas JE, Gastaut H, Edgar GWF (1958) Essai sur la significance des démyelinisations dans l'idiotie amaurotique infantile. Psychiatr Neurol 132:50–93

Bielschowsky M, Henneberg R (1928) Über familiäre diffuse Sklerose (leukodystrophia cerebri progressiva hereditaria). J Psychol Neurol 36:131–181

Blackwood W (1957) The histological classification of diffuse demyelinating cerebral sclerosis. In: Cerebral lipidosis, a symposium. Blackwell Scientific, Oxford, pp 1–10

Carswell R (1838) Pathological anatomy:illustrations of the elementary forms of disease. Longmans Green, London

Challa VR (1987) White matter lesions in MR imaging of elderly subjects. Radiology 164:874–875

Charcot JM (1868) Lectures on the diseases of the nervous system, vol 3. New Sydenham Society, London (Lectures delivered in 1868, English translation published in 1877)

Cruveilhier J (1835–1842) Anatomie pathologique du corps humain, vol II, fascicle XXXII. Bailliere, Paris

Davison AN, Dobbing J (1966) Myelination as vulnerable period in brain development. Br Med Bull 20:40–44

Diezel PB (1955) Histochemische Untersuchungen an den Globoidzellen der familiaeren infantilen diffusen Sklerose vom Typus Krabbe. Virchows Arch Pathol Anat 327:206–228

Edgar GWF (1955) Approche biochimique des lipidoses et des leucodystrophies. Rev Neurol 92:277–284

Fardeau M, Lapresle J (1963) Maladie de Tay-Sachs avec atteinte importante de la substance blanche. A propos de deux observations anatomo-cliniques. Rev Neurol 109:157–175

Fölling A (1934) Ueber Ausscheiding von Phenylbrenztraubensäure in den Harn als Stoffwechselanomalie in Verbindung mit Imbezillität. Z Physiol Chem 227:169–176

George AE, de Leon MJ, Gentes CI, Miller J, London E, Budzilovich GN, Ferris S, Chase N (1986) Leukoencephalopathy in normal and pathologic aging:CT of brain lucencies. AJNR 7:561–566

Gupta SR, Naheedy MH, Young JC, Ghobrial M, Rubino FA, Hindo W (1988) Periventricular white matter changes and dementia. Clinical, neuropsychological, radiological and pathological correlation. Arch Neurol 45:637–641

Hallervorden J (1940) Die zentralen Entmarkungskrankheiten. Dtsch Z Nervenheilkd 150:201–239

Hauw JJ, Delaère P, Seilhean D, Cornu P (1992) Morphology of demyelination in the human central nervous system. J Neuroimmunol 40:139–152

Herschkowitz N, Schulte FJ (1984) The lipidoses:from detect to dysfunction. Neuropediatrics 15:110–111

Heubner O (1897) Über diffuse Hirnsklerose. Charite Ann 22:298–310

Huk WJ, Bydder GM, Curati WL (1990) Degenerative disorders of the brain and white matter diseases. In: Huk WJ, Gademann G, Friedmann G (eds) Magnetic resonance imaging of central nervous system diseases. Springer, Berlin Heidelberg New York, pp 197–224

Jervis GA (1947) Studies on phenylpyruvic oligofrenia:the position of the metabolic error. J Biol Chem 169:651–656

Johnson MA, Pennock JM, Bydder GM, Steiner RE, Thomas DJ, Hayward R, Bryant DRT, Payne JA, Levene MI, Whitelaw A, Dubowitz LMS, Dubowitz V (1983) Clinical NMR imaging of the brain in children: normal and neurologic disease. AJR 141:1005–1018

Krabbe K (1916) A new familial infantile form of diffuse brain-sclerosis. Brain 39:74–114

Lassmann H, Ammerer HP, Kulnig W (1978) Ultrastructural sequence of myelin degradation. Wallerian degeneration in the rat optic nerve. Acta Neuropathol (Berl) 44:91–102

Matthieu JM (1993) An introduction to the molecular basis of inherited myelin diseases. J Inherited Metab Dis 16:724–732

Menkes JH (1990) The leukodystrophies. N Engl J Med 322:54–55

Merzbacher L (1910) Eine eigenartige familiär-hereditäre Erkrankungsform (aplasia axialis extracorticalis congenita). Z Gesamte Neurol Psychiatr 3:1–138

Morell P, Wiesmann U (1984) A correlative synopsis of the leukodystrophies. Neuropediatrics 15 [Suppl]:62–65

Neubürger K (1921) Histologisches zur Frage der diffusen Hirnsklerose. Z Gesamte Neurol Psychiatr 73:336–352

Peiffer J (1962) Differentiation of various types of leukodystrophy. World Neurol 3:580–597

Pelizaeus F (1899) Über eine eigenartige familiäre Entwicklungshemmung vornehmlich auf motorischem Gebiet. Arch Psychiatr Nervenkr 31:100–104

Poser CM (1957) Discussion des rapports sur les maladies demyelinisantes. Proceedings of the 3rd international congress on neuropathology, Brussels. Editions Acta Medica Belgica, pp 106–111

Poser CM (1961) Leukodystrophy and the concept of dysmyelination. Arch Neurol 4:323–332

Poser CM (1978) Dysmyelination revisited. Arch Neurol 35:401–407

Poser CM (1987) The dysmyelinating diseases. In: Baker AB, Joynt RJ (eds) Clinical neurology, vol 3. Harper and Row, Philadelphia, chap 34

Raine CS (1984) The neuropathology of myelin diseases. In: Morell P (ed) Myelin, 2nd edn. Plenum, New York, pp 259–310

Ranvier L (1871) Contribution à l'histologie et à la physiologie des nerfs periphériques. CR Acad Sci 73:1168

Ranvier L (1875) Traité technique d'histologie. Savy, Paris

Schilder P (1912) Zur Kenntnis der sogenannten diffusen Sklerose. Über Encephalitis periaxialis diffusa. Z Gesamte Neurol Psychiatr 10:1–60

Scholz W (1925) Klinische, pathologisch-anatomische und erbbiologische Untersuchungen bei familiärer, diffuser Hirnsklerose im Kindesalter. Z Gesamte Neurol Psychiatr 99:651–717

Seitelberger F (1984) Structural manifestations of leukodystrophies. Neuropediatrics 15 [Suppl]:53–61

Stam FC, Heslinga JM, Deierkauf FA, Booij HL (1962) Leukodystrophy of the Norman-Greenfield and Krabbe type. Psychiatr Neurol Neurosurg 65:254–265

Stam FC (1970) Concept, classification and nosology of the leukodystrophies. In: Vinken PJ, Bruyn GW (eds) Handbook of clinical neurology, vol 10. North Holland, Amsterdam, pp 1–42

Suzuki K, Suzuki Y (1970) Globoid cell leukodystrophy (Krabbe's disease): deficiency of galactocerebroside beta-galactosidase. Proc Natl Acad Sci USA 66:302–309

Thieffry S, Bertrand I, Bargeton E, Edgar GWF, Arthuis M(1960) Idiotie amaurotique infantile ave alterations graves de la substance blanche. Rev Neurol 102:130–152

Virchow R (1854) Ueber das ausgebreitete Vorkommen einer dem Nervenmark analogen Substanz in den thierischen Geweben. Virchows Arch Pathol Anat:562–572

Von Hirsch T, Peiffer J (1955) Über histologische Methoden in der Differentialdiagnose von Leukodystrophien und Lipidosen. Arch Psychiatr Z Neurol 194:88–104

Von Hirsch T, Peiffer J (1957) A histochemical study of the pre-lipid and metachromatic degenerative products in leucodystrophy. In: Cerebral lipidoses, a symposium. Blackwell Scientific, Oxford, pp 68–76

Pasternak JF, Predey TA, Mikhael MA (1991) Neonatal asphyxia: vulnerability of basal ganglia, thalamus, and brainstem. Pediatr Neurol 7:147–149

Pulsinelli WA (1985) Selective neuronal vulnerability: morphological and molecular characteristics. Prog Brain Res 63:29–37

Schmidt R, Offenbacher H, Fazekas F, Payer F, Kleinert R, Porsch G (1991) Magnetic resonance imaging, computed tomography, and autopsy findings after cardiorespiratory arrest. J Neuroimag 1:197–199

Scholz W (1953) Selective neuronal necrosis and its topistic patterns in hypoxemia and oligemia. J Neuropathol Exp Neurol 12:249–261

Scholz W (1963) Topistic lesions. In: Schadé JP, McMenemey WH (eds) Selective vulnerability of the brain in hypoxaemia. Blackwell Scientific, Oxford, pp 257–267

Sims NR (1992) Energy metabolism and selective neuronal vulnerability following global cerebral ischemia. Neurochem Res 17:923–931

Spielmeyer W (1925) Zur Pathogenese örtlich elektiver Gehirnveränderungen. Z Neurol Psychiatr 99:756–777

Vogt C, Vogt O (1937) Sitz und Wesen der Krankheiten im Licht der topistischen Hirnforschung und des Varierens der Tiere. J Psychol Neurol 47:237–457

Yamada M, Inaba A, Yamawaki M, Ishida K, Yokota T, Uchihara T, Eishi Y, Okeda R (1994) Paraneoplastic encephalomyelo-ganglionitis: cellular binding sites of the antineuronal antibody. Acta Neuropathol (Berl) 88:85–92

3 Selective Vulnerability

Barboriak DP, Provenzale JM, Boyko OB (1994) MR diagnosis of Creutzfeldt-Jakob disease: significance of high signal intensity of the basal ganglia. AJR 162:137–140

Brismar J, Ageel A, Brismar G, Coates R, Gascon G, Ozand P (1990) Maple syrup urine disease: findings on CT and MR scans of the brain in 10 infants. AJNR 11:1219–1228

Davison AN, Dobbing J (1966) Myelination as a vulnerable period in brain development. Br Med Bull 22:40–44

Hawker K, Lang AE (1990) Hypoxic-ischemic damage of the basal ganglia. Mov Disord 5:219–224

Kodama T, Numaguchi Y, Gellad FE, Dwyer BA, Kristt DA (1991) Magnetic resonance imaging of limbic encephalitis. Neuroradiology 33:520–523

Lipton SA, Rosenberg PA (1994) Excitatory amino acids as a final common pathway for neurologic disorders. N Engl J Med 330:613–622

Ludolph AC, Riepe M, Ullrich K (1993) Excitotoxicity, energy metabolism and neurodegeneration. J Inherited Metab Dis 16:716–723

Meyer A (1936) The selective regional vulnerability of the brain and its relation to psychiatric problems. Proc R Soc Med 29:1175–1181

Omar R, Pappolla M (1993) Oxygen free radicals as inducers of heat shock protein synthesis in cultured human neuroblastoma cells:relevance to neurodegenerative disease. Clin Neurosci 242:262–267

4 Myelination and Retarded Myelination

Baierl P, Förster C, Fendel H, Naegele M, Fink U, Kenn W (1988) Magnetic resonance imaging of normal and pathological white matter maturation. Pediatr Radiol 18:183–189

Ballesteros MC, Hansen PE, Soila K (1993) MR imaging of the developing human brain, part 2. Postnatal development. Radiographics 13:611–622

Barkovich AJ, Kjos BO, Jackson DE, Norman D (1988) Normal maturation of the neonatal and infant brain: MR imaging at 1.5 T. Radiology 166:173–180

Barkovich AJ, Jackson DE (1989) MRI assessment of normal and abnormal brain myelinization. MRI Dec 3:17–25

Barkovich AJ (1990) Normal development of the neonatal and infant brain. In: Barkovich AJ (ed) Pediatric neuroimaging. Raven, New York, pp 5–34

Barkovich AJ (1992) Normal and abnormal myelination in children. In: Huckman MS, Forbes GS, Harwood-Nash DC (eds) Neuroradiology. Categorical course syllabus, presented at the American Roentgen Ray Society, Orlando, pp 215–222

Dietrich RB, Bradley WG, Zaragoza EJ, Otto RJ, Taira RK, Wilson GH, Kangarloo H (1988) MR evaluation of early myelination patterns in normal and developmentally delayed infants. AJNR 9:69–76

Flechsig P (1920) Anatomie des menschlichen Gehirns und Rückenmarks auf myelogentischer Grundlage. Thieme, Leipzig

Girard N, Raybaud C, Du Lac P (1991) Étude de la myélinisation cerebrale en IRM. J Neuroradiol 18:291–307

Grodd W (1993) Kerspintomographie neuropädiatrischer Erkrankungen. Normale Reifung des kindlichen Gehirns. Klin Neuroradiol 3:13–27

Hashimoto T, Tayama M, Miyazaki M, Kuroda Y (1990) Development of the brainstem: assessment by MR imaging. Neuropediatrics 22:139–146

Holland BA, Haas DK, Norman D, Brant-Zawadzki M, Newton TH (1986) MRI of normal brain maturation. AJNR 7:201–208

Johnson MA, Pennock JM, Bydder GM, Steiner RE, Thomas DJ, Hayward R, Bryant DRT, Payne JA, Levene MI, Whitelaw A, Dubowitz LMS, Dubowitz V (1983) Clinical NMR imaging of the brain in children:normal and neurologic disease. AJR 141:1005–1018

Kamman RL, Go KG, Brouwer W, Berendsen HJC (1988) Nuclear magnetic resonance relaxation in experimental brain edema: effects of water concentration, protein concentration, and temperature. Magn Reson Med 6:265–274

Keene MFL, Hewer EE (1931) Some observations on myelination in the human nervous system. J Anat 6:1–13

Kinney HC, Brody BA, Kloman AS, Gilles FH (1988) Sequence of central nervous system myelination in human infancy. II. Patterns of myelination in autopsied infants. J Neuropathol Exp Neurol 47:217–234

Koenig SH (1991) Cholesterol of myelin is the determinant of gray-white contrast in MRI of brain. Magn Reson Med 20:285–291

Koenig SH, Brown RD, Spiller M, Lundbom N (1990) Relaxometry of brain: why white matter appears bright in MRI. Magn Reson Med 14:482–495

Konishi Y, Kuriyama M, Hayakawa K, Konishi K, Yasujima M, Fujii Y, Sudo M, Ishii Y (1991) Magnetic resonance imaging in preterm infants. Pediatr Neurol 7:191–195

Kucharczyk W, Macdonald PM, Stanisz GJ, Henkelman RM (1994) Relaxivity and magnetization transfer of white matter lipids at MR imaging:importance of cerebrosides and pH^1. Radiology 192:521–529

Lee BCP, Lipper E, Nass R, Ehrlich ME, de Ciccio-Bloom E, Auld PAM (1986) MRI of the central nervous system in neonates and young children. AJNR 7:605–616

Maezawa M, Seki T, Imura S, Akiyama K, Takikawa I, Yuasa Y (1993) Magnetic resonance signal intensity ratio of gray/white matter in children. Brain Dev 15:198–204

Martin E, Kikinis R, Zuerrer M, Boesch C, Briner J, Kewitz G, Kaelin P (1988) Developmental stages of human brain: an MR study. J Comput Assist Tomogr 12:917–922

Martin E, Boesch C, Zuerrer M, Kikinis R, Molinari L, Kaelin P, Boltshauser E, Duc G (1990) MR imaging of brain maturation in normal and developmentally handicapped children. J Comput Assist Tomogr 14:685–692

Martin E, Krassnitzer S, Kaelin P, Boesch C (1991) MR imaging of the brainstem: normal postnatal development. Neuroradiology 33:391–395

Masumura M (1987) Proton relaxation time of immature brain. II. In vivo measurements of proton relaxation times (T_1 and T_2) in pediatric brain by MRI. Childs Nerv Syst 3:6–11

McArdle CB, Richardson CJ, Nicholas DA, Mirfakhraee M, Hayden CK, Amparo EG (1987a) Developmental features of the neonatal brain: MR imaging, part I. Gray-white matter differentiation and myelination. Radiology 162:223–229

McArdle CB, Richardson CJ, Nicholas DA, Mirfakhraee M, Hayden CK, Amparo EG (1987b) Developmental features of the neonatal brain: MR imaging, part II. Ventricular size and extracerebral space. Radiology 162:230–234

Mintz MC, Grossman RI, Isaacson G, Thickman DI, Kundel H, Joseph P, DeSimone D (1987) MR imaging of fetal brain. J Comput Assist Tomogr 11:120–123

Rorke LB, Riggs HE, Showers MJC, Cabrera CV, Cohn M (1969) Myelination of the brain in the newborn. Lippincott, Philadelphia, pp 11–15, 30–63

Staudt M, Schropp C, Staudt F, Obletter N, Bise K, Breit A (1993) Myelination of the brain in MRI: a staging system. Pediatr Radiol 23:169–176

Staudt M, Schropp C, Staudt F, Obletter N, Bise K, Breit A, Weinmann HM (1994) MRI assessment of myelination: an age standardization. Pediatr Radiol 24:122–127

Stricker T, Martin E, Boesch C (1990) Development of the human cerebellum observed with high-field-strength MR imaging. Radiology 177:431–435

Triulzi F (1992) Anatomia funzionale RM dell'encefalo neonatale. Riv Neuroradiol 5 [Suppl 1]:9–18

Valk J (1987) Myelination. In: Valk J (ed) MRI of the brain, head, neck and spine. Nijhoff, Dordrecht, pp 362–397

Van der Knaap MS, Valk J (1990) MR imaging of the various stages of normal myelination during the first year of life. Neuroradiology 31:459–470

Wolff SD, Fralix TA, Balaban RS (1989) Lipid bilayer and water proton magnetization transfer (abstract). In: Society of Magnetic Resonance in Medicine (ed) Works in progress. Society of Magnetic Resonance in Medicine, Berkely, p 1149

Yakovlev PI, Lecours AR (1967) The myelogenetic cycles of regional maturation of the brain. In: Minkowski A (ed) Regional development of the brain in early life. Blackwell, Oxford, pp 3–70

5 Lysosomes and Lysosomal Disorders

Alroy J, Warren CD, Raghavan SS, Kolodny EH (1989) Animal models for lysosomal storage diseases: their past and future contribution. Hum Pathol 20:823–826

Beem EP (1989) Structural aspects of lysosomal enzymes; implications for their cellular localization in normal and pathological tissues. Thesis. Krips, Meppel

Bohley P, Seglen PO (1992) Proteases and proteolysis in the lysosome. Experientia 48:151–157

Dahmst NM, Lobel P, Kornfeld S (1989) Mannose 6-phosphate receptors and lysosomal enzyme targeting. J Biol Chem 264:12115–12118

de Duve C, Pressman BC, Gianetto R, Wattiaux R, Appelmans F (1955) Tissue fractionation studies. Biochem J 60:604–617

Draye JP, Quitart J, Courtoy PJ, Baudhuin P (1987) Relations between plasma membrane and lysosomal membrane. 1. Fate of covalently labelled plasma membrane protein. Eur J Biochem 170:395–403

Fürst W, Sandhoff K (1992) Activator proteins and topology of lysosomal sphingolipid catabolism. Biochim Biophys Acta 1126:1–16

Galjart NJ, Morreau H, Willemsen R, Gillemans N, Bonten EJ, d'Azzo A (1991) Human lysosomal protective protein has cathepsin A-like activity distinct from its protective function. J Biol Chem 266:14754–14762

Glew RH, Basu A, Prence EM, Remaley AT (1985) Biology of disease; lysosomal storage diseases. Lab Invest 53:250–269

Gonzales-Noriega A, Coutino R, Saavedra VM, Barrera R (1989) Adsorptive endocytosis of lysosomal enzymes by human fibroblasts:presence of two different functional systems that deliver an acid hydrolase to lysosomes. Arch Biochem Biophys 268:649–658

Gordon PB, Hoyvik H, Seglen PO (1992) Prelysosomal and lysosomal connections between autophagy and endocytosis. Biochem J 283:361–369

Hasilik A (1992) The early and late processing of lysosomal enzymes:proteolysis and compartmentation. Experientia 48:130–151

Holtzman E, Novikoff AB (1976) Cells and organelles, 3rd edn. Saunders, Philadelphia

Kelly BM, Waheed A, van Etten R, Chang PL (1989) Heterogeneity of lysosomes in human fibroblasts. Mol Cell Biochem 87:171–183

Kornfeld S (1985) Trafficking of lysosomal enzymes in normal and disease states. J Clin Invest 77:1–6

Kornfeld S (1987) Trafficking of lysosomal enzymes. FASEB J 1:462–468

Kornfeld S (1990) Lysosomal enzyme targeting. Biochem Soc Trans 18:367–274

Kornfeld S, Mellman I (1989) The biogenesis of lysosomes. Annu Rev Cell Biol 5:483–525

Lang T, Chastellier de C, Ryter A, Thilo L (1988) Endocytic membrane traffic with respect to phagosomes in macrophages infected with non-pathogenic bacteria: phagosomal membrane acquires the same composition as lysosomal membrane. Eur J Cell Biol 46:39–50

Moser HW (1992) New concepts in the diagnosis and treatment of lysosomal and peroxisomal disorders. Curr Opin Neurol Neurosurg 5:355–258

Neufeld EF (1991) Lysosomal storage diseases. Annu Rev Biochem 60:257–280

O'Brien JS, Kishimoto Y (1991) Saposin proteins: structure, function, and role in human lysosomal storage disorders. FASEB J 5:301–308

Paton BC, Schmid B, Kustermann-Kuhn B, Poulos A, Harzer K (1992) Additional biochemical findings in a patient and fetal sibling with a genetic defect in the sphingolipid activator protein (SAP) precursor, prosaposin. Biochem J 285:481–488

Pfeffer SR (1988) Mannose 6-phosphate receptors and their role in targeting proteins to lysosomes. J Membr Biol 103:7–16

Plomp PJAM, Gordon PB, Meijer AJ, Hoyvik H, Seglen PO (1989) Energy dpendence of different steps in the autophagic-lysosomal pathway. J Biol Chem 264:6699–6704

Storrie B (1988) Assembly of lysosomes: perspectives from comparative molecular cell biology. Int Rev Cytol 11:53–105

Tager JM (1987) Inborn errors of cellular organelles: an overview. J Inherited Metab Dis 10 [Suppl 1]:3–10

Tanaka Y, Yano S, Furuno K, Ishikawa T, Himeno M, Kato K (1990) Transport of acid phosphatase to lysosomes does not involve passage through the cell surface. Biochem Biophys Res Commun 170:1067–1073

Von Figura K, Hasilik A (1986) Lysosomal enzymes and their receptors. Annu Rev Biochem 55:167–193

6 Metachromatic Leukodystrophy

Ameen M, Chang PL (1987) Pseudo arylsulfatase A deficiency: biosynthesis of an abnormal arylsulfatase A. FEBS Lett 219:130–134

Ameen M, Lazzarino DA, Kelly BM, Gabel CA, Chang PL (1990) Deficient glycosylation of arylsulfatase A in pseudo arylsulfatase-A deficiency. Mol Cell Biochem 92:117–127

Aurebeck G, Osterberg K, Blaw M, Chou S, Nelson E (1964) Electron microscopic observations on metachromatic leukodystrophy. Arch Neurol 11:273–288

Austin J, McAfee D, Armstrong D, O'Rourke M, Shearer L, Bachhawat B (1964) Low sulfatase activities in metachromatic leukodystrophy (MLD). Trans Am Neurol Assoc 89:147–150

Bass NH, Witmer J, Dreifuss FE (1970) A pedigree study of metachromatic leukodystrophy. Neurology 20:52–62

Baumann N, Masson M, Carreau V, Lefevre M, Herschkowitz N, Turpin JC (1991) Adult forms of metachromatic leukodystrophy: clinical and biochemical approach. Dev Neurosci 13:211–215

Bohne W, Figura von K, Gieselmann V (1991) An 11-bp deletion in the arylsulfatase A gene of a patient with late infantile metachromatic leukodystrophy. Hum Genet 87:155–158

Clarke JTR, Skomorowski MA, Chang PL (1989) Marked clinical difference between two sibs affected with juvenile metachromatic leukodystrophy. Am J Med Genet 33:10–13

Dayan AD (1967) Peripheral neuropathy of metachromatic leucodystrophy: observations on segmental demyelination and remyelination and the intracellular distribution of sulphatide. J Neurol Neurosurg Psychiatry 30:311–318

Dayan AD, Marsh J, Jackson M, McGuire VM, Vimal C, Nicolaides K, Sheridan R (1988) First-trimester diagnosis of metachromatic leucodystrophy. Clin Genet 34:122–125

Fluharty AL, Fluharty CB, Bohne W, von Figura K, Gieselmann V (1991) Two new arylsulfatase A (ARSA) mutations in a juvenile metachromatic leukodystrophy (MLD) patient. Am J Hum Genet 49:1340–1350

Francis GS, Bonni A, Shen N, Hechtman P, Yamut B, Carpenter S, Karpati G, Chang PL (1993) Metachromatic Leukodystrophy: multiple nonfunctional and pseudodeficiency alleles in a pedigree: problems with diagnosis and counseling. Ann Neurol 34:212–218

Fressinaud C, Vallat JM, Masson M, Jauberteau MO, Baumann N, Hugon J (1992) Adult-onset metachromatic leukodystrophy presenting as isolated peripheral neuropathy. Neurology 42:1396–1398

Fukumizu M, Matsui K, Hanaoka S, Sakutagawa N, Kurokawa T (1992) Partial seizures in two cases of metachromatic leukodystrophy:electrophysiologic and neuroradiologic findings. J Child Neurol 7:381–386

Fullerton PM (1964) Peripheral nerve conduction in metachromatic leucodystrophy (sulphatide lipidosis). J Neurol Neurosurg Psychiatry 27:100–105

Gieselmann V (1991) An assay for the rapid detection of the arylsulfatase A pseudodeficiency allele facilitates diagnosis and genetic counselinf for metachromatic leukodystrophy. Hum Genet 86:251–255

Gieselmann V, Polten A, Kreysing J, von Figura K (1989) Arylsulfatase A pseudodeficiency: loss of a polyadenylylation signal and N-glycosylation site. Proc Natl Acad Sci USA 86:9436–9440

Gieselmann V, Fluharty AL, Tonnesen T, von Figura K (1991a) Mutations in the arylsulfatase A pseudodeficiency allele causing metachromatic leukodystrophy. Am J Hum Genet 49:407–413

Gieselmann V, Polten A, Kreysing J, Kappler J, Fluharty A, Bohne W, von Figura K (1991b) Mutations in arylsulfatase A alleles causing metachromatic leukodystrophy. Brain Dysfunct 4:235–243

Gieselmann V, Polten A, Kreysing J, Kappler J, Fluharty A, von Figura K (1991c) Molecular genetics of metachromatic leukodystrophy. Dev Neurosci 13:222–227

Gieselmann V, Polten A, Kreysing J, von Figura K (1994) Molecular genetics of metachromatic leukodystrophy. J Inherited Metab Dis 17:500–509

Ginsberg L, Gershfeld NL (1991) Membrane bilayer instability and the pathogenesis of disorders of myelin. Neurosci Lett 130:133–136

Grégoire A, Périer O, Dustin P (1966) Metachromatic leukodystrophy, an electron microscopic study. J Neuropathol Exp Neurol 25:617–636

Hagberg B (1963) Clinical symptoms, signs and tests in metachromatic leukodystrophy. In: Folch-Pi J, Bauer H (eds) Brain lipids and lipoproteins and the leukodystrophies. Elsevier, Amsterdam, pp 134–146

Haltia T, Palo J, Haltia M, Icen A (1980) Juvenile metachromatic leukodystrophy:clinical, biochemical, and neuropathologic studies in nine new cases. Arch Neurol 37:42–46

Hohenschutz C, Friedl W, Schlör KH, Waheed A, Conzelmann E, Sandhoff K, Propping P (1988) Probable metachromatic leukodystrophy/pseudodeficiency compound heterozygote at the arylsulfatase A locus with neurological and psychiatric symptomatology. Am J Med Genet 31:169–175

Holtschmidt H, Sandhoff K, Kwon HY, Harzer K, Nakano T, Suzuki K (1991) Sulfatide activator protein. J Biol Chem 266:7556–7560

Hyde TM, Ziegler JC, Weinberger DR (1992) Psychiatric disturbances in metachromatic leukodystrophy: Insights into the neurobiology of psychosis. Arch Neurol 49:401–406

Inui K, Furukawa M, Nishimoto J, Okada S, Yabuuchi H (1987) Metabolism of cerebroside sulphate and subcellular distribution of its metabolites in cultured skin fibroblasts derived from controls, metachromatic leukodystrophy, globoid cell leukodystrophy and Farber disease. J Inherited Metab Dis 10:293–296

Inui K, Furukawa M, Okada S, Yabuuchi H (1988) Metabolism of cerebroside sulfate and subcellular distribution of its metabolites in cultured skin fibroblasts from controls, metachromatic leukodystrophy, and globoic cell leukodystrophy. J Clin Invest 81:310–317

Jayakumar PN, Aroor SR, Jha RK, Arya BYT (1989) Computed tomography (CT) in late infantile metachromatic leucodystrophy. Acta Neurol Scand 79:23–26

Jervis GA (1960) Infantile metachromatic leukodystrophy. J Neuropathol Exp Neurol 19:323–340

Kappler J, Watts RWE, Conzelmann E, Gibbs DA, Propping P, Gieselmann V (1991) Low arylsulphatase A activity and choreoathetotic syndrome in three siblings: differentiation of pseudodeficiency from metachromatic leukodystrophy. Eur J Pediatr 150:287–290

Kappler J, von Figura K, Gieselmann V (1992) Late-onset metachromatic leukodystrophy:molecular pathology in two siblings. Ann Neurol 31:256–261

Kondo R, Wakamatsu N, Yoshino H, Fukuhara N, Miyatake T, Tsuji S (1991) Identification of a mutation in the arylsulfatase A gene of a patient with adult-type metachromatic leukodystrophy. Am J Hum Genet 48:971–978

Kreysing J, von Figura K, Gieselmann V (1990) Structure of the arylsulfatase A gene. Eur J Biochem 191:627–631

Krivit W, Shapiro E, Kennedy W, Lipton M, Lockman L, Smith S, Gail Summers C, Wenger DA, Tsai MY, Ramsay NKC, Kersey JH, Yao JK, Kaye E (1990) Treatment of late infantile metachromatic leukodystrophy by bone marrow transplantation. N Engl J Med 322:28–32

Krivit W, Shapiro E, Hoogerbrugge PM, Moser HW (1992) State of the art review:bone marrow transplantation treatment for storage diseases. Bone Marrow Transpl 10 [Suppl 1]: 87–96

Leroy JG, von Elsen AF, Martin JJ, Dumon JE, Hulet AE, Okada S, Navarro C (1973) Infantile metachromatic leukodystrophy. N Engl J Med 288:1365–1369

Li ZG, Waye JS, Chang PL (1992) Diagnosis of arylsulfatase A deficiency. Am J Med Genet 43:976–982

McKhann GM (1984) Metachromatic leukodystrophy: clinical and enzymatic parameters. Neuropediatrics 15:4–10

Mei Liu H (1968) Ultrastructure of central nervous system lesions in metachromatic leukodystrophy with special reference to morphogenesis. J Neuropathol Exp Neurol 27:624–644

Norman RM, Urich H, Tingey AH (1960) Metachromatic leuco-encephalopathy: a form of lipidosis. Brain 83:369–380

Norton WT, Cammer W (1984) Chemical pathology of diseases involving myelin. In: Morell P (ed) Myelin. Plenum, New York, pp 369–403

Olsson Y, Sourander P (1969) The reliability of the diagnosis of metachromatic leucodystrophy by peripheral nerve biopsy. Acta Paediatr Scand 58:15–24

Penzien JM, Kappler J, Herschkowitz N, Schuknecht B, Keinekugel P, Propping P, Tonnesen T, Lou H, Moser H, Zierz S, Conzelmann E, Gieselmann V (1993) Compound heterozygosity for metachromatic leukodystrophy and arylsulfatase A pseudodeficiency alleles is not associated with progressive neurological disease. Am J Hum Genet 52:557–564

Poenaru L, Castelnau L, Besancon AM, Nicolesco H, Akli S, Theophil D (1988) First trimester prenatal diagnosis of metachromatic leukodystrophy on chorionic villi by immunoprecipitation – electrophoresis. J Inherited Metab Dis 11:123–130

Polten A, Fluharty AL, Fluharty CB, Kappler J, von Figura K, Gieselmann V (1991) Molecular basis of different forms of metachromatic leukodystrophy. N Engl J Med 324:18–22

Rafi MA, Zhang X, de Gala G, Wenger DA (1990) Detection of a point mutation in sphingolipid activator protein-1 mRNA in patients with a cariant form of metachromatic leukodystrophy. Biochem Biophys Res Commun 166:1017–1023

Rafi MA, Amini S, Zhang X, Wenger DA (1992) Correction of sulfatide metabolism after transfer of prosaposin cDNA to cultured cells from a patient with SAP-I deficiency. Am J Hum Genet 50:1252–1258

Reider-Grosswasser I, Bornstein N (1987) CT and MRI in late-onset metachromatic leukodystrophy. Acta Neurol Scand 75:64–69

Résibois-Grégoire A (1967) Electron microscopic studies of metachromatic leucodystrophy II. Compound nature of the inclusions. Acta Neuropathol 9:244–253

Rommerskirch W, Fluharty AL, Peters C, von Figura K, Gieselmann (1991) Restoration of arylsulphatase A activity in human-metachromatic-leucodystrophy fibroblasts via retroviral-vector-mediated gene transfer. Biochem J 280:459–461

Schipper HI, Seidel D (1984) Computed tomography in late-onset metachromatic leucodystrophy. Neuroradiology 26:39–44

Schlote W, Harzer K, Christomanou H, Paton BC, KustermannB, Schmid B, Seeger J, Beudt U, Schuster I, Langenbeck U (1991) Sphingolipid activator protein 1 deficiency in metachromatic leucodystrophy with normal arylsulphatase A activity. A clinical, morphological, biochemical, and immunological study. Eur J Pediatr 150:584–591

Scholz W (1925) Klinische, pathologisch-anatomische und erbbiologische Untersuchungen. Z Neurol Psychiatr 99:651–717

Shapiro EG, Lipton ME, Krivit W (1992) White matter dysfunction and its neuropsychological correlates: a longitudinal study of a case of metachromatic leukodystrophy treated with bone marrow transplant. J Clin Exp Neuropsychol 14:610–624

Skomer C, Stears J, Austin J (1983) Metachromatic leukodystrophy (MLD). Arch Neurol 40:354–355

Slavin S, Naparstek E, Ziegler M, Lewin A (1992) Clinical application of intrauterine bone marrow transplantation for treatment of genetic diseases – feasibility studies. Bone Marrow Transplant 9 [Suppl 1]:189–190

Stevens RL, Fluharty AL, Kihara H, Kaback MM, Shapiro LJ, Marsh B, Sandhoff K, Fischer G (1981) Cerebroside sulfatase activator deficiency induced metachromatic leukodystrophy. Am J Hum Genet 33:900–906

Toda K, Kobayashi T, Goto I, Kurokawa T, Ogomori K (1989) Accumulation of lysosulfatide (sulfogalactosylsphingosine) in tissues of a boy with metachromatic leukodystrophy. Biochem Biophys Res Commun 159:605–611

Waltz G, Harik SI, Kaufman B (1987) Adult metachromatic leukodystrophy: value of computed tomographic scanning and magnetic resonance imaging of the brain. Arch Neurol 44:225–227

Wenger DA, Louie E (1991) Pseudodeficiencies of arylsulfatase A and galactocerebrosidase activities. Dev Neurosci 13:216–221

Wright GDS, Patel MK, Mikel J (1988) An adult onset metachromatic leukodystrophy with dominant inheritance and normal arylsulphatase A levels. J Neurol Sci 87:153–166

Zhang XL, Rafi MA, DeGala G, Wenger DA (1990) Insertion in the mRNA of a metachromatic leukodystrophy patient with sphingolipid activator protein-1 deficiency. Proc Natl Acad Sci USA 87:1426–1430

Zhang X, Rafi MA, Gala de G, Wenger DA (1991) The mechanism for a 33-nucleotide insertion in mRNA causing sphingolipid activator protein (SAP-1)-deficient metachromatic leukodystrophy. Hum Genet 87:211–215

7 Multiple Sulfatase Deficiency

Aqeel AA, Ozand PT, Brismar J, Gascon GG, Brismar G, Nester M, Sakati N (1992) Saudi variant of multiple sulfatase deficiency. J Child Neurol 7:S12-S21

Austin J, Armstrong D, Shearer L (1965) Metachromatic form of diffuse cerebral sclerosis. Arch Neurol 13:593–614

Austin JH (1973) Studies in metachromatic leukodystrophy. Arch Neurol 28:258–264

Basner R, von Figura K, Glössl J, Klein U, Kresse H, Mlekusch W (1979) Multiple deficiency of mucopolysaccharide sulfatases in mucosulfatidosis. Pediatr Res 13:1316–1318

Bateman BJ, Philippart M, Isenberg SJ (1984) Ocular features of multiple sulfatase deficiency and a new variant of metachromatic leukodystrophy. J Pediatr Ophthalmol Strab 21:133–139

Bharucha BA, Nalk G, Savliwala AS, Joshi RM, Kumta NB (1984) Siblings with the Austin variant of metachromatic leukodystrophy multiple sulfatidosis. Indian J Pediatr 51:477–480

Burch M, Fesnom AH, Jackson M, Pitts-Tucker T, Congdon PJ (1986) Multiple sulphatase deficiency presenting at birth. Clin Genet 30:409–415

Burk RD, Valle D, Thomas GH, Miller C, Moser A, Moser H, Rosenbaum KN (1984) Early manifestations of multiple sulfatase deficiency. J Pediatr 104:574–578

Conary JT, Hasilik A, von Figura K (1988) Synthesis and stability of steroid sulfatase in fibroblasts from multiple sulfatase deficiency. Biol Chem Hoppe-Seyler 369:297–302

Constantopoulos G (1988) Multiple sulfatase deficiency with a novel biochemical presentation. Eur J Pediatr 147:634–638

Couchot J, Pluot M, Schmauch MA, Pennaforte F, Fandre M (1974) La Mucosulfatidose. Étude de trois cas familiaux. Arch Franc Pediatr 31:775–795

Eto Y, Gomibuchi I, Umezawa F, Tsuda T (1987) Pathochemistry, pathogenesis and enzyme replacement in multiple-sulfatase deficiency. Enzyme 38:273–279

Fede K, Horwitz AL (1984) Complementation of multiple sulfatase deficiency in somatic cell hybrids. Am J Hum Genet 36:623–633

Fluharty AL, Stevens RL, Davis LL, Shapiro LJ, Kihara H (1978) Presence of arylsulfatase A (ARS A) in multiple sulfatase deficiency disorder fibroblasts. Am J Hum Genet 30:249–255

Guerra WF, Verity A, Fluharty AL, Nguyen HT, Philippart M (1990) Multiple sulfatase deficiency:clinical, neuropathological, ultrastructural and biochemical studies. J Neuropathol Exp Neurol 49:406–423

Harbord M, Buncic JR, Chuang SA, Skomorowski MA, Clarke JTR (1991) Multiple sulfatase deficiency with early severe retinal degeneration. J Child Neurol 6:229–235

Harbord M, Buncic R, Chuang SA, Skomorowski MA, Clarke JTR (1991) Multiple sulfatase deficiency with early severe retinal degeneration. J Child Neurol 6:229–235

Horwitz AL, Warshawsky L, King J, Burns G (1986) Rapid degradation of steroid sulfatase in multiple sulfatase deficiency. Biochem Biophys Res Commun 135:389–396

Kepes JJ, Berry A, Zacharias DL (1988) Multiple sulfatase deficiency: bridge between neuronal storage diseases and leukodystrophies. Pathology 20:285–291

Mossakowski M, Mathieson G, Cumings JN (1961) On the relationship of metachromatic leucodystrophy and amaurotic idiocy. Brain 84:585–604

Nevsimalova S, Elleder M, Smid F, Zemankova M (1984) Multiple sulphatase deficiency in homozygotic twins. J Inherited Metab Dis 7:38–40

Perlmutter-Cremer N, Libert J, Vamos E, Sphel M, Kiebaers I (1981) Unusual early manifestation of multiple sulfatase deficiency. Ann Radiol 24:43–48

Rampini S, Isler W, Baerlocher K, Bischoff A, Ulrich J, Plüss HJ (1970) Die Kombination von metachromatischer Leukodystrophie und Mukopolysaccharidose als selbständiges Krankheitsbild (Mukosulfatidose). Helv Pediatr Acta 5:436–461

Raynaud EJ, Escourolle R, Baumann N, Turpin JC, Dubois G, Malpuech G, Lagarde R (1975) Metachromatic leukodystrophy. Ultrastructural and enzymatic study of a case of variant 0 form. Arch Neurol 32:834–838

Rommerskirch W, von Figura K (1992) Multiple sulfatase deficiency:catalytically inactive sulfatases are expressd from retrovirally introduced sulfatase cDNAs. Proc Natl Acad Sci USA 89:261–265

Soong BW, Casamassima AC, Fink JK, Constantopoulos G, Horwitz AL (1988) Multiple sulfatase deficiency. Neurology 38:1273–1275

Tanaka A, Hirabayashi M, Ishii M, Yamaoka S (1987) Complementation studies with clinical and biochemical characterizations of a new variant of multiple sulphatase deficiency. J Inherited Metab Dis 10:103–110

Vamos E, Lubairs I, Bousard N, Liberi J, Pirimutter N (1981) Multiple sulphatase deficiency with early onset. J Inherited Metab 4:103–104

Waheed A, Hasilik A, Figura von K (1982) Enhanced breakdown of arylsulfatase A in multiple sulfatase deficiency. Eur J Biochem 123:317–321

8 Globoid Cell Leukodystrophy

Andrews JM, Cancilla PA, Grippo J, Menkes JH (1971) Globoid cell leukodystrophy (Krabbe's disease): morphological and biochemical studies. Neurology 21:337–352

Austin J (1963) Studies in globoid (Krabbe) leukodystrophy. Arch Neurol 9:207–231

Austin J (1963) Studies in globoid (Krabbe) leukodystrophy. II. J Neurochem 10:921–930

Austin J, Suzuki K, Armstrong D, Brady R, Bachhawat BK, Schlenker J, Stumpf D (1970) Studies in globoid (Krabbe) leukodystrophy (GLD). Arch Neurol 23:502–512

Baker RH, Trautmann JC, Younge BR, Nelson KD, Zimmerman R (1990) Late juvenile-onset Krabbe's disease. Ophthalmology 97:1176–1180

Baram TZ, Goldman AM, Percy AK (1986) Krabbe disease: specific MRI and CT findings. Neurology 36:111–115

Bischoff A, Ulrich J (1969) Peripheral neuropathy in globoid cell leukodystrophy (Krabbe's disease). Ultrastructural and histochemical findings. Brain 92:861–870

Cavanagh N, Kendall B (1986) High density on computed tomography in infantile Krabbe's disease: a case report. Dev Med Child Neurol 28:799–802

Choi S, Enzmann DR (1993) Infantile Krabbe disease: complementary CT and MR findings. AJNR 14:1164–1166

Cruz-Sanchez FF, Martos JA, Rives A, Ribalta T, Ferrer I, Cardesa A (1991) Adult type of leukodystrophy. Krabbe's disease? Clin Neurol Neurosurg 93-3:217–222

Demaerel Ph, Wilms G, Verdru P, Carton H, Baert AL (1990) MR findings in globoid cell leukodystrophy. Neuroradiology 32:520–522

Dunn HG, Dolman CL, Farrell DF, Tischler B, Hasinoff C, Woolf LI (1976) Krabbe's leukodystrophy without globoid cells. Neurology 26:1035–1041

Ellis WG, Schneider EL, McCulloch JR, Suzuki K, Epstein CJ (1973) Fetal globoid cell leukodystrophy (Krabbe disease). Arch Neurol 29:253–257

Epstein MA, Zimmerman RA, Rorke LB, Sladky JT (1991) Late-onset globoid cell leukodystrophy mimicking an infiltrating glioma. Pediatr Radiol 21:131–132

Eto Y, Suzuki K (1971) Brain spingoglycolipids in Krabbe's globoid cell leucodystrophy. J Neurochem 18:503–511

Eto Y, Suzuki K, Suzuki K (1970) Globoid cell leukodystrophy (Krabbe's disease): isolation of myelin with normal glycolipid composition. J Lipid Res 11:473–479

Farley TJ, Ketonen LM, Bodensteiner JB, Wang DD (1992) Serial MRI and CT findings in infantile Krabbe disease. Pediatr Neurol 8:455–458

Feanny SJ, Chuang SH, Becker LE, Clarke JTR (1987) Intracerebral paraventricular hyperdensities:a new CT sign in Krabbe globoid cell leukodystrophy. J Inherited Metab Dis 10:24–27

Finelli DA, Tarr RW, Sawyer RN, Horwitz SJ (1994) Deceptively normal MR in early infantile Krabbe disease. AJNR 15:167–171

Fiumara A, Pavone L, Siciliano L, Tinè A, Parano E, Innico G (1990) Late-onset globoid cell leukodystrophy:report on seven new patients. Childs Nerv Syst 6:194–197

Giles L, Cooper A, Fowler B, Sardharwalla IB, Donnai P (1987) Krabbe's disease:first trimester diagnosis confirmed on cultured amniotic fluid cells and fetal tissues. Prenat Diagn 7:329–332

Goebel HH, Harzer K, Ernst JP, Bohl J, Klein H (1990) Late-onset globoid cell leukodystrophy:unusual ultrastructural pathology and subtotal β-galactocerebrosidase deficiency. J Child Neurol 5:299–307

Grewal RP, Petronas N, Barton NW (1991) Late onset globoid cell leukodystrophy. J Neurol Neurosurg Psychiatry 54:1011–1012

Hagberg B, Kollberg H, Sourander P, Akesson HO (1969) Infantile globoid cell leucodystrophy. Neuropediatrics 1:74–88

Hagberg B (1984) Krabbe's disease: clinical presentation of neurological variants. Neuropediatrics 15:11–15

Harzer K, Hager HD, Tariverdian G (1987) Prenatal enzymatic diagnosis and exclusion of Krabbe's disease (globoid cell leukodystrophy) using chorionic villi in five risk pregnancies. Hum Genet 77:342–344

Ieshima A, Eda I, Matsui A, Yoshino K, Takashima S, Takeshita K (1983) Computed tomography in Krabbe's disease: comparison with neuropathology. Neuroradiology 25:323–327

Igisu H, Nakamura M (1986) Inhibition of cytochrome C oxidase by psychosine (Galactosylsphingosine). Biochem Biophys Res Commun 137:323–327

Jardin LB, Giugliani R, Fensom AH (1992) Thalamic and basal ganglia hyperdensities – A CT marker for globoid cell leukodystrophy? Neuropediatrics 23:30–31

Kapoor R, McDonald WI, Crockard A, Moseley IF (1992) Clinical onset and MRI features of Krabbe's disease in adolescence. J Neurol Neurosurg Psychiatry 55:331–332

Kobayashi T, Shinoda H, Goto I, Yamanaka T, Suzuki Y (1987) Globoid cell leukodystrophy is a generalized galactosylsphingosine (psychosine) storage disease. Biochem Biophys Res Commun 144:41–46

Kobayashi T, Goto I, Yamanaka T, Suzuki Y, Nakano T, Suzuki K (1988) Infantile and fetal globoid cell leukodystrophy: analysis of galactosylceramide and galactosylsphingosine. Ann Neurol 24:517–522

Kolodny EH, Raghavan S, Krivit W (1991) Late-onset Krabbe disease (globoid cell leukodystrophy):clinical and biochemical features of 15 cases. Dev Neurosci 13:232–239

Krabbe K (1916) A new familial, infantile form of diffuse brain-sclerosis. Brain 39:74–114

Kurokawa T, Chen YJ, Nagata M (1987) Late infantile Krabbe leukodystrophy: MRI and evoked potentials in a Japanese girl. Neuropediatrics 18:182–183

Kwan E, Drace J, Enzmann D (1984) Specific CT findings in Krabbe disease. AJNR 5:453–458

Loonen MCB (1985) Late-onset globoid cell leucodystrophy (Krabbe's disease): clinical and genetic delineation of two forms and their relation to the early-infantile form. Neuropediatrics 16:137–142

Lyon G, Hagberg B, Evrard Ph, Allaire C, Pavone L, Vanier M (1991) Symptomatology of late onset Krabbe's leukodystrophy: the european experience. Dev Neurosci 13:240–244

Malone MJ, Szöke MC, Looney GL (1975) Globoid leukodystrophy: I. Clinical and enzymatic studies. Arch Neurol 32:606–612

McKelvie P, Vine P, Hopkins I, Poulos A (1990) A case of Krabbe's leukodystrophy without globoid cells. Pathology 22:235–238

Mei Liu H (1970) Ultrastructure of globoid leukodystrophy (Krabbe's disease) with reference to the origin of globoid cells. J Neuropathol Exp Neurol 29:441–462

Menkes JH, Duncan C, Moossy J (1966) Molecular composition of the major glycolipids in globoid cell leukodystrophy. Neurology 16:581–593

Mitsuo K, Kobayashi T, Shinnoh N, Goto I (1989) Biosynthesis of galactosylsphingosine (psychosine) in the twitcher mouse. Neurochem Res 14:899–903

Olsson Y, Sourander P, Svennerholm L (1966) Experimental studies on the pathogenesis of leucodystrophies. I. The effect of intracerebrally injected sphingolipids in the rat's brain. Acta Neuropathol (Berl) 6:153–163

Percy AK, Odrezin GT, Knowles PD, Rouah E, Armstrong DD (1994) Globoid cell leukodystrophy:comparison of neuropathology with magnetic resonance imaging. Acta Neuropathol (Berl) 88:26–32

Phelps M, Aicardi J, Vanier MT (1991) Late onset Krabbe's leukodystrophy: a report of four cases. J Neurol Neurosurg Psychiatry 54:293–296

Sasaki M, Sakuragawa N, Takashima S, Hanaoka S, Arima M (1991) MRI and CT findings in Krabbe disease. Pediatr Neurol 7:283–288

Schwankhaus JD, Patronas N, Dorwart R, Eldridge R, Schlesinger S, McFarland H (1988) Computed tomography and magnetic resonance imaging in adult-onset leukodystrophy. Arch Neurol 45:1004–1008

Sourander P, Hansson HA, Olsson Y, Svennerholm L (1966) Experimental studies on the pathogenesis of leucodystrophies. II. The effect of sphingolipids on various cell types in cultures from the nervous system. Acta Neuropathol (Berl) 6:231–242

Sugama S, Eto Y, Yamamoto H, Kim SU (1991) Psychosine cytotoxicity toward rat C6 glioma cells and the protective effects of phorbol ester and dimethylsulfoxide: implications for therapy in Krabbe disease. Brain Dev 13:104–109

Suzuki K, Grover WD (1970) Krabbe's leukodystrophy (globoid cell leukodystrophy). Arch Neurol 22:385–396

Suzuki K, Suzuki Y (1970) Globoid cell leucodystrophy (Krabbe's disease):deficiency of galactocerebroside β-galactosidase. Proc Natl Acad Sci USA 66:302–309

Suzuki Y, Suzuki K (1971) Krabbe's globoid cell leukodystrophy: deficiency of galactocerebrosidase in serum, leukocytes, and fibroblasts. Science 171:73–75

Svennerholm L, Vanier MT, Mansson JE (1980) Krabbe disease:a galactosylsphingosine (psychosine) lipidosis. J Lipid Res 21:53–64

Tada K, Taniike M, Tsukamoto H, Inui K, Okada S (1992) Serial magnetic resonance imaging studies in a case of late onset globoid cell leukodystrophy. Neuropediatrics 23:306–309

Verdru P, Lammens M, Dom R, Van Elsen A (1991) Globoid cell leukodystrophy:a family with both late-infantile and adult type. Neurology 41:1382–1384

Vos AJM, Joosten EMG, Gabreëls-Festen AAWM, Gabreëls FJM (1983) An atypical case of infantile globoid cell leukodystrophy. Neuropediatrics 14:110–112

Wenger DA, Louie E (1991) Pseudodeficiencies of arylsulfatase A and galactocerebrosidase activities. Dev Neurosci 13:216–221

Wenger DA, Riccardi VM (1976) Possible misdiagnosis of Krabbe disease. J Pediatr 88:76–79

Ynis EJ, Lee RE (1969) The ultrastructure of globoid (Krabbe) leukodystrophy. Lab Invest 21:415–419

Zlotogora J, Chakraborty S, Knowlton RG, Wenger DA (1990) Krabbe disease locus mapped to chromosome 14 by genetic linkage. Am J Hum Genet 47:37–44

9 GM$_1$ Gangliosidosis

Beratis NG, Varvarigou-Frimas A, Beratis S, Sklower SL (1989) Angiokeratoma corporis diffusum in GM$_1$ gangliosidosis, type 1. Clin Genet 36:59–64

Cabral A, Portela R, Tasso T, Eusebio F, Moreira A, Marques dos Santos H, Soares J, Moura-Nunes JF (1989) A case of GM$_1$ gangliosidosis type I. Ophthalmic Paediatr Genet 10:63–67

Gascon GG, Ozand PT, Erwin RE (1992) GM$_1$ gangliosidosis type 2 in two siblings. J Child Neurol 7:S41–S50

Goebel HH (1984) Morphology of the gangliosidoses. Neuropediatrics 15:97–106

Guazzi GC, D'Amor I, von Hoof F, Fuschelli C, Alessandrini C, Palmeri S, Federico A (1988) Type 3 (chronic) GM$_1$ gangliosidosis presenting as infanto-choreo-athetotic dementia, without epilepsy, in three sisters. Neurology 38:1124–1127

Ida H, Eto Y, Maekawa K (1989) Fetal GM$_1$-gangliosidosis: morphological and biochemical studies. Brain Dev 11:394–398

Inui K, Namba R, Ihara Y, Nobukuni K, Taniike M, Midorikawa M, Tsukamoto H (1990) A case of chronic GM$_1$ gangliosidosis presenting as dystonia:clinical and biochemical studies. J Neurol 237:491–493

Kasama T, Taketomi T (1986) Abnormalities of cerebral lipids in GM$_1$-gangliosidoses, infantile, juvenile, and chronic type. Jpn J Exp Med 56:1–11

Kaye EM, Alroy J, Raghavan SS, Schwarting GA, Adelman LS, Runge V, Gelblum D, Johann G, Thalhammer DVM, Zuniga G (1992) Dysmyelinogenesis in animal model of GM$_1$ gangliosidosis. Pediatr Neurol 8:255–261

Kobayashi T, Suzuki K (1981) Chronic GM$_1$ gangliosidosis presenting as dystonia:II. Biochemical studies. Ann Neurol 9:476–483

Kohlschütter A (1984) Clinical course of GM$_1$ gangliosidoses. Neuropediatrics 15:71–73

Lake BD (1984) Lysosomal enzyme deficiencies. In: Hume Adams J, Corsellis JAN, Duchen LW (eds) Greenfield's neuropathology, 4th edn. Arnold, London, pp 491–572

Morimoto S, Yamamoto Y, O'Brien JS, Kishimoto Y (1990) Distribution of saposin proteins (sphingolipid activator proteins) in lysosomal storage and other diseases. Proc Natl Acad Sci USA 87:3493–3497

Nardocci N, Bertagnolio B, Rumi V, Combi M, Bardelli P, Angelini L (1993) Chronic GM$_1$ gangliosidosis presenting as dystonia: clinical and biochemical studies in a new case. Neuropediatrics 24:164–166

Nausieda PA, Klawans HI (1977) Generalized gangliosidosis – GM$_1$ disease (muccopolysaccharidosis VII, pseudo-Hurler's disease, Norman Landing disease). In: Vinken PJ, Bruyn GW (eds) Handbook of clinical neurology, vol 29. North Holland, Amsterdam, pp 367–369

Nishimoto J, Nanba E, Inui K, Okada S, Suzuki K (1991) GM$_1$-gangliosidosis (genetic β-galactosidase deficiency): identification of four mutations in different clinical phenotypes among Japanese patients. Am J Hum Genet 49:566–574

O'Brien JS (1970) Generalized gangliosidosis. In: Vinken PJ, Bruyn GW (eds) Handbook of clinical neurology, vol 10. North Holland, Amsterdam, pp 462–483

O'Brien JS (1983) The gangliosidosis. In: Stanbury JB, Wijngaarden JB, Frederickson DS (eds) The metabolic basis of inherited disease, 5th edn. McGraw-Hill, New York, pp 945–967

O'Brien JS, Storb R, Raff RF, Harding J, Appelbaum F, Morimoto S, Kishimoto Y, Graham T, Ahern-Rindell A, O'Brien SL (1990) Bone marrow transplantation in canine GM$_1$ gangliosidosis. Clin Genet 38:274–280

Pampiglione G, Harden A (1984) Neurophysiological investigations in GM$_1$ and GM$_2$ gangliosidoses. Neuropediatrics 15:74–84

Sandhoff K, Conzelmann E (1984) The biochemical basis of gangliosidoses. Neuropediatrics 15:85–92

Schwab ME, Vassella F (1984) Synopsis: gangliosidoses. Neuropediatrics 15:107–109

Suzuki K, Suzuki K, Chen GC (1968) Morphological, histochemical and biochemical studies on a case of systemic late infantile lipidosis (generalized gangliosidosis). J Neuropathol Exp Neurol 27:15–38

Suzuki K, Suzuki K, Kamoshita S (1969) Chemical pathology of GM$_1$ gangliosidosis (generalized gangliosidosis). J Neuropathol Exp Neurol 28:25–73

Suzuki Y, Sakuraba H, Oshima A, Yoshida K, Shimmoto M, Takano T, Fukuhara Y (1991) Clinical and molecular heterogeneity in hereditary β-galactosidase deficiency. Dev Neurosci 13:299–303

Uyama E, Terasaki T, Watanabe S, Naito M, Owada M, Araki S, Ando M (1992) Type 3 GM$_1$ gangliosidosis: characteristic MRI findings correlated with dystonia. Acta Neurol Scand 86:609–615

Walkley SU, Baker HJ, Rattazzi MC, Haskins ME, Wu JY (1991) Neuroaxonal dystrophy in neuronal storage disorders: evidence for major GABAergic neuron involvement. J Neurol Sci 104:1–8

Wood PA, McBride MR, Baker HJ, Christian ST (1985) Fluorescence polarization analysis, lipid composition, and Na$^+$, K$^+$-ATPase kinetics of synaptosomal membranes in feline GM$_1$ and GM$_2$ gangliosidosis. J Neurochem 44:947–956

Yoshida K, Oshima A, Sakuraba H, Nakano T, Yanagisawa N, Inui K, Okada S, Uyama E, Namba R, Kondo K, Iwasaki S, Takamiya K, Suzuki Y (1992) GM$_1$ gangliosidosis in adults: clinical and molecular analysis of 16 Japanese patients. Ann Neurol 31:328–332

10 GM$_2$ Gangliosidosis

Argov Z, Navon R (1984) Clinical and genetic variations in the syndrome of adult GM$_2$ gangliosidosis resulting from hexosaminidase A deficiency. Ann Neurol 16:14–20

Azzo A, Proia RL, Kolodny EH, Kaback MM, Neufeld EF (1984) Faulty association of α-and β-subunits in some forms of β-hexosaminidase A deficiency. J Biol Chem 259:11070–11074

Barnes D, Misra VP, Young EP, Thomas PK, Harding AE (1991) An adult onset hexosaminidase A deficiency syndrome with sensory neuropathy and internuclear ophthalmoplegia. J Neurol Neurosurg Psychiatr 54:1112–1113

Barness LA, Henry K, Kling P, Laxova R, Kaback M, Gilbert-Barness E (1991) Clinico-pathological report: a 7-year old white-male boy with progressive neurological deterioration. Am J Med Genet 40:271–279

Bérard-Badier M, Paillas JE, Gastaut H, Edgar GWF (1958) Essai sur la signification des démyélinisations dans l'idiotie amaurotique infantile. Psychiatr Neurol 132:50–93

Bolhuis PA, Oonk JGW, Kamp PE, Ris AJ, Michalski JC, Overdijk B, Reuser AJJ (1987) Ganglioside storage, hexosaminidase lability, and urinary oligosaccharides in adult Sandhoff's disease. Neurology 37:75–81

Brett EM, Ellis RB, Haas L, Ikonne JU, Lake BD, Patrick AD, Stephens R (1973) Late onset GM$_2$ gangliosidosis: clinical, pathological, and biochemical studies on 8 patients. Arch Dis Child 48:775–785

Brismar J, Brismar G, Coates R, Gascon G, Ozand P (1990) Increased density of the thalamus on CT scans in patients with GM$_2$ gangliosidoses. AJNR 11:125–130

Budde-Steffen C, Steffen M, Siegel DA, Suzuki K (1988) Presence of β-hexosaminidase A α-chain mRNA in two different variants of GM$_2$-gangliosidosis. Neuropediatrics 19:59–61

Burg J, Banerjee A, Sandhoff K (1985) Molecular forms of GM$_2$-activator protein. Biol Chem Hoppe Seyler 366:887–891

Charrow J, Binns HJ (1986) Ganglioside loading of cultured fibroblasts:a provocative method for the diagnosis of the GM$_2$ gangliosidoses. Clin Chim Acta 156:41–50

Conzelmann E, Kytzia HJ, Navon R, Sandhoff K (1983) Ganglioside GM$_2$ N-acetyl-β-D-galactosaminidase activity in cultured fibroblasts of late-infantile and adult GM$_2$ gangliosidosis patients and of healthy probands with low hexosaminidase level. Am J Hum Genet 35:900–913

Conzelmann E, Sandhoff K (1978) AB variant of infantile GM$_2$ gangliosidosis:deficiency of a factor necessary for stimulation of hexosaminidase A-catalyzed degradation of ganglioside GM$_2$ and glycolipid GA$_2$. Proc Natl Acad Sci USA 75:3979–3983

Fardeau M, Lapresle J (1963) Maladie de Tay-Sachs avec atteinte importante de la substance blanche. A propos de deux observations anatomo-cliniques. Rev Neurol 109:157–175

Federico A, Palmeri S, Malandrini A, Fabrizi G, Mondelli M, Guazzi GC (1991) The clinical aspects of adult hexosaminidase deficiencies. Dev Neurosci 13:280–287

Fukumizu M, Yoshikawa H, Takashima N, Kurokawa T (1992) Tay-Sachs disease: progression of changes on neuroimaging in four cases. Neuroradiology 34:483–486

Goebel HH, Stolte G, Kustermann-Kuhn B, Harzer K (1989) B$_1$ variant of GM$_2$ gangliosidosis in a 12-year-old patient. Pediatr Res 25:89–93

Goebel HH (1984) Morphology of the gangliosidoses. Neuropediatrics 15 [Suppl]: 97–106

Goldie WD, Holtzman D, Suzuki K (1977) Chronic hexosaminidase A and B deficiency. Ann Neurol 2:156–158

Gordon BA, Gordon KE, Hinton GG, Cadera W, Feleki V, Bayleran J, Hechtman P (1988) Tay-Sachs disease:B1 variant. Pediatr Neurol 4:54–57

Grabowski GA, Kruse JR, Goldberg JD, Chockkalingam K, Gordon RE, Blakemore KJ, Mahoney MJ, Desnick RJ (1984) First-trimester prenatal diagnosis of Tay-Sachs disease. Am J Hum Genet 36:1369–1378

Gray RGF, Green A, Rabb L, Broadhead DM, Besley GTN (1990) A case of the B$_1$ variant of GM$_2$-gangliosidosis. J Inherited Metab Dis 13:280–282

Hirabayashi Y, Li YT, Li SC (1983) The protein activator specific for the enzymic hydrolysis of GM$_2$ ganglioside in normal human brain and brains of three types of GM$_2$ gangliosidosis. J Neurochem 40:168–175

Johnson WG, Chutorian A, Miranda A (1977) A new juvenile hexosaminidase deficiency disease presenting as cerebellar ataxia: clinical and biochemical studies. Neurology 27:1012–1018

MacLeod PM, Wood S, Jan JE, Applegarth DA, Dolman CL (1976) Progressive cerebellar ataxia, spasticity, psychomotor retardation, and hexosaminidase deficiency in a 10-

year-old child: juvenile Sandhoff disease. Neurology 27:571–573

Karni A, Navon R, Sadeh M (1988) Hexosaminidase A deficiency manifesting as spinal muscular atrophy of late onset. Ann Neurol 24:451–453

Koelfen W, Freund M, Jaschke W, Koenig S, Schultze C (1994) GM$_2$ gangliosidosis (Sandhoff's disease): two year follow-up by MRI. Neuroradiology 36:152–154

Kotagal S (1986) Diagnosis of AB variant, GM$_2$ gangliosidosis. Ann Neurol 19:102

Kotagal S, Wenger DA, Alcala H, Gomez C, Horenstein S (1986) AB variant GM$_2$ gangliosidosis: cerebrospinal fluid and neuropathlogic characteristics. Neurology 36:438–440

Kytzia HJ, Hinrichs U, Sandhoff K (1984) Diagnosis of infantile and juvenile forms of GM$_2$ gangliosidosis variant 0. Resiudal activities toward natural and different synthetic substrates. Hum Genet 67:414–418

Maia M, Alves D, Ribeiro G, Pinto R, Sa Miranda MC (1989) Juvenile GM$_2$ gangliosidosis variant B$_1$: clinical and biochemical study in seven patients. Neuropediatrics 21:18–23

Meek D, Wolfe LS, Andermann E, Andermann F (1984) Juvenile progressive dystonia: a new phenotype of GM$_2$ gangliosidosis. Ann Neurol 15:348–352

Morimoto S, Yamamoto Y, O'Brien JS, Kishimoto Y (1990) Distribution of saposin proteins (sphingolipid activator proteins) in lysosomal storage and other diseases. Proc Natl Acad Sci USA 87:3493–3497

Nardocci N, Betagnolio B, Rumi V, Angelini L (1992) Progressive dystonia symptomatic of juvenile GM$_2$ gangliosidosis. Movement Dis 7:64–67

Navon R (1991) Molecular and clinical heterogeneity of adult GM$_2$ gangliosidosis. Dev Neurosci 13:295–298

Navon R, Proia RL (1989) The mutations in Ashkenazi Jews with adult GM$_2$ gangliosidosis, the adult form of Tay-Sachs disease. Science 243:1471–1474

Navon R, Argov Z, Brand N, Sandbank U (1981) Adult GM$_2$ gangliosidosis in association with Tay-Sachs disease: a new phenotype. Neurology 31:1397–1401

Navon R, Argov Z, Frisch A (1986) Hexosaminidase A deficiency in adults. Am J Med Genetics 24:179–196

Navon R, Kolodny EH, Mitsumoto H, Thomas GH, Proia RL (1990) Ashkenazi-Jewish and non-Jewish adult GM$_2$ gangliosidosis patients share a common genetic defect. Am J Hum Genet 46:817–821

Neote K, Mahuran DJ, Gravel RA (1991) Molecular genetics of β-hexosaminidase deficiencies. Adv Neurol 56:189–207

O'Brien JS (1983) The gangliosidoses. In: Stanbury JB, Wijngaarden JB, Frederickson DS (eds) The metabolic basis of inherited disease, 5th edn. McGraw-Hill, New York, pp 945–967

Oates CE, Bosch EP, Hart MN (1986) Movement disorders associated with chronic GM$_2$ gangliosidosis. Eur Neurol 25:154–159

Ohno K, Suzuki K (1988) Mutation in GM$_2$-gangliosidosis B1 variant. J Neurochem 50:316–318

Oonk JGW, van den Helm HJ, Martin JJ (1979) Spinocerebellar degeneration: hexosaminidase A and B deficiency in two adult sisters. Neurology 29:380–384

Pampiglione G, Harden A (1984) Neurophysiological investigations in GM, and GM$_2$ gangliosidoses. Neuropediatrics 15 [Suppl]:74–84

Paw BH, Moskowitz SM, Uhrhammer N, Wright N, Kaback MM, Neufeld EF (1990) Juvenile GM$_2$ gangliosidosis caused by substitution of histidine for arginine at position 499 or 504 of the α-subunit of β-hexosaminidase. J Biol Chem 265:9452–9457E, Ginsberg N, Verlinksy Y, Cadkin A, Chu L, Trnka L (1983) Prenatal Tay-Sachs diagnosis by chorionic villi sampling. Lancet 30:286

Praamstra P, Wevers RA, Gabreëls FJM, Rotteveel JJ, Renier WO, Sengers RCA, Lamers KJB (1990) GM$_2$-gangliosidosis: clinical and biochemical aspects of four cases. Clin Neurol Neurosurg 92:143–148

Pullarkat RK, Reha H, Beratis NG (1981) Accumulation of ganglioside GM$_2$ in cerebrospinal fluid of a patient with the variant AB of infantile GM$_2$ gangliosidosis. Pediatrics 68:106–108

Rapin I, Suzuki K, Suzuki K, Valsamis MP (1976) Adult (chronic) GM$_2$ gangliosidosis: atypical spinocerebellar degeneration in a Jewish sibship. Arch Neurol 33:120–130

Rubin M, Karpati G, Wolfe LS, Carpenter S, Klavins MH, Mahuran DJ (1988) Adult onset motor neuropathy in the juvenile type of hexosaminidase A and B deficiency. J Neurol Sci 87:103–119

Sandhoff K, Harzer K, Wässle W, Jatzkewitz H (1971) Enzyme alterations and lipid storage in three variants of Tay-Sachs disease. J Neurochem 18:2469–2489

Sandhoff K, Conzelmann E (1984) The biochemical basis of gangliosidoses. Neuropediatrics 15 [Suppl]: 85–92

Schulte FJ (1984) Clinical course of GM$_2$ gangliosidoses: a correlative attempt. Neuropediatrics 15:66–70

Sommer B, Spohr HL (1991) GM$_2$-Gangliosidose, Variante 0 (M. Sandhoff): Verdachtsdiagnose einer Speicherkrankheit durch Ultraschall. Monatsschr Kinderheilkd 139:160–162

Sonderfeld S, Brendler S, Sandhoff K, Galjaard H, Hoogeveen AT (1985) Genetic complementation in somatic cell hybrids of four variants of infantile GM$_2$ gangliosidosis. Hum Genet 71:196–200

Sonderfeld S, Conzelmann E, Scharzmann G, Burg J, Hinrichs U, Sandhoff K (1985) Incorporation and metabolism of ganglioside GM$_2$ in skin fibroblasts from normal and GM$_2$ gangliosidosis subjects. Eur J Biochem 149:247–255

Specula N, Vanier MT, Goutières F, Mikol J, Aicardi J (1990) The juvenile and chronic forms of GM$_2$ gangliosidosis: clinical and enzymatic heterogeneity. Neurology 40:145–150

Stalker HP, Kim Han B (1989) Thalamic hyperdenisty:a previously unreported sign of Sandhoff disease. AJNR 10:S82

Streifler JY, Gornish M, Hadar H, Gadoth N (1993) Brain imaging in late-onset GM$_2$ gangliosidosis. Neurology 43:2055–2058

Suzuki K, Vanier MT (1991) Biochemical and molecular aspects of late-onset GM$_2$-gangliosidosis: B1 variant as a prototype. Dev Neurosci 13:288–294

Swab ME, Vassella F (1984) Synopsis: gangliosidoses. Neuropediatrics 15 [Suppl]:107–109

Thieffry S, Bertrand I, Bargeton E, Edgar GWF, Arthuis M (1960) Idiotie amaurotique infantile avec altérations graves de la substance blanche. Rev Neurol 102:130–152

Thomas PK, Young E, King RHM (1989) Sandhoff disease mimicking adult-onset bulbospinal neuropathy. J Neurol Neurosurg Psychiatry 52:1103–1106

Toma L, Pinto W, Rodrigues VC, Dietrich CP, Nader HB (1990) Impaired sulphated glycosaminoglycan metabolism in a patient with GM$_2$ gangliosidosis (Tay-Sachs disease). J Inherited Metab Dis 13:721–731

Volk BW, Schneck L, Adachi M (1970) Clinic, pathology and biochemistry of Tay-Sachs disease. In: Vinken PJ, Bruyn GW (eds) Handbook of clinical neurology, vol 10. North Holland, Amsterdam, pp 385–426

Walkley SU, Baker HJ, Rattazzi MC, Haskins ME, Wu JY (1991) Neuroaxonal dystrophy in neuronal storage disorders: evidence for major GABAergic neuron involvement. J Neurol Sci 104:1–8

Willner JP, Grabowski GA, Gordon RE, Bender AN, Desnick RJ (1981) Chronic GM$_2$ gangliosidosis masquerading as atypical Friedreich ataxia:clinical, morphologic, and biochemical studies of nine cases. Neurology 31:787–798

Wood PA, McBride MR, Baker HJ, Christian ST (1985) Fluorescence polarization analysis, lipid composition and Na$^+$, K$^+$-ATPase kinetics of synaptosomal membranes in feline GM$_1$ and GM$_2$ gangliosidosis. J Neurochem 44:947–956

Xie B, Wang W, Mahuran DJ (1992) A Cys$_{138}$-to-Arg substitution in the GM$_2$ activator protein is associated with the AB variant form of GM$_2$ gangliosidosis. Am J Hum Genet 50:1046–1052

Yoshikawa H, Yamada K, Sakuragawa N (1992) MRI in the early stage of Tay-Sachs disease. Neuroradiology 34:394–395

11 Fabry's Disease

Beyer E, Djatlovitskaya E, Zairatyants O, Berestova A, Mendelson M, Brook E, Wiederschain G (1990) Identification of Fabry disease in two brothers. J Inherited Metab Dis 13:230–231

Deveber GA, Schwarting GA, Kolodny EH, Kowall NW (1992) Fabry disease:immunocytochemical characterization of neuronal involvement. Ann Neurol 31:409–415

Filling-Katz MR, Merrick HF, Fink JK, Miles RB, Sokol J, Barton NW (1989) Carbamazepine in Fabry's disease: effective analgesia with dose-dependent exacerbation of autonomic dysfunction. Neurology 39:598–600

Grewal RP, Barton NW (1992) Fabry's disease presenting with stroke. Clin Neurol Neurosurg 94:177–179

Grewal RP, McLatchey SK (1992) Cerebrovascular manifestations in a female carrier of Fabry's disease. Acta Neurol Belg 92:36–40

Kaye EM, Kolodny EH, Logigian EL, Ullman MD (1988) Nervous system involvement in Fabry's disease: clinicopathological and biochemical correlation. Ann Neurol 23:505–509

Kleijer WJ, Hussaarts-Odijk LM, Sachs ES, Jahoda MGJ, Niermeijer MF (1987) Prenatal diagnosis of Fabry's disease by direct analysis of chorionic villi. Prenat Diagn 7:283–287

Kornreich R, Bishop DF, Desnick RJ (1990) α-galactosidase A gene rearrangements causing Fabry disease. J Biol Chem 265:9319–9326

MacDermot KD, Morgan SH, Cheshire JK, Wilson TM (1987) Anderson Fabry disease, a close linkage with highly polymorphic DNA markers DXS17, DXS87 and DXS88. Hum Genet 77:263–266

Menzies DG, Campbell IW (1988) Magnetic resonance in Fabry's disease. J Neurol Neurosurg Psychiatry 51:1240–1241

Morgan SH, Rudge P, Smith SJM, Bronstein AM, Kendall BE, Holly E, Young EP, Crawfurd MA, Bannister R (1990) The neurological complications of Anderson-Fabry disease (α-galactosidase A deficiency): investigation of symptomatic and presymptomatic patients. Q J Med New Ser 75:491–504

Moumdjian R, Tampieri D, Melanson D, Ethier R (1989) Anderson-Fabry disease: a case report with MR, CT and cerebral angiography. AJNR 10:S69–S70

Natowicz M, Kelley RI (1987) Mendelian etiologies of stroke. Ann Neurol 22:175–192

Nelis GF, Jacobs GJA (1989) anorexia, weight loss, and diarrhea as presenting symptoms of angiokeratoma corporis diffusum (Fabry-Anderson's disease). Dig Dis Sci 34:1798–1800

Paller AS (1987) Metabolic disorders characterized by angiokeratomas and neurologic dysfunction. Neurol Clin 5:441–446

Rahman AN, Lindenberg R (1963) The neuropathology of hereditary dystopic lipidosis. Arch Neurol 9:373–385

Thomas PK (1988) Inherited neuropathies related to disorders of lipid metabolism. In: DiDonato S (ed) Advances in neurology, molecular genetics of neurological and neuromuscular disease. Raven, New York, pp 133–144

12 Fucosidosis

Allen HJ, Ahmed H, DiCioccio RA (1990) Metabolic correction of fucosidosis lymphoid cells by galaptin-α-L-fucosidase conjugates. Biochem Biophys Res Commun 172:335–340

Darby JK, Willems PJ, Nakashima P, Johnsen J, Ferrell RE, Wijsman EM, Gerhard DS, Dracopoli NC, Housman D, Henke J, Fowler ML, Shows TB, O'Brien JS, Cavalli-Sforza LL (1988) Restrictin analysis of the structural α-L-fucosidase gene and its linkage to fucosidosis. Am J Hum Genet 43:749–755

Dawson G, Lenn NJ (1976) Polysaccharide metabolism. In: Vinken PJ, Bruyn GW (eds) Handbook of clinical neurology, vol 27. North Holland, Amsterdam, pp 143–168

Kretz KA, Cripe D, Carson GS, Fukushima H, O'Brien JS (1992) Structure and sequence of the human α-L-fucosidase gene and pseudogene. Genomics 12:276–280

Lake BD (1984) Lysosomal enzyme deficiencies. In: Hume Adams J, Corsellis JAN, Duchen LW (eds) Greenfield's neuropathology, 4th edn. Arnold, London, pp 491–572

Myrianthopoulos NC (1981) Fucosidosis. In: Vinken PJ, Bruyn GW (eds) Handbook of clinical neurology, vol 42. North Holland, Amsterdam, pp 549–550

Nausieda PA, Klawans HL (1971) Lipid storage disorders. In: Vinken PJ, Bruyn GW (eds) Handbook of clinical neurology, vol 29. North Holland, Amsterdam, pp 345–389

Taylor RM, Farrow BRH, Stewart GJ, Healy PJ, Tiver K (1987) Lysosomal enzyme replacement in neural tissue by allogenic bone marrow transplantation following total lymphoid irradiation in canine fucosidosis. Transplant Proc XIX:2730–2734

Taylor RM, Farrow BRH, Stewart GJ (1992) Amelioration of clinical disease following bone marrow transplantation in fucosidase-deficient dogs. Am J Med Genet 42:628–632

13 Mucopolysaccharidoses

Adinolfi M (1993) Hunter syndrome: cloning of the gene, mutations and carrier detection. Dev Med Child Neurol 35:79–85

Afifi AK, Sato Y, Waziri MH, Bell WE (1990) Computed tomography and magnetic resonance imaging of the brain in Hurler's disease. J Child Neurol 5:235–241

Andria G, di Natale P, del Giudice E, Strisciuglio P, Murino P (1979) Sanfilippo B syndrome (MPS III B): mild and severe forms within the same sibship. Clin Genet 15:500–504

Ballabio A, Pallini R, di Natale P (1984) Mucopolysaccharidosis III B: hybridization studies on fibroblasts from a mild case and fibroblasts from severe patients. Clin Genet 25:191–195

Beck M (1991) Mukopolysaccharidosen; Nosologie – Klinik – Therapieansätze. Monatsschr Kinderheilkd 139:120–127

Beck M, Steglich C, Zabel B, Dahl N, Schwinger E, Hopwood JJ, Gal A (1992) Deletion of the Hunter gene and both DXS466 and DXS304 in a patient with mucopolysaccharidosis. Am J Med Genet 44:100–103

Bernsen PLJA, Wevers RA, Gabreëls FJM, Lamers KJB, Sonnen AEH, Schuurmans Stekhoven JH (1987) Phenotypic expression in mucopolysaccharidosis VII. J Neurol Neurosurg Psychiatry 50:699–703

Besley GTN, Broadhead DM, Ellis PM (1992) First-trimester diagnosis of Hunter syndrome (MPS II). (Letters to the editor). Prenatal Diagnosis 12:72–73

Blaser SI, Harwood-Nash DCF (1992) Radiology of the developing central nervous system. Curr Opin Neurol Neurosurg 5:843–848

Brooks DA (1993) The immunochemical analysis of enzyme from mucopolysaccharidoses patients. J Inherited Metab Dis 16:3–15

Clarke JTR, Greer WL, Strasberg PM, Pearce RD, Skomorowski MA, Ray PN (1991) Hunter disease (mucopolysaccharidosis type II) associated with unbalanced inactivation of the X chromosomes in a karyotypically normal girl. Am J Hum Genet 49:289–297

Clarke JTR, Wilson pJ, Morris CP, Hopwood JJ, Richards RI, Sutherland GR, Ray PN (1992) Characterization of a deletion at Xq27-q28 associated with unbalanced inactivation of the nonmutant X chromosome. Am J Hum Genet 51:316–322

Clarke JTR, Willard HF, Teshima I, Chang PL, Skomorowski MA (1990) Hunter disease (mucopolysaccharidosis type II) in a karyotypically normal girl. Clin Genet 37:355–362

Daria Haust M, Gordon BA, Hong R, Choi JH, Langer LO, Spranger J, Opitz JM (1985) Clinicopathological conference: an adolescent girl with severe mental impairment and mucopolysacchariduria. Am J Med Genet 22:1–27

Dekaban AS, Constantopoulos G (1977) Mucopolysaccharidosis types I, II, III A and V; pathological and biochemical abnormalities in the neural and mesenchymal elements of the brain. Acta Neuropathol (Berl) 39:1–7

de Schrojenstein-de Valk HMJ, Kamp JJP (1987) Follow-up on seven adult patients with mild Sanfilippo B-disease. Am J Med Genet 28:125–129

di Natale P, Annella T, Daniele A, de Luca T, Morabito E, Pallini R, Rosario P, Spagnuolo G (1993) Biochemical diagnosis of mucopolysaccharidoses: experience of 297 diagnoses in a 15-year period (1977–1991). J Inherited Metab Dis 16:473–483

Flomen RH, Green PM, Bentley DR, Giannelli F, Green EP (1992) Detection of point mutations and a gross deletion in six Hunter syndrome patients. Genomics 13:543–550

Fukuda S, Tomatsu S, Sukegawa K, Sasaki T, Yamada Y, Kuwahara T, Okamoto H, Ikedo Y, Yamaguchi S, Orii T (1991) Molecular analysis of mucopolysaccharidosis type VII. J Inherited Metab Dis 14:800–804

Gabrielli O, Salvolini U, Maricotti M (1992) Cerebral MRI in two brothers with mucopolysaccharidosis type I and different clinical phenotypes. Neuroradiology 34:313–315

Giugliani R, Jackson M, Skinner SJ, Vimal CM, Fensom AH, Fahmy N, Sjövall A, Benson PF (1987) Progressive mental regression in siblings with Morquio disease type B (mucopolysaccharidosis IV B). Clin Genet 32:313–325

Gschwind C, Tonkin MA (1992) Carpal tunnel syndrome in children with mucopolysaccharidosis and related disorders. J Hand Surg 17A:44–47

Harwood-Nash DC (1991) MRI and paediatric neuroradiology: a present perspective. Eur Radiol 1:3–18

Herrick IA, Rhine EJ (1988) The mucopolysaccharidoses and anaesthesia: a report of clinical experience. Can J Anaesth 35:67–73

Hoogerbrugge PM, Brouwer OF, Fischer A (1991) Bone marrow transplantation for metabolic diseases with severe neurological symptoms. Bone Marrow Transplant 7 [Suppl 2]: 71

Johnson MA, Desai S, Hugh-Jones K, Starer F (1984) Magnetic resonance imaging of the brain in Hurler syndrome. AJNR 5:816–819

Kulkarni MV, Williams JC, Yeakley JW, Andrews JL, McArdle CB, Narayana PA, Howell RR, Jonas AJ (1987) Magnetic resonance imaging in the diagnosis of the cranio-cervical manifestations of the mucopolysaccharidoses. Magn Reson Imaging 5:317–323

Kyle JW, Birkenmeier EH, Gwynnn B, Vogler C, Hoppe PC, Hoffmann JW, Sly WS (1990) Correction of murine mucopolysaccharidois VII by a human β-glucuronidase transgene. Proc Natl Acad Sci U S A 87:3914–3918

Le Guern E, Couillin P, Oberlé I, Ravise N, Boue J (1990) More precise localization of the gene for Hunter syndrome. Genomics 7:358–362

Lee Ch, Dineen E, Brack M, Kirsch JE, Runge VM (1993) The mucopolysaccharidoses:characterization by cranial MR imaging. AJNR 14:1285–1292

Litjens T, Baker EG, Beckmann KR, Phillip Morris C, Hopwood JJ, Callen DF (1989) Chromosomal localization of ARSB, the gene for human N-acetylgalactosamine-4-sulphatase. Hum Genet 82:67–68

Loeb H, Jonniaux G, Resibois A, Cremer N, Dodion J, Tondeur M, Gregoire, Richard J, Cieters P (1968) Biochemical and ultrastructural studies in Hurler's syndrome. J Pediatr 73:860–874

Martin JJ, Ceuterick C (1988) The contribution of pathology to the study of storage disorders. Pathol Res Pract 183:375–385

Muenzer J, Neufeld EF, Constantopoulos G, Caruso RC, Kaiser-Kupfer MI, Pikus A, Danoff J, Berry RR, McDonald HD, Thompson JN, Rodén L, Zasloff MA (1992) Attempted enzyme replacement using human amnion membrane implantations in mucopolysaccharidoses. J Inherited Metab Dis 15:25–37

Murata R, Nakajima S, Tanaka A, Miyagi N, Matsuoka O, Kogame S, Inoue Y (1989) MR imaging of the brain in patients with mucopolysaccharidosis. AJNR 10:1165–1170

Nelon J, Kinirons M (1988) Clinical findings in 12 patients with MPS IV A (Morquio's disease). Clin Genet 33:121–125

Nelson J, Thomas PS (1988) Clinical findings in 12 patients with MPS IV A (Morquio's disease); further evidence for heterogeneity, part III: odontoid dysplasia. Clin Genet 33:126–130

Nelson J, Shields MD, Connor Mulholland H (1990) Cardiovascular studies in the mucopolysaccharidoses. J Med Genet 27:94–100

Nelson J, Broadhead D, Mossman J (1988) Clinical findings in 12 patients with MPS IV A (Morquio's disease); further evidence for heterogeneity, part I: clinical and biochemical findings. Clin Genet 33:111–120

Nelson J, Grebbell FS (1987) The value of computed tomography in patients with mucopolysaccharidosis. Neuroradiology 29:544–549

Oshima A, Yoshida K, Shimmoto M, Fukuhara Y, Sakuraba H, Suzuki Y (1991) Human β-galactosidase gene mutations in Morquio B disease. Am J Hum Genet 49:1091–1093

Perretti A, Petrillo A, Pelosi L, Balbi P, Parenti G, Riemma A, Strisciuglio P (1989) Detection of early abnormalities in the mucopolysaccharidoses by the use of visual and brainstem auditory evoked potentials. Neuropeadiatrics 21:83–86

Purpura DP, Suzuki K (1976) Distortion of neuronal geometry and formation of aberrant synapses in neuronal storage disease. Brain Res 116:1–21

Rauch RA, Friloux LA III, Lott IT (1989) MR imaging of cavitary lesions in the brain with Hurler/Scheie. AJNR 10:S1-S3

Roberts SH, Upadhyaya M, Sarfarazi M, Harper PS (1989) Further evidence localising the gene for Hunter's syndrome to the distal region of the X chromosome long arm. J Med Genet 26:309–313

Schmidt H, Ullrich K, von Lengerke HJ, Kleine M, Brämswig J (1987) Radiological findings in patients with mucopolysaccharidosis I H/S (Hurler-Scheie syndrome). Pediatr Radiol 17:409–414

Scott HS, Nelson PV, Cooper A, Wraith JE, Hopwood JJ, Phillip Morris C (1992) Mucopolysaccharidosis type I (Hurler syndrome): linkage disequilibrium indicates the presence of a major allele. Hum Genet 88:701–702

Sewell AC, Gehler J, Mittermaier G, Meyer E (1982) Mucopolysaccharidosis type VII (β-glucuronidase deficiency): a report of a new case and a survey of those in the literature. Clin Genet 21:366–373

Shimoda-Matsubayashi S, Kuru Y, Sumie H, Ito T, Hattori N, Okuma Y, Mizuno Y (1990) MRI findings in the mild type of mucopolysaccharidosis II (Hunter's syndrome). Neuroradiology 32:328–330

Shimoda-Matsubayashi S, Kuru Y, Sumie H, Ito T, Hattori N, Okuma Y, Mizuno Y (1990) MRI findings in the mild type of mucopolysaccharidosis II (Hunter's syndrome). Neuroradiology 32:328–330

Stephan MJ, Stevens EL Jr, Wenstrup RJ, Greenberg CR, Gritter HL, Hodges GF, Guller B (1989) Mucopolysaccharidosis

I presenting with endocardial fibroelastosis of infancy. Am J Dis Child 143:782–784

Stevens JM, Kendall BE, Alan Crockard H, Ransford A (1991) The odontoid process in Morquio-Brailsford's disease; the effects of occipitocervical fusion. J Bone Joint Surg 73:851–858

Taccone A, Tortori Donati P, Marzoli A, Dell'Acqua A, Occhi M, Gatti R, Leone D (1992) Mucopolisaccaridosi: valutazione del cranio con tomografia computerizzata e risonanza magnetica. Radiol Med 84:236–241

Tamaki N, Kojima N, Tanimoto M, Suyama T, Matsumoto S (1987) Myelopathy due to diffuse thickening of the cervical dura mater in Maroteaux-Lamy syndrome: report of a case. Neurosurgery 21:416–419

Tomatsu S, Fukuda S, Sukegawa K, Ikedo Y, Yamada S, Yamada Y, Sasaki T, Okamoto H, Kuwahara T, Yamaguchi S, Kiman T, Shintaku H, Isshiki G, Orii T (1991) Mucopolysaccharidosis type VII: characterization of mutations and molecular heterogeneity. Am J Hum Genet 48:89–96

Van den Kamp JJP, Niermeijer MF, von Figura K, Giesberts MAH (1981) Genetic heterogeneity and clinical variability in the Sanfilippo syndrome (types A, B and C). Clin Genet 20:152–160

Vestermark S, Tonnesen T, Schultz Andersen M, Güttler F (1987) Mental retardation in a patient with Maroteaux-Lamy. Clin Genet 31:114–117

Von Figura K, Hasilik A, Steckel F, van den Kamp J (1984) Biosynthesis and maturation of α-N-acetylglucosaminidase in normal and Sanfilippo B-fibroblasts. Am J Hum Genet 36:93–100

Walkley SU, Haskins ME, Shull RM (1988) Alterations in neuron morphology in mucopolysaccharidosis type I: a Golgi study. Acta Neuropathol (Berl) 75:611–620

Watis RWE, Spellacy E, Hume Adams J (1986) Neuropathological and clinical correlations in Hurler disease. J Inherited Metab Dis 9:261–272

Watts RWE, Spellacy E, Kendall BE, du Boulay G, Gibbs DA (1981) Computed tomography studies on patients with mucopolysaccharidoses. Neuroradiology 21:9–23

Wehnert M, Hopwood JJ, Schröder W, Herrmann FH (1992) Structural gene aberrations in mucopolysaccharidosis II (Hunter). Hum Genet 89:430–432

Wende S, Ludwig B, Kishikawa T, Rochel M, Gehler J (1984) The value of CT in diagnosis and prognosis of different inborn neurodegenerative disorders in childhood. J Neurol 231:57–70

Wicker G, Prill V, Brooks D, Gibson G, Hopwood J, Figura von K, Peters C (1991) Mucopolysaccharidosis VI (Maroteaux-Lamy syndrome). J Biol Chem 266:21386–21391

Wilson PJ, Morris CP, Anson DS, Occhiodoro T, Bielicki J, Clements PR, Hopwood JJ (1990) Hunter syndrome: isolation of an iduronate-2-sulfatase cDNA clone and analysis of patient DNA. Proc Natl Acad Sci U S A 87:8531–8535

Wilson PJ, Suthers GK, Callen DF, Baker E, Nelson PV, Cooper A, Wraith JE, Sutherland GR, Phillip Morris C, Hopwood JJ (1991) Frequent deletions at Xq28 indicate genetic heterogeneity in Hunter syndrome. Hum Genet 86:505–508

Winters PR, Harrod MJ, Molenich-Heetred SA, Kirkpatrick J, Rosenberg RN (1976) α-L-iduronidase deficiency and possible Hurler-Scheie genetic compound: clinical, pathologic and biochemical findings. Neurology 26:1003–1007

Wynne-Davies R, Hall CM, Howell CJ, Baker GCW, Crossan J, Evans GA, Fulford GE, Smith MA, Witherow PJ (1989) Instability of the upper cervical spine. Arch Dis Child 64:283–288

Young ID, Harper PS, Archer IM, Newcombe RG (1982) A clinical and genetic study of Hunter's syndrome. I. Heterogeneity. J Med Genet 19:401–407

Zlotogora J (1987) Intrafamilial variablity in lysosomal storage diseases. Am J Med Genet 27:633–638

14 Peroxisomes and Peroxisomal Disorders

Bachir Bioukar E, Deschatrette J (1993) Update on genetic and molecular investigations of diseases with general impairment of peroxisomal functions. Biochimie 75:303–308

Beard ME, Baker R, Conomos P, Pugatch D, Holtzman E (1984) Oxidation of oxalate and polyamines by rat peroxisomes. J Histochem Cytochem 33:460–464

Bennett MJ Pollitt RJ, Goodman SI, Hale DE, Vamecq J (1991) Atypical riboflavon-responsive glutaric aciduria, and deficient peroxisomal glutaryl-CoA oxidase activity: a new peroxisomal disorder. J Inherited Metab Dis 14:165–173

Brul S, Westerveld A, Strijland A, Wanders RJA, Schram AW, Heymans HSA, Schutgens RBH, van den Bosch H, Tager JM (1988) Genetic heterogeneity in the cerebrohepatorenal (Zellweger) syndrome and other inherited disorders with a generalized impairment of peroxisomal functions. J Clin Invest 81:1710–1715

Brul S, Wiemer EAC, Westerveld A, Strijland A, Wanders RJA, Schram AW, Heymans HSA, Schutgens RBH, van den Bosch H, Tager JM (1988) Kinetics of the assembly of peroxisomes after fusion of complementary cell lines from patients with the cerebro-hepato-renal (Zellweger) syndrome and related disorders. Biochem Biophys Res Commun 152:1083–1089

Casteels M, van Roermund CWT, Schepers L, Govaert L, Eyssen HJ, Mannaerts GP, Wanders RJA (1989) Deficient oxidation of trihydroxycoprostanic acid in liver homogenates from patients with peroxisomal diseases. J Inherited Metab Dis 12:415–422

Causeret C, Bentejac M, Bugaut M (1993) Proteins and enzymes of the peroxisomal membrane in mammals. Biol Cell 77:89–104

Clayton PT, Lake BD, Hall NA, Shortland DB, Carruthers RA, Lawson AM (1987) Plasma bile acids in patients with peroxisomal dysfunction syndromes: analysis by capillary gas chromatography – mass spectrometry. Pediatrics 146:166–173

Cook HW, Thomas SE, Xu Z (1991) Essential fatty acids and serine as plasmalogen precursors in relation to competing metabolic pathways. Biochem Cell Biol 69:475–484

Cuezva JM, Floeres AI, Liras A, Santaren JF, Alconada A (1993) Molecular chaperones and the biogenesis of mitochondria and peroxisomes. Biol Cell 77:47–62

de Duve C, Baudhuin P (1966) Peroxisomes (microbodies and related particles). Physiol Rev 46:323–357

Del Rio LA, Sandalio LM, Palma JM, Bueno P, Corpas FJ (1992) Metabolism of oxygen radicals in peroxisomes and cellular implications. Free Radic Biol Med 13:557–580

Diczfafusy U, Frode Kase B, Alexson SEH, Bjoerkhem I (1991) Metabolism of protaglandin $F_{2\alpha}$ in Zellweger syndrome. J Clin Invest 88:978–984

Fingerhut R, Schmitz W, Conzelmann E (1993) Accumulation of phytanic acid α-oxidation intermediates in Zellweger fibroblasts. J Inherited Metab Dis 16:591–594

Frode Kase B, Pedersen JI, Wathne KO, Gustafsson J, Bjoerkhem I(1991) Importance of peroxisomes in the formation of chenodeoxycholic acid in human liver. Metabolism of $3\alpha,7\alpha$-dihydroxy-5β-cholestanoic acid in Zellweger syndrome. Pediatr Res 29:64–69

Guerroui S, Aubourg P, Chen WW, Hashimoto T, Scotto J (1989) Molecular analysis of peroxisomal β-oxidation enzymes in infants with peroxisomal disorders indicates heterogeneity of the primary defect. Biochem Biophys Res Commun 161:242–251

Heikoop JC, van den Berg M, Strijland A, Weijers PJ, Just WW, Meijer AJ, Tager JM (1992) Turnover of peroxisomal vesicles by autophagic proteolysis in cultured fibroblasts from Zellweger patients. Eur J Cell Biol 57:165–171

Hodge VJ, Gould SJ, Subramani S, Moser HW, Krisans SK (1991) Normal cholesterol synthesis in human cells requires functional peroxisomes. Biochem Biophys Res Commun 181:537–541

Kaiser E, Kramar R (1988) Clinical biochemistry of peroxisomal disorders. Clin Chim Acta 173:57–80

Lazarow PB (1987) The role of peroxisomes in mammalian cellular metabolism. J Inherited Metab Dis 10 [Suppl I]:11–22

MacCollin M, de Vivo DC, Moser AB, Beard M (1990) Ataxia and peripheral neuropathy: a benign variant of peroxisome dysgenesis. Ann Neurol 28:833–836

Mayatepek E, Lehmann WD, Fauler J, Talkas D, Frolich JC, Schutgens RBH, Wanders RJA, Keppler D (1993) Impaired degradation of leukotrienes in patients with peroxisome deficiency disorders. J Clin Invest 91:881–888

Molzer B, Gullotta F, Harzer K, Poulos A, Bernheimer H (1993) Unusual orthochromatic leukodystrophy with epitheloid cells (Norman-Gullotta): increase of very long chain fatty acids in brain discloses a peroxisomal disorder. Acta Neuropathol (Berl) 86:187–189

Moser HW (1988) The peroxisome:nervous system role of a previously underrated organelle. Neurology 38:1617–1627

Moser HW, Mihalik SJ, Watkins PA (1989) Adrenoleukodystrophy and other peroxisomal disorders that affect the nervous system, including new observations on L-pipecolic acid oxidase in primates. Brain Dev 11:80–90

Moser HW, Bergin A, Cornblath D (1991) Peroxisomal disorders. Biochem Cell Biol 69:463–474

Osmundsen H, Bremer J, Pedersen JI (1991) Metabolic aspects of peroxisomal β-oxidation. Biochim Biophys Acta 1085:141–158

Osumi T, Tsukamoto T, Hata S, Yokota S, Miura S, Fujiki Y, Hijikata M, Niyazawa S, Hashimoto T (1991) Amino-terminal presequence of the precursor of peroxisomal 3-ketoacyl-CoA thiolase is a cleavable signal peptide for peroxisomal targeting. Biochem Biophys Res Commun 181:947–954

Palosari PM, Kalervo Hiltunen J (1990) Peroxisomal bifunctional protein from rat liver is a trifunctional enzyme possessing 2-enoyl-CoA hydratase, 3-hydroxyacyl-CoA dehydrogenase, and Δ^3,Δ^2-enoyl-CoA isomerase activities. J Biol Neurochem 265:2446–2449

Santos MJ, Imanaka T, Shio H, Small GM, Lazarow PB (1988) Peroxisomal membrane ghosts in Zellweger syndrome – aberrant organelle assembly. Science 239:1536–1538

Schulz H (1991) Beta oxidation of fatty acids. Biochim Biophys Acta 1081:109–120

Schutgens RBH, Wanders RJA, Heymans HSA, Schram AW, Tager JM, Schrakamp G, van den Bosch H (1987) Zellweger syndrome: biochemical procedures in diagnosis, prevention and treatment. J Inherited Metab Dis 10 [Suppl]: 33–45

Shimozawa N, Taukamoto T, Suzuki Y, Orii T, Fujki Y (1992) Animal cell mutants represent two complementation groups of peroxisome-defective Zellweger syndrome. J Clin Invest 90:1864–1870

Shimozawa N, Suzuki Y, Orii T, Moser A, Moser HW, Wanders RJA (1993) Standardization of complementation grouping of peroxisome-deficient disorders and the second Zellweger patient with peroxisomal assembly factor-I defect. Am J Hum Genet 52:843–844

Singh H, Usher S, Johnson D, Poulos A (1990) A comparative study of straight chain and branched chain fatty oxidation in skin fibroblasts from patients with peroxisomal disorders. J Lipid Res 31:217–225

Singh I, Lazo O, Dhausi GS, Contreras M (1992) Transport of fatty acids into human and rat peroxisomes. J Biol Chem 267:13306–13313

Small GM, Santos MJ, Imanaka T, Poulos A, Danks DM, Moser HW, Lazarow PB (1988) Peroxisomal integral membrane proteins in livers of patients with Zellweger syndrome, infantile Refsum's disease and X-linked adrenoleukodystrophy. J Inherited Metab Dis 11:358–371

Ten Brink HJ, Poll-The BT, Saudubray JM, Wanders RJA, Jakobs C (1991) Pristanic acid does not accumulate in peroxisomal acyl-CoA oxidase deficiency: evidence for a distinct peroxisomal pristanyl-CoA oxidase. J Inherited Metab Dis 14:681–684

Ten Brink HJ, Wanders RJA, Stellaard F, Schutgens RBH, Jakobs C (1991) Pristanic acid and phytanic acid in plasma from patients with a single peroxisomal enzyme deficiency. J Inherited Metab Dis 14:345–348

Ten Brink HJ, Schor DSM, Kok RM, Stellaard F, Kneer J, Poll-The BT, Saudubray JM, Jakobs C (1992) In vivo study of phytanic acid alpha-oxidation in classic Refsum's disease and chondrodysplasia punctata. Pediatr Res 32:566–570

Theil AC, Schutgens RBH, Wanders RJA, Heymans HSA (1992) Clinical recognition of patients affected by a peroxisomal disorder: a retrospective study in 40 patients. Eur J Pediatr 151:117–120

Tranchant C, Aubourg P, Mohr M, Rocchiccioli F, Zaenker C, Warter JM (1993) A new peroxisomal disease with impaired phytanic and pipecolic acid oxidation. Neurology 43:2044–2048

Van Roermund CWT, Brul S, Tager JM, Schutgens RBH, Wanders RJA (1991) Acyl-CoA oxidase, peroxisomal thiolase and dihydroxyacetone phosphate acyltransferase: aberrant subcellular localization in Zellweger syndrome. J Inherited Metab Dis 14:152–164

Van Veldhoven PP, Huang S, Eyssen HJ, Mannaerts GP (1993) The deficient degradation of synthetic 2-and 3-methyl-branched fatty acids in fibroblasts from patients with peroxisomal disorders. J Inherited Metab Dis 16:381–391

Wanders RJA, van Roermund CWT, van Wijland MJA, Heikoop J, Schutgens RBH, Schram AW, Tager JM, van den Bosch H, Poll-The BT, Saudubray JM, Moser HW, Moser AB (1987) Peroxisomal very long-chain fatty acid β-oxidation in human skin fibroblasts:activity in Zellweger syndrome and other peroxisomal disorders. Clin Chim Acta 166:255–263

Wanders RJA, Heymans HSA, Schutgens RBH, Barth PG, van den Bosch H, Tager JM (1988) Peroxisomal disorders in neurology. J Neurol Sci 88:1–39

Wanders RJA, van Roermund CWT, Schutgens RBH, Barth PG, Heymans HSA, van den Bosch H, Tager JM (1990) The inborn errors of peroxisomal β-oxidation: a review. J Inherited Metab Dis 13:4–36

Wanders RJA, Tager JM (1991) Peroxisomal fatty acid β-oxidation in relation to adrenoleukodystrophy. Dev Neurosci 13:262–266

Wanders RJA, van Roermund CWT, Jakobs C, ten Brink HJ (1991) Identification of pristanoyl-CoA oxidase and phytanic acid decarboxylation in peroxisomes and mitochondria from human liver:implications for Zellweger syndrome. J Inherited Metab Dis 14:349–352

Wanders RJA, Schutgens RBH, Barth PG, Tager JM, van den Bosch H (1993) Postnatal diagnosis of peroxisomal disorders: a biochemical approach. Biochimie 75:269–279

Wilson GN (1991) Structure-function relationships in the proxisome:implications for human disease. Biochem Med Metab Biol 46:288–298

Zellweger H (1987) The cerebro-hepato-renal (Zellweger) syndrome and other peroxisomal disorders. Dev Med Child Neurol 29:821–829

15   Zellweger Cerebrohepatorenal Syndrome, Neonatal Adrenoleukodystrophy, and Infantile Refsum Disease

Agamanolis DP, Patre S (1979) Glycogen accumulation in the central nervous system in the cerebro-hepato-renal syndrome. J Neurol Sci 41:325–334

Agamanolis DP, Robinson HB, Timmons GD (1976) Cerebrohepato-renal syndrome. Report of a case with histochemical and ultrastructural observations. J Neuropathol Exp Neurol 35:226–246

Aikawa J, Ishizawa S, Narisawa K, Tada K, Yokota S, Hashimoto T (1987) The abnormality of peroxisomal membrane proteins in Zellweger syndrome. J Inherited Metab Dis 10 [Suppl 2]:211–213

Aikawa J, Chen WW, Kelley RI, Tada K, Moser HW, Chen GL (1991) Low-density particles (W-particles) containing catalase in Zellweger syndrome and normal fibroblasts. Proc Natl Acad Sci U S A 88:10084–10088

Aubourg P, Robain O, Rocchiccioli F, Dancea S, Scotto J (1985) The cerebro-hepato-renal (Zellweger) syndrome: lamellar lipid profiles in adrenocortical, hepatic mesenchymal, astrocyte cells and increased levels of very long chain fatty acids and phytanic acid in the plasma. J Neurol Sci 69:9–25

Aubourg P, Scotto J, Rocchiccioli R, Feldmann-Pautrat D, Robain O (1986) Neonatal adrenoleukodystrophy. J Neurol Neurosurg Psychiatry 49:77–86

Bachir Bioukar E, Deschatrette J (1993) Update on genetic and molecular investigations of diseases with general impairment of peroxisomal functions. Biochimie 75:303–308

Balfe A, Hoefler G, Chen WW, Watkins PA (1990) Aberrant subcellular localization of peroxisomal 3-ketoacyl-CoA thiolase in the Zellweger syndrome and rhizomelic chondrodysplasia punctata. Pediatr Res 27:304–310

Barth PG, Schutgens RBH, Bakkeren JAJM, Dingemans KP, Heymans HSA, Douwes AC, van der Klei-van Moorsel JM (1985) A milder variant of Zellweger syndrome. Eur J Pediatr 144:338–342

Beard ME, Moser AB, Sapirstein V, Holtzman E (1986) Peroxisomes in infantile phytanic acid storage disease: a cytochemical study of skin fibroblasts. J Inherited Metab Dis 9:321–334

Benke PJ, Reyes PF, Parker JC Jr (1981) New form of adrenoleukodystrophy. Hum Genet 58:204–208

Bizzozero OA, Zuniga G, Lees MB (1991) Fatty acid composition of human myelin proteolipid protein in peroxisomal disorders. J Neurochem 56:872–878

Bruhn H, Kruse B, Korenke GC, Hanefeld F, Haenicke W, Merboldt KD, Frahm J (1992) Proton NMR spectroscopy of cerebral metabolic alterations in infantile peroxisomal disorders. J Comput Assist Tomogr 16:335–344

Brul S, Westerveld A, Strijland A, Wanders RJA, Schram AW, Heymans HSA, Schutgens RBH, van den Bosch H, Tager JM (1988) Genetic heterogeneity in the cerebrohepatorenal (Zellweger) syndrome and other inherited disorders with a generalized impairment of peroxisomal functions. J Clin Invest 81:1710–1715

Budden SS, Kennaway NG, Buist NRM, Poulos A, Weleber RG (1986) Dysmorphic syndrome with phytanic acid oxidase deficiency, abnormal very long chain fatty acids, and pipecolic acidemia: studies in four children. J Pediatr 108:33–39

Chow CW, Poulos A, Fellenberg AJ, Christodoulou J, Danks DM (1992) Autopsy findings in two siblings with infantile Refsum disease. Acta Neuropathol (Berl) 83:190–195

Clayton PT, Lake BD, Hall NA, Shortland DB, Carruthers RA, Lawson AM (1987) Plasma bile acids in patients with peroxisomal dysfunction syndromes: analysis by capillary gas chromatography mass spectrometry. Eur J Pediatr 146:166–173

Cohen SMZ, Brown FR, Martyn L, Moser HW, Chen W, Kistenmacher M, Punnettt H, de la Cruz ZC, Chan NH, Green RW (1983) Ocular histopathologic and biochemical studies of the cerebrohepatorenal syndrome (Zellweger syndrome) and its relationship to neonatal adrenoleukodystrophy. Am J Ophthalmol 96:488–501

De Leon GA, Grover WD, Huff DS, Moringo-Meure G, Punnett HH, Kistenmacher ML (1977) Globoid cells, glial nodules, and peculiar fibrillary changes in the cerebro-hepato-renal syndrome of Zellweger. Ann Neurol 2:473–484

Dimmick JE, Applegarth DA (1993) Pathology of peroxisomal disorders. Perspect Pediatr Pathol 17:45–98

Dubois J, Sebag G, Argyropoulou M, Brunelle F (1991) MR findings in infantile Refsum disease: case report of two family members. AJNR 12:1159–1160

Evrard P, Caviness VS, Prats-Vinas J, Lyon G (1978) The mechanism of arrest of neuronal migration in the Zellweger malformation: an hypothesis based upon cytoarchitectonic analysis. Acta Neuropathol (Berl) 41:109–117

Folz SJ, Trobe JD (1991) The peroxisome and the eye. Survey Ophthalmol 35:353–368

Gaertner J, Chen WW, Kelly RI, Mihalik SJ, Moser HS (1991) The 22-kD peroxisomal integral membrane protein in Zellweger syndrome – presence, abundance, and association with a peroxisomal thiolase precursor protein. Pediatr Res 29:141–146

Gaertner J, Moser H, Valle D (1992) Mutations in the 70 K peroxisomal membrane protein gene in Zellweger syndrome. Nature Genet 1:16–23

Goldfischer S, Collins J, Rapin I, Schiller C, Chang CH, Nigro M, Black VH, Javitt NB, Moser HW, Lazarow PB (1985) Peroxisomal defects in neonatal-onset and X-linked adrenoleukodystrophies. Science 227:67–70

Govaerts L, Sippell WG, Monnens L (1989) Further analysis of the disturbed adrenocortical function in the cerebro-hepato-renal syndrome of Zellweger. J Inherited Metab Dis 12:423–428

Heikoop JC, van den Berg M, Strijland A, Weijers PJ, Just WW, Meijer AJ, Tager JM (1992) Turnover of peroxisomal vesicles by autophagic proteolysis in cultured fibroblasts from Zellweger patients. Eur J Cell Biol 59:165–171

Hermetter A, Rainer B, Ivessa E, Kalb E, Loidl J, Roscher A, Paltauf F (1989) Influence of plasmalogen deficiency on membrane fluidity of human skin fibroblasts: a fluorescence anisotropy study. Biochim Biophys Acta 978:151–157

Heymans HSA, Schutgens RB, Tan R, van den Bosch H, Borst P (1983) Severe plasmalogen deficiency in tissues of ifants without peroxisomes (Zellweger syndrome). Nature 306:69–70

Holmes RD, Wilson GN, Hajra A (1987) Oral ether lipid therapy in patients with peroxisomal disorders. J Inherited Metab Dis 10 [Suppl 2]:239–241

Holmes RD, Moore KH, Ofenstein JP, Tsatsos P, Kiechle FL (1993) Lactic acidosis and mitochondrial dysfunction in two children with peroxisomal disorders. J Inherited Metab Dis 16:368–380

Hughes JL, Poulos A, Robertson E, Chow CW, Sheffield LJ, Christodoulou J, Carter RF (1990) Pathology of hepatic peroxisomes and mitochondria in patients with peroxisomal disorders. Virchows Arch [A] 416:255–264

Jaffe R, Crumrine P, Hashida Y, Moser HW (1982) Neonatal adrenoleukodystrophy. Clinical, pathologic, and biochemical delineation of a syndrome affecting both males and females. Am J Pathol 108:100–111

Kase BF, Pedersen JI, Wathne KO, Gustafsson J, Bjorkhem I (1991) Importance of perixomes in the formation of chenodexycholic acid in human liver. Metabolism of 3α,7α-dihydroxy-5α-cholestanoid acid in Zellweger syndrome. Pediatr Res 29:64–69

Kelley RI (1983) Review:the cerebrohepatorenal syndrome of Zellweger, morphologic and metabolic aspects. Am J Med Genet 16:503–517

Kelley RI, Datta NA, Dobyns WB, Hajra AK, Moser AB, Noetzel MJ, Zackal EH, Moser HW (1986) Neonatal adrenoleukodystrophy: new cases, biochemical studies, and differentiation from Zellweger and related peroxisomal polydystrophy syndromes. Am J Med Genet 23:869–901

Kendall B (1992) Disorders of lysosomes, peroxisomes, and mitochondria. AJNR 13:621–653

Kerckaert I, Dingemans KP, Heymans HSA, Vamecq J, Roels F (1988) Polarizing inclusions in some organs of children with congenital peroxisomal diseases (Zellweger's, Refsum's, chondrodysplasia punctata (rhizomelic form), X-linked adrenoleukodystrophy). J Inherited Metab Dis 11:372–386

Manz HJ, Schelein M, McCullough DC, Kishimoto Y, Eiben RM (1980) New phenotypic variant of adrenoleukodystrophy. J Neurol Sci 45:245–260

Martinez M (1992) Abnormal profiles of polyunsaturated fatty acids in the brain, liver, kidney and retina of patients with peroxisomal disorders. Brain Res 583:171–182

Martinez M, Pineda M, Vidal R, Conill J, Martin B (1993) Docosahexaenoic acid – a new therapeutic approach to peroxisomal-disorder patients:experience with two cases. Neurology 43:1389–1397

Mei Liu H, Bangaru BS, Kidd J, Boggs J (1976) Neuropathological considerations in cerebro-hepato-renal syndrome (Zellweger's syndrome) Acta Neuropathol (Berl) 34:115–123

Mito T, Takada K, Akaboshi S, Takashima S, Takeshita K, Origuchi Y (1989) A pathological study of a peripheral nerve in a case of neonatal adrenleukodystrophy. Acta Neuropathol (Berl) 77:437–440

Molzer B, Korschinsky M, Bernheimer H, Schmid R, Wolf C, Roscher A (1986) Very long chain fatty acids in genetic peroxisomal disease fibroblasts:differences between the cerebro-hepato-renal (Zellweger) syndrome and adrenoleukodystrophy variants. Clin Chim Acta 161:81–90

Molzer B, Kainz-Korschinsky M, Sundt-Heller R, Bernheimer H (1989) Phytanic acid and very long chain fatty acids in genetic peroxisomal disorders. J Clin Chem Clin Biochem 27:309–314

Moser HW, Birgin A, Cornbeath D (1991) Peroxisomal disorders. Biochem Cell Biol 69:463–474

Mueller-Hoecker J, Walther JU, Bise K, Pongratz D, Huebner G (1984) Mitochondrial myopathy with loosely coupled oxidative phosphorylation in a case of Zellweger syndrome. Virchows Arch [B] 45:125–138

Naidu S, Moser HW (1991) Infantile Refsum disease. AJNR 12:1161–1163

Naidu S, Moser AE, Moser HW (1988) Phenotypic and genotypic variability of generalized peroxisomal disorders. Pediatr Neurol 4:5–12

Ogier H, Roels F, Cornelis A, Poll-The BT, Scotto JM, Oievre M, Saudubray JM (1985) Absence of hepatic peroxisomes in a case of infantile Refsum's disease. Scand J Clin Lab Invest 45:767–768

Passarge E, McAdams AJ (1967) Cerebro-hepato-renal syndrome. J Pediatrics 71:691–702

Poll-The BT, Poulos A, Sharp P, Boue J, Ogier H, Odievre M, Saudubray JM (1985) Antenatal diagnosis of infantile Refsum's disease. Clin Genet 27:524–526

Poll-The BT, Ogier H, Saudubray, Schutgens RBH, Wanders RJA, van den Bosch H, Schrakamp G (1986) Impaired plasmalogen metabolism in infantile Refsum's disease. Eur J Pediatr 144:513–514

Poll-The BT, Saudubray JM, Rocchiccioli F, Scotto J, Roels F, Boue J, Ogier H, Dumez Y, Wanders RJA, Schutgens RBH, Schram AW, Tager JM (1987) Prenatal diagnosis and confirmation of infantile Refsum's disease. J Inherited Metab Dis 10 [Suppl 2]:229–232

Poulos A, Singh H, Paton B, Sharp P, Derwas N (1986) Accumulation and defective β-oxidation of very long chain fatty acids in Zellweger's syndrome, adrenoleukodystrophy and Refsum's disease variants. Clin Genet 29:397–408

Poulos A, Sharp P, Johnson D (1989) Plasma polyenoic very-long-chain fatty acids in peroxisomal disease:biochemical discrimination of Zellweger's syndrome from other phenotypes. Neurology 39:44–47

Powers JM, Tummons RC, Caviness VS, Moser AB, Moser HW (1989) Structural and chemical alterations in the cerebral maldevelopment of fetal cerebro-hepato-renal (Zellweger) syndrome. J Neuropathol Exp Neurol 48:270–289

Raafat F, Smith K, Halloran EA, Lacy D (1991) Zellweger syndrome: a histochemical diagnosis of two cases. Pediatr Pathol 11:413–420

Reubsaet FAG, Bruckwilder MLP, Veerkamp JH, Trijbels JMF, Hashimoto T, Monnens LAH (1991) Immunochemical analysis of the peroxisomal β-oxidation enzymes in rat and human heart and skeletal muscle and in skeletal muscle of Zellweger patients. Biochem Med Metab Biol 45:197–203

Robertson EF, Poulos A, Sharp P, Manson J, Wise G, Jaunzems A, Carter R (1988) Treatment of infantile phytanic acid storage disease: clinical, biochemical and ultrastructural findings in two children treated for 2 years. Eur J Pediatr 147:133--142

Roels F, Cornelis A, Poll-The BT, Aubourg P, Ogier H, Scotto J, Saudubray JM (1986) Hepatic peroxisomes are deficient in infantile Refsum disease:a cytochemical study of 4 cases. Am J Med Genet 25:257–271

Roels F, Espeel M, de Craemer D (1991) Liver pathology and immunocytochemistry in congenital peroxisomal diseases: a review. J Inherited Metab Dis 14:853–875

Roels F, Espeel M, Poggi F, Mandel H, van Maldergem L, Saudubray JM (1993) Human liver pathology in peroxisomal diseases: a review including novel data. Biochimie 75:281–292

Roscher AA, Hoefler S, Hoefler G, Paschke E, Paltauf F, Moser A, Moser H (1989) Genetic and phenotypic heterogeneity in disorders of peroxisme biogenesis – a complementation study involving cell lines from 19 patients. Pediatr Res 6:67–72

Santos MJ, Imanaka T, Shio H, Small GM, Lazarow PB (1988) Peroxisomal membrane ghosts in Zellweger syndrome – abberant organelle assembly. Science 239:1536–1538

Sarnat HB, Trevenen CL, Darwish HZ (1993) Ependymal abnormalities in cerebro-hepato-renal disease of Zellweger. Brain Dev 15:270–277

Schram AW, Strijland A, Hashimoto T, Wanders RJA, Schutgens RBH, van den Bosch H, Tager JM (1986) Biosynthesis and maturation of peroxisomal β-oxidation enzymes in fibroblasts in relation to the Zellweger syndrome and infantile Refsum disease. Proc Natl Acad Sci U S A 83:6156–6158

Schutgens RBH, Wanders RJA, Heymans HSA, Schram AW, Tager JM, Schrakamp G, van den Bosch H (1987) Zellweger syndrome:biochemical procedures in diagnosis, prevention and treatment. J Inherited Metab Dis 10:33–45

Schutgens RBH, Schrakamp G, Wanders RJA, Heymans HSA, Tager JM, van den Bosch H (1989) Prenatal and perinatal diagnosis of peroxisomal disorders. J Inherited Metab Dis 12 [Suppl 1]:118–134

Schutgens RBH, Wanders RJA, Jakobs C, Arslan-Kirchner M, Miller K, Wieacker P, Hunnemann D, Hurter P, von Schutz M (1994) A new variant of Zellweger syndrome with normal peroxisomal functions in cultured fibroblasts. J Inherited Metab Dis 17:319–322

Scotto JM, Hadchouel M, Odievre M, Laudat MH, Saudubray JM, Dulac O, Beucler I, Beaune P (1982) Infantile phytanic acid storage disease, a possible variant of Refsum's disease: three cases, including ultrastructural studies of the liver. J Inherited Metab Dis 5:83–90

Sharp P, Johnson D, Poulos A (1991) Molecular species of phosphatidylcholine containing very long chain fatty acids in human brain:enrichment in X-linked adrenoleukodystrophy brain and diseases of peroxisome biogenesis brain. J Neurochem 56:30–37

Shimozawa N, Taukamoto T, Suzuki Y, Orii T, Fujki Y (1992a) Animal cell mutants represent two complementation groups of peroxisome-defective Zellweger syndrome. J Clin Invest 90:1864–1870

Shimozawa N, Tsukamoto T, Suzuki Y, Orii T, Shirayoshi Y, Mori T, Fujiki Y (1992b) A human gene responsible for Zellweger syndrome that affects peroxisome assembly. Science 255:1132–1134

Shimozawa N, Suzuki Y, Orii T, Tsukamoto T, Fujki Y (1993) Prenatal diagnosis of Zellweger syndrome using DNA analysis. Prenat Diagn 13:149

Small GM, Santos MJ, Imanaka T, Poulos A, Danks DM, Moser HW, Lazarow PB (1988) Peroxisomal integral membrane proteins in livers of patients with Zellweger syndrome, infantile Refsum's disease and X-linked adrenoleukodystrophy. J Inherited Metab Dis 11:358–371

Taukamoto T, Miura S, Fujiki Y (1991) Restoration by a 35 K membrane protein of peroxisome assembly in a peroxisome-deficient mammalian cell mutant. Nature 350:77–81

Torvik A, Torp S, Kase BF, Ek J, Skjeldal O, Stokke O (1988) Infantile Refsum's disease: a generalized peroxisomal disorder. Case report with postmortem examination. J Neurol Sci 85:39–53

Trijbels JMF, Berden JA, Monnens LAH, Willems JL, Janssen AJM, Schutgens RBH, van den Broek-van Essen M (1983) Biochemical studies in the liver and muscle of patients with Zellweger syndrome. Pediatr Res 17:514–517

Vamecq J, Draye JP, van Hoof F, Misson JP, Evrard P, Verellen G, Eyssen HJ, van Eldere J, Schutgens RH, Wanders RJA, Roels F, Goldfischer SL (1986) Multiple peroxisomal enzymatic deficiency disorders. A comparative biochemical and morphologic study of Zellweger cerebrohepatorenal syndrome and neonatal adrenoleukodystrophy. Am J Pathol 125:524–535

Van der Knaap MS, Valk J (1991) The MR spectrum of peroxisomal disorders. Neuroradiology 33:30–37

Van Roermund CWT, Brul S, Tager JM, Schutgens RBH, Wanders RJA (1991) Acyl-CoA oxidase, peroxisomal thiolase and dihydroxyacetone phosphate acyltransferase: aberrant subcellular localization in Zellweger syndrome. J Inherited Metab Dis 14:152–164

Volpe JJ, Adams RD (1972) Cerebro-hepato-renal syndrome of Zellweger: an inherited disorder of neuronal migration. Acta Neuropathol (Berl) 20:175–198

Wanders RJA, Schutgens RBH, Schrakamp G, van den Bosch H, Tager JM, Schram AW, Hashimoto T, Poll-The BT, Saudubray JM (1986) Infantile Refsum disease: deficiency of catalase-containing particles (peroxisomes), alkyldihydroxyacetone phosphate synthases and peroxisomal β-oxidation enzyme proteins. Eur J Pediatr 145:172–175

Wanders RJA, Schutgens RBH, Schrakamp G, van den Bosch H, Tager JM, Moser AB, Moser HW (1987) Generalized loss of peroxisomal functions in neonatal adrenoleukodystrophy: implications for pre- and postnatal detection and relationship to X-linked adrenoleukodystrophy. J Inherited Metab Dis 10 [Suppl 2]: 225–228

Wanders RJA, van Roermund CWT, van Wijland MJA, Heikoop J, Schutgens RBH, Schram AW, Tager JM, van den Bosch H, Poll-The BT, Saudubray JM, Moser HW, Moser AB (1987) Peroxisomal very long-chain fatty acid β-oxidation in human skin fibroblasts:activity in Zellweger syndrome and other peroxisomal disorders. Clin Chim Acta 166:255–263

Wanders RJA, Heymans HSA, Schutgens RBH, Barth PG, van den Bosch H, Tager JM (1988a) Peroxisomal disorders in neurology. J Neurol Sci 88:1–39

Wanders RJA, Heymans HSA, Schutgens RBH, Poll-The BT, Saudubray JM, Tager JM, Schrakamp G, van den Bosch H (1988b) Peroxisomal functions in classical Refsum's disease: comparison with the infantile form of Refsum's disease. J Neurol Sci 84:147–155

Wanders RJA, van Roermund CWT, Schutgens RBH, Barth PG, Heymans HSA, van den Bosch H, Tager JM (1990a) The inborn errors of peroxisomal β-oxidation: a review. J Inherited Metab Dis 13:4–36

Wanders RJA, Boltshauser E, Steinmann B, Spycher MA, Schutgens RBH, Bosch van den H, Tager JM (1990b) Infantile phytanic acid storage disease, a disorder of peroxisome biogenesis: a case report. J Neurol Sci 98:1–11

Wanders RJA, Schutgens RBH, van den Bosch H, Tager JM, Kleijer WJ (1991a) Prenatal diagnosis of inborn errors in peroxisomal β-oxidation. Prenat Diagn 11:253–261

Wanders RJA, van Roermund CWT, Jakobs C, ten Brink HJ (1991b) Identification of pristanoyl-CoA oxidase and phytanic acid decarboxylation in peroxisomes and mitochondria from human liver:implications for Zellweger syndrome. J Inherited Metab Dis 14:349–352

Wanders RJA, Schutgens RBH, Barth PG, Tager JM, van den Bosch H (1993) Postnatal diagnosis of peroxisomal disorders:a biochemical approach. Biochimie 75:269–279

Wiemer EAC, Out M, Schelen A, Wanders RJA, Schutgens RBH, van den Bosch H, Tager JM (1991) Phenotypic heterogeneity in cultured skin fibroblasts from patients with disorders of peroxisome biogenesis belonging to the same complementation group. Biochim Biophys Acta 1097:232–237

Wilson GN, Holmes RG, Custer J, Lipkowitz JL, Stover J, Datta N, Hajra A (l986) Zellweger syndrome: diagnostic assays, syndrome delineation, and potential therapy. Am J Med Genet 24:69–82

Wilson GN, Holmes RD, Hajra AK (1988) Peroxisomal disorders:clinical commentary and future prospects. Am J Med Genet 30:771–792

Wolff J, Nyhan WL, Powell H, Takahashi D, Hutzler J, Hajra AK, Datta NS, Singh I, Moser HW (1986) Myopathy in an infant with a fatal peroxisomal disorder. Pediatr Neurol 2:141–146

Zellweger H (1987) The cerebro-hepato-renal (Zellweger) syndrome and other peroxisomal disorders. Dev Med Child Neurol 29:821–829

16 Rhizomelic Chondrodysplasia Punctata

Balfe A, Hoefler G, Chen WW, Watkins PA (1990) Aberrant subcellular localization of peroxisomal 3-ketoacyl-CoA thiolase in the Zellweger syndrome and rhizomelic chondrodysplasia punctata. Pediatr Res 27:304–310

Barr DGD, Kirk JM, Howassi MA, Wanders RJA, Schutgens RBH (1993) Rhizomelic chondrodysplasia punctata with isolated DHAP-AT deficiency. Arch Dis Child 68:415–417

Clayton PT, Eckhardt S, Wilson J, Hall CM, Yousuf Y, Wanders RJA, Schutgens RBH (1994) Isolated dihydroxyacetone-phosphate acyltransferase deficiency presenting with developmental delay. J Inherited Metab Dis 17:533–540

De Craemer D, Zweens MJ, Lyonnet S, Wanders RJA, Poll-The BT, Schutgens RBH, Waelkens JJJ, Saudubray JM, Roels F (1991) Very large peroxiomes in distinct peroxisomal disorders (rhizomelic chondrodysplasia punctata and acyl-CoA oxidase deficiency):novel data. Virchows Arch [A] 419:523–525

Gilbert EF, Opitz JM, Spranger JW, Langer LO, Wolfson JJ, Viseskul C (1976) Chondrodysplasia punctata – rhizomelic form. Pathologic and radiologic studies of three infants. Eur J Pediatr 123:89–109

Gray RGF, Green A, Schutgens RBH, Wanders RJA, Farndon PA, Kennedy CR (1990) Antenatal diagnosis of rhizomelic chondrodysplasia punctata in the second trimester. J Inherited Metab Dis 13:380–382

Gray RGF, Green A, Chapman S, McKeown C, Schutgens RBH, Wanders RJA (1992) Rhizomelic chondrodysplasia punctata – a new clinical variant. J Inherited Metab Dis 15:931–932

Heikoop JC, van Roermund CWT, Just WW, Ofman R, Schutgens RBH, Heymans HSA, Waders RJA, Tager JM (1990) Rhizomelic chondrodysplasia punctata. J Clin Invest 86:126–130

Heikoop JC, van den Berg M, Strijland A, Weijers PJ, Schutgens RBH, Just WW, Wanders RJA, Tager JM (1991) Peroxisomes of normal morphology but deficient in 3-oxoacyl-CoA thiolase in rhizomelic chondrodysplasis punctata fibroblasts. Biochim Biophys Acta 1097:62–70

Heikoop JC, Wanders RJA, Strijland A, Purvis R, Schutgens RBH, Tager JM (1992) Genetic and biochemical heterogeneity in patients with the rhizomelic form of chondrodysplasia punctata – a complementation study. Hum Genet 89:439–444

Heymans HSA, Oorthuys JWE, Nelck G, Wanders RJA, Schutgens RBH (1985) Rhizomelic chondrodysplasia punctata: another peroxisomal disorder. N Engl J Med 313:187–188

Heymans HSA, Oorthuys JWE, Nelck G, Wanders RJA, Dingemans KP, Schutgens RBH (1986) Peroxisomal abnormalities in rhizomelic chondrodysplasia punctata. J Inherited Metab Dis 9 [Suppl 2]:329–331

Hoefler G, Hoefler S, Watkins PA, Chen WW, Moser A, Baldwin V, McGillivary B, Charrow J, Friedman JM, Rutledge L, Hashimoto T, Moser HW (1988a) Biochemical abnormalities in rhizomelic chondrodysplasia punctata. J Pediatr 112:726–733

Hoefler S, Hoefler G, Moser AB, Watkins PA, Chen WW, Moser HW (1988b) Prenatal diagnosis of rhizomelic chondrodysplasia punctata. Prenat Diagn 8:571–576

Hughes JL, Poulos A, Crane DI, Chow CW, Sheffield LJ, Sillence D (1992) Ultrastructure and immunocytochemistry of hepatic peroxisomes in rhizomelic chondrodysplasia punctata. Eur J Pediatr 151:829–836

Nuoffer JM, Pfammatter JP, Spahr A, Toplak H, Wanders RJA, Schutgens RBH, Wiesmann UN (1994) Chondrodysplasia punctata with a mild clinical course. J Inherited Metab Dis 17:60–66

Poll-The BT, Maroteaux P, Narcy C, Quetin P, Guesnu M, Wanders RJA, Schutgens RBH, Saudubray JM (1991) A new type of chondrodysplasia punctata associated with peroxisomal dysfunction. J Inherited Metab Dis 14:361–363

Poulos A, Sheffield L, Sharp P, Sherwood G, Johnson D, Beckman K, Fellenberg AJ, Wraith JE, Chow CW, Usher S, Singh H (1988) Rhizomelic chondrodysplasia punctata: clinical, pathologic, and biochemical finindings in two patients. J Pediatr 113:685–690

Rizzo WB, Craft DA, Judd LL, Moser HW, Moser AB (1993) Fatty alcohol accumulation in the autosomal recessive form of rhizomelic chondrodysplasia punctata. Biochem Med Metab Biol 50:93–102

Singh I, Lazo O, Contreras M, Stanley W, Hashimoto T (1991) Rhizomelic chondrodysplasia punctata: biochemical studies of peroxisomes isolated from cultured skin fibroblasts. Arch Biochem Biophys 286:277–283

Smeitink JAM, Beemer FA, Espeel M, Donckerwolcke RAMG, Jakobs C, Wanders RJA, Schutgens RBH, Roels F, Duran M, Dorland L, Berger R, Poll-The BT (1992) Bone dysplasia associated with phytanic acid accumulation and deficient plasmalogen synthesis: a peroxisomal entity amendable to plasmapheresis. J Inherited Metab Dis 15:377–380

Sugarman GI (1974) Chondrodysplasia punctata (rhizomelic type): case report and pathologic findings. Birth Defects 10:334–340

Suzuki Y, Shimozawa N, Izai K, Uchida Y, Miura K, Akatsuka H, Nagaya M, Yamaguchi S, Orii T (1993) Peroxisomal 3-ketoacyl-CoA thiolase is partially processed in fibroblasts from patients with rhizomelic chondrodysplasia punctata. J Inherited Metab Dis 16:868–871

Ten Brink HJ, Schor DSM, Kok RM, Stellaard F, Kneer J, Poll-The BT, Saudubray JM, Jakobs C (1992) In vivo study of phytanic acid α-oxidation in classic Refsum's disease and chondrodysplasia punctata. Pediatr Res 32:566–570

Viseskul C, Opitz JM, Spranger JW, Hartmann HA, Gilbert EF (1974) Pathology of chondrodysplasia punctata rhizomelic type. Birth Defects 10:327–333

Wanders RJA, Schumacher H, Heikoop J, Schutgens RBH, Tager JM (1992) Human dihydroxyacetonephosphate acyltransferase deficiency:a new peroxisomal disorder. J Inherited Metab Dis 15:389–391

Wardinsky TD, Pagon RA, Powell BR, McGillivray B, Stephan M, Zonana J, Moser A (1990) Rhizomelic chondrodysplasia punctata and survival beyond one year: a review of the literature and five case reports. Clin Genet 38:84–93

Wells TR, Landing BH, Hines Bostwick F (1992) Studies of vertebral coronal cleft in rhizomelic chondrodysplasia punctata. Pediatr Pathol 12:593–600

Williams DW, Elster AD, David Cox T (1991) Cranial MR imaging in rhizomelic chondrodysplasia punctata. AJNR 12:363–365

17 Zellweger-like Syndrome

Paturneau-Jouas M, Taillard F, Gansmuller A, Schutgens R, Mikol J, Aigrot MS, Sereni C (1987) Clinical, biochemical, pathological „Zellweger-like" disorder with morphologically normal peroxisomes. In: Salvayre R (ed) Lipid storage disorders. Nato-Insern, Toulouse, pp 133–134

Suzuki Y, Shimozawa N, Orii T, Igarashi N, Kono N, Hashimoto T (1988) Molecular analysis of peroxisomal β-oxidation enzymes in infants with Zellweger syndrome and Zellweger-like syndrome: further heterogeneity of the peroxisomal disorder. Clin Chim Acta 172:65–76

Suzuki Y, Shimozawa N, Orii T, Igarashi N, Kono N, Matsui A, Inoue Y, Yokota S, Hashimoto T (1988) Zellweger-like syndrome with detectable hepatic peroxisomes: a variant from of peroxisomal disorder. J Pediatr 113:841–845

18 Pseudo-neonatal Adrenoleukodystrophy, Trifunctional Protein Deficiency, Pseudo-Zellweger Syndrome

Barth PG, Wanders RJA, Schutgens RBJ, Bleeker-Wagemakers EM, van Heemstra D (1990) Peroxisomal β-oxidation defect with detectable peroxisomes: a case with neonatal onset and progressive course. Eur J Pediatr 149:722–726

Bout A, Franse MM, Collins J, Blonden L, Tager JM, Benne R (1991) Characterization of the gene encoding human peroxisomal 3-oxoacyl-CoA thiolase (ACAA). No large DNA rearrangement in a thiolase-deficient patient. Biochim Biophys Acta 1090:43–51

Chen GL, Balfe A, Erwa W, Hoefler G, Gaertner J, Aikawa J, Chen WW (1991) Import of human bifunctional enzyme into peroxisomes of human hepatoma cells in vitro. Biochem Biophys Res Commun 178:1084–1091

Christensen E, Woldseth B, Hagve TA, Poll-The BT, Wanders RJA, Sprecher H, Stokke O, Christophersen BO (1993) Peroxisomal β-oxidation of polyunsaturated long chain fatty acids in human fibroblasts. The polyunsaturated and the saturated long chain fatty acids are retroconverted by the same acyl-CoA oxidase. Scand J Clin Lab Invest 53 [Suppl 215]:61–74

Clayton PT, Lake BD, Hjelm M, Stephenson JBP, Besley GTN, Wanders RJA, Schram AW, Tager JM, Schutgens RBH, Lawson AM (1988) Bile acid analyses in „pseudo-Zellweger" syndrome; clues to the defect in peroxisomal β-oxidation. J Inherited Metab Dis 11 [Suppl 2]:165–168

Espeel M, Roels F, van Maldergem L, de Craemer D, Dacremont G, Wanders RJA, Hashimoto T (1991) Peroxisomal localization of the immunoreactive β-oxidation enzymes in a neonate with a β-oxidation defect. Virchows Arch A Pathol Anat 419:301–308

Goldfischer S, Collins J, Rapin I, Neumann P, Neglia W, Spiro AJ, Ishii T, Roels F, Vamecq J, van Hoof F (1986) Pseudo-Zellweger syndrome:deficiencies in several peroxisomal oxidative activities. J Pediatr 108:25–32

Hughes JL, Poulos A, Robertson E, Chow CW, Sheffield LJ, Christodoulou J, Carter RF (1990) Pathology of hepatic peroxisomes and mitochondria in patients with peroxisomal disorders. Virchows Arch [A] 416:255–264

Kyllerman M, Blomstrand S, Mansson JE, Conradi NG, Hinmarsh T (1989) Central nervous system malformations and white matter changes in pseudo-neonatal adrenoleukodystrophy. Neuropediatrics 21:199–201

Mandel H, Berant M, Aizin A, Gershony R, Hemmli S, Schutgens RBH, Wanders RJA (1992) Zellweger-like phenotype in two siblings: a defect in peroxisomal β-oxidation with elevated very long-chain fatty acids but normal bile acids. J Inherited Metab Dis 15:381–384

Martinez M (1990) Severe deficiency of docosahexaenoic acid in peroxisomal disorders. Neurology 40:1292–1298

McGuiness MC, Moser AB, Poll-The BT, Watkins PA (1993) Complementation analysis of patients with intact peroxisomes and impaired peroxisomal β-oxidation. Biochem Med Metab Biol 49:228–242

Naidu S, Hoefler G, Watkins PA, Chen WW, Moser AB, Hoefler S, Rance NE, Powers JM, Beard M, Green WR, Hashimoto T, Moser HW (1988) Neonatal seizures and retardation in a girl with biochemical features of X-linked adrenoleukodystrophy: a possible new peroxisomal disease entity. Neurology 38:1100–1107

Naidu S, Moser AE, Moser HW (1988) Phenotypic and genotypic variability of generalized peroxisomal disorders. Pediatr Neurol 4:5–12

Nakada Y, Hyakuma N, Suzuki Y, Shimozawa N, Takasu E, Ikema R, Hirayama K (1993) A case of pseudo-Zellweger syndrome with a possible bifunctional enzyme deficiency but detectable enzyme protein. Comparison of two cases of Zellweger syndrome. Brain Dev 15:453–456

Paul DA, Goldsmith LS, Miles DK, Moser AB, Spiro AJ, Grover WD (1993) Neonatal adrenoleukodystrophy presenting as infantile progressive spinal muscular atrophy. Pediatr Neurol 9:496–497

Poll-The BT, Roels F, Ogier H, Scotto J, Vamecq J, Schutgens RBH, Wanders RJA, van Roermund CWT, van Wijland MJA, Schram AW, Tager JM, Saudubray JM (1988) A new peroxisomal disorder with enlarged peroxisomes and a specific deficiency of acyl-CoA oxidase (pseudo-neonatal adrenoleukodystrophy). Am J Hum Genet 41:422–434

Roels F, Pauwels M, Poll-The BT, Scotto J, Ogier H, Aubourg P, Saudubray JM (1988) Hepatic peroxisomes in adrenoleukodystrophy and related syndromes: cytochemical and morphometric data. Virchows Arch [A] 413:275–285

Santer R, Clavie A, Oldigs HD, Schaub J, Schutgens RBH, Wanders RJA (1993) Isolated defect of peroxisomal β-oxidation in a 16-year-old patient. Eur J Pediatr 152:339–342

Schram AW, Goldfischer S, Wanders RJA, Brouwer-Kelder EM, van Roermund CWT, Collins J, Hashimoto T, Heymans HSA, Schutgens RBH, van den Bosch H, Tager JM (1987) A genetic disorder due to the deficiency of the peroxisomal β-oxidation enzyme 3-oxoacyl-CoA thiolase. J Inherited Metab Dis 10 [Suppl 2]:214–216

Schram AW, Goldfischer S, van Roermund CWT, Brouwer-Kelder EM, Collins J, Hashimoto T, Heyumans HSA, van den Bosch H, Schutgens RBH, Tager JM, Wanders RJA (1987) Human peroxisomal 3-oxoacyl-coenzyme A thiolase deficiency. Proc Natl Acad Sci U S A 84:2494–2496

Tager JM, Brul S, Wiemer EAC, Strijland A, van Driel R, Schutgens RBH, van den Bosch H, Wanders RJA, Westerveld A (1990) Genetic relationship between the Zellweger syndrome and other peroxisomal disorders characterized by an impairment in the assembly of peroxisomes. J Prog Clin Biol Res 321:545–558

Van Maldergem L, Espeel M, Wanders RJA, Roels F, Gerard P, Scalais E, Mannaerts GP, Casteels M, Gilleroi Y (1992) Neonatal seizures and severe hypotonia in a male infant suffering from a defect in peroxisomal β-oxidation. Neuromusc Dis 2:217–224

Wanders RJA, van Roermund CWT, Schelen A, Schutgens RBH, Tager JM, Stephenson JBP, Clayton PT (1990) A bifunctional protein with deficient enzymic activity:identification of a new peroxisomal disorder using novel methods to measure the peroxisomal β-oxidation enzyme activities. J Inherited Metab Dis 13:375–379

Wanders RJA, van Roermund CWT, Brul S, Schutgens RBH, Tager JM (1992) Bifunctional enzyme deficiency: identification of a new type of peroxisomal disorder in a patient with an impairment in peroxisomal β-oxidation of unknown aetiology by means of complementation analysis. J Inherited Metab Dis 15:385–388

Wanders RJA, Heymans HSA, Schutgens RBH, Barth PG, van den Bosch H, Tager JM (1988) Peroxisomal disorders in neurology. J Neurol Sci 88:1–39

Wanders RJA, van Roermund CWT, Schutgens RBH, Barth PG, Heymans HSA, van den Bosch H, Tager JM (1990) The inborn errors of peroxisomal β-oxidation: a review. J Inherited Metab Dis 13:4–36

Watkins PA, Chen WW, Harris CJ, Hoeffler G, Hoefler S, Blake DC, Baife A, Kelley RI, Moser AB, Beard ME, Moser HW (1989) Peroxisomal bifunctional enzyme deficiency. J Clin Invest 83:771–777

19 X-linked Adrenoleukodystrophy

Antoku Y, Koike F, Ohtsuka Y, Sakai T, Tsukamoto K, Nagara H, Iwashita H, Goto I (1991) Adrenoleukodystrophy: a correlation between satuated very long-chain fatty acids in mononuclear cells and phenotype. Ann Neurol 30:101–103

Aubourg P, Sellier N, Chaussain JL, Kalifa G (1989) MRI detects cerebral involvement in neurologically asymptomatic patients with adrenoleukodystrophy. Neurology 39:1619–1621

Aubourg P, Blanche S, Jambaqué I, Rocchiccioli F, Kalifa G, Naud-Saudreau C, Rolland MO, Debré M, Chaussain JL,

Griscelli C, Fischer A, Bougnères PF (1990) Reversal of early neurologic and neuroradiologic manifestations of X-linked adrenoleukodystrophy by bone marrow transplantation. N Engl J Med 322:1860–1866

Aubourg P, Adamsbaum C, Lavallard-Rousseau MC, Lemaitre A, Boureau F, Mayer M, Kalifa G (1992) Brain MRI and electrophysiologic abnormalities in preclinical and clinical adrenomyeloneuropathy. Neurology 42:85–91

Bewermeijer H, Bamborschke S, Ebhardt G, Hunermann B, Heiss WD (1985) MR imaging in adrenoleukomyeloneuropathy. J Comput Assist Tomogr 9:793–796

Blaw ME, Osterberg K, Kozak P, Nelson E (1964) Sudanophilic leukodystrophy and adrenal cortical atrophy. Arch Neurol 11:626–631

Boles DJ, Craft DA, Padgett DA, Loria RM, Rizzo WB (1991) Clinical variation in X-linked adrenoleukodystrophy: fatty acid and lipid metabolism in cultured fibroblasts. Biochem Med Metab Biol 45:74–91

Boutin B, Matsuguchi L, Lebon P, Ponsol G, Arthuis C (1989) Immunohistochemical analysis of brain macrophages in adrenoleukodystrophy. Neuropediatrics 20:202–206

Brown FR, Chen WW, Kirschner DA, Frayer KL, Powers JM, Moser AB, Moser HW (1983) Myelin membrane from adrenoleukodystrophy brain white matter -biochemical properties. J Neurochem 41:341–348

Coria F, Garcia-Viejo MA, Delgado JA, Duarte J, Claveria LE, Giros M, Pampols T (1993) Diagnosis of X-adrenoleucodystrophy phenotypic variants. Acta Neurol Scand 87:499–502

Davis LE, Snyder RD, Orth DN, Nicholson WE, Kornfeld M, Seelinger DF (1979) Adrenoleukodystrophy and adrenomyeloneuropathy associated with partial adrenal insufficiency in three generations of a kindred. Am J Med 66:342–347

Demaerel P, Faubert C, Wilms G, Casaer P, Piepgras U, Baert AL (1991) MR findings in leukodystrophy. Neuroradiology 33:368–371

Domagk J, Linke I, Argyrakis A, Spaar FW, Rahlf G, Schulte FJ (1975) Adrenoleukodystrophy. Neuropediatrics 6:41–64

Dumic M, Gubarev n, Sikic N, Roscher A, Plavsic V, Filipovic-Grcic B (1992) Sparse hair and multiple endocrine disorders in two women heterozygous for adrenoleukodystrophy. Am J Med Genet 43:829–832

Elrington GM, Bateman DE, Jeffrey MJ, Flawton N (1989) Adrenoleukodystrophy: heterogeneity in two brothers. J Neurol Neurosurg Psychiatry 52:310–313

Farrell DF, Hamilton SR, Knauss TA, Sanocki E, Deeb SS (1993) X-linked adrenoleukodystrophy:Adult cerebral variant. Neurology 43:1518–1522

Federico A, Dotti MT, Annunziata P, Bonuccelli U, Fenzi G, Ciacci G, Malandrini A, Meucci G, Guazzi GC (1988) Adrenomyeloneurodystrophy with late cerebral involvement and evidence of a multiple autoimmune disorder. J Inherited Metab Dis 11 [Suppl 2]:169–172

Garg BP, Markand ON, DeMeyer WE, Warren C (1983) Evoked response studies in patients with adrenoleukodystrophy and heterozygous relatives. Arch Neurol 40:356–359

Graham GE, MacLeod PM, Lillicrap DP, Bridge PJ (1992) Gonadal mosaicism in a family with adrenoleukodystrophy:molecular diagnosis of carrier status among daughters of a gonadal mosaic when direct detection of the mutation is not possible. J Inherited Metab Dis 15:68–74

Hashimi M, Stanley W, Singh I (1986) Lignoceryol-CoASH ligase:enzyme defect in fatty acid β-oxidation system in X-linked childhood adrenoleukodystrophy. FEBS Lett 196:247–250

Higgens CB, Taketa RM, Halpern SE (1975) Abnormal brain scans in adrenal leukodystrophy. Radiology 114:667–669

Holmberg BH, Hägg E, Duchek M, Hagenfeldt L (1992) Screening of patients with hereditary spastic paraparesis and Addison's disease for adrenoleukodystrophy/adrenomyeloneuropathy. Acta Neurol Scand 85:147–149

Hong-Magno ET, Muraki AS, Huttenlocher PR (1987) Atypical CT scans in adrenoleukodystrophy. J Comput Assist Tomogr 11:333–336

Igarashi M, Belchis D, Suzuki K (1976a) Brain gangliosides in adrenoleukodystrophy. J Neurochem 27:327–328

Igarashi M, Schaumburg HH, Powers J, Kishimoto Y, Kolodny E, Suzuki K (1976b) Fatty acid abnormality in adrenoleukodystrophy. J Neurochem 26:851–860

Igarashi M, Belchis D, Suzuki K (1976c) Brain gangliosides in adrenoleukodystrophy. J Neurochem 27:327–328

Jensen ME, Sawyer RW, Braun IF, Rizzo WB (1990) MR imaging appearance of childhood adrenoleukodystrophy with auditory, visual, and motor pathway involvement. Radiographics 10:53–66

Kaplan PW, Tusa RJ, Shankroff J, Heller J, Moser HW (1993) Visual evoked potentials in adrenoleukodystrophy:a trial with glycerol trioleate and Lorenzo oil. Ann Neurol 34:169–174

Koike R, Tsuji S, Ohno T, Suzuki Y, Orii T, Miyatake T (1991) Physiological significance of fatty acid elongation system in adrenoleukodystrophy. J Neurol Sci 103:188–194

Kukowski B (1991) Magnetic transcranial brain stimulation and multimodality evoked potentials in an adrenoleukodystrophy patient and members of his family. Electroencephalogr Clin Neurophysiol 78:260–262

Kumar AJ, Rosenbaum AE, Naidu S, Wener L, Citrin CM, Lindenberg R, Kim WS, James Zinreich S, Molliver ME, Mayberg HS, Moser HW (1987) Adrenoleukodystrophy:Correlating MR imaging with CT. Radiology 165:497–504

Kurihara M, Kumagai K, Yagishita S, Imai M, Watanabe M, Suzuki Y, Orii T (1993) Adrenoleukomyeloneuropathy presenting as cerebellar ataxia in a young child: a probable variant of adrenoleukodystrophy. Brain Dev 15:377–380

Kusaka H, Imai T (1992) Ataxic variant of adrenoleukodystrophy: MRI and CT findings. J Neurol 239:307–310

Lazo O, Contreras M, Hashmi M, Stanley W, Irazu C, Singh I (1988) Peroxisomal lignoceroyl-CoA ligase deficiency in childhood adrenoleukodystrophy and adrenomyeloneuropathy. Proc Natl Acad Sci U S A 85:7647–7651

Lenard HG (1984) Adrenoleukodystrophy. Neuropediatrics 15:16–19

Loes DJ, Hite S, Moser H, Stillman AE, Shapiro E, Lockman L, Latchaw RE, Krivit W (1994) Adrenoleukodystrophy: a scoring method for brain MR observations. AJNR 15:1761–1766

Loes DJ, Stillman AE, Hite S, Shapiro E, Lockman L, Latchaw RE, Moser H, Krivit W (1994) Childhood cerebral form of adrenoleukodystrophy: short-term effect of bone marrow transplantation on brain MR observations. AJNR 15:1767–1771

Lyon-Caen O, Benoit N, Carreau V, Montreuil M, Menage P, Lubetzki C, Cabanis E, Iba-Zizen MT, Tourbah A, Baumann N (1991) Cognitive function in adult adrenoleukodystrophy: comparison with leukoaraiosis and multiple sclerosis. Dev Neurosci 13:251–253

Maestri NE, Beaty TH (1992) Predictions of a 2-locus model for disease heterogeneity: application to adrenoleukodystrophy. Am J Med Genet 44:576–582

Marsh WW, Hurst DL (1991) Variable phenotypes in a family kindred with adrenoleukodystrophy. Pediatr Neurol 7:50–52

Martin JJ, Ceuterick C, Libert J (1980) Skin and conjunctival nerve biopsies in adrenoleukodystrophy and its variants. Ann Neurol 8:291–295

Molzer B, Bernheimer H, Budka H, Pilz P, Toifl K (1981) Accumulation of very long chain fatty acids is common to 3 variants of adrenoleukodystrophy (ALD). J Neurol Sci 51:301–310

Moser HW (1993) Lorenzo oil therapy for adrenoleukodystrophy: a prematurely amplified hope. Ann Neurol 34:121–122

Moser HW, Moser AB, Kawamura N, Murphy J, Suzuki K, Schaumburg H, Kishimoto Y (1980) Adrenoleukodystrophy: elevated C26 fatty acid in cultered skin fibroblasts. Ann Neurol 7:542–549

Moser HW, Moser AB, Frayer KK, Chen W, Schulman JD, O'Neill BP, Kishimoto Y (1981) Adrenoleukodystrophy:increased plasma content of saturated very long chain fatty acids. Neurology 31:1241–1249HW, Moser AE, Singh I, O'Neill BP (1984) Adrenoleukodystrophy: survey of 303 cases: biochemistry, diagnosis, and therapy. Ann Neurol 16:628–641

Moser HW, Bergin A, Naidu S, Ladenson PW (1991a) Adrenoleukodystrophy. Endocrinol Metab Clin North Am 20:297–318

Moser HW, Moser AB, Naidu S, Bergin A (1991b) Clinical aspects of adrenoleukodystrophy and adrenomyeloneuropathy. Dev Neurosci 13:254–261

Moser HW, Moser AB, Smith KD, Bergin A, Borel J, Shankroff J, Stine OC, Merette C, Ott J, Krivit W, Shapiro E (1992) Adrenoleukodystrophy: phenotypic variability and implications for therapy. J Inherited Metab Dis 15:645–664

Mosser J, Douar AM, Sarde CO, Kioschis P, Feil R, Moser H, Poustka AM, Mandel JL, Aubourg P (1993) Putative X-linked adrenoleukodystrophy gene shares unexpected homology with ABC transporters. Nature 361:726–730

Nishio H, Kodama S, Tsubota T, Takumi T, Takahashi T, Yokoyama S, Matsuo T (1985) Adrenoleukodystrophy without adrenal insufficiency and its magnetic resonance imaging. J Neurol 232:265–270

Notarangelo LD, Parolini O, Baiguini G, Buzi F, Paterlini C, Perini A, Rimoldi M, Tiberti S, Uziel G, Notarangelo L, Camerino G, Ugazio AG (1992) Carrier detection in X-linked adrenoleukodystrophy by determination of very long chain fatty acid levels and by linkage analysis. Eur J Pediatr 151:761–763

O'Neill BP, Forbes GS (1981) Computerized tomography and adrenoleukomyeloneuropathy. Arch Neurol 38:293–296

O'Neill BP, Marmion LC, Feringa ER (1981) The adrenoleukomyeloneuropathy complex: expression in four generations. Neurology 31:151–156

O'Neill BP, Moser HW, Saxena KM (1982) Familial X-linked Addison disease as an expression of adrenoleukodystrophy (ALD): elevated C$_{26}$ fatty acid in cultured skin fibroblasts. Neurology 32:543–547

Pasco A, Kalifa G, Sarrazin JL, Adamsbaum C, Aubourg P (1991) Contribution of MRI to the diagnosis of cerebral lesions of adrenoleukodystrophy. Pediatr Radiol 21:161–163

Powell H, Tindall R, Schultz P, Paa D, O'Brien J, Lampert P (1975) Adrenoleukodystrophy. Electron microscopic findings. Arch Neurol 32:250–260

Powers JM, Schaumburg HH (1974) Adreno-leukodystrophy (sex-linked Schilder's disease). Am J Pathol 76:481–491

Powers JM, Liu Y, Moser AB, Moser HW (1992) The inflammatroy myelinopathy of adreno-leukodystrophy: cells, effector molecules, and pathogenetic implications. J Neuropathol Exp Neurol 51:630–643

Ramsey RB, Banik NL, Scott T, Davison AN (1976) Neurochemical findings in adreno-leukodystrophy. J Neurol Sci 29:277–294

Rizzo WB (1993) Lorenzo's oil – hope and disappointment. N Engl J Med 329:801–802

Rizzo WB, Leshner RT, Odone A, Dammann AL, Craft BS, Jensen ME, Jennings SS, Davis S, Jaitly R, Sgro JA (1989) Dietary erucic acid therapy for X-linked adrenoleukodystrophy. Neurology 39:1415–1422

Romero C, Dietemann JL, Kurtz D, Bataillard M, Christmann D (1990) Adrenoleucodystrophie: intéret de l'IRM avec Gadolinium. J Neuroradiol 17:267–276

Sack GH, Morrell JC (1993) Adrenoleukodystrophy: overlapping deletions point to a gene location in Xq28. Biochem Biophys Res Commun 191:955–960

Sadeghi-Nejad A, Senior B (1990) Adrenomyeloneuropathy presenting as addison's disease in childhood. N Engl J Med 322:13–16

Schaumburg HH, Powers JM, Raine CS, Suzuki K, Richardson EP (1975) Adrenoleukodystrophy: a clinical and pathological study of 17 cases. Arch Neurol 32:577–591

Schaumburg HH, Powers JM, Raine CS, Spencer PS, Griffin JW, Prineas JW, Boehme DM (1977) Adrenomyeloneuropathy: a probable variant of adrenoleukodystrophy. Neurology 27:1114–1119

Scholte W, Molzer B, Peiffer J, Poremba M, Schumm F, Harzer K, Schnabel R, Bernheimer H (1987) Adrenoleukodystrophy in an adult female. A clinical, morphological and neurochemical study. J Neurol 235:1–9

Sharp P, Johnson D, Poulos A (1991) Molecular species of phosphatidylcholine containing very long chain fatty acids in human brain:enrichment in X-linked adrenoleukodystrophy brain and diseases of peroxisome biogenesis brain. J Neurochem 56:30–37

Shimizu H, Moser HW, Naidu S (1988) Auditory brainstem response and audiologic findings in adrenoleukodystrophy: its variant and carrier. Otolaryngol Head Neck Surg 98:215–220

Tanaka K, Koyama A, Koike R, Ohno T, Atsumi T, Miyatake T (1985) Adrenomyeloneuropathy:report of a family and electron microscopical findings in peripheral nerve. J Neurol 232:73–78

Theda C, Moser AB, Powers JM, Moser HW (1992) Phospholipids in X-linked adrenoleukodystrophy white matter: fatty acid abnormalities before the onset of demyelination. J Neurol Sci 110:195–204

Uchiyama M, Hata Y, Tada S (1991) MR imaging of adrenoleukodystrophy. Neuroradiology 33:25–29

Uyama E, Iwagoe H, Maeda J, Nakamura M, Terasaki T, Ando M (1993) Presenile-onset cerebral adrenoleukodystrophy presenting as Balint's syndrome and dementia. Neurology 43:1249–1251

Uziel G, Bertini E, Bardelli P, Rimoldi M, Gambetti M (1991) Experience on therapy of adrenoleukodystrophy and adrenomyeloneuropathy. Dev Neurosci 13:274–279

Valle D, Gärtner J (1993) Penetrating the peroxisome. Nature 361:682–683

Van der Knaap MS, Valk J (1989) MR of adrenoleukodystrophy: histopathologic correlations. AJNR 10:S12-S14

Van Geel BM, Assies J, Haverkort EB, Barth PG, Wanders RJA, Schutgens RBH, Keyser A, Zwetsloot CP (1993) Delay in diagnosis of X-linked adrenoleukodystrophy. Clin Neurol Neurosurg 95:115–120

Van Oost BA, van Zandvoort PM, Tünte W, Brunner HG, Hoogeboom AJM, Maaswinkel-Mooy PD, Bakkeren J, Hamel B, Ropers HH (1991) Linkiage analysis in X-linked adrenoleukodystrophy and application in post- and prenatal diagnosis. Hum Genet 86:404–407

Volkow ND, Patchell L, Kulkarni MV, Reed K et al (1987) Adrenoleukodystrophy: imaging with CT, MRI and PET. J Nucl Med 28:524–527

Wanders RJA, van Roermund CWT, van Wijland MJA, Heikoop J, van den Put A, Bentlage P, Meijboom E, Tager JM, Schram AW, van den Bosch H, Schutgens RBH (1987) Peroxisomal fatty acid β-oxidation in human skin fibroblasts: X-linked adrenoleukodystrophy, a peroxisomal very long chain fatty acyl-CoA synthetase deficiency? J Inherited Metab Dis 10 [Suppl 2]:220–224

Wanders RJA, van Roermund CWT, van Wijland MJA, Schutgens RBH, Schram AW, Tager JM, van den Bosch H, Schalkwijk C (1988) X-linked adrenoleukodystrophy: identification of the primary defect at the level of a deficient peroxisomal very long chain fatty acyl-CoA synthetase using a newly developed method for the isolation of peroxisomes from skin fibroblasts. J Inherited Metab Dis 11 [Suppl 2]:173–177

Watkins PA, Naidu S, Moser HW (1987) Adrenoleukodystrophy: biochemical procedures in diagnosis, prevention and treatment. J Inherited Metab Dis 10:46–53

Weller M, Liedtke W, Petersen D, Opitz H, Poremba M (1992) Very-late-onset adrenoleukodystrophy:Possible precipitation of demyelination by cerebral contusion. Neurology 42L 367–370

Willems PJ, Vits L, Wanders RJA, Coucke PJ, van der Auwera BJ, van Elsen AF, Raeymaekers P, van Broeckhoven C, Schutgens RBH, Dacremont G, Leroy JG, Martin JJ, Dumon JE (1990) Linkage of DNA markers at Xq28 to adrenoleukodystrophy and adrenomyeloneuropathy present within the same family. Arch Neurol 47:665–669

Wilson R, Sargent JR (1993) Lipid and fatty acid composition of brain tissue from adrenoleukodystrophy patients. J Neurochem 61:290–297

Wilson R, Tocher DR, Sargent JR (1992) Effects of exogenous monounsaturated fatty acids on fatty acid metabolism in cultured skin fibroblasts from adrenoleukodystrophy patients. J Neurol Sci 109:207–214

Zwetsloot CP, Padberg GW, van Seters AP, Maaswinkel-Mooy PD, Onkenhout W (1992) Adult adrenoleukodystrophy: the clinical spectrum in a large Dutch family. J Neurol 239:107–111

20 Mitochondria and Mitochondrial Disorders

Agsteribbe E, Huckriede A, Veenhuis M, Ruiters MHJ, Niezen-Koning KE, Skjeldal OH, Skullerud K, Gupta RS, Hallberg R, Van Diggelen OP, Scholte HR (1993) A fatal, systemic mitochondrial disease with decreased mitochondrial enzyme activities, abnormal ultrastructure of the mitochondria and deficiency of heat shock protein 60. Biochem Biophys Res Commun 1:146–154

Attardi G, Schatz G (1988) Biogenesis of mitochondria. Ann Rev Cell Biol 4:289–333

Benz R (1990) Biophysical properties of porin pores from mitochondrial outer membrane of eukaryotic cells. Experientia 46:131–137

Bowling AC, Mutisya EM, Walker LC, Price DL, Cork LC, Flint Beal M (1993) Age-dependent impairment of mitochondrial function in primate brain. J Neurochem 60:1964–1967

Breningstall GN (1993) Approach to diagnosis of oxidative metabolism disorders. Pediatr Neurol 9:81–90

Cheng MY, Ulrich Hartl F, Martin J, Pollock RA, Kalousek F, Neupert W, Hallberg EM, Hallberg RL, Horwich AL (1989) Mitochondrial heat-shock protein hsp60 is essential for assembly of proteins imported into yeast mitochondria. Nature 337:620–625

Clayton DA (1992) Structure and function of the mitochondrial genome. J Inherited Metab Dis 15:439–447

Coates PM, Tanaka K (1992) Molecular basis of mitochondrial fatty acid oxidation defects. J Lipid Res 33:1099–1110

Cote C, Boulet D, Poirier J (1990) Expression of the mammalian mitochondrial genome. J Biol Chem 265:7532–7538

Crimmins D, Morris JGL, Walker GL, Sue CM, Byrne E, Stevens S, Jean-Francis B, Yiannikas C, Pamphlett R (1993) Mitochondrial encephalomyopathy: variable clinical expression within a single kindred. J Neurol Neurosurg Psychiatry 56:900–905

Cuezva JM, Flores AI, Liras A, Santaren JF, Alconada A (1993) Molecular chaperones and the biogenesis of mitochondria and peroxisomes. Biol Cell 77:47–62

De Vries DD, Ruitenbeek W, de Wijs IJ, Trijbels JMF, van Oost BA (1993) Enzymological versus DNA investigations in mitochondrial (encephalo-myopathies). J Inherited Metab Dis 16:534–536

Deshaies RJ, Koch BD, Werner-Washburne M, Craig EA, Schekman R (1988) A subfamily of stress proteins facilitates translocation of secretory and mitochondrial precursor polypeptides. Nature 332:800–805

DeVivo DC (1993) The expanding clinical spectrum of mitochondrial diseases. Brain Dev 15:1–22

DiMauro S, Moraes CT (1993) Mitochondrial encephalomyopathies. Arch Neurol 50:1197–1208

DiMauro S, Bonilla E, Zeviani M, Nakagawa M, DeVivo DC (1985) Mitochondrial myopathies. Ann Neurol 17:521–538

DiMauro S, Bonilla E, Zeviani M, Servidei S, DeVivo DC, Schon EA (1987) Mitochondrial myopathies. J Inherited Metab Dis 10 [Suppl 1]:113–128

DiMauro S, Moraes CT, Shanske S, Lombes A, Nakase H, Mita S, Tritschler HJ, Bonilla E, Miranda AF, Schon EA (1991) Mitochondrial encephalomyopathies: biochemical approach. Rev Neurol 147:443–449

DiMauro S, Simonetti S, Chen X, Petruzzella V, Hirano M, Shanske S, Moraes CT, Schon EA (1993) Mitochondrial dysfunction as a mechanism of CNS injury. In: Waxman SG (ed) Molecular and cellular approaches to the treatment of neurological disease. Raven, New York, pp 67–79

Eymard B, Hauw JJ (1992) Mitochondrial encephalomyopathies. Curr Opin Neurol Neurosurg 5:909–916

Gerbitz KD, Obermaier-Kusser B, Zierz S, Pongratz D, Müller-Höcker J, Lestienne P (1990) Mitochondrial myopathies: divergences of genetic deletions, biochemical defects and the clinical syndromes. J Neurol 237:5–10

Gething MJ, Sambrook J (1992) Protein folding in the cell. Nature 355:33–45

Glick B, Schatz G (1991) Import of proteins into mitochondria. Annu Rev Genet 25:21–44

Glick BS, Beasley EM, Schatz G (1992) Protein sorting in mitochondria. Trends Biochem Sci 17:453–459

Gupta RS (1990) Mitochondria, molecular chaperone proteins and the in vivo assembly of microtubules. Trends Biochem Sci 15:415–418

Guzman M, Geelen MJH (1993) Regulation of fatty acid oxidation in mammalian liver. Biochim Biophys Acta 1167:227–241

Haelestrap AP (1989) The regulation of the matrix volume of mammalian mitochondria in vivo and in vitro and its role in the control of mitochondrial metabolism. Biochim Biophys Acta 973:355–382

Haginoya K, Miyabayashi S, Iinuma K, Tada K (1993) Quantitative evaluation of electron transport system proteins in mitochondrial encephalomyopathy. Acta Neuropathol (Berl) 85:370–377

Hale DE, Bennett MJ (1992) Fatty acid oxidation disorders:a new class of metabolic diseases. J Pediatr 121:1–11

Harding AE, Hammans SR (1992) Deletions of the mitochondrial genome. J Inherited Metab Dis 15:480–486

Hausegger KA, Millner MM, Ebner F, Flückiger F, Justich E (1991) Mitochondrial encephalomyopathy – two years follow-up by MRI. Pediatr Radiol 21:231–233

Hawlitschek G, Schneider H, Schmidt B, Tropschug M, Hartl FU, Neupert W (1988) Mitochondrial protein import: identification of processing peptidase and of PEP, a processing enhancing protein. Cell 53:795–806

Holt IJ, Harding AE, Petty RKH, Morgan-Hughes JA (1990) A new mitochondrial disease associated with mitochondrial DNA heteroplasmy. Am J Hum Genet 46:428–433

Horwich A (1990) Protein import into mitochondria and peroxisomes. Curr Opin Cell Biol 2:625–633

Ishitsu T, Miike T, Kitano A, Haraguchi Y, Ohtani Y, Matsuda I, Shimoji A, Kimura H (1987) Heterogeneous phenotypes of mitochondrial encephalomyopathy in a single kindred. Neurology 37:1867–1869

Kiebler M, Pfaller R, Söllner T, Griffiths G, Horstmann H, Pfanner N, Neupert W (1990) Identification of a mitochondrial receptor complex required for recognition and membrane insertion of precursor proteins. Nature 348:610–616

Kroon AM, van den Bogert C (1987) Biogenesis of mitochondria and genetics of mitochondrial defects. J Inherited Metab Dis 10 [Suppl 1]:54–61

Lightowlers RN (1992) Hereditary disorders including mitochondrial diseases. Curr Opin Neurol Neurosurg 5:368–374

Lombes A, Bonilla E, Dimauro S (1989) Mitochondrial encephalomyopathies. Rev Neurol 145:671–689

Mannella CA (1992) The „ins" and „outs" of mitochondrial membrane channels. Trends Biochem Sci 17:315–320

Meijer AJ, van Noorden CJF (1991) Celbiologie in medisch perspectief. VI. Energievoorziening van de cel. Ned Tijdschr Geneeskd 135:2164–2170

Menkes JH (1987) Genetic disorders of mitochondrial function. J Pediatr 110:255–259

Morgan-Hughes JA (1982) Mitochondrial myopathies. In: Mastaglia FL, Walton J (eds) Skeletal muscle pathology. Churchill Livingstone, Edinburgh, pp 309–339

Munnich A, Rustin P, Rötig A, Chretien D, Bonnefont JP, Nuttin C, Cormier V, Vassault A, Parvy P, Bardet J, Charpentier C, Rabier D, Saudubray JM (1992) Clinical aspects of mitochondrial disorders. J Inherited Metab Dis 15:448–455

Ozawa T, Tanaka M, Suzuki H, Nishikimi M (1987) Structure and function of mitochondria: their organization and disorders. Brain Dev 9:76–81

Pfanner N, Neupert W (1990) The mitochondrial protein import apparatus. Annu Rev Biochem 59:331–353

Poulton J (1992) Duplications of mitochondrial DNA: implications for pathogenesis. J Inherited Metab Dis 15:487–498

Poulton J (1993) Mitochondrial DNA and genetic disease. Dev Med Child Neurol 35:833–840

Przyrembel (1987) Therapy of mitochondrial disorders. J Inherited Metab Dis 10:129–146

Ruitenbeek W, Sengers RCA, Trijbels JMF, Janssen AJM, Bakkeren JAJM (1992) The use of chorionic villi in prenatal diagnosis of mitochondriopathies. J Inherited Metab Dis 15:303–306

Scholte HR, Busch HFM, Luyt-Houwen IEM, Vaandrager-Verduin MHM, Przyrembel H, Arts WFM (1987) Defects in oxidative phosphorylation. Biochemical investigations in skeletal muscle and expression of the lesion in other cells. J Inherited Metab Dis 10 [Suppl 1]:81–97

Schulz H (1991) Beta oxidation of fatty acids. Biochim Biophys Acta 1081:109–120

Sengers RCA, Stadhouders AM (1987) Secondary mitochondrial pathology. J Inherited Metab Dis 10 [Suppl 1]:98–104

Sengers RCA, Stadhouders AM, Trijbels JMF (1984) Mitochondrial myopathies. Eur J Pediatr 141:192–207

Shoffner JM, Wallace DC (1992) Mitochondrial genetics: principles and practice. Am J Hum Genet 51:1179–1186

Siciliano G, Rossi B Angelini C, Martinuzzi A, Carrozzo R, Bevilacqua G, Viacava P, Federico A, Fabrizi GM, Muratorio A (1992) Variability of the expression of muscle mitochondrial damage in ocular mitochondrial myopathy. Neuromusc Dis 2:397–404

Stadhouders AM, Sengers RCA (1987) Morphological observations in skeletal muscle from patients with a mitochondrial myopathy. J Inherited Metab Dis 10 [Suppl 1]:62–80

Tager JM, Aarts JMFG, Van den Bogert C, Wanders RJA (1994) Signals on proteins, intracellular targeting and inborn errors of metabolism. J Inherited Metab Dis 17:459–469

Tritschler HJ, Medori R (1993) Mitochondrial DNA alterations as a source of human disorders. Neurology 43:280–288

Tulinius MH, Holme E, Kristiansson B, Larsson NG, Oldfors A (1991) Mitochondrial encephalomyopathies in childhood.

I. Biochemical and morphologic investigations. J Pediatr 119:242–250

Tulinius MH, Holme E, Kristiansson B, Larsson NG, Oldfors A (1991) Mitochondrial encephalomyopathies in childhood. II. Clinical manifestations and syndromes. J Pediatr 119:251–259

Vianey-Liaud C, Divry P, Gregersen N, Mathieu M (1987) The inborn errors of mitochondrial fatty acid oxidation. J Inherited Metab Dis 10 [Suppl 1]:159–198

Wallace DC (1992) Mitochondrial genetics:a paradigm for aging and degenerative diseases? Science 256:628–632

Wallace DC, Lott MT, Shoffner JM, Brown MD (1992) Diseases resulting from mitochondrial DNA point mutations. J Inherited Metab Dis 15:472–479

Wienhues U, Becker K, Schleyer M, Guiard B, Tropschug M, Horwich AL, Pfanner N, Neupert W (1991) Protein folding causes an arrest of preprotein translocation into mitochondria in vivo. J Cell Biol 115:1601–1609

Zeviani M, Bonilla E, DeVivo DC, DiMauro S (1989) Mitochondrial diseases. Neurol Clin 7:123–156

Zeviani M, DiDonato S (1991) Neurological disorders due to mutations of the mitochondrial genome. Neuromusc Dis 1:165–172

Zeviani M (1992) Nucleus-driven mutations of human mitochondrial DNA. J Inherited Metab Dis 15:456–471

21 Defects of Mitochondrial DNA

MELAS

Abe K, Inui T, Hirono N, Mezaki T, Kobayashi Y, Kameyama M (1990) Fluctuating MR images with mitochondrial encephalopathy, lactic acidosis, stroke-like syndrome (MELAS). Neuroradiology 32:77

Abe K, Fujimura H, Nishikawa Y, Yorifuji S, Mezaki T, Hirono N, Nishitani N, Kameyama M (1991) Marked reduction in CSF lactate and pyruvate levels after CoQ therapy in a patient with mitochondrial myopathy, encephalopathy, lactic acidosis and stroke-like episodes (MELAS). Acta Neurol Scand 83:356–359

Allard JC, Tilak S, Carter AP (1988) CT and MR of MELAS syndrome. AJNR 9:1234–1238

Barkovich AJ, Good WV, Koch TK, Berg BO (1993) Mitochondrial disorders:analysis of their clinical and imaging characteristics. AJNR 14:1119–1137

Breningstall GN, Lockman LA (1988) Massive focal brain swelling as a feature of MELAS. Pediatr Neurol 4:366–370

Ciafaloni E, Ricci E, Shanske S, Moraes CT, Silvestri G, Hirano M, Simonetti S, Angelini C, Donati A, Garcia C, Martinuzzi A, Mosewich R, Servidei S, Zammarchi E, Bonilla E, DeVivo DC, Rowland LP, Schon EA, DiMauro S (1992) MELAS: clinical features, biochemistry, and molecular genetics. Ann Neurol 31:391–398

Degoul F, Diry M, Pou-Serradell A, Lloreta J, Marsac C (1994) Myo-leukoencephaopathy in twins: study of 3243-myopathy, encephalopathy, lactic acidosis, and strokelike episodes mitochondrial DNA mutation. Ann Neurol 35:365–370

Fang W, Huang CC, Lee CC, Cheng SY, Pang CY, Wei YH (1993) Ophthalmologic manifestations in MELAS syndrome. Arch Neurol 50:977–980

Förster C, Hübner G, Müller-Höcker J, Pongratz D, Baierl P, Senger R, Ruitenbeek W (1992) Mitochondrial angiopathy in a family with MELAS. Neuropediatrics 23:165–168

Fujii T, Okuno T, Ito M, Motoh K, Hamazaki S, Okada S, Kusaka H, Mikawa H (1990) CT, MRI, and autopsy findings in brain of a patient with MELAS. Pediatr Neurol 6:253–256

Fujii T, Okuno T, Ito M, Mutoh K, Horiguchi Y, Tashiro H, Mikawa H (1991) MELAS of infantile onset:mitochondrial angiopathy or cytopathy? J Neurol Sci 103:37–41

Goto Y, Nonaka I, Horai S (1990) A mutation in the tRNA$^{Leu(UUR)}$ gene associated with the MELAS subgroup of mitochondrial encephalomyopathies. Nature 348:651–653

Goto Y, Horai S, Matsuoka T, Koga Y, Nihei K, Kobayashi M, Nonaka I (1992) Mitochondrial myopathy, encephalopathy, lactic acidosis, and stroke-like episodes (MELAS): a correlative study of the clinical features and mitochondrial DNA mutation. Neurology 42:545–550

Hamazaki S, Okada S, Kusaka H, Fujii T, Okuno T, Kashu I, Midorikawa O (1989) Mitochondrial myopathy, encephalopathy, lactic acidosis, and stroke-like episodes. Acta Pathol Jpn 39:599–606

Hart ZH, Chang CH, Perrin EVD, Neerunjun JS, Ayyar R (1977) Familial poliodystrophy, mitochondrial myopathy, and lactate acidemia. Arch Neurol 34:180–185

Henkes H, Sperner J, Stoltenburg-Didinger (1987) Kerspintomographischer Aspekt der Enzephalomyopathie. Fortschr Rontgenstr 2:214–216

Hirano M, Ricci E, Koenigsberger R, Defendini R, Pavlakis ST, DeVivo DC, DiMauro S, Rowland LP (1992) MELAS: an original case and clinical criteria for diagnosis. Neuromusc Dis 2:125–135

Huang CC, Chen RS, Chen CM, Wang HS, Lee CC, Pang CY, Hsu HS, Lee HC, Wei YH (1994) MELAS syndrome with mitochondrial tRNA$^{Leu(UUR)}$ gene mutation in a Chinese family. J Neurol Neurosurg Psychiatry 57:586–589

Ihara Y, Namba R, Kuroda S, Sato T, Shirabe T (1989) Mitochondrial encephalomyopathy (MELAS): pathological study and successful therapy with coenzyme Q$_{10}$ and idebenone. J Neurol Sci 90:263–271

Inui K, Fukushima H, Tsukamoto H, Taniike M, Midorikawa M, Tanaka J, Nishigaki T, Okada S (1992) Mitochondrial encephalomyopathies with the mutation of the mitochondrial tRNA$^{Leu(UUR)}$ gene. J Pediatr 120:62–66

Johns DR, Stein AG, Wityk R (1993) MELAS syndrome masquerading as herpes simplex encephalitis. Neurology 43:2471–2473

Kawakami Y, Sakuta R, Hashimoto K, Fujino O, Fujita T, Hida M, Horai S, Goto Y, Nonaka I (1993) Mitochondrial myopathy with progressive decrease in mitochondrial tRNA$^{Leu(UUR)}$ mutant genomes. Ann Neurol 35:370–373

Kishi M, Yamamura Y, Kurihara T, Fukuhara N, Tsuruta K, Matsukura S, Hayashi T, Nakagawa M, Kuriyama M (1988) An autopsy case of mitochondrial encephalomyopathy: biochemical and electron microscopic studies of the brain. J Neurol Sci 86:31–40

Koo B, Becker LE, Chuang S, Merante F, Robinson BH, MacGregor D, Tein I, Ho VB, McGreal DA, Wherrett JR, Logan WJ (1993) Mitochondrial encephalomyopathy, lactic acidosis, stroke-like episodes (MELAS): clinical, radiological, pathological, and genetic observations. Ann Neurol 34:25–32

Kuriyama M, Umezaki H, Fukuda Y, Osame M, Koike K, Tateishi J, Igata A (1984) Mitochondrial encephalomyopathy with lactate-pyruvate elevation and brain infarctions. Neurology 34:72–77

Lertrit P, Noer AS, Jean-Francois MJB, Kapsa R, Dennett X, Thyagarajan D, Lethlean K, Byrne E, Marzuki S (1992) A new disease-related mutation for mitochondrial encephalopathy lactic acidosis and strokelike episodes (MELAS) syndrome affects the ND4 subunit of the respiratory complex I. Am J Hum Genet 51:457–468

Macmillan C, Lach B, Shoubridge EA (1993) Variable distribution of mutant mitochondrial DNAs (tRNA$^{Leu[3243]}$) in tissues of symptomatic relatives with MELAS: the role of mitotic segregation. Neurology 43:1586–1590

Matthews PM, Tampieri D, Berkovic SF, Andermann F, Silver K, Chityat D, Arnold DL (1991) Magnetic resonance imaging shows specific abnormalities in the MELAS syndrome. Neurology 41:1043–1046

Miyabayashi S, Hanamizu H, Nakamura R, Hayashi JI, Tada K (1993) Clinical and biochemical phenotype of the MELAS mutation. J Inherited Metab Dis 16:886–892

Moraes CT, Ciacci F, Silvestri G, Shanske S, Sciacco M, Hirano M, Schon EA, Bonilla E, DiMauro S (1993) Atypical clinical presentations associated with the MELAS mutation at position 3243 of human mitochondrial DNA. Neuromusc Dis 3:43–50

Mosewich RK, Donat JR, DiMauro S, Ciafaloni E, Shanske S, Erasmus M, George D (1993) The syndrome of mitochondrial encephalomyopathy, lactic acidosis, and strokelike episodes presenting without stroke. Arch Neurol 50:275–278

Mukoyama M, Kazui H, Sunohara N, Yoshida M, Nonaka I, Satoyoshi E (1986) Mitochondrial myopathy, encephalopathy, lactic acidosis, and stroke-like episodes with acanthocytosis: a clinicopathological study of a unique case. J Neurol 233:228–232

Ohama E, Ohara S, Ikuta F, Tanaka K, Nishizawa M, Miyatake T (1987) Mitochondrial angiopathy in cerebral blood vessels of mitochondrial encephalomyopathy. Acta Neuropathol (Berl) 74:226–233

Ooiwa Y, Uematsu Y, Terada T, Nakai K, Itakura T, Komai N, Moriwaki H (1993) Cerebral blood flow in mitochondrial myopathy, encephalopathy, lactic acidosis, and strokelike episodes. Stroke 24:304–309

Pavlakis SG, Phillips PC, DiMauro S, DeVivo DC, Rowland LP (1984) Mitochondrial myopathy, encephalopathy, lactic acidosis, and strokelike episodes: a distinctive clinical syndrome. Ann Neurol 16:481–488

Penn AMW, Lee JWK, Thuillier P, Wagner M, Maclure KM, Menard MR, Hall LD, Kennaway NG (1992) MELAS syndrome with mitochondrial tRNA$^{Leu(UUR)}$ mutation: correlation of clinical state, nerve conduction, and muscle ^{31}P magnetic resonance spectroscopy during treatment with nicotinamide and riboflavin. Neurology 42:2147–2152

Przyrembel H (1987) Therapy of mitochondrial disorders. J Inherited Metab Dis 10:129–146

Rosen L, Philips S, Enzmann D (1990) Magnetic resonance imaging in MELAS syndrome. Neuroradiology 32:168–171

Sakuta R, Nonaka I (1989) Vascular involvement in mitochondrial myopathy. Ann Neurol 25:594–601

Satoh M, Ishikawa N, Yoshizawa T, Takeda T, Akisada M (1991) N-isopropyl-p-[^{123}I] Iodoamphetamine SPECT in MELAS syndrome: comparison with CT and MR imaging. J Comput Assist Tomogr 15:77–82

Seyama K, Suzuki K, Mizuno Y, Yoshida M, Tanaka M, Ozawa T (1989) Mitochondrial encephalomyopathy with lactic acidosis and stroke-like episodes with special reference to the mechanism of cerebral manifestations. Acta Neurol Scand 80:561–568

Shoji Y, Sato W, Hayasaka K, Takada G (1993) Tissue distribution of mutant mitochondrial DNA in mitochondrial myopathy, encephalopathy, lactic acidosis and stroke-like episodes (MELAS). J Inherited Metab Dis 16:27–30

Sparaco M, Bonilla E, DiMauro S, Powers JM (1993) Neuropathology of mitochondrial encephalomyopathies due to mitochondrial DNA defects. J Neuropathol Exp Neurol 52:1–10

Suzuki T, Koizumi J, Shiraishi H, Ishikawa N, Ofuku K, Sasaki M, Hori T, Ohkoshi N, Anno I (1990) Mitochondrial encephalomyopathy (MELAS) with mental disorder CT, MRI and SPECT findings. Neuroradiology 32:74–76

Taverni N, Dal Pozzo G, Arnetoli G, Zappoli R (1988) Diagnosis and follow-up of mitochondrial encephalomyopathy:CT and MR studies. J Comput Assist Tomogr 12:696–697

Tokunaga M, Mita S, Sakuta R, Nonaka I, Araki S (1993) Increased mitochondrial DNA in blood vessels and ragged-red fibers in mitochondrial myopathy, encephalopathy, lactic acidosis, and stroke-like episodes (MELAS). Ann Neurol 33:275–280

Tokunaga M, Mita S, Murakami T, Kumamoto T, Uchino M, Nonaka I, Ando M (1994) Single muscle fiber analysis of mitochondrial myopathy, encephalopathy, lactic acidosis, and stroke-like episodes (MELAS). Ann Neurol 35:413–419

Van Hellenberg Hubar JLM, Gabreës FJM, Ruitenbeek W, Sengers RCA, Renier WO, Thijssen HOM, ter Laak HJ (1991) MELAS syndrome. Report of two patients, and comparison with data of 24 patients derived from the literature. Neuropediatrics 22:10–14

Yoneda M, Tanaka M, Nishikimi M, Suzuki H, Tanaka K, Nishizawa M, Atsumi T, Ohama E, Horai S, Ikuta F, Miyatake T, Ozawa T (1989) Pleiotropic molecular defects in energy-transducing complexes in mitochondrial encephalomyopathy (MELAS). J Neurol Sci 92:143–158

LHON

Brown MD, Voljavec AS, Lott MT, MacDonald I, Wallace DC (1992) Leber's hereditary optic neuropathy: a model for mitochondrial neurodegenerative diseases. FASEB J 6:2791–2799

Bu X, Rotter JI (1991) X chromosome-linked and mitochondrial gene control of Leber hereditary optic neuropathy: evidence from segregation analysis for dependence on X chromosome inactivation. Proc Natl Acad Sci USA 88:8198–8202

Cornelissen JC, Wanders RJA, Bolhuis PA, Bleeker-Wagemakers E, Oostra RJ, Wijburg FA (1993) Respiratory chain function in Leber's hereditary optic neuropathy: lack of correlation with clinical disease. J Inherited Metab Dis 16:531–533

Cortelli P, Montagna P, Avoni P, Sangiorgi S, Bresolin N, Moggio M, Zaniol P, Mantovani V, Barboni P, Barbiroli B, Lugaresi E (1991) Leber's hereditary optic neuropathy:genetic, biochemical, and phosphorus magnetic resonance spectroscopy study in an Italian family. Neurology 41:1211–1215

Dotti MT, Caputo N, Signorini E, Federico A (1992) Magnetic resonance imaging findings in Leber's hereditary optic neuropathy. Eur Neurol 32:17–19

Harding AE, Sweeney MG, Miller DH, Mumford CJ, Kellar-Wood H, Menard D, McDonald WI, Compston DAS (1992) Occurrence of a multiple sclerosis-like illness in women who have a Leber's hereditary optic neuropathy mitochondrial DNA mutation. Brain 115:979–989

Hirano M, Cleary JM, Stewart AM, Lincoff NS, Odel JG, Santiesteban R, Santiago Luis R (1994) Mitochondrial DNA mutations in an outbreak of optic neuropathy in Cuba. Neurology 44:843–845

Hume Adams J, Blackwood W, Wilson J (1966) Further clinical and pathological observations on Leber's optic atrophy. Brain 89:15–26

Kermode AG, Moseley IF, Kendall BE, Miller DH, MacManus DG, McDonald WI (1989) Magnetic resonance imaging in Leber's optic neuropathy. J Neurol Neurosurg Psychiatry 52:671–674

Larsson NG, Andersen O, Holme E, Oldfors A, Wahlström J (1991) Leber's hereditary optic neuropathy and complex I deficiency in muscle. Ann Neurol 30:701–708

Lees F, MacDonald AME, Aldren Turner JW (1964) Leber's disease with symptoms resembling disseminated sclerosis. J Neurol Neurosurg Psychiatry 27:415–421

Mackey D, Howell N (1992) A variant of Leber hereditary optic neuropathy characterized by recovery of vision and by an unusual mitochondrial genetic etiology. Am J Hum Genet 51:1218–1228

Newman NJ (1993) Leber's hereditary optic neuropathy. Arch Neurol 50:540–548

Paulus W, Straube A, Bauer W, Harding AE (1993) Central nervous system involvement in Leber's optic neuropathy. J Neurol 240:251–253

Sparaco M, Bonilla E, DiMauro S, Powers JM (1993) Neuropathology of mitochondrial encephalomyopathies due to mitochondrial DNA defects. J Neuropathol Exp Neurol 52:1–10

Wallace DC, Singh G, Lott MT, Hodge JA, Schurr TG, Lezza AMS, Elsas LJ, Nikoskelainen EK (1988) Mitochondrial DNA mutation associated with Leber's hereditary optic neuropathy. Science 242:1427–1430

Weiner NC, Newman NJ, Lessell S, Johns DR, Lott MT, Wallace DC (1993) Atypical Leber's hereditary optic neuropathy with molecular confirmation. Arch Neurol 50:470–473

Wilson J (1963) Leber's hereditary optic atrophy some clinical and aetiological considerations. Brain 86:347–362

MNGIE

Bardosi A, Creutzfeldt W, DiMauro S, Felgenhauer K, Friede RL, Goebel HH, Kohlschütter A, Mayer G, Rahlf G, Servidei S, van Lessen G, Wetterling T (1987) Myo-, neuro-, gastrointestinal encephalopathy (MNGIE syndrome) due to partial deficiency of cytochrome-c-oxidase. A new mitochondrial multisystem disorder. Acta Neuropathol (Berl) 74:248–258

Hirano M, Silvestri G, Blake DM, Lombes A, Minetti C, Bonilla E, Hays AP, Lovelace RE, Butler I, Bertorini TE, Threlkeld AB, Mitsumoto H, Salberg LM, Rowland LP, DiMauro S (1994) Mitochondrial neurogastrointestinal encephalomyopathy (MNGIE): clinical, biochemical, and genetic features of an autosomal recessive mitochondrial disorder. Neurology 44:721–727

Sandhu FS, Dillon WP (1991) MR demonstraton of leukoencephalopathy associated with mitochondrial encephalomyopathy: case report. AJNR 12:375–379

Simon LT, Horoupian DS, Dorfman LJ, Marks M, Herrick MK, Wasserstein P, Smith ME (1990) Polyneuropathy, ophthalmoplegia, leukoencephalopathy, and intestinal pseudo-obstruction: POLIP syndrome. Ann Neurol 28:349–360

Sparaco M, Bonilla E, DiMauro S, Powers JM (1993) Neuropathology of mitochondrial encephalomyopathies due to mitochondrial DNA defects. J Neuropathol Exp Neurol 52:1–10

Uncini A, Servidei S, Silvestri G, Manfredi G, Sabatelli M, Di Muzio A, Ricci E, Mirabella M, DiMauro S, Tonali P (1994) Ophthalmoplegia, demyelinating neuropathy, leukoencephalopathy, myopathy, and gastrointestinal dysfunction with multiple deletions of mitochondrial DNA: a mitochondrial multisystem disorder in search of a name. Muscle Nerve 17:667–674

KSS

Allen RJ, DiMauro S, Coulter DL, Papadimitriou A, Rothenberg SP (1983) Kearns-Sayre syndrome with reduced plasma and cerebrospinal fluid folate. Ann Neurol 13:679–682

Bachynski BN, Flynn JT, Rodrigues MM, Rosenthal S, Cullen R, Curless RG (1986) Hyperglycemic acidotic coma and death in Kearns-Sayre syndrome. Ophthalmology 93:391–396

Barkovich AJ, Good WV, Koch TK, Berg BO (1993) Mitochondrial disorders:analysis of their clinical and imaging characteristics. AJNR 14:1119–1137

Bresolin N, Moggio M, Bet L, Gallanti A, Prelle A, Nobile-Orazio E, Adobbati L, Ferrante C, Pellegrini G, Scarlato G (1987) Progressive cytochrome c oxidase deficiency in a case of Kearns-Sayre syndrome:morphological, immunological, and biochemical studies in muscle biopsies and autopsy tissues. Ann Neurol 21:564–572

Byrne E, Marzuki S, Sattayasai N, Dennett X, Trounce I (1987) Mitochondrial studies in Kearns-Sayre syndrome:normal respiratory chain function with absence of a mitochondrial translation product. Neurology 37:1530–1534

Crisi G, Ferrari G, Merelli E, Cocconcelli P (1994) MRI in a case of Kearns-Sayre syndrome confirmed by molecular analysis. Neuroradiology 36:37–38RG, Flynn J, Bachynski B, Gregorios JB, Benke P, Cullen R (1986) Fatal metabolic acidosis, hyperglycemia, and coma after steroid therapy for Kearns-Sayre syndrome. Neurology 36:872–873

Daroff RB, Solitare GB, Pincus JH, Glaser GH (1966) Spongiform encephalopathy with chronic progressive external ophthalmoplegia. Neurology 16:161–169

Demange P, Pham Gia H, Kalifa G, Sellier N (1989) MR of Kearns-Sayre syndrome. AJNR 10:S91

Dewhurst AG, Hall D, Schwartz MS, McKeran RO (1986) Kearns-Sayre syndrome, hypoarathyroidism, and basal ganglia calcification. J Neurol Neurosurg Psychiatry 149:1323–1324

Elsas T, Rinck PA, Isaksen C, Nilsen G, Schjetne OB (1988) Cerebral nuclear magnetic resonance (MRI) in Kearns syndrome. Acta Ophthalmol (Copenh) 66:469–473

Flynn JT, Bachynski BR, Rodrigues MM, Curless RG, Joshi B (1985) Hyperglycemic acidotic coma and death in Kearns-Sayre syndrome. Trans Am Ophthalmol Soc 83:131–161

Herzberg NH, van Schooneveld MJ, Bleeker-Wagemakers EM, Zwart R, Cremers FPM, van der Knaap MS, Bolhuis PA, de Visser M (1993) Kearns-Sayre syndrome with a phenocopy of choroideremia instead of pigmentary retinopathy. Neurology 43:218–221

Hübner G, Gokel JM, Pongratz D, Johannes A, Park JW (1986) Fatal mitochondrial cardiomyopathy in Kearns-Sayre syndrome. Virchows Arch 408:611–621

Kleber FX, Park JW, Hübner G, Johannes A, Pongratz D, König E (1987) Congestive heart failure due to mitochondrial cardiomyopathy in Kearns-Sayre syndrome. Klin Wochenschr 65:480–486

Kuriyama M, Suehara M, Marume N, Osame M, Igata A (1984) High CSF lactate and pyruvate content in Kearns-Sayre syndrome. Neurology 34:253–255

Larsson NG, Holme E, Kristiansson B, Oldfors A, Tulinius M (1990) Progressive increase of the mutated mitochondrial DNA fraction in Kearns-Sayre syndrome. Pediatr Res 28:131–136

McShane MA, Hammans SR, Sweeney M, Holt IJ, Beattie TJ, Brett EM, Harding AE (1991) Pearson syndrome and mitochondrial encephalomyopathy in a patient with a deletion of mtDNA. Am J Hum Genet 48:39–42

Nakaoka H, Kitahara Y, Imataka K, Fujii J, Ishibashi M, Yamaji T (1987) Atrial natriuretic peptide with artificial pacemakers. Am J Cardiol 60:385–388

Nakano T, Imanaka K, Uchida H, Isaka N, Takezawa H (1987) Myocardial ultrastructure in Kearns-Sayre syndrome. Angiology 38:28–35

Ogasahara S, Yorifuji S, Nishikawa Y, Takahashi M, Wada K, Hazama T, Nakamura Y, Hashimoto S, Kono N, Tarui S (1985) Improvement of abnormal pyruvate metabolism and cardiac conduction defect with coenzyme Q10 in Kearns-Sayre syndrome. Neurology 35:372–377

Ogasahara S, Nishikawa Y, Yorifuji S, Soga F, Nakamura Y, Takahashi M, Hashimoto S, Kono N, Tarui S (1986) Treatment of Kearns-Sayre syndrome with coenzyme Q10. Neurology 36:45–53

Oldfors A, Fyhr IM, Holme E, Larsson NG, Tulinius M (1990) Neuropathology in Kearns-Sayre syndrome. Acta Neuropathol (Berl) 80:541–546

Przyrembel H (1987) Therapy of mitochondrial disorders. J Inherited Metab Dis 10:129–146

Rakovec P, Starc R, Butinar D, Janezic A (1986) Conduction disturbances in the Kearns-Sayre syndrome. Cor Vasa 28:294–297

Rheuban KS, Ayres NA, Sellers TD, DiMarco JP (1983) Near-fatal Kearns-Sayre syndrome. Clin Pediatr 22:822–825

Scully RE, Mark EJ, McNeely WF, McNeely BU (1987) Case records of the Massachusetts General Hospital. Case 34-1987. N Engl J Med 317:493–501

Sparaco M, Bonilla E, DiMauro S, Powers JM (1993) Neuropathology of mitochondrial encephalomyopathies due to mitochondrial DNA defects. J Neuropathol Exp Neurol 52:1–10

Yoda S, Terauchi A, Kitahara F, Akabane T (1984) Neurologic deterioration with progressive CT changes in a child with Kearns-Shy syndrome. Brain Dev 6:322–327

Yorifuji S, Ogasahara S, Takahashi M, Tarui S (1985) Decreased activities in mitochondrial inner membrane electron transport system in muscle from patients with Kearns-Sayre syndrome. J Neurol Sci 71:65–75

22   Leigh Syndrome

Adickes ED, Buehler BA, Sanger WG (1986) Familial lethal sleep apnea. Hum Genet 73:39–43

Anzil AP, Weindl A, Struppler A (1981) Ultrastructure of a cerebral white matter lesion in a 41-year-old man with Leigh's encephalomyelopathy (LEM). Acta Neuropathol (Berl) [Suppl] VII:233–238

Arts WFM, Scholte HR, Loonen MCB, Przyrembel H, Fernandes J, Trijbels JMF, Luyt-Houwen IEM (1987) Cytochrome c oxidase deficiency in subacute necrotizing encephalomyelopathy. J Neurol Sci 77:103–115

Awata H, Endo F, Tanoue A, Kitano A, Matsuda I (1994) Characterization of a point mutation in the pyruvate dehydrogenase $E_{1\alpha}$ gene from two boys with primary lactic acidaemia. J Inherited Metab Dis 17:189–195

Bianco F, Floris R, Pozzessere G, Rizzo PA (1987) Subacute necrotizing encephalomyelopathy (Leigh's disease): clinical correlations with computerized tomography in the diagnosis of the juvenile and adult forms. Acta Neurol Scand 75:214–217

Bourgeois M, Goutieres F, Chretien D, Rustin P, Munnich A, Aicardi J (1992) Deficiency in complex II of the respiratory chain, presenting as a leukodystrophy in two sisters with Leigh syndrome. Brain Dev 14:404–408

Campistol J, Cusi V, Vernet A, Fernandez-Alvarez E (1986) Dystonia as a presenting sign of subacute necrotising encephalomyelopathy in infancy. Eur J Pediatr 144:589–591

Campistol J, Fernandez Alvarex E, Cusi V (1984) CT scan appearance in subacute necrotising encephalomyelopathy. Dev Med Child Neurol 26:509–527

Chi CS, Mak SC, Shian WJ (1994) Leigh syndrome with progressive ventriculomegaly. Pediatr Neurol 10:244–246

Coker SB (1993) Leigh disease presenting as Guillain-Barré syndrome. Pediatr Neurol 9:61–63

Crompton MR (1969) Spongiform subacute necrotising encephalomyelopathy. Acta Neuropathol (Berl) 13:204–208

Cross JH, Connelly A, Gadian DG, Kendall BE, Brown GK, Leonard JV (1994) Clinical diversity of pyruvate dehydrogenase deficiency. Pediatr Neurol 10:276–283

Davis PC, Hoffman JC, Braun IF, Ahmann P, Krawiecki N (1987) MR of Leigh's disease (subacute necrotizing encephalomyelopathy). AJNR 8:71–75

De Vries DD, van Engelen BGM, Gabreëls FJM, Ruitenbeek W, van Oost BA (1993) A second missense mutation in the mitochondrial ATPase 6 gene in Leigh's syndrome. Ann Neurol 34:410–412

Delgado G, Gallego J, Tunon T, Zarranz JJ, Villanueva JA (1987) Necrotising haemorrhagic encephalomyelopathy in an adult: Leigh's disease. J Neurol Neurosurg Psychiatry 50:224–227

Egger J, Wynne-Williams CJE, Erdohazi M (1982) Mitochondrial cytopathy or Leigh's syndrome? Mitochondrial abnormalities in spongiform encephalopathies. Neuropediatrics 13:219–224

Egger J, Pincott JR, Wilson J, Erdohazi M (1984) Cortical subacute necrotizing encephalomyelopathy. A study of two patients with mitochondrial dysfunction. Neuropediatrics 15:150–158

Feigin I, Kim HS (1977) Subacute necrotizing encephalomyelopathy in a neonatal infant. J Neuropathol Exp Neurol 36:364–372

Geyer CA, Sartor KJ, Prensky AJ, Abramson CL, Hodges FJ, Gado MH (1988) Leigh disease (subacute necrotizing encephalomyelopathy): CT and MR in five cases. J Comput Assist Tomogr 12:40–44

Goebel HH, Bardosi A, Friede RL, Kohlschütter A, Albani M, Siemes H (1986) Sural nerve biopsy studies in Leigh's subacute necrotizing encephalomyelopathy. Muscle Nerve 9:165–173

Gray F, Louarn F, Gherardi R, Eizenbaum JF, Marsault C (1984) Adult form of Leigh's disease: a clinico pathological case with CT scan examination. J Neurol Neurosurg Psychiatry 47:1211–1215

Greenberg SB, Faerber EN, Riviello JJ, de Leon G, Capitanio MA (1990) Subacute necrotizing encephalomyelopathy (Leigh disease): CT and MRI appearances. Pediatr Radiol 21:5–8

Heckmann H, Ang LC, Casey R, George DH, Lowry N, Shokeur MHK (1991) Leigh's disease with clinical manifestations of Cornelia de Lange syndrome. Pediatr Neurosurg 17:192–195

Heckmann JM, Eastman R, Handler L, Wright M, Owen P (1993) Leigh disease (subacute necrotizing encephalomyelopathy): MR documentation of the evolution of an acute attack. AJNR 14:1157–1159

Honavar M, Janota I, Neville BGR, Chalmers RA (1992) Neuropathology of biotinidase deficiency. Acta Neuropathol (Berl) 84:461–464

Kimura S, Kobayashi T, Amemiya F (1991) Myelin splitting in the spongy lesion in Leigh encephalopathy. Pediatr Neurol 7:56–58

Kissel JT, Kolkin S, Chakeres D, Boesel C, Weiss K (1987) Magnetic resonance imaging in a case of autopsy-proved adult subacute necrotizing encephalomyelopathy (Leigh's disease). Arch Neurol 44:563–566

Koch TK, Yee MHC, Hutchinson HT, Berg BO (1986) Magnetic resonance imaging in subacute necrotizing encephalomyelopathy (Leigh's disease). Ann Neurol 19:605–607

Kohlschütter A, Kraus-Ruppert R, Rohrer T, Herschkowitz NN (1978) Myelin studies in a case of subacute necrotizing encephalomyelopathy. J Neuropathol Exp Neurol 37:155–164

Kretzschmar HA, DeArmond SJ, Koch TK, Patel MS, Newth CJL, Schmidt KA, Packman S (1987) Pyruvate dehydrogenase complex deficiency as a cause of subacute necrotizing encephalopathy (Leigh disease). Pediatrics 79:370–373

Kustermann-Kuhn B, Harzer K, Schröder R, Permanetter W, Peiffer J (1984) Pyruvate dehydrogenase activity is not deficient in the brain of three autopsied cases with Leigh disease (subacute necrotizing encephalomyelopathy, SNE). Hum Genet 68:51–53

Langes K, Frenzel H, Seitz RJ, Kluitmann G (1985) Cardiomyopathy associated with Leigh's disease. Virchows Arch 407:97–105

Macaya A, Munell F, Burke RE, De Vivo DC (1993) Disorders of movement in Leigh syndrome. Neuropediatrics 21:60–67

Manzi SV, Hager KH, Murtagh FR, Mazalewski JG (1990) MR imaging in a patient with Leigh's disease (subacute necrotizing encephalomyelopathy). Pediatr Radiol 21:62–63

Masó E, Ferrer I, Herraiz J, Roquer J, Serrano S (1984) Leigh's syndrome in an adult. J Neurol 231:253–257

Matsuishi T, Yoshino M, Tokunaga O, Katafuchi Y, Yamashita F (1985) Subacute necrotizing encephalomyelopathy (Leigh disease): report of a case with Lennox-Gastaut syndrome. Brain Dev 7:500–504

Matthews PM, Marchington DR, Squier M, Land J, Brown RM, Brown GK (1993) Molecular genetic characterization of an X-linked form of Leigh's syndrome. Ann Neurol 33:652–655

Medina L, Chi TL, De Vivo DC, Hilal SK (1990) MR findings in patients with subacute necrotizing encephalomyelopathy (Leigh syndrome): correlation with biochemical defect. AJNR 11:379–384

Mitchell G, Ogier H, Munnich A, Saudubray JM (1986) Neurological deterioration and lactic acidemia in biotinidase deficiency. A treatable condition mimicking Leigh's disease. Neuropediatrics 17:129–131

Miyabayashi S, Narisawa K, Linuma K, Tada K, Sakai K, Kobayashi K, Kobayashi Y, Morinaga S (1984) Cytochrome c oxidase deficiency in two siblings with Leigh encephalomyelopathy. Brain Dev 6:362–372

Miyabayashi S, Ito T, Narisawa K, Linuma K, Tada K (1985) Biochemical study in 28 children with lactic acidosis, in relation to Leigh's encephalomyelopathy. Eur J Pediatr 143:278–283

Montpetit VJA, Andermann F, Carpenter S, Fawcett JS, Zborowska-Sluis D, Giberson HR (1971) Subacute necrotizing encephalomyelopathy. A review and a study of two families. Brain 94:1–30

Nagai T, Goto Y, Matsuoka T, Sakuta R, Naito E, Kuroda Y, Nonaka I (1992) Leigh encephalopathy: histologic and biochemical analyses of muscle biopsies. Pediatr Neurol 8:328–332

Onuma A, Miyabayashi S, Linuma K, Tada K, Yamada K, Matsuzawa T (1987) Comparative appraisal of CT scan and MRI in the diagnosis of Leigh encephalomyelopathy in two siblings. J Child Neurol 2:324–326

Paltiel HJ, O'Gorman AM, Meagher-Villemure K, Rosenblatt B, Silver K, Watters GV (1987) Subacute necrotizing encephalomyelopathy (Leigh disease): CT study. Radiology 162:115–118

Pamphlett R, Harper C (1985) Leigh's disease: a cause of arterial hypertension. Med J Aust 143:306–308

Robinson BH, DeMeirleir L, Glerum M, Sherwood G, Becker L (1987) Clinical presentation of mitochondrial respiratory chain defects in NADH-coenzyme Q reductase and cytochrome oxidase:clues to pathogenesis of Leigh disease. J Pediatr 110:216–222

Russman BS, Lang AE, Fahn S, Greene P, Grunner ML (1992) Case 1, 1992: progressive gait deterioration, peripheral neuropathy, optic atrophy, bradykinesia, and dystonia in a young girl. Mov Dis 7:373–379

Santorelli FM, Shanske S, Macaya A, DeVivo DC, DiMauro S (1993) The mutation at nt 8993 of mitochondrial DNA is a common cause of Leigh's syndrome. Ann Neurol 34:827–834

Santorelli FM, Shanske S, Jain KD, Tick D, Schon EA, DiMauro S (1994) A T → C mutation at nt 8993 of mitochondrial

DNA in a child with Leigh syndrome. Neurology 44:972–974

Savoiardo M, Uziel G, Strada L, Visciani A, Grisoli M, Wang G (1991) MRI findings in Leigh's disease with cytochrome-c-oxidase deficiency. Neuroradiology 33 [Suppl]:507–508

Seitz RJ, Langes K, Frenzel H, Kluitmann G, Wechsler W (1984) Congenital Leigh's disease: panencephalomyelopathy and peripheral neuropathy. Acta Neuropathol (Berl) 64:167–171

Shoffner JM, Fernhoff PM, Krawiecki NS, Caplan DB, Holt PJ, Koontz DA, Takei Y, Newman NJ, Ortiz RG, Polak M, Ballinger SW, Lott MT, Wallace DC (1992) Subacute necrotizing encephalopathy: oxidative phosphorylation defects and the ATPase 6 point mutation. Neurology 42:2168–2174

Taccone A, Di Rocco M, Fondelli P, Cottafava F (1989) Leigh disease:value of CT in presymptomatic patients and variability of the lesions with time. J Comput Assist Tomogr 13:207–210

Tatuch Y, Christodoulou J, Feigenbaum A, Clarke JTR, Wherret J, Smith C, Rudd N, Petrova-Benedict R, Robinson BH (1992) Heteroplasmic mtDNA mutation (T → G) at 8993 can cause Leigh disease when the percentage of abnormal mtDNA is high. Am J Hum Genet 50:852–858

Van Coster R, Lombes A, De Vivo DC, Chi TL, Dodson WE, Rothman S, Orrechio EJ, Grover W, Berry GT, Schwartz JF, Habib A, DiMauro S (1991) Cytochrome c oxidase-associated Leigh syndrome: phenotypic features and pathogenetic speculations. J Neurol Sci 104:97–111

Van Erven PMM, Gabreëls FJM, Ruitenbeek W, den Hartog MR, Fischer JC, Renier WO, Trijbels JMF, Slooff JL, Janssen AJM (1985) Subacute necrotizing encephalomyelopathy (Leigh syndrome) associated with disturbed oxidation of pyruvate, malate and 2-oxoglutarate in muscle and liver. Acta Neurol Scand 72:36–42

Van Erven PMM, Fischer JC, Gabreëls FJM, Renier WO, Trijbels JMF, Janssen AJM (1986a) Defect of NADH dehydrogenase in Leigh syndrome. Acta Neurol Scand 74:167

Van Erven PMM, Colon EJ, Gabreëls FJM, Renier WO, Vingerhoets DM (1986b) Neurophysiological studies in the Leigh syndrome. Brain Dev 8:590–595

Van Erven PMM, Ruitenbeek W, Gabreëls FJM, Renier WO, Fischer JC, Jansen AJM (1986c) Disturbed oxidative metabolism in subacute necrotizing encephalomyelopathy (Leigh syndrome). Neuropediatrics 17:28–32

Van Erven PMM, Gabreëls FJM, Ruitenbeek W, Renier WO, Fischer JC (1987a) Mitochondrial encephalomyopathy. Arch Neurol 44:775–778

Van Erven PMM, Gabreëls FJM, Ruitenbeek W, Renier WO, Lamers KJB, Sloof JL (1987b) Familial Leigh's syndrome:association with a defect in oxidative metabolism probably restricted to brain. J Neurol 234:215–219

Van Erven PMM, Cillessen JPM, Eekhoff EMW, Gabreëls FJM, Doesburg WH, Lemmens WAJG, Slooff JL, Renier WO, Ruitenbeek W (1987c) Leigh syndrome, a mitochondrial encephalo(myo)pathy. Clin Neurol Neurosurg 89:217–230

Wallace SJ (1985) Deficiencies within the pyruvate dehydrogenase complex: clinical and pathological correlates. Dev Med Child Neurol 27:249–260

Walter GF, Brucher JM, Martin JJ, Ceuterick C, Pilz P, Freund M (1986) Leigh's disease – several nosological entities with an identical histopathological complex? Neuropathol Appl Neurobiol 12:95–107

Wijburg FA, Barth PG, Bindoff LA, Birch-Machin MA, van der Blij JF, Ruitenbeek W, Turnbull DM, Schutgens RBH (1992) Leigh syndrome associated with a deficiency of the pyruvate dehydrogenase complex:results of treatment with a ketogenic diet. Neuropediatrics 23:147–152

Wyatt DT, Noetzel MJ, Hillman RE (1987) Infantile beriberi presenting as subacute necrotizing encephalomyelopathy. J Pediatr 110:888–892

Yamagata T, Yano S, Okabe I, Miyao M, Momoi MY, Yanagisawa M, Hirata H, Komatsu K (1990) Ultrasonography and magnetic resonance imaging in Leigh disease. Pediatr Neurol 6:326–329

Yoshinaga H, Ogino T, Ohtahara S, Sakuta R, Nonaka I, Horai S (1993) A T-to-G mutation at nucleotide pair 8993 in mitochondrial DNA in a patient with Leigh's syndrome. J Child Neurol 8:129–133

Younossi-Hartenstein A, Vierbuchen M, Roth B, Schroeder R (1986) Renal lesions in subacute encephalomyelopathy (Leigh's disease). Int J Pediatr Nephrol 7:117–120

23 Pyruvate Carboxylase Deficiency

Atkin BM, Buist NRM, Utter MF, Leiter AB, Banker BQ (1979) Pyruvate carboxylase deficiency and lactic acidosis in a retarded child without Leigh's disease. Pediatr Res 13:109–116

Augereau C, Dinh DP, Moncion A, Marsac C, Saudubray JM, Robinson BH (1985) Pyruvate carboxylase deficiencies: complementation studies between „French" and „American" phenotypes in cultured fibroblasts. J Inherited Metab Dis 8:59–62

Baal MG, Gabreëls FJM, Renier WO, Hommes FA, Gijsbers THJ, Lamers KJB, Kok JCN (1981) A patient with pyruvate carboxylase deficiency in the liver: treatment with aspartic acid and thiamine. Dev Med Child Neurol 23:521–530

Bartlett K, Ghneim HK, Stirk JH, Dale G, Alberti GMM (1984) Pyruvate carboxylase deficiency. J Inherited Metab Dis 7 [Suppl 1]:74–78

Farkas-Bargeton E, Goutières F, Richardet JM, Thieffry S, Brissaud HE (1971) Leucoencéphalopathie familiale associée à une acidose lactique congénitale. Acta Neuropathol (Berl) 17:156–168

Feldman GL, Wolf B (1980) Evidence for two genetic complementation groups in pyruvate carboxylase-deficient human fibroblast cell lines. Biochem Genet 18:617–624

Greter J, Gustafsson J, Holme E (1985) Pyruvate-carboxylase deficiency with urea cycle impairment. Acta Paediatr Scand 74:982–986

Hansen TL, Christensen E, Willems JL, Trijbels JMF (1983) A mutation of pyruvate carboxylase in fibroblasts from a patient with severe, chronic lactic acidaemia. Clin Chim Acta 131:39–44

Hansen TL, Christensen E, Brandt NJ (1982) Studies on pyruvate carboxylase, pyruvate decarboxylase and lipoamide dehydrogenase in subacute necrotizing encephalomyelopathy. Acta Paediatr Scand 71:263–267

Higgins JJ, Glasgow AM, Lusk M, Kerr DS (1994) MRI, clinical, and biochemical features of partial pyruvate carboxylase deficiency. J Child Neurol 9:436–439

Maesaka H, Komiya K, Misugi K, Tada K (1976) Hyperalaninemia, hyperpyruvicemia and lactic acidosis due to pyruvate carboxylase deficiency of the liver; treatment with thiamine and lipoic acid. Eur J Pediatr 122:159–168

Murphy JV, Isohashi F, Weinberg MB, Utter MF (1981) Pyruvate carboxylase deficiency: an alleged biochemical cause of Leigh's disease. Pediatrics 68:401–404

Oizumi J, Donnell GN, Ng WG, Mulivor RA, Greene AE, Coriell LL (1984) Congenital lactic acidosis associated with pyruvate carboxylase deficiency. Cytogenet Cell Genet 38:81

Oizumi J, Ng WG, Donnell GN (1986) Pyruvate carboxylase defect: metabolic studies on cultured skin fibroblasts. J Inherited Metab Dis 9:120–128

Perry TL, Haworth JC, Robinson BH (1985) Brain amino acid abnormalities in pyruvate carboxylase deficiency. J Inherited Metab Dis 8:63–66

Pollock MA, Cumberbatch M, Bennett MJ, Gray RGF, Brand M, Hyland K, Congdon PJ, Pitts-Tucker T, Gray S (1986) Pyruvate carboxylase deficiency in twins. J Inherited Metab Dis 9:29–30

Robinson BH (1989) Lactic acidemia: biochemical, clinical, and genetic considerations. Adv Hum Genet 18:151–179, 371–372

Robinson BH, Oei J, Sherwood WG, Applegarth D, Wong L, Haworth J, Goodyer P, Casey R, Zaleski LA (1984) The molecular basis for the two different clinical presentations of classical pyruvate carboxylase deficiency. Am J Hum Genet 36:283–294

Robinson BH, Toone JR, Benedict P, Dimmick JE, Oei J, Applegarth DA (1985) Prenatal diagnosis of pyruvate carboxylase deficiency. Prenat Diagn 5:67–71

Robinson BH, Oei J, Saudubray JM, Marsac C, Bartlett K, Quan F, Gravel R (1987) The French and North American phenotypes of pyruvate carboxylase deficiency, correlation with biotin containing protein by ^{3}H-biotin incorporation, ^{35}S-streptavidin labeling, and northern blotting with a cloned cDNA probe. Am J Hum Genet 40:50–59

Rutledge SL, Snead OC, Kelly DR, Kerr DS, Swann JW, Spink DL, Martin DL (1989) Pyruvate carboxylase deficiency: acute exacerbation after ACTH treatment of infantile spasms. Pediatr Neurol 5:249–252

Sander J, Packman S, Berg BO, Hutchison HT, Caswell N (1984) Pyruvate carboxylase activity in subacute necrotizing encephalopathy (Leigh's disease). Neurology 34:515–516

Saudubray JM, Marsac C, Charpentier C, Cathelineau L, Leaud MB, Leroux JP (1976) Neonatal congenital lactic acidosis with pyruvate carboxylase deficiency in two siblings. Acta Paediatr Scand 65:717–724

Tsuchiyama A, Oyanagi K, Hirano S, Tachi N, Sogawa H, Wagatsuma K, Nakao T, Tsugawa S, Kawamura Y (1983) A case of pyruvate carboxylase deficiency with later prenatal diagnosis of an unaffected sibling. J Inherited Metab Dis 6:85–88

Van Coster RN, Fernhoff PM, De Vivo DC (1991) Pyruvate carboxylase deficiency: a benign variant with normal development. Pediatr Res 30:1–4

Wong LTK, Davidson GF, Applegarth DE, Dimmick JE, Norman MG, Toone JR, Pirie G, Wong J (1986) Biochemical and histologic pathology in an infant with cross-reacting material (negative) pyruvate carboxylase deficiency. Pediatr Res 20:274–279

24 Cerebrotendinous Xanthomatosis

Argov Z, Soffer D, Eisenberg S, Zimmerman Y (1986) Chronic demyelinating peripheral neuropathy in cerebrotendinous xanthomatosis. Ann Neurol 20:89–91

Ballantyne CM, Vega GL, East C, Richards G, Grundy SM (1987) Low-density lipoprotein metabolism in cerebrotendinous xanthomatosis. Metabolism 36:270–276

Bencze KS, Van de Polder DR, Prockop LD (1990) Magnetic resonance imaging of the brain and spinal cord in cerebrotendinous xanthomatosis. J Neurol Neurosurg Psychiatry 53:166–167

Berginer VM, Salen G, Shefer S (1984) Long-term treatment of cerebrotendinous xanthomatosis with chenodeoxycholic acid. N Engl J Med 311:1649–1652

Berginer VM, Salen G, Shefer S (1989) Cerebrotendinous xanthomatosis. Neurol Clin 7:55–74

Berginer VM, Berginer J, Salen G, Shefer S, Zimmerman RD (1981) Computed tomography in cerebrotendinous xanthomatosis. Neurology 31:1463–1465

Berginer VM, Berginer J, Korczyn AD, Tamor R (1994) Magnetic resonance imaging in cerebrotendinous xanthomatosis: a prospective clinical and neuroradiological study. J Neurol Sci 122:102–108

Björkhem I (1992) Mechanism of degradation of the steroid side chain in the formation of bile acids. J Lipid Res 33:455–471

Björkhem I, Skrede S, Buchmann MS, East C, Grundy S (1987) Accumulation of 7α-hydroxy-4-cholesten-3-one and cholesta-4,6-dien-3-one in patients with cerebrotendinous xanthomatosis: effect of treatment with chenodeoxycholic acid. Hepatology 7:266–271

Bouwes Bavinck JN, Vermeer BJ, Gevers Leuven JA, Koopman BJ, Wolthers BG (1986) Capillary gas chromatography of urine samples in diagnosing cerebrotendinous xanthomatosis. Arch Dermatol 122:1269–1272

Canelas HM, Quintao ECR, Scaff M, Vasconcelos KS, Brotto MWI (1983) Cerebrotendinous xanthomatosis: clinical and laboratory study of 2 cases. Acta Neurol Scand 67:305–311

Diedrich U, Ropte S (1989) Cerebrotendinöse Xanthomatose: Beschreibung zweier Fälle und Differentialdiagnose zur Encephalomyelitis disseminata. Nervenarzt 60:444–447

Donaghy M, King RHM, McKeran RO, Schwartz MS, Thomas PK (1990) Cerebrotendinous xanthomatosis:clinical, electrophysiological and nerve biopsy findings, and response to treatment with chenodeoxycholic acid. J Neurol 237:216–219

Dotti MT, Salen G, Federico A (1991) Cerebrotendinous Xanthomatosis as a multisystem disease mimicking premature ageing. Dev Neurosci 13; 371–376

Dotti MT, Federico A, Signorini E, Caputo N, Venturi C, Filosomi G, Guazzi GC (1994) Cerebrotendinous xanthomatosis (van Bogaert-Scherer-Epstein disease): CT and MR findings. AJNR 15:1721–1726

Federico A, Dotti MT, Volpi N (1991) Muscle mitochondrial changes in cerebrotendinous xanthomatosis. Ann Neurol 30:734–735

Fiorelli M, Di Piero V, Bastianello S, Bozzao L, Federico A (1990) Cerebrotendinous xanthomatosis: clinical and MRI study (a case report). J Neurol Neurosurg Psychiatry 53:76–78

Grundy SM (1984) Cerebrotendinous xanthomatosis. N Engl J Med 311:1694–1695

Hokezu Y, Kuriyama M, Kubota R, Nakagawa M, Fujiyama J, Osame M (1992) Cerebrotendinous xanthomatosis: cranial CT and MRI studies in eight patients. Neuroradiology 34:308–312

Koopman BJ, van der Molen JC, Wolthers BG, Waterreus RJ (1987) Screening for cerebrotendinous xanthomatosis by using an enzymatic assay for 7α-hydroxylated steroids in urine. Clin Chem 33:142–143

Koopman BJ, Wolthers BG, van der Molen JC, van der Slik W, Waterreus RJ, van Spreeken A (1988) Cerebrotendinous xanthomatosis: a review of biochemical findings of the patient population in the Netherlands. J Inherited Metab Dis 11:56–75

Kuriyama M, Fujiyama J, Kasama T, Osame M (1991a) High levels of plant sterols and cholesterol precursors in cerebrotendinous xanthomatosis. J Lipid Res 32:223–229

Kuriyama M, Fujiyama J, Yoshidome H, Takenage S, Matsumuro K, Kasama T, Fukuda K, Kuramoto T, Hoshita T, Seyama Y, Okatu Y, Osame M (1991b) Cerebrotendinous xanthomatosis: clinical and biochemical evaluation of eight patients and review of the literature. J Neurol Sci 102:225–232

Leitersdorf E, Reshef A, Meiner V, Levitzki R, Pressman Schwartz S, Dann EJ, Berkman N, Cali JJ, Klapholz L, Berginer VM (1993) Frameshift and splice-junction mutations in the sterol 27-hydroxylase gene cause cerebrotendinous xanthomatosis in Jews of Moroccan origin. J Clin Invest 91:2488–2496

Lewis B, Mitchell WD, Marenah CB, Cortese C, Reynolds EH, Shakir R (1983) Cerebrotendinous xanthomatosis: biochemical response to inhibition of cholesterol synthesis. Br Med J 287:21–22

Meiner V, Marais DA, Reshef A, Björkhem I, Leitersdorf E (1994) Premature termination codon at the sterol 27-hydroxylase gene causes cerebrotendinous xanthomatosis in an Afrikaner family. Hum Mol Genet 3:193–194

Menkes JH (1970) Cerebrotendinous xanthomatosis. In: Vinken PJ, Bruyn GW (eds) Handbook of clinical neurology, vol 10. North Holland, Amsterdam, pp 532–541

Mimura Y, Kuriyama M, Tokimura Y, Fujiyama J, Osame M, Takesako K, Tanaka N (1993) Treatment of cerebrotendinous xanthomatosis with low-density lipoprotein (LDL)-apheresis. J Neurol Sci 114:227–230

Mondelli M, Rossi A, Scarpini C, Dotti MT, Federico A (1992) Evoked potentials in cerebrotendinous xanthomatosis and effect induce by chenodeoxycholic acid. Arch Neurol 49:469–475

Oftebro H, Björkhem I, Skree S, Schreiner A, Pedersen JI (1980) Cerebrotendinous xanthomatosis. J Clin Invest 65:1418–1430

Pedley TA, Emerson RG, Warner CL, Rowland LP, Salen G (1985) Treatment of cerebrotendinous xanthomatosis with chenodeoxycholic acid. Ann Neurol 18:517–518

Peynet J, Laurent A, de Liege P, Lecoz P, Gambert P, Legrand A, Mikol J, Warnet A (1991) Cerebrotendinous xanthomatosis: treatments with simvastatin, lovastatin, an chenodeoxycholic acid in 3 siblings. Neurology 41:434–436

Restuccia D, Di Lazzaro V, Servidei S, Colosimo C, Tonali P (1992) Somatosensory and motor evoked potentials in the assessment of cerebrotendinous xanthomatosis before and after treatment with chenodeoxycholic acid: a preliminary study. J Neurol Sci 112:139–146

Salen G, Zaki G, Sabesin S, Boehme D, Sheper S, Mosbach EH (1978) Intrahepatic pigment and crystal forms in patients with cerebrotendinous xanthomatosis (CTX). Gastroenterology 74:82–89

Salen G, Shefer S, Tint GS, Nicolau G, Dayal B, Batta AK (1985) Biosynthesis of bile acids in cerebrotendinous xanthomatosis. J Clin Invest 76:744–750

Salen G, Shefer S, Berginer V (1991) Biochemical abnormalities in cerebrotendinous xanthomatosis. Dev Neurosci 13:363–370

Schimschock JR, Alvord EC, Swanson PD (1968) Cerebrotendinous xanthomatosis. Arch Neurol 18:688–698

Skrede S, Björkhem I, Kvittingen EA, Buchmann MS, Lie SO, East C, Grundy S (1986) Demonstration of 26-hydroxylation of C_{27}-steroids in human skin fibroblasts, and a deficiency of this activity in cerebrotendinous xanthomatosis. J Clin Invest 78:729–735

Swanson PD, Cromwell LD (1986) Magnetic resonance imaging in cerebrotendinous xanthomatosis. Neurology 36:124–126

Tokimura Y, Kuriyama M, Arimura K, Fujiyama J, Osame M (1992) Electrophysiological studies in cerebrotendinous xanthomatosis. J Neurol Neurosurg Psychiatry 55:52–55

Van Hellenberg Hubar JLM, Joosten EMG, Wevers RA (1992) Cerebrotendinous xanthomatosis. J Neurol Neurosurg 94 [Suppl]:S165-S167

Waterreus RJ, Koopman BJ, Wolthers BG, Oosterhuis HJGH (1987) Cerebrotendinous xanthomatosis (CTX): a clinical survey of the patient population in the Netherlands. Clin Neurol Neurosurg 89:169–175

Wevers RA, Cruysberg JRM, van Heijst AFJ, Janssen-Zijlstra FSM, Renier WO, van Engelen BGM, Tolboom JJM (1992) Paediatric cerebrotendinous xanthomatosis. J Inherited Metab Dis 15:374–376

25 Refsum Disease

Beard ME, Sapirstein V, Kolodny EH, Holtzman E (1985) Peroxisomes in fibroblasts from skin of Refsum's disease patients. J Histochem Cytochem 33:480–484

Cammermeijer J (1956) Neuropathological changes in hereditary neuropathies: manifestation of the syndrome heredopathia atactica polyneuritiformis in the presence of interstitial hypertrophic polyneuropathy. J Neuropathol Exp Neurol 15:340–367

Dick JPR, Meeran K, Gibberd FB, Clifford Rose F (1993) Hypokalaemia in acute Refsum's disease. J R Soc Med 86:171–172

Dickson N, Mortimer JG, Faed JM, Pollard AC, Styles M, Peart DA (1989) A child with Refsum's disease: successful treatment with diet and plasma exchange. Dev Med Child Neurol 31:81–97

Djupesland G, Flottorp G, Refsum S (1983) Phytanic acid storage disease:hearing maintained after 15 years of dietary treatment. Neurology 33:237–240

Dotti MT, Rossi A, Rizzuto N, Hayek G, Bardeelli N, Bardelli AM, Federico A (1985) Atypical phenotype of Refsum's disease: clinical, biochemical, neurophysiological and pathological study. Eur Neurol 24:85–93

Fingerhut R, Schmitz W, Garavaglia B, Reichmann H, Conzelmann E (1994) Impaired degradation of phytanic acid in cells from patients with mitochondriopathies: evidence for the involvement of ETF and the respiratory chain in phytanic acid α-oxidation. J Inherited Metab Dis 17:527–532

Flament-Durand J, Noel P, Rutsaert J, Toussaint D, Malmendier C, Lyon G (1971) A case of Refsum's disease: clinical, pathological, ultrastructural and biochemical study. Pathol Eur 6:172–191

Friedman KJ, Shapiro SS (1985) Changes in sterol and phospholipid fatty acid composition in Refsum's disease fibroblasts grown in the presence of phytol. Clin Physiol Biochem 3:249–256

Gibberd FB, Billimoria JD, Goldman JM, Clemens ME, Evans R, Whitelaw MN, Retsas S, Sherratt RM (1985) Heredopathia atactica polyneuritiformis: Refsum's disease. Acta Neurol Scand 72:1–17

Gordon N, Hudson REB (1959) Refsum's syndrome heredopathia atactica polyneuritiformis. Brain 82:41–55

Hansen RP (1965) 3,7,11,15-tetramethylhexadecanoic acid: its occurrence in the tissues of humans afflicted with Refsum's syndrome. Biochim Biophys Acta 106:304–310

Harari D, Gibberd FB, Dick JPR, Sidey MC (1991) Plasma exchange in the treatment of Refsum's disease (heredopathia atactica polyneuritiformis). J Neurol Neurosurg Psychiatry 54:614–617

Herbert MA, Clayton PT (1994) Phytanic acid α-oxidase deficiency (Refsum disease) presenting in infancy. J Inherited Metab Dis 17:211–214

Hungerbühler JP, Meier C, Rousselle L, Quadri P, Bogousslavsky J (1985) Refsum's disease: management by diet and plasmapheresis. Eur Neurol 24:153–159

Kendall BE (1992) Disorders of lysosomes, peroxisomes and mitochondria. AJNR 13:621–653

Kuntzer T, Ochsner F, Schmid F, Regli F (1993) Quantitative EMG analysis and longitudinal nerve conduction studies in a Refsum's disease patient. Muscle Nerve 16:857–863

Leppert D, Schanz U, Burger J, Gmür J, Blau N, Waespe W (1991) Long-term plasma exchange in a case of Refsum's disease. Eur Arch Psychiatry Clin Neurosci 241:82–84

Macbrinn M, O'Brien JS (1968) Lipid composition of the nervous system in Refsum's disease. J Lipid Res 9:552–561

Petit H, Leys D, Skjeldal OH, Caron JC, Lambert P, Lehembre P, Hache JC (1986) La maladie de Refsum. Rev Neurol 142:500–508

Poll-The BT, Skjeldal OH, Stokke O, Poulos A, Demaugre F, Saudubray JM (1989) Phytanic acid alpha-oxidation and complementation analysis of classical Refsum and peroxisomal disorders. Hum Genet 81:175–181

Poulos A, Pollard AC, Mitchell JD, Wise G, Mortimer G (1984) Patterns of Refsum's disease. Arch Dis Child 59:222–229

Reese H, Bareta J (1975) Heredopathia atactica polyneuritiformis. J Neuropathol Exp Neurol 9:385–395

Refsum S (1975) Heredopathia atactica polyneuritiformis: phytanic acid storage disease. In: Vinken PJ, Bruyn GW (eds) Handbook of clinical neurology, vol 21. North Holland, Amsterdam, pp 181–229

Refsum S (1984) Heredopathia atactica polyneuritiformis, Refsum disease. In: Dyck PJ, Thomas PK, Lambert EH, Bunge R (eds) Pheripheral neuropathy, vol 2. Saunders, Philadelphia, pp 1680–1703

Salisachs P (1982) Ataxia and other data reviewed in Charcot-Marie-Tooth and Refsum's disease. J Neurol Neurosurg Psychiatry 45:1085–1091

Singh I, Lazo O, Kalipada P, Singh AK (1992) Phytanic acid α-oxidation in human cultured skin fibroblasts. Biochim Biophys Acta 1180:221–224

Singh I, Pahan K, Dhaunsi GS, Lazo O, Ozand P (1993) Phytanic acid α-oxidation. J Biol Chem 268:9972–9979

Skjeldal OH, Nyberg-Hansen R, Stokke O (1988) Neurological disorders and phytanic acid metabolism. Acta Neurol Scand 78:324–328

Steinberg D (1978) Elucidation of the metabolic error in Refsum's disease:strategy and tactics. Adv Neurol 21:113–124

Stokke O, Refsum S (1982) Refsum's disease and metabolism of phytanic acid. Lancet 1:906–907

Ten Brink HJ, Schor DSM, Kok RM, Stellaard F, Kneer, J, Poll-The BT, Sandubray JM, Jakobs C (1992) In vivo study of phytanic acid α-oxidation in classic Refsum's disease and chonchodysplasia. Pediatr Res 32:566–570

Wall WJH, Worthington BS (1979) Skeletal changes in Refsum's disease. Clin Radiol 30:657–659

Wanders RJA, van Roermund CWT (1993) Studies on phytanic acid α-oxidation in rat liver and cultured human skin fibroblasts. Biochim Biophys Acta 1167:345–350

Wanders RJA, Heymans HSA, Schutgens RBH, Poll-The BT, Saudubray JM, Tager JM, Schrakamp G, van den Bosch H (1988) Peroxisomal functions in classical Refsum's disease: comparison with the infantile form of Refsum's disease. J Neurol Sci 84:147–155

Wanders RJA, van Roermund CWT, Jakobs C, ten Brink HJ (1991) Identification of pristanoyl-CoA oxidase and phytanic acid decarboxylation in peroxisomes and mitochondria from human liver: implications for Zellweger synchome. J Inherited Metab Dis 14:349–352

Watkins PA, Mihalik SJ (1990) Mitochondrial oxidation of phytanic acid in human and monkey liver: implication that Refsum's disease is not a peroxisomal disorder. Biochem Biophys Res Commun 167:580–586

26 Nucleus, DNA and DNA Repair

Burn J (1994) Relevance of the human genome project to inherited metabolic disease. J Inherited Metab Dis 17:421–429

Cattanach BM, Jones J (1994) Genetic imprinting in the mouse: implications for gene regulation. J Inherited Metab Dis 17:403–420

Craig IW (1994) Organization of the human genome. J Inherited Metab Dis 17:391–402

Edlin G (1990) Human genetics. Jones and Bartlett, Boston

Giannelli F (1986) DNA maintenance and its relation to human pathology. J Cell Sci 4 [Suppl]:383–416

Lambert WC (1987) Genetic diseases associated with DNA and chromosomal instability. Dermatol Clin 5:85–108

Martin JB (1993) Molecular genetics in neurology. Ann Neurol 34:757–773

Mazzarello P, Poloni M, Spadari S, Focher F (1992) DNA repair mechanisms in neurological diseases: facts and hypotheses. J Neurol Sci 112:4–14

Rosenthal N (1994) DNA and the genetic code. N Engl J Med 331:39–41

Rosenthal N (1994) Stalking the gene – DNA libraries. N Engl J Med 331:599–600

Rosenthal N (1994) Regulation of gene expression. N Engl J Med 331:931–933

Tager JM, Aerts JMFG, Van den Bogert C, Wanders RJA (1994) Signals on proteins, intracellular targeting and inborn errors of organellar metabolism. J Inherited Metab Dis 17:459–469

Weatherall DJ (1991) The new genetics and clinical practice. Oxford University Press, Oxford

27 Cockayne's Disease

Boltshauser E, Yalcinkaya C, Wichmann W, Reutter F, Prader A, Valavanis A (1989) MRI in Cockayne syndrome type I. Neuroradiology 31:276–277

Cirillo Silengo M, Franceschini P, Bianco R, Biagioli M, Pastorin L, Vista N, BaldassarA, Benso L (1986) Distinctive skeletal dysplasia in Cockayne syndrome. Pediatr Radiol 16:264–266

Colabucci F, Rossodivita A, Parigi A, Colavita N (1987) A clinical and radiological study of two brothers affected by Cockayne syndrome type II. Rays (Roma) 12:57–63

Dabbagh O, Swaiman KF (1988) Cockayne syndrome: MRI correlates of hypomyelination. Pediatr Neurol 4:113–116

Demaerel P, Kendall BE, Kingsley D (1992) Cranial CT and MRI in diseases with DNA repair defects. Neuroradiology 34:117–121

Demaerel P, Wilms G, Verdru P, Carton H, Baert AL (1990) Apport de l'IRM dans le syndrome de Cockayne type I. J Neuroradiol 17:157–160

Descjavamme K. Chavaudra N, Fertil B, Malaise EP (1984) Abnormal sensitivity of some Cockayne's syndrome cell strains to UV- and gamma rays. Association with a reduced ability to repair potentially lethal damage. Mutat Res 131:61–70

Fryns JP, Bulcke J, Verdu P, Carton H, Kleczkowska A, van den Berghe H (1991) Apparent late-onset Cockayne syndrome and interstitial deletion of the long arm of chromosome 10 (del (10) (q11.23q21.2). Am J Med Genet 40:343–344

Grunnet ML, Zimmerman AW, Lewis RA (1983) Ultrastructure and electrodiagnosis of peripheral neuropathy in Cockayne's syndrome. Neurology 33:1606–1609

Guzzetta F (1972) Cockayne-Neill-Dingwall syndrome. In: Vinken PJ; Bruyn GW (eds) Handbook of clinical neurology, vol 13. North Holland, Amsterdam, pp 431–440

Harbord MG, Finn JP, Hall-Craggs MA, Brett EM, Baraitser M (1989) Early onset leukodystrophy with distinct facial features in 2 siblings. Neuropediatrics 20:154–157

Harbord MG, Finn JP, Hall-Craggs MA, Brett EM, Baraitser M (1989) Early onset leukoystrophy with distinct facial features in 2 siblings. Neuropediatrics 20:154–157

Hayashi M, Hayakawa K, Suzuki F, Sugita K, Satoh J, Morimatsu Y (1992) A neuropathological study of early onset Cockayne syndrome with chromosomal anomaly 47XXX. Brain Dev 14:63–67

Houston CS, Zaleski WA, Rozdilsky B (1982) Identical male twins and brother with Cockayne syndrome. Am J Med Genet 13:211–223

Kawai K, Ikenaga M, Ohtani H, Fukuchi K, Yamamura K, Kumahara Y (1983) Rapid procedures for prenatal diagnosis of Cockayne syndrome. Jpn J Human Genet 28:223–229

Leech RW, Brumback RA, Miller RH, Otsuka F, Tarone RE, Robbins JH (1985) Cockayne syndrome: clinicopathologic and tissue culture studies of affected siblings. J Neuropathol Exp Neurol 44:507–519

Lehmann AR, Francis AJ, Giannelli F (1985) Prenatal diagnosis of Cockayne's syndrome. Lancet I:486

Lehmann AR, Thompson AF, Harcourt SA, Stefanini M, Norris PG (1993) Cockayne's syndrome: correlation of clinical features with cellular sensitivity of RNA synthesis to UV irradiation. J Med Genet 30:679–682

Lowry RB (1982) Early onset of Cockayne syndrome. Am J Med Genet 13:209–210

Moyer DB, Marquis P, Shertzer ME, Burton BK (1982) Cockayne syndrome with early onset of manifestations. Am J Med Genet 13:225–230

Nance MA, Berry SA (1992) Cockayne syndrome:review of 140 cases. Am J Med Genet 42:68–84

Neetens A, van Acker K, Smets RM (1982) Cockayne's syndrome. Bull Soc Belg Ophthalmol 203:85–92

Nishio H, Kodama S, Matsuo T, Ichihashi M, Ito H, Fujiwara Y (1988) Cockayne syndrome:magnetic resonance images of the brain in a severe form with early onset. J Inherited Metab Dis 11:88–102

Norman RM, Tingey AH (1966) Syndrome of micrencephaly, strio-cerebellar calcifications, and leucodystrophy. J Neurol Neurosurg Psychiatry 29:157–163

Ohnishi A, Mitsudome A, Murai Y (1987) Primary segmental demyelination in the sural nerve in Cockayne's syndrome. Muscle Nerve 10:163–167

Otsuka F, Robbins JH (1985) The Cockayne syndrome – an inherited multisystem disorder with cutaneous photosensitivity and defective repair of DNA. Am J Dermatopathol 7:387–392

Patton MA, Giannelli F, Francis AJ, Baraiser M, Harding B, Williams AJ (1989) Early onset Cockayne's syndrome: case reports with neuropathological and fibroblast studies. J Med Genet 26:154–159

Pena SDJ, Shokeir MHK (1974) Autosomal recessive cerebro-oculo-facio-skeletal (COFS) syndrome. Clin Genet 5:285–293

Pena SDJ, Evans J, Hunter AGW (1978) COFS syndrome revisited. Birth Defects XIV:205–213

Sasaki K, Tachi N, Shinoda M, Satoh N, Minami R, Ohnishi A (1992) Demyelinating peripheral neuropathy in Cockayne syndrome: a histopathologic and morphometric study. Brain Dev 14:114–117

Sato H, Saito T, Kurosawa K, Ootaka T, Furuyama T, Yoshinaga K (1988) Renal lesions in Cockayne's syndrome. Clin Nephrol 29:206–209

Schwaiger H, Hirsch-Kauffmann M, Schweiger M (1986) DNA repair in human cells: in Cockayne syndrome cells rejoining of DNA strands is impaired. Eur J Cell Biol 41:352–355

Smits MG, Gabreels FJM, Renier WO, Joosten EMG, Gabreels-Festen AAWM, ter Laak HJ, Pinckers AJL, Hombergen GCJ, Notermans SLH, Thijssen HOM (1982) Peripheral and central myelinopathy in Cockayne's syndrome. Neuropediatrics 13:161–167

Sugita K, Takanashi J, Suzuki N, Niimi H (1991) Comparison of cellular sensitivity to UV killing with neuropsychological impairment in Cockayne syndrome patients. Brain Dev 13:163–166

Sugita K, Takanashi J, Ishii M, Niimi H (1992) Comparison of MRI white matter changes with neuropsychologic impairment in Cockayne syndrome. Pediatr Neurol 8:295–298

Takada K, Becker LE (1986) Cockayne's syndrome: report of two autopsy cases associated with neurofibrillary tangles. Clin Neuropathol 5:64–68

Talwar D, Smith SA (1989) Camfak syndrome: a demyelinating inherited disease similar to Cockayne syndrome. Am J Med Genet 34:194–198

Traboulsi EI, de Becker I, Maumenee IH (1992) Ocular findings in Cockayne syndrome. Am J Ophthalmol 114:579–583

Venema J, Mullenders LHF, Natarajan AT, van Zeeland AA, Mayne LV (1990) The genetic defect in Cockayne syndrome is associated with a defect in repair of UV-induced DNA damage in transcriptionally active DNA. Proc Natl Acad Sci U S A 87:4707–4711

Vos A, Gabreels-Festen A, Joosten E, Gabreels F, Renier W, Mullaart R (1983) The neuropathy of Cockayne syndrome. Acta Neuropathol (Berl) 61:153–156

Wood RD (1991) Seven genes for three diseases. Nature 350:190

28 Pelizaeus-Merzbacher Disease

Andre M, Monin P, Moret C, Braun M, Picard L (1990) Maladie de Pelizaeus-Merzbacher. J Neuroradiol 17:216–221

Apkarain P, Koetsveld-Baart JC, Barth PG (1993) Visual evoked potential characteristics and early diagnosis of Pelizaeus-Merzbacher disease. Arch Neurol 50:981–985

Bargeton-Farkas E, Edgar GWF (1964) Anatomo-chemical studies on a case of congenital sudanophilic leucodystrophy. Acta Neuropathol (Berl) 3:578–587

Begleiter ML, Harris DJ (1989) Autosomal recessive form of connatal Pelizaeus-Merzbacher disease. Am J Med Genet 33:311–313

Boespflug-Tanguy O, Mimault C, Melki J, Cavagna A, Giraud G, Dinh DP, Dastuge B, Dautigny A (1994) Genetic homogeneity of Pelizaeus-Merzbacher disease: tight linkage to the proteolipoprotein locus in 16 affected families. Am J Hum Genet 55:461–467

Boltshauser E, Schinzel A, Wichmann W, Haller D, Valavanis A (1988) Pelizaeus-Merzbacher disease: identification of heterozygotes with magnetic resonance imaging? Hum Genet 80:393–394

Boulloche J, Aicardi J (1986) Pelizaeus-Merzbacher disease: clinical and nosological study. J Child Neurol 1:233–239

Bourre JM, Jacque C, Nguyen-Legros J, Bornhofen JH, Araoz CA, Daudu O, Baumann NA (1978) Pelizaeus-Merzbacher disease: biochemical analysis of isolated myelin (electron-microscopy:protein, lipid and unsubstituted fatty acids analysis). Eur Neurol 17:317–326

Bridge PJ, MacLeod PM, Lillicrap DP (1991) Carrier detection and prenatal diagnosis of Pelizaeus-Merzbacher disease using a combination of anonymous DNA polymorphisms and the proteolipid protein (PLP) gene cDNA. Am J Med Genet 38:616–621

Bruyn GW, Weenink HR, Bots GTAM, Teepen JLJM, Wolferen WJA (1985) Pelizaeus-Merzbacher disease. Acta Neuropathol (Berl) 67:177–189

Caro PA, Marks HG (1990) Magnetic resonance imaging and computed tomography in Pelizaeus-Merzbacher disease. Magn Reson Imaging 8:791–796

Cassidy SB, Sheehan NC, Farrell DF, Grunnet M, Holmes GI, Zimmerman AW (1987) Connatal Pelizaeus-Merzbacher disease:an autosomal recessive form. Pediatr Neurol 3:300–305

Doll R, Natowicz MR, Schiffmann R, Smith FI (1992) Molecular diagnostics for myelin proteolipid protein gene mutations in Pelizaus-Merzbacher disease. Am J Hum Genet 51:161–169

Feldman JI, Kearns DB, Seid AB, Pransky SM, Jones MC (1990) The otolaryngologic manifestations of Pelizaeus-Merzbacher disease. Arch Otolaryngol Head Neck Surg 116:613–616

Garg BP, Markand ON, DeMyer WE (1983) Usefulness of BAER studies in the early diagnosis of Pelizaeus-Merzbacher disease. Neurology 33:955–956

Haenggeli CA, Engel E, Pizzolato GP (1989) Connatal Pelizaeus-Merzbacher disease. Dev Med Child Neurol 31:797–815

Hayashi T, Ichiyama T, Koga M, Okino F, Katayama K, Kobayashi K (1990) A possible Japanese male case of Pelizaeus-Merzbacher disease. Brain Dev 12:439–443

Huygen PLM, Verhagen WLM, Renier WO (1992) Oculomotor and vestibular anomalies in Pelizaeus-Merzbacher disease:a study on a kindred with 2 affected and 3 normal males, 3 obligate and 8 possible carriers. J Neurol Sci 113:17–25

Iyoda K, Tanaka J, Suzuki Y, Nagao Y, Ohtahara S (1988) Histopathologic and biochemical analysis of classic Pelizaeus-Merzbacher disease. Pediatr Neurol 4:252–254

Johnson VP, Carpenter NJ, Alan Kelts K (1991) Pelizaeus-Merzbacher disease: clinical and DNA-linkage study of an extended family. Am J Med Genet 41:355–261

Journel H, Roussey M, Gandon Y, Allaire C, Carsin M, le Marec B (1987) Magnetic resonance imaging in Pelizaeus-Merzbacher disease. Neuroradiology 29:403–405

Kaga M, Murakami T, Naitoh H, Nihei K (1990) Studies on pediatric patients with absent auditory brainstem response (ABR) later components. Brain Dev 12:380–384

Koeppen AH, Ronca NA, Greenfield EA, Hans MB (1987) Defective biosynthesis of proteolipid protein in Pelizaeus-Merzbacher disease. Ann Neurol 21:159–170

Koeppen AH, Barron KD, Csiza CK, Greenfield EA (1988) Comparative immunocytochemistry of Pelizaeus-Merzbacher disease, the jimpy mouse, and the myelin-deficient rat. J Neurol Sci 84:315–327

Konishi Y, Kamoshita S (1975) An autopsy case of classical Pelizaeus-Merzbacher's disease. Acta Neuropathol (Berl) 31:267–270

Manpaa J, Lindahl E, Aula P, Savontaus ML (1990) Prenatal diagnosis in Pelizaus-Merzbacher disease using RFLP analysis. Clin Genet 37:141–146

Mattei MB, Alliel PM, Dauiguy A, Passage E, Pham-Dinh D, Mattei JF, Jolles P (1986) The gene encoding for the major brain proteolipid (PLP) maps on the q-22 band of the human X chromosome. Hum Genet 72:352–353

Merzbacher L (1910) Eine eigenartige familiär-hereditäre Erkrankungsform (aplasia axialis extracorticalis congenita). Z Gesamte Neurol Psychiatr 3:1–138

Novotny EJ (1988) Arthrogryposis associated with connatal Pelizaeus-Merzbacher disease: case report. Neuropediatrics 19:221–223

Pamphlett R, Silberstein P (1986) Pelizaeus-Merzbacher disease in a brother and sister. Acta Neuropathol (Berl) 69:343–346

Pelizaeus F (1899) Ueber eine eigenartige familiäre Entwickelungshemmung vornehmlich auf motorischem Gebiet. Arch Psychiatr Nervenkr 31:100–104

Pratt WM, Trofatter JA, Larsen MB, Hodes ME, Dlouhy SR (1992) New variant in exon 3 of the proteolipid protein (PLP) gene in a family with Pelizaeus-Merzbacher disease. Am J Med Genet 43:642–646

Pratt VM, Trofatter JA, Schinzel A, Dlouhy SR, Conneally PM, Hodes ME (1991) A new mutation in the proteolipid protein (PLP) gene in a german family with Pelizaeus-Merbacher disease. Am J Med Genet 38:136–139

Raskind WH, Williams CA, Hudson LD, Bird TD (1991) Complete deletion of the proteolipid protein gene (PLP) in a family with X-linked Pelizaeus-Merzbacher disease. Am J Hum Genet 49:1355–1360

Renier WO, Gabreeels FJM, Hustinx TWJ, Jaspar HHJ, Geelen JAG, van Haelst UJG, Lommen EJP, ter Haar BGA (1981) Connatal Pelizaeus-Merzbacher disease with congenital stridor in two maternal cousins. Acta Neuropathol (Berl) 54:11–17

Scheffer IE, Baraitser M, Wilson J, Harding B, Kendall B, Brett EM (1991) Pelizaeus-Merzbacher disease:classical or connatal? Neuropediatrics 22:71–78

Schneck L, Adachi M, Volk BW (1971) Congenital failure of myelinization: Pelizaeus-Merzbacher disease? Neurology 21:817–824

Schneider A, Montague P, Griffiths I, Fanarragat M, Kennedy P, Brophyt P, Nave KA (1992) Uncoupling of hypomyelination and glial cell death by a mutation in the proteolipid protein gene. Nature 358:758–761

Seitelberger F (1970) Pelizaeus-Merzbacher disease. In: Vinken PJ, Bruyn GW (eds) Handbook of clinical neurology, vol 10. North Holland, Amsterdam, pp 150–202

Shimomura C, Matsui A, Choh H, Funahashi M, Suzuki Y, Tsuchiya K (1988) Magnetic resonance imaging in Pelizaeus-Merzbacher disease. Pediatr Neurol 4:124–125

Silverstein AM, Hirsh DK, Trobe JD, Gebarski SS (1990) MR imaging of the brain in five members of a family with Pelizaeus-Merzbacher disease. AJNR 11:495–499

Stoffel W, Hillen H, Giersiefen H (1984) Structure and molecular arrangement of proteolipid protein of central nervous system myelin. Proc Natl Acad Sci U S A 81:5012–5016

Strautnieks S, Rutland P, Winter RM, Baraitser M, Malcolm S (1992) Pelizaues-Merzbacher disease: detection of mutations Thr[8] Pro and Leu[223] Pro in the proteolipid protein gene, and prenatal diagnosis. Am J Hum Genet 51:871–878

Sugita K, Ishii M, Takanashi J, Suzuki N, Isogai E, Niimi H (1992) Pelizaeus-Merzbacher disease: cellular hypersensitivity to ultraviolet light. Brain Dev 14:44–47

Ulrich J, Herschkowitz N (1977) Seitelberger's connatal form of Pelizaeus-Merzbacher disease. Acta Neuropathol (Berl) 40:129–136

Van der Knaap MS, Valk J (1989) The reflection of histology in MR imaging of Pelizaeus-Merzbacher disease. AJNR 10:99–103

Vnia O (1978) Congenital Pelizaeus-Merzbacher disease (Seitelberger type), malformation and cystic degeneration of the central nervous system. Neuropediatrics 9:172–184

Watanabe I, Patel V, Goebel HH, Siakotos AN, Zeman W, Demyer W, Schroder Dyer J (1973) Early lesion of Pelizaeus-Merzbacher disease: electron microscopic and biochemical study. J Neuropathol Exp Neurol 32:313–333

Watanabe I, McCaman R, Dyken P, Zeman W (1969) Absence of cerebral myelin sheaths in a case of presumed Pelizaeus-Merzbacher disease. J Neuropathol Exp Neurol 28:243–256

Weimbs T, Dick T, Stoffel W, Boltshauser E (1990) A point mutation at the X-chromosomal proteolipid protein locus in Pelizaeus-Merzbacher disease leads to disruption of myelinogenesis. Biol Chem Hoppe Seyler 371:1175–1183

Willard HF, Riordan JR (1985) Assignment of the gene for myelin proteolipid protein to the X chromosome: implications for X-linked myelin disorders. Science 230:940–942

Witter B, Debuch H, Klein H (1980) Lipid investigation of central and peripheral nervous system in connatal Pelizaeus-Merzbacher's disease. J Neurochem 34:957–962

Yokoi S, Amano N, Hanawa H, Isyama K, Ishikawa A, Ogino T (1985) Postnatal sudanophilic leukodystrophy in two siblings. Acta Neuropathol (Berl) 67:103–113

Zeman W, Demyer W, Falls HF (1964) Pelizaeus-Merzbacher disease. J Neuropathol Exp Neurol 23:334–354

29 18q⁻ Syndrome

Felding I, Kristoffersson U, Sjöström H, Noren O (1987) Contribution to the 18q⁻ syndrome. A patient with del (18) (q22.3qter). Clin Genet 31:206–210

Fryns JP, Logghe N, van Eygen M, van den Berghe H (1979) 18q⁻ syndrome in mother and daughter. Eur J Pediatr 130:189–192

Kamholz J, Spielman R, Gogolin K, Modi W, O'Brien S, Lazzarini R (1987) The human myelin-basic-protein gene: chromosomal localization and RFLP analysis. Am J Hum Genet 40:365–373

Kamholz J, Fischbeck K, Ritter A, Zackai E, McDonald D, Emanuel B (1988) Segmental spinal muscular atrophy associated with a partial deletion of chromosome 18. Am J Hum Genet 43:A110

Kolodny EH (1993) Dysmyelinating and demyelinating conditions in infancy. Curr Opin Neurol Neurosurg 6:379–386

Lemke G (1988) Unwrapping the genes of myelin. Neuron 1:535–543

Loevner LA, Grossman RI, Shapiro R (1994) White matter changes associated with partial deletion of the long arm of chromosome 18 (18q⁻ syndrome): a dysmyelinating disorder? Radiology 193 [Suppl]:214

Miller G, Mowrey PN, Hopper KD, Frankel CA, Ladda RL (1990) Neurologic manifestations in 18q⁻ syndrome. Am J Med Genet 37:128–132

Ono J, Harada K, Yamamoto T, Onoe S, Okada S (1994) Delayed myelination in a patient with 18q⁻ syndrome. Pediatr Neurol 11:64–67

Rodichok L, Miller G (1992) A study of evoked potentials in the 18q⁻ syndrome which includes the absence of the gene locus for myelin basic protein. Neuropediatrics 23:218–220

Saxe DF, Takahashi N, Hood L, Simon MI (1985) Localization of the human myelin basic protein gene (MBP) to region 18q22→qter by in situ hybridization. Cytogenet Cell Genet 39:246–249

Wertelecki W, Gerald PS (1971) Clinical and chromosomal studies of the 18q⁻ syndrome. J Pediatr 78:44–52

Wilson MG, Towner JW, Forsman I, Siris E (1979) Syndromes associated with deletion of the long arm of chromosome 18 [del (18q)]. Am J Med Genet 3:155–174

30 Phenylketonuria

Agrawal HC, Bone AH, Davison AN (1969) Inhibition of brain protein synthesis by phenylalanine. Biochem J 112:27

Alvord EC, Stevenson LD, Vogel FS, Engle RL (1950) Neuropathological findings in phenyl-pyruvic oligophrenia (phenyl-ketonuria). J Neuropathol Exp Neurol 9:298–310

Battistini S, de Stefano N, Parlanti S, Federico A (1991) Unexpected white matter changes in an early treated PKU case and improvement after dietary treatment. Funct Neurol 6:177–180

Bick U, Fahrendorf G, Ludolph AC, Vassallo P, Weglage J, Ullrich K (1991) Disturbed myelination in patients with treated hyperphenylalaninaemia:evaluation with magnetic resonance imaging. Eur J Pediatr 150:185–189

Brismar J, Aqeel A, Gascon G, Ozand P (1989) Malignant hyperphenylalaninemia: CT and MR of the brain. AJNR 11:135–138

Burri R, Steffen CH, Stieger S, Brodbeck U, Colombo JP, Herschkowitz N (1990) Reduced myelinogenesis and recovery in hyperphenylalaninemic rats. Mol Chem Neuropathol 13:57–69

Dhondt JL, Farriaux JP, Boudha A, Largillière C, Ringel J, Roger MM, Leeming RJ (1985) Neonatal hyperphenylalaninemia presumably caused by guanosine triphosphate-cyclohydrolase deficiency. J Pediatr 106:954–956

Eisensmith RC, Woo SLC (1991) Phenylketonuria and the phenylalanine hydroxylase gene. Mol Biol Med 8:3–18

Elliman D, Garner J (1991) Review of neonatal screening programme for phenylketonuria. Br Med J 303:471

Fisch RO, Burke B, Bass J, Ferrara TB, Mastri A (1986) Maternal phenylketonuria – chronology of the detrimental effects on embryogenesis and fetal development: pathological report, survey, clinical application. Pediatr Pathol 5:449–461

Fölling A (1934) Über Ausscheidung von Phenylbrenztraubensäure in den Harn als Stoffwechselanomalie in Verbindung mit Imbezillität. Z Physiol Chem 227:169–176

Gerstl B, Malamud N, Eng LF, Hayman RB (1967) Lipid alterations in human brains in phenylketonuria. Neurology 17:51–57

Giovannini M, Biasucci G, Brioschi M, Ghiglioni D, Riva E (1991) Cofactor defects and PKU: diagnosis and treatment. Int Pediatr 6:26–31

Gudinchet F, Maeder P, Meuli RA, Deonna T, Mathieu JM (1992) Cranial CT and MRI in malignant phenylketonuria. Pediatr Radiol 22:223–224

Güttler F (1980) Hyperphenylalaninemia: diagnosis and classification of the various types of phenylalanine hydroxylase deficiency in childhood. Acta Paediatr Scand 280 [Suppl]:1–80

Harris H, Hirschhorn K (1983) Phenylketonuria and its variants. Adv Hum Genet 13:217–297

Jardim LB, Giugliani R, Coelho JC, Dutra-Filho CS, Blau N (1994) Possible high frequency of tetrahydrobiopterin deficiency in South Brazil. J Inherited Metab Dis 17:223–229

Jervis GA (1947) Studies on phenylpyruvic oligophrenia. The position of the metabolic error. J Biol Chem 169:651–656

Konecki DS, Lichter-Konecki U (1991) The phenylketonuria locus: current knowledge about alleles and mutations of the phenylalanine hydroxylase gene in various populations. Hum Genet 87:377–388

Ledley FD (1991) Clinical application of genotypic diagnosis for phenylketonuria: theoretical considerations. Eur J Pediatr 150:752–756

Leuzzi V, Gualdi GF, Fabbrizi F, Trasimeni G, DiBiasi C, Antonozzi I (1993) Neuroradiological (MRI) abnormalities in phenylketonuric subjects: clinical and biochemical correlations. Neuropediatrics 24:302–306

Levy HL, Lobbregt D, Sansaricq C, Snyderman SE (1992) Comparison of phenylketonuric and nonphenylketonuric sibs from untreated pregnancies in a mother with phenylketonuria. Am J Med Genet 44:439–442

Lou HC, Toft PB, Andressen J, Mikkelsen I, Olsen B, Güttler F, Wieslander S, Henriksen O (1992) An occipito-temporal syndrome in adolescents with optimally controlled hyperphenylalaninaemia. J Inherited Metab Dis 15:687–695

Malamud N (1966) Neuropathology of phenylketonuria. J Neuropathol Exp Neurol 25:254–268

McCombe PA, McLaughlin DB, Chalk JB, Brown NN, McGill JJ, Pender MP (1992) Spasticity and white matter abnormalities in adult phenylketonuria. J Neurol Neurosurg Psychiatry 55:359–361

Menkes JH (1967) The pathogenesis of mental retardation in phenylketonuria and other inborn errors of amino acid metabolism. Pediatrics 39:297–308

Naylor EW, Ennis D, Davidson GF, Wong LTK, Applegarth DA, Niederwieser A (1987) Guanosine triphosphate cyclohydrolase I deficiency: early diagnosis by routine urine pteridine screening. Pediatrics 79:374–378

Niederwieser A, Blau N, Wang M, Joller P, Atares M, Cardesa-Garcia J (1984) GTP cyclohydrolase I deficiency, a new enzyme defect causing hyperphenylalaninemia with neopterin, biopterin, dopamine, and serotonin deficiencies and muscular hypotonia. Eur J Pediatr 141:208–214

Okano Y, Eisensmith RC, Güttler F, Lichter-Konecki U, Konecki DS, Trefz FK, Dasovich M, Wang T, Henriksen K, Lou H, Woo SLC (1991) Molecular basis of phenotypic heterogeneity in phenylketonuria. N Engl J Med 324:1232–1238

Pearsen KD, Gean-Marton AD, Levy HL, Davis KR (1990) Phenylketonuria: MR imaging of the brain with clinical correlation. Radiology 177:437–440

Pietz J, Schmidt E, Matthis P, Kobialka B, Kutscha A, de Sonneville L (1993) EEGs in phenylketonuria. I:Follow up to adulthood. II: Short-term diet-related changes in EEGs and cognitive function. Dev Med Child Neurol 35:54–64

Poser CM, van Bogaert L (1959) Neuropathologic observations in phenylketonuria. Brain 82:1–9

Shaw DWW, Weinberger E, Maravilla KR (1990) Cranial MR in phenylketonuria. J Comput Assist Tomogr 14:458–460

Shaw DWW, Maravilla KR, Weinberger E, Garretson J, Trahms CM, Scott CR (1991) MR imaging in phenylketonuria. AJNR 12:403–406

Silberberg DH (1967) Phenylketonuria metabolites in cerebellum culture morphology. Arch Neurol 17:524–529

Smith I (1991) Review of neonatal screening programme for phenylketonuria. Br Med J 303:333–335

Sugita R, Takahashi S, Ishii K, Matsumoto K, Ishibashi T, Sakamoto K, Narisawa K (1990) Brain CT and MR findings in hyperphenylalaninemia due to dihydropteridine reductase deficiency (variant of phenylketonuria). J Comput Assist Tomogr 14:699–703

Svensson E, Iselius L, Hagenfeldt L (1994) Severity of mutation in the phenylalanine hydroxylase gene influences phenylalanine metabolism in phenylketonuria and hyperphenylalaninaemia heterozygotes. J Inherited Metab Dis 17:215–222

Thompson AJ, Smith I, Brenton D, Youl BD, Rylance G, Davidson DC, Kendall B, Lees AJ (1990) Neurological deterioration in young adults with phenylketonuria. Lancet 336:602–605

Thompson AJ, Tillotson S, Smith I, Kendall B, Moore SG, Brenton DP (1993) Brain MRI changes in phenylketonuria. Brain 116:811–821

Walter JH, Tyfield LA, Holton JB, Johnson C (1993) Biochemical control, genetic analysis and magnetic resonance imaging in patients with phenylketonuria. Eur J Pediatr 152:822–827

Weglage J, Schuierer G, Kurlemann G, Bick R, Ullrich K (1993) Different degrees of white matter abnormalities in untreated phenylketonurics: findings in magnetic resonance imaging. J Inherited Metab Dis 16:1047–1048

31 Glutaric Aciduria Type 1

Altman NR, Rovira MJ, Bauer M (1991) Glutaric aciduria type 1: MR findings in two cases. AJNR 12:966–968

Amir N, Peleg OE, Shalev RS, Christensen E (1987) Glutaric aciduria type I: clinical heterogeneity and neuroradiologic features. Neurology 37:1654–1657

Amir N, Elpeleg ON, Shalev RS, Christensen E (1989) Glutaric aciduria type I: enzymatic and neuroradiologic investigations of two kindreds. J Pediatr 114:983–989

Amit R, Berginer J, Shapira Y (1990) CT in glutaric aciduria. Neurology 40:188–189

Bennett MJ, Marlow N, Pollitt RJ, Wales JKH (1986) Glutaric aciduria type 1: biochemical investigations and postmortem findings. Eur J Pediatr 145:403–405

Bennett MJ, Pollitt RJ, Goodman SI, Hale DE, Vamecq J (1991) Atypical riboflavin-responsive glutaric aciduria, and deficient peroxisomal glutaryl-CoA oxidase activity: a new peroxisomal disorder. J Inherited Metab Dis 14:165–173

Bergman I, Finegold D, Gartner JC, Zitelli BJ, Claassen D, Scarano J, Roe CR, Stanley C, Goodman SI (1989) Acute profound dystonia in infants with glutaric acidemia. Pediatrics 83:228–234

Campistol J, Ribes A, Alvarez L, Christensen E, Millington DS (1992) Glutaric aciduria type I: unusual biochemical presentation. J Pediatr 121:83–86

Chalmers RA, Cheng KN, English NR, Jones MA, Savage W (1989) Glutaric aciduria type I: prenatal exclusion using GC-MS analysis of amniotic fluid and enzymology with oxidation of [6-^{14}C] lysine. J Inherited Metab Dis 12:335–336

Chow CW, Haan EA, Goodman SI, Anderson RMcD, Evans WA, Kleinschmidt-de Masters BK, Wise G, McGill JJ, Danks DM (1988) Neuropathology in glutaric acidaemia type 1. Acta Neuropathol (Berl) 76:590–594

Christensen E (1989) First trimester prenatal exclusion of glutaryl-CoA dehydrogenase deficiency (glutaric aciduria type 1). J Inherited Metab Dis 12 [Suppl 2]:277–279

Francois B, Jaeken J, Gillis P (1990) Vigabatrin in the treatment of glutaric aciduria type I. J Inherited Metab Dis 13:352–354

Goodman SE, Norenberg MD, Shikes RH, Breslich DJ, Moe PG (1977) Glutaric aciduria: biochemical and morphologic considerations. J Pediatr 90:746–750

Gregersen N, Brandt NJ, Christensen E, Grøn I, Rasmussen K, Brandt S (1977) Glutaric aciduria: clinical and laboratory findings in two brothers. J Pediatr 90:740–745

Hald JK, Nakstad PH, Skjeldal OH, Strømme P (1991) Bilateral arachnoid cysts of the temporal fossa in four children with glutaric aciduria type I. AJNR 12:407–409

Haworth JC, Booth FA, Chudley AE, de Groot GW, Dilling LA, Goodman SI, Greenberg CR, Mallory CJ, McClarty BM, Seshia SS, Seargeant LE (1991) Phenotypic variability in glutaric aciduria type I: report of fourteen cases in five Canadian Indian kindreds. J Pediatr 118:52–58

Heyes MP (1987) Hypothesis: a role for quinolinic acid in the neuropathology of glutaric aciduria type I. Can J Neurol Sci 14:441–443

Hoffmann GF, Trefz FK, Barth PG, Böhles HJ, Lehnert W, Christensen E, Valk J, Rating D, Bremer HJ (1991a) Macrocephaly: an important indication for organic acid analysis. J Inherited Metab Dis 329–332

Hoffmann GF, Trefz FK, Barth PG, Böhles HJ, Biggemann B, Bremer HJ, Christensen E, Frosch M, Hanefeld F, Hunneman DH, Jacobi H, Kurlemann G, Lawrenz-Wolf B, Rating D, Roe CR, Schutgens RBH, Ullrich K, Weisser J, Wendel U, Lehnert W (1991b) Glutaryl-coenzyme A dehydrogenase deficiency:a distinct encephalopathy. Pediatrics 88:1194–1203

Kidouchi K, Sugiyama N, Morishita H, Kobayashi M, Wada Y, Nagai S, Sakakibara J (1987) Identification of glutarylcarnitine in glutaric aciduria type 1. J Inherited Metab Dis 10 [Suppl 2]:279–281

Kyllerman M, Skjeldal OH, Lundberg M, Holme I, Jellum E, von Döbeln U, Fossen A, Carlsson G (1994) Dystonia and dyskinesia in glutaric aciduria type I: clinical heterogeneity and therapeutic considerations. Mov Disord 9:22–30

Lafolla AK, Kahler SG (1989) Megalencephaly in the neonatal period as the initial manifestation of glutaric aciduria type I. J Pediatr 114:1004–1006

Land JM, Goulder P, Johnson A, Hockaday J (1992) Glutaric aciduria type 1. An atypical presentation together with some observations upon treatment and the possible cause of cerebral damage. Neuropediatrics 23:322–326

Leibel RL, Shih VE, Goodman SI, Bauman ML, McCabe ERB, Zwerdling RG, Bergman I, Costello C (1980) Glutaric acidemia: a metabolic disorder causing progressive choreoathetosis. Neurology 30:1163–1168

Lipkin PH, Roe CR, Goodman SI, Batshaw ML (1988) A case of glutaric acidemia type I: effect of riboflavin and carnitine. J Pediatr 112:62–65

Mandel H, Braun J, El-Peleg O, Christensen E, Berant M (1991) Glutaric aciduria type I. Brain CT features and a diagnostic pitfall. Neuroradiology 33:75–78

Martinez-Lage JF, Casas C, Fernandez MA, Puche A, Rodriguez Costa T, Poza M (1994) Macrocephaly, dystonia, and bilateral temporal arachnoid cysts:glutaric aciduria type 1. Childs Nerv Syst 10:198–203

Morton DH, Bennett MJ, Seargeant LE, Nichter CA, Kelley RI (1991) Glutaric aciduria type I: a common cause of episodic encephalopathy and spastic paralysis in the amish of Lancaster county, Pennsylvania. Am J Med Genet 4:89–95

Nagasawa H, Yamaguchi S, Suzuki Y, Kobayashi M, Wada Y, Shikura K, Shimao S, Okada T, Orii T (1992) Neuroradiological findings in glutaric aciduria type I: report of four Japanese patients. Acta Paediatr Jpn 34:409–415

Osaka H, Kimura S, Nezu A, Yamazaki S, Saitoh K, Yamaguchi S (1993) Chronic subdural hematoma, as an initial manifestation of glutaric aciduria type-1. Brain Dev 15:125–127

Ribes A, Riudor E, Briones P, Christensen E, Campistol J, Millington DS (1992) Significance of bound glutarate in the diagnosis of glutaric aciduria type I. J Inherited Metab Dis 15:367–370

Soffer D, Amir N, Elpeleg ON, Gomori JM, Shalev RS, Gottschalk-Sabag S (1992) Striatal degeneration and spongy myelinopathy in glutaric acidemia. J Neurol Sci 107:199–204

Stutchfield P, Edwards MA, Gray RGF, Crawley P, Green A (1985) Glutaric aciduria type I misdiagnosed as Leigh's encephalopathy and cerebral palsy. Dev Med Child Neurol 27:514–521

Vamecq J, van Hoof F (1984) Implication of a peroxisomal enzyme in the catabolism of glutaryl-CoA. Biochem J 221:203–211

Vamecq J, de Hoffmann E, van Hoof F (1985) Mitochondrial and peroxisomal metabolism of glutaryl-CoA. Eur J Biochem 146:663–669

Yager JY, McClarty BM, Seshia SS (1988) CT scan findings in an infant with glutaric aciduria type I. Dev Med Child Neurol 30:808–820

32 Propionic Acidemia

Behbehani AW, Lehnert W, Langenbeck U, Luthe H, Baumgartner R (1984) Propionazidämie mit Myelinisierungsstörungen im ZNS. Klin Padiatr 196:106–110

Brismar J, Ozand PT (1994) CT and MR of the brain in disorders of the propionate and methylmalonate metabolism. AJNR 15:1459–1473

Davies SEC, Iles RA, Stacey TE, de Sousa C, Chalmers RA (1991) Carnitine therapy and metabolism in the disorders of propionyl-CoA metabolism studied using ^{1}H-NMR spectroscopy. Clin Chim Acta 204:263–278

Gebarski SS, Gabrielsen TO, Knake JE, Latack JT (1983) Cerebral CT findings in methylmalonic and propionic acidemias. AJNR 4:955–957

Gortner L, Leupold D, Pohlandt F, Bartmann P (1989) Peritoneal dialysis in the treatment of metabolic crises caused by inherited disorders of organic and amino acid metabolism. Acta Paediatr Scand 78:706–711

Gravel RA, Akerman BR, Lamhonwah AM, Loyer M, Léondel-Rio A, Italiano I (1994) Mutations participating in interallelic complementation in propionic acidemia. Am J Hum Genet 55:51–58

Harding BN, Leonard JV, Erdohazi M (1991) Propionic acidaemia:a neuropathological study of two patients presenting in infancy. Neuropathol Appl Neurobiol 17:133–138

Kalloghlian A, Gleispach H, Ozand PT (1992) A patient with propionic acidemia managed with continuous insulin infusion and total parenteral nutrition. J Child Neurol 7:S88–S91

Kendall BE (1992) Disorders of lysosomes, peroxisomes, and mitochondria. AJNR 13:621–653

Lamhonwah AM, Troxel CE, Schuster S, Gravel RA (1990) Two distinct mutations at the same site in the PCCB gene in propionic acidemia. Genomics 8:249–254

Martin JJ, Schlote W (1972) Central nervous system lesions in disorders of amino-acid metabolism. J Neurol Sci 15:49–76

Mirowitz SA, Sartor K, Prensky AJ, Gado M, Hodges FJ (1991) Neurodegenerative diseases of childhood: MR and CT evaluation. J Comput Assist Tomogr 15:210–222

Ogier H, Charpentier C, Saudubray JM (1989) Organic acidemias. In: Fernandes J, Saudubray JM, Tada K (eds) Inborn metabolic diseases, diagnosis and treatment. Springer, Berlin Heidelberg New York, pp 271–299

Ohura T, Miyabayashi S, Narisawa K, Tada K (1991) Genetic heterogeneity of proionic acidemia: analysis of 15 Japanese patients. Hum Genet 87:41–44

Ozand PT, Gascon GG (1991a) Organic acidurias: a review, part 1. J Child Neurol 6:196–219

Ozand PT, Gascon GG (1991b) Organic acidurias: a review, part 2. J Child Neurol 6:288–303

Rolland MO, Divry P, Mandon G, Guibaud P, Mathieu M, Sournies G, Thoulon JM (1990) Early prenatal diagnosis of propionic acidaemia with simultaneous sampling of chorionic villus and amniotic fluid. J Inherited Metab Dis 13:345–348

Sethi KD, Ray R, Roesel RA, Carter AL, Callagher BB, Loring DW, Hommes FA (1989) Adult-onset chorea and dementia with propionic acidemia. Neurology 39:1343–1345

Shigematsu Y, Mori I, Nakai A, Kikawa Y, Kuriyama M, Konishi Y, Fuji T, Sudo M (1990) Acute infantile hemiplegia in a patient with propionic acidaemia. Eur J Pediatr 149:659–660

Shuman RM, Leech RW, Scott CR (1978) The neuropathology of the nonketotic and ketotic hyperglycinemias: three cases. Neurology 28:139–146

Steinman L, Clancy RR, Cann H, Urich H (1983) The neuropathology of propionic acidemia. Dev Med Child Neurol 25:87–94

Surtees RAH, Matthews EE, Leonard JV (1992) Neurologic outcome of propionic acidemia. Pediatr Neurol 8:333–337

Thomas E (1992) Dietary management of inborn errors of amino acid metabolism with protein-modified diets. J Child Neurol 7 [Suppl]:S92–S111

Wolf B, Hsia YE, Sweetman L, Gravel R, Harris DJ, Nyhan WL (1981) Propionic acidemia:a clinical update. J Pediatr 99:835–846

33 Hyperprolinemia

Bellet H, Morin D, Daudet H, Dumas ML, Valette H, Magnan de Bornier B, Dumas R (1991) Type II hyperprolinaemia with renal involvement. J Inherited Metab Dis 14:846–847

Martin JJ, Schlote W (1972) Central nervous system lesions in disorders of amino-acid metabolism. J Neurol Sci 15:49–76

Ozand PT, Gascon GG (1991a) Organic acidurias: a review, part 1. J Child Neurol 6:196–219

Ozand PT, Gascon GG (1991b) Organic acidurias: a review, part 2. J Child Neurol 6:288–303

Phang JM, Scriver CR (1989) Disorders of proline and hydroxyproline metabolism. In: Scriver CR, Beaudet Al, Sly WS, Valle D (eds) The metabolic basis of inherited disease. McGraw-Hill, New York, pp 577–597

Steinlin M, Boltshauser E, Steinmann B, Wichmann W, Niemeyer G (1989) Hyperprolinaemia type I and white matter disease: coincidence or causal relationship? Eur J Pediatr 149:40–42

Wajner M, Wannmacher MD, Purkiss P (1990) High urinary excretion of N-(pyrrole-2-carboxyl) glycine in type II hyperprolinemia. Clin Genet 37:485–489

Woody NC, Snyder CH, Harris JA (1969) Hyperprolinemia: clinical and biochemical family study. Pediatrics 44:554–563

34 Nonketotic Hyperglycinemia

Agamanolis DP, Potter JL, Herrick MK, Sternberger NH (1982) The neuropathology of glycine encephalopathy: a report of five cases with immunohistochemical and ultrastructural observations. Neurology 32:975–985

Agamanolis DP, Potter JL, Lundgren DW (1993) Neonatal glycine encephalopathy: biochemical and neuropathologic findings. Pediatr Neurol 9:140–143

Anderson JM (1969) Spongy degeneration in the white matter of the central nervous system in the newborn: pathological findings in three infants, one with hyperglycinaemia. J Neurol Neurosurg Psychiatry 32:328–337

Kish SJ, Dixon LM, Burnham WM, Perry TL, Becker L, Cheng J, Chang LJ, Rebbetoy M (1988) Brain neurotransmitters in glycine encephalopathy. Ann Neurol 24:458–461

Martin JJ, Schlote W (1972) Central nervous system lesions in disorders of amino-acid metabolism. J Neurol Sci 15:49–76

Ohya Y, Ochi N, Mizutani N, Hayakawa C, Watanabe K (1991) Nonketotic hyperglycinemia: treatment with NMDA antagonist and consideration of neuropathogenesis. Pediatr Neurol 7:65–68

Ozand PT, Gascon GG (1991a) Organic acidurias: a review, part 1. J Child Neurol 6:196–219

Ozand PT, Gascon GG (1991b) Organic acidurias: a review, part 2. J Child Neurol 6:288–303

Press GA, Barshop BA, Haas RH, Nyhan WL, Glass RF, Hesselink JR (1989) Abnormalities of the brain in nonketotic hyperglycinemia: MR manifestations. AJNR 10:315–321

Schmitt B, Steinmann B, Gitzelmann R, Thun-Hohenstein L, Mascher H, Dumermuth G (1993) Nonketotic hyperglycinemia:clinical and electrophysiologic effects of dextromethorphan, an antagonist of the NMDA receptor. Neurology 43:421–424

Shuman RM, Leech RW, Scott CR (1978) The neuropathology of the nonketotic and ketotic hyperglycinemias: three cases. Neurology 28:139–146

Tada K, Kure S (1993) Non-ketotic hyperglycinaemia: molecular lesion, diagnosis and pathophysiology. J Inherited Metab Dis 16:691–703

Zammarchi E, Donati MA, Ciani F, Pasquini E, Pela I, Fiorini P (1994) Failure of early dextromethorphan and sodium benzoate therapy in an infant with nonketotic hyperglycinemia. Neuropediatrics 25:274–276

35 Maple Syrup Urine Disease

Banks WA, Kastin AJ (1988) Review: interactions between the blood-brain barrier and endogenous peptides: emerging clinical implications. Am J Med Sci 295:459–465

Berry GT, Heidenreich R, Kaplan P, Levine F, Mazur A, Palmieri MJ, Yudkoff M, Segal S (1991) Branched-chain amino acid-free parenteral nutrition in the treatment of acute metabolic decompensation in patients with maple syrup urine disease. N Engl J Med 324:175–179

Biggemann B, Zass R, Wendel U (1993) Postoperative metabolic decompensation in maple syrup urine disease is completely prevented by insulin. J Inherited Metab Dis 16:912–913

Brismar J, Aqeel A, Brismar G, Coates R, Gascon G, Ozand P (1990) Maple syrup urine disease: findings on CT and MR scans of the brain in 10 infants. AJNR 11:1219–1228

Chuang DT (1989) Molecular studies of mammalian branched-chain α-keto acid dehydrogenase complexes: domain structures, expression, and inborn errors. Ann NY Acad Sci 573:137–154

Ellerine NP, Herring WJ, Elsas LJ, McKean MC, Klein PD, Danner DJ (1993) Thiamin-responsive maple syrup urine disease in a patient antigenically missing dihydrolipoamide acyltransferase. Biochem Med Metab Biol 49:363–374

Felber SR, Sperl W, Chemelli A, Murr Ch, Wendel U (1993) Maple syrup urine disease: metabolic decompensation monitored by proton magnetic resonance imaging and spectroscopy. Ann Neurol 33:396–401

Fisher CW, Chuang JL, Griffin TA, Lau KS, Cox RP, Chuang DT (1989) Molecular phenotypes in cultured maple syrup urine disease cells. J Biol Chem 264:3448–3453

Fisher CW, Lau KS, Fisher CR, Wynn M, Cox RP, Chuang DT (1991a) A 17-bp insertion and a Phe215 → Cys missense mutation in the dihydrolipoyl transacylase (E$_2$) mRNA from a thiamine-responsive maple syrup urine disease patient WG-34. Biochem Biophys Res Commun 174:804–809

Fisher CR, Fisher CW, Chuang DT, Cox RP (1991b) Occurrence of a Tyr393 → Asn (Y393N) mutation in the E$_1\alpha$ geneof the branched-chain α-keto acid dehydrogenase complex in maple syrup urine disease patients from a mennonite population. Am J Hum Genet 49:429–434

Fisher CW, Fisher CR, Chuang JL, Lau KS, Chuang DT, Cox RP (1993) Occurrence of a 2-bp (AT) deletion allele and a nonsense (G-to-T) mutant allele at the E$_2$ (DBT) locus of six patients with maple syrup urine disease: multiple-exon skipping as a secondary effect of the mutations. Am J Hum Genet 52:414–424

Giacoia GP, Berry GT (1993) Acrodermatitis enteropathica-like syndrome secondary to isoleucine deficiency during treatment of maple syrup urine disease. Am J Dis Child 147:954–956

Harper PAW, Healy PJ, Dennis JA (1990) Animal model of human disease. Maple syrup urine disease (branched chain ketoaciduria). Am J Pathol 136:1445–1446

Herring WJ, Litwer S, Weber JL, Danner DJ (1991) Molecular genetic basis of maple syrup urine disease in a family with two defective alleles for branched chain acyltransferase and localization of the gene to human chromosome 1. Am J Hum Genet 48:342–350

Hilliges C, Awiszus D, Wendel U (1993) Intellectual performance of children with maple syrup urine disease. Eur J Pediatr 152:144–147

Indo Y, Akaboshi I, Nobukumi Y, Endo F, Matsuda I (1988) Maple syrup urine disease: a possible biochemical basis for the clinical heterogeneity. Hum Genet 80:6–10

Kamei A, Takashima S, Chan F, Becker LE (1992) Abnormal dendritic development in maple syrup urine disease. Pediatr Neurol 8:145–147

Kaplan P, Mazur A, Field M, Berlin JA, Berry GT, Heidenreich R, Yudkoff M, Segal S (1991) Intellectual outcome in children with maple syrup urine disease. J Pediatr 119:46–50

Langenbeck U, Wendel U, Mench-Hoinowski A, Kuschel D, Becker K, Przyrembel H, Bremer HJ (1978) Correlations between branched-chain amino acids and branched-chain α-keto acids in blood in maple syrup urine disease. Clin Chim Acta 88:283–291

Levin ML, Scheimann A, Lewis RA, Beaudet AL (1993) Cerebral edema in maple syrup urine disease. J Pediatr 122:167–168

Menkes JH, Solcher H (1967) Maple syrup disease. Arch Neurol 16:486–491

Menkes JH, Hurst PL, Craig JM (1954) A new syndrome: progressive familial infantile cerebral dysfunction associated with an unusual urinary substance. Pediatr 14:462–464

Menkes JH, Philippart M, Fiol RE (1965) Cerebral lipids in maple syrup disease. J Pediatr 66:584–594

Mitsubuchi H, Nobukuni Y, Akaboshi I, Indo Y, Endo F, Matsuda I (1991a) Maple syrup urine disease caused by a partial deletion in the inner E$_2$ core domain of the branched chain α-keto acid dehydrogenase complex due to aberrant splicing. J Clin Invest 87:1207–1211

Mitsubuchi H, Nobukuni Y, Endo F, Matsuda I (1991b) Structural organization and chromosomal localization of the gene for the E$_1$ β subunit of human branched chain α-keto acid dehydrogenase. J Biol Chem 266:14686–14691

Mitsubuchi H, Matsuda I, Nobukuni Y, Heidenreich R, Indo Y, Endo F, Mallee J, Segal S (1992) Gene analysis of Mennonite maple syrup urine disease kindred using primer-specified restriction map modification. J Inherited Metab Dis 15:181–187

Müller K, Kahn T, Wendel U (1993) Is demyelination a feature of maple syrup urine disease? Pediatr Neurol 9:375–382

Nobukuni Y, Mitsubuchi H, Akaboshi I, Indo Y, Endo F, Matsuda I (1991a) Maple syrup urine disease: clinical and biochemical significance of gene analysis. J Inherited Metab Dis 14:787–792

Nobukuni Y, Mistsubuchi H, Akaboshi I, Indo Y, Endo F, Yoshioka A, Matsuda I (1991b) Maple syrup urine disease. J Clin Invest 87:1862–1866

Nobukuni Y, Mitsubuchi H, Ohta K, Akaboshi I, Indo Y, Endo F, Matsuda I (1992) Molecular diagnosis of maple syrup urine disease:screening and identification of gene mutations in the branched-chain α-ketoacid dehydrogenase multienzyme complex. J Inherited Metab Dis 15:827–833

Nord A, van Doorninck WJ, Greene C (1991) Developmental profile of patients with maple syrup urine disease. J Inherited Metab Dis 14:881–889

Northrup H, Sigman ES, Hebert AA (1993) Exfoliative erythroderma resulting from inadequate intake of branched-chain amino acids in infants with maple syrup urine disease. Arch Dermatol 129:384–385

Parini R, Sereni LP, Bagozzi DC, Corbetta C, Rabier D, Narcy C, Hubert P, Saudubray JM (1993) Nasogastric drip feeding as the only treatment of neonatal maple syrup urine disease. Pediatrics 92:280–283

Parsons HG, Carter RJ, Unrath M, Snyder FF (1990) Evaluation of branched-chain amino acid intake in children with maple syrup urine disease and methylmalonic aciduria. J Inherited Metab Dis 13:125–136

Peinemann F, Danner DJ (1994) Maple syrup urine disease 1954 to 1993. J Inherited Metab Dis 17:3–15

Prensky AL, Moser HW (1966) Brain lipids, proteolipids, and free amino acids in maple syrup urine disease. J Neurochem 13:863–874

Prensky AL, Carr S, Moser HW (1968) Development of myelin in inherited disorders of amino acid metabolism. Arch Neurol 19:552–558

Riviello JJ, Rezvani I, DiGeorge AM, Foley CM (1991) Cerebral edema causing death in children with maple syrup urine disease. J Pediatr 119:42–45

Scriver CR, Clow CL, Mackenzie S, Delvin E (1971) Thiamine-responsive maple-syrup-urine disease. Lancet I:310–312

Scriver CR, Clow CL, George H (1985) So-called thiamin-responsive maple syrup urine disease: 15-year follow-up of the original patient. J Pediatr 107:763–765

Silberberg DH (1969) Maple syrup urine disease metabolites studies in cerebellum cultures. J Neurochem 16:1141–1146

Silberman J, Dancis J, Feigin I (1961) Neuropathological observations in maple syrup urine disease. Arch Neurol 5:351–363

Taccone A, Schiaffino MC, Cerone R, Fondelli MP, Romano C (1992) Computed tomography in maple syrup urine disease. Eur J Radiol 14:207–212

Tharp BR (1992) Unique EEG pattern (comb-like rhythm) in neonatal maple syrup urine disease. Pediatr Neurol 8:65–68

Thompson GN, Francis DEM, Halliday D (1991) Acute illness in maple syrup urine disease: dynamics of protein metabolism and implications for management. J Pediatr 119:35–41

Treacy E, Clow CL, Reade TR, Chitayat D, Mamer OA, Scriver CR (1992) Maple syrup urine disease: interrelations between branched-chain amino, oxo- and hydroxyacids; implications for treatment; associations with CNS dysmyelination. J Inherited Metab Dis 15:121–135

Tribble D, Shapira R (1983) Myelin proteins:degradation in rat brain initiated by metabolites causative of maple syrup urine disease. Biochem Biophys Res Commun 114:440–446

Uziel G, Savoiardo M, Nardocci N (1988) CT and MRI in maple syrup urine disease. Neurology 38:486–488

Van Calcar SC, Harding CO, Davidson SR, Barness LA, Wolff JA (1992) Case reports of successful pregnancy in women with maple syrup urine disease and propionic acidemia. Am J Med Genet 44:641–646

Verdu A, Lopez-Herce J, Pascual-Castroviejo I, Martinez-Bermejo A, Ugarte M, Garcia MJ (1985) Maple syrup urine disease variant form: presentation with psychomotor retardation and CT scan abnormalities. Acta Paediatr Scand 74:815–818

Zhang B, Kuntz MJ, Goodwin GW, Edenberg HJ, Crabb DW, Harris RA (1989a) cDNA cloning of the $E_1\alpha$ subunitof the branched-chain α-keto acid dehydrogenase and elucidation of a molecular basis for maple syrup urine disease. Ann NY Acad Sci 573:130–136

Zhang B, Edenberg HJ, Crabb DW, Harris RA (1989b) Evidence for both a regulatory mutation and a structural mutation in a family with maple syrup urine disease. J Clin Invest 83:1425–1429

Zhang B, Wappner RS, Brandt IK, Harris RA, Crabb DW (1990) Sequence of the $E_1\alpha$ subunit of branched-chain α-ketoacid dehydrogenase in two patients with thiamine-responsive maple syrup urine disease. Am J Hum Genet 46:843–846

Zneimer SM, Lau KS, Eddy RL, Shows TB, Chuang JL, Chuang DT, Cox RP (1991) Regional assignment of two genes of the human branched-chain α-keto acid dehydrogenase complex: the E_1 β gene (BCKDHB) to chromosome 6p21-22 and the E_2 gene (DBT) to chromosome 1p31. Genomics 10:740–747

36 Canavan's Disease

Adachi M, Volk BW (1968) Protracted form of spongy degeneration of the central nervous system. Neurology 18:1084–1092

Adachi M, Wallace BJ, Schneck L, Volk BW (1966) Fine structure of spongy degeneration of the central nervous system (van Bogaert and Bertrand type). Neuropathol Exp Neurol 25:598–616

Adachi M, Torii J, Schneck L, Volk BW (1972) Electron microscopic and enzyme histochemical studies of the cerebellum in spongy degeneration. Acta Neuropathol (Berl) 20:22–31

Adachi M, Schneck L, Cara J, Volk BW (1973) Spongy degeneration of the central nervous system (Van Bogaert and Bertrand type; Canavan's disease). Hum Pathol 4:331–347

Austin SJ, Connelly A, Gadian DG, Benton JS, Brett EM (1991) Localized 1H NMR spectroscopy in Canavan's disease: a report of two cases. Magn Reson Med 19:439–445

Banker BQ, Robertson JT, Victor M (1964) Spongy degeneration of the central nervous system in infancy. Neurology 14:981–1001

Barker PB, Bryan RN, Kumar AJ, Naidu S (1992) Proton NMR spectroscopy of Canavan's disease. Neuropediatrics 23:263–267

Bartallini G, Margollicci M, Balestri P, Farnetani MA, Cioni M, Fois A (1992) Biochemical diagnosis of Canavan disease. Childs Nerv Syst 8:468–470

Bennett MJ, Gibson KM, Sherwood WG, Divry P, Rolland MO, Elpeleg ON, Rinaldo P, Jakobs C (1993) Reliable prenatal diagnosis of Canavan disease (aspartoacylase deficiency): comparison of enzymatic and metabolite analysis. J Inherited Metab Dis 16:831–836

Birken DL, Oldendorf WH (1989) N-acetyl-L-aspartic acid:a literature review of a compound prominent in 1H-NMR spectroscopic studies of the brain. Neurosci Biobehav Rev 13:23–31

Brismar J, Brismar G, Gascon G, Ozand P (1990) Canavan disease: CT and MR imaging of the brain. AJNR 11:805–810

Brown LW, Rorke LB, Deray MJ, Smith SB, Altman N (1985–1986) Psychomotor retardation and macrocephaly in an infant. Pediatr Neurosci 12:266–271

De Coo IFM, Gabreëls FJM, Renier WO, de Pont JJHHM, Hälst UJGM, Veerkamp JH, Trijbels JMF, Jaspar HHJ, Renkawek (1991) Canavan disease: neuromorphological and biochemical analysis of a brain biopsy specimen. Clin Neuropathol 10:73–78

Divry P, Vianey-Liaud C, Gay C, Maçabeo V, Rapin F, Echenne B (1988) N-acetylaspartic aciduria: report of three new cases in children with a neurological syndrome associating macrocephaly and leukodystrophy. J Inherited Metab Dis 11:307–308

Echenne B, Divry P, Vlaney-Liaud C (1989) Spongy degeneration of the neuraxis (Canavan-Van Bogaert disease) and N-acetylaspartic aciduria. Neuropediatrics 20:70–81

Gascon GG, Ozand PT, Mahdi A, Jamil A, Haider A, Brismar J, Al-Nasser M (1990) Infantile CNS spongy degeneration – 14 cases: clinical update. Neurology 40:1876–1882

Gascon GG, Youssef NG, Subramanyam SB, Ozand PT (1992) Coincident neuraminidase and aspartoacylase deficiency associated with chromosome 9q paracentric inversion in a Saudi family. J Child Neurol [Suppl 7]:S73–S78

Grod W, Krägeloh-Mann I, Petersen D, Trefz FK, Harzer K (1990) In vivo assessment of N-acetylaspartate in brain in spongy degeneration (Canavan's disease) by proton spectroscopy. Lancet 336:437–438

Hagenfeldt L, Bollgren I, Venizelos N (1987) N-acetylaspartic aciduria due to aspartoacylase deficiency – a new aetiology of childhood leucodystrophy. J Inherited Metab Dis 10:135–141

Hamaguchi H, Nihei K, Nakamoto N, Ezoe T, Naito H, Hara M, Yokota K, Inoue Y, Matsumoto I (1993) A case of Canavan disease: the first biochemically proven case in a Japanese girl. Brain Dev 15:367–371

Jacobs C, ten Brink HJ, Divry P, Rolland MO (1992) Prenatal detection of Canavan disease. Eur J Pediatr 151:620

Jacobs JM, LeQuesne PM (1992) Toxic disorders. In: Adams JH, Duchen LW (eds) Greenfields neuropathology. Arnold, London, pp 881–987

Kamoshita S, Rapin I, Suzuki K, Suzuki K (1968) Spongy degeneration of the brain. Neurology 18:975–985

Kaul R, Gao GP, Balamurugan K, Matalon R (1993) Cloning of the human aspartoacylase cDNA and a predominant missense mutation in Canavan disease. Nature Genet 5:118–123

Kaul R, Gao GP, Balamurugan K, Matalon R (1994) Canavan disease:molecular basis of aspartoacylase deficiency. J Inherited Metab Dis 17:295–297

Kelley RI (1993) Prenatal detection of Canavan disease by measurement of N-acetyl-L-aspartate in amniotic fluid. J Inherited Metab Dis 16:918–919

Kendall BE (1992) Disorders of lysosomes, peroxisomes, and mitochondria. AJNR 13:621–653

Kvittingen EA, Guldal G, Borsting S, Skalpe IO, Stokke O, Jellum E (1986) N-acetylaspartic aciduria in a child with a progressive cerebral atrophy. Clin Chim Acta 158:217–227

Lee JC, Bakay L (1965) Ultrastructural changes in the edematous central nervous system. Arch Neurol 13:48–57

Lo WD, Sander JE, Königsberger MR (1985) Similarity of brain CT appearance in spongy degeneration to that of subacute necrotizing encephalomyelopathy. Ann Neurol 18:352–354

Mahloudji M, Daneshbod K, Karjoo M (1970) Familial spongy degeneration of the brain. Arch Neurol 22:294–298

Marks HG, Caro PA, Wang Z, Detre JA, Bogdan AR, Gusnard DA, Zimmerman RA (1991) Use of computed tomography, magnetic resonance imaging, and localized 1H magnetic resonance spectroscopy in Canavan's disease: a case report. Ann Neurol 30:106–110

Matalon R, Michals K, Sebesta D, Deanching M, Gashkoff P, Casanova J (1988) Aspartoacylase deficiency and N-acetyl-aspartic aciduria in patients with Canavan disease. Am J Med Genet 29:463–471

Matalon R, Kaul R, Casanova J, Michals K, Johnson A, Rapin I, Gashkoff P, Deanching M (1989) Aspartoacylase deficiency: the enzyme defect in Canavan disease. J Inherited Metab Dis 12 [Suppl 2]:329–331

Matalon R, Kaul R, Michals K (1993) Canavan disease: biochemical and molecular studies. J Inherited Metab Dis 16:744–752

Meyding-Lamadé U, Sartor K (1993) Magnetresonanztomographie bei neurodegenerativen Erkrankungen im Kindesalter. Klin Neuroradiol 3:52–61

Ozand PT, Gascon GG, Dhalla M (1990) Aspartoacylase deficiency and Canavan disease in Saudi Arabia. Am J Med Genet 35:266–268

Page McAdams H, Geyer CA, Done SL, Deigh D, Mitchell M, Ghaed VN (1990) CT and MR imaging of Canavan disease. AJNR 11:397–399

Patel TB, Clark JB (1979) Synthesis of N-acetyl-L-aspartate by rat brain mitochondria and its involvement in mitochondrial/cytosolic carbon transport. Biochem J 184:539–546

Paulus W, Peiffer J (1990) Intracerebral distribution of mitochondrial abnormalities in 21 cases of infantile spongy dystrophy. J Neurol Sci 95:49–62

Rolland MO, Divry P, Mandon G, Thoulon JM, Fiumara A, Matthieu M (1993) First-trimester prenatal diagnosis of Canavan disease. J Inherited Metab Dis 16:581–583

Runge VM, Wood ML, Kaufman DM, Trail MR, Nelson KL (1988) The straight and narrow path to good head and spine MRI. Radiographics 8:507–531

Subramanyam SB, Tipirneni A, Youssef N, Gascon GG, Ozand PT (1992) Biochemical heterogeneity of infantile central nervous system spongy degeneration. J Child Neurol [Suppl] 7:S22-S25

Toft PB, Geiss-Holtorff R, Roland MO, Pryd SO, Mueller-Forell W, Christensen E, Lehnert W, Lou HC, Ott D, Hennig J, Henriksen O (1993) Magnetic resonance imaging in juvenile Canavan disease. Eur J Pediatr 152:750–753

Towfighi J, Gonatas NK (1976) Hexachlorophene and the nervous system. Prog Neuropathol 3:101–113

Van Bogaert L, Bertrand I (1933) Les leucodystrophies progressives familiales. Rev Neurol 2:249–286

Van Moers A, Sperner J, Michael Th, Scheffner D, Schutgens RHB (1991) Variable course of Canavan disease in two boys with early infantile aspartoacylase deficiency. Dev Med Child Neurol 33:824–828

Yalaz K, Topcu H, Topaloglu O, Guercay OE, Oezcan B, Oenol B, Renda Y (1990) N-acetylaspartic aciduria in Canavan disease:another proof in two infants. Neuropediatrics 21:140–142

Zelnik N, Amir N, Luder AS, Hemli JA, Elpeleg ON, Fatal A, Gross-Tsur V, Harel S (1993) Protracted clinical course for patients with Canavan disease. Dev Med Child Neurol 35:346–358

37   L-2-Hydroxyglutaric Aciduria

Barth PG, Hoffmann GF, Jaeken J, Lehnert W, Hanefeld F, van Gennip AH, Duran M, Valk J, Schutgens RBH, Trefz FK, Reimann G, Hartung HP (1992) L-2-hydroxyglutaric acidemia: a novel inherited neurometabolic disease. Ann Neurol 32:66–71

Barth PG, Hoffmann GF, Jaeken J, Wanders RJA, Duran M, Jansen GA, Jakobs C, Lehnert W, Hanefeld F, Valk J, Schutgens RBH, Trefz FK, Hartung HP, Chamoles NA, Sfaello Z, Caruso U (1993) L-2-hydroxyglutaric acidaemia: clinical and biochemical findings in 12 patients and preliminary report on L-2-hydroxyacid dehydrogenase. J Inherited Metab Dis 16:753–761

Divry P, Jakobs C, Vianey-Saban C, Gibson KM, Michelakakis H, Papaimitriou A, Divari R, Chabrol B, Cournelle MA, Livet MO (1993) L-2-hydroxyglutaric aciduria: two further cases. J Inherited Metab Dis 16:505–507

Duran M, Kamerling JP (1980) L-2-hydroxyglutaric aciduria. J Inherited Metab Dis 3:109–112

Gibson KM, ten Brink HJ, Schor SM, Kok RM, Bootsma AH, Hoffmann GF, Jakobs C (1993) Stable-isotope dilution analysis of D- and L-2-hydroxyglutaric acid: application to the detection and prenatal diagnosis of D- and L-2-hydroxyglutaric acidemias. Pediatr Res 34:277–280

Jaeken J, Willekens H (1988) Leukodystrophy associated with hyperlysinorhachia and 2-hydroxyglutaric aciduria. Pediatr Res 24:266

Jansen GA, Wanders RJA (1993) L-2-hydroxyglutarate dehydrogenase: identification of a novel enzyme activity in rat and human liver. Implications for L-2-hydroxyglutaric acidemia. Biochim Biophys Acta 1225:53–56

Kaabachi N, Larnaout A, Rabier D, Jakobs C, Belal S, Hentati F, Parvey P, Bardet J, Hamida MB, Mebazaa A, Kamoun P (1993) Familial encephalopathy and L-2-hydroxyglutaric aciduria. J Inherited Metab Dis 16:893

Larnaout A, Hentati F, Belal S, Ben Hamida C, Kaabachi N, Ben Hamida M (1994) Clinical and pathological study of three Tunisian siblings with L-2-hydroxyglutaric aciduria. Acta Neuropathol (Berl) 88:367–370

Wilcken B, Pitt J, Heath D, Walsh P, Wilson G, Buchanan M (1993) L-2-hydroxyglutaric aciduria: three Australian cases. J Inherited Metab Dis 16:501–504

38 Hyperhomocysteinemias

Bartholomew DW, Batshaw ML, Allen RH, Roe CR, Rosenblatt D, Valle DL, Francomano CA (1988) Therapeutic approaches to cobalamin-C methylmalonic acidemia and homocystinuria. J Pediatr 112:32–39

Beckman DR, Hoganson G, Berlow S, Gilbert EF (1987) Pathological findings in 5,10-methylene tetrahydrofolate reductase deficiency. Birth Defects 23:47–64

Bellini C, Cerone R, Bonacci W, Caruso U, Magliano CP, Serra G, Fowler B, Romano C (1992) Biochemical diagnosis and outcome of 2 years treatment in a patient with combined methylmalonic aciduria and homocystinuria. Eur J Pediatr 151:818–820

Beradelli A, Thompson PD, Zaccagnini M, Giardini O, Eufemia PD, Massoud R, Manfredi M (1991) Two sisters with generalized dystonia associated with homocystinuria. Movement Dis 6:163–165

Brattström L, Israelsson B, Lindgärde F, Hultberg B (1988) Higher total plasma homocysteine in vitamin B_{12} deficiency than in heterozygosity for homocystinuria due to cystathionine β-synthase deficiency. Metabolism 37:175–178

Carmel R, Watkins D, Goodman SI, Rosenblatt DS (1988) Hereditary defect of cobalamin metabolism (cblG mutation) presenting as a neurologic disorder in adulthood. N Engl J Med 318:1738–1741

Carmel R (1988) Pernicious anemia. Arch Intern Med 148:1712–1714

Carson NAJ, Dent CE, Field CMB, Gaull GE (1965) Homocystinuria. J Pediatr 66:565–583

Chou SM, Waisman HA (1965) Spongy degeneration of the central nervous system. Arch Pathol Lab Med 79:357–363

Clayton PT, Smith I, Harding B, Hyland K, Leonard JV, Leeming RJ (1986) Subacute combined degeneration of the cord, dementia and Parkinsonism due to an inborn error of folate metabolism. J Neurol Neurosurg Psychiatry 49:920–927

Dayan AD, Ramsey RB (1974) An inborn error of vitamin B_{12} metabolism associated with cellular deficiency of coenzyme forms of the vitamin. J Neurol Sci 23:117–128

Duchen LW, Jacobs JM (1992) Nutritional deficiencies and metabolic disorders. In: Adams JH, Duchen LW (eds) Greenfield's neuropathology, 5th edn. Arnold, London, pp 811–880

Dunn HG, Perry TL, Dolman CL (1966) Homocystinuria. Neurology 16:407–420

Fenton WA, Rosenberg LE (1978) Genetic and biochemical analysis of human cobalamin mutants in cell culture. Annu Rev Genet 12:223–248

Fine EJ, Soria E, Paroski MW, Petryk D, Thomasula L (1990) The neurophysiological profile of vitamin B_{12} deficiency. Muscle Nerve 13:158–164

Flippo TS, Holder WD (1993) Neurologic degeneration associated with nitrous oxide anesthesia in patients with vitamin B_{12} deficiency. Arch Surg 128:1391–1395

Garewal G, Narang A, Das KC (1988) Infantile tremor syndrome: a vitamin B_{12} deficiency syndrome in infants. J Trop Pediatr 34:174–178

Gerritsen T, Waisman HA (1964) Homocystinuria, an error in the metabolism of methionine. Pediatrics 33:413–420

Graham SM, Arvela OM, Wise GA (1992) Long-term neurologic consequences of nutritional vitamin B_{12} deficiency in infants. J Pediatr 121:710–714

Haworth JC, Dilling LA, Surtees RAH, Seargeant LE, Shing HL, Cooper BA, Rosenblatt DS (1993) Symptomatic and asymptomatic methylenetetrahydrofolate reductase deficiency in two adult brothers. Am J Med Genet 45:572–576

Healton EB, Savage DG, Brust JCM, Garrett TJ, Lindenbaum J (1991) Neurologic aspects of cobalamin deficiency. Medicine 70:229–245

Hector M, Burton JR (1988) What are the psychiatric manifestations of vitamin B_{12} deficiency? J Am Geriatr Soc 36:1105–1112

Higginbottom MC, Sweetman L, Nyhan WL (1978) A syndrome of methylmalonic aciduria, homocystinuria, megalobastic anemia and neurologic abnormalities in a vitaman B_{12} deficient breast-fed infant of a strict vegetarian. N Engl J Med 299:317–323

Hoffbrand AV, Jackson BFA (1993) Correction of the DNA synthesis defect in vitamin B_{12} deficiency by tetrahydrofolate: evidence in favour of the methyl-folate trap hypothesis as the cause of megaloblastic anaemia in vitamin B_{12} deficiency. Br J Haematol 83:643–647

Holloway KL, Alberico AM (1990) Postoperative myeloneuropathy:a preventable complication in patients with B_{12} deficiency. J Neurosurg 72:732–736

Hyland K, Smith I, Bottiglieri T, Perry J, Wendel U, Clayton PT, Leonard JV (1988) Demyelination and decreased S-adenosylmethionine in 5,10-methylenetetrahydrofolate reductase deficiency. Neurology 38:459–462

Keskin S, Yalcin E (1994) Case report of homocystinuria:clinical, electroencephalographic, and magnetic resonance imaging findings. J Child Neurol 9:210–211

Kishi T, Kawamura I, Harada Y, Eguchi T, Sakura N, Ueda K, Narisawa K, Rosenblatt DS (1994) Effect of betaine on S-adenosylmethionine levels in the cerebrospinal fluid in a patient with methylenetetrahydrofolate reductase deficiency and peripheral neuropathy. J Inherited Metab Dis 17:560–565

Kraus JP (1994) Molecular basis of phenotype expression in homocystinuria. J Inherited Metab Dis 17:383–390

Kühne T, Bubl R, Baumgartner R (1991) Maternal vegan diet causing a serious infantile neurological disorder due to vitamin B_{12} deficiency. Eur J Pediatr 150:205–208

Lee CC, Surtees R, Duchen LW (1992) Distal motor axonopathy and central nervous system myelin vacuolation caused by cycloleucine, an inhibitor of methionine adenosyltransferase. Brain 115:935–955

Lever EG, Elwes RDC, Williams A, Reynolds EH (1986) Subacute combined degeneration of the cord due to folate deficiency: response to methyl folate treatment. J Neurol Neurosurg Psychiatry 49:1203–1207

Lindenbaum J, Healton EB, Savage DG, Brust JCM, Garrett TJ, Podell ER, Marcell PD, Stabler SP, Allen RH (1988) Neuropsychiatric disorders caused by cobalamin deficiency in the absence of anemia or macrocytosis. N Engl J Med 318:1720–1728

Ludolph AC, Ullrich K, Bick U, Fahrendorf G, Pzyrembel H (1991) Functional and morphological deficits in late-treated patients with homocystinuria: a clinical, electrophysiologic and MRI study. Acta Neurol Scand 83:161–165

Mitchell GA, Watkins D, Melançon SB, Rosenblatt DS, Geoffroy G, Orquin J, Homsy MB, Dallaire L (1986) Clinical heterogeneity in cobalamin C variant of combined homocystinuria and methylmalonic aciduria. J Pediatr 108:410–415

Murata S, Naritomi H, Sawada T (1994) MRI in subacute combined degeneration. Neuroradiology 36:408–409

Narayanan MN, Dawson DW, Lewis MJ (1991) Dietary deficiency of vitamin B_{12} is associated with low serum cobalamin levels in non-vegetarians. Eur J Haematol 47:115–118

Nishimura M, Yoshino K, Tomita Y, Takashima S, Tanaka J, Narisawa K, Kurobane I (1985) Central and peripheral nervous system pathology of homocystinuria due to 5,10-methylenetetrahydrofolate reductase deficiency. Pediatr Neurol 1:375–378

Perry J, Chanarin I, Deacon R, Lumb M (1990) Methylation of DNA in megaloblastic anaemia. J Clin Pathol 43:211–212

Reynolds EH, Bottiglieri T, Laundy M, Stern J, Payan J, Linnell J, Faludy J (1993) Subacute combined degeneration with high serum vitamin B_{12} level and abnormal vitamin B_{12} binding protein. Arch Neurol 50:739–742

Schuh S, Rosenblatt DS, Cooper BA, Schroeder ML, Bishop AJ, Seargeant LE, Haworth JC (1984) Homocystinuria and megaloblastic anemia responsive to vitamin B_{12} therapy. N Engl J Med 310:686–690

Shevell MI, Rosenblatt DS (1992) The neurology of cobalamin. Can J Neurol Sci 19:472–486

Shinnar S, Singer HS (1984) Cobalamin C mutation (methylmalonic aciduria and homocystinuria) in adolescence. N Engl J Med 311:451–454

Shojania AM (1984) Folic acid and vitamin B_{12} deficiency in pregnancy and in the neonatal period. Clin Perinatol 11:433–459

Soria ED, Fine EJ (1992) Somatosensory evoked potentials in the neurological sequelae of treated vitamin B_{12} deficiency. Electromyogr Clin Neurophysiol 32:63–71

Stabler SP, Allen RH, Savage DG, Lindenbaum J (1990) Clinical spectrum and diagnosis of cobalamin deficiency. Blood 76:871–881

Steiner I, Kidron D, Soffer D, Wirguin I, Abramsky O (1988) Sensory peripheral neuropathy of vitamin B_{12} deficiency: a primary demyelinating disease? J Neurol 235:163–164

Surtees R (1993) Biochemical pathogenesis of subacute combined degeneration of the spinal cord and brain. J Inherited Metab Dis 16:762–770

Surtees R, Leonard J, Austin S (1991) Association of demyelination with deficiency of cerebrospinal-fluid-S-adenosylmethionine in inborn errors of methyl-transfer pathway. Lancet 338:1550–1554

Surtees R, Heales S, Bowron A (1994) Association of cerebrospinal fluid deficiency of 5-methyltetrahydrofolate, but not S-adenosylmethionine, with reduced concentrations of the acid metabolites of 5-hydroxytryptamine and dopamine. Clin Sci 86:697–702

Timms SR, Curé JK, Kurent JE (1993) Subacute combined degeneration of the spinal cord:MR findings. AJNR 14:1224–1227

Tracey JP, Schiffman FJ (1992) Magnetic resonance imaging in cobalamin deficiency. Lancet 339:1172–1173

Tuchman M, Kelly P, Watkins D, Rosenblatt DS (1988) Vitamin B_{12}-responsive megaloblastic anemia, homocystinuria, and transient methylmalonic aciduria in cblE disease. J Pediatr 113:1052–1055

Van den Berg M, van der Knaap MS, Boers GHJ, Stehouwer CDA, Rauwerda JA, Valk J (1995) Neuroradiological aspects of hyperhomocysteinemia. Neuroradiology (to be published)

Van Diemen-Steenvoorde R, van Nieuwenhuizen O, de Klerk JBC, Duran M (1990) Quasi-Moyamoya disease and heterozygosity for homocystinuria in a five-year-old girl. Neuropediatrics 21:110–112

Visy JM, le Coz P, Chadefaux B, Fressinaud C, Woimant F, Marquet J, Zittoun J, Visy J, Vallat JM, Haguenau M (1991) Homocystinuria due to 5,10-methylenetetrahydrofolate reductase deficiency revealed by stroke in adult siblings. Neurology 41:1313–1315

Vonsattel JPG, Hedley-Whyte ET (1989) Homocystinuria. In: Toole JF (ed) Handbook of clinical neurology, vol 11. Science, Amsterdam, pp 325–334

Walk D, Kang SS, Horwitz A (1994) Intermittent encephalopathy, reversible nerve conduction slowing, and MRI evidence of cerebral white matter disease in methylenetatrahydrofolate reductase deficiency. Neurology 44:344–347

Watkins D, Rosenblatt DS (1988) Genetic heterogeneity among patients with methylcobalamin deficiency. J Clin Invest 81:1690–1694

Weir DG, Molloy AM, Keating JN, Young PB, Kennedy S, Kennedy DG, Scott JM (1992) Correlation of the ratio of S-adenosyl-L-methionine to S-adenosyl-L-homocysteine in the brain and cerebrospinal fluid of the pig:implications for the determination of this methylation ratio in human brain. Clin Sci 82:93–97

White HH, Rowland LP, Araki S, Thompson HL, Cowen D (1965) Homocystinuria. Arch Neurol 13:455–470

39 Urea Cycle Defects

Aida S, Ogata T, Kamota T, Nakamura N (1989) Primary ornithine transcarbamylase deficiency. Acta Pathol Jpn 39:451–456

Bachmann C (1992) Ornithine carbamoyl transferase deficiency:findings, models and problems. J Inherited Metab Dis 15:578–591

Batshaw ML (1994) Inborn errors of urea synthesis. Ann Neurol 35:133–141

Berrez JM, Bardot O, Thiard MC, Alvarez F, Latruff N (1991) Molecular analysis of a human liver mitochondrial ornithine transcarbamylase deficiency. J Inherited Metab Dis 14:29–36

Brockstedt M, Smit LME, de Grauw AJC, van der Klei-van Moorsel JM, Jakobs C (1990) A new case of hyperargininaemia: neurological and biochemical findings prior to and during dietary treatment. Eur J Pediatr 149:341–343

Bruton CJ, Corsellis JAN, Russell A (1970) Hereditary hyperammonaemia. Brain 93:423–434

Burlina AB, Bachmann C, Wermuth B, Bordugo A, Ferrari V, Colombo JP, Zacchello F (1992) Partial N-acetylglutamate synthetase deficiency:a new case with uncontrollable movement disorders. J Inherited Metab Dis 15:395–398

Carstens RP, Fenton WA, Rosenberg LR (1991) Identification of RNA splicing errors resulting in human ornithine transcarbamylase deficiency. Am J Hum Genet 48:1105–1114

Christodoulou J, Qureshi IA, McInnes RR, Clarke JTR (1993) Ornithine transcarbamylase deficiency presenting with strokelike episodes. J Pediatr 122:423–425

Connelly A, Cross JH, Gadian DG, Hunter JV, Kirkham FJ, Leonard JV (1993) Magnetic resonance spectroscopy shows increased brain glutamine in ornithine carbamoyl transferase deficiency. Pediatr Res 33:77–81

Dolman CL, Clasen RA, Dorovini-Zis K (1988) Severe cerebral damage in ornithine transcarbamylase deficiency. Clin Neuropathol 7:10–15

Donn SM, Thone JG (1985) Prospective prevention of neonatal hyperammonaemia in argininosuccinic acidura by arginine therapy. J Inherited Metab Dis 8:18–20

Feldmann D, Rozet JM, Pelet A, Hentzen D, Briand P, Hubert P, Largilliere C, Rabier D, Farriaux JP, Munnich A (1992) Site specific screening for point mutations in ornithine transcarbamylase deficiency. J Med Genet 29:471–475

Finkelstein JE, Hauser ER, Leonard CO, Brusilow SW (1990) Late-onset ornithine transcarbamylase deficiency in male patients. J Pediatr 117:897–902

Gallagher JV, Rifai N, Conry J, Soldin SJ (1991) Role of the clinical laboratory in evaluation of argininosuccinate lyase deficiency. Clin Chem 37:1384–1389

Gerrits GPJM, Gabreëls FJM, Monnens LAH, De Abreu RA, van Raaij-Selten B, Niezen-Koning KE, Trijbels JMF (1993) Arginiosuccinic aciduria:clinical and biochemical findings in three children with the late onset form, with special emphasis on cerebrospinal fluid findings of amino acids and pyrimidines. Neuropediatrics 21:15–18

Grody WW, Klein D, Dodson AE, Kern RM, Wissmann PB, Goodman BK, Bassand P, Marescau B, Kang SS, Leonard JV, Cederbaum SD (1992) Molecular genetic study of human arginase deficiency. Am J Hum Genet 50:1281–1290

Grody WW, Kern RM, Klein D, Dodson AE, Wissman PB, Barsky SH, Cederbaum SD (1993) Arginase deficiency manifesting delayed clinical sequelae and induction of a kidney arginase isozyme. Hum Genet 91:1–5

Grompe M, Caskey CT, Fenwick RG (1991) Improved molecular diagnostics for ornithine transcarbamylase deficiency. Am J Hum Genet 48:212–222

Harding BN, Leonard JV, Erdohazi M (1984) Ornithine carbamoyl transferase deficiency:a neuropathological study. Eur J Pediatr 141:215–220

Häussinger D, Steeb R, Gerok W (1992) Metabolic alkalosis as driving force for urea synthesis in liver disease: pathogenetic model and therapeutic implications. Clin Invest 70:411–415

Hayakawa C, Aono S, Keino H, Mizutani N, Watanabe K, Ikemoto M, Totani M, Murachi T, Kashiwamata S (1991) Absence of erythrocyte arginase protein in Japanese patients with hyperargininemia. Eur J Pediatr 150:800–803

Hommmes FA, de Groot CJ, Wilmink CW, Jonxis JHP (1969) Carbamylphosphate synthetase deficiency in an infant with severe cerebral damage. Arch Dis Child 44:688–693

Honeycutt D, Callahan K, Rutledge L, Evans B (1992) Heterozygote ornithine transcarbamylase deficiency presenting as symptomatic hyperammonemia during initiation of valproate therapy. Neurology 42:666–668

Hopkins IJ, Connelly JF, Dawson AG, Hird FJR, Maddison TG (1969) Hyperammonaemia due to ornithine transcarbamylase deficiency. Arch Dis Child 44:143–148

Horiuchi M, Imamura Y, Nakamura N, Maruyama I, Saheki T (1993) Carbamoylphosphate synthetase deficiency in an adult: deterioration due to administration of valproic acid. J Inherited Metab Dis 16:39–45

Hudak ML, Douglas Jones M, Brusilow SW (1985) Differentiation of transient hyperammonemia of the newborn and urea cycle enzyme defects by clinical presentation. J Pediatr 107:712–719

Kendall BE (1992) Disorders of lysosomes, peroxisomes, and mitochondria. AJNR 13:621–653

Kobayashi K, Itakura Y, Saheki T, Nakano K, Sase M, Oyanagi K, Okamoto R, Mino M (1986) Absence of argininosuccinate lyase protein in the liver of two patients with argininosuccinic aciduria. Clin Chim Acta 159:59–67

Kornfeld M, Woodfin BM, Papile L, Davis LE, Bernard LR (1985) Neuropathology of ornithine carbamyl transferase deficiency. Acta Neuropathol (Berl) 65:261–264

Levin B, Abraham JM, Oberholzer VG, Burgess EA (1969) Hyperammonaemia: a deficiency of liver ornithine transcarbamylase. Arch Dis Child 44:152–161

Maestri NE, Hauser ER, Bartholomew D, Brusilow SW (1991) Prospective treatment of urea cycle disorders. J Pediatr 119:923–928

Mamourian AC, du Plessis A (1991) Urea cycle defect: a case with MR and CT findings resembling infarct. Pediatr Radiol 21:594–595

Marescau B, de Deyn PP, Lowenthal A, Qureshi IA, Antonozzi I, Bachmann C, Cederbaum SD, Cerone R, Chamoles N, Colombo JP, Hyland K, Gatti R, Kang SS, Letarte J, Lambert M, Mizutani N, Possemiers I, Rezvani I, Snyderman SE, Terheggen HG, Yoshino M (1990) Guanidino compound analysis as a complementary diagnostic parameter for hyperargininemia: follow-up of guanidino compound levels during therapy. Pediatr Res 27:297–303

Martin JJ, Farriaux JP, De Jonghe P (1982) Neuropathology of citrullinemia. Acta Neuropathol (Berl) 56:303–306

Matsuda I, Nagata N, Matsuura T, Oyanagi K, Tada K, Narisawa K, Kitagawa T, Sakiyama T, Yamashita F, Yoshino M (1991) Retrospective survey of urea cycle disorders: part 1. Clinical and laboratory observations of thirty-two Japanese male patients with ornithine transcarbamylase deficiency. Am J Med Genet 38:85–89

Matsuura T, Hoshide R, Fukushima M, Sakiyama T, Owada M, Matsuda I (1993a) Prenatal monitoring of ornithine transcarbamoylase deficiency in two families by DNA analysis. J Inherited Metab Dis 16:31–38

Matsuura T, Hoshide R, Setoyama C, Shimada K, Hase Y, Yanagawa T, Kajita M, Matsuda I (1993b) Four novel gene mutations in five Japanese male patients with neonatal or late onset OTC deficiency:application of PCR-single-strand conformation polymorphisms for all exons and adjacent introns. Hum Genet 92:49–56

Mayatepek E, Kurczynski TW, Hoppel CL, Gunning WT (1991) Carnitine deficiency associated with ornithine transcarbamylase deficiency. Pediatr Neurol 7:196–199

McInnes RR, Shih V, Chilton S (1984) Interallelic complementation in an inborn error of metabolism: genetic heterogeneity in argininosuccinate lyase deficiency. Proc Natl Acad Sci U S A 81:4480–4484

Msali M, Batshaw ML, Suss R, Brusilow SW, Mellits ED (1984) Neurologic outcome in children with inborn errors of urea synthesis. N Engl J Med 310:1500–1505

Olier J, Gallego J, Digon E (1989) Computerized tomography in primary hyperammonemia. Neuroradiology 31:356–257

Qureshi IA, Letarte J, Ouellet R, Larochelle J, Lemieux B (1983) A new French-Canadian family affected by hyperarginiaemia. J Inherited Metab Dis 6:179–182

Simard L, O'Brien WE, McInnes RR (1986) Argininosuccinate lyase deficiency:evidence for heterogeneous structural gene mutations by immunoblotting. Am J Hum Genet 39:38–51

Slomski R, Braulke I, Behrend C, Schröder E, Colombo JP, Reiss J (1992) Ornithine transcarbamylase (OTC) deficiency in a female patient with a de novo deletion of the paternal X chromosome. Hum Genet 89:632–634

Solitare GB, Shih VE, Nelligan DJ, Dolan TF (1969) Argininosuccinic aciduria: clinical, biochemical, anatomical and neuropathological observations. J Ment Defic Res 13:153–170

Strautnicks S, Rutland P, Malcolm S (1991) Arginine 109 to glutamine mutation in a girl with ornithine carbamoyl transferase deficiency. J Med Genet 28:871–874

Travers H, Reed JS, Kennedy JA (1986) Ultrastructural study of the liver in argininosuccinase deficiency. Pediatr Pathol 5:307–318

Tsai MY, Holzknecht RA, Tuchman M (1993) Single-strand conformational polymorphism and direct sequencing applied to carrier testing in families with ornithine transcarbamylase deficiency. Hum Genet 91:321–325

Tuchman M (1992) The clinical, biochemical, and molecular spectrum of ornithine transcarbamylase deficiency. J Lab Clin Med 120:836–850

Tuchman M (1993) Mutations and polymorphisms in the human ornithine transcarbamylase gene. Hum Mutat 2:174–178

Tuchman M, Mauer SM, Holzknecht RA, Summar ML, Vnencak-Jones CL (1992) Prospective versus clinical diagnosis and therapy of acute neonatal hyperammonaemia in two sisters with carbamyl phosphate synthetase deficiency. J Inherited Metab Dis 15:269–277

Uchino T, Haraguchi Y, Aparicio JM, Mizutani N, Higashikawa M, Naitoh H, Mori M, Matsuda I (1992) Three novel mutations in the liver-type arginase gene in three unrelated Japanese patients with argininemia. Am J Hum Genet 51:1406–1412

Walker DC, McCloskey DA, Simard LR, McInnes RR (1990) Molecular analysis of human argininosuccinate lyase: mutant characterization and alternative splicing of the coding region. Proc Natl Acad Sci U S A 87:9625–9629

Widhalm K, Koch S, Scheibenreiter S, Knoll E, Colombo JP, Bachmann C, Thalhammer O (1992) Long-term follow-up of 12 patients with the late-onset variant of argininosuccinic acid lyase deficiency: no impairment of intellectual and psychomotor development during therapy. Pediatrics 87:1182–1184

40 Galactosemia

Beigi B, O'Keefe M, Bowell R, Naughten E, Badawi N, Lanigan B (1993) Ophthalmic findings in classical galactosaemia – prospective study. Br J Ophthalmol 77:162–164

Belman AL, Moshe SL, Zimmerman RD (1986) Computed tomographic demonstration of cerebral edema in a child with galactosemia. Pediatrics 78:606–609

Berry GT, Palmieri M, Gross KC, Acosta PB, Henstenburg JA, Mazur A, Reynolds R, Segal S (1993) The effect of dietary fruits and vegetables on urinary galactitol excretion in galactose-1-phosphate uridyltransferase deficiency. J Inherited Metab Dis 16:91–100

Böhles H, Wenzel D, Shin YS (1986) Progressive cerebellar and extrapyramidal motor disturbances in galactosaemic twins. Eur J Pediatr 145:413–417

Bresolin N, Comi GP, Fortunato F, Meola G, Gallanti A, Tajana A, Velicogna M, Gonano EF (1993) Clinical and biochemical evidence of skeletal muscle involvement in galactose-1-phosphate uridyl transferase deficiency. J Neurol 240:272–277

Brivet M, Raymond JP, Konopka P (1989) Effect of lactation in a mother with galactosemia. J Pediatr 115:280–282

Burke JP, O'Keefe M, Bowell R, Naughten ER (1988) Cataracts in children with classical galactosaemia and in their parents. J Inherited Metab Dis 11 [Suppl 2]:246–248

Burke JP, O'Keefe M, Bowell R, Naughten ER (1989) Ophthalmic findings in classical galactosemia – a screened population. J Pediatr Ophthalmol Strabismus 26:165–168

Cook JGH, Don NA, Mann TP (1971) Hereditary galactokinase deficiency. Arch Dis Child 46:465–469

Crome L (1962) A case of galactosaemia with the pathological and neuropathological findings. Arch Dis Child 37:415–429

Dahlqvist A, Gamstorp I, Madsen H (1970) A patient with hereditary galactokinase deficiency. Acta Paediatr Scand 59:669–675

Donnell GN (ed) (1993) Galactosemia, new frontiers in research. NIH Publ 93.3438

Elsas LJ, Fridovich-Keil JL, Leslie ND (1993) Galactosemia. A molecular approach to the enigma. Int Pediatr 8:101–109

Friedman JH, Levy HL, Boustany RM (1989) Late onset of distinct neurologic syndromes in galactosemic siblings. Neurology 39:741–742

Gitzelmann R (1965) Deficiency of erythrocyte galactokinase in a patient with galactose diabetes. Lancet II:670–671

Gitzelmann R, Steinmann B, Mitchell B, Haigis E (1976) Uridine diphosphate galactose 4-epimerase deficiency. Report of eight cases in three families. Helv Paediatr Acta 31:441–452

Haberland C, Perou M, Brunngraber EG, Hof H (1971) The neuropathology of galactosemia. J Neuropathol Exp Neurol 30:431–447

Henderson MJ, Holton JB (1983) Further observations in a case of uridine diphosphate galactose-4-epimerase deficiency with a severe clinical presentation. J Inherited Metab Dis 6:17–20

Holton JB, Allen JT, Gillett MG (1989) Prenatal diagnosis of disorders of galactose metabolism. J Inherited Metab Dis 12 [Suppl 1]:202–206

Keevill NJ, Holton JB, Allen JT (1994) UDP-glucose and UDP-galactose concentrations in cultured skin fibroblasts of patients with classical galactosaemia. J Inherited Metab Dis 17:23–26

Kliegman RM, Sparks JW (1985) Perinatal galactose metabolism. J Pediatr 107:831–841

Koch TK, Schmidt KA, Wagstaff JE, Won G, Packman S (1992) Neurologic complications in galactosemia. Pediatr Neurol 8:217–220

Landing BH, Ang SM, Villarreal-Engelhardt G, Donnell GN (1993) Galactosemia: clinical and pathologic features, tissue staining patterns with labeled galactose- and galactosamine-binding lectins, and possible loci of nonenzymatic galactosylation. Perspect Pediatr Pathol 17:99–124

Lee RT, Peterson CL, Calman AF, Herskowitz I, O'Donnell JJ (1992) Cloning of a human galactokinase gene (GK2) on chromosome 15 by complementation in yeast. Proc Natl Acad Sci U S A 89:10887–10891

Leslie ND, Immerman EB, Flach JE, Florex M, Fridovich-Keil JL, Elsas LJ (1992) The human galactose-1-phosphate uridyltransferase gene. Genomics 14:474–480

Levy NS, Krill AE, Beutler E (1972) Galactokinase deficiency and cataracts. Am J Ophthalmol 74:41–48

Lo W, Packman S, Nash S, Schmidt K, Ireland S, Diamond I, Donnell G (1984) Curious neurologic sequelae in galactosemia. Pediatrics 73:309–312

Magnani M, Cucchiarine L, Dacha M, Fornaini G (1982) A new variant of galactokinase. Hum Hered 32:329–334

Nelson CD, Waggoner DD, Donnell GN, Tuerck JM, Buist NRM (1991) Verbal dyspraxia in treated galactosemia. Pediatrics 88:346–350

Nelson MD, Wolff JA, Cross CA, Donnell GN, Kaufman FR (1992) Galactosemia: evaluation with MR imaging. Radiology 184:255–261

Olambiwonnu NO, McVie R, Won G, Frasier SD, Donnell GN (1974) Galactokinase deficiency in twins: clinical and biochemical studies. Pediatrics 53:314–318

Ornstein KS, McGuire EJ, Berry GT, Roth S, Segal S (1992) Abnormal galactosylation of complex carbohydrates in cultured fibroblasts from patients with galactose-1-phosphate uridyltransferase deficiency. Pediatr Res 31:508–511

Petry K, Greinix HT, Nudelman E, Eisen H, Hakomori SI, Levy HL, Reichardt JKV (1991) Characterization of a novel biochemical abnormality in galactosemia: deficiency of glycolipids containing galactose or N-acetylgalactosamine and accumulation of precursors in brain and lymphocytes. Biochem Med Metab Biol 46:93–104

Pickering WR, Howell RR (1972) Galactokinase deficiency:clinical and biochemical findings in a new kindred. J Pediatr 81:50–55

Podskarbi T, Reichardt J, Shin YS (1994) Studies of DNA in galactose-1-phosphate uridyltransferase deficiency and the Duarte variant in Germany. J Inherited Metab Dis 17:149–150

Reichardt JKV (1993) The molecular genetic basis of galactosemia. Int Pediatr 8:110–113

Reichardt JKV, Woo SLC (1991) Molecular basis of galactosemia: mutations and polymorphisms in the gene encoding human galactose-1-phosphate uridylyltransferase. Proc Natl Acad Sci U S A 88:2633–2637

Reichardt JKV, Packman S, Woo SL (1991) Molecular characterization of two galactosemia mutations: correlation of mutations with highly conserved domains in galactose-1-phosphate uridyl transferase. Am J Hum Genet 49:860–867

Reichardt JKV, Levy HL, Woo SLC (1992a) Molecular characterization of two galactosemia mutations and one polymorphism: implications for structure-function analysis of human galactose-1-phosphate uridyltransferase. Biochem 31:5430–5433

Reichardt JKV, Belmont JW, Levy HL, Woo SLC (1992b) Characterization of two missense mutations in human galactose-1-phosphate uridyltransferase: different molecular mechanisms for galactosemia. Genomics 12:596–600

Reichardt JKV, Novelli G, Dallapiccola B (1993) Molecular characterization of the H3119Q galactosemia mutation. Hum Mol Genet 2:325–326

Rogers S, Heidenreich R, Mallee J, Segal S (1992) Regional activity of galactose-1-phosphate uridyltransferase in rat brain. Pediatr Res 31:512–515

Sardharwalla IB, Wraith JE, Bridge C, Fowler B, Roberts SA (1988) A patient with severe type of epimerase deficiency galactosaemia. J Inherited Metab Dis 11 [Suppl 2]:249–251

Schwarz HP, Schaefer T, Bachmann C (1985) Galactose and galactitol in the urine of children with compound heterozygosity for Duarte variant and classical galactosemia (Gt^D/gt) after an oral galactose load. Clin Chem 31:420–422

Schweitzer S, Shin Y, Jakobs C, Brodehl J (1993) Long-term outcome in 134 patients with galactosaemia. Eur J Pediatr 152:36–43

Segal S (1993) The challenge of galactosemia. Int Pediatr 8:125–132

Segal S, Rutman JY, Frimptr GW (1979) Galactokinase deficiency and mental retardation. J Pediatr 95:750–753

Shin YS, Endres W, Rieth M, Schaub J (1983) Prenatal diagnosis of galactosemia and properties of galactose-1-phosphate uridyltransferase in erythrocytes of galactosemic variants as well as in human fetal and adult organs. Clin Chim Acta 128:271–281

Smetana HF, Olen E (1962) Hereditary galactose disease. Am J Clin Pathol 38:3–25

Sokol RJ, McCabe ERB, Kotzer AM, Langendoerfer SI (1989) Pitfalls in diagnosing galactosemia: false negative newborn screening following red blood cell transfusion. J Pediatr Gastroenterol Nutr 8:266–268

Thalhammer O, Gitzelmann R, Pantlitschko M (1968) Hypergalactosemia and galactosuria due to galactokinase deficiency in a newborn. Pediatr 42:441–445

Wadelius C, Lagerkvist A, Molin AK, Larsson A, von Döbeln U, Pettersson U (1993) Galactosemia caused by a point mutation that activates cryptic donor splice site in the galactose-1-phosphate uridyltransferase gene. Genomics 17:525–526

Waggoner DD, Buist NRM (1993) Long-term complications in treated galactosemia. Int Pediatr 8:97–100

Waggoner DD, Buist NRM, Donnell GN (1990) Long-term prognosis in galactosaemia:results of a survery of 350 cases. J Inherited Metab Dis 13:802–818

41 Sjögren-Larsson Syndrome

Di Rocco M, Filocamo M, Tortori-Donati P, Veneselli E, Borrone C, Rizzo WB (1994) Sjögren-Larsson syndrome: nuclear magnetic resonance imging of the brain in a 4-year-old boy. J Inherited Metab Dis 17:112–114

Gomori JM, Leibovici V, Zlotogorski A, Wirguin I, Haham-Zadeh S (1987) Computed tomography in Sjögren-Larsson syndrome. Neuroradiology 29:557–559

Judge MR, Lake BD, Smith VV, Besley GTN, Harper JI (1990) Depletion of alcohol (hexanol) dehydrogenase activity in the epidermis and jejunal mucosa in Sjögren-Larsson syndrome. J Invest Dermatol 95:632–634

Kelson TL, Craft DA, Rizzo WB (1992) Carrier detection for Sjögren-Larsson syndrome. J Inherited Metab Dis 15:105–111

Lake BD, Smith VV, Judge MR, Harper JI, Besley GTN (1991) Hexanol dehydrogenase activity shown by enzyme histochemistry on skin biopsies allows differentiation of Sjögren-Larsson syndrome from other ichthyoses. J Inherited Metab Dis 14:338–340

Mulder LJMM, Oranje AP, Loonen MCB (1987) Cranial CT in the Sjogren-Larsson syndrome. Neuroradiology 29:560–561

Richards BW (1960) Sjögren-Larsson syndrome. In: Vinken PJ, Bruyn GW (eds) Handbook of clinical neurology, vol 13. North Holland, Amsterdam, pp 468–482

Rizzo WB, Craft DA (1991) Sjögren-Larsson syndrome. Deficient activity of the fatty aldehyde dehydrogenase component of fatty alcohol: NAD^+ oxidoreductase in cultured fibroblasts. J Clin Invest 88:1643–1648

Scalais E, Verloes A, Sacré JP, Pierard GE, Rizzo WB (1992) Sjögren-Larsson-like syndrome with bone dysplasia and normal fatty alcohol NAD^+ oxidoreductase activity. Pediatr Neurol 8:459–465

Sylvester PE (1969) Pathological findings in Sjögren-Larsson syndrome. J Ment Defic Res 13:267–275

Tabsh K, Rizzo WB, Holbrook K, Theroux N (1993) Sjögren-Larsson syndrome: technique and timing of prenatal diagnosis. Obstet Gynecol 82 (suppl II):700–703

Wester P, Bergström U, Brun A, Jagell S, Karlsson B, Eriksson A (1991) Monoaminergic dysfunction in Sjögren-Larsson syndrome. Mol Chem Neuropathol 15:13–28

42 Lowe Syndrome

Athreya BH, Schumacher HR, Getz HD, Norman ME, Borden S, Witzleben CL (1983) Arthropathy of Lowe's (oculocerebrorenal) syndrome. Arthritis Rheum 26:728–735

Attree O, Olivos IM, Okabe I, Bailey LC, Nelson DL, Lewis RA, McInnes RR, Nussbaum RL (1992) The Lowe's oculocerebrorenal syndrome gene encodes a protein highly homologous to inositol polyphosphate-5-phosphatase. Nature 358:239–242

Carroll WJ, Woodruff WW, Cadman TE (1993) MR findings in oculocerebrorenal syndrome. AJNR 14:449–451

Charnas L, Bernar J, Pezeshkpour GH, Dalakas M, Harper GS, Gahl WA (1988) MRI findings and peripheral neuropathy in Lowe's syndrome. Neuropediatrics 19:7–9

Charnas LR, Bernardini I, Rader D, Hoeg JM, Gahl WA (1991) Clinical and laboratory findings in the oculocerebrorenal syndrome of Lowe, with special reference to growth and renal function. N Engl J Med 324:1318–1325

Cibis GW, Waeltermann JM, Whitcraft CT, Tripathi RC, Harris DJ (1986) Lenticular opacities in carriers of Lowe's syndrome. J Ophthalmol 93:1041–1045

Demmer LA, Wippold FJ, Dowton SB (1992) Periventricular white matter cystic lesions in Lowe (oculocerebrorenal) syndrome. Pediatr Radiol 22:76–77

Fivush BA, Rausen C, Christenson MJ, Olson JL (1992) Acute tubular necrosis associated with Lowe's syndrome: possible role of rhabdomyolysis. Am J Kidney Dis XX:396–399

Garzuly F, Jellinger K, Szabo L, Toth K (1973) Morbid changes in Lowe's oculo-cerebro-renal syndrome. Neuropediatrics 4:304–313

Giannakopoulos P, Bouras C, Vallet P, Constantinidis J (1990) Lowe syndrome: clinical and neuropathological studies of an adult case. J Ment Defic Res 34:491–500

Irvine R (1992) Second messengers and Lowe syndrome. Nature Genet 1:315–316

Kenworthy L, Park T, Charnas LR (1993) Cognitive and behavioral profile of the oculocerebrorenal syndrome of Lowe. Am J Med Genet 46:297–303

Kohyama J, Niimura F, Kawashima K, Iwakawa Y, Nonaka I (1989) Congenital fiber type disproportion myopathy in Lowe syndrome. Pediatr Neurol 5:373–376

Loughead JL, Mimouni F, Schilling S, Feingold M (1991) Lowe's syndrome. Am J Dis Child 145:113–114

Mueller OT, Hartsfield JK, Gallardo LA, Essig YP, Miller KL, Papenhausen PR, Tedesco TA (1991) Lowe oculocerebrorenal syndrome in a female with a balanced X; 20 translocation: mapping of the X chromosome breakpoint. Am J Hum Genet 49:804–810

O'Tuama LA, Laster DW (1987) Oculocerebrorenal syndrome: case report with CT and MR correlates. AJNR 8:555–557

Okabe I, Attree O, Bailey LC, Nelson DL, Nussbaum RL (1992) Isolation of cDNA sequences around the chromosomal breakpoint in a female with Lowe syndrome by direct screening of cDNA libraries with yeast artificial chromosomes. J Inherited Metab Dis 15:526–531

Pueschel SM, Brem AS, Nittoli P (1992) Central nervous system an renal investigations in patients with Lowe syndrome. Childs Nerv Syst 8:45–48

Reilly DS, Lewis RA, Ledbetter DH, Nussbaum RL (1988) Tightly linked flanking markers for the Lowe oculocerebrorenal syndrome, with application to carrier assessment. Am J Hum Genet 42:748–755

Reilly DS, Lewis RA, Nussbaum RL (1990) Genetic and physical mapping of Xq24-q26 markers flanking the Lowe oculocerebrorenal syndrome. Genomics 8:62–70

Savolaine ER, Bielke DJ (1993) Cranial magnetic resonance imaging in Lowe's syndrome. Clin Imaging 17:133–136

Terslev E (1960) Two cases of aminoaciduria, ocular changes and retarded mental and somatic development (Lowe's syndrome). Acta Paediatr 49:635–644

Tripathi RC, Cibis GW, Tripathi BJ (1986) Pathogenesis of cataracts in patients with Lowe's syndrome. J Ophthalmol 93:1046–1051

Wadelius C, Fagerholm P, Pettersson U, Anneren G (1989) Lowe oculocerebrorenal syndrome: DNA-based linkage of the gene to Xq24-q26, using tightly linkedd flanking markers and the correlation to lens examination in carrier diagnosis. Am J Hum Genet 44:241–247

43   Wilson Disease

Aisen AM, Martel W, Gabrielsen TO, Glazer GM, Brewer G, Young AB, Hill G (1985) Wilson disease of the brain: MR imaging. Radiology 157:137–141

Bingle CD, Srai SKS, Epstein O (1992) Copper metabolism in hypercupremic human livers. Studies of its subcellular distribution, association with binding proteins an expression of mRNAs. J Hepatol 15:94–101

Bowcock AM, Tomfohre J, Weissenbach J, Bonne-Tamir B, St George-Hyslop P, Giagheddu M, Cavalli-Sforza LL, Farrer LA (1994) Refining the position of Wilson disease by linkage disequilibrium with polymorphic microsatellites. Am J Hum Genet 54:79–87

Brewer GJ, Yuzbasiyan-Gurkan V (1992) Wilson disease. Medicine 71:139–164

Brewer GJ, Dick RD, Yuzbasiyan-Gurkin V, Tankanow R, Young AB, Kluin KJ (1991) Initial therapy of patients with Wilson's disease with tetrathiomolybdate. Arch Neurol 48:42–47

Brugieres P, Combes C, Ricolfi F, Degos JD, Poirier J, Gaston A (1992) Atypical MR presentation of Wilson disease: a possible consequence of paramagnetic effect of copper? Neuroradiology 34:222–224

Bull PC, Thomas GR, Rommens JM, Forbes JR, Wilson Cox D (1993) The Wilson disease gene is a putative copper transporting P-type ATPase similar to the Menkes gene. Nature Genet 5:327–337

Chelly J, Monaco AP (1993) Cloning the Wilson disease gene. Nature Genet 5:317–318

Chu NS (1989) Clinical, CT and evoked potential manifestations in Wilson's disease with cerebral white matter involvement. Clin Neurol Neurosurg 91:45–51

Cossé P, Pirastu M, Nugaro A, Figus A, Balestrieri A, Borrone C, Giacchino R, Devoto M, Monni G, Cao A (1992) Prenatal diagnosis of Wilson's disease by analysis of DNA polymorphism. N Engl J Med 327:57

Czaja MJ, Weiner FR, Schwarzenberg SJ, Sternlieb I, Scheinberg IH, van Thiel H, LaRusso NF, Giambrone MA, Kirschner R, Koschinsky ML, MacGillivray RTA (1987) Molecular studies of ceruloplasmin deficiency in Wilson's disease. J Clin Invest 80:1200–1204

De Haan J, Grossman RI, Civitello L, Hackney DB, Golberg HI, Bilaniuk LT, Zimmerman RA (1987) High-field magnetic resonance imaging of Wilson's disease. J Comput Tomogr 11:132–135

Dening TR, Berrios GE, Walshe JM (1988) Wilson's disease and epilepsy. Brain 111:1139–1155

Gaffney D, Walker JL, O'Donnell JG, Fell GS, O'Neill KF, Park RHR, Russell RI (1992) DNA-based presymptomatic diagnosis of Wilson disease. J Inherited Metab Dis 15:161–170

Grimm G, Prayer L, Oder W, Ferenci P, Madl C, Knoflach P, Schneider B, Imhof H, Gangl A (1991) Comparison of functional and structural brain disturbances in Wilson's disease. Neurology 41:272–276

Grimm G, Madl C, Katzenschlager R, Oder W, Ferenci P, Gangl A (1992) Detailed evaluation of evoked potentials in Wilson's disease. Electroencephalogr Clin Neurophysiol 82:119–124

Hefter H, Rautenberg W, Kreuzpainter G, Arent G, Freund HJ, Pichlmayr R, Strohmeyer G (1991) Does orthotopic liver transplantation heal Wilson's disease? Clinical follow-up of two liver-transplanted patients. Acta Neurol Scand 84:192–196

Hitoshi S, Iwata M, Yoshikawa K (1991) Mid-brain pathology of Wilson's disease: MRI analysis of three cases. J Neurol Neurosurg Psychiatry 54:624–626

Hoogenraad TU, Koevoet R, de Ruyter-Korver EGWM (1979) Oral zinc sulphate as long term treatment in Wilson's disease. Eur Neurol 18:205–211

Houwen RHJ, Roberts EA, Thomas GR, Cox DW (1993) DNA markers for the diagnosis of Wilson disease. J Hepatol 17:269–276

Imlya M, Ichikawa K, Matsushima H, Kageyama Y, Fujioka A (1992) MR of the base of the pons in Wilson disease. AJNR 13:1009–1012

Ishino H, Mii T, Hayashi Y, Saito A, Otsuki S (1972) A case of Wilson's disease with enormous cavity formation of cerebral white matter. Neurology 22:905–909

Iyengar V, Brewer GJ, Dick RD, Owyang C (1988) Studies of cholecystokinin-stimulated biliary secretions reveal a high molecular weight copper-binding substance in normal subjects that is absent in patients with Wilson's disease. J Lab Clin Med 111:267–274

Lang CJG, Rabs-Kolominsky P, Engelhardt A (1993) Fatal deterioration of Wilson's disease after institution of oral zinc therapy. Arch Neurol 50:1007–1008

Lawler GA, Pennock JM, Steiner RE, Jenkins WJ, Sherlock S, Young IR (1983) Nuclear magnetic resonance (NMR) imaging in Wilson disease. J Comput Assist Tomogr 7:1–8

Linné T, Agartz I, Sääf J, Wahlund LO (1990) Cerebral abnormalities in Wilson's disease as evaluated by ultra-low-field magnetic resonance imaging and computerized image processing. Magn Reson Imaging 8:819–824

Longhi R, Riva E, Rottoli A, Valsasina R, Pinelli P, Giovannini M (1989) Nuclear magnetic resonance brain study in a case of Wilson disease. J Inherited Metab Dis 12 [Suppl]:386–388

Magalhaes ACA, Caramelli P, Menezes JR, Lo LS, Bacheschi LA, Barbosa ER, Rosemberg LA (1994) Wilson's disease: MRI with clinical correlation. Neuroradiology 36:97–100

Mason AL, Marsh W, Alpers DH (1993) Intractable neurological Wilson's disease treated with orthotopic liver transplantation. Dig Dis Sci 38:1746–1750

McQuai A, Laman M, Mason J (1992) The interactions of penicillamine with copper in vivo and the effect on hepatic metallothionein levels and copper/zinc distribution: the implications for Wilson's disease and arthritis therapy. J Lab Clin Med 119:744–750

Meyer BU, Britton TC, Benecke R (1991) Wilson's disease: normalisation of cortically evoked motor responses with treatment. J Neurol 238:327–330

Nazer H, Brismar J, Al-Kawi MZ, Gunasekaran TS, Jorulf KH (1993) Magnetic resonance imaging of the brain in Wilson's disease. Neuroradiology 35:130–133

Oder W, Grimm G, Kollegger H, Ferenci P, Schneider B, Deecke L (1991) Neurological and neuropsychiatric spectrum of Wilson's disease:a prospective study of 45 cases. J Neurol 238:281–287

Oder W, Prayer L, Grimm G, Spatt J, Ferenci P, Kollegger H, Schneider B, Gangl A, Deecke L (1993) Wilson's disease: evidence of subgroups derived from clinical findings and brain lesions. Neurology 43:120–124

Petrukhin K, Fischer SG, Pirastu M, Tanzi RE, Chernov I, Devoto M, Brzustowics LM, Cayanis E, Vitale E, Russo JJ, Matseoane D, Boukhgalter B, Wasco W, Figus AL, Loudianos J, Cao A, Sternlieb I, Evgrafov O, Parano E, Pavone L, Warburton D, Ott J, Penchaszadeh GK, Scheinberg IH, Gilliam TC (1993) Mapping, cloning and genetic characterization of the region containing the Wilson disease gene. Nature Genet 5:338–343

Prayer L, Wimberger D, Kramer J, Grimm G, Oder W, Imhof H (1990) Cranial MRI in Wilson's disease. Neuradiology 32:211–214

Roh JK, Lee TG, Wie BA, Lee SB, Park SH, Chang KH (1994) Initial and follow-up brain MRI findings and correlation with the clinical course in Wilson's disease. Neurology 44:1064–1068

Schagen van Leeuwen JH, Christiaens GCML, Hoogenraad TU (1991) Recurrent abortion and the diagnosis of Wilson disease. Obstet Gynecol 78:547–549

Schulman S, Barbeau A (1963) Wilson's disease: a case with almost total loss of cerebral white matter. J Neuropathol Exp Neurol 22:105–119

Selwa LM, Vanderzant CW, Brunberg JA, Brewer GJ, Drury I, Beydoun A (1993) Correlation of evoked potential and MRI findings in Wilson's disease. Neurology 43:2059–2064

Sener RN (1993a) Wilson's disease: MRI demonstration of cavitations in basal ganglia and thalami. Pediatr Radiol 23:157

Sener RN (1993b) The claustrum on MRI: normal anatomy, and the bright claustrum as a new sign in Wilson's disease. Pediatr Radiol 23:594–596

Siegemund R, Lössner, Günther K, Kühn HJ, Bachmann H (1991) Mode of action of triethylenetetramine dihydrochloride on copper metabolism in Wilson's disease. Acta Neurol Scand 83:356–359

Snow BJ, Bhatt M, Wayne Martin WR, Li D, Calne DB (1991) The nigrostriatal dopaminergic pathway in Wilson's disease studied with positron emission tomography. J Neurol Neurosurg Psychiatry 54:12–17

Starosta-Rubinstein S, Young AB, Kluin K, Hill G, Aisen AM, Gabrielsen T, Brewer GJ (1987) Clinical assessment of 31 patients with Wilson's disease. Correlations with structural changes on magnetic resonance imaging. Arch Neurol 44:365–370

Sternlieb I (1993) The outlook for the diagnosis of Wilson's disease. J Hepatol 17:263–264

Takano K, Kuroiwa Y, Shimada Y, Mannen T, Toyokura Y (1983) CT manifestation of cerebral white matter lesion in Wilson disease. Ann Neurol 13:108–109

Tanzi RE, Petrukhin K, Chernov I, Pellequer JL, Wasco W, Ross B, Romano M, Parano E, Pavone L, Brzustowicz LM, Devoto M, Peppercorn J, Bush AI, Sternlieb I, Pirastu M, Gusella JF, Evgrafov O, Penchaszaeh GK, Honig B, Eelman IS, Soares MB, Scheinberg IH, Gilliam TC (1993) The Wilson disease gene is a copper transporting ATPase with homology to the Menkes disease gene. Nature Genet 5:344–350

Thomas GR, Roberts EA, Rosales TO, Moroz SP, Lambert MA, Wong LTK, Cox DW (1993) Allelic association and linkage studies in Wilson disease. Hum Mol Genet 2:1401–1405

Thomas GR, Bull PC, Roberts EA, Walshe JM, Cox DW (1994) Haplotype studies in Wilson disease. Am J Hum Genet 54:71–78

Thuomas KA, Aquilonius SMA, Bergström K, Westermark K (1993) Magnetic resonance imaging of the brain in Wilson's disease. Neuroradiology 35:134–141

Walshe JM, Yeallan M (1992) Wilson's disease: the problem of delayed diagnosis. J Neurol Neurosurg Psychiatry 55:692–696

Willeit J, Kiechl SG (1991) Wilson's disease with neurological impairment but no Kayser-Fleischer rings. Lancet 337:1426

Williams FJB, Walshe JM (1981) Wilson's disease. An analysis of the cranial computerized tomographic appearances found in 60 patients and the changes in response to treatment with chelating agents. Brain 104:735–752

Yarze JC, Martin P, Munoz SJ, Friedman LS (1992) Wilson's disease:current status. Am J Med 92:643–654

Yuzbasiyan-Gurkan V, Grider A, Nostrant T, Cousins RJ, Brewer GJ (1992) Treatment of Wilson's disease with zinc: X. intestinal metallothionein induction. J Lab Clin Med 120:380–386

44 Neuronal Ceroid Lipofuscinoses

Autti T, Raininko R, Launes J, Nuutila A, Santavuori P (1992) Jansky-Bielschowsky variant disease: CT, MRI, and SPECT findings. Pediatr Neurol 8:121–126

Barohn RJ, Dowd DC, Kagan-Hallet KS (1992) Congenital ceroid-lipofuscinosis. Pediatr Neurol 8:54–59

Bateman JB, Philippart M (1986) Ocular features of the Hagberg-Santavuori syndrome. Am J Ophthalmol 102:262–271

Bennett MJ, Gayton AR, Rittey CDR, Hosking GP (1994) Juvenile neuronal ceroid-lipofuscinosis: developmental progress after supplementation with polyunsaturated fatty acids. Dev med Child Neurol 36:630–638

Berkovic SF, Carpenter S, Andermann F, Andermann E, Wolfe LS (1988) Kufs' disease: a critical reappraisal. Brain 111:27–62

Boustany RMN (1992) Neurology of the neuronal ceroid-lipofuscinoses: late infantile and juvenile types. Am J Med Genet 42:533–535

Boustany RMN, Filipek P (1993) Seizures, depression and dementia in teenagers with Batten disease. J Inherited Metab Dis 16:252–255

Boustany RMN, Kolodny EH (1989) Neurological progress. The neuronal ceroid lipofuscinoses: a review. Rev Neurol 145:105–110

Boustany RMN, Alroy J, Kolodny EH (1988) Clinical classification of neuronal ceroid-lipofuscinosis subtypes. Am J Med Genet 5 [Suppl]:47–58

Brod RD, Packer AJ, Van Dyk HJL (1987) Diagnosis of neuronal ceroid lipofuscinosis by ultrastructural examination of peripheral blood lymphocytes. Arch Ophthalmol 105:1388–1393

Carlesimo M, Giustini S, Rossodivita A, Cardona F, Calvieri S (1993) Late infantile ceroid-lipofuscinoses. Am J Dermatolpathol 15:456–460

Confort-Gouny S, Chabrol B, Vion-Dury J, Mancini J, Cozzone PJ (1993) MRI and localized proton MRS in early infantile form of neuronal ceroid-lipofuscinosis. Pediatr Neurol 9:57–60

Constantinidis J, Wisniewski KE, Wisniewski TM (1992) The adult and a new late adult forms of neuronal ceroid lipofuscinosis. Acta Neuropathol (Berl) 83:461–468

Donnet A, Habib M, Pellissier JF, Régis H, Farnarier G, Pelletier J, Gosset A, Roger J, Khalil R (1992) Kufs' disease presenting as progressive dementia with late-onset generalized seizures: a clinicopathological and electrophysiological study. Epilepsia 33:65–74

Dunn DW (1987) CT in ceroid lipofuscinosis. Neurology 37:1025–1026

Dyken PR (1988) Reconsideration of the classification of the neuronal ceroid-lipofuscinoses. Am J Med Genet [Suppl] 5:69–84

Fueki N, Linuma K, Kojima A, Yanai K, Haginoya K, Tada K, Ido T, Ito M (1990) Reduced regional cerebral metabolic rate for glucose at the terminal stage in a case of late infantile neuronal ceroid lipofuscinosis. J Child Neurol 5:98–100

Goebel HH (1992) Neuronal ceroid-lipofuscinoses:the current status. Brain Dev 14:203–211

Goebel HH, Fix JD, Zeman W (1974) The fine structure of the retina in neuronal ceroid-lipofuscinosis. Am J Ophthalmol 77:25–39

Hall NA, Lake BD, Patrick AD (1991) Recent biochemical and genetic advances in our understanding of Batten's disease (ceroid-lipofuscinosis). Dev Neurosci 13:339–344

Haltia M, Rapola J, Santavuori P (1973a) Infantile type of so-called neuronal ceroid-lipofuscinosis. Acta Neuropathol (Berl) 26:157–170

Haltia M, Rapola J, Santavuori P, Keränen A (1973b) Infantile type of so-called neuronal ceroid-lipofuscinosis, part 2. Morphlogical and biochemical studies. J Neurol Sci 18:269–285

Hellsten E, Vesa J, Speer MC, Mäkelä TP, Järvelä I, Alitalo K, Ott J, Peltonen L (1993) Refined assignment of the infantile neuronal ceroid lipofuscinosis (INCL, CLN1) locus at 1p32:incorporation of linkage disequilibrium in multipoint analysis. Genomics 16:720–725

Hofman IL (1993) Observations in institutionalized neuronal ceroid-lipofuscinosis patients with special reference to involuntary movements. J Inherited Metab Dis 16:249–251

Järvelä I, Rapola J, Peltonen L, Puhakka L, Vesa J, Ammälä P, Salonen R, Ryynänen M, Haring P, Mustonen A, Santavuori P (1991) DNA-based prenatal diagnosis of the infantile form of neuronal ceroid lipofuscinosis (INCL, CLN1). Prenat Diagn 11:323–328

Järvelä I, Vesa J, Santavuori P, Hellsten E, Peltonen L (1992) Molecular genetics of neuronal ceroid lipofuscinoses. Pediatr Res 32:645–648

Jongen PJH, Gabreëls FJM, Schuurmans Stekhoven JH, Renier WO, Le Coultre R, Begeer JH (1987) Early infantile form of neuronal ceroid lipofuscinosis. Clin Neurol Neurosurg 89:161–167

Kimura S, Goebel HH (1988) Light and electron microscopic study of juvenile neuronal cerroid-lipofuscinosis lymphocytes. Pediatr Neurol 4:148–152

Kohlschütter A, Gardiner RM, Goebbel HH (1993) Human forms of neuronal ceroid-lipofuscinosis (Batten disease): consensus on diagnostic criteria, Hamburg 1992. J Inherited Metab Dis 16:241–244

Lake BD (1993) Morphological approaches to the prenatal diagnosis of late-infantile and juvenile Batten disease. J Inherited Metab Dis 16:345–348

Machen BC, Williams JP, Lum GB, Dyken P, Joslyn JN, Harpen MD, Dotson P (1987) Magnetic resonance imaging in neuronal ceroid lipofuscinosis. J Comput Tomogr 11:160–166

Martin JJ (1993) Adult type of neuronal ceroid-lipofuscinosis. J Inherited Metab Dis 16:237–240

Mitchison HM, Taschner PEM, O'Rawe AM, De Vos N, Phillips HA, Thompson AD, Kozman HM, Haines JL, Schlumpf K, D'Arigo K, Boustany RMN, Callen DF, Breuning MH, Gardiner RM, Mole SE, Lerner TJ (1994) Genetic mapping of the Batten disease locus (CLN3) to the interval D16S288-D16S83 by analysis of haplotypes and allelic association. Genomics 22:465–468

Palmer DN, Fearnley IM, Walker JE, Hall NA, Lake BD, Wolfe LS, Haltia M, Martinus RD, Jolly RD (1992) Mitochondrial ATP synthase subunit c storage in the ceroid-lipofuscinoses (Batten disease). Am J Med Genet 42:561–567

Piattella L, Cardinali C, Zamponi N, Papa O (1991) Spielmeyer-Vogt disease: clinical and neurophysiological aspects. Child's Nerv Syst 7:226–230

Raininko R, Santavuori P, Heiskala H, Sainio K, Palo J (1990) CT findings in neuronal ceroid lipofuscinoses. Neuropediatrics 21:95–101

Rapola J, Salonen R, Ammälä P, Santavuori P (1993) Prenatal diagnosis of infantile neuronal ceroid-lipofuscinosis, INCL: morphological aspects. J Inherited Metab Dis 16:349–352

Rider JA, Dawson G, Siakotos AN (1992) Perspective of biochemical research in the neuronal ceroid-lipofuscinosis. Am J Med Genet 42:519–524

Santavuori P (1988) Neuronal ceroid-lipofuscinoses in childhood. Brain Dev 10:80–83

Santavuori P, Haltia M, Rapola J (1974) Infantile type of so-called neuronal ceroid-lipofuscinosis. Dev Med Child Neurol 16:644–653

Santavuori P, Rapola J, Nuutila A, Raininko R, Lappi M, Launes J, Herva R, Sainio K (1991) The spectrum of Jansky-Bielschowsky disease. Neuropediatrics 22:92–96

Santavuori P, Raininko R, Vanhanen SL, Launes J, Sainio K (1992) MRI of the brain, EEG sleep spindles and SPECT in the early diagnosis of infantile neuronal ceroid lipofuscinosis. Dev Med Child Neurol 34:61–79

Santavuori P, Vanhanen SL, Sainio K, Nieminen M, Wallden T, Launes J, Raininko R (1993a) Infantile neuronal ceroid-lipofuscinosis (INCL): diagnostic criteria. J Inherited Metab Dis 16:227–229

Santavuori P, Linnankivi T, Jaeken J, Vanhanen SL, Telakivi T, Heiskala H (1993b) Psychological symptoms and sleep disturbances in neuronal ceroid-lipofuscinoses (NCL). J Inherited Metab Dis 16:245–248

Santavuori P, Rapola J, Raininko R, Autti T, Lappi M, Nuutila A, Launes J, Sainio K (1993c) Early juvenile neuronal ceroid-lipofuscinosis or variant Jansky-Bielschowsky disease: diagnostic criteria and nomenclature. J Inherited Metab Dis 16:230–232

Svennerholm L, Fredman P, Jungbjer B, Mansson JE, Rynmark BM, Boström K, Hagberg B, Noren L, Santavuori P (1987) Large alterations in ganglioside and neutral glycosphingolipid patterns in brains form cases with infantile neuronal ceroid lipofuscinosis/polyunsaturated fatty acid lipidosis. J Neurochem 49:1772–1783

Tyynelä J, Palmer DN, Baumann M, Haltia M (1991) Storage of saposins A and D in infantile neuronal ceroid-lipofuscinosis. FEBS Lett 330:8–12

Uvebrant P, Björck E, Conradi N, Hökegård KH, Martinsson T, Wahlström J (1993) Successful DNA-based prenatal exclusion of juvenile neuronal ceroid lipofuscinosis. Prenat Diagn 13:651–657

Williams R, Vesa J, Järvelä I, McKay T, Mitchison H, Hellsten E, Thompson A, Callen D, Sutherland G, Luna-Battadano D, Stallings R, Peltonen L, Gardiner M (1993) Genetic heterogeneity in neuronal ceroid lipofuscinosis (NCL): evidence that the late-infantile subtype (Jansky-Bielschowsky disease; CLN2) is not an allelic form of the juvenile or infantile subtypes. Am J Hum Genet 53:931–935

Wisniewski KE, Rapin I, Heaney-Kieras J (1988) Clinicopathological variability in the childhood neuronal ceroid-lipofuscinoses and new observations on glycoprotein abnormalities. Am J Med Genet 5 [Suppl]:27–46

Wisniewski KE, Kida E, Patxot OF, Connell F (1992) Variability in the clinical and pathological findings in the neuronal ceroid lipofuscinoses: review of data and observations. Am J Med Genet 42:525–532

Wisniewski KE, Kida E, Connell F, Elleder M, Eviatar L, Konkol RJ (1993) New subform of the late infantile form of neuronal ceroid lipofuscinosis. Neuropediatrics 24:155–163

45 Alexander's Disease

Arend AO, Leary PM, Rutherfoord GS (1991) Alexander's disease: a case report with brain biopsy, ultrasound, CT scan and MRI findings. Clin Neuropathol 3:122–126

Bobele GB, Garnica A, Schäfer B, Leonard JC, Wilson D, Marks WA, Leech RW, Brumback RA (1990) Neuroimaging findings in Alexander's disease. J Child Neurol 5:253–258

Borrett D, Becker LE (1985) Alexander's disease. A disease of astrocytes. Brain 108:367–385

Clifton AG, Kendall E, Kingsley DPE, Cross JH, Andar U (1991) Computed tomography in Alexander's disease. An atypical case with extensive low density in both frontal lobes. Neuroradiology 333:438–440

Dinda AK, Sarkar C, Roy S (1990) Rosenthal fibres: an immunohistochemical, ultrastructural and immunoelectron microscopic study. Acta Neuropathol (Berl) 79:456–460

Farrell K, Chuang S, Becker LE (1984) Computed tomography in Alexander's disease. Ann Neurol 15:605–607

Garcia L, Gascon G, Ozand P, Yaish H (1992) Increased intracranial pressure in Alexander disease: a rare presentation of white-matter disease. J Child Neurol 7:168–171

Goldman JE, Corbin E (1988) Isolation of a major protein component of Rosenthal fibers. Am J Pathol 130:569–578

Goldman JE, Corbin E (1991) Rosenthal fibers contain ubiquinated <a>B-Crystallin. Am J Pathol 139:933–938

Gutmann DH (1991) Chromosome 11q23.3-qter deletion and Alexander disease. Am J Med Genet 39:226

Habib M, Hassoun J, Ali-Cherif A, Alonzo B, Toga M, Khalil R (1984) Maladie d'Alexander de l'adulte. Rev Neurol 140:179–189

Harbord MG, LeQuesne GW (1988) Alexander's disease: cranial ultrasound findings. Pediatr Radiol 18:227–228

Harding BN (1990) Rosenthal fibers in Alexander's disease. J Child Neurol 5:259–260

Hess DC, Fischer AQ, Yaghmai F, Figueroa R, Akamatsu Y (1990) Comparative neuroimaging with pathologic correlates in Alexander's disease. J Child Neurol 5:248–252

Iwaki T, Kume-Iwaki A, Liem RKH, Goldman JE (1989) αB-Crystallin is expressed in non-lenticular tissues and accumulates in Alexander's diseases brain. Cell 57:71–78

Iwaki A, Iwaki T, Goldman JE, Ogomori K, Tateishi J, Sakaki Y (1992) Accumulation of αB-Crystallin in brains of patients with Alexander's disease is not due to an abnormality of the 5′-flanking and coding sequence of the genomic DNA. Neurosci Lett 140 89–92

Iwaki T, Iwaki A, Tateishi J, Sakaki Y, Goldman JE (1993) αB-crystallin and 27-kd heat shock protein are regulated by stress conditions in the central nervous system and accumulate in Rosenthal fibers. Am J Pathol 143:487–495

Nagao H, Kida K, Matsuda H, Shishido T, Matsuoka K, Nonaka I (1981) Alexander disease: clinical, electrodiagnostic and radiographic studies. Neuropediatrics 12:22–32

Neal JW, Cave FM, Singbrao SK, Cole G, Wallace SJ (1992) Alexander's disease in infancy and childhood: a report of two cases. Acta Neuropathol (Berl) 84:322–327

Ochi N, Kobayashi K, Maehara M, Nakayama A, Negoro T, Shinohara H, Watanabe K, Nagatsu T, Kato K (1991) Increment of <a>B-crystallin mRNA in the brain of patient with infantile type Alexander's disease. Biochim Biophys Res Commun 179:1030–1035

Peiffer J (1988) Alexander's disease – really a leucodystrophy? Pathol Eur 305–312

Pridmore CL, Baraitser M, Harding B, Boyd SG, Kendall B, Brett EM (1993) Alexander's disease: clues to diagnosis. J Child Neurol 8:134–144

Riggs JE, Schochet SS, Nelson J (1988) Asymptomatic adult Alexander's disease: entity or nosological misconception? Neurology 38:152–154

Russo LS, Aron A, Anderson PJ (1976) Alexander's disease: a report and reappraisal. Neurology 26:607–614

Sherwin RM, Berthrong M (1970) Alexander's disease with sudanophilic leukodystrophy. Arch Pathol 89:321–328

Stam FC (1970) Megalencephalic type of congenital leucodystrophy. In: Vinken PJ, Bruyn GW (eds) Handbook of clinical neurology, vol 10. North Holland, Amsterdam, pp 94–102

Tomokane N, Iwaki T, Tateishi J, Iwaki A, Goldman JE (1991) Rosenthal fibers share epitopes with αB-crystallin, glial fibrillary acidic protein, and ubiquitin, but not with vimentin. Am J Pathol 138:875–885

Torreman M, Smit LME, van der Valk P, Valk J, Scheltens P (1993) A case of macrocephaly, hydrocephalus, megacerebellum, white matter abnormalities and Rosenthal Fibres. Dev Med Child Neurol 35:727–741

Towfighi J, Young R, Sassani J, Ramer J, Horoupian DS (1983) Alexander's disease: further light- and electron-microscopic observations. Acta Neuropathol (Berl) 61:36–42

Townsend JJ, Wilson JF, Harris T, Coulter D, Fife R (1985) Alexander's disease. Acta Neuropathol (Berl) 67:163–166

Vogel PS, Hallervorden J (1962) Leukodystrophy with diffuse Rosenthal fiber formation. Acta Neuropathol (Berl) 2:126–143

Walls TJ, Jones RA, Cartlidge N, Saunders M (1984) Alexander's disease with Rosenthal fibre formation in an adult. J Neurol Neurosurg Psychiatry 47:399–403

Wardinksky TD, Weinberger E, Pagon RA, Clarren SK, Thuline HC (1990) Partial deletion of the long arm of chromosome 11 with abnormal white matter. Am J Med Genet 35:60–63

Wardkinsky TD, Pagon RA, Weinberger E, Clarren SK (1991) Response to Dr. David Gutmann. Am J Med Genet 39:227

Wohlwill FJ, Bernstein J, Yakovlev PI (1959) Dysmyelinogeneic leukodystrophy. J Neuropathol Exp Neurol 18:359–383

46 Myotonic Dystrophy

Andrew MAJ, Peterson MC, Michael CPT, Dew S, Larry LTC, Powe K (1989) High-resolution magnetic resonance imaging findings in juvenile-onset myotonic dystrophy. Arch Neurol 46:481–482

Brunner HG, Jansen G, Nillesen W, Nelen MR, de Die CEM, Höweler CJ, van Oost BA, Wieringa B, Ropers HH, Smeets HJM (1993) Brief report: reverse mutation in myotonic dystrophy. N Engl J Med 328:476–480

Chang L, Anderson T, Migneco A, Boone K, Mehringer CM, Villanueva-Meyer J, Berman N, Mena I (1993) Cerebral abnormalities in myotonic dystrophy. Arch Neurol 50:917–923

Damian MS, Bachmann G, Trittmacher S, Herrmann D, Dorndorf W (1992) Zerebrale Magnetresonanztomographie bei myotonischer Dystrophie Curschmann-Steinert. Klin Neuroradiol 2:11–16

Damian MS, Bachmann G, Herrmann D, Dorndorf W (1993) Magnetic resonance imaging of muscle and brain in myotonic dystrophy. J Neurol 240:8–12

Fischbeck KH (1994) The mechanism of myotonic dystrophy. Ann Neurol 35:255–256

Garcia-Alix A, Cabanas F, Morales C, Pellicer A, Echevarria J, Paisan L, Quero J (1991) Cerebral abnormalities in congenital myotonic dystrophy. Pediatr Neurol 7:28–32

Glantz RH, Wright RB, Huckman MS, Garron DC, Siegel IM (1988) Central nervous system magnetic resonance imaging findings in myotonic dystrophy. Arch Neurol 45:36–37

Huber SJ, Kissel JT, Shuttleworth EC, Chakeres DW, Clapp LE, Brogan MA (1989) Magnetic resonance imaging and clinical correlates of intellectual impairment in myotonic dystrophy. Arch Neurol 46:536–540

Ptacek LJ, Johnson KJ, Griggs RC (1993) Genetics and physiology of the myotonic muscle disorders. N Engl J Med 328:482–489

Rosman NP, Rebeiz JJ (1967) The cerebral defect and myopathy in myotonic dystrophy. Neurology 17:1106–1112

Shelbourne P, Davies J, Buxton J, Anvret M, Blennow E, Bonduelle M, Schmedding E, Glass I, Lindenbaum R, Lane R, Williamson R, Johnson K (1993) Direct diagnosis of myotonic dystrophy with a disease-specific DNA marker. N Engl J Med 328:471–475

Tanabe Y, Iai M, Tamai K, Fujimoto N, Sugita K (1992) Neuroradiological findings in chilren with congenital myotonic dystrophy. Acta Paediatr 81:613–617

47 Congenital Muscular Dystrophy

General

Arikawa E, Ishihara T, Nonaka I, Sugita H, Arahata K (1991) Immunocytochemical analysis of dystrophin in congenital muscular dystrophy. J Neurol Sci 105:79–87

Cornelio F, Dones I (1984) Muscle fiber degeneration and necrosis in muscular dystrophy and other muscle diseases: cytochemical and immunocytochemical data. Ann Neurol 16:694–701

Dobyns WB (1993) Classification of the cerebro-oculo-muscular syndrome(s). Brain Dev 15:242–244

Dobyns WB, Pagon RA, Armstrong D, Curry CJR, Greenberg F, Grix A, Holmes LB, Laxova R, Michels VV, Robinow M, Zimmerman RL (1989) Diagnostic criteria for Walker-Warburg syndrome. Am J Med Genet 32:195–210

Kihira S, Nonaka I (1985) Congenital muscular dystrophy. A histochemical study with morphometric analysis on biopsie muscles. J Neurol Sci 70:139–149

Kimura S, Sasaki Y, Kobayashi T, Ohtsuki N, Tanaka Y, Hara M, Miyake S, Yamada M, Iwamoto H, Misugi N (1993) Fukuyama-type congenital muscular dystrophy and the Walker-Warburg syndrome. Brain Dev 15:182–189

Knubley WA, Bertorini T (1988) Congenital muscular dystrophy with cerebellar atrophy. Dev Med Child Neurol 30:378–390

Komiyama A, Nonaka I, Hirayama K (1989) Muscle pathology in Marinesco-Sjögren syndrome. J Neurol Sci 89:103–113

Laverda AM, Battaglia MA, Drigo P, Battistella PA, Casara GL, Suppiej A, Casellato R (1993) Congenital muscular dystrophy, brain and eye abnormalities:one or more clinical entities? Childs Nerv Syst 9:84–87

Leyten QH, ter Laak HJ, Gabreëls FJM, Renier WO, Renkawek K, Sengers RCA (1993) Congenital muscular dystrophy. A study on the variability of morphological changes and dystrophin distribution. Acta Neuropathol (Berl) 86:386–392

Sarnat HB (1986) Cerebral dysgeneses and their influence on fetal muscle development. Brain Dev 8:495–499

Sasaki M, Yoshioka K, Yanagisawa T, Nemoto A, Takasago Y, Nagano T (1989) Lissencephaly with congenital muscular dystrophy and ocular abnormalities: cerebro-oculo-muscular syndrome. Childs Nerv Syst 5:35–37

Shuper A, Nissenkorn I, Mimouni M, Shapira I, Weitz R (1989) Muscle, eye and brain syndrome – a distinct type of congenital muscular dystrophy? Isr J Med Sci 25:160–162

Tachi N, Nagata N, Wakai S, Chiba S (1991) Congenital muscular dystrophy in Marinesco-Sjögren syndrome. Pediatr Neurol 7:296–298

Takada K (1993) Fukuyama-type congenital muscular dystrophy and the Walker-Warburg syndrome. Brain Dev 15:244–245

Wargowski DS, Chitayat D, Wes Tyson R, Norman MG, Friedman JM (1991) Lethal congenital muscular dystrophy with cataracts and a minor brain anomaly: new entity or variant of Walker-Warburg syndrome? Am J Med Genet 39:19–24

Fukuyama Type of Congenital Muscular Dystrophy

Aida N, Yagishita A, Takada K, Katsumata Y (1994) Cerebellar MR in Fukuyama congenital muscular dystrophy: polymicrogyria with cystic lesions. AJNR 15:1755–1759

Aihara M, Tanabe Y, Kato K (1992) Serial MRI in Fukuyama type congenital muscular dystrophy. Neuroradiology 34:396–398

Chijiiwa T, Nishimura M, Inomata H, Yamana T, Yamana T, Narazaki O, Kurokawa T (1983) Ocular manifestations of congenital muscular dystrophy (Fukuyama type). Ann Ophthalmol 15:921–923, 926–928

Eda I, Takashima S, Ohno K, Takeshita K (1985) Lipid composition of the cerebral gray and white matter in a case with Fukuyama type congenital muscular dystrophy. Brain Dev 7:523–525

Fukuyama Y, Ohsawa M (1984) A genetic study of the Fukuyama type congenital dystrophy. Brain Dev 6:373–390

Fukuyama Y, Osawa M, Suzuki H (1981) Congenital progressive muscular dystrophy of the Fukuyama type – clinical, genetic and pathological considerations. Brain Dev 3:1–29

Kihira S, Nonaka I (1985) Congenital muscular dystrophy. A histochemical study with morphometric analysis on biopsie muscles. J Neurol Sci 70:139–149

Kinoshita M, Nishina M, Koya N (1986) Ten years follow up study of steroid therapy for congenital encephalomyopathy. Brain Dev 8:280–284

Matsumura K, Toa T, Hasegawa T, Kamei M, Imoto N, Shimizu T (1991) A Japanese family with two types of muscular dystrophy: DNA analysis and the dystrophin test. J Child Neurol 6:251–256

Osawa M, Arai Y, Ikenake H, Murasugi H, Sugahara N, Sumida S, Okada N, Shishikura K, Suzuki H, Hirayama Y, Hirasawa K, Fukuyama Y, Tsutsumi A, Ito K, Uchida Y (1991) Fukuyama type congenital progressive muscular dystrophy. Acta Paediatr Jpn 33:261–269

Stern LM, Albertyn L, Manson JI (1990) Fukuyama congenital muscular dystrophy in two Australian female siblings. Dev Med Child Neurol 32:808–819

Takada K, Nakamura H (1990) Cerebellar micropolygyria in Fukuyama congenital muscular dystrophy: observations in fetal and pediatric cases. Brain Dev 12:774–778

Takada K, Nakamura H, Tanaka J (1984) Cortical dysplasia in congenital muscular dystrophy with central nervous system involvement (Fukuyama type). J Neuropathol Exp Neurol 43:395–407

Takada K, Nakamura H, Takashima S (1988) Cortical dysplasia in Fukuyama congenital muscular dystrophy (FCMD): a Golgi and angioarchitectonic analysis. Acta Neuropathol (Berl) 76:170–178

Takashima S, Becker LE, Chan F, Takada K (1987) A golgi study of the cerebral cortex in Fukuyama-type congenital muscular dystrophy, Walker-type „lissencephaly", and classical lissencephaly. Brain Dev 9:621–626

Toda T, Segawa M, Nomura Y, Nonaka I, Masuda K, Ishihara T, Suzuki M, Tomita I, Origuchi Y, Ohno K, Misugi N,

Sasaki Y, Takada K, Kawai M, Otani K, Murakami T, Saito K, Fukuyama Y, Shimizu T, Kanazawa I, Nakamura Y (1993) Localization of a gene for Fukuyama type congenital muscular dystrophy to chromosome 9q31-33. Nature Genet 5:283–286

Tsutsumi A, Uchida Y, Osawa M, Fukuyama Y (1989) Ocular finings in Fukuyama type congenital muscular dystrophy. Brain Dev 11:413–419

Yoshioka M, Saiwai S (1988) Congenital muscular dystrophy (Fukuyama type) – changes in the white matter low density on CT. Brain Dev 10:41–44

Yoshioka M, Okuno T, Ito M, Konishi Y, Itagaki Y, Sakamoto Y (1980) Congenital muscular dystrophy (Fukuyama type) repeated CT studies in 19 children. Comput Tomogr 5:81–88

Yoshioka M, Saiwai S, Kuroki S, Nigami H (1991) MR imaging of the brain in Fukuyama-type congenital muscular dystrophy. AJNR 12:63–65

Santavuori Type of Congenital Muscular Dystrophy

Goebel HH, Fidzianska A, Lenard HG, Osse G, Hori A (1983) A morphological study of non-Japanese congenital muscular dystrophy associated with cerebral lesions. Brain Dev 5:292–301

Kohrman MH, Picchietti L, Wollmann R, Chelmicka-Schorr EE (1986) A variant of Fukuyama congenital muscular dystrophy in a non-Japanese child. Pediatr Neurol 2:290–293

Korinthenberg R, Palm D, Schlake W, Klein J (1984) Congenital muscular dystrophy, brain malformation and ocular problems (muscle, eye and brain disease) in two German families. Eur J Pediatr 142:64–68

Leyten QH, Gabreëls FJM, Renier WO, ter Laak HJ, Sengers RCA, Mullaart RA (1989) Congenital muscular dystrophy. J Pediatr 115:214–221

Peters ABC, Bots GTAM, Roos RAC, van Gelderen HH (1984) Fukuyama type congenital muscular dystrophy – two Dutch siblings. Brain Dev 6:406–416

Ranta S, Pihko H, Santavuori P, Tahvanainen E, de la Chapelle A (1995) Muscle-eye-brain disease and Fukuyama type congenital muscular dystrophy are not allelic. Neuromusc Dis 5:221–225 under the heading of Santavuori type of congenital muscular dystrophy

Santavuori P, Somer H, Sainio K, Rapola J, Kruus S, Nikitin T, Ketonen L, Leisti J (1989) Muscle-eye-brain disease (MEB). Brain Dev 11:147–153

Valanne L, Pihko H, Katevuo K, Karttunen P, Somer H, Santavuori P (1994) MRI of the brain in muscle-eye-brain (MEB) disease. Neuroradiology 36:473–476

Walker-Warburg Type of Congenital Muscular Dystrophy

Bordarier C, Aicardi J, Goutieres F (1984) Congenital hydrocephalus and eye abnormalites with severe developmental brain defects: Warburg's syndrome. Ann Neurol 16:60–65

Dobyns WB, Kirkpatrick JB, Hittner HM, Roberts RM, Kretzer FL (1985) Syndromes with lissencephaly. II: Walker-Warburg and cerebro-oculo-muscular syndromes and a new syndrome with type II lissencephaly. Am J Med Genet 22:157–195

Dobyns WB, Pagon RA, Armstrong D, Curry CJR, Greenberg F, Grix A, Holmes LB, Laxova R, Michels VV, Robinow M, Zimmerman RL (1989) Diagnostic criteria for Walker-Warburg syndrome. Am J Med Genet 32:195–210

Federico A, Dotti MT, Malandrini A, Guazzi GC, Hayek G, Simonati A, Rizzuto N, Toti P (1988) Cerebro-ocular dysplasia and muscular dystrophy: report of two cases. Neuropediatrics 19:109–112

Gerdin H, Gullotta E, Kuchelmeister K, Busse H (1993) Ocular findings in Walker-Warburg syndrome. Childs Nerv Syst 9:418–420

Heggie P, Grossniklaus HE, Roessmann U, Chou SM, Cruse RP (1987) Cerebro-ocular dysplasia-muscular dystrophy syndrome. Arch Ophthalmol 105:520–524

Heyer R, Ehrich J, Goebel HH, Christen HJ, Hanefeld F (1986) Congenital muscular dystrophy with cerebral and ocular malformations (cerebro-oculo-muscular syndrome). Brain Dev 8:614–619

Krijgsman JB, Barth PG, Stam FC, Slooff JL, Jaspar HHJ (1980) Congenital muscular dystrophy and cerebral dysgenesis in a Dutch family. Neuropediatrics 11:108–120

Levine RA, Gray DL, Gould N, Pergament E, Stillerman ML (1983) Warburg syndrome. Ophthalmology 90:1600–1603

Leyten QH, Renkawek K, Renier WO, Gabreëls FJM, Mooy CM, ter Laak HJ, Mullaart RA (1991) Neuropathological findings in muscle-eye-brain disease (MEB-D). Neuropathological delineation of MEB-D from congenital muscular dystrophy of the Fukuyama type. Acta Neuropathol (Berl) 83:55–60

Leyten QH, Gabreëls FJM, Renier WO, Renkawek K, Laak ter HJ, Mullaart RA (1992) Congenital muscular dystrophy with eye and brain malformations in six Dutch patients. Neuropediatrics 23:316–320

Miller G, Ladda RL, Towfighi J (1991) Cerebro-ocular dysplasia – muscular dystrophy (Walker Warburg) syndrome. Findings in 20-week-old fetus. Acta Neuropathol (Berl) 82:234–238

Murphy KJ, PeBenito R, Storm RL, Ferretti C, Liu DPC (1990) Walker-Warburg syndrome. Case report and literature review. Ophthalmic Paediatr Genet 11:103–108

Pagon RA, Clarren SK, Milam DF, Hendrickson AE (1983) Autosomal recessive eye and brain anomalies: Warburg syndrome. J Pediatr 102:542–545

Pavone L, Gullotta F, Grasso S, Vannucchi C (1986) Hydrocephalus, lissencephaly, ocular abnormalities and congenital muscular dystrophy. A Warburg syndrome variant? Neuropediatrics 17:206–211

Rhodes RE, Hatten HP Jr, Ellington KS (1992) Walker-Warburg syndrome. AJNR 13:123–126

Sasaki M, Yoshioka K, Yanagisawa T, Nemoto A, Takasago Y, Nagano T (1989) Lissencephaly with congenital muscular dystrophy and ocular abnormalities: cerebro-oculo-muscular syndrome. Childs Nerv Syst 5:35–37

Simma B, Felber S, Maurer H, Gassner I, Krassnitzer S (1990) MR and ultrasound findings in a case of cerebro-oculomuscular-syndrome. Pediatr Radiol 20:554–555

Squier MV (1993) Fetal type II lissencephaly: a case report. Childs Nerv Syst 9:400–402

Tachi N, Tachi M, Sasaki K, Tanabe C, Minagawa K (1988) Walker-Warburg syndrome in a Japanese patient. Pediatr Neurol 4:236–240

Takada K, Becker LE, Takashima S (1987) Walker-Warburg syndrome with skeletal muscle involvement. A report of three patients. Pediatr Neurosci 13:202–209

Takashima S, Becker LE, Chan F, Takada K (1987) A Golgi study of the cerebral cortex in Fukuyama-type congenital muscular dystrophy, Walker-type „lissencephaly", and classical lissencephaly. Brain Dev 9:621–626

Toda T, Yoshioka M, Nakahori Y, Kanazawa I, Nakamura Y, Nakagome Y (1995) Genetic identity of Fukuyama-type congenital muscular dystrophy and Walker-Warburg syndrome. Ann Neurol 37:99–101 under the heading of Walker-Warburg type of congenital muscular dystrophy

Towfighi J, Sassani JW, Suzuki K, Ladda RL (1984) Cerebroocular dysplasia – muscular dystrophy (COD-MD) syndrome. Acta Neuropathol (Berl) 65:110–123

Whitley CB, Thompson TR, Mastri AR, Gorlin RF (1983) Warburg syndrome: Lethal neurodysplasia with autosomal recessive inheritance. J Pediatr 102:547–551

Williams RS, Swisher CN, Jennings M, Ambler M, Caviness VS Jr (1984) Cerebro-ocular dysgenesis (Walker-Warburg syndrome): neuropathologic and etiologic analysis. Neurology 34:1531–1541

Yamaguchi E, Hayashi T, Kondoh H, Tashiro N, Tsukahara M, Nagamitsu T, Eguchi Y (1993) A case of Walker-Warburg syndrome with uncommon findings. Brain Dev 15:61–66

Yoshioka M, Kuroki S, Kondo T (1990) Ocular manifestations in Fukuyama type congenital muscular dystrophy. Brain Dev 12:423–426

Yoshioka M, Kuroki S, Nigami H, Kawai T, Nakamura H (1992) Clinical variation within sibships in Fukuyama-type congenital muscular dystrophy. Brain Dev 14:334–337

Fowler Type of Congenital Muscular Dystrophy

Dobyns WB (1993) Classification of the cerebro-oculo-muscular syndrome. Brain Dev 15:242–244

Norman MG, McGillivray B (1988) Fetal neuropathology of proliferative vasculopathy and hydranencephaly – hydrocephaly with multiple limb pterygia. Pediatr Neurosci 14:301–306

Congenital muscular dystrophy with white matter disease and subtle cortical dysplasia

Egger J, Kendall BE, Erdohazi M, Lake BD, Wilson J, Brett EM (1983) Involvement of the central nervous system in congenital muscular dystrophies. Dev Med Child Neurol 25:35–42

Gobernado JM, Gimeno A (1982) Changes in cerebral white matter in a case of congenital muscular dystrophy. Pediatr Radiol 12:201–203

Jervis GA (1955) Progressive muscular dystrophy with extensive demyelination of the brain. J Neuropathol Exp Neurol 14:376–386

Leyten QH, Gabreëls FJM, Renier WO, ter Laak HJ, Sengers RCA, Mullaart RA (1989) Congenital muscular dystrophy. J Pediatr 115:214–221

Martinelli P, Gabellini AS, Ciucci G, Govoni E, Vitali S, Gulli MR (1987) Congenital muscular dystrophy with central nervous system involvement:case report. Eur Neurol 26:17–22

Nogen AG (1980) Congenital muscle disease and abnormal findings on computerized tomography. Dev Med Child Neurol 22:658–663

Streib EW, Lucking CH (1989) Congenital muscular dystrophy with leukoencephalopathy. Eur Neurol 29:211–215

Topaloglu H, Yalaz K, Kale G, Ergin M (1990) Congenital muscular dystrophy with cerebral involvement – report of a case of „occidental type cerebromuscular dystrophy"? Neuropediatrics 21:53–54

Topaloglu H, Yalaz K, Renda Y, Caglar M, Gögüs S, Kale G, Gücüyener K, Nurlu G (1991) Occidental type cerebromuscular dystrophy: a report of eleven cases. J Neurol Neurosurg Psychiatry 54:226–229

Topaloglu H, Kale G, Yalmzoglu D, Tasdemir AH, Karaduman A, Topçu, Kotiloglu E (1994) Analysis of „pure" congenital muscular dystrophies in thirty-eight cases. How different is the classical type 1 from the occidental type cerebromuscular dystrophy? Neuropediatrics 25:94–100

Trevisan CP, Carollo C, Segalla P, Angelini C, Drigo P, Giordano R (1991) Congenital muscular dystrophy: brain alterations in an unselected series of Western patients. J Neurol Neurosurg Psychiatry 54:330–334

Vles JSH, de Krom MCTFM, Visser R, Höweler CJ (1983) Two Dutch siblings with congenital muscular dystrophy (Fukuyama type). Clin Neurol Neurosurg 85:175–180

Congenital Muscular Dystrophy with White Matter Disease and Macrocephaly

Bernier JP, Broke MH, Naidich TP, Carroll JE (1979) Myoencephalopathy: cerebral hypomyelination revealed by CT scan of the head in a muscle disease. Ann Neurol 6:165

Castro Gago M, Pena-Guitian J (1988) Congenital muscular dystrophy of a non-Fukuyama type with characteristic CT images. Brain Dev 10:60

Cook JD, Gascon GG, Haider A, Coates R, Stigsby B, Ozand PT, Banna M (1992) Congenital muscular dystrophy with abnormal radiographic myelin pattern. J Child Neurol 7 [Suppl]:S51–S63

Echenne B, Pages M, Marty-Double C (1984) Congenital muscular dystrophy with cerebral white matter spongiosis. Brain Dev 6:491–495

Echenne B, Arthuis M, Billard C, Campos-Castello J, Castel Y, Dulac O, Fontan D, Gauthier A, Kulakowski S, de Meuron G, Moore JR, Nieto-Barrera M, Pages M, Parain D, Pavone L, Ponsot G (1986) Congenital muscular dystrophy and cerebral CT scan anomalies. J Neurol Sci 75:7–22

Hillaire D, Leclerc A, Fauré S, Topaloglu H, Chiannikulchai N, Guicheney P, Grinas L, Legos P, Philpot J, Evangelista T, Routon MC, Mayer M, Pellissier JF, Estournet B, Barois A, Hentati F, Feingold N, Beckmann JS, Dubowitz V, Tomé FMS, Fardeau M (1994) Localization of merosin-negative congenital muscular dystrophy to chromosome 6q2 by homozygosity mapping. Hum Mol Genet 3: 1657–1661

Kao KP, Lin KP (1992) Congenital muscular dystrophy of a non-Fukuyama type with white matter hyperlucency on CT scan. Brain Dev 14:420–422

Pihko H, Louhimo T, Valanne L, Donner M (1992) CNS in congenital muscular dystrophy without mental retardation. Neuropediatrics 23:116–122

Tanaka J, Mimaki T, Okada S, Fujimura H (1990) Changes in cerebral white matter in a case of congenital muscular dystrophy (non-Fukuyama type). Neuropediatrics 21:183–186

Van Engelen BGM, Leyten QH, Bernsen PLJA, Gabreëls FJM, Barkhof F, Joosten EMG, Hamel BCJ, ter Laak HJ, Ruijs MBM, Cruysberg JRM, Valk J (1992) Familial adult-onset muscular dystrophy with leukoencephalopathy. Ann Neurol 32:577–580

48 Infantile-onset Leukoencephalopathy with Swelling and a Discrepantly Mild Clinical Course

Harbord MG, Harden A, Harding B, Brett EM, Baraitser M (1990) Megalencephaly with dysmyelination, spasticity, ataxia, seizures and distinctive neurophysiological findings in two siblings. Neuropediatrics 21:164–168

Van der Knaap MS, Valk J, Barth PG (1993) Spongy white matter changes – MRI characteristics and description of a new disease. In: Society of Magnetic Resonance in Medicine (ed) Book of abstracts, vol 3. Society of Magnetic Resonance in Medicine, Berkeley, p 1458

Van der Knaap MS, Valk J, Barth PG (1994a) Spongiform white matter abnormalities. Clin Neurol Neurosurg 96:265

Van der Knaap MS, Ross B, Valk J (1994b) Uses of MR in inborn errors of metabolism. In: Kucharczyk J, Moseley M, Barkovich AJ (eds) Magnetic Resonance neuroimaging. CRC Press, Boca Raton, pp 245–318

Van der Knaap MS, Valk J, Barth PG (1994c) Leukoencephalopathy with swelling and mild, slowly progressive neurological dysfunction. In: American Society of Neuroradiology (ed) Book of abstracts, Waverly, Baltimore, p 49

Van der Knaap MS, Barth PG, Stroink H, van Nieuwenhuizen O, Arts WFM, Hoogenraad F, Valk J (1995a) Leukoencephalopathy with swelling and a discrepantly mild clinical course in 8 children. Ann Neurol (in press)

Van der Knaap MS, Valk J, Barth PG, Smit LME, Van Engelen BGM, Tortori Donati P (1995b) Leukoencephalopathy with swelling in children and adults. Magnetic resonance imaging patterns and differential diagnosis. Neuroradiology (to be published)

49 Childhood Ataxia with Diffuse Cerebral Hypomyelination

Hanefeld F, Holzbach U, Kruse B, Wilichowski E, Christen HJ, Frahm J (1993) Diffuse white matter disease in three children: an encephalopathy with unique features on magnetic resonance imaging and proton magnetic resonance spectroscopy. Neuropediatr 24: 244–248

Henkes HE, Deutman AF, Busch HFM (1972) Behr disease. In: Vinken PG, Bruyn GW (eds) Handbook of clinical neurology, vol 13. North Holland, Amsterdam, pp 88–93

Horoupian DS, Zucker DK, Moshe S, Peterson HDC (1979) Behr syndrome: a clinicopathologic report. Neurology 29:323–327

Landrigan PJ, Berenberg W, Bresnan M (1973) Behr's syndrome: familial optic atrophy, spastic diplegia and ataxia. Dev Med Child Neurol 15:41–47

Marzan K, Barron TF (1994) MRI abnormalities in Behr syndrome. Pediatr Neurol 10:247–248

Monaco F, Pirisi A, Sechi GP, Mutani R (1979) Complicated optic atrophy (Behr's disease) associated with epilepsy and amino acid imbalance. Eur Neurol 18:101–105

Schiffmann R, Trapp BD, Moller JR, Kaye EM, Parker CC, Brady RO, Barton NW (1992) Childhood ataxia with diffuse central nervous system hypomyelination. Ann Neurol 32:484

Schiffmann R, Moller JR, Trapp BD, Shih HHL, Farrer RG, Katz DA, Alger JR, Parker CC, Hauer PE, Kaneski CR, Heiss JD, Kaye EM, Quarles RH, Brady RO, Barton NW (1994) Childhood ataxia with diffuse central nervous system hypomyelination. Ann Neurol 35:331–340

50 Leukoencephalopathy, Cerebral Calcifications and Chronic Cerebrospinal Fluid Lymphocytosis (Aicardi-Goutières Syndrome)

Aicardi J, Goutières F (1984) A progressive familial encephalopathy in infancy with calcifications of the basal ganglia and chronic cerebrospinal fluid lymphocytosis. Ann Neurol 15:49–54

Babitt DP, Tang T, Dobbs J, Berk R (1969) Idiopathic familial cerebrovascular ferrocalcinosis (Fahr's disease) and review of differential diagnosis of intracranial calcification in children. Am J Roent Rad Ther Nucl Med 105:352–358

Billard C, Dulac O, Bouloche J, Echenne B, Lebon P, Motte J, Robain O, Santini JJ (1989) Encephalopathy with calcifications of the basal ganglia in children. A reappraisal of Fahr's syndrome with respect to 14 new cases. Neuropediatrics 20:12--19

Boltshauser E, Steinlin M, Boesch C, Martin E, Schubiger G (1991) Magnetic resonance imaging in infantile encephalopathy with cerebral calcification and leukodystrophy. Neuropediatrics 22:33–35

Hallervorden J (1950) Ueber diffuse symmetrische Kalkablagerungen bei einem Krankheitsbild mit Microcephalie und Meningoencephalitis. Arch Psychiatr Z Neurol 14:579–600

Jervis GA (1954) Microcephaly with extensive calcium deposits and demyelination. J Neuropathol Exp Neurol 13:318–329

Koussef BG (1980) Fahr's disease report of a family and a review. Acta Paediatr Belg 33:57–61

Lyon G, Robain O, Philippart M, Sarlieve L (1968) Leucodystrophie avec calcifications strio-cérébelleuses, microcéphalie et nanisme. Rev Neurol 119:197–210

Mehta L, Trounce JQ, Moore JR, Young ID (1986) Familial calcification of the basal ganglia with cerebrospinal fluid pleocytosis. J Med Genet 23:157–160

Melchior JC, Benda CE, Yakovlev PI (1960) Familial idiopathic cerebral calcifications in childhood. Am J Dis Child 99:787–803

Neill CA, Dingwall MM (1950) A syndrome resembling progeria: a review of two cases. Arch Dis Child 25:213–221

Norman RM, Tingey AH (1966) Syndrome of micrencephaly, strio-cerebellar calcifications, and leucodystrophy. J Neurol Neurosurg Psychiatry 29:157–163

Razavi-Encha F, Larroche JC, Gaillard D (1988) Infantile familial encephalopathy with cerebral calcifications and leukodystrophy. Neuropediatrics 19:72–79

Troost D, van Rossum A, Veiga Pires J, Willemse J (1984) Cerebral calcifications and cerebellar hypoplasia in two children: clinical, radiologic and neuropathological studies – a separate neurodevelopmental entity. Neuropediatrics 15:102–109

51 Inflammatory and Infectious Disorders

Al Deeb SM (1993) Herpes simplex encephalitis mimicking mumps. Clin Neurol Neurosurg 95:49–53

Altman NR (1993) Intracranial infection in children. Magn Reson Imag 5:143–160

Bale JF (1984) Human cytomegalovirus infection and disorders of the nervous system. Arch Neurol 41:310–320

Bale JF, Andersen RD, Grose C (1987) Magnetic resonance imaging of the brain in childhood herpesvirus infections. Pediatr Infect Dis J 6:644–647

Barkovich AJ, Lindan CE (1994) Congenital cytomegalovirus infection of the brain: imaging analysis and embryologic considerations. AJNR 15:703–715

Beckman JS (1991) The double edged role of nitric oxide in brain function and super-oxide mediated injury. J Dev Physiol 15:53–59

Belman AL, Coyle PK, Roque C, Cantos E (1992) MRI findings in children infected by Borrelia burgdorferi. Pediatr Neurol 8:428–431

Brownell B, Tomlinson AH (1984) Virus diseases of the central nervous system. In: Hume Adams J, Corsellis JAN, Duchen LW (eds) Greenfield's neuropathology, 4th edn. Arnold, London, pp 260–303

Davidson HD, Steiner RE (1985) Magnetic resonance imaging in infections of the central nervous system. AJNR 6:499–504

De Jong R, Brouwer M, Kuiper HM, Hooibrink B, Mildema F, van Lier RAW (1993) Maturation and differentiation dependent responsiveness of human CD4$^+$ T helper subsets. J Immunol 149:2795–2801

Demaerel P, Wilms G, Robberecht W, Johannik K, van Hecke P, Carton H, Baert AL (1992) MRI of herpes simplex encephalitis. Neuroradiology 34:490–493

Dirr LY, Elster AD, Donofrio PD, Smith M (1990) Evolution of brain MRI abnormalities in limbic encephalitis. Neurology 40:1304–1306

Enzmann D, Chang Y, Augustyn G (1990) MR findings in neonatal herpes simplex encephalitis type II. J Comput Assist Tomogr 14:453–457

Gonzalez-Scarano F, Tyler KC (1987) Molecular pathogenesis of neurotropic viral infections. Ann Neurol 22:565–574

Hartung HP, Jung S, Stoll G, Zielasek J, Schmidt B, Archelos JJ, Toyka KV (1992) Inflammatory mediators in demyelinating disorders of the CNS and PNS. J Neuroimmunol 40:197–210

Henson PM, Murphy RC (1989) Mediators of the inflammatory process. Elsevier, Amsterdam (Handbook of inflammation, vol 6)

Higgins RJ, Child G, Vandevelde M (1989) Chronic relapsing demyelinating encephalomyelitis associated with persistent spontaneous canine distemper virus infection. Acta Neuropathol (Berl) 77:441–444

Hofmann FM, Hinton DR, Johnson K, Merill JE (1989) Tumor necrosis factor identified in multiple sclerosis brain. J Exp Med 170:607–612

Ichiyama T, Hayashi T, Yamaguchi E, Tanaka H, Hagiwara K (1992) Involvement of the white matter in the initial stage of herpes simplex encephalitis. Pediatr Radiol 22:145

Johnson RT (1980) Selective vulnerability of neural cells to viral infections. Brain 103:447–472

Johnson RT (1994) The virology of demyelinating diseases. Ann Neurol 36:S54-S60

Kuroda Y, Shimamoto Y (1991) Human tumor necrosis factor-alpha arguments experimental allergic encephalomyelitis in rats. J Neuroimmunol 34:159–165

Lahat E, Smetana Z, Aladjem M, Leventon-Kriss S (1993) A lesion simulating a cerebellar infarct on CT in a child with herpes simplex encephalitis. Neuroradiology 35:339–340

Lentz D, Jordan JE, Pike GB, Enzmann DR (1993) MRI in varicella-zoster virus leukoencephalitis in the immunocompromised host. J Comput Assist Tomogr 17:313–316

Lewis RA, Austen KF, Soberman RJ (1990) Leukotrienes and other products of the 5-lipoxygenase pathway. N Engl J Med 323:645–655

Linington C, Morgan BP, Scolding NJ, Wilkins P, Pidleston S, Compston DAS (1989) The role of complement in the pathogenesis of experimental allergic encephalomyelitis. Brain 112:895–911

MacMicking JD, Willenborg DO, Weidemann MJ, Rockett KA, Cowden WB (1992) Elevated secretion of nitrogen and oxygen intermediates by inflammatory leukocytes in hyperacute experimental autoimmune encephalomyelitis: enhancement by the soluble products of encephalitogenic T cells. J Exp Med 176:303–307

Maimone D, Gregory S, Arnason BGW, Reder AT (1991) Cytokine levels in the cerebrospinal fluid and serum of patients with multiple sclerosis. J Neuroimmunol 32:67–74

Merrill JE, Gerner RH, Myers LW, Ellison GW (1983) Regulation of natural killer cell cytotoxicty by prostaglandin E in the peripheral blood and cerebrospinal fluid of patients with multiple sclerosis and other neurological diseases. J Neuroimmunol 4:223–237

Merrill JE, Strom SR, Ellison GW, Myers LW (1989) In vitro study of mediators of inflammation in multiple sclerosis. J Clin Immunol 9:84–96

Mims CA (1990) The pathogenesis of infectious disease. Academic, London

Moon WK, Chang KH, Cho SY, Han MH, Cha SH, Chi JG, Han MC (1993) Cerebral sparganosis: MR imaging versus CT features. Radiology 188:751–757

Moskowitz LB, Gregorios JB, Hensley GT, Berger JR (1984) Cytomegalovirus. Arch Pathol Lab Med 108:873–877

Murphy S, Pearce B, Jeremy J, Dandona P (1988) Astrocytes as eicosanoid-producing cells. Glia 1:241–245

Powrie F, Coffman RL (1993) Cytokine regulation of T-cell function:potential for therapeutic intervention. Immunol Today 14:270–276

Roth I (1991) Essential immunology, 7th edn. Blackwell Scientific, London

Shaw DWW, Cohen WA (1993) Viral infections of the CNS in children: imaging features. AJR 160:125–133

Smith RR (1992) Neuroradiology of intracranial infection. Pediatr Neurosurg 18:92–104

Traupe H (1993) Kernspintomographische Diagnostik zerebraler Infektionen im Kindesalter. Klin Neuroradiol 3:73–78

Van der Knaap MS, Valk J, Jansen GH, Kappelle LJ, van Nieuwenhuizen O (1993) Mycotic encephalitis: predilection for grey matter. Neuroradiology 35:567–572

Weiner LP, Johnson RT, Herndon RM (1973) Viral infections and demyelinating diseases. N Engl J Med 288:1103–1110

Whitley RJ (1990) Viral encephalitis. N Engl J Med 323:242–250

Wright SI, Unkeless JC (1993) Innate immunity. Fatal attraction: recognition and killing mechanisms in innate immunity. Curr Opin Immunol 5:57–61

52 Multiple Sclerosis

Multiple Sclerosis

Aita JF, Bennett DR, Anderson RE, Ziter F (1978) Cranial CT appearance of acute multiple sclerosis. Neurology 28:251–255

Alexander JA, Castillo M, Hoffman JC (1991) Magnetic resonance findings in a patient with internuclear ophthalmoplegia. Neuroradiological-clinical correlation. J Clin Neuro Ophthalmol 11:58–61

Antonen J, Syrjaelae P, Oikarinen R, Frey H, Krohn K (1987) Acute multiple sclerosis exacerbations are characterized by low cerebrospinal fluid suppressor/cytotoxic T cells. Acta Neurol Scand 75:156–160

Barkhof F, Frequin STFM, Hommes OR, Lamers K, Scheltens Ph, van Geel WJA, Valk J (1992) A correlative triad of gadolinium-DTPA MRI, EDSS, and CSF-MBP in relapsing multiple sclerosis patients treated with high-dose intravenous methylprednisolone. Neurology 42:63–67

Barrett L, Drayer B, Shin C (1985) High-resolution computed tomography in multiple sclerosis. Ann Neurol 17:33–38

Bastianello S, Pozzilli C, Bernardi S, Bozzao L, Fantozzi LM, Buttinelli C, Fieschi C (1990) Serial study of gadolinium-DTPA MRI enhancement in multiple sclerosis. Neurology 40:591–595

Bornstein MB, Miller A, Slagle S, Weitzman M, Crystal H, Drexler E, Keilson M, Merriam A, Wassertheil-Smoller S, Spada V, Weiss W, Arnon R, Jacobsohn I, Teitelbaum D, Sela M (1987) A pilot trial of cop 1 in exacerbating-remitting multiple sclerosis. N Engl J Med 317:408–414

Brainin M, Neuhold A, Reisner T, Maida E, Lang S, Deecke L (1989) Changes within the „normal" cerebral white matter of multiple sclerosis patients during acute attacks and during high-dose cortisone therapy assessed by means of quantitative MRI. J Neurol Neurosurg Psychiatry 52:1355–1359

Burns J, Krasner J, Guerrero F (1986) Human cellular immune response to copolymer I and myelin basic protein. Neurology 36:92–94

Camenga DL, Johnson KP, Alter M, Engelhardt CD, Fishman PS, Greenstein JI, Haley AS, Hirsch RL, Kleiner JE, Kofie VY, Koski CL, Margulies SL, Panitch HS, Valero R (1986) Systemic recombinant-2 interferon therapy in relapsing multiple sclerosis. Arch Neurol 43:1239–1246

Chiappa KH, Parker SW, Shahani BT (1985) Pathoneurophysiology of multiple sclerosis. In: Koetsier JC (ed) Handbook of clinical neurology, vol 3. Elsevier Science, Amsterdam, pp 131–145

Clausen J (1983) Serum antibodies against cytosol antigens in multiple sclerosis. J Neurol Sci 60:205–216

Comi G, Filippi M, Martinelli V, Sirabian G, Visciani A, Campi A, Mammi S, Rovaris M, Canal N (1993) Brain magnetic resonance imaging correlates of cognitive impairment in multiple sclerosis. J Neurol Sci 115 [Suppl]:S66–S71

Compston DAS, Milligan NM, Hughes PJ, Gibbs J (1987) A double-blind controlled trial of high dose methylprednisolone in patients with multiple sclerosis: 2. laboratory results. J Neurol Neurosurg Psychiatry 50:517–522

Cumings JN, Goodwin H (1968) Sphingolipids and phospholipids myelin in multiple sclerosis. Lancet II:664–665

DeCarli C, Menegus MA, rudick RA (1987) Free light chains in multiple sclerosis and infections of the CNS. Neurology 37:1334–1338

Duggan-Keen M, Roberts DF, Bates D (1986) Cell-mediated immunological status in multiple sclerosis patients. Acta Neurol Scand 73:408–414

Durelli L, Cocito D, Riccio A, Barile C, Bergamasco B, Baggio GF, Perla F, Delsedime M, Gusmaroli G, Bergamini L (1986) High-dose intravenous methylprednisolone in the treatment of multiple sclerosis: clinical-immunologic correlations. Neurology 36:238–243

Ebers GC, Bulman DE, Sadovnick AD, Paty DW, Warren S, Hader W, Jock Murray T, Peter Seland T, DuQuette P, Grey T, Nelson R, Nicolle M, Brunet D (1986) A population-based study of multiple sclerosis in twins. N Engl J Med 315:1638–1642

Ebner F, Millner MM, Justich E (1990) Multiple sclerosis in children: value of serial MR studies to monitor patients. AJNR 11:1023–1027

Edwards MK, Farlow MR, Stevens JC (1986) Multiple sclerosis: MRI and clinical correlation. AJNR 7:595–598

Eisen A, Odusote K, Li D, Robertson W, Purvis S, Eisen K, Paty D (1987) Comparison of magnetic resonance imaging with somatosensory testing in MS suspects. Muscle Nerve 10:385–390

Farlow MR, Markand ON, Edwards MK, Stevens JC, Kolar OJ (1986) Multiple sclerosis:magnetic resonance imaging, evoked responses, and spinal fluid electrophoresis. Neurology 36:828–831

Farlow MR, Edwards MK, Kolar OJ, Stevens JC, Yu PI (1987) Magnetic resonance imaging in multiple sclerosis: analysis of correlations to peripheral blood and spinal fluid abnormalities. Neurology 37:1527–1530

Filippi M, Barker GJ, Horsfield MA, Sacares PR, MacManus DG, Thompson AJ, Tofts PS, McDonald WI, Miller DH (1994a) Benign and secondary progressive multiple sclerosis: a preliminary quantitative MRI study. J Neurol 241:246–251

Filippi M, Horsfield MA, Morrissey SP, MacManus DG, Rudge P, McDonald WI, Miller DH (1994b) Quantitative brain MRI lesion load predicts the course of clinically isolated syndromes suggestive of multiple sclerosis. Neurology 44:635–641

Gean-Marton AD, Vezina LG, Marton KI, Stimac GK, Peyster RG, Taveras JM, Davis KR (1991) Abnormal corpus callosum: a sensitive and specific indicator of multiple sclerosis. Radiology 180:215–221

Gebarski SS, Gabrielsen TO, Gilman S, Knake JE, Latack JT, Aisen AM (1985) The initial diagnosis of multiple sclerosis: clinical impact of magnetic resonance imaging. Ann Neurol 17:469–474

Golden GS, Woody RC (1987) The role of nuclear magnetic resonance imaging in the diagnosis of MS in childhood. Neurology 37:689–693

Gonzalez-Scarano F, Grossman RI, Galetta S, Atlas SW, Silberberg DH (1987) Multiple sclerosis disease activity correlates with gadolinium-enhanced magnetic resonance imaging. Ann Neurol 21:300–306

Goodkin DE, Plencner S, Palmer-Saxerud J, Teetzen M, Hertsgaard D (1987) Cyclophosphamide in chronic progressive multiple sclerosis. Arch Neurol 44:823–827

Hafler DA, Fallis RJ, Dawson DM, Schlossman SF, Reinherz EL, Weiner HL (1986) Immunologic responses of progressive multiple sclerosis patients treated with an anti-T cell monoclonal antibody, anti-T12. Neurology 36:777–784

Haile RW, Hodge SE, Iselius L (1983) Genetic susceptibility to multiple sclerosis: a review. Int J Epidemiol 12:8–16

Harpur GD, Suke R, Bass BH, Bass MJ, Bull SB, Reese L, Noseworthy JH, Rice GPA, Ebers GC (1986) Hyperbaric oxygen therapy in chronic stable multiple sclerosis: double-blind study. Neurology 36:988–991

Harris JO, Frank JA, Patronas N, McFarlin DE, McFarland HF (1991) Serial gadolinium-enhanced magnetic resonance imaging scans in patients with early, relapsing-remitting multiple sclerosis: Implications for clinical trials and natural history. Ann Neurol 29:548–555

Hauser SL, Bresnan MJ, Reinherz EL, Weiner HL (1982) Childhood multiple sclerosis: clinical features and demonstration of changes in T cell subsets with disease activity. Ann Neurol 11:463–468

Hauser SL, Bhan AK, Gilles F, Kemp M, Kerr C, Weiner HL (1986) Immunohistochemical analysis of the cellular infiltrate in multiple sclerosis lesions. Ann Neurol 19:578–587

Herndon RM, Rudick RA (1987) Multiple sclerosis and related conditions. Clin Neurol 3:1–61

Honig LS, Siddharthan R, Sheremata WA, Sheldon JJ, Sazant A (1988) Multiple sclerosis: correlation of magnetic resonance imaging with cerebrospinal fluid findings. J Neurol Neurosurg Psychiatry 51:277–280

Husted C (1994) Contributions of neuroimaging to diagnosis and monitoring of multiple sclerosis. Curr Opin Neurol 7:234–241

Jacobs L, Kinkel PR, Kinkel WR (1986) Silent brain lesions in patients with isolated idiopathic optic neuritis. Arch Neurol 43:452–455

Jacobs L, Salazar AM, Herndon R, Reese PA, Freeman A, Jozefowicz R, Cuetter A, Husain F, Smith WA, Ekes R, O'Malley JA (1987) Intrathecally administered natural human fibroblast interferon reduces exacerbations of multiple sclerosis. Arch Neurol 44:589–595

Jacobs L, Munschauer FE, Kaba SE (1991) Clinical and magnetic resonance imaging in optic neuritis. Neurology 41:15–19

Jacobs L, Goodkin DE, Rudick RA, Herndon R (1994) Advances in specific therapy for multiple sclerosis. Curr Opin Neurol 7:250–254

Johnson RT (1985) Viral aspects of multiple sclerosis. In: Koetsier JC (ed) Handbook of clinical neurology, vol 3. Elsevier Science, Amsterdam, pp 319–336

Johnson MD, Lavin P, Whetsell WO (1990) Fulminant monophasic multiple sclerosis, Marburg's type. J Neurol Neurosurg Psychiatry 53:918–921

Kamp HH, Bär PR, van den Doel EHM, Elderson A (1985) Albumin and immunoglobulin-G in the cerebrospinal fluid and the diagnosis of multiple sclerosis. Clin Neurol Neurosurg 87:3–10

Kempster PA, Balla JI, Iansek R, Dennis PM (1987) Value of visual evoked response and oligoclonal bands in cerebrospinal fluid in diagnosis of spinal multiple sclerosis. Lancet I:769–771

Kermode AG, Tofts PS, Thompson AJ, MacManus DG, Rudge P, Kendall BE, Kingsley DPE, Moseley IF, du Boulay EPGH, McDonald WI (1990) Heterogeneity of blood-brain barrier changes in multiple sclerosis: an MRI study with gadolinium-DTPA enhancement. Neurology 40:229–235

Kirshner HS, Tsai SI, Runger VM, Price AC (1985) Magnetic resonance imaging and other techniques in the diagnosis of multiple sclerosis. Arch Neurol 42:859–863

Koopmans RA, Li DKB, Oger JJF, Mayo J, Paty DW (1989) The lesion of multiple sclerosis:Imaging of acute and chronic stages. Neurology 39:959–963

Kuroda Y, Shibasaki H (1987) CSF mononuclear cell subsets in active MS: lack of disease-specific alteration. Neurology 37:497–499

Kurtzke JF (1985) Epidemiology of multiple sclerosis. In: Koetsier JC (ed) Handbook of clinical radiology, vol 3. Elsevier Science, Amsterdam, pp 259–287

Kurtzke JF (1988) Multiple sclerosis: what's in a name? Neurology 38:309–316

Kurtzke JF (1989) Patterns of neurologic involvement in multiple sclerosis. Neurology 39:1235–1238

Larsson HBW, Frederiksen J, Kjaer L, Henriksen O, Olesen J (1988) In vivo determination of T_1 and T_2 in the brain of patients with severe but stable multiple sclerosis. Magn Reson Med 7:43–55

Lisak RP (1986) Interferon and multiple sclerosis. Ann Neurol 20:273

Lukes SA, Crooks LE, Aminoff MJ, Kaufman L, Panitch HS, Mills C, Norman D (1983) Nuclear magnetic resonance imaging in multiple sclerosis. Ann Neurol 13:592–601

Lynch SG, Rose JW, Smoker W, Petajan JH (1990) MRI in familial multiple sclerosis. Neurology 40:900–903

Maeda Y, Kitamoto I, Kurokawa T, Ueda K, Hasuo K, Fujioka K (1989) Infantile multiple sclerosis with extensive white matter lesions. Pediatr Neurol 5:317–319

Maravilla KR, Weinreb JC, Suss R, Nunnally RL (1984) Magnetic resonance demonstration of multiple sclerosis plaques in the cervical cord. AJNR 5:685–689

Martin-Mondiere, Jacque C, Delassalle A, Cesaro P, Carydakis C, Degos JD (1987) Cerebrospinal myelin basic protein in multiple sclerosis. Arch Neurol 44:276–278

McCallum K, Esiri MM, Tourtellotte WW, Booss J (1987) T cell subsets in multiple sclerosis. Brain 110:1297–1308

McDonald WI (1986) The mystery of the origin of multiple sclerosis. J Neurol Neurosurg Psychiatry 49:113–123

McDonald WI, Halliday AM (1977) Diagnosis and classification of multiple sclerosis. Br Med Bull 33:4–9

McFarlin DE, McFarland HF (1982) Multiple sclerosis. N Engl J Med 307:1181–1188, 1246–1251

McFarland HF, Greenstein J, McFarlin DE, Eldridge R, Xu XH, Krebs H (1984) Family and twin studies in multiple sclerosis. Ann NY Acad Sci 436:118–124

Mertin J (1985) Drug treatment of patients with multiple sclerosis. In: Koetsier JC (ed) Handbook of clinical neurology, vol. 3. Elsevier Science, Amsterdam, pp 187–212

Mickey MR, Ellison GW, Fahey JL, Moody DJ, Myers LW (1987) Correlation of clinical and immunologic states in multiple sclerosis. Arch Neurol 44:371–375

Miller DH, Johnson G, McDonald WI, MacManus D (1986) Detection of optic nerve lesions in optic neuritis with magnetic resonance imaging. Lancet I:1490–1491

Miller DH, Ormerod IEC, Gibson A, du Boulay EPGH, Rudge P, McDonald WI (1987) MR brain scanning in patients with vasculitis:differentiation from multiple sclerosis. Neuroradiology 29:226–231

Miller DH, Rudge P, Johnson G, Kendall BE, MacManus DG, Moseley IF, Barnes D, McDonald WI (1988) Serial gadolinium enhanced magnetic resonance imaging in multiple sclerosis. Brain III:927–939

Miller DH, Barkhof F, Nauta JJP (1993) Gadolinium enhancement increases the sensitivity of MRI in detecting disease activity in multiple sclerosis. Brain 116:1077–1094

Milligan NM, Newcombe R, Compston DAS (1987) A double-blind controlled trial of high dose methylprednisolone in patients with multiple sclerosis: 1. clinical effects. J Neurol Neurosurg Psychiatry 50:511–516

Millner MM, Ebner F, Justich E, Urban C (1990) Multiple sclerosis in childhood: contribution of serial MRI to earlier diagnosis. Dev Med Child Neurol 32:769–777

Möller JR, Yanagisawa K, Brady RO, Tourtellotte WW, Quarles RH (1987) Myelin-associated glycoprotein in multiple sclerosis lesions: a quantitative and qualitative analysis. Ann Neurol 22:469–474

Morimoto C, Hafler DA, Weiner HL, Letvin NL, Hagan M, Daley J, Schlossman SF (1987) Selective loss of the supressor-inducer T cell subset in progressive multiple sclerosis. N Engl J Med 316:67–72

Morrissey SP, Miller DH, Kendall BE, Kingsley DPE, Kelly MA, Francis DA, MacManus DG, McDonald WI (1993) The significance of brain magnetic resonance imaging abnormalities at presentation with clinically isolated syndromes suggestive of multiple sclerosis. Brain 116:135–146

Moscarello MA, Chia LS, Leighton D, Absolom D (1985) Size and surface charge properties of myelin vesicles from normal and diseased (multiple sclerosis) brain. J Neurochem 45:415–421

Moscarello MA, Brady GW, Fein DB, Wood DD, Cruz TF (1986) The role of charge microheterogeneity of basic protein in the formation and maintenance of the multilayered structure of myelin: a possible role in multiple sclerosis. J Neurosci Res 15:87–99

Myrianthopoulos NC (1985) Genetic aspects of multiple sclerosis. In: Koetsier JC (ed) Handbook of clinical radiology, vol 3. Elsevier Science, Amsterdam, pp 289–317

Nesbit GM, Forbes GS, Scheithauer BW, Okazaki H, Rodriguez M (1991) Multiple sclerosis: histopathologic and MR and/or CT correlation in 37 cases at biopsy and three cases at autopsy. Radiology 180:467–474

Oremerod IEC, du Boulay EPGH, Callanan MM, Johnson G (1984) NMR in multiple sclerosis and cerebral vascular disease. Lancet II:1334–1335

Ormerod IEC, McDonald WI, du Boulay GH, Kendall BE, Moseley IF, Halliday AM, Kakigi R, Kriss A, Peringer E (1986) Disseminated lesions at presentation in patients with optic neuritis. J Neurol Neurosurg Psychiatry 49:124–127

Ormerod IEC, Miller DH, McDonald WI, du Boulay EPGH, Rudge P, Kendall BE, Moseley IF, Johnson G, Tofts PS, Halliday AM, Bronstein AM, Scaravilli F, Harding AE, Barnes D, Zilkha KJ (1987) The role of NMR imaging in the assessment of multiple sclerosis and isolated neurological lesions. Brain 110:1579–1616

Osborn AG, Harnsberger HR, Smoker WRK, Boyer RS (1990) Multiple sclerosis in adolescents: CT and MR findings. AJNR 11:489–494

Panitch HS (1987) Systemic α-Interferon in multiple sclerosis. Arch Neurol 44:61–63

Panitch HS, Hirsch RL, Schindler J, Johnson KP (1987) Treatment of multiple sclerosis with gamma interferon: exacerbations associated with activation of the immune system. Neurology 37:1097–1102

Paty DW, Asbury AK, Herndon RM, McFarland HF (1986) Use of magnetic resonance imaging in the diagnosis of multiple sclerosis: policy statement. Magn Reson Med 3:1575

Paty DW, Oger JJF, Kastrukoff LF, Hashimoto SA (1988) MRI in the diagnosis of MS: a prospective study with comparison of clinical evaluation, evoked potential, oligoclonal banding and CT. Neurology 38:180–185

Polman CH, Koetsier JC, Wolters EC (1985) Multiple sclerosis: incorporation of results of laboratory techniques in the diagnosis. Clin Neurol Neurosurg 87:187–192

Poser CM (1979) Diseases of the myelin sheath. In: Houston Merritt H (ed) A textbook of neurology, 6th edn. Lippincott, Philadelphia, pp 767–823

Poser CM (1984) Taxonomy and diagnostic parameters in multiple sclerosis. Ann NY Acad Sci 436:233–246

Poser CM (1987) Diagnostic criteria for multiple sclerosis: An addendum. Ann Neurol 22:773

Poser CM, Paty DW, Scheinberg L, McDonald WI (1983) New diagnostic criteria for multiple sclerosis:guidelines for research protocols. Ann Neurol 13:227–231

Poser S, Poser W, Schlaf G, Firnhaber W, Lauer K, Wolter M, Evers P (1986) Prognostic indicators in multiple sclerosis. Acta Neurol Scand 74:387–392

Poser S, Lüer W, Bruhn H, Frahm J, Brück Y, Felgenhauer K (1992) Acute demyelinating disease. Classification and non-invasive diagnosis. Acta Neurol Scand 86:579–585

Prineas JW (1985) The neuropathology of multiple sclerosis. In: Koetsier JC (ed) Handbook of clinical neurology, vol. 3. Elsevier Science, Amsterdam, pp 213–257

Prineas JW, Barnard RO, Kwon EE, Sharer LR, Cho ES (1993) Multiple sclerosis:remyelination of nascent lesions. Ann Neurol 33:137–151

Quint DJ (1991) Multiple sclerosis and imaging of the corpus callosum. Radiology 180:15–17

Raine CS (1984) Biology of the disease: analysis of autoimmune demyelination: its impact upon multiple sclerosis. Lab Invest 50:608–635

Ransohoff RM, Tuohy V, Lehmann P (1994) The immunology of multiple sclerosis: new intricacies and new insights. Curr Opin Neurol 7:242–249

Rao SM, Glatt S, Hammeke TA, McQuillen MP, Khatri BO, Rhodes AM, Pollard S (1985) Chronic progressive multiple sclerosis: relationship between cerebral ventricular size and neuropsychological impairment. Arch Neurol 42:678–682

Reder AT, Arnason BGW (1985) Immunology of multiple sclerosis. In: Koetsier JC (ed) Handbook of clinical neurology, vol 3. Elsevier Science, Amsterdam, pp 337–395

Riikonen R, Ketonen L, Sipponen J (1988) Magnetic resonance imaging, evoked responses and cerebrospinal fluid findings in a follow-up study of children with optic neuritis. Acta Neurol Scand 77:44–49

Rose AS, Ellison GW, Myers LW, Tourtellotte WW (1976) Criteria for the clinical diagnosis of multiple sclerosis. Neurology 26 [Suppl]:20–22

Rudick RA (1992) The value of brain magnetic resonance imaging in multiple sclerosis. Arch Neurol 49:685–686

Rudick RA, Jacobs L, Kinkel PR, Kinkel WR (1986a) Isolated idiopathic optic neuritis: analysis of free light chains in cerebrospinal fluid and correlation with nuclear magnetic resonance findings. Arch Neurol 43:456–458

Rudick RA, Pallant A, Bidlack JM, Herndon RM (1986b) Free kappa light chains in multiple sclerosis spinal fluid. Ann Neurol 20:63–69

Sadovnick AD, Baird PA, Ward RH (1988) Multiple sclerosis: updated risks for relatives. Am J Med Genet 29:533–541

Sandberg-Wollheim M, Vandvik B, Nadj C, Norrby E (1987) The intrathecal immune response in the early stage of multiple sclerosis. J Neurol Sci 81:45–53

Sandberg-Wollheim M, Bynke H, Cronqvist S, Holtas S, Platz P, Ryder LP (1990) A long-term prospective study of optic neuritis: evaluation of risk factors. Ann Neurol 27:386–393

Sanders EACM, Reulen JPH, van der Velde EA, Hogenhuis LAH (1986) The diagnosis of multiple sclerosis. Contribution of non-clinical tests. J Neurol Sci 72:273–285

Sato S, Inuzuka t, Miyatake T (1986) Anti-myelin associated glycoprotein antibody in sera from patients with demyelinating diseases. Acta Neurol Scand 74:115–120

Scaioli V, Rumi V, Cimino C, Angelini L (1991) Childhood multiple sclerosis (MS): multimodal evoked potentials (EP) and Magnetic Resonance Imaging (MRI) comparative study. Neuropediatrics 22:15–23

Schumacher GA, Beebe G, Kibler RF, Kurland CT (1965) Problems of experimental trials of therapy in multiple sclerosis: report by the panel on the evaluation of experimental trials of therapy in multiple sclerosis. Ann NY Acad Sci 122:552–568

Scolding NJ, Zajicek JP, Wood N, Compston DAS (1994) The pathogenesis of demyelinating disease. Prog Neurobiol 43:143–173

Scotti G, Scialfa G, Biondi A, Landoni L, Caputo D, Cazzullo CL (1986) Magnetic resonance in multiple sclerosis. Neuroradiology 28:319–323

Sharief MK, Phil M, Thompson EJ (1991) The predictive value of intrathecal immunoglobulin synthesis and magnetic resonance imaging in acute isolated syndromes for subsequent development of multiple sclerosis. Ann Neurol 29:147–151

Sheldon JJ, Siddharthan R, Tobias J, Sheremata WA, Soila K, Viamonte M (1985) MR imaging of multiple sclerosis: comparison with clinical and CT examinations in 74 patients. AJNR 6:683–690

Sibley WA, Ebers GC, Panitch HS, Reder AT (1993) Interferon beta-1b is effective in relapsing-remitting multiple sclerosis. 1. Clinical results of a multicenter, randomized, double-blind, placebo-controlled trial. Neurology 43:655–661

Simon JH, Holtas SL, Schiffer RB, Rudick RA, Herndon RM, Kido DK, Utz R (1986) Corpus callosum and subcallosal-periventricular lesions in multiple sclerosis: detection with MR. Radiology 160:363–367

Städt D, Kappos L, Rohrbach E, Heun R, Ratzka M (1990) Occurrence of MRI abnormalities in patients with isolated optic neuritis. Eur Neurol 30:305–309

Stevens JC, Farlow MR, Edwards MK, Yu P (1986) Magnetic resonance imaging: clinical correlation in 64 patients with multiple sclerosis. Arch Neurol 43:1145–1148

Suzuki K, Eto Y, Tourtellotte WW, Gonatas JO (1973) Myelin in multiple sclerosis. Arch Neurol 28:293–297

Troiano R, Cook SD, Dowling PC (1987) Steroid therapy in multiple sclerosis. Arch Neurol 44:803–807

Truyen L, Gheuens J, Vyver vd FL, Parizel PM, Peersman GV, Martin JJ (1990) Improved correlation of magnetic resonance imaging (MRI) with clinical status in multiple sclerosis (MS) by use of an extensive standardized imaging-protocol. J Neurol Sci 96:173–182

Uhlenbrock D, Seidel D, Gehlen W, Beyer HK (1988) MR imaging in multiple sclerosis: comparison with clinical, CSF, and visual evoked potential findings. AJNR 9:59–67

Van den Kaaden AJ, Kamphuis DJ, Nossent JC, Rico RE (1993) Longstanding isolated cerebral systemic lupus erythematosus in an 8-year-old black girl. Resemblance with multiple sclerosis. Clin Neurol Neurosurg 95:241–244

Van Haver H, Lissoir F, Droissart C, Ketelaer P (1986) Transfer factor therapy in multiple sclerosis: a three-year prospective double-blind clinical trial. Neurology 36:1399–1402

Verdru P, Theys P, D'Hooghe MB, Carton H (1994) Pregnancy and multiple sclerosis: the influence on long term disability. Clin Neurol Neurosurg 96:38–41

Warren KG, Catz I (1986) Diagnostic value of cerebrospinal fluid antimyelin basic protein in patients with multiple sclerosis. Ann Neurol 20:20–25

Warren KG, Catz I (1987) A correlation between cerebrospinal fluid myelin basic protein and anti-myelin basic protein in multiple sclerosis patients. Ann Neurol 21:183–189

Weiner HL (1987) Cop 1 therapy for multiple sclerosis. N Engl J Med 317:442–444

Weiner HL, Hafler DA (1988) Immunotherapy of multiple sclerosis. Ann Neurol 23:211–222

Wilms G, Marchal G, Kersschot E, Vanhoenacker P, Demaerel P, Bosmans H, Carton H, Baert AL (1991) Axial vs sagittal T_2-weighted brain MR images in the evaluation of multiple sclerosis. J Comput Assist Tomogr 15:359–364

Willoughby EW, Grochowski E, Li DKB, Oger J, Kastrukoff LF, Paty DW (1989) Serial magnetic resonance scanning in multiple sclerosis: a second prospective study in relapsing patients. Ann Neurol 25:43–49

Yetkin FZ, Haughton VM, Papke RA, Fischer ME, Rao SM (1991) Multiple sclerosis: specificity of MR for diagnosis. Radiology 178:447–451

Young IR, Hall AS, Pallis CA, Legg NJ, Bydder GM, Steiner RE (1981) Nuclear magnetic resonance imaging of the brain in multiple sclerosis. Lancet II: 1333–1334

Baló's Concentric Sclerosis

Baló J (1928) Encephalitis periaxialis concentrica. Arch Neurol Psychiatry 19:242–264

Castaigne P, Escourolle R, Chain F, Foncin JF, Gray F, Sauron B, Duyckaerts C (1984) Sclérose concentrique de Baló. Rev Neurol 140:479–487

Courville CB (1985) Concentric sclerosis. In: Vinken PJ, Bruyn GW (eds) Handbook of clinical neurology, vol 3. Elsevier Science, Amsterdam, pp 437–451

Garbern J, Spence AM, Alvord EC (1986) Baló's concentric demyelination diagnosed premortem. Neurology 36:1610–1614

Gray F, Léger JM, Duyckaerts C, Bor Y (1985) Sclérose concentrique de Baló: lesions uniquement pontines. Rev Neurol 141:1:43–45

Hanemann CO, Kleinschmidt A, Reifenberger G, Freund HJ, Seitz RJ (1993) Balo's concentric sclerosis followed by MRI and positron emission tomography. Neuroradiology 35:578–580

Itoyama Y, Tateishi J, Kuroiwa Y (1985) Atypical multiple sclerosis with concentric or lamellar demyelinated lesions: two Japanese patients studied post mortem. Ann Neurol 17:481–487

Korte JH, Bom EP, Vos LD, Breuer TJM, Wondergem JHM (1994) Baló concentric sclerosis: MR diagnosis. AJNR 15:1284–1285

Moore GRW, Neumann PE, Suzuki K, Lijtmaer HN, Traugott U, Raine CS (1985) Baló's concentric sclerosis: new observations on lesion development. Ann Neurol 17:604–611

Spiegel M, Krüger H, Hofmann E, Kappos L (1989) MRI study of Baló's concentric sclerosis before and after immunosuppressive therapy. J Neurol 236:487–488

Yao DL, Webster HF, Hudson LD, Brenner M, Liu DS, Escobar AI, Komoly S (1994) Concentric sclerosis (Baló): morphometric and in situ hybridization study of lesions in six patients. Ann Neurol 35:18–30

Neuromyelitis Optica – Devic's Disease

Aguilera AJ, Carlow TJ, Smith KJ, Simon TL (1985) Lymphocytaplasmapheresis in Devic's syndrome. Transfusion 25:54–56

Arnold TW, Myers GJ (1987) Neuromyelitis optica (Devic syndrome) in a 12-year-old male with complete recovery following steroids. Pediatr Neurol 3:313–315

Filley CM, Sternberg PE, Norenberg MD (1984) Neuromyelitis optica in the elderly. Arch Neurol 41:670–672

Hainefellner JA, Schmidbauer M, Schmutzhard E, Maier H, Budka H (1992) Devic's neuromyelitis optica and Schilder's myelinoclastic diffuse sclerosis. J Neurol Neurosurg Psychiatry 55:1194–1196

Kuroiwa Y (1985) Neuromyelitis optica. In: Koetsier JC (ed) Handbook of clinical neurology, vol 3. Elsevier Science, Amsterdam, pp 397–408

Lefkowitz D, Angelo JN (1984) Neuromyelitis optica with unusual vascular changes. Arch Neurol 41:1103–1105

Leonardi A, Arata L, Farinelli M, Cocito L, Schenone A, Tabaton M, Mancardi GL (1987) Cerebrospinal fluid and neuropathological study in Devic's syndrome. Evidence of intrathecal immune activation. J Neurol Sci 82:281–290

Mandler RN, Davis LE, Jeffery DR, Kornfeld M (1993) Devic's neuromyelitis optica: a clinicopathological study of 8 patients. Ann Neurol 34:162–168

Miller DH, Johnson G, McDonald WI, MacManus D, du Boulay EPGH, Kendall BE, Moseley IF (1986) Detection of optic nerve lesions in optic neuritis with magnetic resonance imaging. Lancet I: 1490–1491

Misra R, Bajaj S (1986) Neuromyelitis optica: a case report from India. Trop Geogr Med 38:91–93

Piccolo G, Franciotta DM, Camana C, Bergamaschi R, Banfi P, Sandrini G, Citterio A (1990) Devic's neuromyelitis optica: long-term follow-up and serial CSF findings in two cases. J Neurol 237:262–264

Tashiro K, Ito K, Maruo Y, Homma S, Yamada T, Fujiki N, Moriwaka F (1987) MR imaging of spinal cord in Devic disease. J Comput Assist Tomogr 11:516–517

Whitham RH, Brey RL (1985) Neuromyelitis optica: two new cases and review of the literature. J Clin Neuro Opthamol 5:263–269

Schilder's Disease

Afifi AK, Bell WE, Menezes AH, Moore SA (1994) Myelinoclastic diffuse sclerosis (Schilder's disease): report of a case and review of the literature. J Child Neurol 9:398–403

Barth PG, Derix MMA, de Krom MCTFM, Valk J, Theunissen PMVM (1989) Schilder's diffuse sclerosis: case study with three years follow-up and neuroimaging. Neuropediatrics 20:230–233

Bullard WN, Southard EE (1906) Diffuse gliosis of the cerebral white matter in a child. Nerv Ment Dis 33:188–193

Cobb SR, Mehringer CM (1987) Wallerian degeneration in a patient with Schilder disease: MR imaging demonstration. Radiology 162:521–522

Dresser LP, Tourian AY, Anthony DC (1991) A case of myelinoclastic diffuse sclerosis in an adult. Neurology 41:316–318

Eblen F, Poremba M, Grodd W, Opitz H, Roggendorf W, Dichgans J (1991) Myelinoclastic diffuse sclerosis (Schilder's disease): cliniconeuroradiologic correlations. Neurology 41:589–591

Konkol RJ, Bousounis D, Kuban KC (1987) Schilder's disease: additional aspects and a therapeutic option. Neuropediatrics 18:149–152

Martin JJ, Guazzi GC (1991) Schilder's diffuse sclerosis. Dev Neurosci 13:267–273

Mehler MF, Rabinowich L (1989) Inflammatory myelinoclastic diffuse sclerosis (Schilder's disease): neuroradiologic findings. AJNR 10:176–180

Pilz P, Schiener P (1973) Kombination von morbus Addison und morbus Schilder bei einer 43 jährigen Frau. Acta Neuropathol (Berl) 26:357–360

Poser CM (1985) Myelinoclastic diffuse sclerosis. In: Koetsier JC (ed) Handbook of clinical neurology, vol 3. Elsevier Science, Amsterdam, pp 419–428

Poser CM, Goutières F, Carpentier MA, Aicardi J (1986) Schilder's myelinoclastic diffuse sclerosis. Pediatrics 77:107–112

Rodesch G, Avni EF, Parizel P, Detemmerman D, Szliwowski H, Brotchi J, Flament-Durand J, Baleriaux DL (1988) Maladie de Schilder: considerations neuroradiologiques. J Neuroradiol 15:386–393

Schilder P (1912) Zur Kenntnis der sogenannten diffusen sklerose. Z Gesamte Neurol Psychiatr 10:1–60

Sedwick LA, Klingele TG, Burde RM, Fulling KH, Gado MH (1986) Schilder's (1912) disease. Total cerebral blindness due to acute demyelination. Arch Neurol 43:85–87

Suzuki Y, Tucker SH, Rorke LB, Suzuki K (1970) Ultrastructural and biochemical studies of Schilder's disease. J Neuropathol Exp Neurol 29:405–419

Stam FC (1970) Concept, classification and nosology of the leucodystrophies. In: Vinken PJ, Bruyn GW (eds) Handbook of clinical neurology, vol 10. North-Holland, Amsterdam, pp 18–19

Wender M, Goncerezewicz A, Adamczewska-Goncerzewicz Z (1986) Contribution to the problem of diagnosing of cerebral diffuse sclerosis. Neuropathol Pol 24:455–470

53 Conditions Mimicking Multiple Sclerosis on MRI

Belman AL, Coyle PK, Roque C, Cantos E (1992) MRI findings in children infected by borrelia burgdorferi. Pediatr Neurol 8:428–431

Bucher B, Poupard JA, Vernant JC, DeFreitas EC (1990) Tropical neuromyelopathies and retroviruses: a review. Rev Infect Dis 12:890–899

Chang CM, Ng HK, Chan YW, Leung SY, Fong KY, Yu YL (1992) Postinfectious myelitis, encephalitis and encephalomyelitis. Clin Exp Neurol 29:250–262

Cintron R, Pachner AR (1994) Spirochetal diseases of the nervous system. Curr Opin Neurol 7:217–222

Coyle PK (1993) Neurologic complications of Lyme disease. Rheum Dis Clin North Am 19:993–1009

Digre KB, Varner MW, Osborn AG, Crawford S (1993) Cranial magnetic resonance imaging in severe preeclampsia vs eclampsia. Arch Neurol 50:399–406

Feasby TE, Hahn AF, Koopman WJ, Lee DH (1990) Central lesions in chronic inflammatory demyelinating polyneuropathy: an MRI study. Neurology 40:476–478

Fernandez RE, Rothberg M, Ferencz G, Wujack D (1990) Lyme disease of the CNS: MR imaging findings in 14 cases. AJNR 11:479–481

Finkel MJ, Halperin JJ (1992) Nervous system Lyme borreliosis – revisited. Arch Neurol 49:102–107

Futrell N (1994) Connective tissue disease and sarcoidosis of the central nervous system. Curr Opin Neurol 7:201–208

Handler MS, Johnson LM, Dick AR, Batnitzky S (1993) Neurosarcoidosis with unusual MRI findings. Neuroradiology 35:146–148

Hara Y, Takahashi M, Ueno S, Yoshikawa H, Yorifuji S, Tarui S (1988) MR imaging of the brain in myelopathy associated with human T-cell lymphotropic virus type I. J Comput Assist Tomogr 12:750–754

Hawke SHB, Hallinan JM, McLeod JG (1990) Cranial magnetic resonance imaging in chronic demyelinating polyneuropathy. J Neurol Neurosurg Psychiatry 53:794–796

Kira JI, Fujihara K, Itoyama Y, Goto I, Hasuo K (1991) Leukoencephalopathy in HTLV-I-associated myelopathy/tropical spastic paraparesis: MRI analysis and a two year follow-up study after corticosteroid therapy. J Neurol Sci 106:41–49

Krüger H, Heim E, Schuknecht B, Scholz S (1991) Acute and chronic neuroborreliosis with and without CNS involvement: a clinical, MRI, and HLA study of 27 cases. J Neurol 238:271–280

Lynn J, Rammohan KW, Bornstein RA, Kissel JT (1992) Central nervous system involvement in the eosinophilia-myalgia syndrome. Arch Neurol 49:1082–1085

Moore GRW, Traugott U, Scheinberg LC, Raine CS (1989) Tropical spastic paraparesis: a model of virus-induced, cytotoxic T-cell-mediated demyelination? Ann Neurol 26:523–530JA, Wolf MD, Yuh WTC, Peeples ME (1992) Cranial nerve involvement with Lyme borreliosis demonstrated by magnetic resonance imaging. Neurology 42:671–673

Ormerod IEC, Waddy HM, Kermode AG, Murray NMF, Thomas PK (1990) Involvement of the central nervous system in chronic inflammatory demyelinating polyneuropathy: a clinical, electrophysiological and magnetic resonance imaging study. J Neurol Neurosurg Psychiatry 53:789–793

Pfister HW, Wilske B, Weber K (1994) Lyme borrellosis: basic science and clinical aspects. Lancet 343:1013–1016

Rafto SE, Milton WJ, Galetta SL, Grossman RI (1990) Biopsy-confirmed CNS Lyme disease: MR appearance at 1.5 T. AJNR 11:482–484

Scheithauer BW, Rubinstein LJ, Herman MM (1984) Leukoencephalopathy in Waldenström's macroglobulinemia. J Neuropathol Exp Neurol 43:408–425

Sherman JL, Stern BJ (1990) Sarcoidosis of the CNS; comparison of unenhanced and enhanced MR images. AJNR 11:915–923

Uncini A, Gallucci M, Lugaresi A, Porrini AM, Onofrj M, Gambi D (1991) CNS involvement in chronic inflammatory demyelinating polyneuropathy: an electrophysiological and MRI study. Electroencephalogr Clin Neurophysiol 31:365–371

Van Doorn PA, Brand A, Strengers PFW, Meulstee J, Vermeulen M (1990) High-dose intravenous immunoglobulin treatment in chronic inflammatory demyelinating polyneuropathy: a double-blind, placebo-controlled, crossover study. Neurology 40:209–212

Waddy HM, Misra VP, King RHM, Thomas PK, Middleton L, Ormerod IEC (1989) Focal cranial nerve involvement in chronic inflammatory demyelinating polyneuropathy: clinical and MRI evidence of peripheral and central lesions. J Neurol 236:400–405

Williams DW, Elster AD, Kramer SI (1990) Neurosarcoidosis: gadolinium-enhanced MR imaging. J Comput Assist Tomogr 14:704–707

54 Acute Disseminated Encephalomyelitis and Acute Hemorrhagic Encephalomyelitis

Adams RD, Cammermeijer J, Brown DD (1949) Acute necrotizing hemorrhagic encephalopathy. J Neuropathol Exp Neurol 8:1–29

Amit R, Glick B, Itzchak Y, Dgani Y, Meyeir S (1992) Acute severe combined demyelination. Childs Nerv Syst 8:354–356

Atlas SW, Grossman RI, Goldberg HI, Hackney DB, Bilaniuk LT, Zimmerman RA (1986) MR diagnosis of acute disseminated encephalomyelitis. J Comput Assist Tomogr 10:798–801

Baum PA, Barkovich AJ, Koch TK, Berg BO (1994) Deep gray matter involvement in children with acute disseminated encephalomyelitis. AJNR 15:1275–1283

Caldemeyer KS, Harris TM, Smith RR, Edwards MK (1991) Gadolinium enhancement in acute disseminated encephalomyelitis. J Comput Assist Tomogr 15:673–675

Caldemeyer KS, Smith RR, Harris TM, Edwards MK (1994) MRI in acute disseminated encephalomyelitis. Neuroradiology 36:216–220

Cohen IR (1986) Regulation of autoimmune disease physiological and therapeutic. Immunol Rev 94:5–21

Grossman RI, Lisak RP, Macchi PJ, Joseph PM (1987) MR of acute experimental allergic encephalomyelitis. AJNR 8:1045–1048

Hart MN, Earle KM (1975) Haemorrhagic and perivenous encephalitis: a clinical-pathological review of 38 cases. J Neurol Neurosurg Psychiatry 38:585–591

Hawke SHB, Hallinan JM, McLeod JG (1990) Cranial magnetic resonance imaging in chronic demyelinating polyneuropathy. J Neurol Neurosurg Psychiatry 53:794–796

Johnsen SD, Sidell AD, Roger Bird C (1989) Subtle encephalomyelitis in children: a variant of acute disseminated encephalomyelitis. J Child Neurol 4:214–217

Johnson Rt, Griffin DE, Hirsch RL, Wolinsky JS, Roedenbeck S, Lindo de Soriano I, Vaisberg A (1984) Measles encephalomyelitis-clinical and immunologic studies. N Engl J Med 310:137–141

Kappelle LJ, Wokke JHJ, Huynen ChHJN, van Gijn J (1986) Acute disseminated encephalitis documented by magnetic resonance imaging and computed tomography. Clin Neurol Neurosurg 88:197–202

Kepes JJ (1993) Large focal tumor-like demyelinating lesions of the brain: intermediate entity between multiple sclerosis and acute disseminated encephalomyelitis? A study of 31 patients. Ann Neurol 33:18–27

Kesselring J, Miller DH, Robb SA, Kendall BE, Moseley IF, Kingsley D, Du Boulay EPGH, McDonald WI (1990) Acute disseminated encephalomyelitis: MRI findings and the distinction from multiple sclerosis. Brain 113:291–302

Kimura S, Unayama T, Mori T (1992) The natural history of acute disseminated leukoencephalitis. A serial magnetic resonance imaging study. Neuropediatrics 23:192–195

Köning H, Rabinowitz SG, Day E, Miller V (1979) Post-infectious encephalomyelitis afer successful treatment of herpes simplex encephalitis with adenine arabinoside. N Engl J Med 300:1089–1093

Kornips HM, Verhagen WIM, Prick MJJ (1993) Acute disseminated encephalomyelitis probably related to a mycoplasma pneumoniae. Infection 95:59–63

Lebar R (1987) Démyélinisation et autoimmunité. Pathol Biol 35:275–283

Lisak RP, Behan PO, Zweiman B, Shetty T (1974) Cell-mediated immunity to myelin basic protein in acute disseminated encephalomyelitis. Neurology 24:560–564

Lukes SA, Norman D (1983) Computed tomography in acute disseminated encephalomyelitis. Ann Neurol 13:567–572

Lukes SA, Normal D, Mills C (1983) Acute disseminated encephalomyelitis: CT and NMR findings. J Comput Assist Tomogr 7:182

Marks WA, Bodensteiner JB, Bobele GB, Hamza M, Wilson DA (1988) Parainflammatory leukoencephalomyelitis: clinical and magnetic resonance imaging findings. J Child Neurol 3:205–213

Nasralla CW, Pay N, Goodpasture HC, Lin JJ, Svoboda WB (1993) Postinfectious encephalopathy in a child following campylobacter jejuni enteritis. AJNR 14:444–448

Ohtaki E, Murakami Y, Komori H, Yamashita Y, Matsuishi T (1992) Acute disseminated encephalomyelitis after Japanese B encephalitis vaccination. Pediatr Neurol 8:137–139

Okuno T, Fuseya Y, Ito M, Konishi Y, Nakano Y (1981) Reversible multiple hypodense areas in white matter diagnosed as acute disseminated encephalomyelitis. J Comput Assist Tomogr 5:119–121

Ormerod IEC, Waddy HM, Kermode AG, Murray NMF, Thomas PK (1990) Involvement of the central nervous system in chronic inflammatory demyelinating polyneuropathy: a clinical, electrophysiological and magnetic resonance imaging study. J Neurol Neurosurg Psychiatry 53:789–793

Poser CM (1969) Disseminated vasculomyelinopathy. Acta Neurol 45:7–44

Poser CM (1989) Magnetic resonance imaging in asymptomatic disseminated vasculomyelinopathy. J Neurol Sci 94:69–77

Poser CM, Roman G, Emery ES (1978) Recurrent disseminated vasculomyelinopathy. Arch Neurol 35:166–170

Rabinowitz SG, Day ED, Paterson PY, Koening H (1983) Endogenous myelin basic protein-serum factors (MBP-SFS) and anti-MBP antibodies in a patient with post-herpes simplex virus acute disseminated encephalomyelitis. J Neurol Sci 60:393–400

Reich H, Lin SR, Goldblatt D (1979) Computerized tomography in acute hemorrhagic leukoencephalopathy:a case report. Neurology 29:255–258

Reik L (1980) Disseminated vasculomyelinopathy: an immune complex disease. Ann Neurol 7:291–296

Russell DS (1955) The nosological unity of acute hemorrhagic leucoencephalitis and acute disseminated encephalomyelitis. Brain 78:369–376

Saito H, Endo M, Takase S, Itahara K (1980) Acute disseminated encephalomyelitis after influenza vaccination. Arch Neurol 37:564–566

Shoji H, Kusuhara T, Honda Y, Hino H, Kojima K, Abe T, Watanabe M (1992) Relapsing acute disseminated encephalomyelitis associated with chronic Epstein-Barr virus infection: MRI findings. Neuroradiology 34:340–342

Tachi N, Watanabe T, Wakai S, Sato T, Chiba S (1992) Acute disseminated encephalomyelitis following HTLV-I associated myelopathy. J Neurol Sci 110:234–235

Thajeb P, Chen ST (1989) Cranial computed tomography in acute disseminated encephalomyelitis. Neuroradiology 31:8–12

Van der Meyden CH, de Villiers JFK, Middlecote BD, Terblanchè J (1994) Gadolinium ring enhancement and mass effect in acute disseminated encephalomyelitis. Neuroradiology 36:221–223

Ziegler DK (1966) Acute disseminated encephalitis. Arch Neurol 14:476–488

55 Acquired Immunodeficiency Syndrome

Barakos JA, Mark AS, Dillon WP, Norman D (1990) MR imaging of acute transverse myelitis and AIDS myelopathy. J Comput Assist Tomogr 14:45–50

Berger JR, Sheremata WA, Resnick L, Atherton S, Fletcher MA, Norenberg M (1989) Multiple sclerosis-like illness occurring with human immunodeficiency virus infection. Neurology 39:324–329

Berger JR, Tornatore C, Major EO, Bruce J, Shapshak P, Yoshioka M, Houff S, Sheremata W, Horton GF, Landy H (1992) Relapsing and remitting human immunodeficiency virus-associated leukoencephalomyelopathy. Ann Neurol 31:34–38

Brew BJ (1994) The clinical spectrum and pathogenesis of HIV encephalopathy, myelopathy, and peripheral neuropathy. Curr Opin Neurol 7:209–216

Broderick DF, Wippold FJ, Clifford DB, Kido DB, Kido D, Wilson BS (1993) White matter lesions and cerebral atrophy on MR images in patients with and without AIDS dementia complex. AJR 161:177–181

Budka H (1989) Human immunodeficiency virus (HIV)-induced disease of the central nervous system: pathology and implications for pathogenesis. Acta Neuropathol (Berl) 77:225–236

Burns DK (1992) The neuropathology of pediatric acquired immunodeficiency syndrome. J Child Neurol 7:332–346

Chamberlain MC (1993) Pediatric AIDS: a longitudinal comparative MRI and CT brain imaging study. J Child Neurol 8:175–181

Chamberlain MC, Nichols SL, Chase CH (1991) Pediatric AIDS: comparative cranial MRI and CT scans. Pediatr Neurol 7:357–362

Chrysikopoulos HS, Press GA, Grafe MR, Hesselink JR, Wiley CA (1990) Encephalitis caused by human immunodeficiency virus: CT and MR imaging manifestations with clinical and pathologic correlation. Radiology 175:185–191

Curless RG (1989) Congenital AIDS: review of neurologic problems. Child Nerv Syst 5:9–11

DeCarli C, Civitello LA, Brouwers P, Pizzo PA (1993) The prevalence of computed tomographic abnormalities of the cerebrum in 100 consecutive children symptomatic with the human immune deficiency virus. Ann Neurol 34:198–205

De Gans J, Portegies P, Derix MMA, Troost D, Valk J, Goudsmit J (1988) Het AIDS-dementiecomplex: een primaire infectie met humaan immunodeficientievirus type 1. Ned Tijdschr Geneeskd 132:1570–1575

Dickson DW, Belman AL, Kim TS, Horoupian DS, Rubinstein A (1989) Spinal cord pathology in pediatric acquired immunodeficiency syndrome. Neurology 39:227–235

Douek P, Bertrand Y, Tran-Minh VA, Patet JD, Souillet G, Philippe N (1991) Primary lymphoma of the CNS in an infant with AIDS: imaging findings. AJR 156:1037–1038

Fliss DM, Parikh J, Freeman JL (1992) Aids-related Kaposi's sarcoma of the sphenoid sinus. J Otolaryngol 21:235–237

Flowers CH, Mafee MF, Crowell R, Raofi B, Arnold P, Dobben G, Wycliffe N (1990) Encephalopathy in AIDS patients: evaluation with MR imaging. AJNR 11:1235–1245

Geremia GK, McCluney KW, Adler SS, Charletta DA, Hoile RD, Huckman MS, Ramsey RG (1990) The magnetic resonance hypointense spine of AIDS. J Comput Assist Tomogr 14:785–789

Gout O, Gessain A, Bolgert F, Saal F, Tournier-Lasserve E, Lasneret J, Caudie C, Brunet P, Lhermitte F, Lyon-Caen O (1989) Chronic myelopathies associated with human T-lymphotropic virus type I. A clinical, serologic, and immunovirologic study of ten patients in France. Arch Neurol 46:255–260

Grafe MR, Wiley CA (1989) Spinal cord and peripheral nerve pathology in AIDS: the roles of cytomegalovirus and human immunodeficiency virus. Ann Neurol 25:561–566

Grafe MR, Press GA, Berthoty DP, Hesselink JR, Wiley CA (1990) Abnormalities of the brain in AIDS patients: correlation of postmortem MR findings with neuropathology. AJNR 11:905–911

Gray F, Gherardi R, Scaravilli F (1988) The neuropathology of the acquired immune deficiency syndrome (AIDS). A review. Brain 111:245–266

Gray F, Haug H, Chimelli L, Geny C, Gaston A, Scaravilli F, Budka H (1991a) Prominent cortical atrophy with neuronal loss as correlate of human immunodeficiency virus encephalopathy. Acta Neuropathol (Berl) 82:229–233

Gray F, Chimelli L, Mohr M, Clavelou P, Scaravilli F, Poirier J (1991b) Fulminating multiple sclerosis-like leukoencephalopathy revealing human immunodeficiency virus infection. Neurology 41:105–109

Gray F, Lescs MC, Keohane C, Paraire F, Marc B, Durigon M, Gherardi R (1992) Early brain changes in HIV infection:Neuropathological study of 11 HIV seropositive, non-AIDS cases. J Neuropathol Exp Neurol 51:177–185

Greene WC (1991) The molecular biology of human immunodeficiency virus type 1 infection. N Engl J Med 324:308–317

Haney PJ, Yale-Loehr AJ, Nussbaum AR, Gellad FE (1989) Imaging of infants and children with AIDS. AJR 152:1033–1041

Hénin D, Smith TW, de Girolami U, Sughayer M, Hauw JJ (1992) Neuropathology of the spinal cord in the acquired immunodeficiency syndrome. Hum Pathol 23:1106–1114

Ho DD, Pomerantz RJ, Kaplan JC (1987) Pathogenesis of infection with human immunodeficiency virus. N Engl J Med 317:278–286

Holland NR, Power C, Mathews VP, Glass JD, Forman M, McArthur JC (1994) Cytomegalovirus encephalitis in acquired immunodeficiency syndrome (AIDS). Neurology 44:507–514

Holliday RA (1993) Manifestations of AIDS in the oromaxillofacial region. The role of imaging. Radiol Clin North Am 31:45–60

Igloffstein J, Vogel P (1991) Subacute AIDS-related lumbosacral radiculopathy: a bacterial infection? J Neurol 238:239–241

Janssen RS, Cornblath DR, Epstein LG, McArthur J, Price RW (1989) Human immunodeficiency virus (HIV) infection and the nervous system:Report from the American Academy of Neurology AIDS task force. Neurology 39:119–122

Jarvik JG, Hesselink JR, Kennedy C, Teschke R, Wiley C, Spector S, Richman D, McCutchan JA (1988) Acquired immunodeficiency syndrome: Magnetic resonance patterns of brain involvement with pathologic correlation. Arch Neurol 45:731–736

Jensen MC, Brant-Zawadzki M (1993) MR imaging of the brain in patients with AIDS: value of routine use of IV Gadopentetate dimeglumine. AJR 160:153–157

Jones HR, Ho DD, Forgacs P, Adelman LS, Silverman ML, Baker RA, Locuratolo P (1988) Acute fulminating fatal leukoencephalopathy as the only manifestation of human immunodeficiency virus infection. Ann Neurol 23:519–522

Kalayjian RC, Cohen ML, Bonomo RA, Flanigan TP (1993) Cytomegalovirus ventriculoencephalitis in AIDS. A syndrome with distinct clinical and pathologic features. Medicine 72:67–77

Kauffman WM, Sivit CJ, Fitz CR, Rakusan TA, Herzog K, Chandra RS (1992) CT and MR evaluation of intracranial involvement in pediatric HIV infection: a clinical-imaging correlation. AJNR 13:949–957

Kieburtz KD, Ketonen L, Zettelmaier AE, Kido D, Caine ED, Simon JH (1990) Magnetic resonance imaging findings in HIV cognitive impairment. Arch Neurol 47:643–645

Kira J, Minato S, Itoyama Y, Goto I, Kato M, Hasuo K (1988) Leukoencephalopathy in HTLV-I-associated myelopathy: MRI and EEG data. J Neurol Sci 87:221–232

Kirshenbaum KJ, Nadimpalli SR, Friedman M, Kirshenbaum GL, Cavallino RP (1991) Benign lymphoepithelial parotid tumors in AIDS patients: CT and MR findings in nine cases. AJNR 12:271–274

Kovacs JA (1992) Efficacy of atovaquone in treatment of toxoplasmosis in patients with AIDS. Lancet 340:637–638

Kovner R, Perecman E, Lazar W, Hainline B, Kaplan MH, Lesser M, Beresford R (1989) Relation of personality and attentional factors to cognitive deficits in human immunodeficiency virus-infected subjects. Arch Neurol 46:274–277

Kupfer MC, Zee CS, Colletti PM, Boswell WD, Rhodes R (1990) MRI evaluation of AIDS-related encephalopathy: toxoplasmosis vs. lymphoma. Magn Reson Imaging 8:51–57

Lang W, Miklossy J, Deruaz JP, Pizzolato GP, Probst A, Schaffner T, Gessaga E, Kleihues (1989) Neuropathology of the acquired immune deficiency syndrome (AIDS): a report of 135 consecutive autopsy cases from Switzerland. Acta Neuropathol (Berl) 77:379–390

Leger JM, Bolgert F, Bouche P (1988) Peripheral nervous system and HIV infection. 13 cases. Rev Neurol 144:789–795

Leger JM, Bouche P, Bolgert F, Chaunu MP, Rosenheim M, Cathala HP, Gentilini M, Hauw JJ, Brunet P (1989) The spectrum of polyneuropathies in patients infected with HIV. J Neurol Neurosurg Psychiatry 52:1369–1374

Li J, Xiong L, Jinkins JR (1993) Gadolinium-enhanced MRI in a patient with AIDS and the Ramsay-Hunt syndrome. Neuroradiology 35:269

Llewelyn JG, Valentine AR, Bradley C, King K, Gross MLP (1990) Multifocal central nervous system lesions and retropharyngeal lymphadenopathy on magnetic resonance imaging:an association that suggested progressive multifocal leukoencephalopathy in a patient with acute aphasia. Br J Radiol 63:897–899

Lüer W, Gerhards J, Poser S, Weber T, Felgenhauer K (1944) Acute diffuse leukoencephalitis in HIV-1 infection. J Neurol Neurosurg Psychiatry 57:105–107.

Manji H, Connolly S, McAllister R, Valentine AR, Kendall BE, Fell M, Durrance P, Thompson AJ, Newman S, Weller IVD, Harrison MJG (1994) Serial MRI of the brain in asymptomatic patients infected with HIV: results from the UCMSM/Medical Research Council neurology cohort. J Neurol Neurosurg Psychiatry 57:144–149

Mundinger A, Adam T, Ott D, Dinkel E, Beck A, Peter HH, Volk B, Schumacher M (1992) CT and MRI: prognostic tools in patients with AIDS and neurological deficits. Neuroradiology 35:75–78

Nisce LZ, Kaumann T, Metroka C (1992) Radiation therapy in patients with AIDS-related central nervous system lymphomas. JAMA 267:1921–1922

Olsen WL, Longo FM, Mills CM, Norman D (1988) White matter disease in AIDS: findings at MR imaging. Radiology 169:445–448

Pedersen C, Thomsen C, Arlien-Soborg P, Prestholm J, Kjoer L, Boesen F, Hansen HS, Nielsen JO (1991) Central nervous system involvement in human immunodeficiency virus disease. Dan Med Bull 38:374–379

Poon TP, Tchertkoff V, Pares GF, Masangkay AV, Daras M, Marc J (1992) Spinal cord toxoplasma lesion in AIDS: MR findings. J Comput Assist Tomogr 16:817–819

Portegies P, Epstein LG, Hung STA, de Gans J, Goudsmit J (1989) Human immunodeficiency virus type 1 antigen in cerebrospinal fluid. Correlation with clinical neurologic status. Arch Neurol 46:261–264

Portegies P, Algra PR, Hollak CEM, Prins JM, Reiss P, Valk J, Lange JMA (1991) Response to cytarabine in progressive multifocal leucoencephalopathy in AIDS. Lancet 337:680–681

Portegies P, Enting RH, de Gans J, Algra PR, Derix MMA, Lange JMA, Goudsmit J (1993) Presentation and course of AIDS dementia complex: 10 years of follow-up in Amsterdam, the Netherlands. AIDS 7:669–675

Porter SB, Sande MA (1992) Toxoplasmosis of the central nervous system in the acquired immunodeficiency syndrome. N Engl J Med 327:1643–1648

Post DMJ, Tate LG, Quencer RM, Hensley GT, Berger JR, Sheremata WA, Maul G (1988) CT, MR, and pathology in HIV encephalitis and meningitis. AJNR 9:469–476

Post DMJ, Levin BE, Berger JR, Duncan R, Quencer RM, Calabro G (1992) Sequential cranial MR findings of asymptomatic and neurologically symptomatic HIV$^+$ subjects. AJNR 13:359–370

Power C, Kong PA, Crawford TO, Wesselingh S, Glass JD, McArthur JC, Trapp BD (1993) Cerebral white matter changes in acquired immunodeficiency syndrome dementia: alterations of the blood-brain barrier. Ann Neurol 34:339–350

Ramsey RG (1992) Update on neuroradiologic imaging of complications of AIDS. Categorical Course Syllabus; American Roentgen Ray Society; 91st annual meeting, Orlando, Florida

Ramsey RG, Geremia GK (1988) CNS complications of AIDS: CT and MR findings. AJR 151:449–454

Reeders JWAJ (1992) Diagnostic imaging of AIDS. Thieme, Stuttgart

Rodesch G, Parizel PM, Farber CM, Lalmand B, Przedborski S, Haens JD, van Calck M, Vanderhofstadt A, Taelman H, Baleriaux D (1989) Nervous system manifestations and neuroradiologic findings in acquired immunodeficiency syndrome (AIDS). Neuroradiology 31:33–39

Schmitt B, Seeger J, Kreuz W, Enenkel S, Jacobi G (1991) Central nervous system involvement of children with HIV infection. Dev Med Child Neurol 33:535–540

Shabas D, Gerard G, Cunha B, Malhotra V, Leeds N (1989) MR imaging of AIDS myelitis. AJNR 10:S51-S52

Shugar JMA, Som PM, Jacobson AL, Ryan JR, Bernard PJ, Dickman SH (1988) Multicentric parotid cysts and cervical adenopathy in AIDS patients. A newly recognized entity: CT and MR manifestations. Laryngoscope 98:772–775

Sönnerborg A, Sääf J, Alexius B, Strannegard O, Wahlund LO, Wetterberg L (1990) Quantitative detection of brain aberrations in human immunodeficiency virus type 1-infected individuals by magnetic resonance imaging. J Infect Dis 162:1245–1251

Talpos D, Tien RD, Hesselink JR (1991) Magnetic resonance imaging of AIDS-related polyradiculopathy. Neurology 41:1996–1997

Tien RD, Chu PK, Hesselink JR, Duberg A, Wiley C (1991) Intracranial cryptococcosis in immunocompromised patients: CT and MR findings in 29 cases. AJNR 12:823–829

Trenkwalder P, Trenkwalder C, Feiden W, Vogl TJ, Einhäupl KM, Lydtin H (1992) Toxoplasmosis with early intracerebral hemorrhage in a patient with the acquired immunodeficiency syndrome. Neurology 42:436–438

Tucker T (1989) Central nervous system AIDS. J Neurol Sci 89:119–133

Tuite M, Ketonen L, Kieburtz K, Handy B (1993) Efficacy of gadolinium in MR brain imaging of HIV-infected patients. AJNR 14:257–263

Varma VA, Hunter S, Tickman R, Srinivasan A, Swan D (1989) Acute fatal HIV encephalitis with negative serologic assays for antibody and antigen: diagnosis by polymerase chain reaction. N Engl J Med 320:1494

Villoria MF, de la Torre J, Fortea F, Munoz L, Hernandez T, Alarcon JJ (1992) Intracranial tuberculosis in AIDS: CT and MRI findings. Neuroradiology 34:11–14

Von Einsiedel RW, Fife TD, Aksamit AJ, Cornford ME, Secor DL, Tomiyasu U, Itabashi HH, Vinters HV (1993) Progressive multifocal leukoencephalopathy in AIDS: a clinicopathologic study and review of the literature. J Neurol 240:391–406

Wehn SM, Heinz ER, Burger PC, Boyko OB (1989) Dilated Virchow-Robin spaces in cryptococcal meningitis associated with AIDS: CT and MR findings. J Comput Assist Tomogr 13:756–762

Yankner BA, Skolnik PR, Shoukimas GM, Gabuzda DH, Sobel RA, Ho DD (1986) Cerebral granulomatous angiitis associated with isolation of human T-lymphotropic virus type III from the central nervous system. Ann Neurol 20:362–364

Zimmer C, Märzheuser S, Patt S, Rolfs A, Gottschalk J, Weigel K, Gosztonyi G (1992) Stereotactic brain biopsy in AIDS. J Neurol 239:394–400

56 Progressive Multifocal Leukoencephalitis

Achim CL, Wiley CA (1992) Expression of major histocompatibility complex antigens in the brains of patients with progressive multifocal leukoencephalopathy. J Neuropathol Exp Neurol 51:257–263

Aksamit AJ, Sever JL, Major EO (1986) Progressive multifocal leukoencephalopathy: JC virus detection by in situ hybridization compared with immunohistochemistry. Neurology 36:499–504

Appen RE, Roth H, ZuRhein GM, Varakis JN (1977) Progressive multifocal leukoencephalopathy. Arch Ophthalmol 95:656–659

Atwood WJ, Amemiya K, Traub R, Harms J, Major EO (1992) Interaction of the human polyomavirus, JCV, with human B-lymphocytes. Virology 190:716–723

Ault GS, Stoner GL (1993) Human polyomavirus JC promoter/enhancer rearrangement patterns from progressive multifocal leukoencephalopathy brain are unique derivatives of a single archetypal structure. J Gen Virol 74:1499–1507

Bedri J, Weinstein W, DeGregorio P (1983) Progressive multifocal leukoencephalopathy in acquired immunodeficiency syndrome. N Engl J Med 309:492–493

Bernick C, Gregorios JB (1984) Progressive multifocal leukoencephalopathy in a patient with acquired immune deficiency syndrome. Arch Neurol 41:780–782

Blum LW, Chambers RA, Schwartzman RJ, Streletz LJ (1985) Progressive multifocal leukoencephalopathy in acquired immune deficiency syndrome. Arch Neurol 42:137–139

Bosch EP, Cancilla PA, Cornell SH (1976) Computerized tomography in progressive multifocal leukoencephalopathy. Arch Neurol 33:216

Brun A, Nordenfelt E, Palm L (1976) Clustering progressive multifocal cases of leukoencephalopathy. N Engl J Med 295:1537

Buckman R, Wiltshaw E (1976) Progressive multifocal leucoencephalopathy successfully treated with cytosine arabinoside. Br J Haematol 34:153–158

Carroll BA, Lane B, Norman D, Enzmann D (1977) Diagnosis of progressive multifocal leukoencephalopathy by computed tomography. Radiology 122:137–141

Choy DSJ, Weiss A, Lin PT (1992) Progressive multifocal leukoencephalopathy following treatment for Wegener's granulomatosis. JAMA 268:600–601

England JD, Hsu CY, Garen PD, Goust JM, Biggs PJ (1984) Progressive multifocal leukoencephalopathy occurring with the acquired immune deficiency syndrome. South Med J 77:1041–1043

Gillespie SM, Chang Y, Lemp G, Arther R, Buchbinder S, Steimle A, Baumgartner J, Rando T, Neal D, Rutherford G, Schonberger L, Janssen R (1991) Progressive multifocal leukoencephalopathy in persons infected with human immunodeficiency virus, San Francisco, 1981–1989. Ann Neurol 30:597–604

Grinnell BW, Padgett BL, Walker DL (1983) Distribution of nonintegrated DNA from JC papovavirus in organs of patients with progressive multifocal leukoencephalopathy. J Infect Dis 147:669–675

Hansman Whiteman ML, Donovan Post MJ, Berger JR, Tate LG, Bell MD, Limonte LP (1993) Progressive multifocal leukoencephalopathy in 47 HIV-seropositive patients: neuroimaging with clinical and pathologic correlation. Radiology 187:233–240

Hawkins CP, McLaughlin JE, Kendall BE, McDonald WI (1993) Pathological finings correlated with MRI in HIV infection. Neuroradiology 35:264–268

Henson J, Saffer J, Furneaux H (1992) The transcription factor Sp 1 binds to the JC virus promoter and is selectively expressed in glial cells in human brain. Ann Neurol 32:72–77

Ho JL, Poldre PA, McEniry D, Howley PM, Snydman DR, Rudders RA, Worthington M (1984) Acquired immunodeficiency syndrome with progressive multifocal leukoencephalopathy and monoclonal B-cell proliferation. Ann Intern Med 100:693–696

Houff SA, Major EO, Katz DA, Kufta CV, Sever JL, Pittaluga S, Roberts JR, Gitt J, Saini N, Lux W (1988) Involvement of JC virus-infected mononuclear cells from the bone marrow and spleen in the pathogenesis of progressive multifocal leukoencephalopathy. N Engl J Med 318:301–305

Iida T, Kitamura T, Guo J, Taguchi F, Aso Y, Nagashima K, Yogo Y (1993) Origin of JC polyomavirus variants associated with progressive multifocal leukoencephalopathy. Proc Natl Acad Sci U S A 90:5062–5065

Kaye BR, Neuwelt CM, London SS, DeArmond SJ (1992) Central nervous system systemic lupus erythematosus mimicking progressive multifocal leucoencephalopathy. Ann Rheum Dis 51:1152–1156

Kirsh J, Rosenthall L, Finlayson MH, Wee R (1976) Progressive multifocal leukoencephalopathy. Radiology 119:399–400

Koeppen S, Lehmann HJ (1987) Progressive multifocal leukoencephalopathy: neurological findings and evaluation of magnetic resonance imaging and computed tomography. Neurosurg Rev 10:127–132

Ksamit AJ, Gendelman HE, Orenstein JM, Pezeshkpour GH (1990) AIDS-associated progressive multifocal leukencephalopathy (PML): comparison to non-AIDS PML with in situ hybridization and immunohistochemistry. Neurology 40:1073–1078

Kuchelmeister K, Gullotta F, Bergmann M, Angeli G, Masini T (1993) Progressive multifocal leukoencephalopathy (PML) in the acquired immunodeficiency syndrome (AIDS). A neuropathological autopsy study of 21 cases. Pathol Res Pract 189:163–173

Mark AS, Atlas SW (1989) Progressive multifocal leukoencephalopathy in patients with AIDS: appearance on MR images. Radiology 173:517–520

Newton P, Aldridge RD, Lessells AM, Best PV (1986) Progressive multifocal leukoencephalopathy complicating systemic lupus erythematosus. Arthritis Rheum 29:337–343

Nicoli F, Chave B, Peragut JC, Gastaut JL ((1992) Efficacy of cytarabine in progressive multifocal leucoencephalopathy in AIDS. Lancet 339:306

Padgett BL, Walker DL, ZuRhein GM, Hodach AE, Chou SM (1976) JC papovavirus in progressive multifocal leukoencephalopathy. J Infect Dis 133:686–690

Peters ACB, Versteeg J, Bots GTAM, Boogerd W, Vielvoye GJ (1980) Progressive multifocal leukoencephalopathy. Immunofluorescent demonstration of simian virus 40 antigen in CSF cells and response to cytarabine therapy. Arch Neurol 37:497–501

Richardson EP (1970) Progressive multifocal leukoencephalopathy. In: Vinken PJ, Bruyn GW (eds) Handbook of clinical neurology, vol 9. North Holland, Amsterdam, pp 485–499

Richardson EP (1988) Progressive multifocal leukoencephalopathy 30 years later. N Engl J Med 318:315–316

Rockwell D, Ruben FL, Winkelstein A, Mendelow H (1976) Absence of immune deficiencies in a case of progressive multifocal leukoencephalopathy. Am J Med 61:433–436

Rosenbloom MA, Uphoff DF (1983) The association of progressive multifocal leukoencephalopathy and sarcoidosis. Chest 83:572–575

Sandyk R (1983) Progressive multifocal leucoencephalopathy. S Afr Med J 64:320–321

Sangaland VE, Embil JA (1982) Recovery of papovavirus in cell culture explants of brain tissue from case of progressive multifocal leukoencephalopathy. Lancet 2:329–330

Sangaland VE, Embil JA (1984) Emergence of papovavirus in long-term cultures of astrocytes from progressive multifocal leukoencephalopathy patients. J Neuropathol Exp Neurol 43:553–567

Sima AAF, Finkelstein SD, McLachlan DR (1983) Multiple malignant astrocytomas in a patient with spontaneous progressive multifocal leukoencephalopathy. Ann Neurol 14:183–188

Singer C, Berger JR, Bowen BC, Bruce JH, Weiner WJ (1993) Akinetic-rigid syndrome in a 13-year-old girl with HIV-related progressive multifocal leukoencephalopathy. Mov Disord 8:113–116

Smith CR, Sima AAF, Salit IE, Gentili F (1982) Progressive multifocal leukoencephalopathy:failure of cytarabine therapy. Neurology 32:200–203

Sponzilli EE (1976) Progressive multifocal leukoencephalopathy: complication of immunosuppression. Arthritis Rheum 19:267

Steiger MJ, Tarnesby G, Gabe S, McLaughlin J, Schapira AHV (1993) Successful outcome of progressive multifocal leukoencephalopathy with cytarabine and interferon. Ann Neurol 33:407–411

Takemoto KK (1978) Human papovaviruses. Int Rev Exp Pathol 18:281–301

Trotot PM, Vazeux R, Yamashita HK, Sandoz-Tronca C, Mikol J, Vedrenne C, Thiebaut JB, Gray F, Cikurel M, Pialoux G, Levillain R (1990) MRI pattern of progressive multifocal leukoencephalopathy (PML) in AIDS. J Neuroradiol 17:233–254

Vazeux R, Cumont M, Girard PM, Nassif X, Trotot P, Marche C, Matthiessen L, Vedrenne C, Mikol J, Henin D, Katlama C, Bolgert F, Montagnier L (1990) Severe encephalitis resulting from coinfections with HIV and JC virus. Neurology 40:944–948

Zachoval R, Hunstein W, Ho AD (1980) Progressive multifocal leukoencephalopathy in a patient with Hodgkin's disease. Blut 41:451–454

57 Subacute Sclerosing Panencephalitis

Beersma MF, Galama JMD, van Druten HAM, Renier WO, Lucas CJ, Kapsenberg JG (1992) Subacute sclerosing panencephalitis in the Netherlands – 1976–1990
Int J Epidemiol 21:583–588

Bohlega S, Al-Kawi MZ (1994) Subacute sclerosing panencephalitis. J Neuroimag 4:71–76

Brown HR, Goller NL, Rudelli RD, Dymecki J, Wisniewski HM (1989) Postmortem detection of measles virus in non-neural tissues in subacute sclerosing panencephalitis. Ann Neurol 26:263–268

Choppin PW (1981) Measles virus and chronic neurological diseases. Ann Neurol 9:17–20

Dhib-Jalbut S, Haddad FS (1984) Subacute sclerosing panencephalitis in one member of identical twins. Neuropediatrics 15:49–51

Dyken PR (1985) Subacute sclerosing panencephalitis. Neurol Clin 3:179–196

Dyken PR, Cunningham SC, Charles Ward L (1989) Changing character of subacute sclerosing panencephalitis in the United States. Pediatr Neurol 5:339–341

Fournier JG, Tardieu M, Lebon P, Robain O, Ponsot G, Rozenblatt S, Bouteille M (1985) Detection of measles virus RNA in lymphocytes from peripheral blood and brain perivascular infiltrates of patients with subacut sclerosing panencephalitis. N Engl J Med 313:910–915

Geller TJ, Vern BA, Sarwar M (1987) Focal MRI findings in early SSPE. Pediatr Neurol 3:310–312

Griffith JF (1985) Subacute sclerosing panencephalitis and lymphocytes. N Engl J Med 313:952–954

Hall WW, Choppin PW (1981) Measles-virus proteins in the brain tissue of patients with subacute sclerosing panencephalitis. N Engl J Med 304:1152–1155

Iwasaki Y, Sako K, Tsunoda I, Ohara Y (1993) Phenotypes of mononuclear cell infiltrates in human central nervous system. Acta Neuropathol (Berl) 85:653–657

Jabbour JT, Garcia JH, Lemmi H, Ragland J, Duenas DA, Sever JL (1969) Subacute sclerosing panencephalitis. JAMA 207:2248–2254

Johnson KP, Byington DP, Gaddis L (1974) Subacute sclerosing panencephalitis. Adv Neurol 6:77–86

Lum GB, Williams JP, Dyken PR, Machen BC, Dotson PM, Harpen MD, McLeod N (1986) Magnetic resonance and CT imaging correlated with clinical status in SSPE. Pediatr Neurol 2:75–79

Modi G, Campbell H, Bill P (1989) Subacute sclerosing panencephalitis: changes on CT scan during acute relapse. Neuroradiology 31:433–434

Noetzel MJ, Dodson WE (1983) Progressive CT abnormalities despite clinical improvement in SSPE treated with inosiplex. Ann Neurol 13:457–460

Ohya T, Martinez AJ, Jabbour JT, Lemmi, Duenas DA (1974) Subacute sclerosing panencephalitis. Neurology 24:211–218

Payne FE, Baublis JV, Itabashi HH (1969) Isolation of measles virus from cell cultures of brain from a patient with subacute sclerosing panencephalitis. N Engl J Med 281:585–589

Poser CM (1990) Notes on the pathogenesis of subacute sclerosing panencephalitis. J Neurol Sci 95:219–224

Riekkinen P, Palo J, Arstila A, Rinne UK, Frey H, Savolainen H, Kivalo E (1970) Protein composition of white matter myelin in subacute sclerosing panencephalits. J Neurol Sci 14:15–20

Scully RE, Mark EJ, McNeely BU (1986) Case records of the masschusetts general hospital. N Engl J Med 314:1689–1700

Takayama S, Iwasaki Y, Yamanouchi H, Sugai K, Takashima S, Iwasaki A (1994) Characteristic clinical features in a case of fulminant subacute sclerosing panencephalitis. Brain Dev 16:132–135

Tan E, Namer IJ, Ciger A, Zileli T, Kucukali T (1991) The prognosis of subacute sclerosing panencephalitis in adults. Clin Neurol Neurosurg 93–3:205–209

Ter Meulen V, Hall WW (1978) Slow virus infections of the nervous system:virological immunological and pathogenetic considerations. J Gen Virol 41:1–25

Tsuchiya K, Yamauchi T, Furui S, Suda Y, Takenaka E (1988) MR imaging vs CT in subacute sclerosing panencephalitis. AJNR 9:943–946

Winer JB, Pires M, Kermode A, Ginsberg L, Rossor M (1991) Resolving MRI abnormalities with progression of subacute sclerosing panencephalitis. Neuroradiology 33:178–180

Yagi S, Miura Y, Mizuta S, Wakunami A, Kataoka N, Morita T, Morita K, Ono S, Fukunaga M (1993) Chronological SPECT studies of a patient with subacute sclerosing panencephalitis. Brain Dev 15:141–145

Yalaz K, Anlar B, Oktem F, Aysun S, Ustacelebi S, Gurcay O, Gurcay O, Gucuyener K, Renda Y (1992) Intraventricular interferon and oral inosiplex in the treatment of subacute sclerosing panencephalitis. Neurology 42:488–491

58 Progressive Rubella Panencephalitis

Bitzan M (1987) Rubella myelitis and encephalitis in childhood; a report of two cases with magnetic resonance imaging. Neuropediatrics 18:84–87

Coyle PK, Wolinsky JS (1981) Characterization of immune complexes in progressive rubella panencephalitis. Ann Neurol 9:557–562

Gilden DH (1983) Slow virus diseases of the CNS. Postgrad Med 73:99–101, 104–108

Hofman FM, Hinton DR, Baemayr J, Weil M, Merrill JE (1991) Lymphokines and immunoregulatory molecules in subacute sclerosing panencephalitis. Clin Immunol Immunopathol 58:331–342

Lebon P, Lyon G (1974) Non-congenital rubella encephalitis. Lancet 24:468

Sugita K, Ando M, Makino M, Takanashi J, Fujimoto N, Niimi H (1991) Magnetic resonance imaging of the brain in congenital rubella virus and cytomegalovirus infections. Neuroradiology 33:239–242

Townsend JJ, Baringer JR, Wolinsky JS, Malamud N, Mednick JP, Panitch HS, Scott RAT, Oshiro LS, Cremer NE (1975) Progressive rubella panencephalitis. N Engl J Med 8:990–993

Townsend JJ, Stroop WG, Baringer JR, Wolinsky JS, McKerrow JH, Berg BO (1982) Neuropathology of progressive rubella panencephalitis after childhood rubella. Neurology 32:185–190

Vandvik B, Weil ML, Grandien M, Norby E (1978) Progessive rubella virus panencephalitis:synthesis of oligoclonal virus-specific IgG antibodies and homogeneous free light chains in the central nervous system. Acta Neurol Scand 57:53–64

Weil ML, Itabashi HH, Cremer NE, Oshiro LS, Lennette EH, Carnay L (1975) Chronic progressive panencephalitis due to rubella virus simulating subacute sclerosing panencephalitis. N Engl J Med 292:994–998

Wolinsky JS, Berg BO, Maitland CJ (1976) Progressive rubella panencephalitis. Arch Neurol 33:722–723

Wolinsky JS, Dau PC, Buimovici-Klein E, Mednick J, Berg BO (1979) Progressive rubella panencephalitis: immunovirological studies and results of isoprinosine therapy. Clin Exp Immunol 35:397–404

59 Toxic Encephalopathy

Barron TF, Devenyi AG, Mamourian AC (1994) Symptomatic manganese neurotoxicity in a patient with chronic liver disease; correlation of clinical symptoms with MRI findings. Pediatr Neurol 10:145–148

Bontozoglou NP, Chakeres DW, Martin GF, Brogan MA, McGhee RB (1991) Cerebellorubral degeneration after resection of cerebellar dentate nucleus neoplasms:evaluation with MR imaging. Radiology 180:223–228

Brismar J, Aqeel A, Gascon G, Ozand P (1990) Malignant hyperphenylalaninemia. AJNR 11:135–138

Brown GK (1994) Metabolic disorders of embryogenesis. J Inherited Metab Dis 17:448–458

Chamuleau RAFM, Bosman DK, Bovee WMMJ, Luyten PR, den Hollander JA (1991) What the clinician can learn from MR glutamine/glutamate assays. NMR Biomed 4:103–108

Crapper McLachlan DR, de Boni U (1980) Aluminum in human brain disease. An overview. Neurotoxicology 1:3–16

Davis LE, Kornfeld M, Mooney HS, Fiedler KJ, Haaland KY, Orrison WW, Cernichiari E, Clarkson TW (1994) Methylmercury poisoning: long-term clinical, radiological, toxicological, and pathological studies of an affected family. Ann Neurol 35:680–688

Dobbing J (1968) Vulnerable periods in developing brain. In: Davison AN, Dobbing J (eds) Applied neurochemistry. Blackwell, Oxford, pp 287–316

Donnal JF, Heinze RE, Burger PC (1990) MR of reversible thalamic lesions in Wernicke syndrome. AJNR 11:893–894

Drayer BP, Bird CR, Williams K, Keller P (1989) Systemic metabolic disease and the globus pallidus: an MRI approach. AJNR 10:902–911

Escobar A, Aruffo C (1980) Chronic thinner intoxication: clinicopathologic report of a human case. J Neurol Neurosurg Psychiatry 43:986–994

Flechsig P (1920) Anatomie des menslichen Gehirns und Rückenmarks auf myelogenetischer Grundlage. Thieme, Leipzig

Galle P, Mey Rignac C, Heine P (1984) Toxicologie. C R Acad Sci (Paris) III:535–539

Galluci M, Bozzao A, Splendiani A, Masciocchi C, Passariello R (1990) Wernicke encephalopathy: MR findings in five patients. AJNR 11:887–892

Glauser TA, Pachter LM, Zimmerman RA (1992) Abnormal magnetic resonance images in hemorrhagic shock and encephalopathy syndrome. J Child Neurol 7:371–374

Heier LA, Carpanzano CR, Mast J, Brill PW, Winchester P, Deck MDF (1991) Maternal cocaine abuse:the spectrum of radiologic abnormalities in the neonatal CNS. AJNR 12:951–956

Hormes JT, Filey CM, Rosenberg NL (1986) Neurologic sequelae of chronic solvent vapor abuse. Neurology 36:698–702

Ikeda M, Tsukagoshi H (1990) Encephalopathy due to toluene sniffing: report of a case with magnetic resonance imaging. Eur Neurol 30:347–349

Kelly CTW (1975) Prolonged cerebellar dysfunction associated with paintsniffing. Pediatrics 56:605–606

Koehler PJ, Twijnstra A (1993) Paraneoplastische neurologische syndromen; nieuwe diagnostische mogelijkheden met antilichaambepalingen. Ned Tijdschr Geneeskd 137:1334–1337

Kornfeld M, Moser AB, Moser HW, Kleinschmidt-DeMasters BK, Nolte K, Phelps A (1994) Solvent vapor abuse leukoencephalopathy. Comparison to adrenoleukodystrophy. J Neuropathol Exp Neurol 53:389–398

Kulisevsky J, Ruscalleda J, Grau JM (1991) MR imaging of acquired hepatocerebral degeneration. AJNR 12:527–528

Lemoine P, Herousseau H, Bortegru J (1968) Children of alcoholic parents; observed anomalies (127 cases). Quest Med 21:476–482

Levy LM, Yang A, Hennigar R, Rothstein J, Bryan RN (1989) The brain and hepatic encephalopathy MR abnormalities. AJNR 10:900–905

Luyten PR, den Hollander JA, Bovee WMMJ, Ross BD, Bosman DK, Chamuleau RAFM. ^{31}P and ^{1}H NMR spectroscopy of the human brain in chronic hepatic encephalopathy (abstract). In: Society of Magnetic Resonance in Medicine (ed) Book of abstracts, vol 1. Society of Magnetic Resonance in Medicine, Berkeley, p 375

McConnell J, Castaldo P (1990) Striatal hyperemia, transient liver failure and chorea after liver transplantation. J Hepatol 10 [Suppl 1]:16–23

Okada J, Yoshikawa K, Matsuo H, Kanno K, Oouchi M (1991) Reversible MRI and CT findings in uremic encephalopathy. Neuroradiology 33:524–526

Powell H, Swarner O, Gluck L, Lampert P (1973) Hexachlorophene myelinopathy in premature infants. J Pediatr 82:976–981

Ross BD (1991) Biochemical considerations in ^{1}H spectroscopy: glutamate and glutamine; myo-inositol and related metabolites. NMR Biomed 4:59–63

Schroth G, Wichmann W, Valavanis A (1991) Blood-brain-barrier disruption in acute Wernicke encephalopathy: MR findings. J Comput Assist Tomogr 15:1059–1061

Sedman AB, Wilkening GN, Warady BA, Lum GM, Alfrey AC (1984) Encephalopathy in childhood secondary to aluminum toxicity. Clin Lab Observations 105:836–838

Shepard TH (1986) Catalog of teratogenic agents. Johns Hopkins University Press, Baltimore

Singer DB, Sung LJ, Wigglesworth RJS (1991) Fetal growth and maturation. In: Wigglesworth RJS, Singer DB (eds) Textbook of fetal and perinatal pathology. Blackwell, Oxford, pp 11–47

Spencer P, Hugen J, Ludolph A (1987) Discovery and partial characterization of primate motor system toxins. Ciba Found Symp 126:221–238

Tokuomi H, Okajuma T, Kanai J, Tsimoda M (1961) Minamata disease: an unusual neurological disorder occurring in Minamata. Kurume Med J 14:47–64

Towfighi J, Gonatas NK (1976) Hexachlorophene and the nervous system. In: Zimmerman HM (ed) Progress in neuropathology, vol III. Grune and Stratton, New York, pp 297–317

Troncoso JC, Price DL, Griffin JW, Parhad IM (1982) Neurofibrillary axonal pathology in aluminum intoxication. Ann Neurol 12:278–283

Valk J, van der Knaap MS (1992) Toxic encephalopathy. AJNR 13:747–760

Van der Knaap MS, Valk J (1988) Classification of congenital abnormalities of the CNS AJNR 9:315–326

Vernadakis A, Parker KK (1980) Drugs and the developing central nervous system. Pharmacol Ther 11:593–647

Vinken PJ, Bruyn GW (1979) Intoxications of the central nervous system. In: Vinken PJ, Bruyn GW (eds) Handbook of clinical neurology, vol 36 and 37. North Holland, New York

Volpe JJ (1987) Drugs and the developing nervous system. In: Volpe JJ (ed) Neurology of the newborn. Saunders, Philadelphia, pp 664–697

Volpe JJ (1992) Effect of cocaine use on the fetus. N Engl J Med 327:399–407

Wiggins RC (1986) Myelination: a critical stage in development. Neurotoxicology 7:103–120

Wolters EC, van Wijngaarden GK, Stam FC (1982) Leukoencephalopathy after inhaling „heroin" pyrolysite. Lancet 1:1233–1236

Xiong L, Matthes JD, Li J, Jinkins JR (1993) MR imaging of „spray heads": toluene abuse via aerosol paint inhalation. AJNR 14:1195–1199

Zeneroli ML, Cioni C, Vezzelli C (1987) Prevalence of brain atrophy in liver cirrhosis patients with chronic persistent encephalopathy. J Hepatol 4:283–292

Zeneroli ML, Cioni G, Crisi G, Vezzelli C, Ventura E (1991) Globus pallidus alterations and brain atrophy in liver cirrhosis patients with encephalopathy: an MR imaging study. Magn Reson Imaging 9:295–302

60 Central Pontine and Extrapontine Myelinolysis

Adams RD, Victor M, Mancall EL (1959) Central pontine myelinolysis. Arch Neurol Psychiatry 81:154–172

Alberca R, Iriarte LM, Rasero P, Villalobos F (1985) Brachial diplegia in central pontine myelinolysis. J Neurol 231:345–346

Arieff AI, Ayus JC (1993) Pathogenesis of hyponatremic encephalopathy:current concepts. Chest 103:607–610

Ayus JC, Krothapalli RK, Arieff AI (1987) Treatment of symptomatic hyponatremia and its relation to brain damage. N Engl J Med 317:1190–1195

Bergin PS, Harvey P (1992) Wernicke's encephalopathy and central pontine myelinolysis associated with hyperemesis gravidarum. Br Med J 305:517–518

Boon AP, Carey MP, Adams DH, Buckels J, McMaster P (1991) Central pontine myelinolysis in liver transplantation. J Clin Pathol 44:909–914

Brunner JE, Redmond JM, Haggar AM, Kruger DF, Elias SB (1990) Central pontine myelinolysis and pontine lesions after rapid correction of hyponatremia: a prospective magnetic resonance imaging study. Ann Neurol 27:61–66

Burcar PJ, Norenberg MD, Yarnell PR (1977) Hyponatremia and central pontine myelinolysis. Neurology 27:223–226

Clifford DB, Gado MH, Levy BK (1989) Osmotic demyelination syndrome: lack of pathologic and radiologic imaging correlation. Arch Neurol 46:343–347

Cunha CD, Bertorini TE, Lawrence J, Witherington JM (1986) Central pontine myelinolysis - a preventable condition. Two case reports and review of the literature. J Tenn Med Assoc 79:469–472

Da Cunha C, Bertorini TE, Lawrence J, Witherington JM (1986) Central pontine myelinolysis: a preventable condition. J Tenn Med Assoc 79:469–472

De Witt LD, Buonanno FS, Kistler P, Zeffiro T, de La Paz RL, Brady TJ, Rosen BR, Pykett IL (1984) Central pontine myelinolysis: demonstration by nuclear magnetic resonance. Neurology 34:570–576

De Zegers Beyl D, Flament-Durand J, Borenstein S, Brunko E (1983) Ocular bobbing and myoclonus in central pontine myelinolysis. J Neurol Neurosurg Psychiatry 46:564–565

Gallucci M, Amicarelli I, Rossi A, Stratta P, Maciocchi C, Zobel BB, Casacchia M, Passariello R (1989) MR imaging of white matter lesions in uncomplicated chronic alcoholism. J Comput Assist Tomogr 13:395–398

Gerber O, Geller M, Stiller J, Yang W (1983) Central pontine myelinolysis. Arch Neurol 40:116–118

Giannetti AV, Pittella JEH (1993) Ischemic and hemorrhagic necrosis of the pons with anatomical location similar to that of central pontine myelinolysis in a chronic alcoholic patient. Clin Neuropathol 12:156–159

Gocht A, Löhler J (1990) Changes in glial cell markers in recent and old demyelinated lesions in central pontine myelinolysis. Acta Neuropathol (Berl) 80:46–58

Goldman JE, Horoupian DS (1981) Demyelination of the lateral geniculate nucleus in central pontine myelinolysis. Ann Neurol 9:185–189

Greenberg WM, Shah PJ (1993) CPM in polydipsic psychiatric patients. Am J Psychiatry 150:842–843

Hardjasudarma M, Husain F, Fowler M, Eisenberg RL, Mirfakhraee M (1992) Central pontine myelinolysis as a manifestation of the paraneoplastic syndrome. South Med J 85:419–421

Harris CP, Townsend JJ, Baringer JR (1993) Symptomatic hyponatraemia: can myelinolysis be prevented by treatment? J Neurol Neurosurg Psychiatry 56:626–632

Hasan D, Wijdicks EFM, Vermeulen M (1990) Hyponatremia is associated with cerebral ischemia in patients with aneurysmal subarachnoid hemorrhage. Ann Neurol 27:106–108

Ho VB, Ritz CR, Yoder CC, Geyer CA (1993) Resolving MR features in osmotic myelinolysis (central pontine and extrapontine myelinolysis). AJNR 14:163–167

Ingram DA, Traub M, Kopelman PG, Summers BA, Swash M (1986) Brain-stem auditory evoked responses in diagnosis of central pontine myelinolysis. J Neurol 233:23–24

Karp BI, Laureno R (1993) Pontine and extrapontine myelinolysis: a neurlogic disorder following rapid correction of hyponatremia. Medicine 72:359–373

Keating JP, Schears GJ, Dodge PR (1991) Oral water intoxication in infants; an American epidemic. Am J Dis Child 145:985–990

Kendall BE (1993) Inborn errors and demyelination: MRI and the diagnosis of white matter disease. J Inherited Metab Dis 16:771–786

Kleinschmidt-de Masters BK, Norenberg MD (1981) Rapid correction of hyponatremia causes demyelination: relation to central pontine myelinolysis. Science 21:1068–1070

Kleinshmidt-de Masters BK, Norenberg MD (1982) Neuropathologic observations in electrolyte-induced myelinolysis in the rat. J Neuropathol Exp Neurol 41:67–80

Kobuke T (1985) Central pontine myelinolysis accompanied by multifocal pseudocalcifications. Acta Pathol Jpn 35:1279–1284

Koci TM, Chiang F, Chow P, Wang A, Chiu LC, Itabashi H, Mehringer CM (1990) Thalamic extrapontine lesions in central pontine myelinolysis. AJNR 11:1229–1233

Kold A (1986) Hyponatremia: cerebral symptoms and role in central pontine myelinolysis. Acta Neurol Scand 73:200–202

Korogi Y, Takahashi M, Shinzato J, Sakamoto Y, Mitsuzaki K, Hirai T, Yoshizumi K (1993) MR findings in two presumed cases of mild central pontine myelinolysis. AJNR 14:651–654

Laureno R (1983) Central pontine myelinolysis following rapid correction of hyponatremia. Ann Neurol 13:232–242

Laureno R (1993) Myelinolysis is due to rapid correction of hyponatremia. Am J Med 94:225–226

Laureno R, Karp BI (1988) Pontine and extrapontine myelinolysis following rapid correction of hyponatremia. Lancet 25:1439–1440

Maraganore DM, Folger WN, Swanson JW, Ahlskog JE (1992) Movement disorders as sequelae of central pontine myelinolysis: report of three cases. Mov Dis 7:142–148

Marra TR (1983) Hemiparesis apparently dueto central pontine myelinolysis following hyponatremia. Ann Neurol 14:687–688

Mascheli M, Cincotta M, Piazinni M (1993) Case report. MRI demonstration of pontine and thalamic myelinolysis in an alcoholic. Clin Radiol 47:137–138

McColl P, Kelly C (1992) A misleading case of central pontine myelinolysis. Risk factors for psychiatric patients. Br J Psychiatry 160:550–552

Messert B, Orrison WW, Hawkins MJ, Quaglieri CE (1979) Central pontine myelinolysis. Neurology 29:147–160

Miller GM, Baker HL Okazaki H, Whisnant JP (1988) Central pontine myelinolysis and its imitators: MR findings. Radiology 168:795–802

Mossuto L, Fattapposta F, Rossi F (1986) Central pontine myelinolysis: diagnosis by computed tomography, magnetic resonance and evoked potentials. Ital J Neurol Sci 7:591–596

Narins RG (1986) Therapy of hyponatremia. Does haste make waste? N Engl J Med 314:1573–1575

Norenberg MD (1983) A hypothesis of osmotic endothelial injury: a pathogenetic mechanism in central pontine myelinolysis. Arch Neurol 40:66–69

Norenberg MD, Leslie KO, Robertson AS (1982) Association between rise in serum sodium and central pontine myelinolysis. Ann Neurol 11:128–135

Okeda R, Kitano M, Sawabe M, Yamada I, Yamada M (1986) Distribution of demyelinating lesions in pontine and extrapontine myelinolysis – three autopsy cases including one case devoid of central pontine myelinolysis. Acta Neuropathol (Berl) 69:259–266

Ragland RL, Duffis AW, Gendelman S, Som PM, Rabinowitz JG (1989) Central pontine myelinolysis with clinical recovery: MR documentation. J Comput Assist Tomogr 13:316–318

Rosenbloom S, Buchholz D, Kumar AJ, Kaplan RA, Moses H, Rosenbaum AE (1984) Evolution of central pontine myelinolysis on CT. AJNR 5:110–112

Rouanet F, Tison F, Dousset V, Corand V, Orgogozo JM (1994) Early T_2 hypointense signal abnormality preceding clinical manifestations of central pontine myelinolysis. Neurology 44:979–980

Sadeh M, Goldhammer Y (1993) Extrapyramidal syndrome responsive to dopaminergic treatment following recovery from central pontine myelinolysis. Eur Neurol 33:48–50

Schroth G (1984) Clinical and CT confirmed recovery from central pontine myelinolysis. Neuroradiology 26:149–151

Slager UT (1985) Central pontine myelinolysis and abnormalities in serum sodium. Clin Neuropathol 5:252–256

Stam J, van Oers MHJ, Verbeeten B Jr (1984) Recovery after central pontine myelinolysis. J Neurol 231:52–53

Sterns RH, Riggs JE, Schochet SS (1986) Osmotic demyelination syndrome following correction of hyponatremia. N Engl J Med 24:1535–1542

Sztencel J, Baleriaux D, Borenstein S, Brunko E, Zegers de Beyl D (1983) Central pontine myelinolysis: correlation between CT and electrophysiologic data. AJNR 4:529–530

Takeda K, Sakuta M, Saeki F (1985) Central pontine myelinolysis diagnosed by magnetic resonance imaging. Ann Neurol 17:310–311

Taylor AL (1993) Postoperative hyponatermia in menstruant women. Ann Intern Med 118:984

Tien R, Arieff AL, Kucharczyk W, Wasik A, Kucharczyk J (1992) Hyponatremic encephalopathy: is central pontine myelinolysis a component? Am J Med 92:513–522

Tinker R, Anderson MG, Anand P, Kermode A, Harding AE (1990) Pontine myelinolysis presenting with acute parkinsonism as a sequel of corrected hyponatremia. J Neurol Neurosurg Psychiatry 53:87–89

Wright DG, Laureno R, Victor M (1979) Pontine and extrapontine myelinolysis. Brain 102:361–385

61 Marchiafava-Bignami Syndrome

Baron R, Heuser K, Marioth G (1989) Marchiafava-Bignami disease with recovery diagnosed by CT and MRI: demyelination affects several CNS structures. J Neurol 236:364–366

Bracard S, Claude D, Vespignani H, Almeras M, Carsin M, Lambert H, Picard L (1986) Computerized tomography and MRI in Marchiafava-Bignami disease. J Neuroradiol 13:87–94

Caparros-Lefebvre D, Pruvo JP, Josien E, Pertuzon B, Clarisse J, Petit H (1994) Marchiafava-Bignami disease: use of contrast media in CT and MRI. Neuroradiology 36:509–511

Chang KH, Cha SH, Han MH, Park SH, Nah DL, Hong JH (1992) Marchiafava-Bignami disease: serial changes in corpus callosum on MRI. Neuroradiology 34:480–482

Clavier E, Thiebot J, Delangre T, Hannequin D, Samson M, Benozio M (1986) Marchiafava-Bignami disease. Neuroradiology 28:376

Hauw JJ, de Baeque C, Hausser-Hauw C, Serdaru M (1988) Chromatolysis in alcoholic encephalopathies. Pellagra-like changes in 22 cases. Brain 111:843–857

Heepe P, Nemeth L, Brune F, Grant JW, Kleihues P (1988) Marchiafava-Bignami disease: a correlative computed tomography and morphological study. Eur Arch Psychiatr Neurol Sci 237:74–79

Humbert T, Guilhermier de P, Maktouf C, Grasset G, Lopez FM, Chabrand P (1992) Marchiafava-Bignami disease. A case studied by structural and functional brain imaging. Eur Arch Psychiatry Clin Neurosci 242:69–71

Izquierdo G, Quesada MA, Chacon J, Martel J (1992) Neuroradiologic abnormalities in Marchiafava-Bignami disease of benign evolution. Eur J Radiol 15:71–74

Mayer JW, De Liège P, Netter JM, Danzé F, Reizine D (1987) Computerized tomography and nuclear magnetic resonance imaging in Marchiafava-Bignami disease. J Neuroradiol 14:152–158

Rosa A, Demiati M, Cartz L, Mizon JP (1991) Marchiafava-Bignami disease, syndrome of interhemispheric disconnection, and right-handed agraphia in a left-hander. Arch Neurol 48:986–988

Serdaru M, Hausser-Hauw C, LaPlane D, Buge A, Castaigne P, Goulon M, Lhermitte F, Hauw JJ (1988) The clinical spectrum of alcoholic pellagra encephalopathy. Brain 111:829–842

62 Posthypoxic-Ischemic Damage

Beal MF (1992) Does impairment of energy metabolism result in excitotoxic neuronal death in neurodegenerative illnesses? Ann Neurol 31:119–130

Berdichevsky E, Riveros N, Sanchez-Armass S, Orrego F (1983) Kainate, N-methylaspartate and other excitatory amino acids increase calcium influx into rat brain cortex cells in vitro. Neurosci Lett 36:75–80

Chan PH, Fishman RA (1980) Transient formation of superoxide radicals in polyunsaturated fatty acid-induced brain swelling. J Neurochem 35:1004–1007

Chan PH, Fishman RA (1982) Alterations of membrane integrity and cellular constituents by arachidonic acid in neuroblastoma and glioma cells. Brain Res 248:151–157

Chan PH, Fishman RA (1985) Free fatty acids, oxygen free radicals, and membrane alterations in brain ischemia and injury. In: Plum F, Pulsinelli W (eds) Cerebrovascular diseases. Raven, New York, pp 161–168

Chan PH, Yurko M, Fishman RA (1982) Phospholipid degradation and cellular edema induced by free radicals in brain cortical slices. J Neurochem 38:525–531

Chan PH, Schmidley JW, Fishman RA, Longar SM (1984) Brain injury, edema, and vascular permeability changes induced by oxygen-derived free radicals. Neurology 34:315–320

Chen M, Bullock R, Graham DI, Frey P, Lowe D, McCulloch J (1991) Evaluation of a competitive NMDA antagonist (D-CPPene) in feline focal cerebral ischemia. Ann Neurol 30:62–70

Clark GD (1989) Role of excitatory amino acids in brain injury caused by hypoxia-ischemia, status epilepticus, and hypoglycemia. Clin Perinatol 16:459–474

Coker SB, Beltran RS, Myers TF, Hmura L (1988) Neonatal stroke: description of patients and investigation into pathogenesis. Pediatr Neurol 4:219–223

Cotman CW, Monaghan DT, Ottersen OP, Storm-Mathisen J (1987) Anatomical organizatin of excitatory amino acid receptors and their pathways. Trends Neurosci 10:273–280

DiFiglia M (1990) Excitotoxic injury of the neostriatum: a model for Huntington's disease. Trends Neurosci 13:286–289

Doble A, Perrier ML (1989) Pharmacology of excitatory amino acid receptors coupled to inositol phosphate metabolism in neonatal rat striatum. Neurochem Int 15:1–8

Dure LSIV, Young AB, Penney JB (1991) Excitatory amino acid binding sites in the caudate nucleus and frontal cortex of Huntington's disease. Ann Neurol 30:785–793

Flamm ES, Demopoulos HB, Seligman ML, Poser RG, Ransohoff J (1978) Free radicals in cerebral ischemia. Stroke 9:445–447

Foster AC, Donald AE, Willis CL, Tridgett R, Kemp JA, Priestley T (1990) The glycine site on the NMDA receptor: pharmacology and involvement in NMDA receptor-mediated neurodegeneration. In: Ben-Ari Y (ed) Excitatory amino acids and neuronal plasticity. Plenum, New York, pp 93–100

Freund TF, Buzsaki G, Leon A, Baimbridge KG, Somogyi P (1990) Relationship of neuronal vulnerability and calcium binding protein immunoreactivity in ischemia. Exp Brain Res 83:55–66

Goldberg MP, Choi DW (1990) Intracellular free calcium increases in cultured cortical neurons deprived of oxygen and glucose. Stroke 21 [Suppl III]:75–77

Hasegawa K, Yoshioka H, Sawada T, Nishikawa H (1991) Lipid peroxidation in neonatal mouse brain subjected to two different types of hypoxia. Brain Dev 13:101–103

Hattori H, Wasterlain CG (1990) Excitatory amino acids in the developing brain: ontogeny, plasticity, and excitotoxicity. Pediatr Neurol 6:219–228

Hertz L (1979) Functional interactions between neurons and astrocytes I. Turnover and metabolism of putative amino acid transmitters. Prog Neurobiol 13:277–323

Ikeda Y, Long DM (1990) The molecular basis of brain injury and brain edema: the role of oxygen free radicals. Neurosurgery 27:1–11

Ikeda J, Nagashima G, Saito N, Nowak TS, Joo F, Mies G, Lohr JM, Ruetzler CA, Klatzo I (1990) Putative neuroexcitation in cerebral ischemia and brain injury. Stroke 21 [Suppl III]: 65–70

Jarvis MF, Wagner GC (1990) 1-methyl-4-phenyl-1,2,3,6-tetrahydropyridine-induced neurotoxicity in the rat: characterization and age-dependent effects. Synapse 5:104–112

Jorgensen MB, Diemer NH (1982) Selective neuron loss after cerebral ischemia in the rat: possible role of transmitter glutamate. Acta Neurol Scand 66:536–546

Kucharczyk J, Mintorovitch J, Moseley ME, Asgari HS, Sevick RJ, Derugin N, Norman D (1991) Ischemic brain damage: reduction by sodium-calcium ion channel modulator RS-87476. Radiology 179:221–227

Koroshetz WJ, Freese A, DiFiglia M (1990) The correlation between excitatory amino acid-induced current responses and excitotoxicity in striatal cultures. Brain Res 521:265–272

Levin SD (1991) Mechanisms of damage in the developing brain. Curr Opin Neurol Neurosurg 4:371–376

Lockerbie RO (1990) Neurotrophic factors and development. Curr Opin Neurol Neurosurg 3:955–958

Lundgren J, Zhang H, Agardh CD, Smith ML, Evans PJ, Halliwell B, Siesjö BK (1991) Acidosis-induced ischemic brain damage: are free radicals involved? J Cereb Blood Flow Metab 11:587–596

Mattson MP (1989) Cellular signaling mechanisms common to the development and degeneration of neuroarchitecture. A review. Mech Ageing Dev 50:103–157

Mattson MP (1990) Excitatory amino acids, growth factors, and calcium: a teeter-totter model for neural plasticity and degeneration. In: Ben-Ari Y (ed) Excitatory amino acids and neuronal plasticity. Plenum, New York, pp 211–220

McCord JM (1985) Oxygen-derived free radicals in postischemic tissue injury. N Engl J Med 312:159–163

McDonald JW, Silverstein FS, Johnston MV (1987) MK-801 protects the neonatal brain from hypoxic-ischemic damage. Eur J Pharmacol 140:359–361

McDonald JW, Johnston MV, Young AB (1990) Differential ontogenic development of three receptors comprising the NMDA receptor/channel complex in the rat hippocampus. Exp Neurol 110:237–247

Myers RE (1979) A unitary theory of causation of anoxic and hypoxic brain pathology. Adv Neurol 26:195–213

Odeh M (1991) The role of reperfusion-induced injury in the pathogenesis of the Crush syndrome. N Engl J Med 324:1417–1422

Olney JW, Ho OL, Rhee V (1971) Cytotoxic effects of acidic and sulphur containing amino acids on the infant mouse central nervous system. Exp Brain Res 14:61–76

Pulsinelli WA (1985) Deafferentation of the hippocampus protects CA1 pyramidal neurons against ischemic injury. Stroke 16:144

Raichle ME (1983) The pathophysiology of brain ischemia. Ann Neurol 13:2–10

Riikonen RS, Kero PO, Simell OG (1992) Excitatory amino acids in cerebrospinal fluid in neonatal asphyxia. Pediatr Neurol 8:37–40

Rothman SM (1983) Synaptic activity mediates death of hypoxic neurons. Science 220:536–537

Rothman S (1984) Synaptic release of excitatory amino acid neurotransmitter mediates anoxic neuronal death. J Neurosci 4:1884–1891

Rothman SM, Olney JW (1986) Glutamate and the pathophysiology of hypoxic-ischemic brain damage. Ann Neurol 19:105–111

Rothman SM, Olney JW (1987) Excitotoxicity and the NMDA receptor. Trends Neurosci 10:299–302

Rothman SM, Thurston JH, Hauhart RE (1987) Delayed neurotoxicity of excitatory amino acids in vitro. Neurosci 22:471–480

Sauer D, Allegrini PR, Thedinga KH, Massieu L, Amacker H, Fagg GE (1992) Evaluation of quinolinic acid induced excitotoxic neurodegeneration in rat striatum by quantitative magnetic resonance imaging in vivo. J Neurosci Methods 42:69–74

Schwarcz R, Meldrum B (1985) Excitatory aminoacid antagonists provide a therapeutic approach to neurological disorders. Lancet II:140–143

Shaw PJ (1992) Excitatory amino acid neurotransmission, excitotoxicity and excitotoxins. Curr Opin Neurol Neurosurg 5:383–390

Siesjö BK (1981) Cell damage in the brain:a speculative synthesis. J Cereb Blood Flow Metab 1:155–185

Siesjö BK (1984) Cerebral circulation and metabolism. J Neurosurg 60:883–908

Siesjö BK (1992) Pathophysiology and treatment of focal cerebral ischemia, part I: pathophysiology. J Neurosurg 77:169–184

Siesjö BK (1992) Pathophysiology and treatment of focal cerebral ischemia, part II: mechanisms of damage and treatment. J Neurosurg 77:337–354

Simon RP, Swan JH, Griffiths T, Meldrum BS (1984) Blockade of N-methyl-D-aspartate receptors may protect against ischemic damage in the brain. Science 226:850–852

Stephenson FA (1990) Neurotransmitter receptors. Curr Opin Neurol Neurosurg 3:951–954

Storm-Mathisen J, Opsahl MW (1978) Asparate and/or glutamate may be transmitters in hippocampal efferents to septum and hypothalamus. Neurosci Lett 9:65–70

Stys PK, Waxman SG, Ransom BR (1991) Na^+-Ca^{2+} exchanger mediates Ca^{2+} influx during anoxia in mammalian central nervous system white matter. Ann Neurol 30:375–380

Turski L, Turski WA (1993) Towards an understanding of the role of glutamate in neurodegenerative disorders:energy metabolism and neuropathology. Experientia 49:1064–1072

Wieloch T (1990) Neuronal injury and cerebrovascular disorders. Curr Opin Neurol Neurosurg 3:944–950

Yoshida S, Abe K, Busto R, Watson BD, Kogure K, Ginsberg MD (1982) Influence of transient ischemia on lipid-soluble antioxidants, free fatty acids and energy metabolites in rat brain. Brain Res 245:307–316

Young RSK, Petroff OAC, Aquila WJ, Yates J (1991) Effects of glutamate, quisqualate, and N-methyl-D-aspartate in neonatal brain. Exp Neurol 111:362–368

63 Posthypoxic-Ischemic Leukoencephalopathy of Neonates

Alberman E, Benson J, Evans S (1982) Visual defects in children of low birthweight. Arch Dis Child 57:818–822

Atkinson J (1984) Human visual development over the first 6 months of life. A review and a hypothesis. Hum Neurobiol 3:61–74

Azzarelli B, Meade P, Muller J (1980) Hypoxic lesions in areas of primary myelination. A distinct pattern in cerebral palsy. Child Brain 7:132–145

Baenziger O, Martin E, Steinlin M, Good M, Largo R, Burger R, Fanconi S, Duc G, Buchli R, Rumpel H (1993) Early pattern recognition in severe perinatal asphyxia: a prospective MRI study. Neuroradiology 35:437–442

Baker LL, Stevenson DK, Enzmann DR (1988) End-stage periventricular leukomalacia: MR evaluation. Radiology 168:809–815

Barkovich AJ (1992) MR and CT evaluation of profound neonatal and infantile asphyxia. AJNR 13:959–972

Barkovich AJ, Truwit CL (1990) Brain damage from perinatal asphyxia: correlation of MR findings with gestational age. AJNR 11:1087–1096

Barth PG, Valk J, Olislagers-de Slegte R (1984) Aspect scanographique des zones corticales et sous-corticales centrales dans les paralysies cerebrales. J Neuroradiol 11:65–71

Brazy JE, Lewis DV, Mitnick MH, van der Vliet FFJ (1985) Noninvasive monitoring of cerebral oxygenation in preterm infants:preliminary observations. Pediatrics 75:217–225

Byrne P, Welch R, Johnson MA, Darrah J, Piper M (1990) Serial magnetic resonance imaging in neonatal hypoxic-ischemic encephalopathy. J Pediatr 117:694–700

Candy EJ, Hoon AH, Capute AJ, Bryan RN (1993) MRI in motor delay: important adjunct to classification of cerebral palsy. Pediatr Neurol 9:421–429

Carson SC, Hertzberg BS, Bowie JD, Burger PC (1990) Value of sonography in the diagnosis of intracranial hemorrhage and periventricular leukomalacia:a postmortem study of 35 cases. AJNR 11:677–683

Carter BS, Haverkamp AD, Merenstein GB (1993) The definition of acute perinatal asphyxia. Clin Perinatol 20:287–304

Cope M, Delpy DT (1988) System for long-term measurement of cerebral blood and tissue oxygenation on newborn infants by near infra-red transillumination. Med Biol Eng Comput 26:289–294

Courville CB, Myers RO (1958) The process of demyelination in the central nervous system. J Neuropathol Exp Neurol 17:158–173

De Vries LS, Connell JA, Dubowitz LMS, Oozeer RC, Dubowitz V (1987) Neurological, electrophysiological and MRI abnormalities in infants with extensive cystic leukomalacia. Neuropediatrics 18:61–66

De Vries LS, Wigglesworth JS, Regev R, Dubowitz LMS (1988) Evolution of periventricular leukomalacia during the neonatal period and infancy: correlation of imaging and postmortem findings. Early Hum Dev 17:205–219

De Vries LS, Regev R, Dubowitz LMS, Whitelaw A, Aber VR (1988) Perinatal risk factors for the development of extensive cystic leukomalacia. Am J Dis Child 142:732–735

De Vries LS, Pierrat V, Eken P, Minami T, Daniels H, Casaer P (1991) Prognostic value of early somatosensory evoked potentials for adverse outcome in full-term infants with birth asphyxia. Brain Dev 13:320–325

De Vries LS, Eken P, Dubowitz LMS (1992) The spectrum of leukomalacia using cranial ultrasound. Behav Brain Res 49:1–6

De Vries LS, Eken P, Groenendaal F, van Haastert IC, Meiners LC (1993) Correlation between the degree of periventricular leukomalacia diagnosed using cranial ultrasound and MRI

later in infancy in children with cerebral palsy. Neuropediatrics 24:263–268

DeReuck J (1971) The human periventricular arterial blood supply and the anatomy of cerebral infarctions. Eur Neurol 5:321–334

DeReuck JL (1984) Cerebral angioarchitecture and perinatal brain lesions in premature and full-term infants. Acta Neurol Scand 70:391–395

DeReuck J, Chattha AS, Richardson EP (1972) Pathogenesis and evolution of periventricular leukomalacia in infancy. Arch Neurol 27:229–236

Dietrich RB, Bradley WG (1988) Iron accumulation in the basal ganglia following severe ischemic-anoxic insults in children. Radiology 168:203–206

Donovan DE, Coues P, Paine RS (1962) The prognostic implications of neurologic abnormalities in the neonatal period. Neurology 12:910–914

Dubowitz LMS, Dubowitz V, Palmer PG, Miller G, Fawer CL, Levene MI (1984) Correlation of neurologic assessment in the preterm newborn infant with outcome at 1 year. J Pediatr 105:452–456

Dubowitz LMS, Bydder GM, Mushin J (1985) Developmental sequence of periventricular leukomalacia. Arch Dis Child 60:349–355

Feldman HM, Scher MS, Kemp SS (1990) Neurodevelopmental outcome of children with evidence of periventricular leukomalacia on late MRI. Pediatr Neurol 6:296–302

Fernell E, Hagberg G, Hagberg B (1993) Infantile hydrocephalus in preterm, low-birth-weight infants – nationwide Swedish cohort study 1979–1988. Acta Paediatr 82:45–48

Flodmark O, Roland EH, Hill A, Whitfield MF (1987) Periventricular leukomalacia:radiologic diagnosis. Radiology 162:119–124

Flodmark O, Lupton B, Li D, Stimac GK, Roland EH, Hill A, Whitfield MF, Norman MG (1989) MR imaging of periventricular leukomalacia in childhood. AJR 152:583–590

Gabrielli O, Coppa GV, Giorgi P, Salvolini U (1990) Brain maturation and magnetic resonance imaging. J Pediatr 117:675

Grunnet ML (1979) Periventricular leukomalacia complex. Arch Pathol Lab Med:103:6–10

Hagberg B, Hagberg G, Olow I (1984) The changing panorama of cerebral palsy in Sweden. Acta Paediatr Scand 73:433–440

Hagberg B, Hagberg G, Zetterström R (1989) Decreasing perinatal mortality. Increase in cerebral palsy morbidity? Acta Paediatr Scand 78:664–670

Heibel M, Heber R, Bechinger D, Kornhuber HH (1993) Early diagnosis of perinatal cerebral lesions in apparently normal full-term newborns by ultrasound of the brain. Neuroradiology 35:85–91

Hill A (1991) Current concepts of hypoxic-ischemic cerebral injury in the term newborn. Pediatr Neurol 7:317–325

Johnson MA, Pennock JM, Bydder GM, Dubowitz LMS, Thomas DJ, Young IR (1987) Serial MR imaging in neonatal cerebral injury. AJNR 8:83–92

Johnson MH (1990) Cortical maturation and the development of visual attention in early infancy. J Cogn Neurosci 2:81–95

Keeney SE, Adcock EW, McArdle CB (1991) Prospective observations of 100 high-risk neonates by high-field (1.5 Tesla) magnetic resonance imaging of the central nervous system.

II. Lesions associated with hypoxic-ischemic encephalopathy. Pediatrics 87:431–438

Keller MS, DiPietro MA, Telle RL, White SJ, Chawla HS, Curtis-Cohen M, Blane CE (1987) Periventricular cavitations in the first week of life. AJNR 8:291–295

Koeda T, Takeshita K (1992) Visuo-perceptual impairment and cerebral lesions in spastic diplegia with preterm birth. Brain Dev 14:239–244

Koeda T, Suganuma I, Kohno Y, Takamatsu T, Taeshita K (1990) MR imaging of spastic diplegia. Comparative study between preterm and term infants. Neuroradiology 32:187–190

Konishi Y, Kuriyama M, Hayakawa K, Konishi K, Yasujima M, Fujii Y, Sudo M (1990) Periventricular hyperintensity detected by magnetic resonance imaging in infancy. Pediatr Neurol 6:229–232

Konishi Y, Kuriyama M, Hayakawa K, Konishi K, Yasujima M, Fujii Y, Sudo M, Ishii Y (1991) Magnetic resonance imaging in preterm infants. Pediatr Neurol 7:191–195

Krägeloh-Mann I, Hagberg B, Petersen D, Riethmüller J, Gut E, Michaelis R (1991) Bilateral spastic cerebral palsy – pathogenetic aspects from MRI. Neuropediatrics 23:46–48

Krägeloh-Mann I, Olofsson KE, Hagberg G, Selbmann HK, Meisner C, Hagberg B, Schelp B, Michaelis R, Haas G (1993) Bilateral spastic cerebral palsy. A comparative study between South-West Germany and western Sweden. I: clinical patterns and disabilities. Dev Med Child Neurol 35:1037–1047

Kushner M, Nencini P, Reivich M, Rango M, Jamieson D, Fazekas F, Zimmerman R, Chawluk J, Alavi A, Alves W (1990) Relation of hyperglycemia early in ischemic brain infarction to cerebral anatomy, metabolism, and clinical outcome. Ann Neurol 28:129–135

Lanzi G, Fazzi E, Gerardo A, Ometto A, Piazza F, Rondini G (1990) Early predictors of neurodevelopmental outcome at 12–36 months in very low-birthweight infants. Brain Dev 12:482–487

Levene MI (1986) Non-invasive assessment of neonatal cerebral function. Dev Med Child Neurol 28:364–374

Mayer PL, Kier EL (1991) The controversy of the periventricular white matter circulation:a review of the anatomic literature. AJNR 12:223–228

McArdle CB, Richardson CJ, Hayden CK, Nicholas DA, Crofford MJ, Amparo EG (1987) Abnormalities of the neonatal brain: MR imaging, part I. Intracranial hemorrhage. Radiology 163:387–394

Mito T, Koyama K, Houdou S, Takashima S, Suzuki S (1990) Response on near-infrared spectroscopy and of cerebral blood flow to hypoxemia induced by N_2 and CO_2 in young rabbits. Brain Dev 12:408–411

Monset-Couchard M, de Bethmann O, Radvanyi-Bouvet MF, Pain C, Bordarier C, Relier JP (1988) Neurodevelopmental outcome in cystic periventricular leukomalacia (CPVL) (30 cases). Neuropediatrics 19:124–131

Moore JB, Parker CP, Smith RJ, Goethe BD (1987) Concealment of neonatal cerebral infarction on MRI by normal brain water. Pediatr Radiol 17:314–315

Muttitt SC, Taylor MJ, Kobayashi JS, MacMillan L, Whyte HE (1991) Serial visual evoked potentials and outcome in term birth asphyxia. Pediatr Neurol 7:86–90

Nakamura Y, Okudera T, Hashimoto T (1994) Vascular architecture in white matter of neonates: its relationship to periventricular leukomalacia. J Neuropathol Exp Neurol 53:582–589

Nelson MD, Gonzalez-Gomez I, Gilles FH (1991) The search for human telencephalic ventriculofugal arteries. AJNR 12:215–222

Parmelee AH, Minkowski A, Dargassies SSA, Dryfus-Brisac C, Lezine I, Berges J, Chervin G, Stern E (1970) Neurological evaluation of the premature infant. A follow-up study. Biol Neonate 15:65–78

Pasternak JF, Predy TA, Mikhael MA (1991) Neonatal asphyxia: vulnerability of basal ganglia, thalamus, and brainstem. Pediatr Neurol 7:147–149

Robinson RO, Trounce JQ, Janota I, Cox T (1993) Late fetal pontine destruction. Pediatr Neurol 9:213–215

Roland EH, Hill A (1992) MR and CT evaluation of profound neonatal and infantile asphyxia. AJNR 13:973–975

Rorke LB, Zimmerman RA (1992) Prematurity, postmaturity, and destructive lesions in utero. AJNR 13:517–536

Roth SC, Azzopardi D, David Edwards A, Baudin J, Cady EB, Townsend J, Delpy DT, Stewart AL, Wyatt JS, Osmund E, Reynolds R (1992) Relation between cerebral oxidative metabolism following birth asphyxia, and neurodevelopmental outcome and brain growth at one year. Dev Med Child Neurol 34:285–295

Rutherford MA, Pennock JM, Murdoch-Eaton DM, Cowan FM, Dubowitz LMS (1992) Athetoid cerebral palsy with cysts in the putamen after hypoxic-ischaemic encephalopathy. Arch Dis Child 67:846–850

Sarnat HB, Sarnat MS (1976) Neonatal encephalopathy following fetal distress. Arch Neurol 33:696–705

Sawada H, Udaka F, Seriu N, Shindou K, Kameyama M, Tsujimura M (1990) MRI demonstration of cortical laminar necrosis and delayed white matter injury in anoxic encephalopathy. Neuroradiology 32:319–321

Schellinger D, Grant EG, Richardson JD (1994) Cystic periventricular leukomalacia: sonographic and CT findings. AJNR 5:439–445

Schenk-Rootlieb AJF, van Nieuwenhuizen O, van der Graaf Y, Wittebol-Post D, Willemse J (1992) The prevalence of cerebral visual disturbance in children with cerebral palsy. Dev Med Child Neurol 34:473–480

Scher MS, Dobson V, Carpenter NA, Guthrie RD (1989) Visual and neurological outcome of infants with periventricular leukomalacia. Dev Med Child Neurol 31:353–365

Schouman-Claeys E, Henry-Feugeas MC, Roset F, Larroche JC, Hassine D, Sadik JC, Frija G, Gabilan JC (1993) Periventricular leukomalacia: correlation between MR imaging and autopsy findings during the first 2 months of life. Radiology 189:59–64

Shah AR, Kurth CD, Gwiazdowski SG, Chance B, Delivoria-Papadopoulos M (1992) Fluctuations in cerebral oxygenation and blood volume during endotracheal suctioning in premature infants. J Pediatr 120:769–774

Skranes JS, Nilsen G, Smevik O, Vik T, Rinck P, Brubakk AM (1992) Cerebral magnetic resonance imaging (MRI) of very low birth weight infants at one year of corrected age. Pediatr Radiol 22:406–409

Squier M, Kelling JW (1991) The incidence of prenatal brain injury. Neuropathol Appl Neurobiol 17:29–38

Steinlin M, Dirr R, Martin E, Boesch C, Largo RH, Fanconi S, Boltshauser E (1991) MRI following severe perinatal asphyxia: preliminary experience. Pediatr Neurol 7; 164–170

Steinlin M, Good M, Martin E, Bänziger O, Largo RH, Boltshauser E (1993) Congenital hemiplegia: morphology of cerebral lesions and pathogenetic aspects from MRI. Neuropediatrics 24:224–229

Stewart A, Thorburn RJ, Lipscomb AP, Amiel-Tison C (1983) Neonatal neurologic examinations of very preterm infants: comparison of results with ultrasound diagnosis of periventricular hemorrhage. Am J Perinatol 1:6–11

Stewart A, Hope PL, Hamilton P, Costello AML, Baudin J, Bradford B, Amiel-Tison C, Reynolds EOR (1988) Prediction in very preterm infants of satisfactory neurodevelopmental progress at 12 months. Dev Med Child Neurol 30:53–63

Takashima S, Tanaka K (1978) Development of cerebrovascular architecture and its relationship to periventricular leukomalacia. Arch Neurol 35:11–16

Thun-Hohenstein L, Forster I, Künzle C, Martin E, Boltshauser E (1994) Transient bifrontal solitary periventricular cysts in term neonates. Neuroradiology 36:241–244

Triulzi F (1994) Ruolo della RM nella sindrome anossicoemorragica del neonato. Riv Neuroradiol 7:163–170

Truwit CL, Barkovich AJ, Koch TK, Ferriero DM (1992) Cerebral palsy: MR findings in 40 patients. AJNR 13:67–78

Uauy R, Birch E, Birch D, Peirano P (1992) Visual and brain function measurements in studies of n-3 fatty acid requirements of infants. J Pediatr 120:S168–S180

Valk J, van der Knaap MS, de Grauw T, Taets van Amerongen AHM (1991) The role of imaging modalities in the diagnosis of posthypoxic-ischemic and hemorrhagic conditions of infants, part I. Klin Neuroradiol 1:72–79

Valk J, van der Knaap MS, de Grauw T, Taets van Amerongen AHM (1991) The role of imaging modalities in the diagnosis of posthypoxic-ischemic and hemorrhagic conditions of infants, part II. Klin Neuroradiol 2:127–138

Van der Eecken HM, Adams RD (1953) The anatomy and functional significance of the meningeal arterial anastomoses of the human brain. J Neuropathol Exp Neurol 12:132–157

Van de Bor M, den Ouden L, Guit GL (1992) Value of cranial ultrasound and magnetic resonance imaging in predicting neurodevelopmental outcome in preterm infants. Pediatrics 90:196–199

Van Bogaert P, Baleriaux D, Christophe C, Szliwowski HB (1992) MRI of patients with cerebral palsy and normal CT scan. Neuroradiology 34:52–56

Van Bel F, den Ouden L, van de Bor M, Stijnen T, Baan J, Ruys JH (1989) Cerebral blood-flow velocity during the first week of life of preterm infants and neurodevelopment at two years. Dev Med Child Neurol 31:320–328

Voit T, Lemburg P, Neuen E, Lumenta C, Stork W (1987) Damage of thalamus and basal ganglia in asphyxiated fullterm neonates. Neuropediatrics 18:176–181

Volpe JJ (1989) Current concepts of brain injury in the premature infant. AJR 153:243–251

Volpe JJ (1992) Value of MR in definition of the neuropathology of cerebral palsy in vivo. AJNR 13:79–83

Welch RJ, Byrne P (1990) Periventricular leukomalacia (PVL) and myelination. Pediatrics 86:1002–1003

Wilson DA, Steiner RE (1986) Periventricular leukomalacia: evaluation with MR imaging. Radiology 160:507–511

Wray S, Cope M, Delpy DT, Wyatt JS, Osmund E, Reynolds R (1988) Characterization of the near infrared absorption spectra of cytochrome aa$_3$ and haemoglobin for the non-invasive monitoring of cerebral oxygenation. Biochim Biophys Acta 933:184–192

Yamamoto N, Watanabe K, Sugiura J, Okada J, Nagae H, Fujimoto Y (1990) Marked latency change of auditory brainstem response in preterm infants in the early postnatal period. Brain Dev 12:766–769

Yokochi K, Aiba K, horie M, Inukai K, Fujimoto S, Kodama M, Kodama K (1991) Magnetic resonance imaging in children with spastic diplegia:correlation with the severity of their motor and mental abnormality. Dev Med Child Neurol 33:18–25

Zuerrer M, Martin E, Boltshauser E (1991) MR imaging of intracranial hemorrhage in neonates and infants at 2.35 Tesla. Neuroradiology 33:223–229

64 Delayed Posthypoxic Leukoencephalopathy of Maturity

De Reuck J, van der Eecken H (1974) Periventricular leukoencephalopathy and meningo-cortical arterio-venous malformation. Acta Neurol Belg 74:276–283

Elovaara E, Rantanen J (1983) Carbon monoxide-induced brain injury:neurochemical studies after single and repeated exposures. J Appl Toxicol 3:154–160

Feigin I, Budzilovich G, Weinberg S, Ogata J (1973) Degeneration of white matter in hypoxia, acidosis and edema. J Neuropathol Exp Neurol 32:125–143

Garland H, Pearce J (1967) Neurological complications of carbon monoxide poisoning. Q J Med 36:445–455

Ginsberg MD, Myers RE, McDonagh BF (1974) Experimental carbon monoxide encephalopathy in the primate. Arch Neurol 30:209–216

Ginsberg MD, Hedley-Whyte ET, Richardson EP (1976) Hypoxic-ischemic leukoencephalopathy in man. Arch Neurol 33:5–14

Illum F (1980) Calcification of the basal ganglia following carbon monoxide poisoning. Neuroradiology 19:213–214

Kamada K, Houkin K, Aoki T, Koiwa M, Kashiwaba T, Iwasaki Y, Abe H (1994) Cerebral metabolic changes in delayed carbon monoxide sequelae studied by proton MR spectroscopy. Neuroradiology 36:104–106

Klawans HL, Stein RW, Tanner CM, Goetz CG (1982) A pure parkinsonian syndrome following acute carbon monoxide intoxication. Arch Neurol 39:302–304

Koehler RC, Jones MD, Traystman RJ (1982) Cerebral circulatory response to carbon monoxide and hypoxic hypoxia in the lamb. Am J Physiol 243:H27–H32

Kono E, Kono R, Shida K (1983) Computerized tomographies of 34 patients at the chronic stage of acute carbon monoxide poisoning. Arch Psychiatr Nervenkr 233:271–278

Lee MS, Marsden CD (1994) Neurological sequelae following carbon monoxide poisoning clinical course and outcome according to the clinical types and brain computed tomography scan findings. Mov Disord 9:550–558

Lumsden CE (1970) Glia and myelin in ischaemia, blood disorders and intoxications. In: Vinken PJ, Bruyn GW (eds) Handbook of clinical neurology, vol 9. North Holland, Amsterdam, pp 572–663

Nardizzi LR (1979) Computerized tomographic correlate of carbon monoxide poisoning. Arch Neurol 36:38–39

Okeda R, Funata N, Takano T, Miyazaki Y, Higashino F, Yokoyama K, Manabe M (1981) The pathogenesis of carbon monoxide encephalopathy in the acute phase – physiological and morphological correlation. Acta Neuropathol (Berl) 54:1–10

Okeda R, Song SY, Funta N, Higashino F (1983) An experimental study of the pathogenesis of Grinker's myelinopathy in carbon monoxide intoxication. Acta Neuropathol (Berl) 59:200–206

Plum F, Posner JB, Hain RF (1962) Delayed neurological deterioration after anoxia. Arch Intern Med 110:18–25

Posse S, Cuenod CA, Le Bihan D (1993) Human brain: proton diffusion MR spectroscopy. Radiology 188:719–725

Sawa GM, Watson CPN, Terbrugge K, Chiu M (1981) Delayed encephaopathy following carbon monoxide intoxication. J Can Sci Neurol 8:77–79

Sawada Y, Sakamoto T, Nishide K, Sadamitsu D, Fusamoto H, Yoshioka T, Sugimoto T, Onishi S (1983) Correlation of pathological findings with computed tomographic findings after acute carbon monoxide poisoning. N Engl J Med 26:1296

Sawada Y, Takahashi M, Ohashi N, Fusamoto H, Maemura K, Kobayashi H, Yoshioka T, Sugimoto T (1980) Computerised tomography as an indication of long-term outcome after acute carbon monoxide poisoning. Lancet I:783–784

Silverman CS, Brenner J, Murtagh FR (1993) Hemorrhagic necrosis and vascular injury in carbon monoxide poisoning: MR demonstration. AJNR 14:168–170

Taylor R, Holgate RC (1988) Carbon monoxide poisoning: asymmetric and unilateral changes on CT. AJNR 9:975–977

Uchino A, Hasuo K, Shida K, Matsumoto S, Yasumori K, Masuda K (1994) MRI of the brain in chronic carbon monoxide poisoning. Neuroradiology 36:399–401

Vieregge P, Klostermann W, Blümm RG, Borgis KJ (1989) Carbon monoxide pisoning: clinical, neurophysiological, and brain imaging observations in acute disease and follow-up. J Neurol 236:478–481

Vion-Dury J, Jiddane M, van Bunnen Y, Rumeau C, Lavielle J (1987) Etude IRM des séquelles d'intoxication au monoxyde de carbone:à propos de deux cas. J Neuroradiol 14:60–65

Zagami AS, Lethlean AK, Mellick R (1993) Delayed neurological deterioration following carbon monoxide poisoning: MRI findings. J Neurol 240:113–116

65 Subcortical Arteriosclerotic Encephalopathy

Aharon-Peretz J, Cummings JL, Hill MA (1988) Vascular dementia and dementia of the Alzheimer type. Arch Neurol 45:719–721

Appel B, Muller RN, Collard M, Moens E, Mortelmans L, Martin JJ, Lowenthal A (1985) NMR approach of the periventricular white matter. Arch Int Physiol Biochim 93:19–26

Awad IA, Johnson PC, Spetzler RF, Hodak JA (1986a) Incidental subcortical lesions identified on magnetic resonance imaging in the elderly. II. Postmortem pathological correlations. Stroke 17:1090–1097

Awad IA, Spetzler RF, Hodak JA, Awad CA, Carey R (1986b) Incidental subcortical lesions identified on magnetic reso-

nance imaging in the elderly. 1. Correlation with age and cerebrovascular risk factors. Stroke 17:1084–1089

Baudrimont M, Dubas F, Joutel A, Tournier-Lasserve E, Bousser MG (1993) Autosomal dominant leukoencephalopathy and subcortical ischemic stroke. A clinicopathological study. Stroke 24:122–125

Binswanger O (1894) Die Abgrenzung des allgemeinen progressiven Paralyse. Berl Klin Wochenschr 31:1103–1137

Bradley WG Jr, Waluch V, Brant-Zawadzki M, Yadley RA, Wycoff RR (1984) Patchy, periventricular white matter lesions in the elderly: a common observation during NMR imaging. Noninv Med Imaging 1:35–41

Brant-Zawadski M, Fein G, van Dyke C, Kierman R, Davenport L, de Groot J (1985) MR imaging of the aging brain: patchy white matter lesions and dementia. AJNR 6:675–682

Challa VR (1987) White matter lesions in MR imaging of elderly subjects. Radiology 164:874–875

Del Ser T, Bermejo F, Portera A, Arredondo JM, Bouras C, Constantindis J (1990) Vascular dementia: a clinicopathological study. J Neurol Sci 96:1–17

De Reuck J, Schaumburg HH (1972) Periventricular artherosclerotic leukoencephalopathy. Neurology 22:1094–1097

De Reuck J, Crevits L, de Coster W, Sieben G, van den Eecken H (1980) Pathogenesis of Binswanger chronic progressive subcortical encephalopathy. Neurology 30:920–928

Drayer BP (1988a) Imaging of the aging brain, part I. Normal findings. Radiology 166:785–796

Drayer BP (1988b) Imaging of the aging brain, part II. Pathologic conditions. Radiology 166:797–806

Earnest MP, Fahn S, Karp JH, Rowland LW (1974) Normal pressure hydrocephalus and hypertensive cerebrovascular disease. Arch Neurol 31:262–266

George AE, de Leon MJ, Gentes CI, Miller J, London E, Budrilovich GN, Ferris S, Chase N (1986) Leukoencephalopathy in normal and pathologic aging: 1. CT of brain lucencies. AJNR 7:561–566

Gerard G, Weisberg LA (1986) MRI periventricular lesions in adults. Neurology 36:998–1001

Gupta SR, Naheedy MH, Young JC, Ghobrial M, Rubino FA, Hindo W (1988) Periventricular white matter changes and dementia. Arch Neurol 45:637–641

Hachinski VC, Potter P, Merskey H (1987) Leuko-araiosis. Arch Neurol 44:21–23

Inzitari D, Diaz F, Fox A, Hachinski VC, Steingart A, Lau C, Donald A, Wade J, Mulic H, Merskey H (1987) Vascular risk factors and leukoaraiosis. Arch Neurol 44:42–47

Junqué C, Pujol J, Vendreel P, Bruna O, Jodar M, Ribas JC, Vinas J, Capdevilla A, Mari-Vilalta JL (1990) Leuko-Araiosis on magnetic resonance imaging and speed of mental processing. Arch Neurol 47:151–156

Kertesz A, Black SE, Tokar G, Benke T, Carr T, Nicholson L (1988) Periventricular and subcortical hyperintensities on magnetic resonance imaging. Arch Neurol 45:404–408

Kinkel WR, Jacobs L, Polachini I, Bates V, Heffner RR (1985) Subcortical arteriosclerotic encephalopathy (Binswanger's disease). Arch Neurol 42:951–959

Kirkpatrick JB, Hayman LA (1987) White matter lesions in MR imaging of clinically healthy brains of elderly subjects: possible pathologic basis. Radiology 162:509–511

Kobari M, Meyer JS, Ichijo M, Oravez WT (1990) Leukoaraiosis: correlation of MR and CT findings with blood flow, atrophy, and cognition. AJNR 11:273–281

Kobari M, Meyer JS, Ichijo M (1990) Leuko-araiosis, cerebral atrophy, and cerebral perfusion in normal aging. Arch Neurol 47:161–165

Lee D, Fox A, Vinuela F, Pelz D, Lau C, Donald A, Merskey H (1987) Interobserver variation in computed tomography of the brain. Arch Neurol 44:30–31

Lee A, Yu YL, Tsoi M, Woo E, Chang CM (1989) Subcortical arteriosclerotic encephalopathy – a controlled psychometric study. Clin Neurol Neurosurg 91:235–241

Leifer D, Buonanno FS, Richardson EP (1990) Clinicopathologic correlations of cranial magnetic resonance imaging of periventricular white matter. Neurology 40:911–918

Loizou LA, Kendall BE, Marshall J (1981) Subcortical arteriosclerotic encephalopathy: a clinical and radiological investigation. J Neurol Neurosurg Psychiatry 44:294–304

Lotz PR, Ballinger WE, Quisling RG (1986) Subcortical arteriosclerotic encephalopathy: CT spectrum and pathologic correlation. AJNR 7:817–822

Malone MJ, Szoke MC (1985) Neurochemical changes in white matter. Aged human brain and Alzheimer's disease. Arch Neurol 42:1063–1066

Marshall VG, Bradley WG, Marshall CE, Bhoopat T, Rhodes RH (1988) Deep white matter infarction:correlation of MR imaging and histopathologic findings. Radiology 167:517–522

McQuinn BA, O'Leary DH (1987) White matter lucencies on computed tomography, subacute arteriosclerotic encephalopathy (Binswanger's disease), and blood pressure. Stroke 18:900–905

Meyer JS, McClintic KI, Rogers RI, Sims P, Mortel KF (1988) Aetiological considerations and risk factors for multi-infarct dementia. J Neurol Neurosurg Psychiatry 51:1489–1497

Miller Fisher C (1989) Binswanger's encephalopathy: a review. J Neurol 236:65–79

Olszewski J (1962) Subcortical arterio-sclerotic encephalopathy. World Neurol 3:359–375

Prencipe M, Marini C (1989) Leuko-araiosis: definition and clinical correlates – an overview. Eur Neurol 29 [Suppl 2]:27–29

Rao SM, Mittenberg W, Bernadin L, Haughton V, Leo GJ (1989) Neuropsychological test findings in subjects with leukoaraiosis. Arch Neurol 46:40–44

Roman GC (1987) Senile Dementia of the Binswanger type. A vascular form of dementia in the elderly. JAMA 258:1782–1788

Sandijk R (1983) Subcortical arteriosclerotic encephalopathy (Binswanger's disease). S Afr Med J 63:204–205

Sacquegna T, Guttmann S, Giuliani S, Agati R, Daidone R, Morreale A, Ambrosetto G, Gallassi R (1989) Binswanger's disease: a review of the literature and a personal contribution. Eur Neurol 29 [Suppl 2]:20–22

Steingart A, Hachinski VC, Lau C, Fox AJ, Diaz F, Cape R, Lee D, Inzitari D, Merskey H (1987) Cognitive and neurologic findings in subjects with diffuse white matter lucencies on computed tomographic scan (leuko-araiosis). Arch Neurol 44:32–35

Sullivan P, Pary R, Telang F, Hind Rifai A, Zubenko GS (1990) Risk factors for white matter changes detected by magnetic resonance imaging in elderly. Stroke 21:1424–1428

Tomonage M, Yamanouchi H, Tohgi H, Kameyama M (1982) Clinicopathologic study of progressive subcortical vascular encephalopathy (Binswanger type) in the elderly. J Am Geriatr Soc 30:524–529

Tournier-Lasserve E, Iba-Zizen MT, Romero N, Bousser MG (1991) Autosomal dominant syndrome with strokelike episodes and leukoencephalopathy. Stroke 22:1297–1302

Tournier-Lasserve E, Joutel A, Melki J, Weissenbach J, Lathrop GM, Chabriat H, Mas JL, Cabanis EA, Baudrimont M, Maciazek J, Bach MA, Bousser MG (1993) Cerebral autosomal dominant arteriopathy with subcortical infarcts and leukoencephalopathy maps to chromosome 19q12. Nature Genet 3:256–259

Van Swieten JC, van den Hout JHW, van Ketel BA, Hijdra A, Wokke JHJ, Van Gijn J (1991) Periventricular lesions in the white matter on magnetic resonance imaging in the elderly. Brain 114:761–774

Van Swieten JC, Hijdra A, Koudstaal PJ, Van Gijn (1990) Grading white matter lesions on CT or MRI, a simple scale. J Neurol Neurosurg Psychiatry 53:1080–1083

Van Swieten JC, Geyskes GG, Derix MMA, Ramos LMP, Van Latum JC, Van Gijn J (1991) Hypertension in the elderly is associated with diffuse lesions of the cerebral white matter and with cognitive decline. Ann Neurol 30:825–830

Verny M, Duyckaerts C, Pierot L, Hauw JJ (1991) Leuko-araiosis. Dev Neurosci 13:245–250

Zeumer H, Schonsky B, Sturm KW (1980) Predominant white matter involvement in subcortical arteriosclerotic encephalopathy (Binswanger disease). J Comput Assist Tomogr 4:14–19

66 Vasculitis

Anderson JR (1981) Intracerebral calcification in a case of systemic lupus erythematosus with neurological manifestations. Neurpathol Appl Neurobiol 7:161–166

Baum KA, Hopf U, Nehrig C, Stoever M, Schoerner W (1993) Systemic lupus erythematosus: neuropsychiatric signs and symptoms related to cerebral MRI findings. Clin Neurol Neurosurg 95:29–34

Besana C, Comi G, DelMaschio A, Praderio L, Vergani A, Medaglini S, Martinelli V, Triulzi F, Locatelli T (1989) Electrophysiological and MRI evaluation of neurological involvement in Behçet's disease. J Neurol Neurosurg Psychiatry 52:749–754

Elinson P, Foster KW, Kaufman DB (1990) Magnetic resonance imaging of central nervous system vasculitis. Acta Paediatr Scand 79:710–713

Gobernado JM, Leiva C, Rabano J, Alvarez-Cermeno JC, Fernandez-Molina A (1984) Recovery from rheumatoid cerebral vasculitis. J Neurol Neurosurg Psychiatry 47:410–413

Greenan TJ, Grossman RI, Goldberg HI (1992) Cerebral vasculitis: MR imaging and angiographic correlation. Radiology 182:65–72

Hiraiwa M, Nonaka C, Abe T, Iio M (1983) Positron emission tomography in systemic lupus erythematosus: relation of cerebral vasculitis to PET findings. AJNR 4:541–543

Ishikawa O, Ohnishi K, Miyachi Y, Ishizaka H (1994) Cerebral lesions in systemic lupus erythematosus detected by magnetic resonance imaging. Relationship to anticardiolipin antibody. J Rheumatol 21:87–90

Kendall B (1984) Cerebral angiography in vasculitis affecting the nervous system. Eur Neurol 23:400–406

Koo EH, Massey EW (1986) Therapy for granulomatous angiitis. Clin Neuropharmacol 9:132–137

Mas JL, Louarn F, Degos JD (1983) Revue generale. Angiitis nonspecifique de systeme nerveux central. Rev Neurol 139:467–484

McAbee GN, Barasch ES (1990) Resolving MRI lesions in lupus erythematosus selectively involving the brainstem. Pediatr Neurol 6:186–189

Miller DH, Ormerod IEC, Gibson A, du Boulay EPGH, Rudge P, McDonald WI (1987) MR brain scanning in patients with vasculitis: differentiation from multiple sclerosis. Neuroradiology 29:226–231

Miller DH, Buchanan N, Barker G, Morrissey SP, Kendall BE, Rudge P, Khamashta M, Hughes GRV, McDonald WI (1992) Gadolinium-enhanced magnetic resonance imaging of the central nervous system in systemic lupus erythematosus. J Neurol 239:460–464

Mills JA (1994) Systemic lupus erythematosus. N Engl J Med 330:1871–1879

Nagaoka S, Matsunaga K, Chiba J, Ishigatsubo Y, Tani K (1982) Five cases of systemic lupus erythematosus with intracranial calcification. Clin Neurol 22:635–643

Pierot L, Sauve C, Leger JM, Martin N, Koeger AC, Wechsler B, Chiras J (1993) Asymptomatic cerebral involvement in Sjogren's syndrome: MRI findings of 15 cases. Neuroradiology 35:378–380

Sigal LH (1987) The neurologic presentation of vasculitic and rheumatologic syndromes. Medicine 66:157–180

Van der Kaaden AJ, Kamphuis DJ, Nossent JC, Rico RE (1993) Longstanding isolated cerebral systemic lupus erythematosus in an 8-year-old black girl. Clin Neurol Neurosurg 95:241–244

Wechsler B, Dell'Isola B, Vidaihet M, Dormont D, Piette JC, Bletry O, Godeau P (1993) MRI in 31 patients with Behçet's disease and neurological involvement:prospective study with clinical correlation. J Neurol Neurosurg Psychiatry 56:793–798

Yamamoto K, Nogaki H, Takase Y, Morimatsu M (1992) Systemic lupus erythematosus associated with marked intracranial calcification. AJNR 13:1340–1342

Zuheir Al Kawi M, Bohlega S, Banna M (1991) MRI findings in neuro-Behçet's disease. Neurology 41:405–408

67 Leukoencephalopathy After Chemotherapy and/or Radiotherapy

Asato R, Akuyama Y, Ito M, Kubota M, Okumura R, Miki Y, Konishi J, Mikwawa H (1992) Nuclear magnetic resonance abnormalities of the cerebral white matter in children with acute lymphoblastic leukemia and malignant lymphoma during and after central nervous system prophylactic treatment with intrathecal methotrexate. Cancer 70:1997–2004

Bates S, McKeever P, Masur H, Levens D, Macher A, Armstrong G, Magrath IT (1985) Myelopathy following intrathe-cal chemotherapy in a patient with extensive Burkitt's lymphoma and altered immune status. Am J Med 78:697–702

Breuer AC, Blank NK, Schoene WC (1978) Multifocal pontine lesions in cancer patients treated with chemotherapy and CNS radiotherapy. Cancer 41:2112–2120

Burger PC, Mahaley MS, Dudka L, Vogel FS (1979) The morphologic effects of radiation administered therapeutically for intracranial gliomas. A postmortem study of 25 cases. Cancer 44:1256–1272

Burger PC, Kamenar E, Schold SC, Fay JW, Phillips GL, Herzig GP (1981) Encephalomyelopathy following high-dose BC-NU therapy. Cancer 48:1318–1327

Catane R, Schwade JG, Yarr I, Lichter AS, Tepper JE, Dunnick NR, Brody L, Brereton HD, Cohen M, Glatstein E (1981) Follow-up neurological evaluation in patients with small cell lung carcinoma treated with prophylactic cranial irradiation and chemotherapy. Int J Radiat Oncol Biol Phys 7:105–109

Craig JB, Jackson DV, Moody D, Cruz JM, Pope EK, Powell BL, Spurr CL, Capizzi RL (1984) Prospective evaluation of changes in computed cranial tomography in patients with small cell lung carcinoma treated with chemotherapy and prophylactic cranial irradiation. J Clin Oncol 2:1151–1156

Courtville CB, Myers RO (1958) The process of demyelination in the central nervous system. J Neuropathol Exp Neurol 17:158–173

Curnes JT, Laster DW, Ball MR, Moody DM, Witcofski RL (1986) Magnetic resonance imaging of radiation injury to the brain. AJNR 7:389–394

DiChiro G, Oldfield E, Wright DC, DeMichele D, Katz DA, Patronas NJ, Doppman JL, Larson SM, Ito M, Kufta CV (1987) Cerebral necrosis after radiotherapy and/or intraarterial chemotherapy for brain tumors: PET and neuropathologic studies. AJNR 8:1083–1091

Dooms GC, Hecht S, Brant-Zawadzki M, Berthiaume Y, Norman D, Newton TH (1986) Brain radiation lesions: MR imaging. Radiology 158:149–155

Flament-Durand J, Ketelbant-Balasse P, Maurus R, Regnier R, Spehl M (1975) Intracerebral calcifications appearing during the course of acute lymphocytic leukemia treated with methotrexate and X rays. Cancer 35:319–325

Fukamachi A, Wakao T, Akai J (1982) Brain stem necrosis after irradiation of pituitary adenoma. Surg Neurol 18:343–350

Haymaker W, Ibrahim MZM, Miquel J, Call N (1968) Delayed radiation effects in the brains of monkeys exposed to X- and γ-rays. J Neuropathol Exp Neurol 27:50–79

Hecht-Leavitt C, Grossman RI, Curran WJ, McGrath JT, Biery DN, Joseph PM, Nelson DF (1987) MR of brain radiation injury: experimental studies in cats. AJNR 8:427–430

Hook CC, Kimmel DW, Kvols LK, Scheithauer BW, Forsyth PA, Rubin J, Moertel CG, Rodriguez M (1992) Multifocal inflammatory leukoencephalopathy with 5-fluorouracil and levamisole. Ann Neurol 31:262–267

Johnson BE, Becker B, Goff WB, Petronas N, Krehbiel MA, Makuch RW, McKenna G, Glatstein E, Ihde DC (1985) Neurologic, neuropsychologic, and computed cranial tomography scan abnormalities in 2- to 10-year survivors of small-cell lung cancer. J Clin Oncol 3:1659–1667

Lampert PW, Davis RL (1964) Delayed effects of radiation on the human central nervous system. Neurology 14:912–917

Lee YY, Nauert C, Glass JP (1986) Treatment-related white matter changes in cancer patients. Cancer 57:1473–1482

Leibel SA, Sheline GE (1987) Radiation therapy for neoplasms of the brain. J Neurosurg 66:1–22

Martins AN, Johnston JS, Henry JM, Stoffel TJ, Di Chiro G (1977) Delayed radiation necrosis of the brain. J Neurosurg 47:336–345

Mikhael MA (1979) Radiation necrosis of the brain: correlation between patterns on computed tomography and dose of radiation. J Comput Assist Tomogr 3:241–249

Miyatake S, Kikuchi H, Oda Y, Ishikawa M, Kojima M, Matsubayashi K, Minamikawa J, Yamagata S, Asato R (1992) A case of treatment-related leukoencephalopathy: sequential MRI, CT and PET findings. J Neuro Oncol 14:143–149

Pääkko E, Vainiompaa L, Lanning M, Laitinen J, Pyhtinen J (1992) White matter changes in children treated for acute lymphoblastic leukemia. Cancer 70:2728–2733

Peterson K, Rosenblum MK, Powers JM, Alvord E, Walker RW, Posner JB (1993) Effect of brain irradiation on demyelinating lesions. Neurology 43:2105–2112

Pratt RA, Di Chiro G, Weed JC (1977) Cerebral necrosis following irradiation and chemotherapy for metastatic choriocarcinoma. Surg Neurol 7:117–120

Price RA, Jamieson PA (1975) The central nervous system in childhood leukemia. II. Subacute leukoencephalopathy. Cancer 35:306–318

Rizzoli HV, Pagnanelli DM (1984) Treatment of delayed radiation necrosis of the brain. A clinical observation. J Neurosurg 60:589–594

Rottenberg DA, Chernik NL, Deck MDF, Ellis F, Posner JB (1977) Cerebral necrosis following radiotherapy of extracranial neoplasms. Ann Neurol 1:339–357

Rottenberg DA, Horten B, Kim JH, Posner JB (1980) Progressive white matter destruction following irradiation of an extracranial neoplasm. Ann Neurol 8:76–78

Rubinstein LJ, Herman MM, Long TF, Wilbur JR (1975) Disseminated necrotizing leukoencephalopathy: a complication of treated central nervous system leukemia and lymphoma. Cancer 35:291–305

Safdari H, Fuentes JM, Dubois JB, Alirezai M, Castan P, Vlahovitch B (1985) Radiation necrosis of the brain: time of onset and incidence related to total dose and fractionation of radiation. Neuroradiology 27:44–47

Sheline G (1980) Irradiation injury of the human brain: a review of clinical experience. In: Gilbert HA, Kagan AR (eds) Radiation damage to the nervous system. Raven, New York, pp 39–58

So NK, O'Neill BP, Frytak S, Eagan RT, Earnest F, Lee RE (1987) Delayed leukoencephalopathy in survivors small cell lung cancer. Neurology 37:1198–1201

Stemmer SM, Stears JC, Burton BS, Jones RB, Simon JH (1994) White matter changes in patients with breast cancer treated with high-dose chemotherapy and autologous bone marrow support. AJNR 15:1267–1273

Tsuruda JS, Kortman KE, Bradley WG, Wheeler DC, van Dalsem W, Bradley TP (1987) Radiation effects on cerebral white matter: MR evaluation. AJNR 8:431–437

Valk PE, Dillon WP (1991) Radiation injury of the brain. AJNR 12:45–62

Wang AM, Skias DD, Rumbaugh CL, Schoene WC, Zamani A (1983) Central nervous system changes after radiation therapy and/or chemotherapy: correlation of CT and autopsy findings. AJNR 4:466–471

Wilson WB, Perez GM, Kleinschmidt-DeMasters BK (1987) Sudden onset of blindness in patients treated with oral CCNU and low-dose cranial irradiation. Cancer 59:901–907

Wilson DA, Nitschke R, Bowman ME, Chaffin MJ, Sexauer CL, Prince JR (1991) Transient white matter changes on MR images in children undergoing chemotherapy for acute lymphocytic leukemia: correlation with neuropsychologic deficiencies. Radiology 180:205–209

68 Cerebral Edema and Fluid Compartments in the CNS

Baugh JR, Krug EF, Weir MR (1983) Punishment by salt poisoning. South Med J 76:540–541

Bradac GB, Ferszt R, Bender A, Schörner W (1986) Peritumoral edema in meningiomas. Neuroradiology 28:304–312

Bradley WG, Whittemore AR, Watanabe AS, Davis SJ, Teresi LM, Homyak M (1991) Association of deep white matter infarction with chronic communicating hydrocephalus: implications regarding the possible origin of normal-pressure hydrocephalus. AJNR 12:31–39

Calvin ME, Knepper R, Robertson WO (1964) Hazards to health: salt poisoning. N Engl J Med 270:625–626

Elton NW, Elton WJ, Nazareno JP (1963) Pathology of acute salt poisoning in infants. Am J Clin Pathol 39:252–264

Finberg L, Harrison HE (1955) Hypernatremia in infants – evolution of clinical and biochemical findings, accompanying this state. Pediatrics 16:1–12

George AE (1991) Chronic communicating hydrocephalus and periventricular white matter disease: a debate with regard to cause and effect. AJNR 12:42–44

Gilbert JJ, Paulseth JE, Coates RK, Malott D (1983) Cerebral edema associated with meningiomas. Neurosurgery 12:599–605

Go KG, Wilmink JT, Molenaar WM (1988) Peritumoral brain edema associated with meningiomas. Neurosurgery 23:175–179

Golder W, Felgenhauer N, von Einsiedel H, von Clarmann M (1992) Ausgedehnte Kleinhirnblutungen nach Kochsalzvergiftung. Klin Neuroradiol 2:21–23

Habbick BF, Hill A, Tchang SPK (1984) Computed tomography in an infant with salt poisoning: relationship of hypodense areas in basal ganglia to serum sodium concentration. Pediatrics 74:1123–1125

Hakim S (1964) Some observations on CSF pressure: hydrocephalic syndrome in adults with „normal" CSF pressure. Thesis no. 957. Javerzian University School of Medicine, Bogota, Columbia

Hamza M, Bodensteiner JB, Noorani PA, Barnes PD (1987) Benign extracerebral fluid collections: a cause of macrocrania in infancy. Pediatr Neurol 3:218–221

Ito U, Reulen HJ, Huber P (1986) Spatial and quantitative distribution of human peritumoural brain oedema in computerized tomography. Acta Neurochir (Wien) 81:53–60

Laursen H, Hansen AJ, Sheardown M (1993) Cerebrovascular permeability and brain edema after cortical photochemical infarcts in the rat. Acta Neuropathol (Berl) 86:378–385

Lutrell CN, Finberg L (1974) Hemorrhagic encephalopathy induced by hypernatremia. I. Clinical, laboratory and pathological observations. Arch Neurol 81:424–432

Milhorat TH (1992) Classification of the cerebral edemas with reference to hydrocephalus and pseudotumor cerebri. Childs Nerv Syst 8:301–306

Naidich TP (1994) Hydrocephalus. Core Curriculum Course in Neuroradiology of the ASNR, pp 31–41

Ohno K, Matsushima Y, Aoyagi M, Ikeda J, Suzuki R, Ichimura K, Tamaki M, Hirakawa K (1992) Peritumoral cerebral edema in meningiomas:the role of the tumor-brain interface. Clin Neurol Neurosurg 94:291–295

Raimondi AJ (1994) A unifying theory for the definition and classification of hydrocephalus. Childs Nerv Syst 10:2–12

Roman GC (1991) White matter lesions and normal-pressure hydrocephalus: Binswanger disease or Hakim syndrome? AJNR 12:40–41

Sato O, Takei F, Yamada S (1994) Hydrocephalus:is impaired cerebrospinal fluid circulation only one problem involved? Childs Nerv Syst 10:151–155

Schoeman JF (1994) Childhood pseudotumor cerebri:clinical and intracranial pressure response to acetazolamide and furosemide treatment in a case series. J Child Neurol 9:130–134

Sheridan M, Johnston I (1994) Hydrocephalus and pseudotumour cerebri in the mucopolysaccharidoses. Childs Nerv Syst 10:148–150

Smith HP, Challa VR, Moody DM, Kelly DL (1981) Biological features of meningiomas that determine the production of cerebral edema. Neurosurgery 8:428–433

Stevens JM, Ruiz JS, Kendall BE (1983) Observation on peritumoural oedema in meningioma, part I: distribution, spread and resolution of vasogenic oedema seen on computed tomography. Neuroradiology 25:71–80

Valk J (1993) Compartimentalization of fluids in the CNS under different conditions; various kinds of cerebral edema. 3rd Refresher Course of the ESNR in Bruges, pp 77–85

Walter GF, Maresch W (1987) Irrtümliche Kochsalzintoxikation bei Neugeborenen. Morphologische Befunde und pathogenetische Diskussion. Klin Padiatr 199:269–273

Weller RO, Wisniewski H (1969) Histological and ultrastructural changes with experimental hydrocephalus in adult rabbits. Brain 92:819–828

Weller RO, Wisniewski H, Shulman K, Terry RD (1971) Experimental hydrocephalus in young dogs: histological and ultrastructural study of the brain tissue damage. J Neuropathol Exp Neurol 30:613–627

69 Wallerian Degeneration and Myelin Loss Secondary to Neuronal and Axonal Degeneration

Bignami A, Eng LF (1973) Biochemical studies of myelin in wallerian degeneration of rat optic nerve. J Neurochem 20:165–173

Bignami A, Ralston HJ (1969) The cellular reaction to wallerian degeneration in the central nervous system of the cat. Brain Res 13:444–461

Bots GTAM (1970) Wallerian degeneration in peripheral nerves. In: Vinken PJ, Bruyn GW (eds) Handbook of clinical neurology, vol 7. North Holland, Amsterdam, pp 202–219

Bouchareb M, Moulin T, Cattin F, Dietemann JL, Racle A, Verdot H, Bonneville JF (1988) Wallerian degeneration of the descending tracts. J Neuroradiol 15:238–252

Cook RD, Wisniewski HM (1973) The role of oligodendroglia and astroglia in wallerian degeneration of the optic nerve. Brain Res 61:191–206

Duchen LW (1992) Anterograde (Wallerian) degeneration in the central nervous system. In: Adams HJ, Duchen LW (eds) Greenfield's neuropathology, 5th edn. Arnold, London, pp 16–54

Girard PF, Tommasi M, Rochet M, Boucher M (1968) Leucoencéphalopathie avec cavitations massives, bilatérales et symétriques. Presse Med 76:163–166

Griffin JW, George R, Lobato C, Tyor WR, Yan LC, Glass JD (1992) Macrophage responses and myelin clearance during Wallerian degeneration: relevance to immune-mediated demyelination. J Neuroimmunol 40:153–166

Inoue Y, Matsumura Y, Fukuda T, Nemoto Y, Shirahata N, Suzuki T, Shakudo M, Yawata S, Tanaka S, Takemoto K, Onoyama Y (1990) MR imaging of wallerian degeneration in the brainstem:temporal relationships. AJNR 11:897–903

Kuhn JM, Johnson KA, Davis KR (1988) Wallerian degeneration: evaluation with MR imaging. Radiology 168:199–202

Kuhn MJ, Mikulis DJ, Ayoub DM, Kosofsky BE, Davis KR, Taveras, JM (1989) Wallerian degeneration after cerebral infarction: evaluation with sequential MR imaging. Radiology 172:179–182

Lassmann H, Ammerer HP, Jurecka W, Kulnig W (1978) Ultrastructural sequence of myelin degradation. Acta Neuropathol (Berl) 44:103–109

Lexa FJ, Grossman RI, Rosenquist AC (1994) MR of wallerian degeneration in the feline visual system:characterization by magnetization transfer rate with histopathologic correlation. AJNR 15:201–212

Ludwin SK (1990) Oligodendrocyte survival in wallerian degeneration. Acta Neuropathol (Berl) 80:184–191

Malamud N, Haymaker W (1947) Cranial trauma and extrapyramidal involvement: cerebral changes simulating those of anoxia. J Neuropathol Exp Neurol 6:271–226

Martin JJ (1983) Secondary demyelination. Bull Soc Belge Ophtalmol 208:473–478

Mascalchi M, Slavi F, Bartolozzi C (1993) MRI of wallerian degeneration in the cervical spinal cord. J Comput Assist Tomogr 17:824–831

Orita T, Tsurutani T, Izumihara A, Matsunaga T (1991) Coronal MR imaging for visualization of wallerian degeneration of the pyramidal tract. J Comput Assist Tomogr 15:802–804

Pennock JM, Rutherford MA, Cowan FM, Bydder GM (1993) MRI: early onset of changes in wallerian degeneration. Clin Radiol 47:311–314

Pujol J, Martí-Vilalta JL, Junqué C, Vendrell P, Fernández J, Capdevila (1990) Wallerian degeneration of the pyramidal tract in capsular infarction studied by magnetic resonance imaging. Stroke 21:404–409

Raitta C (1983) Ophthalmologic features of secondary demyelination. Bull Soc Belge Ophtalmol 208:483–487

Reigner J, Matthieu JM, Kraus-Ruppert R, Lassmann H, Poduslo J (1981) Myelin proteins, glycoproteins, and myelin-related enzymes in experimental demyelination of the rabbit optic nerve: sequence of events. J Neurochem 36:1986–1995

Savoidardo M, Parevson D, Grisoli M, Forester M, D'Incerti L, Farina L (1992) The effects of wallerian degeneration of the optic radiations demonstrated by MRI. Neuroradiology 34:323–325

Seitz RJ, Reiners K, Himmelmann F, Heininger K, Hartung HP, Toyka KV (1989) The blood-nerve barrier in wallerian degeneration: a sequential long-term study. Muscle Nerve: 627–635

Sonoda S, Tsubahara A, Saito M, Chino N (1992) Extent of pyramidal tract Wallerian degeneration in the brain stem on MRI and degree of motor impairment after supratentorial stroke. Disabil Rehabil 14:89–92

Strich SJ (1956) Diffuse degeneration of the cerebral white matter in severe dementia following head injury. J Neurol Neurosurg Psychiatry 19:163–185

Strich SJ (1961) Shearing of nerve fibres as a cause of brain damage due to head injury. Lancet II:443–448

Terae S, Taneichi H, Abumi K (1993) MRI of wallerian degeneration of the injured spinal cord. J Comput Assist Tomogr 17:700–703

Uchino A, Imada H, Ohno M (1990) MR imaging of wallerian degeneration in the human brain stem after ictus. Neuroradiology 32:191–195

Udaka F, Sawada H, Seriu N, Shindou K, Nishitani N, Kameyama M (1992) MRI and SPECT findings in amyotrophic lateral sclerosis. Demonstration of upper motor neurone involvement by clinical neuroimaging. Neuroradiology 34:389–393

Waragai M, Watanabe H, Iwabuchi S (1994) The somatotopic localisation of the descending cortical tract in the cerebral peduncle: a study using MRI of changes following Wallerian degeneration in the cerebral peduncle after a supratentorial vascular lesion. Neuroradiology 36:402–404

Wolman, M (1970) Histochemistry of myelination and demyelination. In: Vinken PJ, Bruyn GW (eds) Handbook of clinical neurology, vol 9. North Holland, Amsterdam, pp 23–44

70 Pattern Recognition in White Matter Disorders

Ball WS, Prenger EC, Ballard ET (1992) Neurotoxicity of radio/chemotherapy in children: pathologic and MR correlation. AJNR 13:761–776

Ford CC, Ceckler TL, Karp J, Herndon RM (1990) Magnetic resonance imaging of experimental demyelinating lesions. Magn Reson Med 14:461–481

Getty DJ, Pickett RM, D'Orsi CJ, Swets JA (1988) Enhanced interpretation of diagnostic images. Invest Radiol 23:240–252

Hanefeld F, Holzbach U, Kruse B, Wilichowski E, Christen HJ, Frahm J (1993) Diffuse white matter disease in three children: an encephalopathy with unique features on magnetic resonance imaging and proton magnetic resonance spectroscopy. Neuropediatrics 24:244–248

McAdams HP, Geyer CA, Done SL, Deigh D, Mitchell M, Ghaed VN (1990) CT and MR imaging of Canavan disease. AJNR 11:397–399

Miller DH, Robb SA, Ormerod IEC, Pohl KRE, MacManus DG, Kendall BE, Moseley IF, McDonald WI (1990) Magnetic resonance imaging of inflammatory and demyelinating white matter diseases of childhood. Dev Med Child Neurol 32:97–107

Osaka H, Kimura S, Nezu A, Yamazaki S, Saitoh K, Yamaguchi S (1993) Chronic subdural hematoma, as an initial manifestation of glutaric aciduria type 1. Brain Dev 15:125–127

Révész T, Hawkins CP, Du Boulay EPGH, Barnard RO, McDonald WI (1989) Pathological findings correlated with magnetic resonance imaging in subcortical arteriosclerotic encephalopathy (Binswanger's disease). J Neurol Neurosurg Psychiatry 52:1337–1344

Sackett DL, Haynes RB, Tugwell P (1985) Clinical epidemiology:a basic science for clinical medicine. Little Brown, Boston

Sartor K, Meyding U (1993) Magnetresonanztomographie bei neurodegenerativen Erkrankungen im Kindesalter. Klin Neuroradiol 3:52–61

Van der Knaap MS, Valk J (1991) Pattern recognition in magnetic resonance imaging of white matter disorders in children and young adults. Neuroradiology 33:478–493

71 Magnetic Resonance Spectroscopy

Arnold DL, Matthews PM, Francis GS, O'Connor J, Antel JP (1992) Proton magnetic resonance spectroscopic imaging for metabolic characterization of demyelinating plaques. Ann Neurol 31:235–241

Arnold DL, Riess GT, Matthews PM, Francis GS, Collins DL, Wolfson C, Antel JP (1994) Use of proton magnetic resonance spectroscopy for monitoring disease progression in multiple sclerosis. Ann Neurol 36:76–82

Austin SJ, Connelly A, Gadian DG, Benton JS, Brett EM (1991) Localized ^{1}H NMR spectroscopy in Canavan's disease: a report of two cases. Magn Reson Med 19:439–445

Azzopardi D, Wyatt JS, Hamilton PA, Cady EB, Delpy DT, Hope PL, Reynolds EOR (1989a) Phosphorus metabolites and intracellular pH in the brains of normal and small for gestational age infants investigated by magnetic resonance spectroscopy. Pediatr Res 25:440–444

Azzopardi D, Wyatt JS, Cady EB, Delpy DT, Baudin J, Stewart AL, Hope PL, Hamilton PA, Reynolds EOR (1989b) Prognosis of newborn infants with hypoxic-ischemic brain injury assessed by phosphorus magnetic resonance spectroscopy. Pediatr Res 25:445–451

Barbiroli B, Montagna P, Martinelli P, Lodi R, Iotti S, Cortelli P, Funicello R, Zaniol P (1993) Defective brain energy metabolism shown by in vivo ^{31}P MR spectroscopy in 28 patients with mitochondrial cytopathies. J Cereb Blood Flow Metab 13:469–474

Barker PB, Bryan RN, Kumar AJ, Naidu S (1992) Proton NMR spectroscopy of Canavan's disease. Neuropediatrics 23:263–267

Bates TE, Williams SR, Gadian DG, Bell JD, Small RK, Iles RA (1989a) ^{1}H NMR study of cerebral development in the rat. NMR Biomed 2:225–229

Bates TE, Williams SR, Gadian DG (1989b) Phosphodiesters in the liver: the effect of field strength on the ^{31}P signal. Magn Reson Med 12:145–150

Behar KL, Boehm D (1994) Measurement of GABA following GABA-transaminase inhibition by gabaculine: a ^{1}H and ^{31}P NMR spectroscopic study of rat brain in vivo. Magn Reson Med 31:660–667

Bessman SP, Carpenter CL (1985) The creatine-creatine phosphate energy shuttle. Annu Rev Biochem 54:831–862

Birken DL, Oldendorf WH (1989) N-acetyl-L-aspartic acid:a literature review of a compound prominent in ^{1}H-NMR spectroscopic studies of brain. Neurosci Biobehav Rev 13:23–31

Bloch F, Hansen WW, Packard M (1946) The nuclear induction experiment. Phys Rev 70:474–485

Boesch C, Gruetter R, Martin E, Duc G, Wüthrich K (1989) Variations in the in vivo P-31 MR spectra of the developing human brain during postnatal life. Radiology 172:197–199

Bottomley PA (1989) Human in vivo NMR spectroscopy in diagnostic medicine: clinical tool or research probe? Radiology 170:1–15

Bottomley PA (1992) Proton MR spectroscopy for diagnosing hepatic encephalopathy? Radiology 182:6–7

Bottomley PA, Hardy CJ, Cousins JP, Armstrong M, Wagle WA (1990) AIDS dementia complex: brain high-energy phosphate metabolite deficits. Radiology 176:407–411

Brenner RE, Munro PMG, Williams SCR, Bell JD, Barker GJ, Hawkins CP, Landon DN, McDonald WI (1993) The proton NMR spectrum in acute EAE: the significance of the change in the Cho:Cr ratio. Magn Reson Med 29:737–745

Bresolin N, Martinelli P, Barbiroli B, Zaniol P, Ausenda C, Montagna P, Gallanti A, Comi GP, Scarlato G, Lugaresi E (1991) Muscle mitochondrial DNA deletion and ^{31}P-NMR spectroscopy alterations in a migraine patient. J Neurol Sci 104:182–189

Bruhn H, Kruse B, Korenke GC, Hanefeld F, Hänicke W, Merboldt KD, Frahm J (1992) Proton NMR spectroscopy of cerebral metabolic alterations in infantile peroxisomal disorders. J Comput Assist Tomogr 16:335–344

Bruhn H, Frahm J, Merboldt KD, Hänicke W, Hanefeld F, Christen HJ, Kruse B, Bauer HJ (1992) Multiple sclerosis in children:cerebral metabolic alterations monitored by localized proton magnetic resonance spectroscopy in vivo. Ann Neurol 32:140–150

Buchli R, Boesiger MP, Rumpel H (1994) Developmental changes of phosphorus metabolite concentrations in the human brain: a ^{31}P magnetic resonance spectroscopy study in vivo. Pediatr Res 35:431–435

Burri R, Lazeyras F, Aue WP, Straehl P, Bigler P, Althaus U, Herschkowitz N (1988) Correlation between ^{31}P NMR phosphomonoester and biochemically determined phosphorylethanolamine and phosphatidylethanolamine during development of the rat brain. Dev Neurosci 10:213–221

Cady EB, de Costello AML, Dawson MJ, Delpy DT, Hope PL, Reynolds EOR, Tofts PS, Wilkie DR (1983) Non-invasive investigation of cerebral metabolism in newborn infants by phosphorus nuclear magnetic resonance spectroscopy. Lancet I:1059–1062

Cerdan S, Subramanian HV, Hilberman M, Cone J, Egan J, Chance B, Williamson JR (1986) ^{31}P NMR detection of mobile dog brain phospholipids. Magn Reson Med 3:432–439

Chamuleau RAFM, Bosman DK, Bovee WMMJ, Luyten PR, den Hollander JA (1991) What the clinician can learn from MR glutamine/glutamate assays. NMR Biomed 4:103–108

Chance B, Leigh JS, Clark BJ, Maris J, Kent J, Nioka S, Smith D (1985) Control of oxidative metabolism and oxygen delivery in human skeletal muscle: a steady-state analysis of the work/energy cost transfer function. Proc Natl Acad Sci U S A 82:8384–8388

Chong WK, Sweeney B, Wilkinson ID, Paley M, Hall-Craggs MA, Kendall BE, Shepard JK, Beecham M, Miller RF, Weller IVD, Newman SP, Harrison MJG (1993) Proton spectroscopy of the brain in HIV infection: correlatin with clinical, immunologic, and MR imaging findings. Radiology 188:119–124

Chong WK, Paley M, Wilkinson ID, Hall-Craggs MA, Sweeney B, Harrison MJG, Miller RF, Kendall BE (1994) Localized cerebral proton MR spectroscopy in HIV infection and AIDS. AJNR 15:21–25

Confort-Gouny S, Vion-Dury J, Nicoli F, Dano P, Donnet A, Grazziani N, Gastaut JL, Grisoli F, Cozzone PJ (1993) A multiparametric data analysis showing the potential of localized proton MR spectroscopy of the brain in the metabolic characterization of neurological diseases. J Neurol Sci 118:123–133

Connelly A, Cross JH, Gadian DG, Hunter JV, Kirkham FJ, Leonard JV (1993) Magnetic resonance spectroscopy shows increased brain glutamine in ornithine carbamoyl transferase deficiency. Pediatr Res 33:77–81

Corbett RJT (1990) In vivo multinuclear magnetic resonance spectroscopy investigations of cerebral development and metabolic encephalopathy using neonatal animal models. Semin Perinatol 14:258–271

Corbett RJT, Laptook AR, Garcia D, Ruley JI (1993) Energy reserves and utilization rates in developing brain measured in vivo by ^{31}P and ^{1}H nuclear magnetic resonance spectroscopy. J Cereb Blood Flow Metab 13:235–246

Cross JH, Gadian DG, Connelly A, Leonard JV (1993) Proton magnetic resonance spectroscopy studies in lactic acidosis and mitochondrial disorders. J Inherited Metab Dis 16:800–811

Daly PF, Lyon RC, Faustino PJ, Cohen JS (1987) Phospholipid in cancer cells monitored by ^{31}P NMR spectroscopy. J Biol Chem 262:14875–14878

Davie CA, Hawkins CP, Barker GJ, Brennan A, Tofts PS, Miller DH, McDonald WI (1993) Detection of myelin breakdown products by proton magnetic resonance spectroscopy. Lancet 341:630–631

Davie CA, Hawkins CP, Barker GJ, Brennan A, Tofts PS, Miller DH, McDonald WI (1994) Serial proton magnetic resonance spectroscopy in acute multiple sclerosis lesions. Brain 117:49–58

Dawson RMC (1985) Enzymic pathways of phospholipid metabolism in the nervous system. In: Eichberg J (ed) Phospholipids in nervous tissues. Wiley, New York, pp 45–78

De Graaf AA, Deutz NEP, Bosman DK, Chamuleau RAFM, de Haan JG, Bovee WMMJ (1991) The use of in vivo proton

NMR to study the effects of hyperammonemia in the rat cerebral cortex. NMR Biomed 4:31–37

Detre JA, Wang Z, Bogdan AR, Gusnard DA, Bay CA, Bingham PM, Zimmerman RA (1991) Regional variation in brain lactate in Leigh syndrome by localized ^{1}H magnetic resonance spectroscopy. Ann Neurol 29:218–221

Edzes HT, Teerlink T, van der Knaap MS, Valk J (1992) Analysis of phospholipids in brain tissue by ^{31}P NMR at different compositions of the solvent system chloroform-methanol-water. Magn Reson Med 26:46–59

Eleff SM, Barker PB, Blackband SJ, Chatham JC, Lutz NW, Johns DR, Bryan RN, Hurko O (1990) Phosphorus magnetic resonance spectroscopy of patients with mitochondrial cytopathies demonstrates decreased levels of brain phosphocreatine. Ann Neurol 27:626–630

Felber SR, Sperl W, Chemelli A, Murr Ch, Wendel U (1993) Maple syrup urine disease: metabolic decompensation monitored by proton magnetic resonance imaging and spectroscopy. Ann Neurol 33:396–401

Goplerud JM, Delivoria-Papadopoulos M (1993) Nuclear magnetic resonance imaging and spectroscopy following asphyxia. Clin Perinatol 20:345–367

Grodd W, Krägeloh-Mann I, Klose U, Sauter R (1991) Metabolic and destructive brain disorders in children: findings with localized proton MR spectroscopy. Radiology 181:173–181

Groenendaal F, Veenhoven RH, van der Grond J, Jansen GH, Witkamp TD, de Vries LS (1994) Cerebral lactate and N-acetyl-aspartate/choline ratios in asphyxiated full-term neonates demonstrated in vivo using proton magnetic resonance spectroscopy. Pediatr Res 35:148–151

Gruetter R, Fusch C, Martin E, Boesch C (1993) Determination of saturation factors in ^{31}P NMR spectra of the developing human brain. Magn Reson Med 29:7–11

Hamilton PA, Hope PL, Cady EB, Delpy DT, Wyatt JS, Reynolds EOR (1986) Impaired energy metabolism in brains of newborn infants with increased cerebral echodensities. Lancet I:1242–1246

Hanefeld F, Kruse B, Bruhn H, Frahm J (1994) In vivo proton magnetic resonance spectroscopy of the brain in a patient with L-2-hydroxyglutaric acidemia. Pediatr Res 35:614–616

Heindel W, Kugel H, Roth B (1993) Noninvasive detection of increased glycine content by proton MR spectroscopy in the brains of two infants with nonketotic hyperglycinemia. AJNR 14:629–635

Herzberg NH, van Schooneveld MJ, Bleeker-Wagemakers E, Zwart R, Cremers FPM, van der Knaap MS, Bolhuis PA, de Visser M (1993) Kearns-Sayre syndrome with a phenocopy of choroideremia instead of pigmentary retinopathy. Neurology 43:218–221

Holtzman D, McFarland EW, Jacobs D, Offutt MC, Neuringer LJ (1991) Maturational increase in mouse brain creatine kinase reaction rates shown by phosphorus magnetic resonance. Dev Brain Res 58:181–188

Hope PL, de Costello AML, Cady EB, Delpy DT, Tofts PS, Chu A, Hamilton PA, Reynolds EOR (1984) Cerebral energy metabolism studied with phosphorus NMR spectroscopy in normal and birth-asphyxiated infants. Lancet II:366–369

Hüppi PS, Posse S, Lazeyras F, Burri R, Bossland E, Herschkowitz N (1991) Magnetic resonance in preterm and term newborns: ^{1}H-spectroscopy in developing human brain. Pediatr Res 30:574–578

Husted CA, Goodin DS, Hugg JW, Maudsley AA, Tsuruda JS, de Bie SH, Fein G, Matson GB, Weiner MW (1994a) Biochemical alterations in multiple sclerosis lesions and normal-appearing white matter detected by in vivo ^{31}P and ^{1}H spectroscopic imaging. Ann Neurol 36:157–165

Husted CA, Matson GB, Adams DA, Goodin DS (1994b) In vivo detection of myelin phospholipids in multiple sclerosis with phosphorus magnetic resonance spectroscopic imaging. Ann Neurol 36:239–241

Kilby PM, Allis JL, Radda GK (1990) Spin-spin relaxation of the phosphodiester resonance in the ^{31}P NMR spectrum of human brain. The determination of the concentrations of phosphodiester components. FEBS Lett 272:163–165

Kilby PM, Bolas NM, Radda GK (1991) ^{31}P-NMR study of brain phospholipid structures in vivo. Biochim Biophys Acta 1085:257–264

Koller KJ, Zaczek R, Coyle JT (1984) N-acetyl-aspartyl-glutamate:regional levels in rat brain and the effects of brain lesions as determined by a new HPLC method. J Neurochem 43:1136–1142

Koopmans RA, Li DKB, Zhu G, Allen PS, Penn A, Paty DW (1993) Magnetic resonance spectroscopy of multiple sclerosis: in-vivo detection of myelin breakdown products. Lancet 341:631–632

Krägeloh-Mann I, Grodd W, Niemann G, Haas G, Ruitenbeek W (1992) Assessment and therapy monitoring of Leigh disease by MRI and proton spectroscopy. Pediatr Neurol 8:60–64

Krägeloh-Mann I, Grodd W, Schöning M, Marquard K, Nägele T, Ruitenbeek W (1993) Proton spectroscopy in five patients with Leigh's disease and mitochondrial enzyme deficiency. Dev Med Child Neurol 35:769–776

Kreis R, Farrow N, Ross BD (1991) Localized ^{1}H NMR spectroscopy in patients with chronic hepatic encephalopathy. Analysis of changes in cerebral glutamine, choline and inositols. NMR Biomed 4:109–116

Kreis R, Ross BD, Farrow NA, Ackerman Z (1992) Metabolic disorders of the brain in chronic hepatic encephalopathy detected with ^{1}H MR spectroscopy. Radiology 182:19–27

Kreis R, Ernst T, Ross BD (1993) Development of the human brain:in vivo quantification of metabolite and water content with proton magnetic resonance spectroscopy. Magn Reson Med 30:424–437

Kruse B, Hanefeld F, Christen HJ, Bruhn H, Michaelis T, Hänicke W, Frahm J (1993) Alterations of brain metabolites in metachromatic leukodystrophy as detected by localized proton magnetic resonance spectroscopy in vivo. J Neurol 241:68–74

Kruse B, Hanefeld F, Holzbach U, Wilichowski E, Christen HJ, Merboldt KD, Hänicke W, Frahm J (1994a) Proton spectroscopy in patients with Leigh's disease and mitochondrial enzyme deficiency. Dev Med Child Neurol 36:839–845

Kruse B, Barker PB, Van Zijl PCM, Duyn JH, Moonen CTW, Moser HW (1994b) Multislice proton magnetic resonance spectroscopic imaging in X-linked adrenoleukodystrophy. Ann Neurol 36:595–608

Kuwabara T, Watanabe H, Tanaka K, Tsuji S, Ohkubo M, Ito T, Sakai K, Yuasa T (1994) Mitochondrial encephalomyopathy:

elevated visual cortex lactate unresponsive to photic stimulation – a localized ^{1}H-MRS study. Neurology 44:557–559

Lee JH, Arcinue E, Ross BD (1994) Brief report: organic osmolytes in the brain of an infant with hypernatremia. N Engl J Med 331:439–442

Lien YHH, Michaelis T, Moats RA, Ross BD (1994) Scyllo-inositol depletion in hepatic encephalopathy. Life Sci 54:1507–1512

Lolley RN, Balfour WM, Samson FE (1961) The high-energy phosphates in developing brain. J Neurochem 7:289–297

Marks HG, Caro PA, Wang Z, Detre JA, Bogdan AR, Gusnard DA, Zimmerman RA (1991) Use of computed tomography, magnetic resonance imaging, and localized ^{1}H magnetic resonance spectroscopy in Canavan's disease: a case report. Ann Neurol 30:106–110

Matthews PM, Berkovic SF, Shoubridge EA, Andermann F, Karpati G, Carpenter S, Arnold D (1991) In vivo magnetic resonance spectroscopy of brain and muscle in a type of mitochondrial encephalomyopathy (MERRF). Ann Neurol 29:435–438

Matthews PM, Andermann F, Silver K, Karpati G, Arnold DL (1993) Proton MR spectroscopic characterization of differences in regional brain metabolic abnormalities in mitochondrial encephalomyopathies. Neurology 43:2484–2490

McNamara R, Arias-Mendoza F, Brown TR (1994) Investigation of broad resonances in ^{31}P NMR spectra of the human brain in vivo. NMR Biomed 7:237–242

Menon DK, Ainsworth JG, Cox IJ, Coker RC, Sargentoni J, Coutts GA, Baudouin CJ, Kocsis AE, Harris JRW (1992) Proton MR spectroscopy of the brain in AIDS dementia complex. J Comput Assist Tomogr 16:538–542

Meyerhoff DJ, MacKay S, Bachman L, Poole N, Dillon WP, Weiner MW, Fein G (1993) Reduced brain N-acetylaspartate suggests neuronal loss in cognitively impaired human immunodeficiency virus-seropositive individuals:in vivo ^{1}H magnetic resonance spectroscopic imaging. Neurology 43:509–515

Michaelis T, Merboldt KD, Hänicke W, Gyngell ML, Bruhn H, Frahm J (1991) On the identification of cerebral metabolites in localized ^{1}H NMR spectra of human brain in vivo. NMR Biomed 4:90–98

Michaelis T, Helms G, Merboldt KD, Hänicke W, Bruhn H, Frahm J (1993) Identification of scyllo-inositol in proton NMR spectra of human brain in vivo. NMR Biomed 6:105–109

Miller AL, Shamban A (1977) A comparison of methods for stopping intermediary metabolism of developing rat brain. J Neurochem 28:1327–1334

Miller BL (1991) A review of chemical issues in ^{1}H NMR spectroscopy: N-acetyl-L-aspartate, creatine and choline. NMR Biomed 4:47–52

Moon RB, Richards JH (1973) Determination of intracellular pH by ^{31}P magnetic resonance. J Biol Chem 248:7276–7278

Moorcraft J, Bolas NM, Ives NK, Sutton P, Blackledge MJ, Rajagopalan B, Hope PL, Radda GK (1991a) Spatially localized magnetic resonance spectroscopy of the brains of normal and asphyxiated newborns. Pediatrics 87:273–282

Moorcraft J, Bolas NM, Ives NK, Ouwerkerk R, Smyth J, Rajagopalan B, Hope PL, Radda GK (1991b) Global and depth resolved phosphorus magnetic resonance spectroscopy to predict outcome after birth asphyxia. Arch Dis Child 66:1119–1123

Murphy EJ, Rajagopalan B, Brindle KM, Radda GK (1989) Phospholipid bilayer contribution to ^{31}P NMR spectra in vivo. Magn Reson Med 12:282–289

Nadler JV, Cooper JR (1972) N-acetyl-L-aspartic acid content of human neural tumours and bovine peripheral nervous tissues. J Neurochem 19:313–319

Nakada T, Kwee IL (1993) ^{31}P localized spectroscopy of fetal brain in utero. Magn Reson Med 29:122–124

Patel TB, Clark JB (1979) Synthesis of N-acetyl-L-aspartate by rat brain mitochondria and its involvement in mitochondrial/cytosolic carbon transport. Biochem J 184:539–546

Peden CJ, Cowan FM, Bryant DJ, Sargentoni J, Cox IJ, Menon DK, Gadian DG, Bell JD, Dubowitz LM (1990) Proton MR spectroscopy of the brain in infants. J Comput Assist Tomogr 14:886–894

Peden CJ, Rutherford MA, Sargentoni J, Cox IJ, Bryant DJ, Dubowitz LMS (1993) Proton spectroscopy of the neonatal brain following hypoxic-ischaemic injury. Dev Med Child Neurol 35:502–510

Petroff OAC, Prichard JW, Behar KL, Alger JR, den Hollander JA, Shulman RG (1985) Cerebral intracellular pH by ^{31}P nuclear magnetic resonance spectroscopy. Neurology 35:781–788

Petroff OAC, Spencer DD, Alger JR, Prichard JW (1989) High-field proton magnetic resonance spectroscopy of human cerebrum obtained during surgery for epilepsy. Neurology 39:1197–1202

Porcellati G, Arienti G (1983) Metabolism of phosphoglycerides. In: Lajtha A (ed) Metabolism in the nervous system. Plenum, New York, pp 133–161 (Handbook of neurochemistry, vol 3)

Prichard JW (1991) What the clinician can learn from MRS lactate measurements. NMR Biomed 4:99–102

Purcell EM, Torrey HC, Pound RV (1946) Resonance absorption by nuclear magnetic moments in a solid. Phys Rev 69:37–38

Richards TL (1991) Proton MR spectroscopy in multiple sclerosis: value in establishing diagnosis, monitoring progression, and evaluating therapy. AJR 157:1073–1078

Ross B, Kreis R, Ernst T (1992) Clinical tools for the 90s: magnetic resonance spectroscopy and metabolite imaging. Eur J Radiol 14:128–140

Ross BD (1991) Biochemical considerations in ^{1}H spectroscopy. Gutamate and glutamine; myo-inositol and related metabolites. NMR Biomed 4:59–63

Roth SC, Azzopardi D, Edwards AD, Baudin J, Cady EB, Townsend J, Delpy DT, Stewart AL, Wyatt JS, Osmund E, Reynolds R (1992) Relation between cerebral oxidative metabolism following birth asphyxia, and neurodevelopmental outcome and brain growth at one year. Dev Med Child Neurol 34:285–295

Rothman DL, Hanstock CC, Petroff OAC, Novotny EJ, Prichard JW, Shulman RG (1992) Localized ^{1}H NMR spectra of glutamate in the human brain. Magn Reson Med 25:94–106

Rothman DL, Ognen A, Petroff C, Behar KL, Mattson RH (1993) Localized ^{1}H NMR measurements of γ-aminobutyric acid in human brain in vivo. Proc Natl Acad Sci U S A 90:5662–5666

Samson FE, Balfour WM, Dahl NA (1960) Rate of cerebral ATP utilization in rats. Am J Physiol 198:213–216

Sappey-Marinier D, Calabrese G, Hetherington HP, Fisher SNG, Deicken R, van Dyke C, Fein G, Weiner MW (1992) Proton magnetic resonance spectroscopy of human brain: applicatons to normal white matter, chronic infarction, and MRI white matter signal hyperintensities. Magn Reson Med 26:313–327

Stöckler S, Holzbach U, Hanefeld F, Marquardt I, Helms G, Requart M, Hänicke W, Frahm J (1994) Creatine deficiency in the brain: a new, treatable inborn error of metabolism. Pediatr Res 36:409–413

Sun GY, Foudin LL (1985) Phospholipid composition and metabolism in the developing and aging nervous system. In: Eichberg J (ed) Phospholipids in nervous tissues. Wiley, New York, pp 79–134

Szigety SK, Allen PS, Huyser-Wierenga D, Urtasun RC (1993) The effect of radiation on normal human CNS as detected by NMR spectroscopy. Int J Radiat Oncol Biol Phys 25:695–701

Toft PB, Leth H, Lou HC, Pryds O, Henriksen O (1994) Metabolite concentrations in the developing brain estimated with proton MR spectroscopy. J Magn Reson Imaging 4:674–680

Tofts P, Wray S (1985) Changes in brain phosphorus metabolites during the post-natal development of the rat. J Physiol (Lond) 359:417–429

Tzika AA, Ball WS, Vigneron DB, Dunn RS, Kirks DR (1993a) Clinical proton MR spectroscopy of neurodegenerative disease in childhood. AJNR 14:1267–1281

Tzika AA, Vigneron DB, Ball WS, Scott Dunn R, Kirks DR (1993b) Localized proton MR spectroscopy of the brain in children. J Magn Reson Imaging 3:719–729

Tzika AA, Ball WS, Vigneron DB, Dunn RS, Nelson SJ, Kirks DR (1993c) Childhood adrenoleukodystrophy: assessment with proton MR spectroscopy. Radiology 189:467–480

Urenjak J, Williams SR, Gadian DG, Noble M (1992) Specific expression of N-acetylaspartate in neurons, oligodendro-cyte-type-2 astrocyte progenitors, and immature oligodendrocytes in vitro. J Neurochem 59:55–61

Van der Grond J, Dijkstra G, Roelofsen B, Mali WPTM (1991) ^{31}P-NMR determinatin of phosphomonoesters in relation to phospholipid biosynthesis in testis of the rat at different ages. Biochem Biophys Acta 1074:189–194

Van der Knaap MS, van der Grond J, van Rijen PC, Faber JAJ, Valk J, Willemse K (1990) Age-dependent changes in localized proton and phosphorus MR spectroscopy of the brain. Radiology 176:509–515

Van der Knaap MS, van der Grond J, Luyten PR, den Hollander JA, Nauta JJP, Valk J (1992) ^{1}H and ^{31}P magnetic resonance spectroscopy of the brain in degenerative cerebral disorders. Ann Neurol 31:202–211

Van der Knaap MS, Ross B, Valk J (1994) Uses of MR in inborn errors of metabolism. In: Kucharczyk J, Moseley M, Barkovich AJ (eds) Magnetic resonance neuroimaging. CRC Press, Boca Raton, pp 245–318

Veech RL (1991) The metabolism of lactate. NMR Biomed 4:53–58

Vion-Dury J, Meyerhoff DJ, Cozzone PJ, Weiner MW (1994) What might be the impact on neurology of the analysis of brain metabolism by in vivo magnetic resonance spectroscopy? J Neurol 241:354–371

Younkin DP, Delivoria-Papadopoulos M, Leonard JC, Subramanian VH, Eleff S, Leigh JS, Chance B (1984) Unique aspects of human newborn cerebral metabolism evaluated with phosphorus nuclear magnetic resonance spectroscopy. Ann Neurol 16:581–586

Yousem DM, Lenkinski RE, Evans S, Allen D, O'Brien R, Curran W, Schnall M, Bennett M, Wehrli SL, Grossman RI (1992) Proton MR spectroscopy of experimental radiation-induced white matter injury. J Comput Assist Tomogr 16:543–548

Zimmerman RA, Valk J, Wang Z (1993) Clinical proton MR spectroscopy of neurodegenerative disease in childhood. AJNR 14:1282–1284

Subject Index